MICROBIOLOGY

MICROBIOLOGY

T. STUART WALKER, Ph.D.

Professor of Medical Education/Microbiology
Muncie Center for Medical Education
Ball State University and Indiana University School of Medicine
Muncie, Indiana
and
Adjunct Professor
Department of Microbiology and Immunology
Indiana University School of Medicine
Indianapolis, Indiana

W.B. SAUNDERS COMPANY
A Division of Harcourt Brace & Company
Philadelphia London Toronto Montreal Sydney Tokyo

W.B. SAUNDERS COMPANY
A Division of Harcourt Brace & Company

The Curtis Center
Independence Square West
Philadelphia, Pennsylvania 19106

Library of Congress Cataloging-in-Publication Data

Walker, T. Stuart.

  Microbiology / T. Stuart Walker.

    p.   cm.

  Includes index.

  ISBN 0–7216–4641–7

  1. Medical microbiology.   2. Microbiology.   I. Title.

QR46.W245   1998

616′.01—dc21   97-9774

Microbiology   ISBN 0–7216–4641–7

Printed in the United States of America.

Last digit is the print number: 9   8   7   6   5   4   3   2   1

PREFACE

Microbiology is an extremely diverse discipline, requiring the mastery and integration of data concerning biochemistry, molecular biology, pharmacology, immunology, pathology, basic microbiology, and clinical bacteriology, mycology, virology, and parasitology. Because the amount of information on microbes is so vast, microbiology books have generally followed one of two main tracks. The traditional books have tended to be exhaustive encyclopedias of microbiologic facts. Although these books may serve as excellent reference works, they are too long and detailed to be read by the typical medical student who is trying to keep up with several classes simultaneously. Moreover, the traditional texts usually emphasize data from the basic sciences while providing only a brief description of microbial diseases and their diagnoses. In reaction to the encyclopedic texts, a newer wave of short microbiology books has emerged. The primary weakness of these books is that they are too cursory—often so cursory that the amount of material covered in them is considerably less than that provided in the lectures of a typical medical microbiology course. Some of the newer texts achieve brevity by emphasizing the clinical sciences but providing insufficient information on basic microbiology. Others achieve brevity by focusing on a few "model" organisms, but they fail to familiarize readers with a wide range of microbial pathogens and infectious diseases.

The microbiology text presented here was written after 18 years of teaching medical students and searching for a book that was both readable and complete enough to meet their needs. The current text is considerably shorter and more conversational in tone than the encyclopedic texts, yet it contains all of the information that is pertinent to medical students who are learning microbiology. It also provides a solid background of basic microbiology while describing the organisms in a manner that is clinically relevant. By focusing on the molecular processes that are believed to be responsible for microbial diseases, the text spans the gap between basic microbiology and clinical microbiology. Figures, tables, and short narratives about the discovery of microbes and diseases are interspersed throughout the text to help readers understand and retain information.

Although the text was designed to teach first- and second-year medical students, it should also serve as a review tool for individuals who are taking medical board examinations or wish to update their knowledge of pathogens and infectious diseases.

The text is divided into four sections, based on the four major disciplines included within microbiology: bacteriology, mycology, virology, and parasitology. Each section begins with an overview of information in the discipline and then presents a series of chapters that discuss specific organisms. In Section I, for example, Chapters 1 through 3 present basic information on the classification, structure, function, growth, metabolism, and molecular genetics of bacteria; Chapter 4 discusses antibacterial agents; and Chapters 5 through 15 provide more detailed information on specific pathogenic bacteria and the diseases they cause. Each pathogen is described in terms of its general features and mechanisms of pathogenicity, and then the epidemiology, diagnosis, treatment, and prevention of its associated diseases are reviewed. This consistent pattern of presenting the material should help students locate information quickly about any pathogen or infectious disease of interest.

This book was two years in writing but a lifetime in preparation. I would like to thank those whose example, teaching, and prodding helped me develop a thirst for knowledge as well as methods for quenching that thirst. They include Dr. Larry Helmick, my organic chemistry professor; Dr. Warner Wegener, my M.S. adviser; Dr. William Sawyer, my Ph.D. adviser; and Dr. Herbert Winkler, who supervised me during my postdoctoral years. Each of these men contributed in a unique fashion to my development as a scientist and as a writer. This book could not have been written, of course, without the interest and support of my editors at W.B. Saunders, Bill Schmitt and Anne-Marie Shaw. Sharon Maddox deserves special praise for her tireless efforts to turn me into a writer through her encouragement, advice, and developmental work on the manuscript. Timothy Mullican and his colleagues at Observatory Group, Inc., also deserve recognition for their art work.

In addition to thanking the friends who encouraged me, I would like to thank my family for patiently enduring the writing of this book, which seemed at times to be an endless process. I am especially grateful to my wife for her support and to two special children, who occasionally pulled me away from the book to go hiking or biking or to watch a movie so I could retain my sanity. Finally, I would like to express my gratitude to my parents for their contributions to this book. I thank my mother, who was the most thorough thinker I have ever known and showed me what careful and insightful thinking can be at its best. Most of all, I thank my father, Dr. Thomas M. Walker, for inspiring me. It was his courage and compassion that took him as a medical missionary to the jungles of northeastern India. It was there during my childhood that I began to learn about an incredible variety of pathogens and infectious diseases. As I traveled with him down the jungle track from village to village, I saw lives ravaged by leprosy, tuberculosis, cholera, dengue fever, kala-azar, malaria, and other diseases. I watched raptly as he sewed up limbs mauled by tigers or crocodiles and returned sight to eyes blinded by cataracts. As all these things passed before me, they planted within me a desire to understand why and how microbes cause disease. But above all, with his life my father showed me what hard work and commitment can accomplish and that a life that matters requires taking risks.

T. STUART WALKER

CONTENTS

SECTION II

FUNGI AND FUNGAL DISEASES

SECTION III

VIRUSES AND VIRAL DISEASES

SECTION IV

PARASITES AND PARASITIC DISEASES

SECTION I

BACTERIA AND

BACTERIAL DISEASES

BACTERIAL CLASSIFICATION,

STRUCTURE, AND FUNCTION

Microbiology had its origin in 1677, when Antonie van Leeuwenhoek first observed microscopic organisms with a primitive lens. His letters to the Royal Society of London chronicled his early observations, but he kept his lens-making methods secret, and much of the technology that he developed died with him. Ninety years later, using more sophisticated compound lenses, Carolus Linnaeus described six bacterial species, but no solid connection was made between the presence of microbes and the occurrence of disease.

The first indications that microbes might cause disease came from epidemiologic studies. In 1546, Girolamo Fracastoro presented a strong case for the communicability of disease and the existence of seeds of contagion in his classic book, *De Contagione.* Ignaz Semmelweis and Oliver Wendell Holmes crusaded during the 1840s against "childbed fever," which they believed was transmitted via the unwashed hands of physicians. In 1854, John Snow halted an epidemic of cholera in London by showing that its source was the Broad Street pump, whose water was heavily contaminated with sewage. David Livingstone reported in 1858 that he believed nagana (African sleeping sickness) was transmitted by tsetse flies and that the contagion could be eradicated with arsenical treatments.

Veterinary diseases were the first to yield solid evidence of a microbial origin. In 1836, Agosto Bassi showed that a fungus was the cause of a silkworm disease, and in 1865, Louis Pasteur discovered a protozoan that was a deadly pathogen of silkworms. The first human disease discovered to have a microbial etiology was favus (honeycomb ringworm), shown by Johann Schönlein in 1839 to be due to a fungus. In 1850, Casimir Davaine discovered that sheep dying of anthrax had rod-shaped bacteria in their blood. But it was Robert Koch who finally completed the etiologic cycle in 1876 by showing that anthrax bacilli cultured from infected animals could cause anthrax when introduced into uninfected animals and by demonstrating that the bacilli were always found in the secondarily infected animals. During the 1890s, Dmitri Ivanovski and Martinus Beijerinck independently discovered the first virus (tobacco mosaic virus), and the US Army Commission under Walter Reed demon-

strated in 1900 that yellow fever was caused by a virus.

Today, microbiology is one of the broadest and most diverse scientific disciplines. Not only has it grown to include bacteriology, molecular biology, immunology, mycology, virology, and parasitology, but also it has given birth to the revolution in bioengineering and molecular genetics. Investigators have discovered a wide range of bacteria, fungi, viruses, and parasites that cause human disease, and these medically significant organisms are the focus of this book.

CLASSIFICATION OF BACTERIA

Classification as Prokaryotes

The bacterium is a simple, single-celled organism that, unlike the human cell, does not have intracellular membrane-bound organelles such as a nucleus, Golgi apparatus, endoplasmic reticulum, or mitochondrion. Therefore, the bacterium's essential metabolic and biosynthetic activities must be carried out within the cytoplasm and the cell envelope. Because the cells of protozoa, fungi, plants, humans, and other animals have organized, membrane-bound nuclei, these organisms are classified as **eukaryotes** (from Greek *eu,* meaning "true," and *karyon,* meaning "nucleus"). In contrast, bacteria lack a true nucleus and are classified as **prokaryotes** (from *pro,* meaning "before"). The differences between human cells and bacteria go far beyond the presence or absence of a true nucleus, however. As Table 1–1 shows, bacteria differ from eukaryotes in the structure and composition of their cell envelopes, in the machinery of protein synthesis, in the site of various key cellular activities, in the structure of cellular appendages such as flagella, and in their metabolic activities. These differences between human cells and bacteria are important because they provide unique targets for antibiotic action, thereby ensuring that antibiotics are selectively toxic. A good antibiotic kills targeted bacteria without harming the patient.

Classification by Genus and Species

Each bacterium has a taxonomic classification and is known generally by its genus and species name—for example, *Escherichia coli.* **Taxonomic**

TABLE 1–1. A Comparison of the Structures and Activities of Bacteria With Those of Human Cells

Bacteria	Human Cells
Nuclear material is relatively disorganized and not enclosed in a nucleus. There is one chromosome with multiple replicative forks.	Cells have a membrane-bound nucleus with 22 autosomal pairs plus X and Y chromosomes.
All bacteria but mycoplasmas have a trilaminar cell membrane plus a mucopolysaccharide cell wall. Gram-negative bacteria have an outer membrane.	Cells have a trilaminar cell membrane with no cell wall.
Protein synthesis is carried out by 70S ribosomes.	Protein synthesis is carried out by 80S ribosomes.
Cell membranes of all bacteria but mycoplasmas lack steroids.	Cell membranes contain steroids to confer osmotic stability.
Electron transport occurs at the cytoplasmic membrane. Some cellular processes are driven directly by proton translocation.	Electron transport occurs at the mitochondrial membrane. Cellular functions are driven by adenosine triphosphate (ATP).
Cellular functions are not segregated by membranes.	Membrane-bound organelles segregate and carry out cellular functions.
Extracellular appendages are made of simple helical proteins.	Extracellular appendages such as flagella contain microtubules arranged in a 9 + 2 manner.
There is a wide range of metabolic activity with diverse energy sources. Aerobic respiration, anaerobic respiration, and fermentation occur.	There is limited metabolic variability.

classifications traditionally have been based on descriptive characteristics of the bacteria, such as their structure and morphology, staining characteristics, and metabolic activities. With the recent advent of sophisticated molecular biology techniques, taxonomy has become an exercise in comparing DNA and transfer RNA (tRNA) gel patterns, gene sequencing, and percentages of guanine and cytosine in the chromosome. In some cases, bacteria are further divided into serotypes or subspecies on the basis of surface antigens, abilities to be infected by specific bacteriophages, uniquely associated disease states, or metabolic and biosynthetic characteristics. There are, for example, hundreds of *Salmonella* serotypes, and *Treponema pallidum* has recently been divided into the subspecies *pallidum*, *endemicum*, and *pertenue*. Clinicians use taxonomy primarily as a handle for identifying organisms so that they can predict the course of disease, understand the underlying disease process, and devise appropriate treatment strategies. Table 1–2 lists the clinically important bacteria and their associated diseases.

Classification by Size and Shape

Bacteria come in many sizes and shapes, ranging from spirochetes, which may be up to 250 μm long, to spherical mycoplasmas that are 0.15 μm in diameter and can barely be seen by light microscopy. Most of the medically important bacteria are rods (bacilli) or spheres (cocci), but others occur as spirals (spirochetes), as short and fat rods that are almost indistinguishable from cocci (coccobacilli), or as comma-shaped bacteria that are actually truncated helices (vibrios). Fig. 1–1 shows some typical bacterial morphologies.

When bacilli or cocci occur as chains, they are called streptobacilli or streptococci (from Greek *streptos,* meaning "a twisted chain"). Clusters of cocci are called staphylococci (from Greek *staphylē,* "a cluster of grapes"); pairs of cocci are called diplococci; and tetrads of cocci are called sarcinae (from Latin *sarcina,* "a package"). Some bacteria vary in shape or size as they age or as their environment changes. Cultures of these bacteria may contain rods of varying lengths, which are referred to as pleomorphic bacilli. Finally, there are some bacteria with unusual morphologies. *Caulobacter* organisms, for example, are so named because they have a stalklike protuberance at one pole (from Latin *caulis,* "a plant stalk"). Organisms of the genus *Actinomyces* look superficially like fungi, forming moldlike colonies filled with elongated rods that look like fungal hyphae.

Classification by Gram-Staining Characteristics

Most bacteria obtained from clinical samples are identified initially by growing them in pure culture on an artificial medium and then examining the shape and color of the bacteria when a sample of the culture is placed on a microscope slide and stained. In most cases, the key initial procedure uses Gram's stain.

The Gram-Staining Procedure

The Gram-staining procedure was developed in the 1880s by Christian Gram, a Danish pathologist. A minute amount of the bacteria to be stained is placed in a drop of liquid on a slide and is air-dried. The dried droplet should appear to be barely cloudy; if too many bacteria are used, the stain is not reliable. The slide is then gently heat-fixed, so that it is cool enough to touch the back of the hand without causing a burn. The slide is stained with **crystal violet** and washed, and a mordant known as **Lugol's solution** (3% I_2/KI) is added to set the stain. The slide is washed again and is then decolorized briefly with an alcohol-acetone mixture. Finally, the slide is counterstained with **safranin,** washed, and blotted dry.

When the stained bacteria are examined under an oil-immersion lens, **gram-positive** bacteria appear blue or purple, but **gram-negative** bacteria appear red or pink. Stained samples taken from aging cultures of gram-positive bacteria contain a mixture of blue and pink bacteria and are said to

TABLE 1–2. Clinically Important Bacteria and Their Associated Diseases

Bacteria	Associated Disease or Diseases
Gram-positive pyogenic cocci (see Chapter 5)	
Enterococcus faecalis	Endocarditis, intra-abdominal infections, neonatal meningitis, primary bacteremia, and urinary tract infections.
Enterococcus faecium	Endocarditis, intra-abdominal infections, neonatal meningitis, primary bacteremia, and urinary tract infections.
Staphylococcus aureus	Burn infections, carbuncles, endocarditis, enteritis, folliculitis, food poisoning, furuncles, impetigo, osteomyelitis, pneumonia, pyoarthrosis, scalded skin syndrome, toxic shock syndrome, and wound infections.
Staphylococcus epidermidis	Endocarditis; infections in patients with implanted devices; and urinary tract infections.
Staphylococcus saprophyticus	Urinary tract infections in women.
Streptococcus agalactiae	Arthritis, early-onset and delayed-onset neonatal disease (hyaline membrane–like disease and meningitis), endocarditis, meningitis, opportunistic infections, osteomyelitis, perinatal infections, pneumonia, skin infections, and soft tissue infections.
Streptococcus groups C and G	Cellulitis, endocarditis, erysipelas, glomerulonephritis, impetigo, meningitis, neonatal sepsis, pharyngitis, septic arthritis, and wound infections.
Streptococcus intermedius group	Abdominal and brain abscesses, endocarditis, and sinusitis.
Streptococcus mutans	Dental caries and endocarditis.
Streptococcus pneumoniae	Conjunctivitis, meningitis, otitis media, pneumonia, and sinusitis.
Streptococcus pyogenes	Erysipelas, glomerulonephritis, impetigo, necrotizing fasciitis, pharyngitis, pneumonia, puerperal sepsis, rheumatic fever, scarlet fever, and toxic streptococcal syndrome.
Streptococcus sanguis	Endocarditis.
Gram-negative pyogenic bacteria (see Chapter 6)	
Bordetella pertussis	Pertussis (whooping cough).
Haemophilus aegyptius	Brazilian purpuric fever and epidemic conjunctivitis.
Haemophilus ducreyi	Chancroid.
Haemophilus influenzae	Bronchitis, cellulitis, endocarditis, endometritis, epiglottitis, meningitis, neonatal sepsis, otitis media, pneumonia, primary pediatric bacteremia, puerperal sepsis, purulent pericarditis, salpingitis, and sinusitis.
Haemophilus parainfluenzae	Endocarditis and meningitis.
Moraxella catarrhalis	Bronchitis and sinusitis.
Neisseria gonorrhoeae	Disseminated gonococcal infection, gonococcal arthritis-dermatitis syndrome, gonococcal pharyngitis, gonorrhea, ophthalmia neonatorum, and pelvic inflammatory disease.
Neisseria meningitidis	Meningitis and meningococcemia.
Enterobacteriaceae and associated bacteria (see Chapter 7)	
Campylobacter fetus subspecies *fetus*	Acute primary bacteremia, neonatal meningitis, and respiratory infections.
Campylobacter jejuni	Acute enteritis.
Citrobacter species	Diarrhea, neonatal brain abscess, and neonatal meningitis.
Edwardsiella species	Liver abscess, primary bacteremia, and water-associated wound infections.
Enterobacter species	Opportunistic nosocomial infections (such as pneumonia, sepsis, urinary tract infections, and wound infections).
Escherichia coli	Diarrhea, hemolytic-uremic syndrome, neonatal meningitis, opportunistic infections, sepsis, and urinary tract infections.
Hafnia species	Wound infections.
Helicobacter pylori	Active chronic gastritis, chronic superficial gastritis, and peptic ulcers; risk factor for adenocarcinoma of the stomach.
Klebsiella species	Atrophic rhinitis, ozena, pneumonia, rhinoscleroma, and urinary tract infections.
Morganella species	Diarrhea, urinary tract infections, and wound infections.
Pantoea species	Septicemia.
Proteus species	Nosocomial pneumonia, sepsis, urinary tract infections, and wound infections.
Providencia species	Urinary tract infections.
Salmonella species	Enteritis, primary septicemia, and typhoid.
Serratia marcescens	Nosocomial infections (such as pneumonia, sepsis, urinary tract infections, and wound infections).
Shigella species	Bacillary dysentery.
Yersinia enterocolitica	Acute gastroenteritis; diarrhea with arthritis and erythema nodosum; liver abscess; mesenteric lymphadenitis; and terminal ileitis.
Yersinia pseudotuberculosis	Acute gastroenteritis; diarrhea with arthritis and erythema nodosum; liver abscess; mesenteric lymphadenitis; and terminal ileitis.
Pseudomonadaceae (see Chapter 8)	
Burkholderia (Pseudomonas) cepacia	Cepacia syndrome in cystic fibrosis patients; endocarditis; jungle rot; neonatal meningitis; and nosocomial urinary tract infections.
Burkholderia (Pseudomonas) pseudomallei	Melioidosis.

Continued

TABLE 1–2. Clinically Important Bacteria and Their Associated Diseases *(Continued)*

Bacteria	Associated Disease or Diseases
Pseudomonas aeruginosa	Bone and joint infections; brain abscess; burn infections; chronic pneumonia in cystic fibrosis patients; ecthyma gangrenosum; endocarditis; enterocolitis; green nail syndrome; hot tub dermatitis; keratitis; mastoiditis; meningitis; nosocomial urinary tract infections; otitis externa; otitis media; panophthalmitis; primary bacteremic pneumonia; primary nonbacteremic pneumonia; primary nosocomial bacteremia; Shanghai fever; and toe web infection.
Pseudomonas stutzeri	Conjunctivitis, otitis media, pneumonia, and septic arthritis.
Stenotrophomonas (Xanthomonas) maltophilia	Pneumonia, primary bacteremia, and urinary tract infections.
Funguslike bacteria (see Chapter 9)	
Actinomadura species	Madura foot.
Actinomyces israelii	Deep abscesses.
Mycobacterium avium-intracellulare	Subacute lymphadenitis; systemic infections associated with acquired immunodeficiency syndrome (AIDS); and tuberculosislike pulmonary disease.
Mycobacterium kansasii	Disseminated disease in patients with AIDS; and pulmonary infections.
Mycobacterium leprae	Leprosy.
Mycobacterium marinum	Swimming pool granuloma.
Mycobacterium scrofulaceum	Cervical lymphadenitis (scrofula).
Mycobacterium tuberculosis	Tuberculosis.
Nocardia asteroides	Brain abscess, kidney infections, pneumonia, and pneumonitis.
Nocardia brasiliensis	Lymphocutaneous infections and Madura foot.
Streptomyces species	Farmer's lung and mycetoma.
Tropheryma whippelii	Whipple's disease.
Zoonotic bacteria (see Chapter 10)	
Brucella species	Brucellosis.
Capnocytophaga canimorsus	Cellulitis after dog or cat bite; and sepsis.
Capnocytophaga cynodegmi	Cellulitis after dog or cat bite; and sepsis.
Erysipelothrix rhusiopathiae	Erysipeloid.
Francisella tularensis	Tularemia.
Listeria monocytogenes	Brain abscess; gastroenteritis; meningitis in neonates and immunocompromised patients; and sepsis in neonates.
Pasteurella multocida	Infections after cat or dog bite; sepsis; and suppurative respiratory tract infections.
Spirillum minus	Rat-bite fever (sodoku).
Streptobacillus moniliformis	Haverhill fever and rat-bite fever.
Yersinia pestis	Plague.
Mycoplasmas, rickettsiae, and other unusual bacteria (see Chapter 11)	
Bartonella bacilliformis	Carrión's disease (Oroya fever and verruga peruana).
Bartonella (Rochalimaea) henselae	Bacillary angiomatosis, cat-scratch disease, and peliosis hepatis.
Bartonella (Rochalimaea) quintana	Bacillary angiomatosis, intraocular inflammation, relapsing febrile bacteremia, and trench fever.
Chlamydia pneumoniae	Atypical pneumonia, bronchitis, pharyngitis, and sinusitis.
Chlamydia psittaci	Psittacosis (ornithosis).
Chlamydia trachomatis	Inclusion conjunctivitis, lymphogranuloma venereum, neonatal pneumonia, nongonococcal urethritis, pelvic inflammatory disease, Reiter's syndrome, and trachoma.
Coxiella burnetii	Q fever.
Ehrlichia species	Human granulocytic ehrlichiosis, human monocytic ehrlichiosis, and Sennetsu mononucleosis.
Mycoplasma fermentans	Infections associated with AIDS.
Mycoplasma hominis	Chorioamnionitis, endometritis, neonatal meningitis, nongonococcal urethritis, pelvic inflammatory disease, and postpartum fever.
Mycoplasma pneumoniae	Atypical pneumonia and tracheobronchitis.
Rickettsia akari	Rickettsialpox.
Rickettsia prowazekii	Brill-Zinsser disease and epidemic typhus.
Rickettsia rickettsii	Rocky Mountain spotted fever.
Rickettsia tsutsugamushi	Scrub typhus.
Rickettsia typhi	Endemic (murine) typhus.
Ureaplasma urealyticum	Chorioamnionitis, endometritis, neonatal chronic lung disease, neonatal meningitis, nongonococcal urethritis, pelvic inflammatory disease, and postpartum fever.
Spirochetes (see Chapter 12)	
Borrelia burgdorferi	Lyme disease.
Borrelia hermsii	Endemic relapsing fever.
Borrelia recurrentis	Epidemic relapsing fever.
Leptospira interrogans	Leptospirosis, pretibial fever, and Weil's syndrome.
Treponema carateum	Pinta.

Continued

TABLE 1–2. **Clinically Important Bacteria and Their Associated Diseases** *(Continued)*

Bacteria	Associated Disease or Diseases
Spirochetes *(continued)*	
Treponema pallidum	Bejel, syphilis, and yaws.
Legionellae (see Chapter 13)	
Legionella pneumophila	Legionnaires' disease and Pontiac fever.
Toxigenic bacteria (see Chapter 14)	
Aeromonas hydrophila	Watery diarrhea.
Arcanobacterium haemolyticum	Pharyngitis.
Bacillus anthracis	Anthrax.
Bacillus cereus	Food poisoning.
Clostridium botulinum	Botulism.
Clostridium difficile	Pseudomembranous colitis.
Clostridium perfringens	Food poisoning, gas gangrene, and pig-bel.
Clostridium septicum	Cancer-associated bacteremia.
Clostridium tetani	Tetanus.
Corynebacterium diphtheriae	Diphtheria.
Corynebacterium jeikeium	Various infections in patients with neutropenia or leukemia, including bacteremia, pneumonia, prosthetic valve endocarditis, and skin infections.
Corynebacterium minutissimum	Erythrasma.
Plesiomonas shigelloides	Bloody diarrhea.
Vibrio cholerae	Bloody diarrhea and cholera.
Vibrio fluvialis	Bloody diarrhea.
Vibrio mimicus	Watery diarrhea.
Vibrio parahaemolyticus	Japanese summer diarrhea.
Vibrio vulnificus	Sepsis in alcoholics after marine wound.
Nonsporulating anaerobic bacteria (see Chapter 15)	
Bacteroides fragilis	Deep abscesses, especially in the abdomen; genital tract infections in women; and sepsis.
Bifidobacterium species	Polymicrobial lung infections.
Eubacterium species	Periodontitis.
Fusobacterium necrophorum	Deep abscesses, especially in the abdomen.
Fusobacterium nucleatum	Abdominal infections, amniotic infections, brain and lung abscesses, chronic sinusitis, metastatic osteomyelitis, oral infections, and pneumonia.
Gemella species	Intra-abdominal, oral, and urogenital abscesses.
Lactobacillus species	Pleuropulmonary infections.
Mobiluncus species	Bacterial vaginosis.
Peptostreptococcus species	Aspiration pneumonia, brain and lung abscesses, chronic otitis media, gynecologic and obstetric infections, and wound infections.
Porphyromonas species	Aspiration pneumonia; deep abscesses, especially in the abdomen; dental, head, neck, and lung abscesses; and empyema.
Prevotella melaninogenica	Aspiration pneumonia; deep abscesses, especially in the abdomen; dental, head, neck, and lung abscesses; and empyema.
Propionibacterium species	Central nervous system shunt infections, cervicofacial and pulmonary abscesses, and endocarditis.
Streptococcus species	Intra-abdominal, oral, and urogenital abscesses.
Veillonella species	Dental and urogenital abscesses.

be **gram-variable.** The Gram-staining procedure differentiates between two major groups of bacteria whose cell envelopes differ vastly from one another.

Gram-Positive Versus Gram-Negative Bacteria

Structural Differences. Figs. 1–2 and 1–3 show the **cell envelopes** of typical gram-positive and gram-negative bacteria. The cell envelope of a bacterium is the set of integral layers that surround the bacterium, specifically its **cell membranes** and **cell wall.** The typical gram-positive bacterium has a two-layer envelope, consisting of an inner cytoplasmic membrane and a thick, multilayered, highly cross-linked cell wall composed of **peptidoglycan.** In contrast, the typical gram-negative bacterium has a cell envelope consist-

ing of a cytoplasmic membrane, a thin cell wall, and an outer membrane with an outer leaflet composed mostly of a phospholipidlike molecule called **lipopolysaccharide.**

These differences between gram-positive and gram-negative bacteria have a tremendous effect on the ways in which the two groups of organisms interact with their world. In the case of the Gram stain, the differences in the amount of lipid in the two cell envelopes is the key to their differential abilities to be stained. When the mordant is added during the Gram-staining procedure, crystal violet (CV) and iodine (I) form complexes that are largely within the cell. Because the gram-positive cell envelope has relatively little lipid but has a thick cell wall, the acetone-alcohol decolorizing agent dehydrates the cell wall,

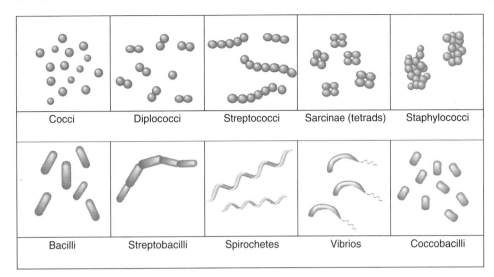

FIGURE 1–1. Morphologies of some of the commonly encountered bacteria.

trapping the CV-I complexes within the cell and making the bacterium appear blue or purple. In contrast, the gram-negative bacterium has an outer membrane that is composed of lipids and lipoproteins, and its cell wall is thin. The decolorizer extracts the outer membrane lipids without causing the wall to form an impermeable barrier. Thus, the color leaks out of the bacterium at this point, and the cell has to be counterstained with safranin to be visualized.

Clinical Differences.   Table 1–3 lists the clinically important gram-positive and gram-negative bacteria. Gram-positive bacteria are found in greatest numbers on the skin and on mucosal surfaces. Most are cocci, although a few (such as diphtheroids and mycobacteria) are bacilli. The most prevalent medi-

cally important gram-positive bacteria are the streptococci, staphylococci, and pneumococci. These bacteria possess **antiphagocytic capsules** and may cause acute pyogenic (pus-forming) infections, such as pneumonia, boils, pharyngitis, and meningitis. Gram-positive bacteria are more sensitive to the lytic actions of lysozyme and penicillin G than are gram-negative bacteria. This is largely because gram-positive bacteria have no outer membrane to restrict the access of these agents to the cell wall.

Most medically important gram-negative bacteria are rods or diplococci, and many are permanent residents of the gastrointestinal tract. They are prevalent causes of infections of wounds and of the urinary tract, lungs, and meninges, as well as the gastrointes-

FIGURE 1–2. Cell envelope of a gram-positive bacterium. Gram-positive bacteria typically have a two-layer cell envelope, composed of an inner cytoplasmic membrane and a multilayered peptidoglycan cell wall. Most gram-positive bacteria have teichoic acids attached to both the cytoplasmic membrane (lipoteichoic acid) and the cell wall (wall teichoic acid). Some gram-positive bacteria have additional layers of protein or waxes (not pictured).

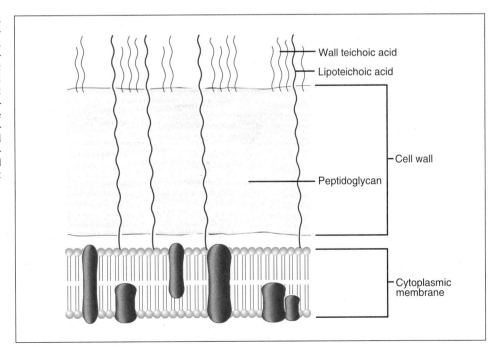

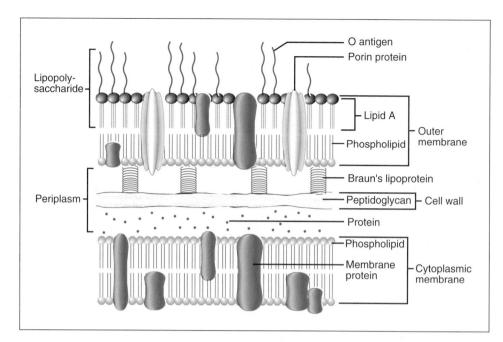

FIGURE 1–3. Cell envelope of a gram-negative bacterium. Gram-negative bacteria typically have a cell envelope consisting of a cytoplasmic membrane, a thin cell wall, and an outer membrane. The outer membrane is attached to the cell wall via Braun's lipoprotein. The outer leaflet of the outer membrane is composed primarily of lipopolysaccharide. Substrate-specific permeases are located in the cytoplasmic membrane, and the outer membrane contains protein pores that allow large molecules to diffuse into the periplasm.

tinal tract. The outer membrane of gram-negative bacteria contains **lipopolysaccharide,** a substance often called **endotoxin** because it elicits systemic toxic effects. A few gram-negative bacteria (usually *Neisseria* and *Haemophilus*) cause acute pyogenic infections.

TABLE 1–3.   Classification of Clinically Important Bacteria by Their Shape and Gram-Staining Characteristics

Gram-positive cocci
Enterococcus, Gemella, Peptostreptococcus, Staphylococcus, and *Streptococcus*

Gram-positive coccobacilli or rods
Actinomadura, Actinomyces, Arcanobacterium, Bacillus, Bifidobacterium, Clostridium, Corynebacterium, Erysipelothrix, Eubacterium, Lactobacillus, Listeria, Mycobacterium, Nocardia, Propionibacterium, Streptomyces, and *Tropheryma*

Gram-negative cocci
Moraxella, Neisseria, and *Veillonella*

Gram-negative coccobacilli or rods
Bacteroides, Bartonella, Bordetella, Brucella, Burkholderia, Capnocytophaga, Citrobacter, Coxiella, Edwardsiella, Enterobacter, Escherichia, Francisella, Fusobacterium, Haemophilus, Hafnia, Klebsiella, Legionella, Mobiluncus, Moraxella, Morganella, Pantoea, Pasteurella, Porphyromonas, Prevotella, Proteus, Providencia, Pseudomonas, Rickettsia, Salmonella, Serratia, Shigella, Stenotrophomonas, Streptobacillus, and *Yersinia*

Gram-negative spirochetes
Borrelia, Leptospira, Spirillum, and *Treponema*

Gram-negative vibrios
Aeromonas, Campylobacter, Helicobacter, Plesiomonas, and *Vibrio*

Other gram-negative bacteria
Chlamydia and *Ehrlichia*

Bacteria that resist Gram's stain
Mycoplasma and *Ureaplasma*

In general, gram-negative bacteria are more sensitive to the lytic action of antibody and complement than are gram-positive bacteria. This is because the outer membrane can be lysed by the terminal membrane attack complex that is formed when complement is activated.

Bacteria That Resist Gram's Stain

Some bacteria are considered to fall outside the realm of classification by Gram's stain, either because they are difficult to stain or because they lack cell walls. Among the bacteria that resist Gram's stain are members of the genera *Mycobacterium* and *Mycoplasma.*

Mycobacteria are gram-positive bacteria that are extremely difficult to stain because their cell envelopes contain large amounts of **waxes.** Suspected mycobacteria are stained using special procedures, such as the **Ziehl-Neelsen procedure,** and are considered to be **acid-fast organisms** because they resist decolorization with mineral acids or acidic methanol. Mycobacteria cause slowly progressive diseases such as tuberculosis and leprosy.

Mycoplasmas are the smallest bacteria known. They do not have a cell wall and therefore cannot be stained by the Gram procedure. The mycoplasmal cytoplasmic membrane contains **steroids,** which replace the usual cell wall functions of providing cellular rigidity and osmotic stability. Because mycoplasmas lack a cell wall, antibiotics that interfere with cell wall synthesis (such as penicillins and cephalosporins) are useless in the treatment of mycoplasmal diseases.

Mycoplasmas are similar in general appearance and structure to wall-less variants of other bacteria that occasionally arise naturally during human infections. These so-called **L forms** multiply slowly, are insensitive to the action of cell wall–reactive antibiotics such as penicillins and cephalosporins, and sometimes arise when an infection is being treated with penicillins or cephalosporins. When the antibiotic course is completed, the selective pressure to persist in a wall-less form is removed. At this point, the bacterium reverts to its normal state, and the patient's disease relapses. L forms are associated with infections caused by *Streptobacillus moniliformis,* one of the agents of rat-bite fever.

COMPONENTS OF THE BACTERIAL CELL ENVELOPE

In order to understand how bacteria interact with their environment, how they cause disease, and how antibiotics work, it is important to understand the structures, activities, synthesis, and control of the various bacterial parts. Because bacteria interact with their world through the cell envelope and its associated structures, each part of the cell envelope will be examined in detail. Figs. 1–2, 1–3, and 1–4 show the structures typically associated with gram-positive and gram-negative bacteria.

The Cytoplasmic Membrane
Structure

The cytoplasmic membranes of gram-positive and gram-negative bacteria are indistinguishable. Each has a trilaminar cytoplasmic membrane that is composed of protein (60–70%), lipids and phospholipids (20–30%), and a small amount of carbohydrate. The phospholipids form a bilayer with the polar ends pointing out, and membrane proteins float within the lipid bilayer.

General Functions

The principal functions of the cytoplasmic membrane are (1) to act as an osmotic barrier, (2) to serve as the site of selective permeability and carrier-mediated transport, (3) to serve as the site of cytochrome activity and proton motive force (PMF) generation, (4) to synthesize the cell wall, and (5) to provide a site for implantation of the chromosome.

Because the cytoplasmic membrane is a lipid film, it forms an osmotic barrier that allows only molecules smaller than glycerol to diffuse into the cytoplasm. Glycerol and larger molecules enter the cytoplasm only if their entry is mediated by **permeases,** which are highly specific transport proteins that span the cytoplasmic membrane. Thus, the cytoplasmic membrane is the site of selective permeability and carrier-mediated transport.

The cytoplasmic membrane is also the site of synthesis. It is here that the single chromosome is implanted. The enzymes for complex lipid biosynthesis are located in the cytoplasmic membrane, as are the enzymes that synthesize the cell wall. In some bacteria, the cytoplasmic membrane invaginates to form **mesosomes.** Mesosomes that occur along the long axis of a bacillus are known as **lateral mesosomes** and are believed to be involved in the secretion of extracellular proteins. Other mesosomes, called **septal mesosomes,** occur at the septum between adjacent connected bacteria and are believed to be involved in segregating copies of the chromosome into daughter cells during cell division.

Carrier-Mediated Transport

The cytoplasmic membrane is the key bacterial osmotic barrier. Ions and nonionic substances the

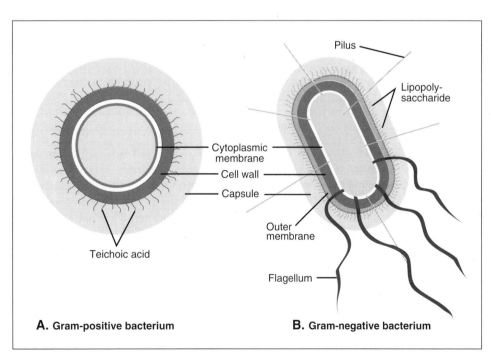

FIGURE 1–4. A comparison of the structures of typical gram-positive (A) and gram-negative (B) bacteria. The gram-positive bacterium has a cytoplasmic membrane; a thick, multilayered cell wall; teichoic acid (wall teichoic acid and lipoteichoic acid) extending from the surface of the bacterium; and a capsule. In contrast, the gram-negative bacterium has a cytoplasmic membrane; a thin cell wall; an outer membrane containing porins (not shown) and lipopolysaccharide; pili and flagella anchored in the cytoplasmic membrane and extending into the environment; and a capsule. Individual gram-positive and gram-negative bacteria may lack one or more of these structures, and some gram-positive bacteria have additional protein or waxy layers.

size of glycerol or larger diffuse slowly through the cytoplasmic membrane unless their movement into the cell is facilitated by permeases. There are at least three important carrier-mediated transport mechanisms found among bacteria: facilitated diffusion, active transport, and group translocation.

Facilitated Diffusion. Bacteria assimilate many substrates from their environment, using processes that involve specific permeases and exhibit Michaelis saturation kinetics. When energy is expended in moving the substrate across the cytoplasmic membrane, the process is called active transport, but when a substrate is accumulated without expending energy, the process is known as facilitated diffusion. Facilitated diffusion involves a carrier whose affinity (K_t) for its substrate is the same on both sides of the membrane. When the concentration of the substrate approaches the affinity of the carrier, the substrate is bound and moved to the opposite side of the membrane. Because the affinity of the carrier is the same on both sides of the cytoplasmic membrane, the substrate can be moved into or out of the bacterium equally well. Thus, molecules transported by facilitated diffusion cannot be accumulated against a concentration gradient.

At first glance, this characteristic of facilitated diffusion would seem to limit its usefulness to situations in which there are high concentrations of a desired substrate outside the bacterium. There are, however, tricks that some bacteria use to accumulate substrate against an *apparent* concentration gradient. The key to this approach is to rapidly alter the substrate once it enters the cell so it never accumulates in a form that the active site of the permease recognizes. For example, as shown in Fig. 1–5A, the gram-negative bacterium *Escherichia coli* transports glycerol via facilitated diffusion by rapidly phosphorylating glycerol after it enters the cytoplasm. By linking glycerol transport to metabolism, the cell accumulates much glycerol 3-phosphate but little genuine glycerol. Because the permease does not recognize glycerol 3-phosphate, it believes that the intracellular concentration of glycerol is perpetually low, and it continues to transport glycerol into the cell. It could be said that the bacterium, in effect, is accumulating glycerol against a concentration gradient, but it is doing so only by subterfuge. Because the accumulated substrate has been disguised by phosphorylating it, the permease is actually continuing to transport glycerol from an area of high concentration (outside) to one of low concentration (inside) where there is much glycerol 3-phosphate but no detectable free glycerol.

Another variant mechanism of facilitated diffusion is shown in Fig. 1–5B. The obligate intracellular bacterium *Rickettsia prowazekii* multiplies only within host cells (usually endothelial cells), where there is an abundance of adenosine triphosphate (ATP) in the cytoplasm. Rickettsiae assimilate ATP from their host by using a specialized facilitated diffusion mechanism that exchanges ATP or adenosine diphosphate (ADP) on one side of their cytoplasmic membrane for a molecule of ATP or ADP on the other side of the membrane. ATP and ADP are recognized equally well, but a molecule cannot move out of the bacterium unless it is exchanged for a molecule from the environment. Thus, for an ATP or ADP molecule to exit the bacterium, another ATP or ADP molecule must be transported into the cell. This allows rickettsiae to equilibrate themselves to the energy charge (the ratio of ATP/ADP/AMP) of the host cell without expending any of their own energy to do so. When the host cell dies and the rickettsiae are released into the blood, they are now temporarily placed into an environment in which there is little or no extracellular ATP or ADP. Thus, because the ATP permease cannot detect any extracellular substrate, no ATP or ADP diffuses out of the rickettsiae. This process of rickettsial ATP transport is an example of **obligate exchange-facilitated diffusion.**

Active Transport. Most people think of active transport when they think of carrier-mediated transport across a membrane. Active transport is similar to facilitated diffusion in that it requires the participation of a specific permease and its activity obeys Michaelis saturation kinetics. Active transport differs from facilitated diffusion in at least two ways: (1) active transport requires the direct or indirect expenditure of energy, and (2) active transport accumulates substrate against a severe concentration gradient. It is the expenditure of energy that drives the movement of the substrate against its concentration gradient. This energy expenditure may be in the form of ATP hydrolysis, or it may be indirect through coupling substrate transport to the movement of ions across the membrane. As discussed in further detail below, active transporters fall into two major groups: (1) primary active transporters, which are driven by ATP hydrolysis and are linked to periplasmic binding proteins, and (2) secondary active transporters, which cotransport substrates with hydrogen ion or sodium ion against phosphate.

Because of the difficulty of crystallizing permeases, surprisingly little is known of the details of how permeases transport their substrates or how these processes are linked to energy expenditure. Substrates bind to permeases at the outer face of the cytoplasmic membrane when the concentration of the substrate approaches the permease affinity. Then, in an energy-dependent process, the substrate is translocated to the inner face of the membrane and is released into the cytoplasm. It appears that the energy expenditure alters the conformation of the permease and that this conformation change allows the permease to release its substrate into the cytoplasm. Early studies of lactose permease suggested that the affinity of LacY permease for its substrate is dramatically reduced when its active site faces the cytoplasm. Thus, the permease always believes that the intracellular concentration of lactose is low and the extracellular concentration is high, because the perception of substrate concentration by the permease is always relative to its affinity. This allows the permease to accumulate lactose against a

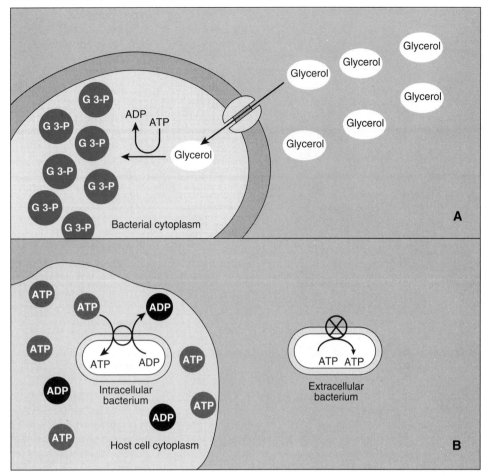

FIGURE 1–5. Two variant mechanisms for transporting molecules via facilitated diffusion. Diagram **A** shows that glycerol transport in *Escherichia coli* is coupled to metabolism, so that the transported glycerol is rapidly phosphorylated by enzymes involved in metabolism. Because glycerol 3-phosphate (G 3-P) is not recognized by the glycerol permease, there is no net accumulation of glycerol. Thus, glycerol continues to be transported, and the bacterium accumulates G 3-P. Diagram **B** illustrates adenosine triphosphate (ATP) transport by *Rickettsia prowazekii*. When the bacterium is within a host cell, ATP or adenosine diphosphate (ADP) is exchanged for ATP or ADP from the host cell cytoplasm. The extracellular bacterium is in an environment that contains no detectable ATP or ADP, so no exchange of substrate occurs.

severe concentration gradient. Other active transport systems do not work this way, however. In some systems, energy-linked transport involves altering the conformation of a membrane channel, which allows the substrate to be released in the direction of the cytoplasm instead of the environment. In either case, the permease changes conformation when energy is expended, and this allows its substrate to flow into the cell against a concentration gradient. This process is extremely efficient. *R. prowazekii,* for example, transports lysine rapidly when the concentration of lysine is 5 μmol/L outside the bacterium but is 1 mmol/L in the bacterial cytoplasm—that is, when there is a 200-fold concentration gradient.

(1) Primary Active Transporters. Primary active transporter systems have been most thoroughly studied in the enteric bacteria *E. coli* and *Salmonella* serotype *typhimurium*. These transport systems were first described more than 20 years ago as high-affinity transport systems whose activity was abolished when the outer membrane was removed from the bacteria by cold osmotic shock. These systems are also known as **ATP-binding cassette (ABC) transport systems** or **traffic ATPases** because their activity depends on the hydrolysis of ATP. ABC systems depend on outer membrane integrity because their substrate is presented to them by periplasmic binding proteins.

ABC systems consist of at least three proteins: a high-affinity **periplasmic binding protein** that is attached to lipids in the cytoplasmic membrane; a **hydrophobic permease** that spans the cytoplasmic membrane, receives the substrate from the binding protein, and is the channel for substrate movement across the membrane; and a **hydrophilic membrane-bound ATPase** that hydrolyzes ATP to allow the translocation of the substrate by the permease.

As Fig. 1–6 shows, substrates that have diffused through outer membrane channels are recognized by the high-affinity binding sites of the periplasmic binding proteins. The substrates are bound by hydrogen bonding, and the binding protein folds around the substrate molecule. The ligated binding protein is recognized by a receptor that is part of the permease, and the substrate is donated to the permease. The cytoplasmic face of the permease is associated with a hydrophilic ATPase protein. This membrane-bound ATPase now hydrolyzes ATP, which allows the substrate to be translocated to the cytoplasm and released. On average, two ATP molecules are expended for each molecule of substrate that is transported. In enteric bacteria, ABC systems translocate sugars, amino acids, and ions, and their high affinity is apparently conferred upon them by the affinity of their associated periplasmic binding proteins. There

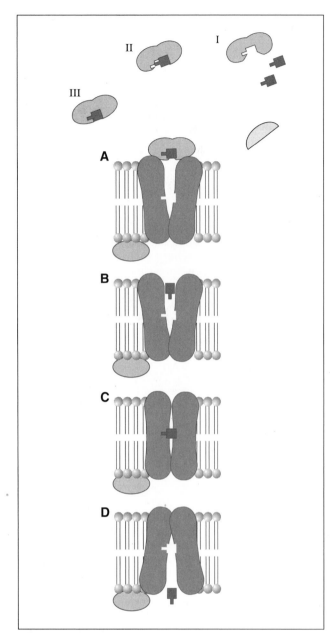

FIGURE 1–6. Linkage of active transport to the activity of high-affinity periplasmic binding proteins. Substrate molecules that have diffused through outer membrane channels (I) are bound by specific periplasmic binding proteins in a two-step process (II and III). The ligated binding protein is then recognized by a substrate-specific permease **(A),** and the substrate is donated to the permease by the binding protein **(B).** The permease then releases the substrate into the cytoplasm when a cytoplasmic protein associated with the permease hydrolyzes one molecule of ATP **(C** and **D).** (Redrawn and reproduced, with permission, from Quiocho, F. A. Atomic structures of periplasmic binding proteins and the high-affinity active transport systems in bacteria. Philos Trans R Soc Lond B Biol Sci 326:341–351, 1990.)

gram-positive bacteria have no outer membrane. However, similar systems coupled to binding proteins have now been described in *Streptococcus pneumoniae* and *Bacillus,* which are gram-positive bacteria. The *Bacillus* binding proteins are released into the environment, where they scavenge substrate to present to their associated permeases.

(2) Secondary Active Transporters. Secondary active transporters move substrate molecules into the cytoplasm by linking their translocation to the flux of ions across the membrane. Here, the movement of ions down their concentration and electrochemical gradient allows the linked substrate to accumulate against its chemical gradient. Examples of secondary active transport systems are symporters that cotransport hydrogen ion with simple sugars, oligosaccharides, or Krebs cycle intermediates. Other examples are antiporters that couple the transport of sugar phosphates into the cell with the export of phosphate ions. These systems are considered to be secondary active transporters because substrate translocation is linked indirectly to metabolism through ion translocation, rather than directly through ATP expenditure. The precise mechanism by which this process is linked to ion translocation is poorly understood.

In enteric bacteria, the secondary active transporters are low-affinity carriers (with a K_t often greater than 100 μmol/L) and are not linked to the activity of periplasmic binding proteins. In some other types of bacteria, however, there are PMF-dependent translocation systems that have affinities of 1 μmol/L or less. When active transport is driven by PMF, about 0.5 ATP equivalents are expended for each molecule of substrate that crosses the cytoplasmic membrane.

Secondary active transport systems have been described in both gram-positive and gram-negative bacteria and are a characteristic of bacteria that generate energy via aerobic or anaerobic respiration.

Group Translocation. Some bacteria transport sugars and glycols via a third transport system known as group translocation. For example, although the gram-negative bacterium *E. coli* transports lactose via active transport, it transports glucose, maltose, mannose, trehalose, fructose, cellobiose, and glucitol via group translocation. Group translocation systems occur primarily among facultative and obligate anaerobes and have been described in both gram-positive and gram-negative bacteria.

(1) Mechanisms of Group Translocation. The key characteristic of group translocation is that energy is not expended to change the conformation of the permease. Instead, the permease system alters the substrate during the translocation process by phosphorylating it. After phosphorylation, the sugar is not recognized by the carrier and is released into the cytoplasm. This differs from facilitated diffusion systems that are coupled to metabolism in that the group translocation permease system itself phosphorylates the substrate as part of the translocation process. Because the substrates translocated are

are relatively few ABC permeases per cell (50–100 molecules), but there may be thousands of copies of each substrate-specific binding protein in the periplasm of enteric bacteria.

Until recently, it was assumed that ABC systems could be found only in gram-negative bacteria, since

phosphorylated, group translocation systems are referred to as **phosphotransferase (PTS) systems.**

A model of group translocation is presented in Fig. 1–7. Three proteins are involved: histidine protein (HPr), a cytoplasmic protein; enzyme I (EI), another cytoplasmic protein; and enzyme II (EII), a multimeric membrane-bound protein. Depending on the PTS system, EII may have three or four domains or subunits, with one set of domains (either C or a combination of C and D) being a carrier that traverses the cytoplasmic membrane. Group translocation involves transferring a phosphate group from protein to protein and finally transferring it to the substrate as it enters the cytoplasm. Phosphoenolpyruvate (PEP) donates its phosphate to EI, which then donates the phosphate to HPr. EI and HPr are referred to as the "general" PTS proteins because the same EI and HPr are utilized in a single bacterium to transport many substrates. HPr now donates its phosphate to the A subunit of EII (EIIA); the phosphate next moves to the B subunit of EII (EIIB); and then as the C subunit of EII (EIIC) moves the substrate into the cytoplasm, EIIB phosphorylates the substrate. Because the phosphorylated substrate is not recognized by EIIC, it is released, and EIIC continues to facilitate the movement of substrate molecules into the cell. The net PTS reaction is simply the following:

$$PEP + sugar_{outside} \rightarrow pyruvate + sugar\text{-}P_{inside}$$

(2) Group Translocation and Regulation of Active Transport Systems. Because the transport of sugars by a PTS system requires no net energy expenditure, it is advantageous for the bacterium to preferentially utilize sugars that enter via a PTS system rather than via an active transport system when both types of systems are present. As Fig. 1–8 shows, PTS systems regulate active transport systems in two ways. First, unphosphorylated EIIA interacts with active transport sugar permeases in an unknown fashion and inhibits their activity. Second, phosphorylated EIIA (P-EIIA) stimulates the generation of cyclic AMP (cAMP) by increasing the activity of a membrane-bound adenylate cyclase. The synthesis of some active transport sugar permeases is inhibited when cAMP levels are low, so the lack of P-EIIA will concomitantly decrease both the amount of cAMP in the cell and the synthesis of these permeases. When the PTS reaction occurs, most of the EIIA is unphosphorylated (because it is rapidly donating phosphate to EIIB), so intracellular cAMP levels will be low, and much EIIA will be available to interact with active transporters. The net result is that the synthesis of active transport sugar permeases ceases and the ac-

FIGURE 1–7. Transport of mannitol, mannose, and glucose via a group translocation system, or phosphotransferase (PTS) system. A phosphate (P) from phosphoenolpyruvate (PEP) is transferred sequentially to enzyme I (EI) and histidine protein (HPr), which are the general PTS proteins. HPr then transfers the phosphate to a sugar or glycol-specific EII, and the A subunit of enzyme II (EIIA) receives the phosphate and transfers it to the EIIB domain. Then, as the substrate passes through the hydrophobic membrane–bound EIIC or EIIC-EIID, the transported substrate is phosphorylated and released into the cytoplasm. (Redrawn and reproduced, with permission, from Postma, P. W., J. W. Lengeler, and G. R. Jacobson. Phosphoenolpyruvate:carbohydrate phosphotransferase systems of bacteria. Microbiol Rev 57:543–594, 1993.)

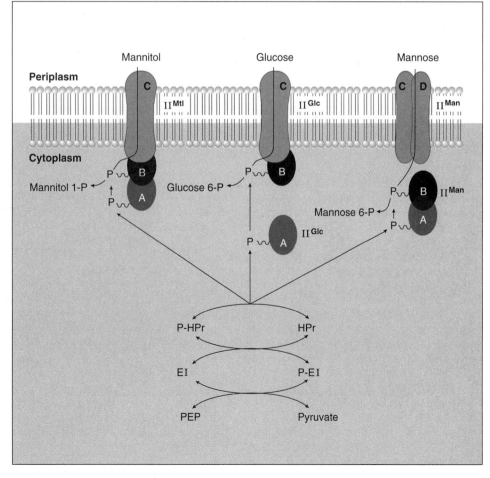

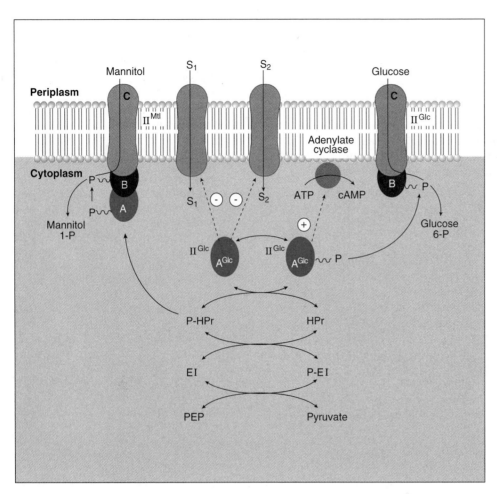

FIGURE 1–8. Regulation of active transport by phosphotransferase (PTS) systems. Two PTS systems are pictured: one for mannitol and one for glucose. When a sugar or glycol is transported via a PTS system, the amount of unphosphorylated EIIA increases as it donates its phosphate group to EIIB. Unphosphorylated EIIA interacts with active transport sugar permeases and inhibits their activity. Phosphorylated EIIA (P-EIIA) increases the activity of a membrane-bound adenylate cyclase. Because sufficient P-EIIA is not present when the PTS system is active, the activity of the adenylate cyclase is low. This reduces the amount of cAMP available. Because cAMP is required to initiate the synthesis of active transport sugar permeases, the synthesis of these molecules halts when glucose is transported via the PTS system. PEP = phosphoenolpyruvate; EI = enzyme I; Hpr = histidine protein; EIIA, EIIB, and EIIC = the A, B, and C subunits of a glycol-specific enzyme; S_1 = substrate 1; S_2 = substrate 2; ATP = adenosine triphosphate; and cAMP = cyclic adenosine monophosphate. (Redrawn and reproduced, with permission, from Postma, P. W., J. W. Lengeler, and G. R. Jacobson. Phosphoenolpyruvate:carbohydrate phosphotransferase systems of bacteria. Microbiol Rev 57:543–594, 1993.)

tivity of existing active transport sugar permeases is inhibited. When the substrate for the PTS system is exhausted, P-EIIA levels rise, and both the synthesis and activity of the active transport permeases rapidly increase.

Through their effects on intracellular cAMP levels, the PTS systems alter the reading of permease genes. This phenomenon, known as catabolite repression, is discussed more completely with regard to the lactose operon in Chapter 2.

(3) Group Translocation and Chemotaxis. PTS-mediated transport is also an important part of the chemotaxis system of motile bacteria. The PTS carrier modules serve as chemoreceptors, and their activity results in movement of a bacterium toward the site of greatest concentration of PTS substrates. This process is described in greater detail when the flagella and pili of motile bacteria are discussed (see Bacterial Cell Appendages, below).

(4) Efficiency of Group Translocation. The free energy released by the hydrolysis of phosphate from PEP is –14.7 kcal/mol (–61.7 kJ/mol), while the free energy of the phosphate bond in a phosphorylated sugar is only –3 kcal/mol (–12.6 kJ/mol). Yet PEP is equivalent in energy to ATP, and ATP-mediated active

transport of sugars requires the expenditure of at least two ATP molecules for each molecule transported: one ATP is expended in changing the permease conformation, and another is used to phosphorylate the transported sugar. Thus, sugars transported by group translocation use only one ATP equivalent to generate an intracellular sugar phosphate, while those transported by primary active transport require at least two ATP equivalents to obtain the same result.

The Periplasm

As Figs. 1–2 and 1–3 show, because only gram-negative bacteria have both an inner membrane (the cytoplasmic membrane) and an outer membrane, only they have a periplasm. This periplasm is more than merely a space between two membranes. It is the anteroom to the cytoplasm, where nutritional and biosynthetic precursors and antibiotics must wait before they enter the cytoplasm. Large molecules that enter the periplasm are broken down here to their constituent parts by periplasmic enzymes. The resultant amino acids or monosaccharides are then transported into the cytoplasm by permeases located in the cytoplasmic membrane. The transport of some of these molecules is facilitated by high-affinity substrate-specific binding proteins that are located in the periplasm (as discussed above). The periplasm also allows gram-negative bacteria to fully protect themselves from the action of some antibiotics by concentrating a small number of molecules of antibiotic hydrolases in this small space. For example, some gram-negative bacteria protect themselves from the lytic action of beta-lactam antibiotics (such as penicillins and cephalosporins) by accumulating beta-lactamase molecules in their periplasms. Finally, the cell wall of gram-negative bacteria lies entirely within the periplasm. Because of the significance of the cell wall and because the gram-positive cell wall does not lie within a periplasm, the structure and synthesis of the cell wall will be discussed separately, below.

The Cell Wall
General Characteristics

The bacterial cell wall (see Figs. 1–2, 1–3, and 1–4) is a sacculus that surrounds the cell like a webbed bag. Sometimes called the **murein sacculus,** it is composed mainly of a unique polysaccharide called peptidoglycan, and it is found in all bacteria except mycoplasmas and halophilic bacteria that live in hypertonic, hyperosmotic environments. The cell wall provides the cell with rigidity (hence, its shape) and prevents osmotic lysis. If the cell wall of a bacterium is removed, two things will happen: the bacterium will revert to a sphere if it was a rod, and the bacterium will lyse if it is placed into a hypotonic environment.

Cell Wall Constituents
Peptidoglycan

(1) Structure. Peptidoglycan is constructed from repeating disaccharide units of **N-acetylglucosamine (GlcNAc)** and **N-acetylmuramic acid (MurNAc)**. The fundamental disaccharide unit is shown in Fig. 1–9. Within each unit, GlcNAc is attached to MurNAc by a β1,4-glycosidic bond. The GlcNAc-MurNAc units are also interconnected by β1,4-glycosidic bonds, and it is these bonds which are broken by the action of lysozyme.

MurNAc is a GlcNAc that has added to it an O-lactyl group to which is attached a series of amino acids. The MurNAc peptide contains novel amino acids, including D-alanine and D-glutamate. Gram-negative bacteria typically have meso-diaminopimelic acid (meso-DAP) as the penultimate amino acid of the MurNAc peptide, as do some gram-positive bacteria. DAP is lysine with an added carboxyl group.

As shown in Fig. 1–9, the MurNAc peptide can be cross-linked to peptides on other GlcNAc-MurNAc units. When peptidoglycan is assembled, the disaccharides are first linked linearly via β1,4-bonds and are then cross-linked through these peptide bonds. Cross-linking makes the cell wall strong and rigid in

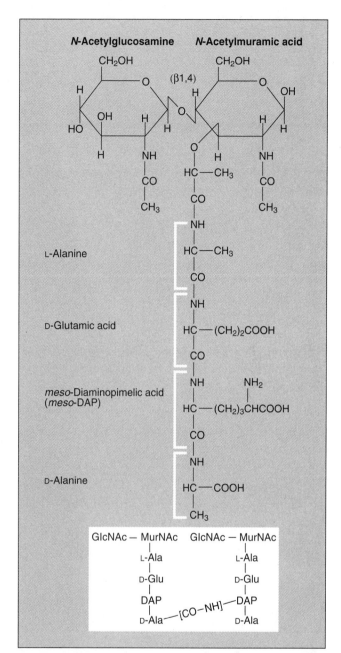

FIGURE 1–9. **The fundamental unit of peptidoglycan, consisting of N-acetylglucosamine (GlcNAc) and N-acetylmuramic acid (MurNAc).** Each disaccharide GlcNAc-MurNAc unit is attached to other disaccharide units by β1,4-glycosidic bonds, and the MurNAc peptides are cross-linked with the peptides of other MurNAcs via a peptide bond.

the face of osmotic pressure by allowing the peptidoglycan to form a web around the bacterium.

The murein sacculus in gram-negative bacteria differs significantly from that in gram-positive bacteria. Fig. 1–10 shows how the sacculus is constructed in E. coli. This model is typical for gram-negative bacteria, in which there is usually only a single layer of peptidoglycan, the cross-linking is lateral, and the cross-link is always between a D-alanine and DAP. In contrast, gram-positive bacteria typically have thick cell walls and may have as many as 40 layers of highly

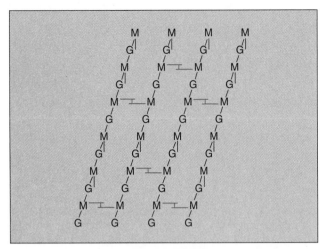

FIGURE 1–10. The murein sacculus. The cell wall is a sacculus composed of linearly linked GlcNAc-MurNAc disaccharide units with peptide cross-links. It is this cross-linking that gives peptidoglycan its tensile strength. G = GlcNAc, or N-acetylglucosamine. M = MurNAc, or N-acetylmuramic acid.

cross-linked peptidoglycan. As shown in Fig. 1–11, to facilitate this more extensive cross-linking, gram-positive bacteria vary the substituents of their MurNAc peptide at positions 2 and 3. These variations allow for cross-links that differ from those seen in the gram-negative cell wall. Additionally, rather than linking DAP and D-alanine directly by a peptide bond, many gram-positive bacteria construct cross-links that contain intervening peptides. For example, in *Staphylococcus aureus,* a lysine at position 3 is linked to the terminal D-alanine on another MurNAc unit via an intervening pentaglycine bridge. This allows longer cross-links to be established, including cross-links between layers.

Peptidoglycan serves as an anchor for unique molecules in gram-positive and gram-negative bacteria. Attached to occasional 6-hydroxyl groups on GlcNAc units of gram-positive bacteria are highly substituted polyol chains that are known as **teichoic acids.** These important antigenic components of gram-positive bacteria are discussed more fully below. Gram-negative bacteria do not have teichoic acids. Instead, attached to the terminal carboxyl group of about one-tenth of the DAP molecules is a lipoprotein known as **Braun's lipoprotein.** Braun's lipoprotein extends into the lipid bilayer of the outer membrane (see Fig. 1–3) and anchors the outer membrane to the cell wall. Braun's lipoprotein has been found in all gram-negative bacteria examined except *Pseudomonas* species.

(2) Cell Wall Synthesis. Figs. 1–12, 1–13, and 1–14 show how the cell wall of the gram-positive bacterium *S. aureus* is constructed. Cell wall synthesis

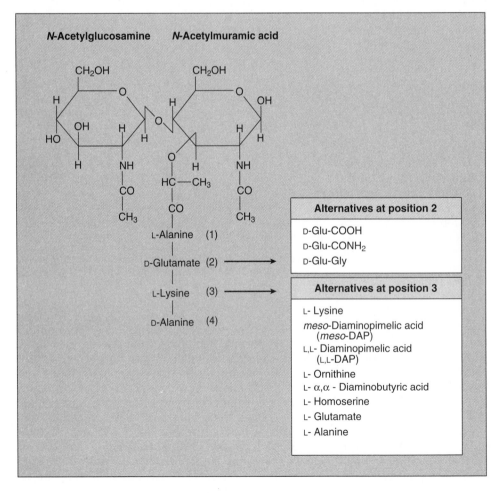

FIGURE 1–11. The peptidoglycan of gram-positive bacteria. Unlike the peptidoglycan of gram-negative bacteria, whose chemical structure is consistent, the peptidoglycan of gram-positive bacteria shows variations in the structure of the N-acetylmuramic acid (MurNAc) peptide at both the second and third amino acid positions.

N-Acetylglucosamine   **N-Acetylmuramic acid**

L-Alanine   (1)

D-Glutamate (2) ⟶

L-Lysine   (3) ⟶

D-Alanine   (4)

Alternatives at position 2
D-Glu-COOH
D-Glu-CONH$_2$
D-Glu-Gly

Alternatives at position 3
L- Lysine
meso-Diaminopimelic acid (*meso*-DAP)
L,L- Diaminopimelic acid (L,L-DAP)
L- Ornithine
L- α,α - Diaminobutyric acid
L- Homoserine
L- Glutamate
L- Alanine

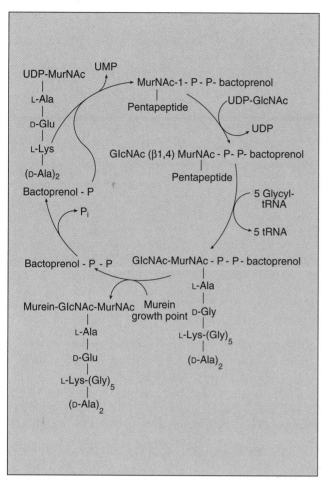

FIGURE 1–12. Cell wall synthesis. The diagram shows how *Staphylococcus aureus* completes its synthesis of the GlcNAc-MurNAc disaccharide unit, using a bactoprenyl phosphate carrier molecule, and inserts the disaccharide into the murein (peptidoglycan) growth point. Vancomycin and ristocetin block donation of the dipeptide to the murein growth point, and bacitracin blocks the dephosphorylation of the carrier molecule that is required to regenerate active bactoprenyl phosphate. GlcNAc = *N*-acetylglucosamine; MurNAc = *N*-acetylmuramic acid; UDP = uridine diphosphate; UMP = uridine monophosphate; bactoprenol-P = bactoprenyl monophosphate; and bactoprenol-P-P = bactoprenyl diphosphate.

begins with the conversion of fructose 6-phosphate to glucosamine 6-phosphate, and an acetate is then added to convert the molecule to *N*-acetylglucosamine 6-phosphate. After the phosphate is moved, *N*-acetylglucosamine 1-phosphate is attached to uridine diphosphate (UDP). Next, PEP is added to convert the molecule to UDP-MurNAc, and the individual amino acids of the MurNAc peptide are then added sequentially to the *O*-lactyl group. This process yields a molecule of UDP-MurNAc-pentapeptide, with the peptide composed of L-alanine, D-glutamic acid, L-lysine, D-alanine, and D-alanine.

Fig. 1–12 shows that the next key step is the displacement of uridine monophosphate (UMP) from UDP-MurNAc-pentapeptide by a 55-carbon isoprenoid lipid carrier molecule called **bactoprenol** or **undecaprenol**. Bactoprenol is composed of 11 isoprene units (see Fig. 1–13) and is anchored to the cytoplasmic membrane. MurNAc-bactoprenyl diphosphate (MurNAc-P-P-bactoprenol) serves as the backbone structure for the next series of events. GlcNAc is added to the MurNAc via a β1,4-glycosidic bond, and the five glycines that will serve as a bridge between MurNAcs are added as five individual glycyl-tRNAs. This forms the fundamental disaccharide unit that will be added to the murein sacculus. Bactoprenol takes the disaccharide to a cell wall growth point. Here, autolytic enzymes (such as amidases) cut the existing peptidoglycan, and the new disaccharide unit is added to the existing sacculus by forming β1,4-glycosidic bonds. The bactoprenyl diphosphate carrier is released and is then dephosphorylated to yield bactoprenyl monophosphate. If dephosphorylation of the carrier does not occur, cell wall synthesis is halted, because there is no available carrier to accept new GlcNAc or MurNAc units. Three antibiotics block cell wall synthesis by interfering with the supply of bactoprenyl phosphate. Vancomycin and ristocetin block the transfer of the disaccharide from bactoprenyl diphosphate to the murein growth site, and bacitracin blocks the dephosphorylation of bactoprenyl diphosphate that is necessary to regenerate the carrier molecule.

FIGURE 1–13. The 55-carbon isoprenoid lipid carrier molecule known as bactoprenol or undecaprenol.

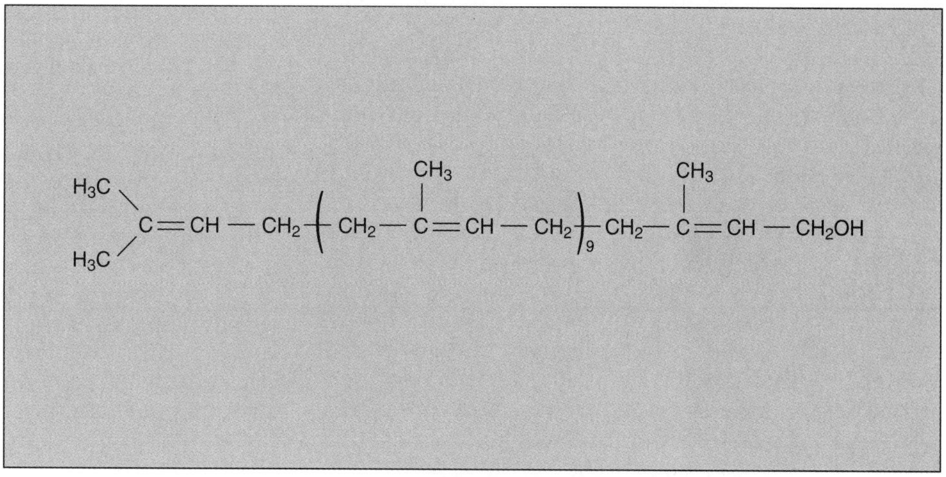

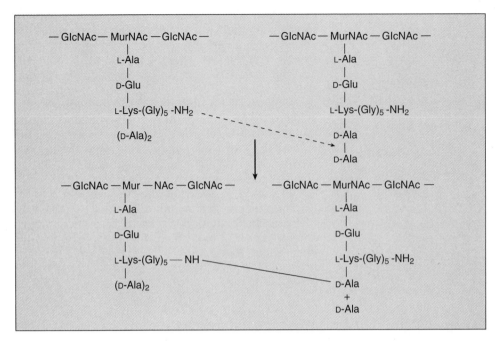

FIGURE 1–14. Transpeptidation during cell wall synthesis. Peptidoglycan is cross-linked when the amino group of the cross-link emanating from the 3 position (here, a glycine) attacks and breaks the peptide bond between the terminal D-alanines. A transpeptidase enzyme catalyzes the formation of a new peptide bond between the glycine and D-alanine. GlcNAc = N-acetylglucosamine; and MurNAc = N-acetylmuramic acid.

Fig. 1–14 depicts the final steps of peptidoglycan synthesis. Each bacterium has one or more **transpeptidases** that catalyze the cross-linking of the cell wall. There are two D-alanines at the end of the MurNAc O-lactyl peptide. The amino group of the terminal glycine in the cross-link peptide attacks the bond between the two D-alanines. Aided by a transpeptidase, the terminal D-alanine is displaced and is replaced by a peptide bond between the glycine of the cross-link and the penultimate D-alanine. This cross-link completes the insertion of the disaccharide unit into the expanding murein sacculus.

Each bacterium has multiple types of transpeptidases because different transpeptidases are used to repair or extend the sacculus and because different wall sites (such as the tip versus the long side of a bacillus) sometimes utilize unique transpeptidases. Transpeptidases are also known as **penicillin-binding proteins** (PBPs) because they are the primary targets of beta-lactam antibiotics such as penicillins, cephalosporins, and monobactams. These antibiotics will be discussed fully in Chapter 4. Their general mode of action relies on their similarity to the peptide composed of amino acid and two D-alanines, which allows them to competitively inhibit the transpeptidation reaction. When the transpeptidase binds a beta-lactam antibiotic, the antibiotic is bound tightly and cell wall cross-linking stops. Meanwhile, autolytic enzymes continue to open up sites in the cell wall for insertion of new disaccharide units. Units are added linearly to these sites, but no cross-linking occurs. As a result, the number of cross-links in the wall decreases, and the tensile strength of the wall diminishes accordingly. Eventually, the wall becomes very weak, and the cell is lysed by osmotic pressure. Obviously, the faster an organism is multiplying, the faster the cell wall is being replaced. Thus, penicillins

and cephalosporins are effective only against growing bacteria, and their efficacy is related to the amount of antibiotic that is able to reach the growth site, the relative affinity of the PBPs for the antibiotic, and the rate at which the culture is multiplying.

(3) The Bacterial Cell Wall and Disease.   Little pathogenic activity has been associated with the release of standard peptidoglycan units during infection. Recent studies have shown, however, that MurNAc residues of some bacteria are O-acetylated at the C-6 hydroxyl group, as shown in Fig. 1–15. The O-acetylated MurNAc residues resist the hydrolytic action of lysozyme and glycosidases produced by phagocytic cells, allowing bacteria with **O-acetylated peptidoglycan** to resist enzymatic lysis. The percentage of MurNAc residues that are O-acetylated varies from 10% to 100%, depending on the bacterial species, but is most commonly between 30% and 50%.

Among the gram-positive and gram-negative bacterial species that have been shown to have O-acetylated peptidoglycan are *Bordetella pertussis, Enterococcus faecalis, Neisseria gonorrhoeae, Proteus mirabilis, Proteus vulgaris,* and *S. aureus.* The bacteria release O-acetylated peptidoglycan fragments of varying sizes during their growth, following their destruction by phagocytic cells, and as a consequence of antibiotic action. These fragments, which may persist in the blood for some time, induce slow-wave sleep, activate complement, elicit fever, and are associated with the onset of attacks of infection-associated arthritis. The results of some studies have suggested that O-acetylated peptidoglycan fragments also precipitate attacks of rheumatoid arthritis. Recently, investigators have shown that a cytolytic toxin which is released by *B. pertussis* and causes massive destruction of ciliated epithelia in patients with pertussis (whooping cough) is identical to O-acetylated peptidoglycan.

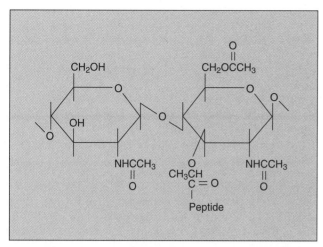

FIGURE 1–15. The structure of O-acetylated peptidoglycan.

It is not known how the peptidoglycan fragments elicit such a variety of responses. Effects such as somnolence and fever have been attributed by some investigators to the ability of O-acetylated peptidoglycan fragments to elicit the production of interleukin-1.

Teichoic Acids and Lipoteichoic Acids

(1) Structure of Teichoic Acids. The cell envelope of gram-positive bacteria contains chains of up to 30 glycerol or ribitol phosphates that are linked by phosphodiester bonds and extend from the cell envelope into the environment (see Fig. 1–2). These polyol chains are referred to as teichoic acids. The alcohol groups of teichoic acids are substituted with sugars, choline, or alanine, making these molecules highly antigenic. In some cases, up to 50% of the cell wall complex is teichoic acid. Teichoic acids may exist as lipoteichoic acids or wall teichoic acids.

(a) Lipoteichoic Acids. All gram-positive bacteria have teichoic acids that are attached to lipids in the cytoplasmic membrane, traverse the cell wall, and extend into the environment. These are known as lipoteichoic acids and are usually composed of highly substituted chains of glycerol phosphate. Lipoteichoic acids are major antigenic determinants in some bacteria. For example, the D polysaccharide of *E. faecalis* is a lipoteichoic acid.

(b) Wall Teichoic Acids. Some gram-positive bacteria have teichoic acids that are attached to occasional 6-OH groups on N-acetylmuramic acid. These wall teichoic acids are not as well understood as lipoteichoic acids, but they also may serve as major antigenic determinants of gram-positive bacteria. For example, the C carbohydrate of *S. pneumoniae* is a wall teichoic acid. In most cases, the wall teichoic acid and the lipoteichoic acid of a single bacterium are structurally unrelated.

(2) Synthesis of Teichoic Acids. The individual units of teichoic acids are assembled on an undecaprenyl phosphate carrier in a manner analogous to that of peptidoglycan synthesis, and they are then transferred to the cytoplasmic membrane or peptidoglycan growth site. The individual alcohols are added to the lipid carrier as cytidine diphosphate alcohols. Teichoic acid synthesis is blocked by antibiotics that interfere with transfer of materials from the lipid carrier or with dephosphorylation of the carrier molecule.

(3) Role of Teichoic Acids in Disease. Although investigators have long known of teichoic acids, surprisingly little is known about why they are important to gram-positive bacteria. Teichoic acids are believed to regulate the activities of amidases and glycosidases that participate in cell wall synthesis as autolysins. Teichoic acids may affect the **competence** of some bacteria—that is, their ability to take up DNA fragments from the environment—as well as their ability to resist lysis by lysozyme and other glycosidases and to attract and transport magnesium. Teichoic acids play two important roles in the pathogenesis of diseases caused by gram-positive bacteria: they promote bacterial survival by serving as **adhesins,** and they can promote a sepsislike syndrome by causing host cells to release inflammatory mediators such as **monokines** and **cytokines.**

Adherence is an important characteristic for bacteria that live on mucosal surfaces. Nonadherent bacteria are easily eliminated from mucosal surfaces by fluid flow and desquamation of the epithelium, so the **virulence** (ability to cause disease) of bacteria is usually dependent on their ability to adhere to the mucosae; strains that lose their ability to adhere become avirulent. The ability of *S. aureus* and *Streptococcus bovis* to adhere to mucosae involves both lipoteichoic acid and a protein adhesin, and *Staphylococcus epidermidis* adheres to fibrin-platelet clots via lipoteichoic acid. Thus, lipoteichoic acid is probably an important oral adhesin for at least two genera of pathogenic bacteria, and it may promote infective endocarditis by mediating the adherence of staphylococci to clots on damaged heart valves.

Patients may develop systemic disease when large numbers of bacteria and their products circulate in the blood. This phenomenon, which is called **sepsis,** is usually caused by the lipopolysaccharide of gram-negative bacteria and can result in death in up to 50% of affected patients. Patients with sepsis are acutely ill, with tachycardia, tachypnea, hypotension, and either fever or hypothermia. They may also suffer from disseminated intravascular coagulation, acute renal failure, and other signs of cardiovascular dysfunction.

Multiplying gram-positive bacteria release blebs of cell membrane and cell wall fragments that are impregnated with teichoic acids. Because, like lipopolysaccharide, teichoic acids are amphipathic, the teichoic acids bind to **lipopolysaccharide-binding protein** (LBP), and a cascade of inflammatory mediators is elicited from host cells.

Lipoteichoic acid and gram-positive organisms are between 20-fold and 100-fold less potent than are lipopolysaccharide and gram-negative bacteria in eliciting the release of inflammatory mediators or causing hypotension. This correlates well with the observation that sepsis is most often associated with infections caused by gram-negative bacteria. Nevertheless, gram-positive sepsis is an important clinical phenomenon, and the ability of teichoic acids to elicit inflammatory mediators is clinically significant.

Other Cell Wall–Associated Structures. There are other layers associated with the cell walls of some gram-positive bacteria. Streptococci and staphylococci have **protein layers,** and streptococci have type-specific **carbohydrate layers.** The protein or carbohydrate molecules are major immunologic characteristics of the cells, and some of them function as antiphagocytic structures. For example, streptococcal M protein acts somewhat like a capsule in its ability to protect the bacteria from phagocytosis, and staphylococcal protein A inhibits phagocytosis by serving as a receptor for the Fc portion of IgG. Mycobacteria have a series of **waxes** and **peptides** that are associated with their peptidoglycan and protect them from destruction by phagocytes. These structures will be discussed fully in the sections that examine the individual pathogens.

The Outer Membrane
General Characteristics

Gram-negative bacteria are the only bacteria that have a membrane lying outside the cell wall complex (see Figs. 1–3 and 1–4). Like the cytoplasmic membrane, the outer membrane is a trilaminar membrane consisting largely of phospholipids oriented with the polar ends out and the hydrophobic regions in the middle of the bilayer. Floating in this bilayer are lipoproteins. **Porins** and **porinlike proteins** in the outer membrane allow the membrane to serve as a molecular sieve, restricting the access of some molecules to the cell wall and cytoplasmic membrane and allowing the entry of only those molecules which can pass through **outer membrane channels.**

In all gram-negative bacteria except *Pseudomonas* species, the outer membrane is anchored to the cell wall via a lipoprotein called **Braun's lipoprotein.** The outer membrane dominates the social activities of gram-negative bacteria, providing structures and receptors that affect adhesion to host cells, resistance to phagocytosis, and susceptibility to bacteriophages. The most clinically significant component of the outer membrane is a phospholipidlike molecule called lipopolysaccharide.

Outer Membrane Constituents
Lipopolysaccharide

(1) Structure. Unlike the cytoplasmic membrane, the outer membrane is asymmetric. That is, while the inner leaflet is composed of phospholipids, lipoproteins, and hydrophobic proteins, the outer leaflet is composed primarily of the membrane channels that span the outer membrane and of a pharmacologically active, phospholipidlike molecule called lipopolysaccharide (LPS). Fig. 1–16 shows that LPS has three distinguishable regions, known as the O antigen, core, and lipid A. The core can be further

subdivided into an inner and outer core. The O antigen extends from the surface of the bacterium into the environment; the outer and inner cores anchor the O antigen to lipid A; and lipid A floats in the outer leaflet of the outer membrane (see Figs. 1–3 and 1–16).

(a) The O Antigen. The O antigen is also known as **bacterial somatic antigen** (from Greek *sōma,* meaning "body") because it is so immunologically prominent. It is composed of a series of repeating units of linear trisaccharides or branched tetra- or pentasaccharides, and it extends from the cell surface into the environment. The O antigen may be up to 40 units in length, but the lengths of individual O antigens on a single bacterium are highly variable. Each gram-negative bacterium has a characteristic O antigen that can be used to identify (or "type") the bacterium. This is a commonly used epidemiologic tool and is especially helpful in identifying strains of enteric bacteria such as *Salmonella* or *E. coli.* For example, among the salmonellae there are more than 1000 antigenic types of O antigen. Because bacteriophages or plasmids (extrachromosomal DNA) may introduce a piece of DNA into a bacterium that codes for an O antigen, individual bacteria may simultaneously express more than one antigenic type of O antigen.

It is evident that the O antigen is not necessary for survival, because some bacteria do not have O antigen. In some cases, these bacteria are "rough" variants of wild-type "smooth" bacteria that have O antigen. (These bacteria were first called "rough" because the loss of expression of O antigen made the bacteria clump in suspension.) Rough bacteria are classified according to how much of the LPS structure is still expressed. Bacteria that express only lipid A and the inner core are referred to as "severe rough" bacteria. Other bacterial species never express O antigen. The LPS of these naturally rough bacteria is called **lipooligosaccharide** (LOS) to denote the natural absence of O antigen.

O antigen has been shown to serve as a receptor that allows some bacteria to adhere to host surface structures. O antigen moderately affects the ability of bacteria to resist phagocytosis by polymorphonuclear leukocytes, and studies have shown that rough bacteria are typically more susceptible to phagocytosis than are their smooth counterparts. O antigen serves as a receptor for some bacteriophages, and loss of O antigen expression allows the bacterium to resist bacteriophage infection. During many gram-negative infections, a strong antibody response is elicited against the O antigen. Thus, efforts to identify the cause of disease sometimes include the use of diagnostic techniques to assess whether antibody to O antigen is present.

(b) The LPS Core. The O antigen is attached to lipid A via the LPS core. The core can be divided into two portions, known as the inner and outer cores. Among the bacterial species, the **outer core** is fairly variable in its structure, containing an assortment of sugars and amino sugars. Almost all outer core

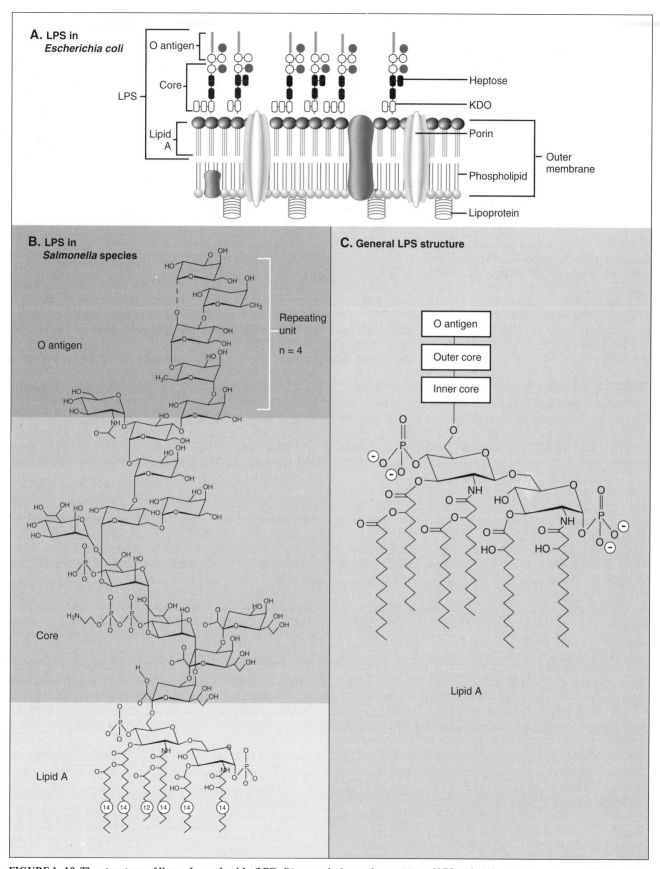

A. LPS in *Escherichia coli*

O antigen

Core

LPS

Lipid A

Heptose

KDO

Porin

Phospholipid

Lipoprotein

Outer membrane

B. LPS in *Salmonella* species

O antigen

Repeating unit

n = 4

Core

Lipid A

C. General LPS structure

O antigen

Outer core

Inner core

Lipid A

FIGURE 1–16. The structure of lipopolysaccharide (LPS). Diagram **A** shows the position of LPS within the outer membrane of *Escherichia coli*, a gram-negative organism. Diagram **B** shows the molecular structure of LPS in *Salmonella* species, which are also gram-negative. Diagram **C** shows the general structure of LPS, emphasizing the structure of lipid A. LPS is composed of three major regions: the type-specific O antigen, which extends into the external environment from the bacterial surface; the core, which consists of an inner and outer core and which anchors the O antigen to the membrane; and lipid A, which is a phospholipidlike molecule that floats in the outer leaflet of the outer membrane. All of the significant pharmacologic activity of LPS resides in the lipid A moiety. KDO = 2-keto-3-deoxyoctulosonic acid.

molecules contain the unusual 7-carbon sugar, **heptose.** The most severe rough mutants (known in salmonellae as R_e mutants) lack the outer core but retain the inner core. The **inner core** is composed mostly of a single sugar known as **2-keto-3-deoxyoctulosonic acid** (KDO). Chemical tests used to detect the presence of LPS most often test for this unique sugar or for heptose. The only known function of the core is to anchor the O antigen to lipid A.

(c) Lipid A. Lipid A is a glycophospholipid composed of a chain of highly substituted D-glucosamine disaccharide units connected by 1,4′-pyrophosphate bridges. All of the hydroxyl units of the glucosamines are substituted, with most of the substitutions being long-chain fatty acids. Lipid A typically contains the unusual fatty acid β-hydroxymyristic acid. One of the glucosamine hydroxyl groups is substituted with the LPS inner core. Lipid A behaves as a phospholipid with six fatty acids and two phosphates.

(2) Synthesis of LPS Components. UDP-GlcNAc is a key precursor for synthesis of both peptidoglycan and the lipid A portion of LPS. Fatty acids are added to UDP-GlcNAc to make UDP-2,3-diacyl-GlcNAc. This molecule is then condensed with a unique lipid known as lipid X and is phosphorylated to yield lipid IV_A. Two KDO molecules of the inner core are added sequentially to lipid IV_A, and then the complex of lipid A and inner core is completed by attaching additional fatty acids.

The individual units of the O antigen are constructed on the bactoprenyl diphosphate carrier by sequentially adding the sugars that form the fundamental O antigen unit. The newly generated tetrasaccharide is then incorporated at the reducing end of the growing O antigen chain by a process known as head condensation. Finally, a ligase transfers the O antigen to the outer core by displacing the bactoprenyl diphosphate.

LPS is synthesized at the cytoplasmic membrane and then migrates to the outer leaflet of the outer membrane. This process is incompletely understood, but it is generally believed that the completed LPS molecule migrates through sites called **Bayer's junctions,** where the cytoplasmic membrane and outer membrane interconnect through the cell wall.

(3) Role of LPS in Disease. Lipid A is a B cell mitogen, is directly toxic to certain host cells, and is an activator surface for the alternative complement activation pathway. Its greatest clinical importance is that it is the molecule responsible for gram-negative **sepsis.** Although the entire LPS molecule is often referred to as **endotoxin,** it is actually the lipid A portion of LPS that is the endotoxin. In animals, injection of LPS results in dramatic systemic toxic effects such as fever, hypotension, and rapid death. Humans with large numbers of circulating gram-negative bacteria develop sepsis and are in danger of dying of septic shock.

Each year in the USA, approximately 400,000 individuals suffer from life-threatening sepsis when gram-negative bacteria enter the blood and elicit systemic disease that can result in vascular collapse and death.

Although gram-positive bacteria occasionally elicit a similar syndrome, most septic shock occurs when gram-negative bacteria enter the blood, often as a consequence of urinary tract infections, meningitis, cellulitis, or pneumonia. Since many of these infections are acquired in the nursing home or hospital (via catheters or surgery) and occur in patients who are already debilitated or immunodepressed, the mortality rate associated with sepsis is high. About 50% of treated patients die, and more than 80% of patients with prolonged tachycardia die.

The clinical definition of sepsis is outlined in Table 1–4. Although the diagnostic criteria seem rather straightforward, studies have shown that about 60% of patients in whom sepsis is diagnosed do not in fact have sepsis. It is important to recognize sepsis as early as possible because a delay in initiating treatment substantially increases the risk of death.

Over the past few years, both the number of patients with sepsis and the mortality rate have continued to climb. This trend has been attributed to an increase in the number of individuals in high-risk groups, including elderly individuals who are institutionalized or hospitalized, transplantation patients, cancer patients receiving chemotherapy, individuals with acquired immunodeficiency syndrome (AIDS), and individuals who have had major surgery. At least one study has shown that when physicians use invasive monitoring techniques aggressively, the incidence of sepsis rises.

It appears that the molecular basis of sepsis is extremely complicated. If there is one central principle, however, it is that lipid A causes host cells to produce abnormal amounts of products that they normally produce to regulate vascular permeability, blood pressure, coagulation, and the immune response. These products include monokines, cytokines, proteases, prostaglandins, eicosanoids, endorphins, and cell surface molecules. Fig. 1–17 provides a simplified schematic of the molecular and cellular events that lead to sepsis. As gram-negative bacteria grow, they release blebs of LPS-impregnated membrane that are potent activator surfaces for the alternative pathway of complement activation. The split complement products that are generated are able to damage host cells, increase vascular permeability,

TABLE 1–4. Clinical Definition of Sepsis

(1) Suspected or documented gram-negative bacteremia
(2) Fever or hypothermia
(3) Tachycardia
(4) Tachypnea
(5) Hypotension or at least two of the following six signs:
    (a) Unexplained metabolic acidosis
    (b) Arterial hypoxia
    (c) Acute renal failure
    (d) Recent unexplained coagulation abnormalities, such as increased prothrombin time, increased partial thromboplastin time, or thrombocytopenia
    (e) Sudden decrease in mental acuity
    (f) Elevated cardiac index with low systemic vascular resistance

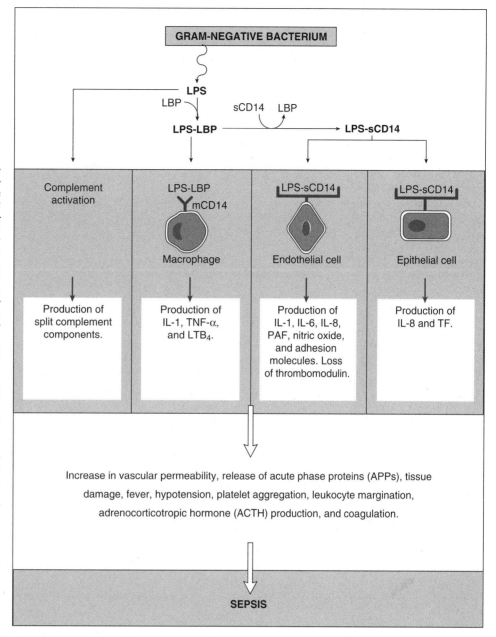

FIGURE 1–17. Molecular processes that occur during gram-negative sepsis. Gram-negative bacteria release blebs of outer membrane filled with lipopolysaccharide (LPS). These blebs may activate complement, or they may bind to a serum protein known as LPS-binding protein (LBP). Some LPS-LBP complexes bind to membrane-bound CD14 (mCD14) on the surface of monocytes and macrophages, and this results in cell activation and production of effectors such as interleukin-1 (IL-1), the alpha form of tumor necrosis factor (TNF-α), and leukotriene B₄ (LTB₄). Alternatively, LBP may be displaced by soluble CD14 (sCD14) in the blood, and LPS-CD14 complexes may bind to endothelial and epithelial cells. When endothelial cells are activated in this fashion, they produce soluble effectors—such as IL-1, IL-6, IL-8, platelet-activating factor (PAF), and nitric oxide—and express new cellular adhesion molecules that cause polymorphonuclear leukocytes to adhere to the endothelium. Endothelial cells can also be activated by TNF released by activated macrophages and monocytes. When epithelial cells are activated by LPS-sCD14 complexes, they produce IL-8 and tissue factor (TF).

cause a drop in blood pressure, elicit platelet aggregation, and summon leukocytes into the blood from the bone marrow. LPS (via lipid A) binds specifically to a serum protein called **lipopolysaccharide-binding protein** (LBP). LBP-bound LPS can then bind to a membrane-bound macrophage receptor called **mCD14,** or it can be displaced by soluble CD14, which is referred to as **sCD14.** The LPS-sCD14 complexes bind a yet-undefined receptor on the surfaces of endothelial and epithelial cells. In each case, the cell that receives the complexed LPS is activated, and it produces a series of soluble products and surface receptors, as outlined in Fig. 1–17 and described in Table 1–5.

LPS-activated macrophages produce three substances—**interleukin-1** (IL-1), the alpha form of **tumor necrosis factor** (TNF-α), and **leukotriene B₄**

(LTB₄)—each of which activates other cells and contributes to hypotension and tissue damage. IL-1 and TNF-α also elicit a group of proteins from the liver called type I **acute phase proteins** (APPs). LPS-activated endothelial cells and epithelial cells express **tissue factor** (TF), which promotes coagulation, and they also release **interleukin-8** (IL-8), which attracts leukocytes, causing them to adhere to the endothelium and to release toxic materials from their lysosomes. In addition, the LPS-activated endothelial cells do the following: release **interleukin-6** (IL-6), a substance that elicits type I and II APPs and promotes tissue damage; express a series of receptors—including **intercellular adhesion molecule 1** (ICAM-1), **vascular cell adhesion molecule 1** (VCAM-1), and **E-selectin**—that cause various types of leukocytes to adhere to vessel walls; and lose their ability to down-

TABLE 1–5. Description and Activities of Molecules Reported to Be Generated During Sepsis

Molecule	Description and Activities
Acute phase proteins (APPs)	
Type I APPs	Are inflammatory proteins released by hepatocytes. Include α_1-acid glycoprotein, C3, and haptoglobin.
Type II APPs	Are inflammatory proteins released by hepatocytes. Include α_1-proteinase inhibitor (α_1-antitrypsin), α_1-antichymotrypsin, hemopexin, fibrinogen, C-reactive protein, factor B of the alternative complement pathway, and serum amyloid protein A.
Complement components	Promote cell damage by generating the terminal membrane attack complex (C5b,6,7,8-polyC9) and by generating chemotactic factors (C5a and C5a-des-arg). Promote vascular permeability by generating anaphylatoxins (C3a and C5a). Promote platelet aggregation (C3a). Elicit release of polymorphonuclear leukocytes from the bone marrow (C3e).
Endothelial cellular adhesion molecules	Include intercellular adhesion molecule 1 (ICAM-1), which is the adhesion molecule for polymorphonuclear leukocytes, monocytes, and natural killer cells; vascular cell adhesion molecule 1 (VCAM-1), which is the adhesion molecule for lymphocytes, monocytes, basophils, and eosinophils; and E-selectin, which is the adhesion molecule for monocytes and memory cells.
Interleukins	
Interleukin-1 (IL-1)	Enhances thrombin-stimulated prostaglandin secretion. Induces basophils and mast cells to release histamine. Elicits type I APPs. Is an endogenous pyrogen involved in fever production. Induces TF expression in several cell types. Induces release of IL-2 and IL-6. Increases vascular permeability. Stimulates release of adrenocorticotropic hormone (ACTH) by causing increased secretion of corticotropin-releasing factor (CRF). Causes endothelial cells to activate and to express ICAM-1, VCAM-1, and E-selectin. Stimulates T cells and B cells.
Interleukin-6 (IL-6)	Elicits type I and II APPs. Stimulates differentiation and proliferation of T cells. Stimulates differentiation of B cells to plasma cells.
Interleukin-8 (IL-8)	Is a chemoattractant for polymorphonuclear leukocytes, basophils, and lymphocytes. Regulates adhesion of polymorphonuclear leukocytes to endothelial cells by promoting expression of leukocytic adhesion molecules in the cluster designation 11–18 (CD11–CD18) family. Causes polymorphonuclear leukocytes to shed L-selectin from their surface. Promotes tissue damage by causing polymorphonuclear leukocytes to release lysosomal enzymes such as elastase.
Leukotriene B$_4$ (LTB$_4$)	Increases vascular permeability. Is chemotactic for polymorphonuclear leukocytes.
Platelet-activating factor (PAF)	Activates platelets, causing them to aggregate and adhere to the endothelium. Activates polymorphonuclear leukocytes. Is a hypotensive agent. Promotes cells to secrete TNF and IL-1.
Thrombomodulin (TM)	Binds thrombin. TM-bound thrombin activates the anticoagulant protein C, which down-regulates thrombosis by cleaving coagulation factors V and VIIIa.
Tissue factor (TF)	Initiates coagulation by activating factors IX and X.
Tumor necrosis factor (TNF)	Elicits type I APPs. Potentiates lipopolysaccharide-dependent IL-6 release. Causes endothelial cells to express ICAM-1, VCAM-1, and E-selectin; to stop expressing surface TM; to secrete nitric oxide; and to release IL-1.

regulate thrombosis by shedding or internalizing **thrombomodulin** (TM). Further information on the activities associated with these products of LPS-activated cells is presented in Table 1–5.

Recent studies have suggested that LPS elicits the release of serum **β-endorphin, nitric oxide,** and various **eicosanoids.** It is currently believed that TNF-α and IL-1 are the central mediators of sepsis. Animals administered high doses of TNF-α experience a syndrome that is almost indistinguishable from sepsis, and this syndrome can be blocked by soluble TNF receptors or monoclonal antibody to TNF. Moreover, the generation of TNF-induced or LPS-induced shock requires that peripheral blood leukocytes and endothelial cells interact directly through their β_2 integrin adhesion molecules. Thus, the processes generating endotoxic shock are complex and multifactorial.

The complexity of the pathogenesis of sepsis has made the search for a "silver bullet" against septic shock elusive. Current strategies for management of sepsis have included removing the bacterium that is the source of LPS (with antibiotics and, if necessary, surgery), administering intravenous fluids to correct hypovolemia, and giving inotropic agents to augment cardiac output and dilate mesenteric and renal arterioles. Yet the mortality rate continues to persist at about 50%, so new strategies are being tried, including the experimental strategies of administering monoclonal antibody directed against either TNF or LPS. Monoclonal antibody to LPS has shown some modest promise as a drug against sepsis, but the results have not been overwhelmingly positive, partially because of the difficulty in identifying early sepsis. Prevention of sepsis, then, becomes a primary goal, making it critical that physicians and other health care professionals follow the precautions of maintaining proper aseptic techniques and taking proper care of catheters, endotracheal tubes, and wounds.

Outer Membrane Channels

(1) Structure and Forms.   Floating in the lipids of the outer membrane of each gram-negative bacterium are more than 100,000 individual protein channels, most of which are porins and porinlike proteins. These proteins differ from the permeases in the cytoplasmic membrane in that outer membrane channels are β-barrels rather than helical proteins, and most are aggregated as trimers with a central pore that allows solutes to diffuse into the periplasm. There are three groups of outer membrane channels: porins, porinlike proteins, and TonB-dependent receptors.

(a) Porins.   Porins are trimeric proteins that form large, water-filled channels which allow ions and hydrophilic molecules that are small (≤600 daltons) to pass through the outer membrane. Porins are also known as **matrix proteins** and as **principal outer membrane proteins** (POMPs). In *E. coli,* three porins have been studied extensively and are known as PhoE, OmpF, and OmpC. PhoE, which is produced when the bacterium is starved for phosphate, has a preference for anions, while OmpF preferentially transports cations. Porins are nonspecific, however, selecting molecules only on the basis of size and charge. The porins have a pore size of 1.1–1.2 nm but have a constriction inside their channel that reduces their effective channel size to 0.8–1.0 nm. OmpF forms a slightly larger pore than does OmpC, and the synthesis of these two porins is coordinated by changes in osmolarity (discussed below).

(b) Porinlike Proteins.   The best-studied porinlike protein is LamB, so called because it also serves as a receptor for the bacteriophage lambda. LamB specifically facilitates the diffusion of maltodextrin polysaccharide chains. It has a specific binding site for maltose, but it also allows other small solutes to diffuse.

(c) TonB-Dependent Receptors.   Although the porins and porinlike proteins are channels that allow molecules to diffuse passively into the periplasm, TonB-dependent receptors are highly specific receptors that are linked to an energy-dependent protein which is called TonB and is located in the cytoplasmic membrane. TonB-dependent receptors specifically bind scarce, large molecules, such as vitamin B_{12} and Fe^{3+}-chelator complexes, and facilitate their movement into the periplasm. TonB-dependent receptors are not well understood.

(2) Synthesis of Porins.   The enteric bacillus *E. coli* can live in two very different environments. When it is in the gastrointestinal tract, where it grows at 37 °C and under conditions in which the environmental osmolarity is high, OmpC (the smaller porin) is preferentially synthesized. It is believed that OmpC protects the organism from the toxic effects of bile salts while allowing nutrients to enter the cell. When *E. coli* is in water, where it must grow at lower temperatures and under conditions in which the osmolarity is low and both toxic substances and nutrients are scarce, OmpF is preferentially synthesized.

The key to this differential expression of porins is the ability of EnvZ, an osmosensor that is located in the cytoplasmic membrane, to regulate the transcription of porin genes and the translation of messenger RNA (mRNA). Fig. 1–18 shows that osmotic pressure influences the ATP-dependent phosphorylation of EnvZ, which in turn phosphorylates a cytoplasmic protein, OmpR. When the external osmolarity is low, small amounts of phosphorylated OmpR (OmpR-P) bind to a high-affinity DNA site upstream from the *omp*F gene, causing the gene to be transcribed. When the external solute concentration is high, the phosphorylation of EnvZ and OmpR increases concomitantly. Because more OmpR-P is now available, it binds to lower-affinity sites upstream from the *omp*F and *omp*C genes. This binding blocks the transcription of the *omp*F gene while stimulating the reading of the *omp*C gene. Additionally, a segment of the DNA adjacent to the *omp*C gene is read in the opposite direction to yield *mic*F mRNA. The *mic*F mRNA acts as a translational repressor, binding to a segment of *omp*F mRNA and preventing it from being translated.

BACTERIAL CELL APPENDAGES

Extending from the surfaces of many bacteria are appendages that mediate locomotion or adherence to host surfaces. There are two major protein cellular appendages: flagella and pili. Flagella are locomotor appendages. The various types of pili (fimbriae) act as cellular adhesins, are involved in transfer of DNA during conjugation, or mediate resistance to phagocytosis.

Flagella

Most motile bacteria swim because they have protein filaments that are called flagella and extend from their surfaces into the medium. Some bacteria, such as the extremely motile *Proteus* strains that "swarm" across agar medium, are surrounded by dozens of flagella and are said to be peritrichous (literally meaning surrounded by hairs), while other bacteria have tufts of flagella at both poles, a tuft at one pole, or a single flagellum at one pole. Spirochetes wrap themselves around specialized flagella that are known as axial filaments and lie under an outer membrane. Fig. 1–19 shows an example of a bacterium with flagella.

Structure

The flagella of bacteria differ from those of eukaryotes. Eukaryotic flagella are composed of tubulin strands arranged in a 9 + 2 pattern. In contrast, the filament of a bacterial flagellum is a left-handed helix of repeating units of a simple protein called **flagellin.** Fig. 1–20 shows that the flagellar filament is anchored in the cell envelope by a series of proteins that form

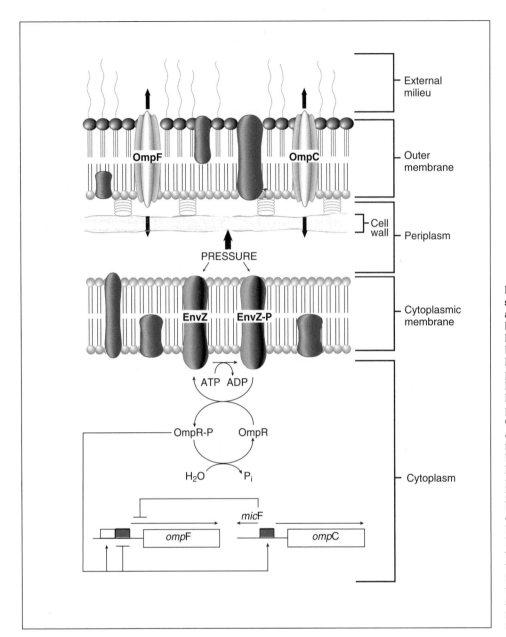

FIGURE 1–18. Regulation of the synthesis of the porins OmpF and OmpC in *Escherichia coli*. EnvZ is an osmosensor protein located in the cytoplasmic membrane. When the osmolarity is low, EnvZ uses adenosine triphosphate (ATP) to phosphorylate itself, and the resulting EnvZ-P then phosphorylates a cytoplasmic regulator protein called OmpR. OmpR-P binds to a low-affinity regulatory site upstream from the *ompF* gene, causing it to be transcribed. When the osmolarity increases, the rate of phosphorylation of EnvZ and OmpR increases, allowing OmpR-P to bind to lower-affinity sites on the chromosome upstream from both *ompF* and *ompC*. These sites block the transcription of *ompF* while increasing the transcription of *ompC*. Additionally, binding of OmpR-P near *ompC* causes transcription of *micF* in the opposite direction. This mRNA segment binds to existing *ompF* mRNA and blocks its translation.

rings through which a rod passes. At the base of the flagellum, in the cytoplasmic membrane, are the proteins that serve as the switch and motor of the flagellum. The motor (Mot) proteins act as a channel that links the passage of protons across the cytoplasmic membrane to the rotation of the flagellum. The flagellum does not beat or wave; rather, it is a rigid helix that rotates like a propeller.

Recent studies have shown that the rotation of the flagellum is driven directly by proton motive force and that one revolution of the flagellum requires that about 1000 protons return through the MotA protein to the cytoplasm. *Escherichia coli* flagella can rotate up to 300 times per second. This process is extremely efficient. Some bacteria that are 1 μm long can travel up to 200 μm per second. This is analogous to a 6-foot-tall man running 1200 feet per second, or 820 miles per hour.

Synthesis

Genes that encode the synthesis of the flagella of *E. coli* and *Salmonella* serotype *typhimurium* are arranged into four regions on the chromosome and are expressed as a **regulon.** That is, these genes exist as sets of **operons** that are coordinated by the same sets of signals. The flagellar operons are expressed in a hierarchical manner. This means that for a given set of operons to be read and expressed as mRNA and proteins, a previous set of operons must first be read. The first genes read are those of the **master operon** (expression class 1 genes). RNA polymerase cannot read the master operon unless it first binds both cyclic AMP (cAMP) and cAMP-binding protein (CAP). Thus, like the lactose operon (see Chapter 2), the synthesis of flagella is subject to catabolite repression.

As noted earlier in the discussion of group trans-

plenty of glucose is available, conditions are satisfactory, so the bacterium does not want to leave the vicinity. The rest of the flagellar genes are read in a coordinated fashion that is reminiscent of the early and late genes of viruses. DNA-dependent RNA polymerases contain a subunit that is called sigma and allows the polymerase to recognize specific sites (promoters) where RNA synthesis should be initiated. The reading of the last set of flagellar genes depends on the production of a new sigma factor that is synthesized among one of the earlier sets of operons. This phenomenon of controlling RNA synthesis by varying sigma factors is discussed at length below in the section concerning genetic control of sporulation.

The filament of the flagellum is constructed at the distal end. Export proteins located at the base of the flagellum pass the flagellin subunits into the hollow core of the flagellum. After the proteins pass through the core to the tip, they are spontaneously assembled at the tip without expending any energy.

Functions

Bacteria move toward substances that are known as chemoattractants. This phenomenon, known as **chemotaxis,** does not occur by sensing a gradient of chemoattractants across the surface of the bacterium, because the bacterial surface is too small. Rather, the bacterium swims for 1 second, tumbles for 0.1 second, and then swims for another second in whatever direction it has reoriented itself during tumbling. When chemoattractants are present, the bacterium will swim longer in the direction of the attractant, giving it a net movement toward the chemotactic agent, as shown in Fig. 1–21.

The means by which a bacterium responds to

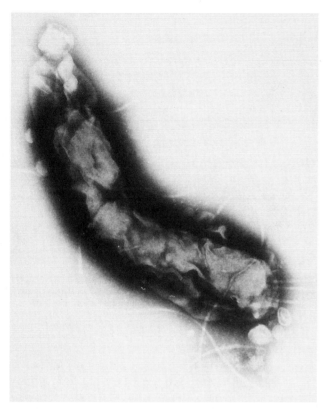

FIGURE 1–19. Photomicrograph of a bacterium with flagella. The bacterium shown is *Bartonella bacilliformis.*

location, when glucose is transported by the phosphotransferase system, cAMP levels drop precipitously owing to the lack of phosphorylated EIIA. Thus, when *E. coli* is growing in a medium containing glucose, the flagellar master operon cannot be read and the synthesis of flagella is halted. Apparently, when

FIGURE 1–20. The structure of the bacterial flagellum. The flagellum is embedded in the cell envelope and extends to the cytoplasmic membrane. At the base of the flagellum are the Mot (motor) proteins that anchor the flagellum to the membrane and rotate the flagellum as protons return to the cytoplasm. The switch proteins control the rotational sense of the flagellum in response to chemotactic agents.

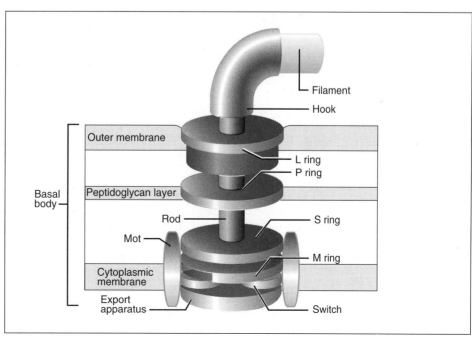

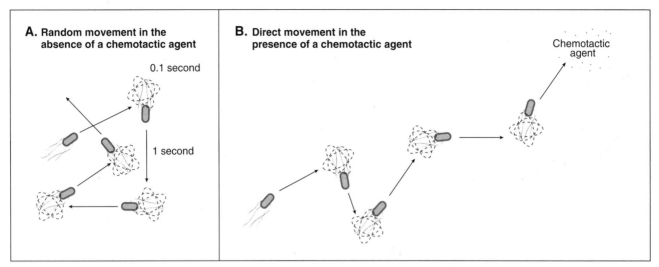

A. Random movement in the absence of a chemotactic agent

0.1 second

1 second

B. Direct movement in the presence of a chemotactic agent

Chemotactic agent

FIGURE 1–21. Patterns of bacterial motility in the absence (A) and presence (B) of a chemotactic agent. In the absence of a chemotactic agent, a motile bacterium will swim for 1 second, tumble randomly for 0.1 second, and then swim for another second in whatever direction it has reoriented itself during tumbling. Because the direction of each new swim is randomly generated, there is no net movement of the bacterium. In the presence of a chemotactic agent, the bacterium continues to alternate between swimming and tumbling, but it swims longer in the direction of the chemoattractant. This causes the bacterium to exhibit a net movement toward the attractant.

chemorepellents and **chemoattractants** is presented in Fig. 1–22. The cytoplasmic membrane of the motile bacterium contains a series of receptors called **methyl-accepting chemotaxis proteins** (MCPs). The MCPs have a receptor in the periplasm, are able to traverse the membrane, and have a module that is located at the inner face of the cytoplasm and converses with proteins inside the bacterium. At least some MCPs are linked to high-affinity periplasmic binding proteins (see the earlier discussion of active transport). When a chemorepellent is present, it interacts with the MCP and affects its degree of methylation. With the assistance of CheW protein, the MCP influences CheA protein to phosphorylate itself, using ATP as a phosphate source. Phosphorylated CheA (P-CheA) then phosphorylates CheY and CheB. CheB resets the MCP by demethylating it, while P-CheY is the key signaling agent to the flagellum. P-CheY interacts with the switch proteins located at the base of the flagellum (FliG, FliM, and FliN) and causes the flagellum to rotate in a *clockwise* direction. Because of the pitch of the flagellin helix, clockwise rotation causes the flagellum to entangle, and the bacterium tumbles aimlessly. Certain phosphorylated compounds, such as acetyl phosphate, carbamoyl phosphate, and phosphoramidate, can also directly phosphorylate CheY and cause the bacterium to tumble. In contrast, attractants that interact with MCPs cause an increase in the activity of CheZ, a substance that dephosphorylates P-CheY. CheY interacts with the switch proteins and then causes the flagellum to rotate in a *counterclockwise* manner. When this happens, the flagellum streams out behind the bacterium, thereby enabling the bacterium to swim smoothly. The transport of sugars and glycols via phosphotransferase systems also increases the amount of CheY and enables the bacterium to swim smoothly,

possibly by stimulating the activity of CheZ. Finally, via a process that is not well understood, the switch proteins receive two signals, one fast and the other longer-lasting and delayed, allowing the bacterium to compare signals over time. This gives the bacterium a sort of "memory" of chemoattractants and enables it to swim longer in the direction of attractants.

Pili (Fimbriae)

Structure and Synthesis

A pilus (from the Latin word for "hair") is a stiff protein appendage that is thinner than a flagellum and looks like a long hair projecting from the bacterium. A single bacterium may have only one pilus or up to hundreds of pili. The surfaces of some bacteria are covered with tiny protein fibrils referred to as fimbriae (from the Latin word for "fringe"). Pili and fimbriae are hollow and are made up of repeating subunits of a protein called **pilin.** Like flagella, pili are assembled at their tips by passing the pilin subunits through the hollow core; the subunits are then assembled spontaneously at the pilus tip.

Functions

Although there are many types of pili, there appear to be two major functional types: common pili and sex pili.

Common pili, which are also called **somatic pili,** are thinner than sex pili and are usually present in high numbers on a cell (Fig. 1–23). The most important function of common pili is to serve as **adhesins,** and their presence is responsible for the ability of many bacteria to adhere to and colonize mucosal surfaces (Fig. 1–24). Pili behave like lectins in that they are proteins that bind specifically to carbohy-

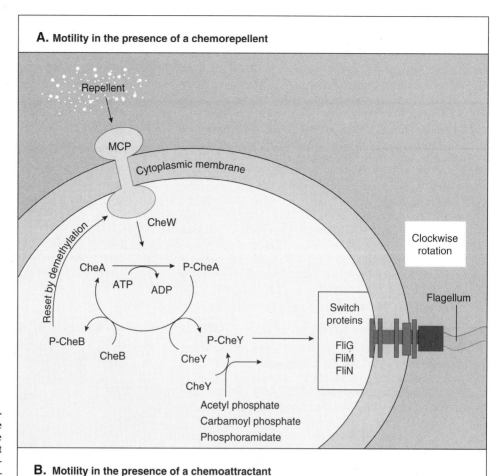

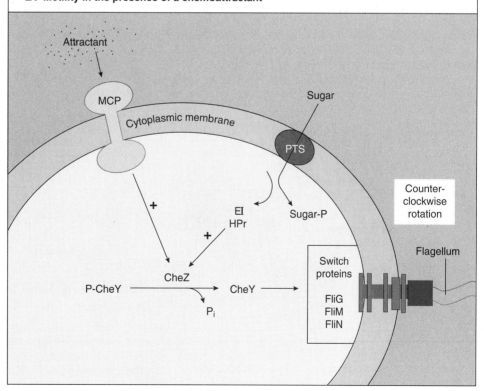

FIGURE 1–22. Molecular control of motility in the presence of a chemorepellent (A) or in the presence of a chemoattractant (B). In the presence of a chemorepellent, a methyl-accepting chemotactic protein (MCP) located in the membrane activates the CheW protein, which catalyzes the phosphorylation of CheA. Phosphorylated CheA (P-CheA) donates its phosphate to CheY and CheB. P-CheB resets the MCP by demethylating it, while P-CheY interacts with three flagellum switch proteins (FliG, FliM, and FliN) and causes the flagellum to rotate in a clockwise fashion. This causes the flagellum to entangle and the bacterium to tumble. CheY can also be directly phosphorylated by substrates such as acetyl phosphate, carbamoyl phosphate, and phosphoramidate. In the presence of a chemoattractant, MCP activates CheZ, which dephosphorylates CheY, causing the flagellum to rotate in a counterclockwise fashion and to swim smoothly. Counterclockwise flagellar rotation and swimming are also promoted when substrates are transported by phosphotransferase (PTS) systems. ADP = adenosine diphosphate; ATP = adenosine triphosphate; EI = enzyme I; and HPr = histidine protein.

drate residues. For this reason, pili are sometimes classified by the types of sugars that inhibit their adherence to host cells. Most enteric bacilli express type I pili, and because the adherence of these pili is blocked in the presence of mannose, type I pili are classified as mannose-sensitive pili. *E. coli* organisms that cause urinary tract infections, however, adhere to renal cells via thinner pili that are called mannose-insensitive pili. A number of pathogenic bacteria have type IV pili. These pili are adhesins for host cells and are also known as bundle-forming pili because they tend to autoaggregate when separated from the bacterium.

Some common pili do more than mediate adherence. For example, type IV pili have been shown to protect *Neisseria gonorrhoeae* (the organism that causes gonorrhea) from being phagocytosed by polymorphonuclear leukocytes. Other bacteria grow as pellicles on top of fluids because their pili allow them to form a mat on the fluid surface. This characteristic is important to strictly aerobic bacteria growing in a liquid medium because it keeps them at the aerobic interface of the liquid.

Sex pili are thicker than common pili, and each "male" bacterium (a bacterium with a sex pilus) typically exhibits only a few such pili (see Fig. 1–23). Sex pili are encoded on pieces of extrachromosomal DNA called **conjugative plasmids** or **fertility factors,** and the sex pili facilitate the transfer of these plasmids from "fertile" donor bacteria to "nonfertile" recipients. The best-studied sex pilus is the F pilus (see Chapter 3). Sex pili bring the bacterium into jeopardy of being infected with a group of temperate (lysogenic) bacteriophages known as **male-specific phages.** These bacteriophages recognize receptors on the sex pilus, adhere, and inject their DNA either into the core of the pilus or at the base of the pilus where it intersects with the outer membrane.

Most piliated bacteria are gram-negative, but a few piliated gram-positive organisms have been identified.

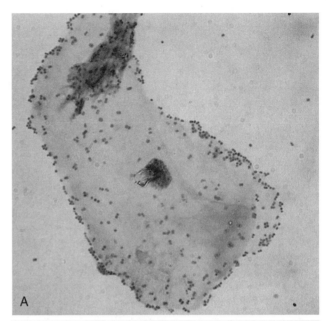

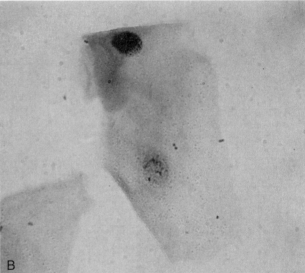

FIGURE 1–24. Photomicrographs showing the effect of piliation on bacterial adherence to epithelial cells. Greater adherence was shown by a piliated variant of *Neisseria subflava* biovar *perflava* **(A)** than by a nonpiliated variant of *N. subflava* biovar *perflava* **(B)** when both were incubated with buccal epithelial cells.

OTHER BACTERIAL STRUCTURES

Capsules, slime layers, and endospores are additional structures found in some bacteria.

Capsules and Slime Layers
Structure and Methods of Identification

Many gram-positive and gram-negative bacteria are surrounded by a mucopolysaccharide or peptide layer of protective material called a capsule. When the capsular material is so loosely associated with the bacterium that it can be easily washed away, this layer is called a slime layer. Some capsules are large and can be easily recognized microscopically using

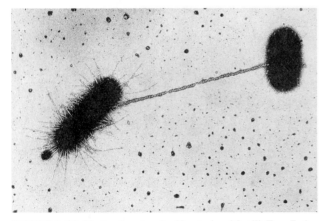

FIGURE 1–23. Photomicrograph of bacteria with pili. Two *Escherichia coli* organisms are shown. The one on the left has many common pili and a single sex pilus attaching it to the nonpiliated one on the right. (Courtesy of Charles C. Brinton, Jr., and Judith Carnahan.)

standard **capsule stains,** while others are so small that they can be visualized only by **electron microscopy.** These very tiny capsules are known as **microcapsules.**

Because most standard bacteriologic stains do not stain capsules, special capsule stains are used to visualize capsules. Most capsule stains take advantage of the colloid nature of **India ink.** Typically, bacteria are suspended in India ink and then counterstained with a standard stain, such as **safranin.** If there is a capsule present, the capsule will be unstained by the safranin and will appear as a clear zone around the stained bacterium. Unfortunately, microcapsules may not be seen by this method and may need to be visualized by electron microscopy after staining the mucopolysaccharides with **ruthenium red.** If the bacterium is coated with acidic mucopolysaccharides, the ruthenium red will form a precipitate on the cell surface.

The **quellung reaction** is a variation of the India ink staining method and is commonly used in the laboratory to identify specific bacterial strains. A sample of the bacterium is incubated with specific anticapsular antibody and then is stained by an India ink method; control bacteria are stained after being incubated with normal serum. If the specific antibody reacts with the capsule, the capsules in the sample incubated with antibody will appear swollen (quellung is from the German word for "swelling") in comparison with those incubated with normal serum. Quellung reactions are used often for epidemiologic purposes, when there are multiple capsule types of a given organism that could be responsible for an outbreak of similar infections. Examining the quellung reactions of each isolate allows laboratory technicians to identify the capsular serotype of the organism responsible for each patient's infection.

Synthesis

Most capsules are repeating units of simple sugars, but some contain repeating units of branched polysaccharides. For example, the type 3 pneumococcal capsule is composed of repeating units of a glucose–glucuronic acid disaccharide. A few capsules, such as that of *Bacillus anthracis* (the anthrax bacillus), are composed of peptides. Polysaccharide capsules are synthesized as individual subunits that are transferred to the outside of the bacterium by bactoprenyl diphosphate. Thus, antibiotics that interfere with bactoprenol function will block the synthesis of polysaccharide capsules and slime layers.

Functions

The capsules of the clinically significant bacteria have three main functions. First, they allow some bacteria to resist being phagocytosed by polymorphonuclear leukocytes. Most encapsulated bacteria cause acute pyogenic (pus-forming) infections. Because of the preponderance of polymorphonuclear leukocytes at the infection site, bacteria that cannot resist phagocytosis will be eliminated. Capsules are the most important of the bacterial antiphagocytic

structures. In some cases, capsules prevent opsonization by interfering with complement activation or deposition of complement split products. Second, capsules or slime layers allow some bacteria to adhere to host surfaces. Pili are the key adhesin for most mucosal bacteria, but some oral streptococci promote their persistence on dental surfaces by expressing a slime layer. Third, capsules allow some bacteria to persist in their environment by keeping them from drying out when they are on exposed surfaces, such as on the surfaces of catheters and other fomites.

Endospores

A small number of gram-positive bacteria escape adverse conditions by differentiating into dormant, highly resistant cells that are called endospores. These resting bacterial forms resist the bactericidal effects of heat, drying, radiation, freezing, and toxic chemicals (such as disinfectants). The ubiquity and persistence of bacterial spores were illustrated by a group of investigators who cultured soil samples taken from a container that had been sealed for 300 years. Since the spores that were found in the dry dust germinated, the investigators concluded that bacterial spores can persist for hundreds of years under extremely harsh conditions.

Endospores play a major role in the epidemiology of some diseases. Some types of infections occur only when endospores are introduced into a site where they can germinate, such as a wound site. In many of these infections, the vegetative forms (metabolically active forms) of the bacterium are not normally able to initiate infection.

Spore-Forming Bacteria

There are two clinically important groups of endospore formers. The first consists of members of the aerobic genus *Bacillus* and includes *B. anthracis, Bacillus cereus,* and *Bacillus subtilis.* The second consists of members of the anaerobic genus *Clostridium* and includes *Clostridium botulinum, Clostridium difficile, Clostridium perfringens,* and *Clostridium tetani.* Among the diseases caused by these organisms are anthrax, food poisoning, botulism, tetanus, gas gangrene, and pseudomembranous colitis.

In almost every case, the spores formed by the organism play a key role in the initiation of human infection. For example, it is because *C. tetani* spores are found everywhere in the soil—but especially in feces-contaminated soil—that dirty penetrating wounds are so dangerous. When tetanus spores are placed into a deep wound that contains devitalized, anaerobic tissue, they germinate and the anaerobic clostridia multiply and release tetanus toxin. To reduce the risk of tetanus from such wounds, the wound must be rid of spores or be made a place where endospores cannot germinate, and the patient must be protected from tetanus toxin produced by germinating endospores. To this end, patients with tetanus-prone wounds are immunized with tetanus toxoid (toxoids are inactivated toxins) and may be given tetanus antitoxin. In addition, their wounds are cleansed thoroughly and debrided.

Structure of Endospores

Bacterial spores look quite different from vegetative bacteria in that they are surrounded by several thick layers. These layers are responsible for most of the resistance of the spores to environmental conditions. The dormant bacterial cytoplasm is called the **core.** It contains only a single copy of the chromosome, no mRNA, little tRNA, and only a few enzymes. Amino acids are stored as low-molecular-weight cytoplasmic proteins that are called **small acid-soluble proteins** (SASPs). Some SASPs contribute to the ability of the spore to resist ultraviolet radiation (and, possibly, heat) by stably increasing the negative superhelix activity (underwinding) of the chromosome. There is no ongoing metabolic activity in the mature spore, and energy is stored as 3-phosphoglycerate, which is more stable than ATP.

The spore's core is surrounded first by a cell membrane and a thin cell wall and then by a thick, concentrically laminated layer called the **cortex.** The cortex is made of a **peptidoglycan** that is much like conventional peptidoglycan except that it contains many unusual cross-links, such as **muramic lactam rings.** But most important, the cortex contains **dipicolinic acid** (DPA), or pyridine-2,6-dicarboxylic acid. DPA, which is also found in the core, is a calcium chelator and may make up as much as 15% of the spore's weight. When DPA deposited in the cortex chelates calcium, it brings the calcium into close contact with the loose, polyanionic peptidoglycan of the cortex. The ionic cross-linking that results causes the peptidoglycan to contract and to expel water in a process similar to that involved in wringing the water out of a wet washcloth. This process is extremely effective. Vegetative bacteria typically consist of about 77.5% water, but only about 15% of the endospore is water. This makes the spore as dry as casein or wool. It is generally believed that the dryness makes the spore heat-resistant, even to the point of being able to survive hours of boiling.

The cortex is surrounded by the inner and outer **spore coats.** The spore coats are concentric layers of at least 15 different proteins, several of which are keratinlike proteins with numerous disulfide bonds. The spore coats are believed to make the spore resistant to chemicals and lysozyme, and they probably contribute to the ability of the spore to resist being killed by ultraviolet or ionizing radiation.

Sporulation

Bacteria sporulate to escape adverse conditions. After all, a "sleeping" bacterium does not need to "eat," and if it is well protected, it will be oblivious to heat, dryness, and other conditions. Fig. 1–25 shows a schematic drawing of the sporulation process.

Requirements for Sporulation. Sporulation is initiated when three requirements are fulfilled. First, the bacterium must be starved for key nutrients. Most often, it is starved for a key carbon-, nitrogen-, or phosphorus-containing compound. Second, the bacterium must be at high density to allow secretion and recognition of **extracellular differentiation factor 1** (EDF-1), a factor believed to be a small peptide that binds to the starved bacterium and signals it to initiate sporulation. Finally, the bacterium must be in the stationary phase.

The actual intracellular signal that initiates sporulation is not certain, but many believe it to be guanosine triphosphate (GTP) or guanosine diphosphate (GDP), possibly through the cellular signals guanosine 3'-diphosphate-5'-diphosphate (ppGpp) and guanosine 3'-triphosphate-5'-diphosphate (pppGpp). The initiation process results in the bacterium dividing asymmetrically and forming a **prespore** and a **mother cell.** Over several hours, the mother cell builds protective walls (the cortex and spore walls) around the prespore while the prespore's metabolic machinery is transformed for dormancy.

Genetic Regulation of Sporulation. The process of sporulation has some puzzling elements. It begins with one bacterium that becomes two bacteria with identical genomes, yet one bacterium dedicates itself entirely to transforming the exterior of the other cell. Then there is the "time" problem; the spore is constructed over several hours, and there are distinctive stages in which entirely new sets of genes are being expressed in the mother cell and the prespore. The explanation for these puzzling elements is that sporulation is under transcriptional control.

Transcription in all bacteria is carried out by an RNA polymerase that consists of a set of subunits known as $\alpha\beta\beta'\sigma$. The last subunit—the **sigma factor** (σ)—allows the RNA polymerase to recognize promoters and read the DNA at appropriate sites. Vegetative genes are read by RNA polymerase molecules that contain σ^A as their recognition factor; the entire enzymatic complex is usually designated as $E\sigma^A$. When the signal for sporulation appears, a few sporulation genes will be read by $E\sigma^A$, but a new sigma factor that is called σ^H and is specific for the first set of sporulation genes will also appear. Moreover, the signal for sporulation will activate the **phosporelay system**—consisting of a series of sensor or transmitter protein kinases—and lead to the phosphorylation of SpoOA. SpoOA is a DNA-binding protein that is called a **response regulator** because it regulates the reading of DNA in response to external signals. Together, $E\sigma^H$ and SpoOA allow a specific set of "early" sporulation **operons** to be read. Two of these early gene products are two more sigma factors called σ^E and σ^F. When the septum is completed, σ^E is partitioned into the mother cell, and σ^F is packaged into the prespore. Because the mother cell and prespore have different sigma factors, they will derepress different **regulons** (a regulon is a group of operons that are controlled by the same signal) and the fates of the two cells will be different.

As Fig. 1–25 shows, early prespore genes are read by $E\sigma^F$. Only two $E\sigma^F$-dependent genes have been identified, one of which is the gene for the next pre-

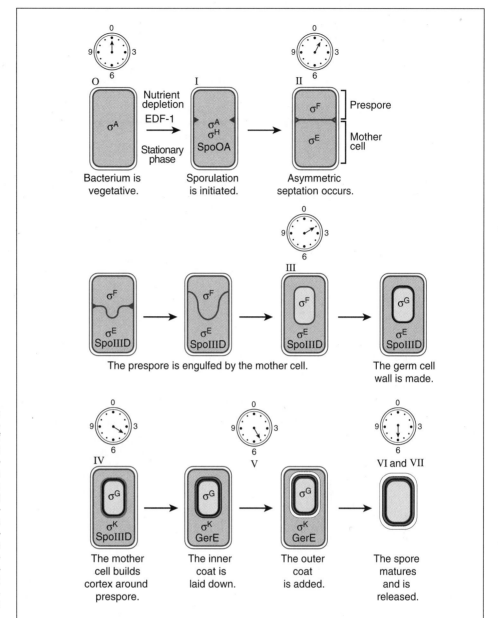

FIGURE 1–25. Morphologic changes that occur during sporulation and the genetic control of these changes. The clocks depict the elapsed time (in hours) at various stages as a single bacillus divides asymmetrically and then is transformed into a developing spore and a mother cell. The Roman numerals above the bacteria signify the stages of development. Inside each cell is the name of the sigma factor and any DNA-binding protein that controls expression of sporulation genes at that stage of development. EDF-1 = extracellular differentiation factor 1.

spore sigma factor, σ^G. The rest of the changes that transform the prespore's metabolism are due to genes in the $E\sigma^G$ regulon. In contrast, the mother cell goes through four sets of genetic control. Genes that are read just after septation are controlled by σ^E alone. During engulfment, new operons are derepressed under the coordinate control of σ^E and a DNA-binding protein called SpoIIID, but the building of the cortex is controlled by σ^K and SpoIIID. The final steps of sporulation (coat production and maturation) are performed by gene products of operons expressed under the control of σ^K and another DNA-binding protein known as GerE. In all, more than 50 operons will be sequentially derepressed, with some of the operons coding for multiple enzymes or structural proteins. These operons include the *spo* (sporulation) operons, *ger* (germination) operons, genes for

cell wall enzymes, and several other assorted operons. Although the *ger* operons were so named because they participate in the germination process, many of these enzymes also play important roles in forming the endospore.

In summary, the reason that the mother cell and prespore follow different paths is that they recognize different sets of genes. The prespore reads the σ^F and σ^G regulons and transforms itself into a dormant cell, while the mother cell reads the σ^E and σ^K regulons under the influence of SpoIIID and GerE and dedicates itself to building the walls that will make the spore almost impervious to the outside world. During this process, the sequence of events is ordered partially in response to signals that go from the mother cell to the prespore and vice versa. This communication between the prespore and mother cell ensures that the events occurring in the two cells are perfectly co-ordinated.

Germination of the Spore

The entire sporulation process takes about 6 hours, but only about 90 minutes are needed for germination to occur. This disparity in time occurs because germination is not sporulation in reverse. Rather, it is a three-stage process that is not under transcriptional control.

The first stage, which is called **activation,** occurs when heat or one of several chemicals activates an L-alanine receptor that is also a protease. The second stage, which is called **initiation,** follows when the activated cell is exposed to L-alanine, certain other amino acids, or glucose. The activated protease cleaves germination-specific cortex lytic enzyme and converts the enzyme to its active form, which degrades the cortex and allows water and nutrients to enter the germinating spore. It is during this second stage that the spore loses its resistance and refractivity and becomes metabolically active. At this point, when the germination process is irreversibly committed, the third stage, which is called **outgrowth,** begins. The outgrowth stage returns the spore to its vegetative morphology. Studies using protein synthesis inhibitors show that while the first and second stages use preformed materials, the third stage involves de novo protein synthesis.

Elimination of Endospores

Because endospores are so resistant to environmental conditions and some spore-formers are highly pathogenic, special procedures must be used to eliminate all bacterial spores. Clinical instruments and materials are often heat-sterilized in an autoclave, which, like a pressure cooker, uses highly pressurized steam. This is necessary because endospores can survive several hours of boiling. To be certain that endospores are eliminated, all parts of the sample to be sterilized must be heated to 121 °C at 1.05 kg/cm^2 (15 lb/in^2) above atmospheric pressure for at least 10–15 minutes. Because it can be difficult to reach endospores in the center of a packet of heavily wrapped instruments, a spore detector of some sort is placed among the instruments and the packet is autoclaved for a longer period (30 minutes or more). Often, the detector is a vial of spores that will be broken open and placed into a growth medium after the autoclaving is complete. If the spores from the vial germinate, this indicates that the packet of instruments was not adequately sterilized.

Selected Readings

Anderson, M. S., et al. Biosynthesis of lipid A in *Escherichia coli*: identification of UDP-3-*O*-[(*R*)-3-hydroxymyristoyl]-α-D-glucosamine as a precursor of UDP-*N*^{2},*O*^{3}-bis[(*R*)-3-hydroxymyristoyl]-α-D-glucosamine. Biochemistry 27:1908–1917, 1988.

Cabellos, C., et al. Differing roles for platelet-activating factor during inflammation of the lung and subarachnoid space: the special case of *Streptococcus pneumoniae*. J Clin Invest 90:612–618, 1992.

Clarke, A. J., and C. Dupont. *O*-Acetylated peptidoglycan: its occurrence, pathobiologic significance, and biosynthesis. Can J Microbiol 38:85–91, 1992.

Errington, J. *Bacillus subtilis* sporulation: regulation of gene expression and control of morphogenesis. Microbiol Rev 57:1–33, 1993.

Higgins, C. F., et al. Periplasmic binding protein-dependent transport systems: the membrane-associated components. Philos Trans R Soc Lond B Biol Sci 326:353–365, 1990.

Johannsen, L., et al. Somnogenic activity of *O*-acetylated and dimeric muramyl peptides. Infect Immun 57:2726–2732, 1989.

Johannsen, L., et al. Somnogenic, pyrogenic, and hematologic effects of bacterial peptidoglycan. Am J Physiol 259:182–186, 1990.

Jones, C. J., and S. I. Aizawa. The bacterial flagellum and flagellar motor: structure, assembly, and function. Adv Microb Physiol 32:109–172, 1991.

Kastowsky, M., T. Gutberlet, and H. Bradaczek. Molecular modeling of the three-dimensional structure and conformational flexibility of bacterial lipopolysaccharide. J Bacteriol 174:4798–4806, 1992.

Keller, R., et al. Macrophage response to bacteria: induction of marked secretory and cellular activities by lipoteichoic acids. Infect Immun 60:3664–3672, 1992.

Losick, R., P. Youngman, and P. J. Piggot. Genetics of endospore formation in *Bacillus subtilis*. Annu Rev Genet 20:625–669, 1986.

Martin, M. A. Epidemiology and clinical impact of gram-negative sepsis. Infect Dis Clin North Am 5:739–753, 1991.

Mayoral, J. L., C. J. Schweich, and D. L. Dunn. Decreased tumor necrosis factor production during the initial stages of infection correlates with survival during murine gram-negative sepsis. Arch Surg 125:24–28, 1990.

Monefeldt, K., and T. Tollefsen. Effects of a streptococcal lipoteichoic acid on complement activation in vitro. J Clin Periodontol 20:186–192, 1993.

Mukaida, N., et al. Novel insight into molecular mechanisms of endotoxic shock: biochemical analysis of lipopolysaccharide signaling in a cell-free system targeting NF-$\kappa\beta$ and regulation of cytokine production and action through β_2 integrin in vivo. J Leukoc Biol 59:145–151, 1996.

Murray, M. J., and M. Kumar. Sepsis and septic shock: deadly complications that are on the rise. Postgrad Med 90:199–208, 1991.

Nikaido, H., and M. H. Saier, Jr. Transport systems in bacteria: common themes in their design. Science 258:936–942, 1992.

Postma, P. W., J. W. Lengeler, and G. R. Jacobson. Phosphoenolpyruvate: carbohydrate phosphotransferase systems of bacteria. Microbiol Rev 57:543–594, 1993.

Quiocho, F. A. Atomic structures of periplasmic binding proteins and the high-affinity active transport systems in bacteria. Philos Trans R Soc Lond B Biol Sci 326:341–351, 1990.

Raetz, C. R. Biochemistry of endotoxins. Annu Rev Biochem 59:129–170, 1990.

Rietschel, E. T., et al. Bacterial endotoxin: molecular relationships between structure and activity. Infect Dis Clin North Am 5:753–779, 1991.

Schnaitman, C. A., and J. D. Klena. Genetics of lipopolysaccharide biosynthesis in enteric bacteria. Microbiol Rev 57:655–682, 1993.

Schultz, G. E. Bacterial porins: structure and function. Curr Opinion Cell Biol 5:701–707, 1993.

Stock, J. B., A. J. Ninfa, and A. M. Stock. Protein phosphorylation and regulation of adaptive responses in bacteria. Microbiol Rev 53:450–490, 1989.

Waage, A., et al. Current understanding of the pathogenesis of gram-negative shock. Infect Dis Clin North Am 5:781–791, 1991.

Wakabayashi, G., et al. *Staphylococcus epidermidis* induces complement activation, tumor necrosis factor and interleukin-1, a shocklike state, and tissue injury in rabbits without endotoxemia: comparison to *Escherichia coli*. J Clin Invest 87:1925–1935, 1991.

Warren, H. S., R. L. Danner, and R. S. Munford. Anti-endotoxin monoclonal antibodies. N Engl J Med 326:1153–1157, 1992.

Wenzel, R. P. Anti-endotoxin monoclonal antibodies: a second look. N Engl J Med 326:1151–1153, 1992.

Winkler, H. H. Rickettsial permeability: an ADP-ATP transport system. J Biol Chem 251:389–396, 1976.

Wright, S. D., et al. CD14, a receptor for complexes of lipopolysac-charide (LPS) and LPS-binding protein. Science 249:1431–1433, 1990.

Ziegler, E. J., et al. Treatment of gram-negative bacteremia and septic shock with HA-1A human monoclonal antibody against endotoxin. N Engl J Med 324:429–436, 1991.

CHAPTER TWO

BACTERIAL GROWTH

AND METABOLISM

An understanding of bacterial multiplication, growth requirements, and metabolism is essential to an understanding of the functions of bacteria and the dynamics and treatment of bacterial infections.

BACTERIAL MULTIPLICATION
Multiplication by Transverse Binary Fission

Most of the medically important bacteria multiply by transverse binary fission (Fig. 2–1). In this process, a bacterium elongates and forms a septum, which divides the bacterium into two approximately equal segments. As the septum is completed, a daughter chromosome is segregated into each daughter cell, and the cells separate. Thus, bacteria multiply logarithmically: one bacterium yields two bacteria, two yield four, four yield eight, and so forth.

Fission is an asexual process. Bacteria do not multiply sexually, although there is a process of exchanging genetic information that involves specific "mating types" and is described in what sounds like sexual terms. However, this process, which is called conjugation and is discussed in Chapter 3, does not involve meiosis or the formation of zygotes or gametes and is not a means of reproduction.

The Standard Bacterial Growth Curve

If a bacterial culture were to double once every 20 minutes (as many do) and were to continue to multiply unabated for 48 hours, one *Escherichia coli* would produce 2^{144} bacteria. *E. coli* is a fairly small bacterium, with a mass of about 1×10^{-12} g. Thus, at the end of 48 hours, there would be a bacterial colony with a mass of 2.2×10^{31} g, or about 4000 times the mass of the earth. Fortunately, however, bacterial growth is self-limiting. Even under ideal conditions, most bacterial cultures multiply logarithmically for only 3–5 hours. They quickly run out of essential nutrients and accumulate toxic by-products of metabolism. For this reason, the growth curve of a bacterium multiplying in a liquid medium generally looks like the curve depicted in Fig. 2–2. Here, the *y*-axis represents the log number of bacteria, while the *x*-axis represents time; bacterial growth is plotted semilogarithmically.

Phases of Growth

Bacteria typically undergo the four phases of growth shown in Fig. 2–2.

Lag Phase. When bacteria are transferred to a new growth medium, there is an initial period during which the bacteria must adjust to the new growth conditions. There may be changes in the temperature, availability of nutrients, level of trace metals, or concentration of waste products. Any of these new conditions may call for repression or derepression of genes. The production of enzymes needed to grow in this new environment may take only seconds or may require many minutes. During this lag phase, the bacteria are not multiplying, so there is no increase in the number of bacteria.

Log Phase (Exponential Phase). Once multiplication begins, the number of bacteria increases logarithmically (to either the base 2 or the base 10) throughout the log phase. Because the bacteria in the suspension are now fairly uniform in shape and size, the cell number and cell mass increase in parallel. It is during the log phase that the **bacterial growth rate** can be determined. Each bacterial species has its own characteristic growth rate, but this rate varies with the nutritional state of the medium and with temperature. Under optimal conditions, some bacteria divide as rapidly as once every 10–11 minutes, while others divide only once every 20 hours.

The growth rate or the doubling time can be easily determined using the following formula:

$$K = \frac{\log_{10}(N_t/N_o)}{0.301\ t}$$

where K is the **exponential growth rate** (as generations per hour), t is the elapsed time (in hours), N_t is the number of bacteria after the elapsed time, and N_o is the original number of bacteria.

The formula can be rearranged to determine the **generation time** (G), which is the time it takes for the bacterial population to double in number:

$$G = \frac{t}{3.3\ \log(N_t/N_o)}$$

If a culture has 100 (that is, 1×10^2) bacteria per milliliter at the beginning of the log phase and the

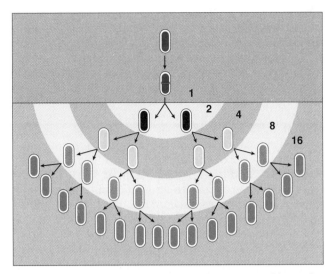

FIGURE 2–1. Bacterial multiplication by transverse binary fission. During the log (exponential) phase of growth, each bacterium yields two identical progeny when it divides asexually.

suspension contains 1×10^9 bacteria per milliliter 10 hours later, the exponential growth rate (K) of the bacterial suspension would be calculated as:

$$K = \frac{\log(10^9/10^2)}{0.301 \times 10 \text{ hours}}$$

$$= \frac{9 - 2}{3.01} = 2.33 \text{ generations per hour}$$

Similarly, the generation time would be calculated as:

$$G = \frac{10 \text{ hours}}{3.3 \log(10^9/10^2)} = 0.433 \text{ hour} = 26 \text{ minutes}$$

Stationary Phase. Eventually, the culture will run out of key nutrients and will accumulate toxic by-products of metabolism. When this occurs, the bacterial generation time will lengthen considerably,

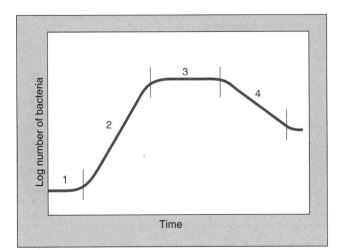

FIGURE 2–2. The standard bacterial growth curve. There are four phases in the standard growth curve: (1) the lag phase, (2) the log (exponential) phase, (3) the stationary phase, and (4) the death phase.

and the rate of bacterial multiplication and death will balance. In Fig. 2–2, the flattened portion of the growth curve is the stationary phase. The metabolic and biosynthetic activities of bacteria in this phase differ considerably from those of bacteria in the log phase.

The stationary phase can greatly alter the susceptibility of bacteria to specific antibiotics. This is why boils and other infections that involve stationary phase bacteria can be difficult to treat. Because the bacteria in a boil are in the stationary phase, they do not replace their cell walls rapidly. For this reason, antibiotics that interfere with cell wall synthesis (such as penicillins and cephalosporins) are not very effective unless the bacteria in the boil can be induced to once more begin growing logarithmically. The therapeutic challenge of dealing with boils is exacerbated by the thick wall that surrounds a boil and inhibits the penetration of antibiotics into the lesion. The physician must drain the boil to bring the bacteria back into log phase. The surface of a boil that has been drained is fairly clean, and bacteria in the boil will rapidly seek to repopulate the area. Once they begin to multiply rapidly, the bacteria are susceptible to appropriate beta-lactam antibiotics.

Death Phase. During the final phase of growth, the lack of key nutrients and the accumulation of toxic by-products of metabolism (including fatty acids released from the cell envelope) cause the bacteria in the suspension to die rapidly. In many instances, this phase is accompanied by activation of amidases and other enzymes that lyse the cell wall.

Alternative Types of Multiplication

Although most medically significant bacteria multiply by transverse binary fission, a few have unusual replicative schemes. Mycoplasmas, which have no cell walls, multiply by budding. Some intracellular bacteria—particularly members of the genera *Chlamydia, Ehrlichia,* and *Coxiella*—have complex life cycles. These cycles are not analogous to viral replication patterns (there is no uncoating event, for example); however, they involve intracellular intermediate forms that multiply rapidly but are noninfectious for other cells. Finally, members of the genus *Streptomyces* are funguslike in that their growth involves formation of small cell types that are known as conidiospores and grow out into elongated hyphalike cells. The terminology used to describe *Streptomyces* is similar to that used to describe the structures and multiplication of fungi. It should be remembered, however, that *Streptomyces* species are prokaryotes, while fungi are eukaryotes, and there are very real differences between the mycelia and spores of *Streptomyces* and those of fungi.

Methods of Enumerating Bacteria

Many procedures performed in the clinical or research laboratory require that bacteria be enumerated. There are two basic methods of determining how many bacteria are in a culture. The first method involves counting the **absolute or total number of bacterial particles** in a suspension and does not distinguish between living and dead bacteria. Counts are usually obtained by using a special counting chamber (a Petroff-Hauser chamber) or by using a spectrophotometer to measure the amount of light scattered by the bacteria in suspension. The second method involves determining the **number of viable or active bacteria** by measuring the amount of some energy-dependent bacterial activity resident in a suspension of bacteria. For example, counts can be obtained by measuring hemolytic or enzyme activities; by determining the number of colonies that arise from an aliquot of a bacterial suspension; or by determining the amount of a bacterial suspension needed to infect, to kill, or to produce fever in 50% of a population of test animals (the ID_{50}, LD_{50}, and FP_{50}, respectively).

The first and second methods may produce fairly equivalent results, but if a large percentage of the bacteria in the culture are dead, the numbers will be widely discordant.

BACTERIAL GROWTH REQUIREMENTS

Human cells show little variation in metabolic characteristics or biochemical activities. Bacteria, however, live under a wide variety of conditions, and they vary considerably in their abilities to occupy specialized ecologic niches. As discussed below, bacteria can be characterized in terms of their temperature, oxygen, and nutrient requirements.

Variations in Temperature Requirements

Based on their temperature requirements for growth, bacteria may be classified as psychrophiles, mesophiles, thermophiles, or stenothermophiles.

There are many environmental bacteria capable of growing in the arctic tundra or in a refrigerator. When their optimal temperature for growth is under 20 °C, they are termed **psychrophiles** (cold-lovers). Remember that two-thirds of the earth is covered by water with temperatures under 10 °C.

Most of the medically important bacteria are **mesophiles.** They grow between 20 °C and 45 °C but have an optimal temperature range of 35–37 °C.

Some bacteria grow in hot springs or other high-temperature environments. If their optimal temperature is between 45 °C and 60 °C, they are called **thermophiles.** If they grow best above 60 °C, they are considered to be **stenothermophiles**. The stenothermophiles have heat-stable tertiary enzyme structures.

Variations in Oxygen Requirements

Based on their oxygen requirements, bacteria may be classified as aerobic, anaerobic, or microaerophilic.

Many bacteria are **aerobes** and grow only in the presence of atmospheric oxygen. Often, these bacteria are respiratory or mucosal pathogens, such as *Neisseria* species or *Mycobacterium tuberculosis*.

Other aerobic bacteria, such as *Pseudomonas aeruginosa,* are opportunistic pathogens that are capable of causing numerous types of infections.

Some bacteria are **anaerobes,** which means that they do not use oxygen, while others are **strict anaerobes,** which means that they can be killed by atmospheric oxygen. Most anaerobic bacteria live in the human gastrointestinal tract and cause deep abscesses (as do *Bacteroides* species), but some are present in the environment as spores and cause disease when introduced into an anaerobic environment (as do *Clostridium* species). It may seem odd, but there are anaerobes in the human mouth. **Facultative anaerobes,** such as *Escherichia coli,* are capable of growing under either aerobic or anaerobic conditions. Many of them are found in the gastrointestinal tract and can cause infections of wounds or lesions of the gastrointestinal or urinary tract.

Finally, some bacteria need oxygen but cannot grow in atmospheric air; they require a reduction in oxygen partial pressure (Po_2) and can be cultured in a medium using N_2 as the nitrogen source. These **microaerophiles** include species of *Campylobacter,* which cause diarrhea and sepsis.

Most community-acquired disease is caused by aerobes or facultative organisms, but as microbiologic techniques improve, the medical importance of anaerobes and microaerophiles is becoming evident. Diseases caused by these organisms were long unrecognized because special media and incubation conditions are needed to grow them. Anaerobes must be transported and grown in prereduced media, and special incubators or devices (such as anaerobe jars or gas packs) are needed for their culture. Anaerobes are often found in deep abscesses, where they are in mixed culture with aerobes or facultative organisms. Thus, clinicians often recognized and treated only the aerobic organisms.

The key to whether an anaerobe is aerotolerant seems to be whether the enzyme **superoxide dismutase** is present. While facultative organisms typically ferment sugars under anaerobic conditions (an organic molecule is the final electron acceptor), many anaerobes typically respire anaerobically. The concept of anaerobic respiration may seem to be an oxymoron, but it is not. The anaerobes generate proton motive force through electron transfer and proton extrusion, but their terminal electron acceptor is a molecule such as sulfate, nitrate, or nitrite. When oxygen is present, the electrons are transferred; but highly cytotoxic intermediates—including superoxide—are made. Because these organisms lack a surface superoxide dismutase, the superoxide is not detoxified, and the superoxide and its products carry out toxic oxygenation reactions. The process of anaerobic respiration is discussed in further detail below.

Variations in Nutrient Requirements

Bacteria are involved in a variety of metabolic schemes and are able to metabolize an incredible number of substances. Some bacteria can grow on a simple medium consisting of salts, ammonium chloride, and glycerol. Other bacteria are extremely fastidious and have complicated growth requirements. For example, gram-negative enteric organisms (such as *E. coli*) have simple nutrient requirements, while organisms that grow on mucosae or within host cells often have a complex set of requirements.

Many types of bacteria have not been grown on a defined medium—that is, a medium in which all of the chemical constituents are precisely known. Instead, they must be grown on an undefined medium, such as one containing blood (blood agar), serum, yeast extract, peptone, or other undefined addition.

The obligately intracellular rickettsiae and the chlamydiae have never been grown on artificial media and must be cultured in eukaryotic cell lines (such as mouse fibroblasts or chicken embryo cells) or in eggs. This does not make them viruses (they are in fact gram-negative bacteria), but it does make them extremely difficult to work with. Clinical laboratories usually do not have facilities to culture these organisms.

BACTERIAL METABOLISM
Energy Production

There are three critical processes of bacterial energy production: aerobic respiration, anaerobic respiration, and fermentation. In this section, the discussion of these processes follows the convention of assuming that each metabolic pathway is being used to produce energy from glucose. In reality, bacteria metabolize a tremendous array of substrates, and these feed into the metabolic cycles at a number of sites. For example, there are bacteria that produce energy from dicarboxylic acids, from phenolic compounds, or from acetate. Metabolic cycles must be available to convert these to products that can be further metabolized by one of the central metabolic pathways, such as the **Embden-Meyerhof pathway** (glycolysis) or the **tricarboxylic acid cycle** (the **TCA cycle,** also called the **Krebs cycle**).

The processes of aerobic respiration, anaerobic respiration, and fermentation are primarily differentiated on the basis of what molecule or molecules serve as the terminal electron acceptor. **Aerobic respiration** uses one of several schemes to convert glucose to pyruvate and then uses the TCA cycle to produce the reduced form of nicotinamide adenine dinucleotide (NADH). Reducing equivalents generated by this pathway are donated to cytochromes in the cytoplasmic membrane, and oxygen serves as the terminal electron acceptor. Proton motive force generated by the movement of protons across the cytoplasmic membrane then drives a membrane-bound adenosine triphosphatase (ATPase) that converts adenosine diphosphate (ADP) to adenosine triphosphate (ATP). **Anaerobic respiration** is similar to aerobic respiration except that it uses a separate set of cytochromes, which donates electrons to an inorganic molecule such as sulfate, nitrate, nitrite, or carbonate. **Fermentation** is the least efficient means of metabolism. During fermentation, glucose is converted to pyruvate via glycolysis. NADH is then recycled back to NAD by converting pyruvate to any of several organic acids (such as lactate, formate, or propionate), and this organic acid serves as the terminal electron acceptor.

Aerobic Respiration

Aerobes and facultative anaerobes metabolize glucose aerobically by aerobic respiration. Facultative anaerobes and some aerobes convert each molecule of glucose to two molecules of pyruvate via glycolysis. Pyruvate is then metabolized via the **TCA cycle,** thereby producing ATP, reducing equivalents (the reduced form of NAD [NADH] and of flavin adenine dinucleotide [FADH]), and six molecules of CO_2. The reducing equivalents donate electrons to the cytochrome system, and a membrane-bound ATPase makes ATP as protons return to the cytoplasm. This scheme produces 38 molecules of ATP, with a net $\Delta G^{o'}$ of 688 kcal (2890 kJ) at an efficiency of 40%. The net result is that bacteria produce two more molecules of ATP than do mammalian systems. The reason is that no ATP is expended moving molecules across the mitochondrial membrane; all the reactions take place in the same compartment.

Some strict aerobes diverge from the upper part of this scheme. There are two common divergences. Some aerobes convert glucose to fructose 6-phosphate (fructose 6-P) and glyceraldehyde 3-phosphate (glyceraldehyde 3-P) via the **pentose phosphate shunt,** which is also called the **6-phosphogluconate pathway** (Fig. 2–3). This pathway generates the reduced form of nicotinamide adenine dinucleotide phosphate (NADPH), and the fructose 6-P and glyceraldehyde 3-P are subsequently metabolized by glycolysis. NADPH can be used for energy production or for fatty acid synthesis, and the five-carbon sugars generated can be used to synthesize nucleic acids. Other strict aerobes (such as *Pseudomonas* and *Neisseria*) convert glucose to pyruvate and glyceraldehyde 3-P by the **Entner-Doudoroff pathway** (see Fig. 2–3). After these compounds are further metabolized via glycolysis, they may be used to generate energy via the TCA cycle, or they may be converted to ethanol.

One of the more unusual metabolic schemes is that used by some aerobes to catabolize acetate. Humans cannot live on acetate alone, because biosynthetic needs drain four-carbon compounds from the TCA cycle. Fig. 2–4 shows the **glyoxylate cycle.** This cycle is an example of an anaplerotic cycle (anaplerotic means "filling up"). Isocitrate is cleaved by a unique enzyme called isocitrate lyase to yield succinate and glyoxylate. An acetate is then fused with the glyoxylate to yield malate. This set of reactions produces some energy, but the key role of this cycle is to replace the carbons drawn off from the TCA cycle by the loss, to biosynthetic pathways, of α-ketoglutarate, succinate, and oxaloacetate. The glyoxylate cycle ensures that there are sufficient carbons available to allow the TCA cycle to continue to function with acetate as the only carbon source.

When bacteria grow on a rich medium that allows

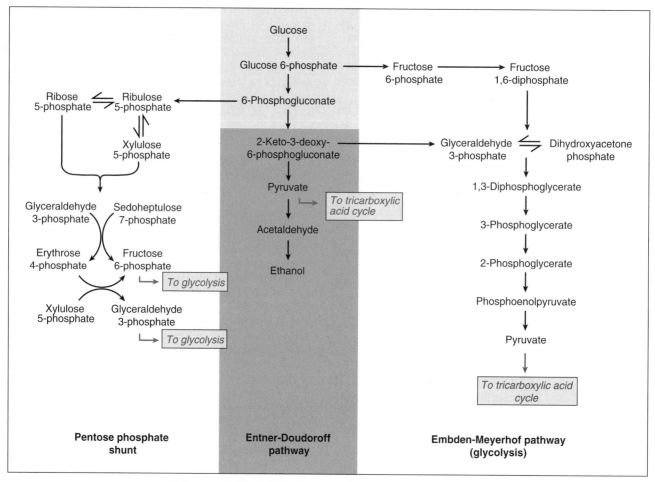

FIGURE 2–3. Three schemes for aerobic metabolism of glucose.

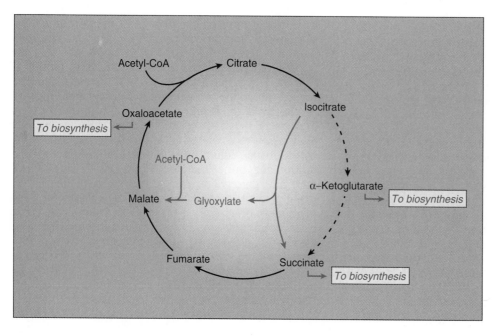

FIGURE 2–4. The glyoxylate cycle. Human cells cannot subsist on acetate, since biosynthetic drain of four-carbon intermediates depletes the tricarboxylic acid cycle. The glyoxylate cycle replenishes these intermediates by splitting isocitrate to form glyoxylate and succinate, and the glyoxylate is condensed with acetate to form malate.

accumulation of excess acetyl coenzyme A (acetyl-CoA), a second anaplerotic reaction is activated. Excess acetyl-CoA allosterically activates the biotin-dependent enzyme pyruvate carboxylase, which in turn condenses phosphoenolpyruvate (PEP) with CO_2 to form oxaloacetic acid.

Anaerobic Respiration

Some anaerobes and facultative anaerobes metabolize sugars anaerobically via glycolysis and the TCA cycle. This may seem unusual because human cells are not capable of using the TCA cycle under anaerobic conditions. These bacteria have unique cytochrome chains that are able to use a variety of inorganic molecules as their terminal electron acceptor. When the electrons are donated to oxygen, superoxide is generated. Because strict anaerobes lack superoxide dismutase, they are rapidly killed by oxygen. Some of the cytochrome systems used by anaerobes are relatively inefficient, with fewer than 30 molecules of ATP being formed from glucose. Although anaerobes metabolize glucose via glycolysis, they seem to be unable to use the pentose phosphate shunt and the Entner-Doudoroff pathway.

Some facultative and anaerobic organisms use nitrate as a final electron acceptor under anaerobic conditions, converting it to nitrite. Under these conditions, *Escherichia coli* produces about half as many molecules of ATP as it does under aerobic conditions. Some other nitrate reducers are *Klebsiella, Pseudomonas aeruginosa, Clostridium perfringens, Enterobacter,* and *Staphylococcus aureus.* Clinical laboratories use a **nitrate reduction test** to determine whether this property is present and to help identify the organisms (in conjunction with other biochemical tests).

Fermentation

Fermentation was discovered by Louis Pasteur, who described it as the consequence of life without air. Fermentation occurs among facultative and some anaerobic organisms growing in the absence of atmospheric oxygen. Its key characteristic is that an organic acid acts as the terminal electron acceptor.

Glucose is converted to pyruvate via anaerobic glycolysis. At this point, the cycle has generated two molecules of ATP via substrate-level phosphorylation and has also generated two molecules of NADH. The NADH must be converted to NAD or the cycle will grind to a halt. As Fig. 2–5 shows, bacteria accomplish this by a variety of means. Human cells typically convert pyruvate to lactate under anaerobic conditions. Some bacteria also do this, but others convert pyruvate to products as diverse as formate, butanediol, ethanol, acetic acid, butyric acid, butanol, acetone, and isopropanol. Each of these schemes recycles NADH back to NAD, allowing glycolysis to continue.

Each fermentation scheme is associated with one or more types of bacteria. For this reason, evolution of specific fermentation products is used to identify many types of bacteria. While some schemes generate gas (CO_2 or H_2) when the medium is acidified by fermentation, others do not. The clinical laboratory identifies many bacteria by growing them in a **Durham tube** (a small inverted test tube used to capture gas) and a culture medium that contains a single sugar and phenol red. The medium will become yellow if the bacterium ferments the sugar, and the Durham tube will contain a tiny bubble if gas is also produced.

Some anaerobes (particularly members of the genus *Clostridium*) ferment amino acids, producing substances such as cadaverine and putrescine as end products. Thus, abscesses caused by these organisms exhibit a foul odor. The key reaction in this process is the **Stickland reaction,** in which one amino acid donates electrons to another. For example, alanine and glycine are fermented by the following reaction:

$$\text{Alanine} + 2\ \text{Glycine} + 2\ H_2O \rightarrow 3\ \text{Acetic acid}$$
$$+\ 3\ NH_3 + CO_2$$

Table 2–1 compares the key characteristics of aerobic respiration, anaerobic respiration, and fermentation. Of the three processes, fermentation is the least efficient.

Oxidative Phosphorylation

Bacteria make ATP via the process of oxidative phosphorylation. This process in bacteria is analogous in some ways to the process in eukaryotic mitochondria but differs in several key components.

Most redox reactions contribute protons and electrons to the pyridine nucleotide NAD, but some reactions involve hydrogenation of NADP or a flavin nucleotide (either flavin adenine dinucleotide [FAD] or flavin mononucleotide [FMN]). When NADH is used, for example, the electrons are donated to a flavoprotein and are passed to a soluble quinone compound (ubiquinone, or coenzyme Q) floating in the cytoplasmic membrane. The electrons are subsequently passed through a series of increasingly electropositive cytochromes that are located within the cytoplasmic membrane. The final cytochrome donates its electrons to molecular oxygen. The energy generated by this electron transfer sequence is used to extrude protons through the membrane.

As protons accumulate outside the cytoplasmic membrane, a **proton motive force** (Δp) is generated. This force consists of an electrical potential difference ($\Delta\psi$) and a pH gradient (ΔpH). The relationship of these factors in the electrochemical gradient is shown in the following formula, in which p is expressed in volts:

$$\Delta p = \Delta\psi + 0.06\ \Delta\text{pH}$$

Protons return to the cytoplasm through specialized proton channels, and their return can be directly linked to three activities: (1) the formation of ATP by a membrane-bound ATPase; (2) the comovement of solutes across the cytoplasmic membrane (see Chapter 1); and (3) the rotation of the bacterial flagellum (see Chapter 1). In eukaryotic systems, three protons

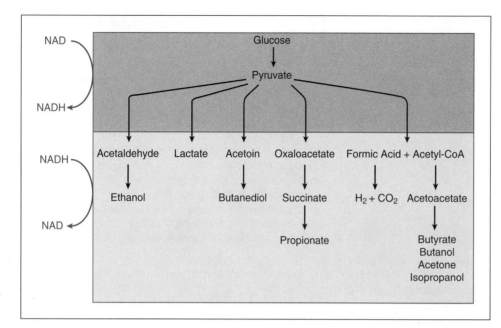

FIGURE 2–5. Alternative fates of pyruvate. Bacteria growing by fermentation generate the reduced form of nicotinamide adenine dinucleotide (NADH) during glycolysis. NADH must be recycled back to NAD after completion of glycolysis, or the glycolytic pathway will halt. Bacteria exhibit a wide variety of schemes to recycle their NADH.

return to the cytoplasm for each NADH molecule generated, so that three molecules of ATP are formed. Bacterial cytochromes vary, however, in their electronegativity. In some bacteria, for example, only one or two molecules of ATP are formed for each molecule of NADH generated.

There are other differences. Human cytochromes interact with ubiquinone, and many bacterial cytochromes do as well. However, most gram-positive bacteria contain menaquinone instead of ubiquinone, and *E. coli* organisms contain both compounds. In *E. coli,* the ratio of ubiquinone to menaquinone varies with the availability of oxygen. When oxygen is limited, the relative amount of menaquinone increases dramatically. Oxygen also affects the

type of terminal cytochrome oxidase present. In some bacteria, cytochrome *b* serves as the terminal cytochrome oxidase when oxygen is plentiful, but it is replaced by cytochrome *o* when little oxygen is present. Furthermore, some bacteria have branched-chain cytochrome systems, while others have terminal cytochromes that preferentially donate electrons to nitrate, nitrite, carbonate, sulfate, or fumarate during anaerobic respiration.

Biosynthesis

Many of the biosynthetic pathways followed by bacteria are similar or identical to those followed by eukaryotic cells. Some of the pathways, particularly

TABLE 2–1. A Comparison of Key Characteristics of Aerobic Respiration, Anaerobic Respiration, and Fermentation*

Characteristic	Aerobic Respiration Processes		Anaerobic Respiration	Fermentation
Pathway	Embden-Myerhof pathway (see Fig. 2–3)	Pentose phosphate shunt or Entner-Doudoroff pathway (see Fig. 2–3)	Embden-Myerhof pathway (see Fig. 2–3)	Various pathways (see Fig. 2–5)
Source of energy	PMF and SLP	PMF and SLP	PMF and SLP	SLP
Source of biosynthetic intermediates	TCA cycle	TCA cycle	TCA cycle	Split TCA cycle (see Fig. 2–6)
Cytochrome involvement	Yes	Yes	Yes, but not with same cytochromes as in aerobic respiration	No
Terminal electron acceptor	O_2	O_2	NO_2, NO_3, SO_4, CO_3, and fumarate	Organic acids
Number of ATP molecules produced	38	Varies	16–38 (usually fewer than 30)	2
Organism involvement				
Strict aerobes	Yes	Yes	No	No
Facultative anaerobes	Yes	No	Yes[†]	Yes[†]
Strict anaerobes	No	No	Yes[†]	Yes[†]

* ATP = adenosine triphosphate; PMF = proton motive force; SLP = substrate-level phosphorylation; and TCA = tricarboxylic acid.
† Individual facultative and strict anaerobes vary in their abilities to ferment or to respire anaerobically. Some can do both, while others can only ferment or respire anaerobically.

those used to synthesize cell wall and cell membrane components, are discussed in Chapter 1. A few general comments are made here about the unique aspects of bacterial biosynthesis.

First, the TCA cycle provides many key biosynthetic intermediates, particularly for the synthesis of amino acids and porphyrins. This raises a problem for *E. coli* and other bacteria that grow by fermentation. During fermentation, α-ketoglutarate oxidase is nonfunctional, so the TCA cycle should not be available. But as Fig. 2–6 shows, *E. coli* that are growing by fermentation utilize a **split TCA cycle** to synthesize amino acids and hemin. Oxaloacetate is converted reductively to fumarate and then succinate, while it is also converted oxidatively to citrate, isocitrate, and α-ketoglutarate. The reductive branch is possible because the NAD-linked succinate dehydrogenase is replaced by fumarate reductase. By having reductive and oxidative branches, the reducing equivalents are balanced out, and there is no net change in the ratio of NAD to NADH.

Second, many bacteria do not import folic acid from exogenous sources but instead synthesize it themselves. Tetrahydrofolate is needed for a number of biosynthetic reactions, including those involved in synthesis of purines and vitamins. Scientists have taken advantage of this biochemical quirk in the development of antibiotics known as sulfonamides. Folic acid is a condensation of pteridine, glutamic acid, and *p*-aminobenzoic acid (PABA). The sulfonamides competitively inhibit folic acid synthesis by acting as an analogue of PABA. A second step in tetrahydrofolate synthesis can be inhibited by the antibiotic trimethoprim. When used together, trimethoprim and sulfonamides act synergistically to inhibit bacterial growth. Unfortunately, if the end products of folic acid utilization (such as purines and vitamins) are available because of tissue damage, folic acid is no longer needed, and the bacteria will not be affected by sulfonamides (see Chapter 4).

Auxotrophy

The discussion of bacterial genetics below and in Chapter 3 requires an understanding of a bacterial metabolic phenomenon known as auxotrophy. Bacteria exist as either **prototrophs** (the parental metabolic type) or **auxotrophs.** Auxotrophs have a genetic lesion that causes them to differ metabolically from their prototrophic counterparts.

If a bacterium is an auxotroph for an amino acid, it has lost the ability to synthesize that amino acid de novo and cannot survive unless the amino acid is provided in the growth medium. If a bacterium is an auxotroph for a carbohydrate, it has lost the ability to catabolize a sugar and cannot survive if that sugar is the sole carbon and energy source. Thus, an *E. coli* strain that is auxotrophic for maltose and leucine (a *mal⁻leu⁻* strain) is unable to grow on a medium that contains maltose as the sole carbon and energy source, and it must be provided with leucine from an exogenous source because it cannot make leucine de novo. In contrast, the parental strain (the *mal⁺leu⁺* strain) of *E. coli* can be grown on a medium that contains maltose but no leucine. Auxotrophs are used to map the location of genes on the bacterial chromosome.

Control of Bacterial Metabolism

Bacteria control enzyme activity and enzyme synthesis in a variety of ways. **Enzyme activity** is regulated directly by feedback **allosteric control.** This is often referred to as **fine control** because the effects of the allosteric inhibition or stimulation can be seen immediately. In addition, enzyme activity is regulated by standard control mechanisms such as competitive, noncompetitive, and uncompetitive inhibition. **Enzyme synthesis** is regulated either by **transcriptional control** or **translational control.** Control at the transcriptional or translational level is often called **coarse control** because it takes some time for the effects of the control to be observed. If, for instance, the synthesis of an enzyme is halted, the effects will not be evident until the preexisting enzyme molecules are metabolized.

Allosteric Control of Enzyme Activity

Bacteria can control enzyme activity either by stimulating it or by inhibiting it.

Positive control is most often seen in catabolic and amphibolic pathways. A chemical binds to an allosteric site on the enzyme, changes its conformation, and increases its activity. An example of this is the ability of the cellular energy charge—that is, the concentration of ATP, ADP, and adenosine monophosphate (AMP)—to regulate energy supply by turning on key catabolic enzymes.

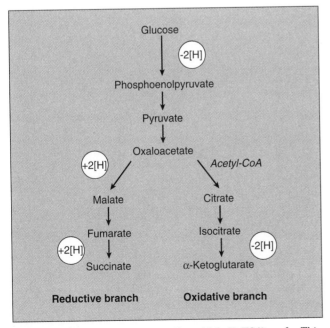

FIGURE 2–6. The split tricarboxylic acid (split TCA) cycle. This cycle is used by *Escherichia coli* organisms to provide for their biosynthetic needs during fermentative growth.

Negative control is exerted most often on anabolic pathways and at branch points between catabolic and anabolic pathways. In a given pathway, not all of the enzymes will be susceptible to feedback inhibition. Instead, the enzymes subject to control are most often those at key spots along the pathway, such as at the beginning and at branch points.

An interesting example of feedback allosteric control is that exerted on the pathway that converts L-aspartate to lysine, methionine, threonine, and isoleucine (Fig. 2–7). This pathway has feedback loops to each of the branch points in the system to keep from wasting substrate. For example, when *E. coli* has sufficient methionine, it may still need isoleucine. Therefore, the methionine feeds back and shuts off the first enzyme in its synthesis but does not impede the conversion of homoserine to isoleucine. This pathway has another interesting feature. Notice that there are three aspartokinase (AK) isozymes: AK1 is inhibited by threonine, AK3 is inhibited by lysine, and AK2 is not subject to feedback inhibition. This scheme is designed to prevent **pseudoauxotrophy.** Recall that amino acid auxotrophy is a genetic change that results in the loss of the ability to make a particular amino acid. The auxotroph cannot survive unless the amino acid is provided in the growth medium, even though the parent (prototroph) was fully able to synthesize the amino acid de novo. A pseudoauxotroph is a bacterium that *temporarily* loses the ability to make a needed amino acid when another amino acid is present in excess.

There are some pathways in which isozymes of a single enzyme are subject to contradictory control mechanisms. One of these is illustrated in Fig. 2–8. In this pathway, acetolactate synthetase converts active acetaldehyde and pyruvate to acetolactate. This can then be used to synthesize valine (anabolism) or to make energy by conversion to butylene glycol. In this case, one isozyme is inhibited when there is excess valine, while the other is stimulated by fermentative conditions.

Transcriptional Control of Enzyme Synthesis

The enzymes and transport proteins of many bacterial metabolic pathways are controlled at the transcriptional level. When the genes for a single pathway are controlled coordinately, they are referred to as an **operon.** When several pathways are under coordinate control by a single regulator gene, they are referred to as a **regulon.** It is important to note that not all bacterial enzymes are subject to transcriptional control. Bacterial enzymes are said to be **constitutive enzymes** if they are synthesized at a steady rate throughout the growth cycle and are under no coordinate transcriptional control.

Positively controlled operons, also called **inducible operons,** are usually those which code for a **catabolic pathway.** When no substrate is available for the pathway, an active repressor binds to the operator site and blocks reading of the operon. When the substrate for the pathway appears in sufficient quantity, an **inducer** is generated for the purpose of binding to and inactivating (releasing) the repressor. After the repressor is released from the operator site of the operon, the DNA-dependent RNA polymerase is able to read the operon. Inducible operons make sense because when a catabolic pathway has no substrate available, there is no need for the enzymes to be synthesized.

Negatively controlled operons are subject to feedback repression. These operons usually code for the enzymes of an **anabolic pathway.** Under normal circumstances, a bacterium needs to synthesize products of the operon. A **repressor** is made, but it becomes active only when the end product of the pathway reaches a critically high level. At this point, the end product binds to the repressor and activates it. Because of its role, the end product is called a

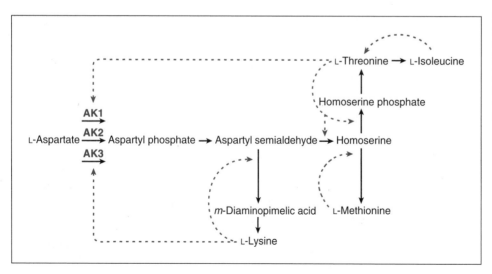

FIGURE 2–7. Allosteric control of the anabolic conversion of L-aspartate to amino acids. The existence of three aspartokinase isozymes (AK1, AK2, and AK3), each with unique allosteric control sites, prevents pseudoauxotrophy. Dotted lines indicate negative feedback loops.

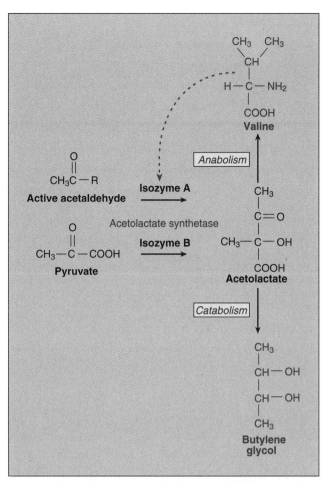

FIGURE 2–8. Control of the conversion of active acetaldehyde and pyruvate to acetolactate by acetolactate synthetase. The activity of isozyme A is under negative feedback allosteric control (dotted lines), while the activity of isozyme B is stimulated by fermentative conditions.

in the medium, the DNA-dependent RNA polymerase combines with a cyclic AMP–binding protein (CAP) and cyclic AMP (cAMP) to form an active polymerase complex. The polymerase binds to the *lac* promoter and begins to travel down the DNA. When it reaches the operator site, the repressor prevents the DNA from being unwound, so the polymerase stops reading and falls off; the structural genes will not be read. At this time, there are only one or two lactose permease molecules in the bacterial cytoplasmic membrane. When lactose is added to the medium as the only sugar, a few molecules enter the cell, and a **natural inducer** called allolactose is formed. Allolactose binds to the repressor and inactivates it by changing its form, thereby tremendously reducing its affinity for DNA. As a result, the repressor will fall off the DNA. Now the RNA polymerase will be able to pass through the operator site and transcribe the structural genes. Within minutes, there will be a 1000-fold increase in the number of β-galactosidase and lactose permease molecules in the bacterium.

Scientists have devised a number of inducers that are analogues of allolactose and are capable of inactivating the repressor. Some of these analogues cannot be metabolized and are known as **gratuitous inducers.** Others are readily broken down by β-galactosidase but are extremely poor inducers. The key to being a good inducer does not lie in the ability to be metabolized but, rather, in the ability to reduce the affinity that the repressor has for the DNA.

(2) Catabolite Repression. Scientists studying the genetic regulatory mechanisms in protein synthesis found that when *lac*⁺ *E. coli* was grown in a medium that contained just two sugars—glucose and lactose—the bacteria exhibited a biphasic growth

corepressor. The operon cannot be read again until the concentration of product falls significantly.

The lactose operon and the tryptophan operon provide examples of the types of transcriptional control involved in catabolic and anabolic pathways.

The Lactose Operon. The best understood catabolic operon is the lactose operon, which is often called the *lac* operon. As shown in Fig. 2–9, this operon consists of five discrete sites: the *lac* promoter (P_{lac}); the *lac* operator (O); and the genes for β-galactosidase (z), lactose permease (y), and transacetylase (a). The *lac* operon is controlled by a single repressor known as the *lac* repressor (R). The repressor protein gene is separate from the *lac* operon and has its own promoter (P_r). It is a tetrameric protein that fits into a three-dimensional groove in the O region of the *lac* operon and prevents unwinding of the DNA during messenger RNA (mRNA) synthesis. The *lac* operon is involved in catabolite activation and repression and is also part of a larger global regulatory network.

(1) Operon Activation. Transcriptional control follows a series of steps. When no lactose is present

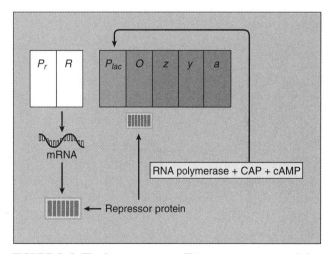

FIGURE 2–9. The lactose operon. This operon consists of the *lac* promoter (P_{lac}); the *lac* operator (O); and the genes for β-galactosidase (z), lactose permease (y), and transacetylase (a). The operon is controlled by a single repressor (R), which has its own promoter (P_r). R produces an active repressor protein, which binds to P_{lac} unless its conformation is changed by binding to an inducer. The DNA-dependent RNA polymerase synthesizes messenger RNA (mRNA) when it complexes with cyclic AMP–binding protein (CAP) and cyclic AMP (cAMP) and initiates reading at the O site.

curve. That is, the bacterial mass increased for a time, leveled off, and then began increasing again, as shown in Fig. 2–10. This phenomenon is called **diauxie.**

Further investigation revealed that the bacteria were metabolizing only glucose during the first growth phase and metabolizing only lactose during the second growth phase. What happened was that glucose entered the bacterium via group transloca-tion, a process that causes levels of cAMP to be de-pressed (see Chapter 1 for details). As cAMP levels dropped, there was insufficient cAMP to form the active RNA polymerase–CAP–cAMP complexes nec-essary to initiate transcription of the operon. Even though there was enough lactose to bind to the re-pressor and derepress the operon, the operon could not be read, because no DNA-dependent RNA poly-merase could bind to the *lac* promoter. Thus, only glucose was metabolized during the initial phase. When the last of the glucose was expended, causing a lag in growth, the cAMP levels began to climb. Fi-nally, the RNA polymerase–CAP–cAMP complexes began to form and bind to the *lac* promoter, and the derepressed operon was read. During the second growth phase only lactose was metabolized.

This process is called catabolite repression be-cause cAMP is a catabolite and its fluctuation is re-sponsible for the ability and inability of the operon to be read. The system for catabolite activation and repression is only one of several types of global regu-latory systems, as discussed later in this chapter.

The Tryptophan Operon. The tryptophan op-eron is probably the best-understood anabolic op-eron. It is sometimes referred to as the *trp* operon, and it codes for enzymes used in the synthesis of L-tryptophan. As shown in Fig. 2–11, the *trp* operon consists of the following: a combined promoter-operator site (*P-O*); a 162-nucleotide-pair leader re-gion that contains an attenuator sequence (*a*); five

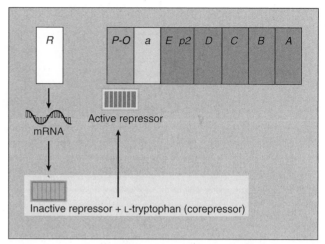

FIGURE 2–11. The tryptophan operon. This operon consists of a combined promoter-operator site (*P-O*); a 162-nucleotide-pair leader region that contains an attenuator sequence (*a*); five struc-tural genes (*E, D, C, B,* and *A*); and a low-efficiency internal pro-moter (*p2*) that allows for sporadic low-level reading of structural genes even when the operon is repressed. The repressor (*R*) is inactive unless it binds to L-tryptophan (the corepressor) to block reading of the operon.

structural genes (*E, D, C, B,* and *A*); and a low-efficiency internal promoter (*p2*) that allows for spo-radic low-level reading of structural genes even when the operon is repressed. Two unusual features of the *trp* operon are this process of low-level reading, which is called **promoter variation,** and the process of at-tenuation, which is described below. Like the *lac* re-pressor, the *trp* repressor (*R*) is coded for by a gene at a distal site. Unlike the *lac* repressor, however, the *trp* repressor is *inactive* unless excess L-tryptophan is present. The activities of the *trp* repressor and operon change as the available amounts of L-tryptophan change (Table 2–2).

(1) Response to a High Concentration of L-Tryptophan. When the concentration of L-tryptophan in a bacterium approaches the K_m of the *trp* repressor, the L-tryptophan becomes a corepres-sor, binding to the repressor and making it active. The active repressor binds to the combined *P-O* site on the *trp* operon, acting as a competitive inhibitor

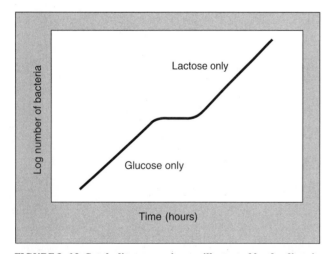

FIGURE 2–10. Catabolite repression, as illustrated by the diauxie phenomenon. *Escherichia coli* grown in a medium that contains equimolar concentrations of glucose and lactose will first metabo-lize glucose, then enter a lag phase while the catabolite repression is eased, and then metabolize lactose. Glucose transport inhibits reading of the lactose operon by depressing the levels of cyclic AMP (cAMP).

TABLE 2–2. The Effects of Changes in the Concentration of L-Tryptophan on the Activity of the Tryptophan Operon

L-Tryptophan Concentration	Effects
High	Repressor is activated; neither transcription nor translation takes place.
Low	Operon is not repressed but is attenuated; about 15% of messages started are completed.
Extremely low (tryptophan starvation)	Attenuation is eased; about 25% of messages started are completed.

to the DNA-dependent RNA polymerase. As a result, no transcription or translation can take place.

(2) Response to a Low Concentration of L-Tryptophan. When the concentration of L-tryptophan is low in a bacterium, the process of **attenuation** begins. Although eukaryotic cells have at least three RNA polymerases, bacterial cells have only one. In eukaryotes, the mRNA is capped, spliced, and exported to the cytoplasm, where it is translated in the rough endoplasmic reticulum. In bacteria, however, the mRNA is translated as it is being transcribed, with *no* posttranscriptional modification or transport, and the mRNA messages are **polycistronic messages** (that is, there are many genes on one continuous message). The bacterial RNA polymerase has four subunits, $\alpha\beta\beta'\sigma$. The β subunit binds to the nucleotides; β' binds to the DNA; and σ is required for recognition of promoters.

The RNA polymerase will stop transcribing if one of two things happens: if rho (ρ) protein binds to the newly transcribed RNA or if a stop signal consisting of a stem-loop mRNA structure forms. It is this second mechanism that is involved in attenuation.

Keep in mind that transcription and translation are physically linked. There is a region that consists of 42 nucleotide pairs (residues 27–68) and codes for a 14-residue leader peptide. When the L-tryptophan concentration is low but the cell is not experiencing L-tryptophan starvation, the repressor will not be activated. Thus, the RNA polymerase will bind to the *P-O* site and will begin to transcribe. The first segment transcribed will be the leader peptide. Within the leader region are two consecutive *trp* codons (UGG sites). If there is enough L-tryptophan to charge the tryptophanyl transfer RNA (tRNA), this section will be translated and the leader peptide will be completed. The failure of the ribosome to be held up here will allow the newly formed mRNA downstream (between the ribosome and the RNA polymerase) to form a stem-loop structure that looks like a rho termination signal. This structure is depicted in Fig. 2–12B, and its formation results in the termination of transcription at nucleotide pair 141 (np 141).

If, however, the bacterium is starved for L-tryptophan, there will not be enough charged tryptophanyl tRNA to quickly "fill the order" for the two consecutive *trp* codons. As a result, translation will stall while transcription continues unabated. When the transcriptional machinery reaches the series of uracils at np 141, there will be no stop signal generated upstream to halt the polymerase, so the RNA polymerase will continue on and read the structural genes.

The key to attenuation is that transcription and translation are linked and that when *translation* fails to stall at the two UGG codons, the mRNA between the ribosome and the RNA polymerase makes a shape that stops transcription at np 141. If the bacterium has a low concentration of L-tryptophan, about 15% of the messages begun are completed and translated, owing to the effects of attenuation. If the bacterium is starved for L-tryptophan, attenuation is eased, allowing about 25% of the messages begun to be completed and translated.

Global Regulatory Networks. Networks that are controlled by the same regulon and thus respond in a coordinated manner to changes in environmental conditions are referred to as global regulatory networks. There are at least four types of system responses in a network.

(1) Repression and Activation of Catabolic Operons. Fluctuation of cAMP affects the activity of various catabolic operons. This process is best understood from its effects on the lactose operon, as described above.

(2) Replacement of Sigma Factors. In response to environmental changes such as loss of energy supply, vegetative RNA polymerase sigma factors can be replaced by one or more sigma factors that recognize specific sets of sporulation operons. For additional information, see the discussion of sporulation in Chapter 1.

(3) Formation of Stringent Factor. When amino acid levels drop dangerously low, some bacteria express the so-called stringent response to cope with amino acid starvation. When amino acid levels drop, uncharged tRNA binds to the translational machinery and causes the formation of an enzyme called stringent factor. Stringent factor causes the bacterium to accumulate guanosine 3'-diphosphate-5'-diphosphate (ppGpp), which in turn causes ribosomal RNA (rRNA) and tRNA synthesis to decrease. Additionally, proteins are broken down to provide amino acids, and amino acid synthesis pathways are stimulated. When amino acid levels reach an acceptable level, the *spoT* gene product degrades ppGpp and the cell returns to its normal functions.

(4) Signal Transduction. The signal transduction system responds to several environmental changes by phosphorylating proteins. A sensor molecule detects the environmental change (such as nitrogen or phosphate deprivation) and then phosphorylates a specific effector protein. The phosphorylated effector protein now activates transcription for its regulon. For additional information, see the discussion of metabolic control of motility in Chapter 1.

Transcriptional Control of Metabolism by the Fumarate-Nitrate Regulator Protein

When facultative bacteria are grown anaerobically, a transcriptional regulator known as the fumarate-nitrate regulator (FNR) protein controls the expression of genes needed during anaerobic growth. The FNR protein has five cysteine residues, four of which are in a cluster, and the residues bind iron and sense the presence of molecular oxygen. When oxygen is not present, the FNR protein will activate the expression of a series of anaerobiosis-specific enzymes and will repress the expression of enzymes needed only during aerobic growth.

Translational Control of Protein Synthesis

Although the synthesis of proteins is controlled most often at the transcriptional level, several bacterial proteins have been shown to be regulated

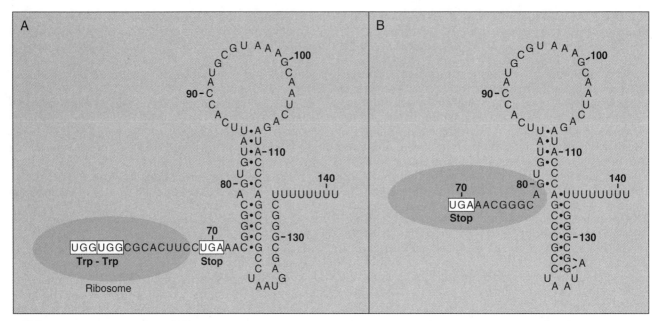

FIGURE 2–12. The hypothesized mechanism of attenuation in the tryptophan operon. If sufficient L-tryptophan is available to rapidly fill the two consecutive UGG sites, the leader peptide is completed, the messenger RNA (mRNA) assumes the structure seen in diagram **B,** and transcription halts at nucleotide 141. If L-tryptophan is scarce, however, the ribosome stalls at the two consecutive UGG sites, causing the stem-loop structure in diagram **A** to form. No stop signal is generated, and the RNA polymerase will read through the end of the attenuator region. (Redrawn and reproduced, with permission, from Lee, F., and C. Yanofsky. Transcription termination at the Trp operon attenuators of *Escherichia coli* and *Salmonella typhimurium:* RNA secondary structure and regulation of termination. Proc Natl Acad Sci U S A 74:4365–4369, 1977.)

at the translational level. Three examples are presented.

Ribosomal Protein Synthesis. The synthesis of ribosomal proteins in at least some bacteria is under operon control. Each operon codes for a protein that is a **translational repressor** for that operon. As Fig. 2–13 shows, when excess rRNA is present and the bacterium wants to synthesize ribosomes, the repressor is inactivated by binding to a portion of rRNA. When rRNA levels drop, the repressor binds instead to a portion of mRNA that encodes ribosomal proteins, and this brings the protein synthesis to a halt. The key to the system is that rRNA and mRNA compete for the repressor. If rRNA outcompetes its rival, ribosomal protein is made.

Inducible Resistance to Erythromycin. The mRNA that codes for erythromycin resistance has a structure that is similar to an attenuator. When there is no erythromycin present, there is no reason for the resistance gene to be read; therefore, an attenuatorlike structure forms on the mRNA, and the resistance gene cannot be translated. When erythromycin is added to the environment, the ribosomes stall in the leader region and the attenuator structure is not formed. As a result, the mRNA is read. Note that this attenuation effect is on translation, not on transcription.

Antisense RNA. *E. coli* has two major types of outer membrane proteins coded for by the genes *omp*C and *omp*F. The ratio of these proteins in the outer membrane is affected by the osmolarity of the growth medium. The *omp*C mRNA and the *omp*F anti-

sense mRNA are synthesized coordinately. When *omp*C is induced, both *omp*C mRNA and a segment of *omp*F antisense mRNA (called *mic*F) are produced. The *omp*C mRNA will be translated, but the *mic*F will bind to the translational initiation site for *omp*F by

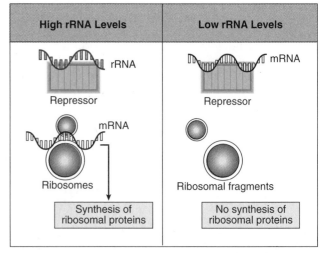

FIGURE 2–13. Translational control of ribosomal protein synthesis. When excess ribosomal RNA (rRNA) is present, the repressor is inactivated by binding to a portion of rRNA. This allows synthesis of ribosomal proteins to continue. When rRNA levels become extremely low, the repressor instead binds to a portion of the messenger RNA (mRNA) that encodes ribosomal proteins, and no synthesis of ribosomal proteins occurs.

base-pairing and will block the initiation of translation of *omp*F mRNA. This process is described more completely in Chapter 1.

Selected Readings

Ferguson, S. J. Similarities between mitochondrial and bacterial electron transport with particular reference to the action of inhibitors. Biochem Soc Trans 22:181–183, 1994.

Meister, M., S. R. Caplan, and H. C. Berg. Dynamics of a tightly coupled mechanism for flagellar rotation: bacterial motility, chemiosmotic coupling, and proton motive force. Biophys J 55:905–914, 1989.

Moodie, A. D., and W. J. Ingledew. Microbial anaerobic respiration. Adv Microb Physiol 31:225–269, 1990.

Poolman, B. Energy transduction in lactic acid bacteria. FEMS Microbiol Rev 12:125–147, 1993.

Reddy, P. S., et al. Evidence for a ppGpp-binding site on *Escherichia coli* RNA polymerase: proximity relationship with the rifampicin-binding domain. Mol Microbiol 15:255–265, 1995.

Skulachev, V. P. Chemiosmotic systems in bioenergetics: H($^+$) cycles and Na($^+$) cycles. Biosci Rep 11:387–441, 1991.

Smith, D. G., et al. Hydrolysis of urea by *Ureaplasma urealyticum* generates a transmembrane potential with resultant ATP synthesis. J Bacteriol 175:3253–3258, 1993.

Unden, G., and M. Trageser. Oxygen-regulated gene expression in *Escherichia coli:* control of anaerobic respiration by the FNR protein. Antonie Van Leeuwenhoek 59:65–76, 1991.

Vogel, U., and K. F. Jensen. Effects of the antiterminator BoxA on transcription elongation kinetics and ppGpp inhibition of transcription elongation in *Escherichia coli.* J Biol Chem 270:18335–18340, 1995.

Yanofsky, C., et al. The complete nucleotide sequence of the tryptophan operon of *Escherichia coli.* Nucleic Acids Res 9:6647–6668, 1981.

CHAPTER THREE

BACTERIAL GENETICS

The scientific conceptualization of the nature of the basic unit of inheritance has changed rather dramatically during the past few years as a result of the vast explosion of information concerning **deoxyribonucleic acid** (DNA), **ribonucleic acid** (RNA), and the molecular processes involved in **inheritance.** For many years, a **gene** was defined as the unit of DNA that coded for one enzyme. This definition lost some meaning when biochemists determined that there are **multimeric enzymes** containing unique subunits encoded by discrete segments of DNA. Then came the discovery of **immunoglobulins** with multiple DNA segments coding for a single peptide. These types of discoveries led to the development of the term **cistron,** which was meant to define the segment of DNA that encodes a single polypeptide chain. As the genetic picture has become even more detailed with the discovery of **introns** (noncoding intervening sequences in genes), **exons** (coding sequences in genes), and **overlapping genes,** geneticists have now largely returned to speaking of a gene as the element that codes for a discrete peptide. Thus, the synthesis of an immunoglobulin is encoded by several genes whose products are used to construct a single functional protein that contains multiple subunits.

A gene is much larger than the protein for which it codes. For example, a protein of about 50 kD is constructed from about 500 amino acids. Given that each amino acid is encoded by three nucleotides, that there are two DNA strands, and that each nucleotide has a molecular weight of about 330 daltons, the molecular weight of the double strand that encodes the protein is about 990 kD. Thus, the molecular weight of the DNA segment is about 20 times that of the protein it encodes. This is not wasteful, because this single gene will be read many times. In some cases, thousands of protein molecules will be synthesized by reading one gene.

THE BACTERIAL CHROMOSOME

The bacterial chromosome is circular, but it has a definite orientation—that is, the genes occur in sequence. This orderliness of the genome has allowed the bacterial chromosome to be mapped. Other characteristics of bacteria facilitate the use of these organisms as genetic models.

Use of Bacteria for Genome Mapping

Mapping has been carried out most completely in *Escherichia coli.* In these bacteria, the order in which genes occur is largely determined by the order in which they are transferred during conjugation. In the process of conjugation, which is described in detail later in this chapter, a copy of the chromosome can be passed directly from one bacterium to another. The chromosome is always passed in the same orientation, and the genes go into the recipient cell in a time-dependent process. Because the rate of transfer is constant, investigators can determine the order in which the genes appear in recipient cells by varying the duration of conjugation. A period of about 100 minutes is required to transfer the entire chromosome, and the genes are mapped by minutes. Genes that are very close together (closer than 1 minute) are mapped by crossover frequency.

Mechanisms of Genetic Change in Bacteria

Bacteria can change their characteristics at the chromosomal level by at least five mechanisms: (1) mutation of existing genes; (2) acquisition of genes from an external source, such as a bacteriophage or another bacterium; (3) rearrangement of existing genes to allow inactivation of one gene in favor of the expression of another; (4) repression and derepression of operons; and (5) control of the expression of regulons through sigma proteins and DNA binding proteins. Operon control is discussed in Chapter 2 (the lactose and tryptophan operons), and gene control through sigma factors is discussed in Chapter 1 (control of sporulation).

The first three means of differential gene expression differ from the last two in that they involve an actual change in the content of the bacterial DNA. These changes are important because they result in a permanent alteration in the characteristics of the bacterium. When genes are introduced from the outside (from a bacteriophage or another bacterium), the recipient bacterium may begin to express completely new characteristics, some of which can have a major clinical impact. A specific characteristic (such as lipopolysaccharide, an exotoxin, or an antibiotic resistance mechanism) often appears only after a piece of DNA encoding the characteristic is introduced from the outside via conjugation, transduction, transformation, or phage conversion, as discussed in greater detail below (see Exchange of Bacterial DNA).

GENETIC PROCESSES

Six processes are described in this section of the chapter: DNA replication, DNA mutation, DNA repair,

DNA recombination, exchange of bacterial DNA, and gene expression.

DNA Replication

The Rate of Replication

The bacterial chromosome is a negative superhelix of two complementary strands of DNA. The negative superhelical tension is maintained by DNA gyrase in a process that expends adenosine triphosphate (ATP).

Unlike eukaryotic cells, bacteria replicate their DNA continuously throughout the cell division cycle, and initiation of DNA replication is coordinated with cell division. The chromosome, which is replicated semiconservatively, is replicated fully about every 40 minutes. During logarithmic growth, the DNA replicative rate is constant no matter what the rate of cell division is. Once the chromosome is replicated, another 20 minutes is required to construct the septum and complete cell division. Thus, the entire replicative cycle is about 40 plus 20 minutes, or a total of 60 minutes. The construction of the septum that will create two daughter cells is controlled by the balance between two nonspecific division inhibitors (the MinC and MinD proteins) and a protein that determines where septation will occur (the MinE protein).

Initiation of DNA replication is coordinated with the growth rate, so a bacterium multiplying faster than once every 60 minutes must initiate a new cycle of DNA replication before the preceding cycle is completed. For this reason, a rapidly growing bacterium has multiple replicative forks. Thus, while the rate of DNA replication is constant, the number of replicative forks in the cell is directly related to the rate of cell division. This principle is illustrated in Fig. 3–1. Not much is understood about how cell division and DNA replication are coordinated, but investigators have noted that protein synthesis is required for initiation to occur. This has led to the hypothesis that growth rate–dependent accumulation of an initiator protein triggers each round of DNA replication.

The Process of Replication

All DNA segments that can be replicated autonomously within a bacterium are referred to as **replicons** and contain a site called the replication origin. Chromosomes, plasmids, and bacteriophages all are replicons, and their replication entails four steps: initiation of the process, elongation of the chromosome, proofreading of the product of replication, and termination of the replication process.

Initiation of the Replication Process. The initiation process is summarized in Fig. 3–2. Each circular chromosome has a **replication origin,** such as *ori*C, and the DNA replication proceeds bidirectionally from it. The *ori*C has 245 **base pairs** (bp), is rich in adenine and thymine, and contains sites called **DnaA boxes,** where **DnaA protein** binds in the presence of ATP. DnaA protein first binds to four 9-bp repeat sequences on the right side of *ori*C, accumulating

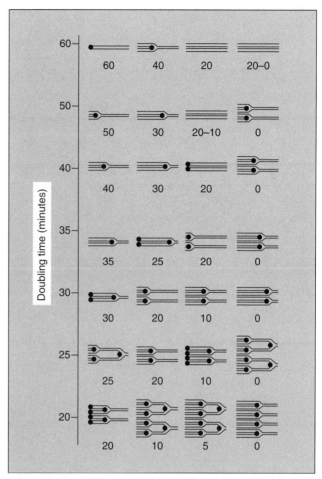

FIGURE 3–1. **Relationship between bacterial doubling time and the initiation of DNA synthesis.** About 40 minutes is required to replicate the chromosome, and another 20 minutes is needed to complete the septum. As the doubling time decreases, the rate of initiation and the number of replicative forks in each bacterium increase concomitantly. (Source: Cooper, S., and C. E. Helmstetter. Chromosome replication and the division cycle of *Escherichia coli.* J Mol Biol 31:519–540, 1968. Redrawn and reproduced, with permission, from Academic Press.)

between 20 and 40 molecules of DnaA at these sites. DnaA then binds to three 13-mer tandem repeats on the left side of *ori*C. When all seven sites are filled, the DNA strands separate to form an open complex.

Once DnaA protein has bound to the chromosome, a protein known as **helicase** or **DnaB protein** unwinds the DNA in the origin in an energy-dependent process, and **single-strand binding protein** (SSBP) attaches to each strand in the open area to keep the strands separate. SSBP coats the entire length of the single-stranded DNA segment without interfering with DNA replication. As this is occurring, the helicase begins to open the DNA adjacent to the *ori*C. This could jeopardize the status of the helix, so **DNA gyrase** stabilizes the helix by binding to the chromosome at distal sites. The DNA site opened for initiation is about 60 bp long.

Now the replicative process begins. **DnaG primase** synthesizes a short **RNA primer** (15–50 bp long) and, in doing so, completes construction of a complex

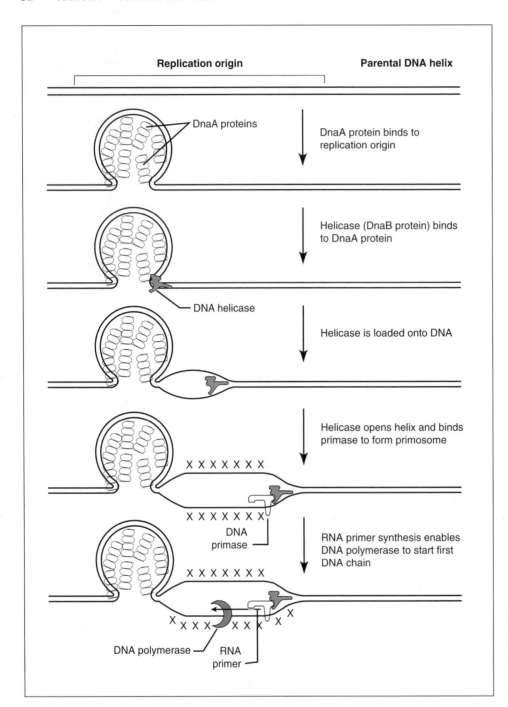

FIGURE 3–2. Initiation of the DNA replication process. X = single-strand binding protein. (Redrawn and reproduced, with permission, from Alberts, B., et al. Molecular Biology of the Cell, 3rd ed. New York, Garland Publishing, 1994.)

Within figure: Replication origin | Parental DNA helix; DnaA proteins — DnaA protein binds to replication origin; Helicase (DnaB protein) binds to DnaA protein; DNA helicase — Helicase is loaded onto DNA; Helicase opens helix and binds primase to form primosome; DNA primase — RNA primer synthesis enables DNA polymerase to start first DNA chain; DNA polymerase — RNA primer

called the **primosome.** An RNA primer is needed because bacterial DNA polymerases cannot synthesize DNA from free nucleotides; they must begin at a 3'-OH of RNA or DNA. **DNA polymerase III** begins to synthesize DNA starting at the RNA primer, synthesizing from 5' to 3'. (Unlike eukaryotic cells, bacteria have three DNA polymerases. **DNA polymerase I** helps complete the lagging strand and is a repair enzyme, and **DNA polymerase II** is involved in DNA repair.) DNA synthesis is bidirectional, so replicative forks travel down the chromosome in opposite directions, each carrying out semiconservative replication of the chromosome.

Elongation of the Chromosome. Figs. 3–3, 3–4, and 3–5 show how the DNA chain is elongated. Because DNA polymerase III synthesizes DNA from 5' to 3', the **leading strand** is synthesized continuously while the **lagging strand** is synthesized discontinuously. The lagging strand is synthesized as short segments of DNA called **Okazaki fragments** (see Figs. 3–3 and 3–5). Each Okazaki fragment is about 1000–2000 bp long and concludes at the preceding priming RNA fragment. DNA polymerase I excises the 10-bp RNA primer and fills the gap with DNA. The segments of nascent DNA in the lagging strand are then annealed by polynucleotide ligase. The lagging strand

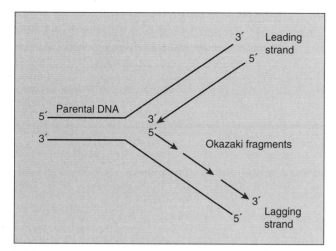

FIGURE 3–3. Comparison of synthesis of the two DNA strands. The leading strand is synthesized continuously, but the lagging strand is copied discontinuously to form Okazaki fragments.

is continuously folded back like a safety pin (see Fig. 3–5) to allow a single DNA polymerase III complex to synthesize the leading strand and the lagging strand simultaneously and in the same spatial orientation. Thus, a new DNA polymerase III will not have to be assembled on the lagging strand to synthesize each Okazaki fragment. DNA synthesis is rapid, replicating about 50,000 bp per minute. This is possible because the β subunit of DNA polymerase III forms a clamp around the DNA strand, and this clamp allows the enzyme to slide rapidly along the DNA.

Proofreading the Product of Replication. DNA replication is precise, with errors occurring only once every 10^7–10^{11} bp, which is equivalent to about one

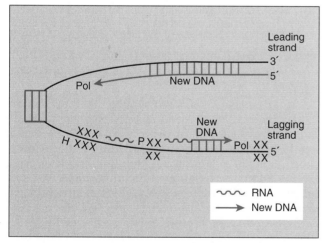

FIGURE 3–4. A simplified model of DNA replication. The leading strand is synthesized continuously by DNA polymerase III. The lagging strand is synthesized discontinuously as Okazaki fragments. Each Okazaki fragment is preceded by synthesis of a short RNA primer. The primers will later be degraded by DNA polymerase I and replaced with DNA segments that will be annealed by a ligase. Pol = DNA polymerase III; H = helicase; P = primase; and X = single-strand binding protein.

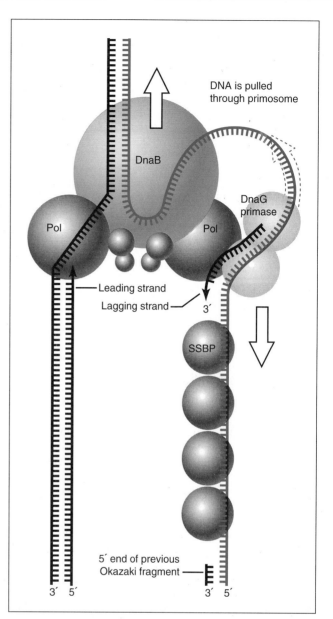

FIGURE 3–5. Chromosomal replication by DNA polymerase III. As the helicase (DnaB protein) opens the replicative fork, a single DNA polymerase III complex (Pol) replicates both strands simultaneously. This can occur because the lagging strand is folded back on itself like a safety pin to spatially reorient the DNA. SSBP = single-strand binding protein. (Source: Lewin, B. Genes V. Oxford, Oxford University Press, 1994. Redrawn and reproduced by permission of Oxford University Press.)

mistake per cycle of replication. This process is so exact for two reasons. First, the DNA polymerase III proofreads its own product. If the nucleotide incorporated does not pair properly, the 5'-3' exonuclease activity of DNA polymerase III deletes the error and inserts the proper base. Second, another repair system rechecks the newly synthesized strands for mistakes and repairs them. An enzyme known as the **dam methylase** methylates adenines within GATC sequences in each new strand to signify that this strand belongs to the bacterium (rather than to a bacteriophage). The repair system precedes the dam methylase, so it recognizes the unmethylated strand as being newly synthesized. After it completes its examination and repair of the strand, the methylase places its signature on the nascent DNA strands.

Termination of the Replication Process. The means by which bacteria terminate DNA replication are poorly understood. Two **termination sites,** called *ter*D,A and *ter*C,B, have been identified and are located about 100,000 bp (100 kilobase pairs) on either side of where the two replicative forks meet, which is about halfway around the chromosome. Each termination region is specific for one direction of fork movement, and each fork must pass through the opposite fork's terminator to reach its own. The terminator regions contain a 23-bp consensus sequence, and the *tus* gene product is required to terminate DNA replication.

DNA Mutation

Types of Mutation

Despite the precision of DNA replication and the presence of proofreading mechanisms, mistakes are made. When they persist, they are called mutations. A mutation is a change in the sequence of bases. There are at least four types of mutations that can occur: deletions, insertions, transitions, and transversions.

As shown in Fig. 3–6, a **deletion** occurs when one or more base pairs is deleted, and an **insertion** involves the addition of one or more base pairs. Because each codon contains three bases (a triplet code), if the number of bases inserted or deleted is not a multiple of three, there will be a shift in the reading frame—that is, a **frameshift mutation.** When a frameshift occurs, the protein synthesized downstream from the frameshift will be totally changed. The usual result of a frameshift is that a **nonsense codon** will appear soon after the altered region, and the protein will be terminated early. Thus, the protein will be shortened or truncated.

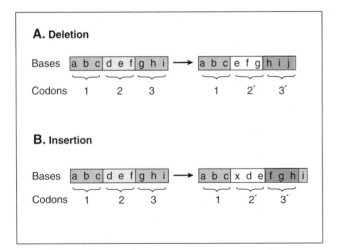

FIGURE 3–6. Deletion (A) and insertion (B) mutations. Deletion or insertion of bases causes the reading frame of DNA to shift unless a multiple of three bases is deleted or inserted.

A **transition** occurs when one purine base is exchanged for another (for example, A is exchanged for G), whereas a **transversion** involves interconverting a purine for a pyrimidine (for example, A is exchanged for C). When this happens, if the new base causes the codon to call for a new amino acid, **missense** is said to occur.

Causes of Mutation

In most cases, mutations are extremely rare events. Mutations can be caused, however, by adding agents that directly alter bacterial DNA. Ultraviolet radiation can act as a **physical mutagen** by causing pyrimidine dimers to form and is often used to mutagenize small aliquots of bacterial suspensions. When larger amounts of bacteria must be mutagenized, **chemical mutagens** are most often used. These fall into three major categories: covalent modifiers, intercalating agents, and base analogues.

Covalent modifiers usually alkylate or deaminate a base on the DNA. For example, alkylating agents (such as nitrosoguanidine) alkylate the O^6 of guanine, causing it to mispair with thymine. Thus, a GC becomes an AT. Nitrous acid, on the other hand, deaminates C to U, changing CG to TA.

Examples of **intercalating agents** are acridine orange and ethidium bromide. These substances, which are fluorescent dyes, intercalate between the stacked bases of the supercoiled DNA. Because intercalation alters the stacking of the bases, the bases are misread. Intercalating dyes can also shift the reading frame of a chromosome, causing a frameshift mutation.

Some antiviral drugs are **base analogues** that are preferentially inserted into viral DNA, resulting in missense mutations. There are also base analogues that are used to synthesize bacterial DNA. An example of this type of analogue is 5-bromouracil. In the keto form, 5-bromouracil pairs with A; however, in the enol form, it pairs with G.

Expression and Consequences of Mutation

Any of several consequences may follow a single mutational event.

First, because of the "wobble" of the genetic code (more than one codon per amino acid), there may be no change in the protein at all. If a new amino acid is inserted because of a missense and the mutation occurs in a structural region that has no bearing on the folding or function of the molecule, there may be no effect, in which case the phenomenon is called a **silent mutation.**

Second, if the mutation affects the secondary or tertiary structure, the protein may react differently to environmental changes. For example, the protein may become more susceptible to temperature changes, becoming more thermolabile. A change such as increased thermolability can be lethal for the bacterium under certain conditions and is therefore called a **conditionally lethal mutation.**

Third, if a mutation occurs in the vicinity of an

active site or at a site of allosteric control, the protein may change its activity or regulatory response significantly. If it is an enzyme, it may now be inactivated, or it may be no longer subject to feedback allosteric control. In some cases, the mutation may inactivate a repressor or change a site in an operon that was subject to a repressor, and the synthesis of the enzyme may now become constitutive.

Fourth, if a mutation results in an altered protein (owing to transition or transversion), antibody directed against the original protein will, in most cases, still recognize the altered protein. The altered protein may be nonfunctional, but if it is sufficiently similar to the original protein in terms of folding and other characteristics, it will cross-react with antibody directed against the original, and the bacterium may produce normal levels of cross-reactive material. In this case, the mutation will not be detected by immunologic means but will have to be detected by an assay that measures the activity of the product.

Fifth, a single mutation may affect the expression of more than one protein. This process, called **pleiotropic mutation,** occurs because RNA transcription and translation are coupled, and bacterial transcription generates polycistronic messages. When an early stop signal is generated by a mutation, the DNA-dependent RNA polymerase pauses at the stop signal during transcription. This causes ribosome dissociation and a halt in coupled protein synthesis. The rho protein will now bind to any rho-dependent terminator on the messenger RNA (mRNA) downstream from the stop signal, and both transcription and translation will terminate.

Suppression of Mutation

Not all mutations are expressed. Some are suppressed by undergoing a second mutational event that restores the original amino acid to the site. Others are suppressed by a mechanism called **suppressor mutation.** There are three types of suppressor mutation: **missense suppression,** which occurs when the active conformation of the protein is restored by substituting a second amino acid; **frameshift suppression,** which involves the occurrence of a second, compensating frameshift mutation; and **nonsense suppression,** which occurs when a mutation in the transfer RNA (tRNA) anticodon causes nonsense to be read as sense. Nonsense suppression works only when there are multiple copies of the tRNA gene. Otherwise, sense would now be read as nonsense for the correct codon of an affected amino acid.

Mutation and Acquired Antibiotic Resistance

Possible Explanations for Acquired Resistance.   It is not uncommon for a patient to suffer a clinical relapse during antibiotic therapy. Even if the bacterium causing the patient's illness was shown initially to be sensitive to the antibiotic being used, subsequent testing may reveal that the organism is now resistant. There are several possible reasons for this change.

First, the bacterium may have received a piece of DNA (usually a plasmid) from another bacterium that contains genes for antibiotic resistance; these genes could enter via transduction, conjugation, or transformation. Usually, the bacterium receives an **R plasmid** (resistance plasmid) that carries genes which encode an enzyme that inactivates the antibiotic being used. A common example of this is the entry of an R plasmid that codes for a penicillinase enzyme. Penicillinases inactivate penicillins by cleaving a bond in the beta-lactam ring of the antibiotic.

Second, the antibiotic may have caused derepression of an already-present operon that codes for a product conferring antibiotic resistance. This occasionally occurs when a penicillin analogue derepresses a chromosomal penicillinase gene that encodes an enzyme capable of inactivating many types of penicillins.

Third, there may have been a mutation of a gene already present on the chromosome that codes for a target of the antibiotic. The product of the mutated gene is altered in a manner that makes it become relatively unresponsive to the action of the antibiotic. This often occurs during therapy with nalidixic acid and its relatives, the fluoroquinolone antibiotics (ciprofloxacin, ofloxacin, and others). These antibiotics inhibit DNA synthesis by blocking the formation of a phosphodiester bond by **DNA gyrase.** DNA gyrase has two subunits, encoded by the gyrA and gyrB genes. The gyrA gene often mutates to produce a gyrase A subunit that no longer binds avidly to nalidixic acid or a fluoroquinolone. Thus, the bacterium may be sensitive to a fluoroquinolone at the beginning of therapy, as demonstrated by the fact that the treated patient shows improvement. But after several days, the infection seems to return, and now the bacterium is fluoroquinolone-resistant. The following question must then be asked: Did the fluoroquinolone cause the bacterium to become resistant, or did the fluoroquinolone only reveal what had already occurred and merely act as an agent of selective pressure? This question can be answered through the classic Luria-Delbrück experiment.

Fluctuation Analysis.   The **Luria-Delbrück experiment** is based on a concept called fluctuation analysis. This concept is depicted in Fig. 3–7, which outlines the steps that were followed in an experiment concerning the susceptibility of *Escherichia coli* to ampicillin. In this experiment, if mutations to antibiotic resistance occurred because antibiotic was present, then all of the plates from both tubes would have had the same number of resistant colonies (with only small variations), because they all were exposed to ampicillin for the same amount of time. In contrast, if mutations occurred randomly and were revealed (selected for) only when ampicillin was present, then there would have been a wide fluctuation in the number of resistant colonies in the samples from the 50 tubes. This is because resistant mutants would have arisen spontaneously at different times in each of the 50 tubes. Thus, if a bacterium mutated during the first hour after inoculation and the tubes were

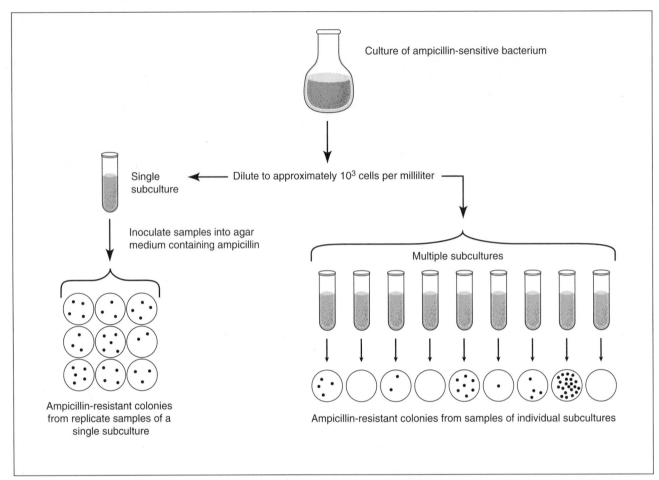

FIGURE 3–7. An example of the Luria-Delbrück experiment (fluctuation analysis). A flask containing 100 mL of an *Escherichia coli* strain that was sensitive to killing by ampicillin was grown to confluency. Two small aliquots of the suspension were then removed and placed into two 10-mL tubes of a growth medium. The tube on the left was grown to confluency, and then 50 Petri dishes containing ampicillin-impregnated agar were each inoculated with a sample from this tube. The plates were incubated, and each plate exhibited a small number of colonies that were resistant to the ampicillin. In contrast, the tube on the right was used to inoculate each of 50 tubes containing a growth medium but *no* ampicillin. These tubes were incubated until the bacteria were confluent, and then one sample from each tube was used to inoculate one plate with agar that contained ampicillin; 50 tubes were used to inoculate 50 plates. These plates were incubated and were found to contain some colonies that were resistant to ampicillin. Unlike in the other set of plates, however, in this set there was tremendous variation in the number of resistant colonies found in the plates. This experiment showed that mutations arise spontaneously and are revealed by selective pressure (here, the ampicillin).

incubated for 5 hours, the mutants could produce progeny for 4 more hours. In another tube, a mutant could spontaneously arise 3 hours into the incubation and multiply for only 2 more hours. This would cause wide fluctuation when the bacteria were plated onto the ampicillin-containing medium, where only the ampicillin-resistant bacteria could survive.

The results of the experiment depicted in Fig. 3–7 show that mutations to resistance occur spontaneously and that antibiotics do not cause the bacteria to become resistant. When the antibiotic is present, the sensitive bacteria are killed. The only bacteria that remain alive in the culture are the few bacteria that have previously mutated to resistance, and since they represent such a small portion of the bacteria, the patient seems to recover in response to the antibiotic. Gradually, however, the resistant bacteria multiply and repopulate the sites once held by the sensitive bacteria, with the result that the disease relapses.

DNA Repair

DNA that is altered by a mutagen can undergo repair by direct reversal, repair by excision, or repair by the SOS regulon.

Repair by Direct Reversal

There are several systems that mediate repair by direct reversal. The best understood of these systems involves photoreactivation. Here, an enzyme called **photolyase** is activated in the presence of light to repair damaged DNA. This system is particularly capable of repairing thymine dimers induced by ultraviolet (UV) light.

Repair by Excision

Excision repair is the most important means of DNA repair. This system depends on the products of the genes *uvr*A, *uvr*B, and *uvr*C, which form an endonuclease complex. The endonuclease complex merges with other enzymes to form a **repairosome** to resynthesize and correct UV-induced dimers. A DNA glycosylase cleaves the DNA at the site of the damage, and the UvrABC endonuclease completes the repair.

Repair by the SOS Regulon

The SOS regulon is a key "global" DNA repair system. In this system, there are two important gene products: the products of the genes *rec*A and *lex*A. The RecA protein is a multifunctional protein. In addition to repairing DNA, it triggers endogenous protease activity that causes LexA protein to degrade itself. This second function is important because LexA protein is a repressor that shuts off the reading of the SOS regulon. Fig. 3–8 shows that the SOS regulon is repressed by the *lex*A gene product until there is DNA damage. When the chromosome is damaged, the RecA protein triggers the protease activity of LexA, and the LexA protein is degraded. This allows the SOS regulon to be read, and the gene products of the regulon repair the chromosome.

The SOS regulon repairs the chromosome in several ways. Sometimes the damaged region is skipped during replication. Later, this region is repaired by splicing a good region from a good parental strand. This process, called **recombinational repair,** causes the donor strand to be lost. Alternatively, the damaged site may be repaired by a process that almost ignores the normal rules of base pairing. This process, called **error-prone repair,** does not work well, however, because it may result either in the generation of a nonsense codon or in the construction of a nonfunctional protein containing many amino acid mistakes.

DNA Recombination

The previous discussion introduced the concept that one bacterium (the recipient bacterium) can receive genes from other bacteria (donor bacteria) and that the donated genes can become part of the genome of and be expressed by the recipient bacterium. This is possible not only because genes can be passed among bacteria but also because genes that enter a bacterium can recombine with the existing genome.

Bacteria possess two general classes of DNA: replicons and nonreplicons. A **replicon** is a DNA segment that is able to be replicated autonomously because it has a replication origin, such as *ori*C. Bacterial replicons include chromosomes, plasmids, and bacteriophages. A **nonreplicon** is a DNA segment that lacks a replication origin and can be replicated only if it is recombined into a replicon. The bacterial nonreplicon may be a transposon or may be a chromosomal fragment that lacks the *ori*C region and enters a bacterium via conjugation, transformation, or transduction.

Recombination may be heterologous or homologous. **Heterologous recombination** involves introducing new genes into a replicon, whereas **homologous recombination** involves repositioning existing genes within a replicon.

Heterologous Recombination

New genes can be introduced into a replicon via generalized recombination, site-specific recombination, or transpositional recombination.

Generalized Recombination. Generalized recombination occurs when a piece of donor DNA contains a polynucleotide sequence homologous to a DNA segment found within a recipient chromosome or plasmid. The **RecA protein** facilitates exchange between reciprocal sites, resulting in formation of a

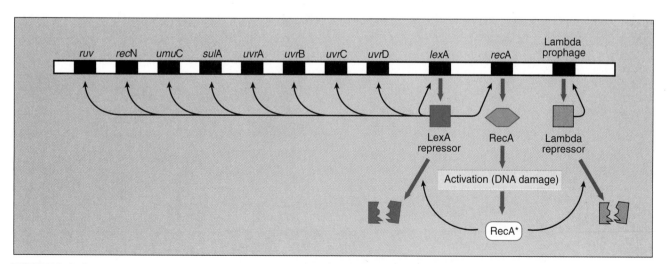

FIGURE 3–8. Control of expression of the SOS regulon. Under normal conditions, the LexA protein represses expression of the SOS regulon. When DNA damage occurs, the RecA protein is activated and causes the LexA protein to degrade itself. This allows the SOS regulon to be read, and its gene products repair the chromosome. (From: DNA Replication [supplement] by Kornberg, Copyright © 1982 by W. H. Freeman and Company. Redrawn and used with permission.)

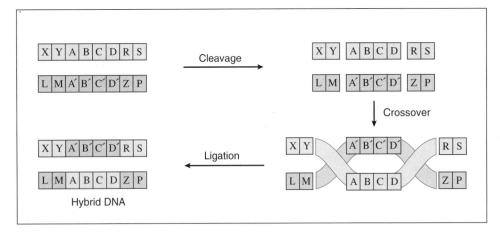

FIGURE 3–9. Generalized recombination. Reciprocal sites on DNA strands synapse, and the strands are cleaved at one or two sites. Genes are then exchanged between the strands, and the recombined segments are ligated. These processes are mediated by the RecA protein.

hybrid replicon. A simplified schematic of this process is presented in Fig. 3–9.

Site-Specific Recombination. Site-specific recombination involves introduction of a DNA segment that can be inserted only at a discrete site within the recipient replicon. An example of this is the lambda bacteriophage, which always inserts itself between the *gal* and *bio* genes of *E. coli* (Fig. 3–10). Instead of using the RecA protein, this process uses various gene products of the lambda phage. Insertion involves the use of the lambda *int* gene product, and excision of the phage genome from that of the host requires the use of lambda *int* and *xis* gene products.

Transpositional Recombination. Transpositional recombination is the process by which small nonreplicon gene segments called **transposons** are moved from site to site on a single genome or are moved from one replicon to another (such as from

a plasmid to a chromosome). Transposons, which are also called **transposable elements** or **Tn elements,** are segments of double-stranded DNA that cannot be replicated unless they are within a replicon. One of the reasons that transposons are important is that genes encoding for **virulence characteristics** (characteristics that allow the bacterium to cause disease) and genes encoding for **drug resistance** are often carried on transposons.

Three types of transposons have been described: insertion sequences, composite transposons, and Tn A–type transposons.

Insertion sequences, which are also called **IS elements,** were discovered as novel segments that inactivated the *gal* operon of *E. coli*. They range in size from 700 to 1500 bp, carry a single gene (for a transposase enzyme), and exhibit short, inverted complementary nucleotide sequences at each end.

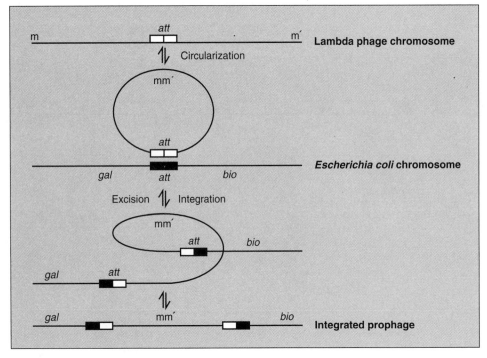

FIGURE 3–10. Insertion of the lambda phage into an *Escherichia coli* chromosome. Inverted repeat segments in the circular lambda genome (denoted *att*) recognize compatible sites between *gal* and *bio* in the *E. coli* chromosome. In a process mediated by phage Int protein, the phage genome is integrated into the chromosome and is decircularized. The integrated phage genome is known as a prophage. The letters m and m′ denote the free ends of the phage chromosome when it is linear. (Redrawn and reproduced, with permission, from Baron, S. Medical Microbiology, 3rd ed. New York, Churchill Livingstone, 1991.)

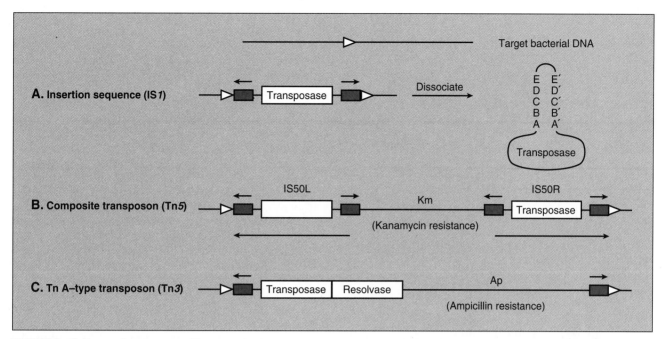

FIGURE 3–11. Types of transposons. There are three types of transposons: the insertion sequence, shown in diagram **A;** the composite transposon, shown in diagram **B;** and the Tn A–type transposon, shown in diagram **C.** Some bacteriophages, such as mu, are believed to be transposons. IS = insertion sequence; Tn = transposon; Km = kanamycin; and Ap = ampicillin. (Redrawn and reproduced, with permission, from Baron, S. Medical Microbiology, 3rd ed. New York, Churchill Livingstone, 1991.)

For this reason, when insertion sequences are dissociated, they form unique stem-loop structures that can be seen by electron microscopy (Fig. 3–11A).

Composite transposons range in size from 2000 to 40,000 bp, carry several genes, and have an insertion sequence on each end (Fig. 3–11B). The composite transposons are the transposons most often associated with virulence genes or antibiotic resistance. For example, Tn*1681* carries genes for *E. coli* heat-stable enterotoxin, and Tn*10* carries the gene for tetracycline resistance.

Tn A–type transposons have no insertion sequence at the ends but have short terminal inverted repeat sequences. These transposons encode a transposase, a resolvase, and several ancillary genes. Tn*3*, which is the prototypic transposon of the **Tn A family** (Fig. 3–11C), carries the gene for ampicillin resistance. It appears that *Haemophilus influenzae* (a bacterium that causes meningitis, epiglottitis, and otitis media) and *Neisseria gonorrhoeae* (the bacterium that causes gonorrhea) first developed resistance to ampicillin when they obtained Tn*3* from enteric bacteria, such as *E. coli*.

Transpositional recombination is not a form of generalized recombination, and it does not involve the activity of the RecA protein. As shown in Figs. 3–12 and 3–13, there are two different mechanisms of transpositional recombination.

Fig. 3–12 depicts the means by which insertion sequences and composite transposons are believed to move. Here, the recipient DNA is cleaved in such a way as to result in staggered DNA sequences in the opposing pieces of paired DNA. The transposon is then cleaved from its original site; the donor DNA will

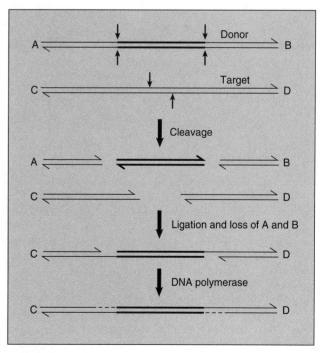

FIGURE 3–12. Movement of insertion sequences and composite transposons. These transposons are cleaved from a donor site and are inserted into another site on the same or another chromosomal strand. This process can result in loss of the originating DNA strand. (Redrawn and reproduced, with permission, from Joklik, W. K., et al. Zinsser Microbiology, 20th ed. East Norwalk, Conn., Appleton and Lange, 1992.)

to B. The transposon segments are then replicated, and a final series of crossover events returns the strands to their original orientation, but now each double-stranded DNA replicon contains a copy of the transposon.

Homologous Recombination

A small number of bacteria change their characteristics when existing genes on a replicon are rearranged. This homologous recombination can occur via site-specific inversion or via gene conversion.

Site-Specific Inversion.   Site-specific inversion is best understood from studies of the mechanism by which *Salmonella* species alter their flagellar antigens. Salmonellae undergo phase variation, a process that allows them to express either H1 or H2 flagellar antigens. H antigens are different antigenic types of flagellin, and their production is encoded by the H1 and H2 genes. As Fig. 3–14 shows, these genes are located on a segment of the chromosome that also contains a promoter and the *rh*1 gene; *rh*1 codes for a repressor for the H1 gene. When the promoter adjacent to H2 is properly oriented, both H2 and *rh*1 are read, and the *rh*1 gene product represses the expression of H1. When the P2 gene is inverted, however, transcription begins at P1, and the H1 gene is read.

Inversion occurs because the segment of DNA that contains the H genes also contains short inverted repeat sequences similar to those found in transposons. Sites that undergo inversion (such as H antigen genes) are controlled by a protein called the **factor for inversion stimulation protein** or the **Fis protein.** This protein binds to so-called enhancer regions in the chromosome and causes the frequency of reversion to be from 10^3 to 10^7 times greater than the frequency of spontaneous mutation.

Gene Conversion.   The ability of *N. gonorrhoeae* to cause gonorrhea at least partially depends on pili that mediate attachment to mucosal epithelia and allow the bacteria to resist phagocytosis by polymorphonuclear leukocytes. Much of the effective immune response is attributable to antipilus antibody, which blocks mucosal adherence and opsonizes the gonococci. To counteract this, gonococci change the immunodominant region of each pilus by expressing a new pilus protein antigen at the site. The gonococci accomplish this largely through the process of gene conversion, although additional mechanisms are also involved.

Each gonococcal chromosome contains a series of pilus antigen genes, consisting of many defective pilus genes in addition to one good pilus gene that will be expressed. During gonococcal growth, the genes periodically undergo rearrangement because of the appearance of multiple crossover events between good and defective genes. These rearrangements render the good gene defective and reassign its function to a gene whose formerly defective region has been corrected. Then the immunodominant region of the gonococcal pilus expresses new antigens. When this occurs, the patient with gonorrhea soon becomes

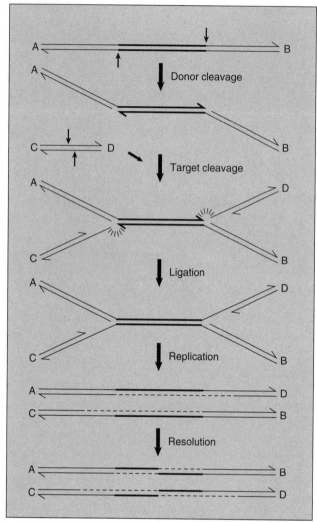

FIGURE 3–13. Movement of Tn A–type transposons. The process known as duplicative transposition results in a copy of the transposon being found in both the donor and the recipient DNA. (Redrawn and reproduced, with permission, from Shapiro, J. A. Molecular model for the transposition and replication of bacteriophage mu and other transposable elements. Proc Natl Acad Sci U S A 76:1933–1937, 1979.)

eventually be degraded because it has been seriously damaged. The transposon is inserted between the areas of staggered cleavage in the recipient DNA, and a DNA polymerase copies the staggered ends to yield double-stranded DNA with direct repeats at each end of the transposon. Thus, this method of transposition removes the transposon from one site and places it in another. If the transposon is inserted into the middle of a gene, that gene may be inactivated.

Fig. 3–13 shows how the Tn A–type transposons are thought to move. This process, which is known as **duplicative transposition,** results in a copy of the transposon being found in both the donor DNA and the recipient DNA. The donor DNA is cleaved at both sides of the transposon, and a site in the recipient DNA is cleaved. The segments are brought into proximity, and then a crossover event occurs: A is annealed to D through the transposon, and C is attached

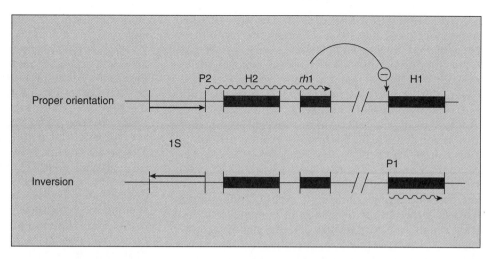

FIGURE 3-14. Site-specific inversion in *Salmonella*. When the promoter for flagellar genes adjacent to the H2 gene is properly oriented, the H2 gene is read and the *rh*1 repressor blocks the reading of the H1 gene. When the P2 gene is inverted, the H2 and *rh*1 genes are not transcribed and the P1 promoter initiates expression of the H1 gene. (Source: Davis, B. D., et al. Microbiology, 4th ed. Philadelphia, J. B. Lippincott Co., 1990. Redrawn and reproduced, with permission, from Lippincott-Raven Publishers.)

populated by a new serotype of gonococci. This means that as antibody forms against one serotype, the organisms of that serotype will be gradually eliminated, only to be replaced by organisms of a new serotype. This propensity for antigenic variation of gonococcal pilus antigens has made development of a vaccine against *N. gonorrhoeae* extremely difficult.

A similar process occurs in *Borrelia hermsii*, a spirochete that is responsible for relapsing fever. The process in *Borrelia* involves the exchange of information between coexisting linear plasmids in the organism and is discussed in Chapter 12.

Exchange of Bacterial DNA

Exchange of bacterial DNA is accomplished via conjugation, transformation, or transduction.

Conjugation

Conjugation is a means by which DNA is passed directly from one bacterium to another through a **conjugal bridge.** Although the conjugal bridge has not been identified with certainty, some believe it is the **sex pilus** and others hypothesize that it is the **TraD protein.** Note that the use of the concept of sex is an anthropomorphism. Bacteria do not truly mate, form zygotes, or undergo meiosis.

Most conjugation occurs among gram-negative enteric bacteria (*E. coli, Salmonella, Shigella,* and others), but a process analogous to conjugation was described recently among gram-positive bacteria. Conjugation among gram-positive bacteria probably does not involve sex pili.

Types of Conjugation.   There are three types of conjugation. The first results in the transfer of plasmid genes, the second results in the transfer of chromosomal genes, and the third results in the transfer of both plasmid and chromosomal genes.

(1) Conjugation Resulting in Transfer of Plasmid Genes.   In 1946, Joshua Lederberg and Edward Tatum found that when two strains of *E. coli* were mixed in a single flask, bacteria with mixed heredity soon appeared. They determined that bacteria were ex-

changing genes, and they called the process conjugation. At least three general principles are followed during conjugation.

First, conjugation occurs when bacteria of two mating types meet and are connected by a conjugal bridge such as a sex pilus. The **donor bacterium** is designated as F$^+$ (fertile), and the **recipient bacterium** is designated as F$^-$ (nonfertile). Each F$^+$ bacterium has an average of 23 sex pili, and each pilus is 2–3 μm long and has a central pore. Unlike the F$^-$ bacterium, the F$^+$ bacterium has a structure that is about 100,000 bp (100 kilobase pairs) long, consists of more than 60 genes, and is called a **fertility factor,** an **F factor,** or an **F plasmid.** An F plasmid is one of several known types of **conjugative plasmids,** each of which has a cluster of 25 *tra* (transfer) and *trb* genes that are required for conjugation. The *tra*A gene codes for the synthesis of the sex pilus, and about 12 other *tra* genes control pilus expression. Plasmids that lack these genes are nonconjugative; that is, they do not code for a pilus and are not routinely spread to other bacteria via conjugation. The F plasmid has its own replication origin, called *ori*V, and is replicated coordinately with the chromosome. Each fertile bacterium carries only one copy of the F plasmid. Studies in *E. coli* have shown that F$^+$ bacteria cannot mate with other F$^+$ bacteria, because the genes *tra*S and *tra*T encode surface exclusion proteins that make the surface of an F$^+$ bacterium a poor receiver for the sex pilus.

Second, when bacteria conjugate, there is one-way transfer of DNA from the donor bacterium (here, F$^+$) to the recipient (F$^-$). The genes are always passed at the same rate (expressed in terms of genes transferred per minute) and in the same order. That is, if the order of the genes is ABCDE, the genes will always be passed in this order and never, for example, as EDCBA.

Third, when an F$^+$ bacterium mates with an F$^-$ bacterium, a copy of the F plasmid is passed to the recipient, but the F$^+$ bacterium retains a copy of the plasmid. Thus, an F$^+$ and F$^-$ mating will yield two F$^+$ bacteria. If mating occurs for 10 minutes, the entire plasmid will be passed.

(2) Conjugation Resulting in Transfer of Chromosomal Genes. In 1953, scientists observed a new type of mating in which chromosomal genes pass from the donor cell to the recipient cell at high frequency but the recipient remains nonfertile. Thus, the recipient receives new genes from the donor's chromosome but does not receive the F plasmid (or at least not the *tra* genes). In this form of conjugation, the donor cell is called a high-frequency recombination cell, or **Hfr cell.**

When an Hfr bacterium mates with an F⁻ bacterium, a copy of the entire chromosome passes to the recipient if mating continues for about 100 minutes. This is a rare event because the conjugal bridge is fragile and is easily broken by the slightest movement. Normally, a piece of the chromosome enters the recipient, and the recipient becomes partially diploid (merozygotic). If there is sufficient homology with a region of the recipient chromosome, the newly entered DNA will synapse with the chromosome, and recombination can occur. If recombination does not occur, the newly transferred DNA will be lost (will not pass to progeny of the bacterium) because it is not a replicon. Thus, it will stay in a single cell and will eventually be degraded. If recombination occurs, the new genes will become part of the recipient's genome, and all of its progeny will express any characteristics brought in on that piece of DNA.

The **Hfr genome** is formed when the F plasmid is inserted into the chromosome of the donor cell (Fig. 3–15). This is possible because the F plasmid has an insertion sequence that matches a specific insertion sequence in the chromosome. There are several different F plasmids, and each has a specific site on the chromosome where it is inserted. For example, Hfr H always inserts itself next to the gene *pyr*B, while Hfr 7 always inserts itself between the genes *ton*A and *pro*A. This observation may seem at first to be of little consequence, but it is partially this stability of insertion sites that has allowed the mapping of bacterial genes—a necessary first step toward the genetic engineering that today is used to manufacture many human proteins for use by the clinician.

Fig. 3–16 is a schematic diagram of the conjugal process. Conjugation begins when the sex pilus of the donor bacterium attaches to a specific receptor on the surface of the recipient bacterium, bringing the two cells into close proximity. The DNA is now nicked by the TraY/TraI endonuclease complex at a specific site called the *ori*T (for origin of transfer). The *ori*T site is just downstream from the *tra* genes. As a result, the first genes transferred are those just downstream from *ori*T, and the last ones passed are the *tra* genes. This is why Hfr recipients almost always remain F⁻, even though they receive new genes. It would take 100 minutes of conjugation to reach the *tra* genes, and this occurs only rarely. As the TraY/TraI complex begins to unwind the DNA at a rate of about 1200 bp per minute, one strand of the chromosome is passed through the conjugal bridge to the recipient. This transferred piece of DNA is copied asymmetrically as it enters the recipient cell. The remaining strand is also copied asymmetrically. Thus, the donor retains a double-stranded chromosome, and the recipient gains a double-stranded piece of DNA. The genes always enter in the same order and begin at the same point for each Hfr strain.

(3) Conjugation Resulting in Transfer of Plasmid and Chromosomal Genes. Studies of bacteria have shown that there is a third mating type of cell, the **F′ cell.** During the process of F′ conjugation, which is sometimes called F-duction or sex-duction, the F′ donor is able to pass both the F plasmid and a small number of chromosomal genes to the recipient at high frequency.

F′ bacteria contain a plasmid that has been excised from an Hfr chromosome. When the plasmid "pops out" of the chromosome, the excision machinery sometimes cuts out more than it should. The result is the excision of a piece of the chromosome that contains the F plasmid and some genes that were immediately adjacent to the F plasmid in the chromosome (Fig. 3–17). When these F′ factors are passed to recipients, the recipients become both fertile and

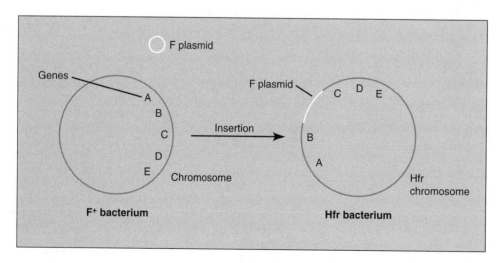

FIGURE 3–15. Generation of an Hfr genome by inserting the F plasmid (fertility factor) into an *Escherichia coli* chromosome.

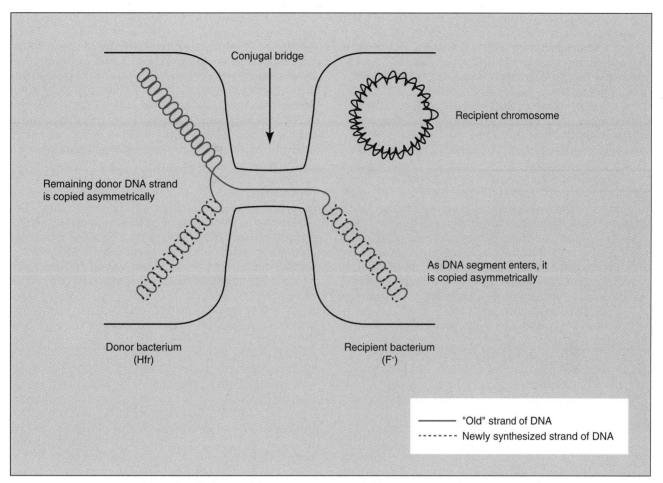

FIGURE 3–16. Movement of DNA between an Hfr and F⁻ bacterium during conjugation.

stably diploid for some chromosomal genes. If, for instance, the *lac* operon is on the F′ plasmid, the recipient may make incredible amounts of β-galactosidase in the presence of lactose (up to 8% of the total cell protein).

Conjugation and Antibiotic Resistance.   There are at least three reasons to be interested in conjuga-

tion. First, conjugation and the recognition of mating types provide a tool by which the bacterial chromosome can be mapped, with all its implications for genetic engineering. Second, it is via conjugation and the passage of plasmids that some virulence factors (such as toxin genes) enter certain bacteria. Third, some plasmids carry drug resistance genes, and

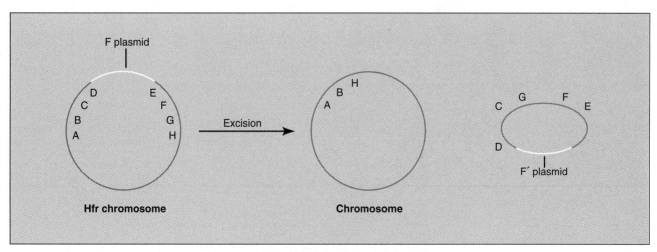

FIGURE 3–17. Creation of an F′ plasmid by incorrect excision of the fertility factor from an Hfr bacterium.

many of the R factors (drug resistance plasmids) are passed among bacteria via conjugation.

(1) Characteristics of the R Factor.   Many pathogens are resistant to multiple drugs and are able to pass this **multiple drug resistance** to other bacteria. It is because these bacteria predominate within hospitals that **nosocomial infections** (hospital-acquired infections) are so dangerous. Multiple drug resistance is almost always due to the presence of **drug resistance plasmids,** or **R factors.** Those R factors which can be passed among bacteria via conjugation are called **conjugative R factors,** whereas those which are passed via transformation or transduction are called **nonconjugative R factors.** Among gram-negative enteric bacteria, conjugal passage of R factors is a major problem. These bacteria, along with staphylococci, enterococci, and pseudomonads, are the primary causes of nosocomial infections, and some of them have been reported to carry R factors for resistance against almost every known antibiotic.

Conjugative R factors are constructed by attaching to a fertility plasmid one or more genes encoding antibiotic resistance. The fertility factor is referred to as the **resistance transfer factor** (RTF), and the portion of the plasmid that encodes drug resistance is called the **resistance determinant segment,** or **r-determinant.** The r-determinants are often added as transposons. Fig. 3–18 depicts a typical R factor, called R1. The R1 plasmid initially contained an F factor (the *tra* gene region, which is the RTF) to which was added Tn*4*; Tn*4* contained resistance genes for streptomycin and sulfonamides. Tn*4* was then modified by adding Tn*3*, which encoded resistance to ampicillin. Finally, three nontransposon genes were added: genes for resistance to chloramphenicol, kanamycin, and neomycin. Thus, any bacterium that receives this conjugative plasmid will become fertile and will also become resistant to multiple drugs.

(2) Processes of R Factor Transfer.   In gram-negative bacteria, R factors can be passed among distantly related organisms via conjugation. Within the Enterobacteriaceae family, for example, this means that a nonpathogenic *E. coli* that is resistant to numerous drugs can conjugate with a pathogenic *Salmonella* serotype *typhi* or with a pathogenic *Shigella dysenteriae* and pass the drug resistance to the pathogenic organism. After an R factor is transmitted to other cells at high frequency for several generations, conjugation will halt. This is because the RTF codes not only for a pilus but also for a repressor protein that builds up inside each fertile bacterium. When repressor protein levels become sufficiently elevated, the synthesis of pilin is repressed. This is advantageous to the bacterium because there are lytic phages that attach specifically to the pilin of "male" cells. To protect themselves from these male-specific phages, the donor cells limit their expression of sex pili.

A few gram-positive bacteria can also pass genes via conjugation, but in this case there is no involvement of pili. Instead, pheromone-like peptides induce bacteria to aggregate, and the aggregated bacteria exchange genetic material. Among the gram-positive species reported to contain conjugative plasmids are *Bacillus, Clostridium, Streptococcus,* and *Streptomyces.*

The R1 plasmid shown in Fig. 3–18 is a conjugative R factor and is typical of those found in enteric bacteria and in pseudomonads. Yet staphylococci also have R factors that are transmitted by transduction (via bacteriophages) rather than conjugation, and the R factors of some enteric bacteria are not passed conjugatively. Conjugative plasmids can revert to a nonconjugative form, or vice versa. Because the r-determinants have elements that are similar to insertion sequences, they can join or leave replicons. Sometimes the r-determinants exit a plasmid, leaving

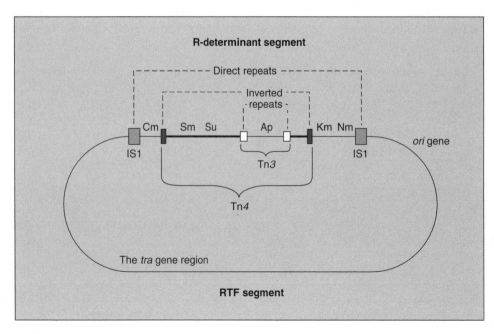

FIGURE 3–18. **The R1 antibiotic resistance plasmid.** In addition to having a resistance determinant (r-determinant) region, R1 contains a resistance transfer factor (RTF) segment that has been fused with Tn*4*, Tn*3*, and some ancillary antibiotic resistance genes. Cm = chloramphenicol; Sm = streptomycin; Su = sulfonamides; Ap = ampicillin; Km = kanamycin; Nm = neomycin; IS = insertion sequence; and Tn = transposon. (Adapted from Cohen, S. N. Appendix B, Map B. *In* Bukhari, A. I., et al., eds.: DNA Insertion Elements, Plasmids, and Episomes. New York, Cold Spring Harbor Laboratory, 1977. Redrawn and reproduced, with permission, from Cold Spring Harbor Laboratory.)

the cell with a separate F factor and nonconjugative R factor. Alternatively, an F factor and a nonconjugative R factor may join to form a conjugative R factor. Finally, polygenic plasmids can be formed when nonconjugative plasmids containing r-determinants join with already-constructed conjugative R factors.

Conjugation and Genetic Mapping.   Conjugation has long been a useful tool for mapping genes in bacteria. During conjugation, genes are passed consecutively, at a constant rate, and always in the same order relative to one another. This allows investigators to look for the consecutive appearance of genes in a culture of bacteria and then to map the genes according to both the **order of transfer** and the **time of appearance** after initiation of conjugation.

Genes that are closer together than 1 minute cannot be distinguished by this method and must be mapped instead on the basis of their **crossover frequency.** The crossover method takes advantage of the fact that when two genes enter a cell, the farther apart they are (up to a limit), the greater the probability is that there will be a crossover between them and they will not be combined in the chromosome. This principle is called the **law of genetic recombination.**

Transformation

While most gene transfer among gram-negative bacteria occurs via conjugation, most gene transfer among gram-positive bacteria occurs via transformation or transduction. Transformation is the uptake of naked DNA by a bacterium. The DNA transferred during conjugation cannot be degraded by adding DNAase to the suspending medium, because this DNA is never outside a cell. In contrast, the DNA taken up during transformation is sensitive to DNAase, because this DNA comes from the environment. Transforming DNA originates from lysed bacteria, and the fragment that is taken up is small, consisting of about 5–20 genes.

Mechanisms in Gram-Positive Bacteria.   Transformation was discovered in 1928 by Frederick Griffith, who worked with two strains of pneumococci. One was a "rough" (unencapsulated) strain that was avirulent and thus unable to cause disease in mice, and the other was a "smooth" (encapsulated) strain that was fully virulent. Fig. 3–19 summarizes the Griffith experiment in which live and killed pneumococci of these rough (R) and smooth (S) strains were used. All mice that were injected with live R pneumococci survived; all mice that were injected with live S pneumococci died rapidly; and all mice that were injected with killed R or S pneumococci survived. However, when live R were mixed with killed S pneumococci and injected into mice, the mice died and live S were recovered from these mice. Griffith thus surmised that something was being transferred from the dead bacteria to the living ones. Years later, Oswald Avery demonstrated that the dead bacteria released DNA, the living bacteria took up fragments of the DNA,

the genes recombined, and the recombinant bacteria developed capsules.

In addition to pneumococci, a number of other gram-positive bacteria can be transformed, including staphylococci, streptococci, and *Bacillus* species. The ability of gram-positive bacteria to be transformed ("competence") depends on the presence of a peptide that is called **competence factor** and is produced only during the late log phase and early stationary phase of growth. Competence factor binds to specific receptors on the cell surface, induces the expression of about 10 new proteins, and causes the bacterium to become competent to take up DNA.

Fig. 3–20 shows the general mechanism of transformation. Donor DNA binds to the cell loosely at first, and then the binding becomes tight, as evidenced by the fact that it cannot be washed off the bacterium. The DNA interacts with a protein that denatures and fragments the DNA, and single-stranded pieces of DNA enter the cell. If there is sufficient homology with the host DNA, synapse and recombination will occur. Plasmid DNA, or phage DNA, can also be taken up this way, in a process referred to as **transfection.** If transfection occurs, it is not necessary for synapse and recombination to occur, since the plasmid is a replicon.

Mechanisms in Gram-Negative Bacteria.   Few gram-negative bacteria are capable of being naturally transformed. Some gram-negative organisms can be forced to accept DNA by treating them with $CaCl_2$, but this is a laboratory tool used primarily in genetic engineering.

Among the gram-negative bacteria, only *Neisseria* and *Haemophilus* are believed to routinely undergo transformation, and these organisms are competent only when piliated. Transformation among gram-negative bacteria does not involve competence factor, and it is more selective than transformation among gram-positive bacteria. Specific oligonucleotide sequences are recognized, so only closely related DNA can be taken up. DNA enters as double-stranded fragments. The strands are subsequently unwound, and only one strand is incorporated.

Application and Significance of Transformation.   Avery's experiment showed that transformation could introduce virulence genes or correct defective virulence genes, making a previously innocuous bacterium dangerous. Transposons that carry drug resistance genes can also enter a bacterium via transformation. Finally, transformation is a key tool in genetic engineering. Bacteria can be induced to accept eukaryotic genes spliced into plasmids (vectors), with the result that the transformed bacteria may synthesize human proteins.

Transduction

Bacteria can obtain new genes when bacteriophages inject DNA that includes one or more bacterial genes. There are two transductive processes: generalized transduction and specialized transduction.

Generalized Transduction.   Generalized trans-

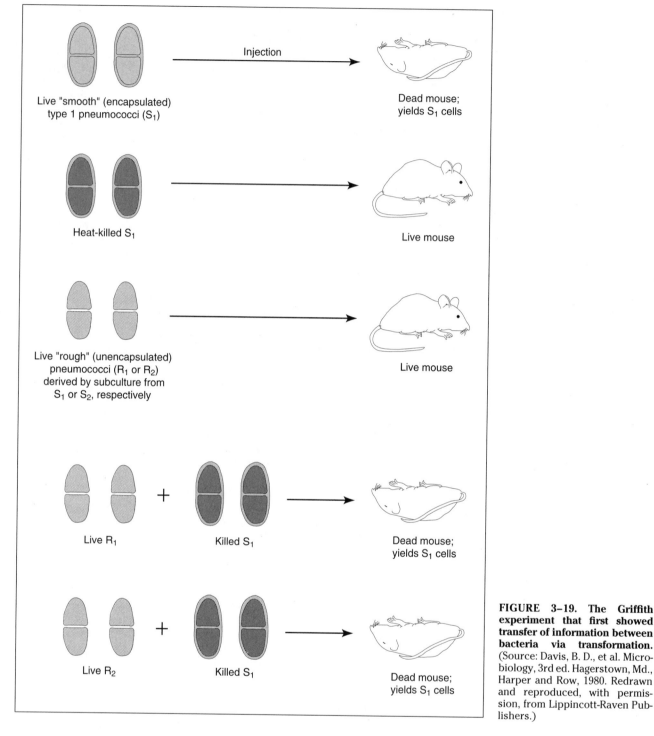

Live "smooth" (encapsulated)
type 1 pneumococci (S$_1$)

Injection

Dead mouse;
yields S$_1$ cells

Heat-killed S$_1$

Live mouse

Live "rough" (unencapsulated)
pneumococci (R$_1$ or R$_2$)
derived by subculture from
S$_1$ or S$_2$, respectively

Live mouse

Live R$_1$ + Killed S$_1$

Dead mouse;
yields S$_1$ cells

Live R$_2$ + Killed S$_1$

Dead mouse;
yields S$_1$ cells

FIGURE 3–19. The Griffith experiment that first showed transfer of information between bacteria via transformation. (Source: Davis, B. D., et al. Microbiology, 3rd ed. Hagerstown, Md., Harper and Row, 1980. Redrawn and reproduced, with permission, from Lippincott-Raven Publishers.)

duction is a process by which bacterial genes are introduced randomly into another bacterium by a bacteriophage. The random nature of the introduction process means that one gene is just as likely as another to be introduced. The transduction can be achieved by either a lysogenic phage or a lytic phage.

Some **lysogenic phages,** such as phage P1, insert their DNA randomly into the bacterial chromosome. When the signal for excision occurs, the phage DNA will be cut out of the chromosome, and some fragments will be excised incorrectly. In some cases, the phage heads will be packaged with a piece of DNA that contains both phage genes and bacterial genes. This is a rare event, and although most of the progeny phage heads will be functional, a few of them will be defective. The defective phage will adsorb normally to another bacterium, but because the DNA that is injected does not contain a full phage genome, the injection will not result in production of more phage. Instead, the recipient of the DNA will become a recombinant for the bacterial genes introduced. This type of transduction is termed "generalized" transduction

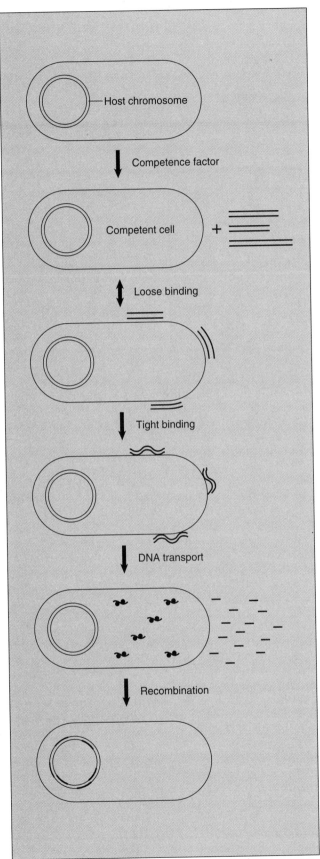

FIGURE 3–20. Transformation among gram-positive bacteria. Double-stranded DNA binds loosely to competent bacteria. DNA binding then becomes tight, the DNA is denatured and fragmented, and single-stranded pieces of DNA enter the bacterium. If sufficient

because the phage is not restricted to inserting itself at a particular site. The phage could insert itself next to any gene, so any gene could be transduced.

Some **lytic phages** will fragment the host DNA during their infection cycle. Occasionally, a fragment of the host DNA will be packaged into a phage head by mistake. This fragment may be quite large, with up to 2% of the genome packaged in one phage head. Again, the defective phage will inject the bacterial DNA into a target bacterium, and recombination will occur if there is sufficient homology.

Specialized Transduction. Some lysogenic phages have a single, discrete insertion site in the bacterial chromosome. The best studied of these is the lambda phage, which is always inserted between the *gal* gene and the *bio* gene, although there may be intervening genes between these two genes. When the signal for a switch from lysogeny to the lytic cycle occurs, the lambda prophage is excised. In about 1 out of every 1000 excisions, there is an error, and some of the genes around the lambda prophage will be excised, leaving part of the lambda genome behind. These defective genes will be packaged into phage heads, and the defective phages will inject their DNA into another target. The mechanism of incorrect excision is illustrated in Fig. 3–21.

Application and Significance of Transduction. Transduction is significant for at least three reasons.

First, many R factors are disseminated by transduction. This is especially important among the gram-positive organisms, in which conjugation is a rare event. Many *Staphylococcus aureus* strains, for example, show multiple drug resistance, and this resistance is encoded on plasmids that are disseminated by lysogenic phages.

Second, a process that is analogous to transduction and is called **phage conversion** is responsible for the ability of several bacteria to produce toxins. Phage conversion differs from transduction in that the toxin genes are part of the phage genome and apparently were transferred to the phage genome by transposition (the toxin gene is on a transposon). For example, the agent of diphtheria, *Corynebacterium diphtheriae,* produces diphtheria toxin only when it has been infected by a lysogenic phage (such as beta) that carries the diphtheria toxin gene.

Third, transduction has been a useful tool in mapping closely grouped bacterial genes. Well-spaced genes can be mapped on the basis of their order of transfer and time of appearance after initiation of conjugation, but closely grouped genes cannot be distinguished in this fashion. One method of mapping closely grouped genes is to look for the percentage of the time that these genes are cotransduced—that is, the percentage of time that they are transduced on the same piece of DNA. The closer these genes

homology exists, the fragments are incorporated into the genome of the recipient bacterium. (Redrawn and reproduced, with permission, from Joklik, W. K., et al. Zinsser Microbiology, 20th ed. East Norwalk, Conn., Appleton and Lange, 1992.)

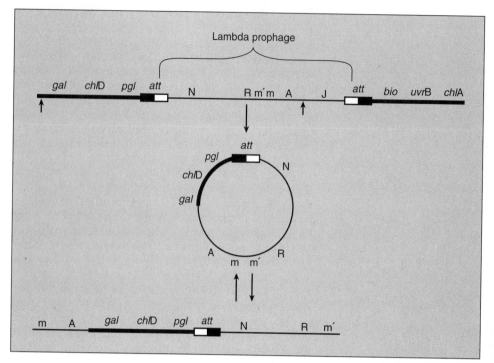

FIGURE 3–21. Incorrect excision of the lambda prophage in *Escherichia coli*. Excision of the prophage is usually performed correctly, but cleavage may occur at the indicated sites (arrows), yielding defective progeny that contain host genes. Inverted repeat segments in the circular lambda genome are denoted by *att*. The letters m and m′ denote the free ends of the phage chromosome when it is linear. (From Campbell, A. Genetic structure. *In* Hershey, A. D., ed. The Bacteriophage Lambda. New York, Cold Spring Harbor Laboratory, 1971. Redrawn and reproduced, with permission, from Cold Spring Harbor Laboratory.)

are to one another, the more likely they are to be cotransduced. Conversely, the farther apart they are, the less likely they are to be excised together from the chromosome.

Gene Expression

Transcription in Bacterial Versus Eukaryotic Cells

People usually think of the chromosome as a series of genes on two strands of DNA, one of which is anticomplementary to the other. It therefore appears that one strand contains the genetic information and is read to synthesize RNA, while the other strand serves as a structural complement to the template strand. This is not, however, the case. Rather, each strand contains readable genes, some genes overlap, and the reading of the genes is controlled by the occurrence of promoters along each strand of the chromosome.

Eukaryotic cells utilize several DNA-dependent RNA polymerases to synthesize RNA. In contrast, bacteria have a single **RNA polymerase** whose activity is governed by its association with an initiating factor (sigma factor, or σ) and is influenced by a wide variety of transcription control proteins. (For additional information concerning transcription control proteins, see the discussion of the genetic regulation of sporulation in Chapter 1.) Each RNA polymerase consists of two α chains, one β chain, one β' chain, and the sigma factor. The core enzyme therefore consists of $\alpha\alpha\beta\beta'$, and addition of sigma completes the **RNA polymerase holoenzyme complex.** Bacteria synthesize unique sigma factors to recognize and transcribe specific sets of operons, but most transcription in *E. coli* involves the 70-kD sigma factor, or σ^{70}.

The steps involved in transcription are shown in

Fig. 3–22. Free RNA polymerase molecules continually collide with the DNA template without binding tightly. When, however, the holoenzyme collides with a promoter, the sigma factor binds tightly to the chromosome. The holoenzyme fits into a groove about 50 bp in length, unwinds the DNA about one and one-half turns, and opens a segment about 12 bp long; this is the **transcription bubble.** An RNA strand about 10 bp long is synthesized, and then the sigma factor is displaced by the NusA protein. The sigma factor can now join with another RNA polymerase core to initiate a new round of transcription. Unlike DNA polymerase, RNA polymerase can initiate synthesis using nucleoside triphosphate sugars and needs no priming template. Like DNA polymerase, RNA polymerase synthesizes the new RNA strand in a 5′ to 3′ direction.

Unlike transcription in eukaryotes, transcription in bacteria generates polycistronic messages. Transcription continues until it reaches an appropriate strong or weak terminator signal. **Strong (type I) terminator signals** usually occur at the ends of operons, contain a hairpin turn followed by a series of 6–8 uracils, and cause transcription to halt. The uracil series causes the newly synthesized RNA to dissociate from the DNA template because uracil forms weak hydrogen bonds. **Weak (type II) terminator signals** often occur within operons, have smaller hairpin turns, and may cause transcription to pause rather than halt. When RNA polymerase stalls at a weak terminator, it will be dislodged if it engages the **rho protein.** Rho protein is a large hexameric protein that binds to 80-bp segments of mRNA. When transcription pauses at a weak terminator, rho moves along the mRNA strand to the paused polymerase if there are no intervening ribosomes. Rho binds to the DNA-polymerase complex, hydrolyzes ATP, and displaces

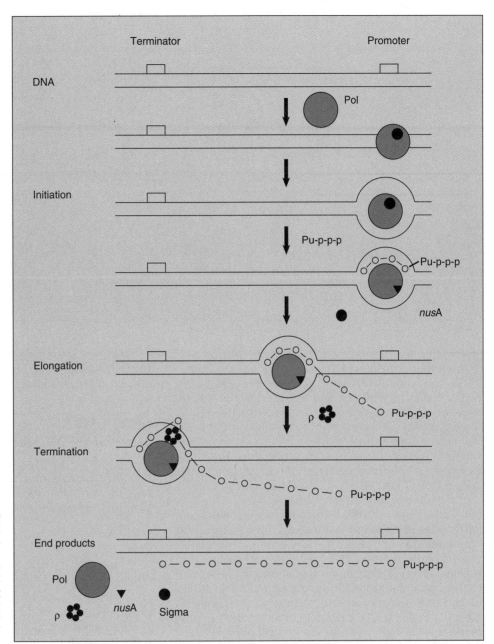

FIGURE 3–22. An overview of transcription of the bacterial chromosome. Pol = DNA-dependent RNA polymerase; Pu-p-p-p = purine triphosphate; and ρ = rho protein. (Source: Davis, B. D., et al. Microbiology, 4th ed. Philadelphia, J. B. Lippincott Co., 1990. Redrawn and reproduced, with permission, from Lippincott-Raven Publishers.)

the RNA polymerase. This completes the synthesis of mRNA. Rho protein also accentuates the action of strong terminators.

Translation in Bacterial Versus Eukaryotic Cells

Eukaryotic transcription results in the formation of monocistronic mRNA messages in the nucleus. The mRNA must be capped and transported to the cytoplasm, where 80S ribosomes translate the messages into proteins. In contrast, bacterial transcription and translation take place in the same compartment. Polycistronic messages are constructed and are translated by polysomes even as transcription continues. There is no intervening capping of the mRNA, and transcription and translation are physically linked

(Fig. 3–23). Because of this linkage, processes that directly affect transcription or translation may also affect the corresponding linked synthesis of RNA or protein. It is this linkage that allows attenuation to occur (see the discussion of the tryptophan operon in Chapter 2).

Bacterial translation can be described briefly as follows. The mRNA complexes with 70S ribosomes that are composed of a 50S and a 30S subunit. Because the ribosomes in bacterial cells have different proteins and sizes of ribosomal RNA (rRNA) segments than do their counterparts in eukaryotic cells, they serve as excellent antibiotic targets. In bacterial cells, mRNA is initially bound by the small ribosomal fragment only after the peptidyl (P) site is filled by aminoformyl methionine tRNA, which serves as the initiator

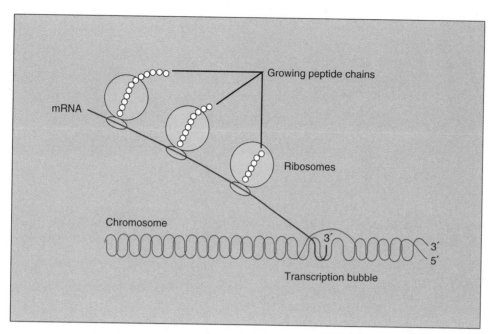

FIGURE 3–23. Transcription of the bacterial chromosome yields polycistronic messages, and transcription and translation are physically linked.

tRNA. Initiation requires the occurrence of the initiating codon, which is usually AUG (but is occasionally GUG). Once the 50S fragment is added to the mRNA-30S ribosome complex, protein synthesis begins.

Fig. 3–24 summarizes the translation process. Each incoming aminoacyl tRNA (AA-tRNA) complexes with elongation factor and guanosine triphosphate (GTP). It is this complex that initially binds to the codon in the acceptor (A) site. This causes translation to pause briefly. If the codon matches the anticodon, GTP is hydrolyzed, elongation factor is released, and the peptide bond is formed. If the codon and anticodon do not match, the tRNA complex will dissociate from the codon and leave the ribosome. This process ensures that the correct amino acid is added to the growing peptide. The growing peptide is added to the end of each entering amino acid. Finally, G factor expends a GTP molecule to move the growing peptide from the A site to the P site, allowing new AA-tRNA–elongation factor complexes to enter the A site. This process continues until it reaches a terminator signal. Two protein release factors facilitate termination. **Release factor 1** (RF1) recognizes UAG or UAA, while **release factor 2** (RF2) recognizes UAA or UGA. Each hydrolyzes the bond between the peptide and RNA and allows release of the peptide from the ribosome. This cycle occurs simultaneously in a series of ribosomes over the length of the polycistronic mRNA molecule.

Translation thus involves three discernible processes: an **initiation process,** a three-step **elongation process,** and a **termination process.** Translation is initiated by the binding of F-met-tRNA and the addition of the first amino acid. Each round of peptide elongation involves entry of the AA-tRNA to the A site (recognition), formation of the peptide bond (peptidyl transfer), and movement of the nascent peptide from the A site to the P site (translocation). Finally,

the peptide, mRNA, and ribosomal fragments dissociate during termination.

GENETIC TOOLS
Recombinant DNA Technology

Transduction and transformation can be used to introduce pieces of DNA into recipient bacteria via recombinant DNA technology, which is often called **genetic engineering** or **biotechnology.**

Uses

The purpose of recombinant techniques is to introduce a human or animal gene into a microbe such as a bacterium or a yeast and have that microbe produce animal products.

Plasmids are frequently referred to as **vectors.** A **shuttle vector** is a plasmid that can be introduced into either a bacterium or a eukaryotic cell, and a **cosmid vector** is a plasmid that contains the *cos* site, which allows it to be packaged efficiently into phage heads.

Recombinant DNA technology is not without its limitations. One problem is that some proteins cannot be made by bacteria, because of the types of disulfide bonds that must be completed to construct the active protein. Another problem is that it is difficult to introduce unmethylated animal DNA into a bacterium without having it degraded by **restriction endonucleases.** Fortunately, this second problem can be avoided by using restriction endonucleases to cleave plasmids and animal DNA, insert pieces of animal DNA into the plasmid, and then anneal them. When this is done, the bacterium should be able to accept the plasmid by transformation or transduction.

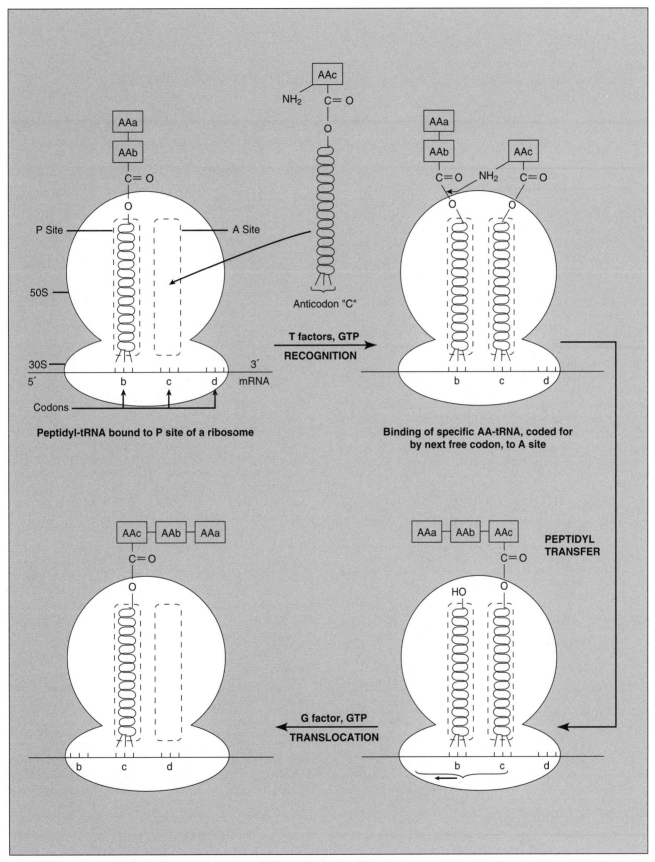

FIGURE 3–24. An overview of translation of bacterial proteins. See text for details. AAa = amino acid a; AAb = amino acid b; AAc = amino acid c; P site = peptidyl site; A site = acceptor site; AA-tRNA = aminoacyl tRNA; and GTP = guanosine triphosphate. (Source: Davis, B. D., et al. Microbiology, 4th ed. Philadelphia, J. B. Lippincott Co., 1990. Redrawn and reproduced, with permission, from Lippincott-Raven Publishers.)

Procedures

Restriction endonucleases cleave **palindromic sequences** in double-stranded DNA. Table 3–1 shows some of the cleavage sites recognized by these enzymes. For example, *Eco*RI, which is widely used, cleaves the following:

GAATTC
CTTAAG

to yield sites with ends that are staggered:

AATTC
CTTAA

These staggered ends are called **sticky ends** because they will match up with any other piece of DNA similarly cleaved to form a piece of hybrid DNA. A ligase is then used to anneal these sites covalently.

The general procedure, as depicted in Fig. 3–25, is to treat a suspension of host DNA with an endonuclease and to treat a suspension of a plasmid (vector) the same way. The two are mixed to allow matching of sticky ends, and a ligase is then added to reform plasmids. In many cases, plasmids will have already randomly picked up various pieces of the other DNA. Next, transduction or transformation is used to introduce the plasmid into a culture of bacteria. Finally, samples of the bacteria are grown, and each sample is screened for production of the protein of interest. This may require the screening of thousands of bacterial colonies. If a bacterium is found to produce active product, its progeny will be grown in pure culture in

TABLE 3–1. Cleavage Sites of Several Widely Used Restriction Endonucleases

Restriction Endonuclease*	Recognition Sequence†
Bgl II	A/GATCT
*Bsa*AI	YAC/GTR
*Bsi*YI	CCNNNN/NNGG
*Bsp*MII	T/CCGGA
Cfr I	Y/GGCCR
*Eco*RI	G/AATTC
*Eco*RII	/CCWGG
*Hind*II	GTY/RAC
*Hind*III	A/AGCTT
Hpa II	C/CGG
Mae I	C/TAG
Mbo I	/GATC
Msp I	C/CGG
Mwo I	GCNNNNN/NNGC
Not I	GC/GGCGGC
Pst I	CTGCA/G

*Endonucleases are designated on the basis of the organisms from which they are isolated, with letters and roman numerals indicating genus, species, strain (if any), and series number. For example, in *Eco*RII, the *Eco* stands for *Escherichia coli*, the R is the strain designation, and the II indicates the series number. If there is no strain, the series number is preceded by a space.

†The slash mark (/) indicates the site of cleavage within the recognition sequence. A = adenine; C = cytosine; G = guanine; T = thymine; R = adenine or guanine; W = adenine or thymine; Y = cytosine or thymine; and N = adenine, cytosine, guanine, or thymine.

a chemostat to produce vast amounts of the product, and lawyers will be summoned to start the patenting process.

The Polymerase Chain Reaction

During the mid-1980s, scientists with the Cetus Corporation stumbled upon a novel technique that is now beginning to revolutionize molecular biology by making it possible to locate trace amounts of specific DNA segments in large samples. This new technology is based on the polymerase chain reaction (PCR).

Uses

Scientists had long believed that infectious and genetic diseases could be diagnosed more rapidly and effectively if there were a method that allowed them to locate unique disease-specific pieces of DNA in samples from patients. In the case of tuberculosis, for example, the usual method of diagnosis entails culturing the responsible organism, *Mycobacterium tuberculosis,* from sputum samples. Unfortunately, because *M. tuberculosis* grows extremely slowly, cultures must be incubated for up to a month before samples with no growth can be declared to be negative. If, instead, a piece of *M. tuberculosis*–specific DNA could be located in the sputum, the diagnosis might be able to be confirmed rapidly. Some groups had been moderately successful in using DNA gels and hybridization techniques to find bacteria in diarrheal samples containing DNA segments that coded for enterotoxins. In general, however, techniques such as this enjoyed only limited success because most clinical samples contained too little bacterial or viral DNA and too much host DNA.

The solution to the problem was to develop a technique that was capable of finding and multiplying only the DNA segments of interest. This is exactly what the PCR assay does. Some have called it "a photocopy machine for DNA," while others have said that it "finds a needle in a haystack and then makes a stack of needles."

Procedures

Suppose a team of laboratory technicians was asked to report whether a patient has urethritis caused by *Chlamydia trachomatis*. They would obtain a sample of urethral exudate and extract the DNA. In their efforts to locate the chlamydial DNA, they would take advantage of the following known information. If the patient has chlamydial urethritis (also called nongonococcal urethritis, or NGU), the sample will contain segments of human DNA and a small amount of chlamydial DNA. Each piece of chlamydial DNA will contain several series of bases that are unique to that DNA fragment. If a small piece of DNA can be made to match one of the existing segments and can be added to a single-stranded piece of chlamydial DNA, it will pair with the existing segment of DNA, and the double-stranded segment will serve as a primer to

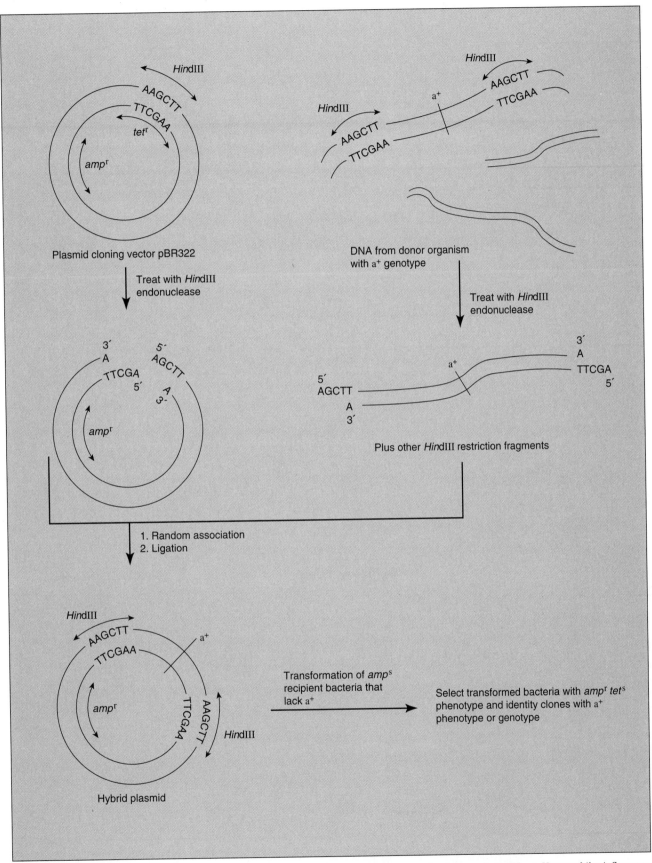

FIGURE 3–25. Recombinant DNA technology. See text for details. *Hind*III = restriction endonuclease derived from *Haemophilus influenzae*; *amp*ʳ and *amp*ˢ = genes for ampicillin resistance and sensitivity, respectively; *tet*ʳ and *tet*ˢ = genes for tetracycline resistance and sensitivity, respectively; and aᐩ = the targeted gene. (Redrawn and reproduced, with permission, from Baron, S. Medical Microbiology, 3rd ed. New York, Churchill Livingstone, 1991.)

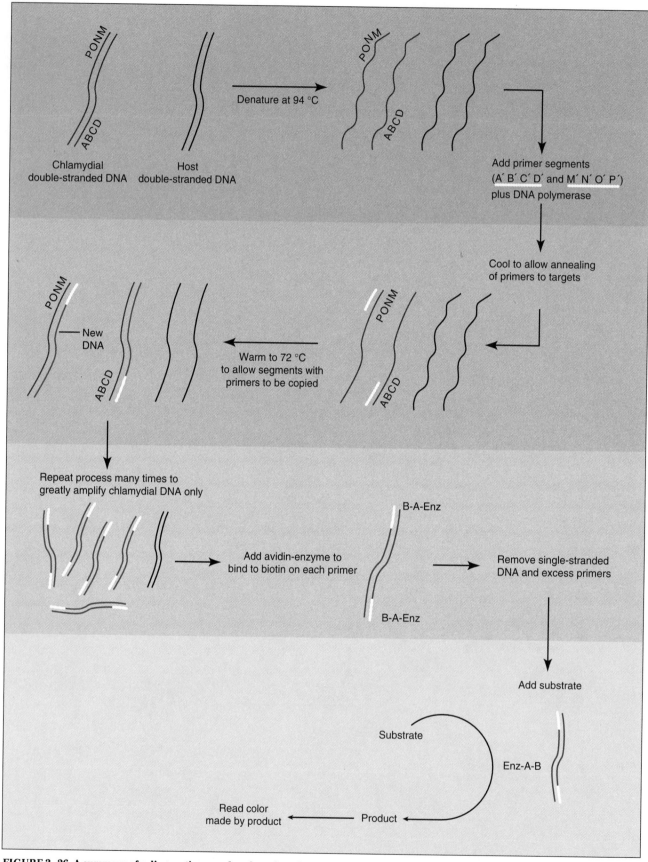

FIGURE 3–26. A summary of a diagnostic procedure based on the polymerase chain reaction (PCR). B-A-Enz = biotin plus avidin enzyme.

allow a DNA polymerase to copy the rest of the single strand of DNA.

The steps of the procedure are illustrated in Fig. 3–26. The sample is heated to 94 °C to denature the DNA and separate the strands. The sample now contains single strands of chlamydial and host DNA. Next, primer segments are added. These primer segments match the segments on both the positive and negative strands of the chlamydial DNA and are at the ends of the highly specific regions. The DNA suspension is cooled to a temperature that will allow the primer segments to anneal rapidly to their matching sites on the chlamydial DNA but will not allow efficient annealing of the larger fragments of DNA. In many cases, this temperature is around 60 °C. At this time, a DNA polymerase is also added.

Once the primers have annealed to their specific sites, the suspension is heated to 72 °C to allow the DNA polymerase to copy single-stranded pieces of chlamydial DNA that have short double-stranded sites where the primer segments have annealed. The polymerase used (Taq DNA polymerase) is from a thermophilic bacterium, so it works best at high temperatures, which keep the large DNA segments from annealing.

Each time the suspension goes through the replicative cycle, the number of chlamydial DNA fragments will be doubled. To maximize the detection of the DNA, the process is repeated 30–40 times over 3–4 hours, and millions of copies of the chlamydial DNA are made. Finally, the amplified DNA segments must be identified. In some cases, this is done by running the samples on a gel and then staining the gel for characteristic bands. A popular recent approach has been to attach a molecule of biotin to each primer segment. This means that each amplified DNA segment will not only contain at least one primer segment but will also have a biotin molecule attached to it. The double-stranded DNA segments can be partially purified by passing the suspension through a resin column or by incubating them in a well that is coated with DNA segments that will bind the double-stranded DNA segments. Finally, the biotin-containing amplified segments will be detected by adding avidin complexed with alkaline phosphatase. The biotin and avidin will bind to each other, and the substrate for alkaline phosphatase will be added. Thus, for each molecule of amplified DNA, there will be a molecule of alkaline phosphatase that will convert its substrate to a product that will be detected colorimetrically.

PCR assays have already been developed for a number of bacterial, viral, and protozoal diseases, and more are being developed almost daily. Additionally, the PCR technique has been used to detect the presence of inherited diseases, and it will likely be used to diagnose malignant neoplasms. Some investigators have claimed that PCR assays will soon replace culture techniques in the hospital laboratories. Because of the cost of PCR assays, however, this transformation may not be as rapid as some have envisioned.

Selected Readings

Alberts, B., et al. Molecular Biology of the Cell, 3rd ed. New York, Garland Publishing, 1994.

Allen, G. C., and A. Kornberg. Fine balance in the regulation of DnaB helicase by DnaC protein in the replication of *Escherichia coli.* J Biol Chem 266:22096–22101, 1991.

Erlich, H. PCR Technology: Principles and Application for DNA Amplification. New York, Stockton Press, 1989.

Herendeen, D. R., and T. J. Kelly. DNA polymerase III: running rings around the fork. Cell 84:5–8, 1996.

Hwang, D. S., and A. Kornberg. Opposed actions of regulatory proteins, DnaA and IciA, in opening of the replication origin of *Escherichia coli.* J Biol Chem 267:23087–23091, 1992.

Kelman, Z., and M. O'Donnell. DNA replication: enzymology and mechanisms. Curr Opinion Genet Dev 4:185–195, 1994.

Kong, X. P., et al. Three-dimensional structure of the β subunit of *Escherichia coli* DNA polymerase III holoenzyme: a sliding DNA clamp. Cell 69:425–437, 1992.

Lewin, B. Genes V. Oxford, Oxford University Press, 1994.

O'Donnell, M., et al. The sliding clamp of DNA polymerase III holoenzyme encircles DNA. Mol Biol Cell 3:953–957, 1992.

Polyakov, A., et al. Three-dimensional structure of *Escherichia coli* core RNA polymerase: promoter binding and elongation conformations of the enzyme. Cell 83:365–373, 1995.

Rothfield, L. I., and C. R. Zhao. How do bacteria decide where to divide? Cell 84:183–186, 1996.

Skarstad, K., et al. A novel binding protein of the origin of the *Escherichia coli* chromosome. J Biol Chem 268:5365–5370, 1993.

CHAPTER FOUR

ANTIBACTERIAL AGENTS

THE DEVELOPMENT AND NATURE OF ANTIBIOTICS
History of Antibiotic Development

The development of antibiotics is one of the truly significant achievements of the 20th century. Although some early remedies contained antimicrobial chemicals and were effective, their application was generally limited to a small number of diseases. Probably the best known of these remedies was cinchona bark, which contained quinine and was chewed by people suffering from malaria.

The first antibacterial substance to be used on a widespread basis by Western cultures was mercury, whose use in the treatment of syphilis gave rise to the following nursery rhyme: "Rub a dub dub, three men in a tub, / And who do you think they be? / The butcher, the baker, the candlestick maker, / Throw them out, knaves all three!" Tubbing and rubbing were two methods of treatment, consisting either of having the patients (the "knaves" in this nursery rhyme) soak in a tub of mercury or of rubbing mercury into the gummatous lesions of syphilis. Treatment with mercury had three major drawbacks. First, it was not always effective. Second, the mercury was a narrow-spectrum drug, since it was useful only against the bacterium that caused syphilis. Third, mercury was toxic to both the bacterium and the patient. Mercury damages the nervous system, a phenomenon that was immortalized in Lewis Carroll's tale about Alice and a mad hatter. Hats were once handmade from mercury-treated felt, and the hatmakers' long-term exposure to mercury damaged their nervous systems, with the result that most hatters eventually became "mad." This introduces a critical concept in antibiotic development, that of **selective toxicity.** For an antibiotic to be useful it must be effective but must also be selective in its toxicity, killing infectious agents but not patients.

The search for antibiotics began in earnest during the late 19th century, when many diseases were discovered to be caused by bacteria, viruses, and parasites. The chemist Paul Ehrlich, in particular, searched for a "silver bullet" that would kill all pathogens. Because he owned a dye factory, he screened hundreds of dyes for antibacterial activity. His greatest success came in 1905, when the 606th compound tested was found to kill treponemes. This arsenical dye, called salvarsan, was marketed as an antibiotic for the treatment of syphilis.

The first major breakthrough in modern antibiotic development came in the early 1930s, when Gerhard Domagk discovered the first **sulfonamide,** which he called Prontosil. The mechanism of action of the sulfonamides was worked out by D. D. Woods, who discovered that the inhibitory effects of sulfonamides on bacterial growth could be reversed by adding **p-aminobenzoic acid** (PABA) to the growth medium. This led to the conclusion that **sulfanilamide** (an early sulfonamide antibiotic) acted as a structural analogue of PABA.

Alexander Fleming discovered **penicillin G** in 1929, but because he had little success or encouragement in studying this unstable substance, he discontinued his work. He had largely failed to understand the implications of his discovery. It was not until 1939 that the British scientists H. W. Florey and E. B. Chain isolated and purified penicillin. By this time, England was involved in World War II, so British and American scientists collaborated to develop penicillin for clinical use. By 1942, their efforts were successful, and the development of penicillin as an effective therapeutic agent was a boon for Allied forces.

Today, there is a bewildering array of antibiotics. Pharmaceutical firms continue in their efforts to develop antibiotics with greater efficacy, wider spectrums of activity, and lower levels of toxicity. Competition results not only in the discovery of new drugs but also in the proliferation of "me too" antibiotics. After one firm makes a significant development, other firms may follow suit, changing a moiety on the antibiotic structure so as not to be guilty of patent infringement. The structural change alters some property of the drug—such as rate of metabolism, penetration into tissues, site of inactivation, or spectrum of use—and the change in activity becomes the focal point of sales efforts. The changes are sometimes useful, but the modifications are often minimal, and hospital formularies restrict which form of the drug is made routinely available.

General Concepts of Antibiotic Activity
Bactericidal Versus Bacteriostatic Antibiotics

Key Differences. Although bactericidal antibiotics kill bacteria, bacteriostatic antibiotics merely halt the growth of bacteria. In an ideal world, all antibiotics would be "cidal," yet "static" antibiotics have proved to be quite useful because halting bacterial growth allows the immune system the time and opportunity it needs to eliminate the infecting agent.

This last statement hints at a key difference between static and cidal antibiotics: if a static antibiotic is removed from a culture, the bacteria will resume growth, but the effects of cidal antibiotics are irreversible. It is not always easy to determine whether a given antibiotic will be static or cidal in its effects. It is obvious that antibiotics that lyse bacteria are cidal, but not all cidal antibiotics are lytic.

As shown in Fig. 4–1, the effects of various antibiotics on the growth of a particular bacterial species can be determined by using a spectrophotometer to compare the absorbance (density or turbidity) of suspensions of bacteria exposed to the antibiotics or by using plate counts to compare the number of viable bacteria in the suspensions. In Fig. 4–1, which compares the effects that four antibiotics have on *Escherichia coli,* **penicillin** is cidal, causing a drop in both the absorbance and the number of viable bacteria. **Chloramphenicol** and **streptomycin** both halt growth immediately after being added to the culture, as shown by their absorbance. Unlike chloramphenicol, however, streptomycin is cidal, as demonstrated by the drop in the number of viable bacteria. **Sulfanilamide** is static and allows some bacterial multiplication to occur after it is added to the culture.

Clinical Considerations. Two groups of patients cannot be treated successfully with static antibiotics: (1) immunodeficient patients with acute infections and (2) patients with infections in immunologically privileged sites. This can be illustrated with two examples. First, severely neutropenic patients with bacteremic pneumonia are not likely to survive without intensive therapy with cidal antibiotics. This is because recovery from bacterial pneumonia depends on vigorous neutrophil activity. Second, patients with bacterial meningitis are at high risk because the subarachnoid space is not well served by

the immune response. If these patients receive a static antibiotic, there is little phagocytic response available to eliminate the bacteria. Once the static antibiotic is removed, the bacteria will multiply rapidly, resulting in grave consequences.

Whether an antibiotic is static or cidal depends on the amount of drug that can reach the target site. Some antibiotics are cidal at high concentrations and static at low concentrations. As a result, they may be static against bacteria in a boil, where antibiotic access is poor, even though they are cidal against bacteria in the blood. If an antibiotic is toxic to a patient at a cidal concentration, it may not be possible to use the antibiotic as a cidal agent. Moreover, because the targets for the action of each antibiotic vary somewhat among bacteria, some antibiotics are cidal against one bacterial species and static against another. The safe and effective treatment of patients requires an understanding of what an antibiotic will do at various concentrations, at various sites of infection, and against various infectious agents.

Narrow-Spectrum Versus Broad-Spectrum Antibiotics

The antimicrobial spectrum of an antibiotic is the range of organisms that can be killed or harmed by that antibiotic. For example, **penicillin G,** which is primarily used for treatment of gram-positive bacteria, is effective against only a few gram-negative pathogens and is therefore considered to have a fairly narrow spectrum of activity. In contrast, the **tetracyclines,** which are effective against many gram-positive and gram-negative pathogens, are considered to be broad-spectrum antibiotics.

It may be tempting to think that the tetracyclines should be used preferentially because of their broad antimicrobial spectrum, but several other factors

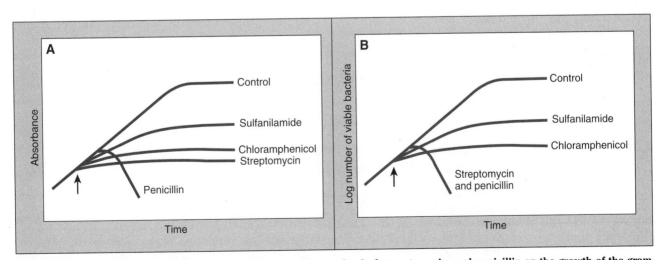

FIGURE 4–1. Comparison of the effects of sulfanilamide, chloramphenicol, streptomycin, and penicillin on the growth of the gram-negative bacterium *Escherichia coli.* Diagram A compares the absorbance (density or turbidity) of suspensions of bacteria exposed to the antibiotics, as measured in a spectrophotometer. Diagram B compares the log number of viable bacteria in the suspensions, as measured by plate counts. Arrows indicate when the antibiotics were added to the suspensions.

must be considered when devising a rational approach to antibiotic usage. For example, some antibiotics are more toxic that others, and when the use of a more toxic drug is necessary, it is advantageous to use lower concentrations if therapeutic considerations allow. Some antibiotics do not reach the infection site in adequate amounts, and the half-life of some antibiotics is too short for their intended use. Many types of infections require the use of cidal antibiotics.

Multiple-Drug Therapy

Physicians often use antibiotics in combination (1) to prevent the onset of disease in immunosuppressed or debilitated patients, (2) to treat chronic diseases in which bacteria may develop resistance to an antibiotic during the course of therapy, (3) as empiric therapy when the specific agent of disease is unknown, (4) to treat infections that involve more than one bacterial species, and (5) to treat infections caused by bacteria that are difficult to eradicate. The central goal of multiple-drug therapy in most cases is to broaden the antimicrobial spectrum or to increase the efficacy of antibiotics against a single bacterial species.

Synergistic Effects.   A common therapeutic approach is to combine antibiotics that act synergistically. Generally, antibiotics are considered to act synergistically if their effect when they are used in combination is four or more times as great as the sum of their individual effects. Synergism results when a **penicillin** or a **cephalosporin** is given in combination with an **aminoglycoside.** Synergism also results with the use of a combination of **trimethoprim** (TMP) and **sulfamethoxazole** (SMX).

Penicillins and cephalosporins kill bacteria by inhibiting cell wall synthesis, while aminoglycosides block protein synthesis. In some cases, a bacterium that is only marginally sensitive to these antibiotics when they are used individually is extremely sensitive to them when they are used in combination. It is believed that inhibition of cell wall synthesis by a penicillin or cephalosporin makes the bacterium more permeable to the aminoglycoside. With more of the aminoglycoside accumulating within the bacterium, the bacterium is rapidly killed by the aminoglycoside. This allows small amounts of the relatively toxic aminoglycoside to be used in treating the patient. Combining the use of an aminoglycoside with a penicillin or cephalosporin has proved helpful in treating infections caused by gram-negative bacilli, including *Pseudomonas aeruginosa,* an organism particularly difficult to manage.

TMP and SMX act synergistically because the two antibiotics block separate steps of the pathway that converts PABA and pteridine to tetrahydrofolate. The TMP/SMX combination is used to treat a wide variety of bacterial and parasitic infections.

Antagonistic Effects.   Unfortunately, not all antibiotic combinations have synergistic or additive effects. Some combinations are antagonistic, with one antibiotic inhibiting the activity of the other. An example of this is the combination of **chloramphenicol** with a **penicillin** such as ampicillin. **Ampicillin** inhibits cell wall synthesis, a process that requires rapidly growing bacteria. When bacteria are simultaneously exposed to chloramphenicol and ampicillin, the bacteriostatic chloramphenicol not only stops the multiplication of bacteria but also halts the need for cell wall synthesis. Because cell wall synthesis is no longer needed, ampicillin has no effect on the bacteria. Thus, the bactericidal activity of ampicillin is completely blocked by the bacteriostatic activity of chloramphenicol. In general, it is recommended that static and cidal antibiotics not be used in combination.

BACTERIAL SENSITIVITY AND RESISTANCE TO ANTIBIOTICS
Selective Toxicity

A major factor that has allowed the development of antibiotics against bacteria is that bacteria are **prokaryotes** and, as such, differ significantly from human cells. It is against the differences in cellular structure and function that antibiotics are directed, and it is this concept that allows antibiotics to be selectively toxic. As outlined in Table 4–1 and discussed in detail later in this chapter, there are four main types of antibiotics, each of which attacks a different target: (1) antibiotics that affect the cell envelope, (2) antibiotics that inhibit protein synthesis, (3) antibiotics that affect nucleic acid synthesis and structure, and (4) antimetabolite antibiotics. In general, antibiotics of the first and third categories are cidal, those of the second category may be static or cidal, and those of the fourth category are static.

The number of antibiotics against bacteria is far greater than the number against fungi, parasites, and viruses. This is because fungi and parasites have more in common with human cells and because viruses utilize the replicative machinery available in human cells. Unfortunately, because of the great similarity among all eukaryotic cells, antibiotics directed against fungi, parasites, and viruses tend to be rather toxic to humans. Even those antibiotics that are directed against bacteria have some toxicity for humans. With a number of drugs, such as the aminoglycosides, the **therapeutic margin** (the margin between the effective dose and the toxic dose) is small, so the blood levels of these antibiotics must be carefully monitored.

Sensitivity to Antibiotics

Some bacteria are fairly uniform in their response to antimicrobial agents, but the following organisms isolated from blood, urine, sputum, or cerebrospinal fluid should be tested for susceptibility to

TABLE 4–1. Classification of Antibiotics by Target of Action

ANTIBIOTICS THAT AFFECT THE CELL ENVELOPE
  Agents That Inhibit Cell Wall Synthesis
    Beta-lactam antibiotics
      Natural penicillins
        (1) Penicillin G
        (2) Penicillin V
      Semisynthetic penicillins and analogues
        (1) Penicillinase-resistant penicillins (cloxacillin, dicloxacillin, flucloxacillin, methicillin, nafcillin, and oxacillin)
        (2) Extended-spectrum penicillins (amdinocillin, amoxicillin, ampicillin, and bacampicillin)
        (3) Antipseudomonal penicillins (azlocillin, carbenicillin, piperacillin, mezlocillin, and ticarcillin)
        (4) Analogues (clavulanic acid, sulbactam, and tazobactam)
      Other penicillinlike antibiotics
        (1) Carbapenems (imipenem and meropenem)
        (2) Monobactams (aztreonam)
      Cephalosporins, cephamycins, and related antibiotics
        (1) First-generation cephalosporins (cefadroxil, cefazolin, cefprozil, cephalexin, cephalothin, cephapirin, and cephradine)
        (2) Second-generation cephalosporins (cefaclor, cefamandole, cefonicid, ceforanide, and cefuroxime)
        (3) Third-generation cephalosporins (cefixime, cefoperazone, cefotaxime, cefpodoxime, ceftazidime, ceftizoxime, and ceftriaxone)
        (4) "Fourth-generation" cephalosporins (cefepime and cefpirome)
        (5) Cephamycins (cefmetazole, cefotetan, and cefoxitin)
        (6) Related antibiotics (loracarbef and moxalactam)
    Glycopeptide antibiotics (teicoplanin and vancomycin)
    Bacitracin
    Cycloserine
  Agents That Disturb Cell Membrane Integrity
    Polymyxin B
    Polymyxin E

ANTIBIOTICS THAT INHIBIT PROTEIN SYNTHESIS
  Agents That Affect the 50S Ribosomal Fragment
    Chloramphenicol
    Macrolides (azithromycin, clarithromycin, dirithromycin, erythromycin, and troleandomycin)
    Lincosamides (clindamycin and lincomycin)
  Agents That Affect the 30S Ribosomal Fragment
    Aminoglycosides (amikacin, gentamicin, kanamycin, netilmicin, spectinomycin, streptomycin, and tobramycin)
    Tetracyclines (chlortetracycline, demeclocycline, doxycycline, minocycline, oxytetracycline, and tetracycline)
  Other Agents That Inhibit Protein Synthesis
    Mupirocin and others

ANTIBIOTICS THAT AFFECT NUCLEIC ACID SYNTHESIS AND STRUCTURE
    Rifamycins (rifabutin and rifampin)
    Nalidixic acid
    Fluoroquinolones (ciprofloxacin, enoxacin, lomefloxacin, norfloxacin, and ofloxacin)
    Novobiocin
    Metronidazole
    Clofazimine

ANTIMETABOLITE ANTIBIOTICS
    Sulfonamides (sulfacytine, sulfadiazine, sulfamerazine, sulfamethazine, sulfamethizole, sulfamethoxazole, sulfasalazine, and sulfisoxazole)
    Trimethoprim
    Aminosalicylate sodium
    Dapsone
    Isoniazid
    Ethionamide
    Ethambutol

OTHER ANTIBACTERIAL AGENTS
    Methenamine
    Nitrofurantoin
    Pyrazinamide

---

appropriate antibiotics: gram-negative enteric bacteria (including *Enterobacter, Escherichia coli, Klebsiella, Proteus, Salmonella, Serratia, Shigella,* and *Yersinia*), *Enterococcus faecalis, Haemophilus influenzae, Pseudomonas aeruginosa,* and *Staphylococcus aureus.*

In addition, blood isolates of coagulase-negative staphylococci and pneumococci are often tested for antibiotic sensitivity, and other bacteria are tested when the physician determines that such testing is needed.

Testing Procedures

The Microdilution Method. The microdilution method is the most commonly used method to test the antibiotic sensitivity of bacteria. Microtiter wells containing serial twofold dilutions of antibiotics are inoculated with a standard inoculum of the bacterium in question, the plates are incubated overnight, and the wells are then examined for the presence of bacterial growth. The lowest concentration of each antibiotic dilution series that prevents bacterial growth is considered to be the **minimum inhibitory concentration** (MIC) of the antibiotic.

The **minimum bactericidal concentration** (MBC) of each antibiotic is not routinely determined in most hospitals, but it can be determined for individual samples of bacteria when requested by a physician. The MBC is determined by plating out standard aliquots of the supernatant from each well that shows no visible bacterial growth. The MBC is then defined as the lowest concentration of each antibiotic that kills 99.9% of the bacteria in the original inoculum. In many cases, the MIC and MBC of cidal antibiotics are equivalent—that is, all wells that show no growth do so because all the bacteria in the well have been killed. Some bacteria, however, are deficient in autolytic enzymes, and the concentration of antibiotic needed to kill them is at least 32-fold greater than that needed to halt their growth. These bacteria are said to be **tolerant** of the antibiotic.

A variation of the microdilution method can also be used to test serum samples for the presence of bactericidal levels of antibiotics being used to treat individual patients.

The Disk Diffusion Method (Kirby-Bauer Test). If bacteria grow poorly in the medium used in the microdilution test, their antibiotic sensitivity can be tested using a disk diffusion method known as the Kirby-Bauer test. In this case, a standard inoculum of the bacterium is spread onto a large Petri dish containing Mueller-Hinton agar. Filter paper disks impregnated with standard amounts of antibiotics are then pressed onto the agar surface, and the plate is incubated appropriately. The bacteria grow as a lawn across the surface of the agar, but circular zones appear around each antibiotic disk where the growth of the bacteria is inhibited. The microbiologist measures the diameter of the zone of inhibition and compares this zone with a published standard. Bacteria are classified as being **sensitive, intermediate,** or **resistant** to each antibiotic.

Colorimetric Tests. For the testing of some bacterial species, such as *Neisseria gonorrhoeae,* a full spectrum of antibiotic sensitivities is not needed, but it is important to know if the isolate has **beta-lactamase activity.** Simple colorimetric tests are available to rapidly identify beta-lactamase–producing strains of a bacterial species.

Interpretation of Results

Sensitivity testing has proved to be of great benefit to clinicians, but there are several reasons why the test results should be interpreted with caution. First, the tests are sensitive to technical variations. A small change in temperature, pH, or inoculum size, for example, can affect the outcome of the test, and the results are often irreproducible when the same isolate is tested by multiple laboratories. Second, antibiotic sensitivity tests are performed under standard conditions that may be quite different from in vivo conditions. For example, since the efficacy of aminoglycosides varies with pH, it should be no surprise when bacteria that are found to be sensitive to aminoglycosides at pH 7.4 in vitro are not so sensitive in an acidic environment in vivo. Third, the standard values used to determine susceptibility and resistance are related to achievable in vivo blood levels of the antibiotic. Thus, sensitivity tests often underestimate the efficacy of antibiotics against pathogens in the urinary tract, where many drugs concentrate. Fourth, susceptibility in vitro is not the only factor that affects the outcome of antibiotic therapy in vivo. Other factors include the location and extent of the infection, the presence of underlying immunocompromising disease or mixed infection, the accuracy of diagnosis, the adequacy of the dosage, the age and compliance of the patient, the bacterial acquisition of resistance during infection, and the need for surgical intervention or drainage.

Resistance to Antibiotics

Patterns of Resistance

Despite the existence of so many antibiotics and a multi-billion-dollar pharmaceutical industry, bacterial diseases are far from being eliminated. A major reason for this is that so many bacteria resist the effects of antibiotics. Consider what an antibiotic must do to exert its effect. It must recognize a suitable target, reach that target, achieve a sufficient concentration, and maintain that concentration for an adequate period of time.

Some treatment problems occur when the antibiotic of choice is unable to reach its target because it cannot cross the blood-brain barrier or cannot reach bacteria within an abscess. Other problems are related to antibiotic concentration. In some cases, the antibiotic is rapidly excreted or metabolized, causing peak blood levels of the drug to be maintained only briefly. This makes the antibiotic ineffective for treating infections caused by bacteria that are killed only when exposed to prolonged high levels of the drug. In other cases, the antibiotic is rapidly concentrated within a particular organ or tissue, and other sites of infection may be relatively inaccessible to the antibiotic.

Nongenetic Mechanisms of Resistance

Bacteria resist the actions of antibiotics via at least three commonly occurring means. First, some bacteria produce enzymes that inactivate an antibiotic by attaching a group (methyl, acetyl, or phosphate) or by cleaving a key bond (for example, the beta-lactam ring of penicillins). Second, some bacteria become relatively resistant to an antibiotic when their permeability to the antibiotic is changed, often because of alterations in porin molecules or in lipopolysaccharide constituents. Lipopolysaccharide changes affect permeability by altering the organism's net surface charge. In the case of resistance to **tetracycline,** for example, efflux of the drug is greatly increased. Third, the target of the antibiotic may be altered such that it now recognizes the antibiotic poorly. Two important examples of this mechanism are (1) the ability of staphylococci to resist the action of **methicillin** when their penicillin-binding proteins (PBPs) lose their affinity for methicillin and (2) the ability of some *E. coli* to become resistant to **streptomycin** when their S12 protein is altered.

These changes have radically altered the susceptibility patterns of many bacteria and have had a tremendous impact on therapeutics. Consider the following historical progression. During the 1960s, the standard therapy for gonorrhea was injection of 1.2 million units of **penicillin G.** During the early 1970s, gonococci became progressively less permeable to the drug, so the dosage was raised to 2.4 million units. Subsequently, the recommendation was to give 4.8 million units of penicillin G, along with probenecid, an agent that prolongs the peak blood levels of penicillin by slowing its excretion. Penicillinase-producing strains of *N. gonorrhoeae* first appeared during the late 1970s and are now so prevalent that penicillin G is no longer routinely used to treat gonorrhea. Instead, the disease is treated with third-generation **cephalosporins** (usually ceftriaxone or cefixime), **fluoroquinolones,** or **spectinomycin.** The penicillinase-producing organisms are believed to have arisen because an R factor (TEM-1) was transferred to gonococci from enteric bacteria.

Genetic Mechanisms of Resistance

The example of *N. gonorrhoeae* illustrates how bacteria often initially express one type of resistance mechanism (here, permeability changes) and later acquire a second resistance mechanism (in this case, formation of a beta-lactamase) through gene transfer. Not only has transformation been implicated in the acquisition of penicillin resistance by pneumococci, but staphylococci have been found to transfer beta-lactamase–containing **R factors** via transduction. Moreover, many gram-negative bacteria have been reported to exchange R factors via conjugation. Some R factors have a very narrow host range, such as those found in *Salmonella* serotype *typhi* and in *Vibrio cholerae,* but other R factors have been found in a wide variety of bacteria. For example, the resistance plasmid pAMB1 has been reported in isolates of *Bacillus, Clostridium, Enterococcus, Lactobacillus, Staphylococcus,* and *Streptococcus,* and another R factor (RP4) has been located within *Acinetobacter, Pseudomonas,* and a variety of enteric bacilli.

Some antibiotic resistance genes are found on **nonconjugative plasmids,** which can be mobilized by **conjugative plasmids** (the wrong plasmid is transferred during conjugation). These genes may also move from one plasmid to another, via either RecA-dependent recombination or transposition. It is believed that TEM-1 genes were transferred from enteric bacteria to gonococci via transpositional recombination. In this case, an enteric plasmid containing the TEM-1 transposon was believed to have entered a gonococcus. The enteric plasmid could not be replicated there, but the TEM-1 genes "jumped" from the enteric plasmid to a gonococcal plasmid. This "rescued" the resistance genes and allowed them to perpetuate within a new population.

Investigators once thought that resistance could not be passed between gram-negative and gram-positive bacteria, but cloning experiments have now shown that such transfer can occur, and there is inferential evidence that this has occurred in vivo. First, the R factor TetM was originally found only in enterococci (which are gram-positive), but it is now also found in gonococci and *Haemophilus* (which are gram-negative). Second, enterococcal transposon tn*917* contains a gene for resistance to **erythromycin.** This gene, known as *erm*B, seems to be identical to the *erm*BC gene of *E. coli* and *Klebsiella,* the tn*1545* gene of *Streptococcus pneumoniae,* and the *erm*AM gene of *Streptococcus sanguis.* Finally, tn*4400,* which carries a gene for resistance to **clindamycin,** has been transferred from *Bacteroides fragilis* to *E. coli.* This transfer worries many infectious disease specialists because it suggests that *B. fragilis* genes which encode beta-lactamases that degrade **cefoxitin** and **imipenem** might be able to be transferred in the same fashion.

ANTIBIOTICS THAT AFFECT THE CELL ENVELOPE
General Principles

The structure and synthesis of the cell envelopes of gram-positive and gram-negative bacteria are described in Chapter 1. **Gram-positive bacteria** (see Fig. 1–2) have an inner cytoplasmic membrane and a multilaminate peptidoglycan cell wall, and teichoic acids are attached to each of these structures. In contrast, **gram-negative bacteria** (see Fig. 1–3) have an inner cytoplasmic membrane, a thin cell wall, and an outer membrane that is impregnated with porins and lipopolysaccharide. Because their cell wall is so accessible, gram-positive bacteria tend to be quite susceptible to antibiotics that block various steps of peptidoglycan synthesis. Some agents that inhibit cell wall synthesis are also useful against gram-negative bacteria, but they must be designed to allow them to pass through the outer membrane pores to gain access to the cell wall synthesis machinery. Gram-negative bacteria are also susceptible to detergent-like antibiotics that dissolve the outer membrane.

Recommended antibiotics for the treatment of diseases caused by bacteria are listed in Table 4–2 and discussed in detail below.

TABLE 4–2. Recommended Antibiotics for the Treatment of Diseases Caused by Bacteria

Bacteria	Effective Antibiotic Treatments*
Gram-positive pyogenic cocci (see Chapter 5)	
Enterococcus faecalis	Ampicillin; vancomycin; penicillin/gentamicin; vancomycin/aminoglycoside.
Enterococcus faecium†	Ampicillin; vancomycin; penicillin/gentamicin; vancomycin/aminoglycoside.
Staphylococcus aureus	Penicillinase-resistant penicillin; first-generation cephalosporin; vancomycin; clindamycin.
Staphylococcus epidermidis	Vancomycin.
Staphylococcus saprophyticus	TMP/SMX; ampicillin; amoxicillin; fluoroquinolone.
Streptococcus agalactiae	Penicillin; ampicillin.
Streptococcus groups C and G	Penicillin; vancomycin; first- or second-generation cephalosporin.
Streptococcus intermedius group	Penicillin; vancomycin.
Streptococcus mutans	Penicillin/gentamicin; vancomycin/gentamicin/rifampin.
Streptococcus pneumoniae	Penicillin; cefotaxime; ceftriaxone; vancomycin; imipenem.
Streptococcus pyogenes	Penicillin G or V; oral first-generation cephalosporin; erythromycin.
Streptococcus sanguis	Penicillin/gentamicin; vancomycin/gentamicin/rifampin.
Gram-negative pyogenic bacteria (see Chapter 6)	
Bordetella pertussis	Erythromycin; TMP/SMX; ampicillin.
Haemophilus aegyptius	BPF strains: amoxicillin; amoxicillin/clavulanate; TMP/SMX; cefuroxime; cefixime. Other strains: neomycin/polymyxin.
Haemophilus ducreyi	Azithromycin; ceftriaxone.
Haemophilus influenzae	Ceftriaxone; cefotaxime; amoxicillin/clavulanate; oral second- or third-generation cephalosporin; macrolide; ampicillin/sulbactam.
Haemophilus parainfluenzae	Ceftriaxone; cefotaxime; amoxicillin/clavulanate; oral second- or third-generation cephalosporin; macrolide; ampicillin/sulbactam.
Moraxella catarrhalis	Amoxicillin/clavulanate; oral second- or third-generation cephalosporin; azithromycin; TMP/SMX.
Neisseria gonorrhoeae	Ceftriaxone; cefotaxime; ceftizoxime; amoxicillin/probenecid.
Neisseria meningitidis	Penicillin; ceftriaxone.
Enterobacteriaceae and associated bacteria (see Chapter 7)	
Campylobacter fetus subspecies *fetus*	Imipenem; gentamicin.
Campylobacter jejuni	Fluoroquinolone; erythromycin.
Citrobacter species	Imipenem; fluoroquinolone; antipseudomonal aminoglycoside.
Edwardsiella species	Ampicillin.
Enterobacter species	Imipenem; antipseudomonal penicillin/antipseudomonal aminoglycoside.
Escherichia coli	Ampicillin/gentamicin; TMP/SMX; fluoroquinolone; third-generation cephalosporin; ticarcillin/clavulanate; antipseudomonal penicillin/antipseudomonal aminoglycoside.
Hafnia species	Antipseudomonal aminoglycoside; imipenem.
Helicobacter pylori	Metronidazole/amoxicillin/bismuth subsalicylate; metronidazole/tetracycline/bismuth subsalicylate.
Klebsiella species	Ozena and rhinoscleroma strains: rifampin/TMP/SMX. Other strains: parenteral third-generation cephalosporin; ciprofloxacin.
Morganella species	Imipenem; antipseudomonal aminoglycoside; fluoroquinolone.
Pantoea species	Antipseudomonal penicillin/antipseudomonal aminoglycoside; imipenem.
Proteus mirabilis	Ampicillin; TMP/SMX.
Proteus vulgaris	Parenteral third-generation cephalosporin; fluoroquinolone.
Providencia species	Amikacin; fluoroquinolone; TMP/SMX.
Salmonella serotype *typhi*	Amoxicillin; TMP/SMX; chloramphenicol; ciprofloxacin; third-generation cephalosporin.
Serratia marcescens	Gentamicin; parenteral third-generation cephalosporin; imipenem; fluoroquinolone.
Shigella species	Fluoroquinolone; TMP/SMX; ampicillin.
Yersinia enterocolitica	Parenteral third-generation cephalosporin/antipseudomonal aminoglycoside; doxycycline; TMP/SMX.
Yersinia pseudotuberculosis	Parenteral third-generation cephalosporin/antipseudomonal aminoglycoside; doxycycline; TMP/SMX.
Pseudomonadaceae (see Chapter 8)	
Burkholderia (Pseudomonas) cepacia	TMP/SMX; ceftazidime; ciprofloxacin.
Burkholderia (Pseudomonas) pseudomallei	Ceftazidime; wide variety of secondary options.
Pseudomonas aeruginosa	Antipseudomonal penicillin; parenteral antipseudomonal third-generation cephalosporin; imipenem; antipseudomonal aminoglycoside; beta-lactam antibiotic/antipseudomonal aminoglycoside.
Pseudomonas stutzeri	Wide variety of broad-spectrum antibiotics.
Stenotrophomonas (Xanthomonas) maltophilia	Chloramphenicol; minocycline; TMP/SMX; ticarcillin/clavulanate.

Continued

TABLE 4–2. Recommended Antibiotics for the Treatment of Diseases Caused by Bacteria (Continued)

Bacteria	Effective Antibiotic Treatments*
Funguslike bacteria (see Chapter 9)	
Actinomadura species	Streptomycin/TMP/SMX; streptomycin/dapsone.
Actinomyces israelii	Penicillin; ampicillin; doxycycline; ceftriaxone.
Mycobacterium avium-intracellulare	Clarithromycin/ethambutol; clarithromycin/clofazimine; clarithromycin/ciprofloxacin; rifabutin/ethambutol.
Mycobacterium kansasii	Rifampin/INH/ethambutol.
Mycobacterium leprae	Multiple drug regimen involving dapsone, clofazimine, rifampin, and ethionamide.
Mycobacterium marinum	Rifampin/ethambutol; minocycline; TMP/SMX.
Mycobacterium scrofulaceum	INH/rifampin/cycloserine; streptomycin/rifampin/cycloserine.
Mycobacterium tuberculosis	Multiple drug regimen involving primary and secondary drugs. Primary drugs include INH, rifampin, ethambutol, pyrazinamide, and streptomycin. Secondary drugs include amikacin, capreomycin, ciprofloxacin, clofazimine, dapsone, ethionamide, ofloxacin, PAS, and rifabutin.
Nocardia asteroides	High-dose sulfonamide; TMP/SMX; TMP/ceftriaxone/amikacin.
Nocardia brasiliensis	Amoxicillin/clavulanate; amikacin/ceftriaxone.
Streptomyces species	None (surgery required).
Tropheryma whippelii	Penicillin/streptomycin followed by tetracycline, chloramphenicol, or TMP/SMX.
Zoonotic bacteria (see Chapter 10)	
Brucella species	Tetracycline/streptomycin; doxycycline/rifampin; doxycycline; ceftriaxone/rifampin; streptomycin/doxycycline; streptomycin/minocycline.
Capnocytophaga species	Penicillin; amoxicillin; erythromycin; cefoxitin; clindamycin.
Erysipelothrix rhusiopathiae	Penicillin; ampicillin; first-generation cephalosporin.
Francisella tularensis	Streptomycin; gentamicin.
Listeria monocytogenes	Ampicillin; TMP/SMX.
Pasteurella multocida	Penicillin; doxycycline; amoxicillin/clavulanate.
Spirillum minus	Ampicillin; penicillin; streptomycin.
Streptobacillus moniliformis	Ampicillin; penicillin; streptomycin.
Yersinia pestis	Streptomycin; chloramphenicol; tetracycline; gentamicin.
Mycoplasmas, rickettsiae, and other unusual bacteria (see Chapter 11)	
Bartonella bacilliformis	Tetracycline; penicillin; chloramphenicol.
Bartonella (Rochalimaea) henselae	Rifampin; ciprofloxacin; gentamicin; TMP/SMX; erythromycin; doxycycline.
Bartonella (Rochalimaea) quintana	Tetracycline; many secondary options.
Chlamydia pneumoniae	Tetracycline; doxycycline.
Chlamydia psittaci	A tetracycline.
Chlamydia trachomatis	Doxycycline; azithromycin; erythromycin; fluoroquinolone; sulfisoxazole.
Coxiella burnetii	Acute infection: doxycycline. Chronic infection: fluoroquinolone; fluoroquinolone/rifampin.
Ehrlichia species	A tetracycline.
Mycoplasma fermentans	No recommendation.
Mycoplasma hominis	Erythromycin; doxycycline.
Mycoplasma pneumoniae	Macrolide; doxycycline.
Rickettsia akari	A tetracycline; chloramphenicol.
Rickettsia prowazekii	Doxycycline; chloramphenicol.
Rickettsia rickettsii	Chloramphenicol; doxycycline.
Rickettsia tsutsugamushi	A tetracycline; chloramphenicol.
Rickettsia typhi	Doxycycline; chloramphenicol.
Ureaplasma urealyticum	Erythromycin; doxycycline.
Spirochetes (see Chapter 12)	
Borrelia burgdorferi	Doxycycline; amoxicillin; ceftriaxone.
Borrelia hermsii	Doxycycline; erythromycin; penicillin.
Borrelia recurrentis	Doxycycline; erythromycin; penicillin.
Leptospira interrogans	Doxycycline; penicillin.
Treponema carateum	Penicillin.
Treponema pallidum	Penicillin; penicillin/probenecid.
Legionellae (see Chapter 13)	
Legionella species	Erythromycin; erythromycin/rifampin; extended-spectrum macrolide; tetracycline; doxycycline.
Toxigenic bacteria (see Chapter 14)	
Aeromonas hydrophila	Rehydration/fluoroquinolone.
Arcanobacterium haemolyticum	Penicillin G; erythromycin.
Bacillus anthracis	Penicillin G or V; ciprofloxacin; doxycycline; erythromycin.
Bacillus cereus	None (rehydration required).
Clostridium botulinum	Antitoxin.

Continued

TABLE 4–2. Recommended Antibiotics for the Treatment of Diseases Caused by Bacteria *(Continued)*

Bacteria	Effective Antibiotic Treatments*
Toxigenic bacteria *(continued)*	
Clostridium difficile	Metronidazole; vancomycin.
Clostridium perfringens	Penicillin/surgery.
Clostridium septicum	Penicillin.
Clostridium tetani	Antitoxin/surgery/penicillin/toxoid; antitoxin/surgery/metronidazole/toxoid.
Corynebacterium diphtheriae	Erythromycin/antitoxin; penicillin/antitoxin.
Corynebacterium jeikeium	Vancomycin; ciprofloxacin.
Corynebacterium minutissimum	Erythromycin.
Plesiomonas shigelloides	Fluoroquinolone; TMP/SMX.
Vibrio cholerae	Rehydration/TMP/SMX; rehydration/fluoroquinolone; rehydration/tetracycline.
Vibrio fluvialis	None (rehydration required).
Vibrio mimicus	Rehydration/tetracycline; rehydration/fluoroquinolone.
Vibrio parahaemolyticus	Rehydration/tetracycline; rehydration/fluoroquinolone.
Vibrio vulnificus	Tetracycline/antipseudomonal aminoglycoside; doxycycline/ceftazidime.
Nonsporulating anaerobic bacteria (see Chapter 15)	
Bacteroides fragilis	Metronidazole; clindamycin; cefoxitin; imipenem; cefmetazole; cefotetan; penicillin/beta-lactamase inhibitor.
Bifidobacterium species	Penicillin; clindamycin.
Eubacterium species	Ampicillin; penicillin.
Fusobacterium necrophorum	Penicillin; clindamycin; third-generation cephalosporin; cephamycin.
Fusobacterium nucleatum	Penicillin; clindamycin; third-generation cephalosporin; cephamycin.
Gemella species	Penicillin; clindamycin.
Lactobacillus species	Ampicillin; penicillin; clindamycin; chloramphenicol.
Mobiluncus species	No recommendation.
Peptostreptococcus species	Penicillin; clindamycin.
Porphyromonas species	Metronidazole; clindamycin; cefotaxime; cefoperazone; ampicillin/sulbactam.
Prevotella melaninogenica	Metronidazole; clindamycin; cefoxitin; ampicillin.
Propionibacterium species	Penicillin; ampicillin; third-generation cephalosporin; cephamycin.
Streptococcus species	Penicillin; vancomycin; ampicillin.
Veillonella species	Metronidazole; ampicillin; cefoxitin.

*Antibiotics are listed in their general order of recommended use, with the drug or drug combination used most often listed first. Antibiotics used in combination are separated by the symbol /, such as the combination of penicillin and gentamicin, which is listed as penicillin/gentamicin. Abbreviations are as follows: INH = isoniazid, or isonicotinic acid hydrazide; PAS = aminosalicylate sodium, or *p*-aminosalicylate; TMP = trimethoprim; and SMX = sulfamethoxazole.
†Some strains of *E. faecium* are unresponsive to treatment.

Agents That Inhibit Cell Wall Synthesis

Without doubt, the most important antibiotics have been those that inhibit cell wall synthesis. These antibiotics include the **beta-lactam antibiotics** (carbapenems, cephalosporins, cephamycins, monobactams, and penicillins), the **glycopeptide antibiotics** (teicoplanin and vancomycin), and the antibiotics **bacitracin** and **cycloserine.**

As described in Chapter 1, cell wall synthesis involves the construction of an *N*-acetylglucosamine-*N*-acetylmuramic acid (GlcNAc-MurNAc) disaccharide unit that is attached to a bactoprenol lipid carrier molecule in the cytoplasmic membrane (see Figs. 1–12 and 1–13). Autolytic enzymes open sites in the cell wall where the new disaccharide units will be placed. The bactoprenol donates its GlcNAc-MurNAc moiety to the peptidoglycan growth site, and the newly donated disaccharide unit is attached to the sacculus via β1,4-glycosidic bonds. Transpeptidase enzymes then cross-link the peptide of the newly inserted GlcNAc-MurNAc to that of another GlcNAc-MurNAc (see Fig. 1–14). As this happens, the bactoprenyl diphosphate carrier is dephosphorylated to provide a bactoprenyl monophosphate capable of receiving a new GlcNAc-MurNAc unit (see Fig. 1–12). The key targets of antibiotic action in this process are (1) the transfer of the GlcNAc-MurNAc molecule from the lipid carrier to the growing peptidoglycan chain, (2) the transpeptidation reaction, and (3) the dephosphorylation of bactoprenyl diphosphate to regenerate the carrier. The **glycopeptide antibiotics** inhibit transfer of the disaccharide to the wall growth site; **beta-lactam antibiotics, glycopeptide antibiotics,** and **cycloserine** inhibit the transpeptidation reaction (albeit by different mechanisms); and **bacitracin** blocks dephosphorylation of the lipid carrier.

Antibiotics that block cell wall synthesis are lytic in most bacteria. This is because autolytic enzymes continue to cleave the peptidoglycan sacculus even when GlcNAc-MurNAc units are not being inserted or cross-linked. In fact, it appears that cellular autolysins are activated by at least some beta-lactam antibiotics. Thus, when these antibiotics are present, autolysins continue to weaken the peptidoglycan sacculus until osmotic pressure makes the wall first bulge and then burst.

Beta-Lactam Antibiotics

The beta-lactam antibiotics derive their name from the fact that each has a **beta-lactam ring** that is the active site of the antibiotic. The beta-lactam ring acts as an analogue of acyl-D-alanine-D-alanine and binds tightly to the active site of transpeptidase enzymes that catalyze the transpeptidation of MurNAc units within the cell wall. Transpeptidation is important because cross-linking completes the murein sacculus and provides it with the tensile strength needed to resist osmotic lysis.

The enzymes that bind beta-lactam antibiotics are known as **penicillin-binding proteins** (PBPs) because they were initially identified by their ability to complex with various penicillins. PBPs are a diverse group of transpeptidases and carboxypeptidases, each involved in a different aspect of cell wall synthesis. In *Escherichia coli,* PBP-1a and PBP-1b elongate the cylinder of the rod, while PBP-2 establishes the rod shape of the bacterium. Beta-lactam antibiotics that bind to PBP-1a and PBP-1b cause *E. coli* to lyse rapidly, while those that preferentially bind to PBP-2 cause the bacteria to round up before they lyse. PBP-3 constructs the septum in dividing *E. coli,* and sublethal concentrations of beta-lactams that bind to this enzyme cause *E. coli* to grow as long filaments. PBP-1, PBP-2, and PBP-3 are double-headed enzymes with two active sites; one head is a transglycosylase, and the other is a transpeptidase. PBP-4, PBP-5, and PBP-6 are D,D-carboxypeptidases that cleave the terminal D-alanine during cell wall synthesis to allow the subterminal D-alanine to participate in the cross-link.

Each beta-lactam antibiotic preferentially binds to certain PBPs. For example, **amdinocillin** (a carbapenem also known as **pivmecillinam**) inhibits the action of PBP-2, whereas **aztreonam** (a monobactam) has PBP-3 as its target. Each bacterium has its own mix of PBPs. The type and amount of PBPs present will determine whether the bacterium is resistant or susceptible to a particular beta-lactam antibiotic.

Two classes of **autolysins** seem to be responsible for the lytic action of beta-lactam antibiotics. **Amidases** split the bonds between tetrapeptides and the glycan, while **glycosidases** cleave the β1,4-glycosidic bonds between disaccharide units. These enzymes are activated when cell wall synthesis is incomplete, and mutant strains that lack these enzymes are not lysed by beta-lactam antibiotics. Because the growth of these mutant strains is inhibited but there is no lysis, the strains are said to be tolerant of beta-lactam antibiotics.

Four groups of beta-lactam antibiotics are discussed below: natural penicillins; semisynthetic penicillins and analogues; two penicillinlike antibiotics (the carbapenems and the monobactams); and cephalosporins, cephamycins, and related antibiotics.

Natural Penicillins.   Fig. 4–2 shows the structures of penicillin G and penicillin V, which are natural penicillins.

(1) Penicillin G.   The penicillin discovered in 1929 by Alexander Fleming and subsequently developed by H. W. Florey and E. B. Chain was penicillin G. As Fig. 4–2 shows, its nucleus is a double-ring structure consisting of a thiazolidine ring and a beta-lactam ring, and the phenylacetic acid is attached to the beta-lactam ring via a peptide bond. The active site of the penicillin is the beta-lactam ring. When a

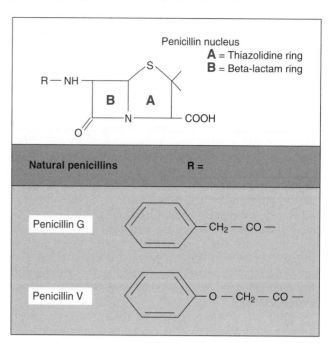

FIGURE 4–2. Structures of the natural penicillins G and V.

molecule of penicillin encounters a PBP, the bond between the CO and N in the beta-lactam ring is broken, and the transpeptidase binds covalently to the CO. This makes the transpeptidase unavailable for peptidoglycan synthesis, and the cross-linking of peptidoglycan is halted. The accumulation of non–cross-linked peptidoglycan precursors further activates autolytic enzymes, and the combination of lack of cross-linking and heightened autolysin activity makes the bacterium osmotically fragile.

Penicillin G has primarily been used as treatment against gram-positive bacteria such as pneumococci, staphylococci, and streptococci. It has also been used to treat infections caused by *Neisseria gonorrhoeae* and *Neisseria meningitidis,* which are gram-negative organisms. Unfortunately, infections caused by many of these bacteria cannot today be reliably treated with penicillin G, because so many isolates have acquired mechanisms to resist the action of penicillin G (see Bacterial Resistance to Beta-Lactam Antibiotics, below).

The beta-lactam ring of penicillin G is strained, making it sensitive to acid hydrolysis. Only about one-fifth of a dose of penicillin G is absorbed, so penicillin G is not a good candidate for oral administration. For this reason, it is commonly administered parenterally (by injection).

The penicillin G mixtures available commercially are excellent allergens. The allergenic component consists not of the penicillin G itself but of the many incomplete penicillin molecules present in the mixture. Some molecules arise from spontaneous degradation of penicillin G during storage, while others are incomplete molecules excreted by the fungus. These molecules act as haptens on serum proteins and can elicit a vigorous immune response.

The most dramatic **immune responses to peni-**

cillin are IgE-mediated, and they range from a wheal and flare at the injection site to massive and immediate systemic **anaphylaxis** resulting in death within seconds after administering the antibiotic. Early exposures may elicit milder reactions, such as hives, asthma, and itching, but systemic anaphylaxis may occur as early as the second or third exposure to penicillin. Systemic anaphylaxis is a terrifying situation. For this reason, physicians commonly ask about the patient's history of reactions to penicillin, have the patient wait in the office for some time after receiving an injection of penicillin, and keep the appropriate emergency equipment and drugs on hand at all times. IgE reactions require that IgE be elicited by a primary exposure and be attached to mast cells in the subcutaneous tissues. This means that a patient never before exposed to penicillin cannot have an IgE-mediated reaction. It is critical to understand, however, that *all* penicillins are cross-sensitizing and cross-reacting.

Not all adverse reactions to penicillin are IgE-mediated. Patients may suffer from **serum sickness–type reactions** with urticaria, pruritus, joint swelling, and respiratory problems up to 12 days after receiving an injection of penicillin, and these reactions can occur following the first exposure to penicillin. Some patients develop an IgG-mediated hemolytic anemia due to complement-mediated lysis of erythrocytes that are coated with penicillin molecules. Nurses, pharmacy workers, and other individuals who frequently handle penicillins may develop a form of contact dermatitis that represents a cell-mediated immune response and is similar in appearance and mechanism to allergic dermatitis following exposure to poison ivy.

Because an estimated 1–5% of adults are allergic to penicillins, each patient must be questioned carefully about a possible history of **penicillin allergy.** If a patient has an uncertain history and it is important that penicillin be administered, the patient can undergo testing for IgE-mediated sensitivity by intradermally injecting a tiny amount of one of several commercially available preparations of penicillin breakdown products. If the patient is allergic to penicillin, he or she will develop a wheal and flare reaction. This procedure is dangerous, however, and another type of antibiotic can usually be substituted to treat the infection. If the patient is penicillin-allergic and the choice is between penicillin administration and death, the patient can be desensitized by sequential oral or parenteral administration of small penicillin doses over several hours.

It appears that about 5% of patients allergic to penicillins are also allergic to **cephalosporins.** Patients with non–IgE-mediated hypersensitivity to penicillins can be treated with a cephalosporin, but patients with IgE-mediated penicillin allergy should not be given a cephalosporin, because of the severity of adverse reactions.

(2) Penicillin V. During the 1950s, investigators discovered that the type of penicillin excreted by *Penicillium* varied with the constituents of the growth medium. By supplementing the medium with any of a variety of organic acids, they were able to produce different types of penicillins. While penicillin G was produced by a medium containing phenylacetic acid, penicillin V was produced by a medium containing phenoxymethyl donors. Penicillin V represented a major advance because it was much more stable than penicillin G in stomach acid. Thus, unlike penicillin G, which had to be administered parenterally, penicillin V could be given orally. Today, penicillin V is widely used in pediatric care.

Semisynthetic Penicillins and Analogues. The discoveries about the medium in which *Penicillium* was grown led to the idea that penicillins with a wide variety of new properties could be developed by changing the penicillin R groups. Investigators soon found that a highly reactive precursor of penicillin, 6-aminopenicillanic acid, could be obtained either by treating penicillin G with an amidase (Fig. 4–3) or by growing *Penicillium* in a medium that contained no acyl donors. Any of an almost infinite number of synthetically generated organic acids could then be fused with 6-aminopenicillanic acid to produce semisynthetic penicillins.

At least three major goals drove the development of semisynthetic penicillins. First, there was a desire to produce more acid-stable penicillins that could be administered orally, rather than parenterally. Infections treatable with penicillins occur most commonly in young children, and oral administration is less objectionable to the children and their parents. Second, some bacterial strains that originally had been susceptible to penicillin therapy later became resistant to it. This **acquired resistance** was due to the ability of bacteria to produce an enzyme (a penicillinase) that inactivates penicillin G by cleaving the beta-lactam ring. **Penicillinase enzymes** are now known to be members of a large group of **beta-lactamase enzymes** that inactivate a wide variety of beta-lactam antibiotics. Investigators sought to attach R groups onto penicillins that would protect the penicillin from beta-lactamase hydrolysis but allow the antibiotic to reach its target transpeptidase. Third, penicillin G and V had a fairly narrow spectrum of activity. While they were effective against many gram-positive organisms, they were only effective against a handful of gram-negative organisms. Investigators searched for R group substitutions that would allow penicillins to kill gram-negative enteric rods and *Pseudomonas aeruginosa.*

Three groups of semisynthetic penicillins were subsequently developed: penicillinase-resistant penicillins, extended-spectrum penicillins, and antipseudomonal penicillins.

(1) Penicillinase-Resistant Penicillins. To treat emerging strains of staphylococci that were resistant to penicillin G, a series of penicillinase-resistant penicillins were designed. The series (Fig. 4–4) includes **methicillin, nafcillin,** and the **isoxazolyl penicillins (oxacillin, cloxacillin, dicloxacillin,** and **flucloxacillin).** These penicillins are more toxic and less active than penicillin G, but they resist being hydrolyzed

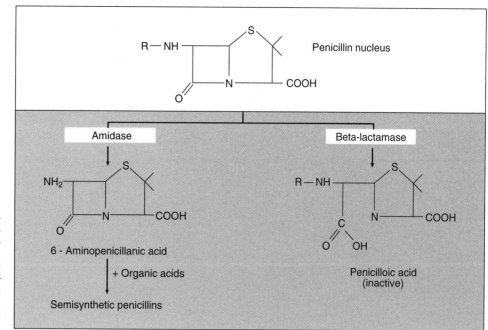

FIGURE 4–3. Enzymatic alteration of the structure of penicillin. Amidases can be used to create 6-aminopenicillanic acid, which can be fused with organic acids to synthesize semisynthetic penicillins. Many bacteria produce beta-lactamases, which inactivate penicillins by cleaving the beta-lactam ring.

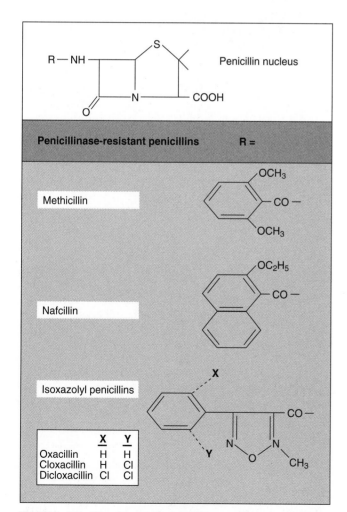

FIGURE 4–4. Structures of penicillinase-resistant penicillins. These semisynthetic penicillins were created for the treatment of staphylococcal infections.

by the beta-lactamases of staphylococci. Although methicillin has been the mainstay of therapy against staphylococci, its usefulness has decreased with the expanding presence of methicillin-resistant *Staphylococcus aureus.*

(2) **Extended-Spectrum Penicillins.** A second group of semisynthetic penicillins was developed to extend the spectrum of penicillins to include gram-negative bacteria. This group (Fig. 4–5) includes the **aminopenicillins (ampicillin, amoxicillin, and bacampicillin)** and **amdinocillin (pivmecillinam).**

The aminopenicillins are effective against many gram-negative bacteria and are about one-half as effective against gram-positive bacteria as is penicillin G. Their amino group allows them to readily traverse the negatively charged outer membrane of gram-negative bacteria. Thus, they are excellent broad-spectrum penicillins. They are also acid-stable and can be administered orally. Their principal limitations are that they are readily hydrolyzed by beta-lactamases and that they are not effective against *P. aeruginosa.* The aminopenicillins are effective against non–beta-lactamase–producing strains of *E. coli, Haemophilus influenzae, Proteus, Salmonella,* and *Shigella.*

Amdinocillin is unusual in that it is extremely active against *E. coli, Enterobacter,* and *Klebsiella* but is relatively inactive against gram-positive bacteria. Studies have shown that the dose of amdinocillin needed to kill some gram-positive bacteria is 60 times as high as that needed to kill *E. coli.* Amdinocillin is inactive against *P. aeruginosa.*

(3) **Antipseudomonal Penicillins.** Three types of penicillins have been developed to attack *P. aeruginosa:* the **carboxypenicillins,** the **piperazine penicillins,** and the **ureidopenicillins.**

Carbenicillin and **ticarcillin** (Fig. 4–6), which are

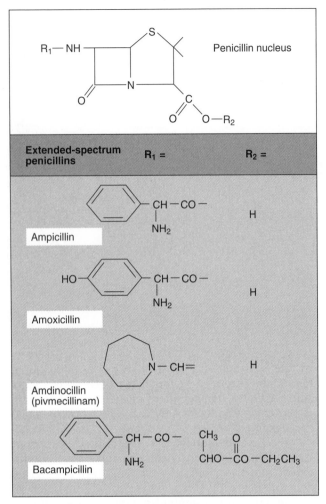

FIGURE 4–5. Structures of extended-spectrum penicillins. These semisynthetic aminopenicillins were created for the treatment of infections caused by gram-negative bacteria. Although they have a broader spectrum of activity than their predecessors, they are sensitive to inactivation by beta-lactamases.

carboxypenicillins, were the first antipseudomonal penicillins. They are not effective against gram-positive bacteria but have excellent activity against gram-negative enteric rods and *Pseudomonas*. The piperazine penicillins, such as **piperacillin,** and the ureidopenicillins, such as **mezlocillin** and **azlocillin,** are even more effective than the carboxypenicillins against enteric bacteria and *Pseudomonas,* owing to their greater affinity for gram-negative PBPs, and they are also more effective than the carboxypenicillins in treating gram-positive infections. Unfortunately, the antipseudomonal penicillins are sensitive to beta-lactamases, must be administered parenterally, and are generally more toxic than are their predecessors.

(4) Combinations and Analogues. Any discussion of extended-spectrum and antipseudomonal penicillins must address two schemes that have extended the usefulness of these antibiotics.

The first scheme involves administering antipseudomonal penicillins with aminoglycoside antibiotics. The aminoglycosides are relatively toxic antibiotics that inhibit protein synthesis and are most

effective against gram-negative rods. Their efficacy is directly proportional to the amount of the antibiotic that accumulates within a susceptible bacterium. Even if an infection caused by a gram-negative rod is relatively insensitive to treatment with either a penicillin or an aminoglycoside, it may respond well to a combination of the two antibiotics, which act synergistically when administered together. It is believed that the penicillin increases the permeability of the bacterium for the aminoglycoside and that the aminoglycoside is the bactericidal agent. This synergistic activity allows the aminoglycoside to be administered at a concentration well below its toxic threshold for the patient.

The second scheme centers around the development of penicillinlike molecules that have relatively little antibacterial activity but can inactivate beta-

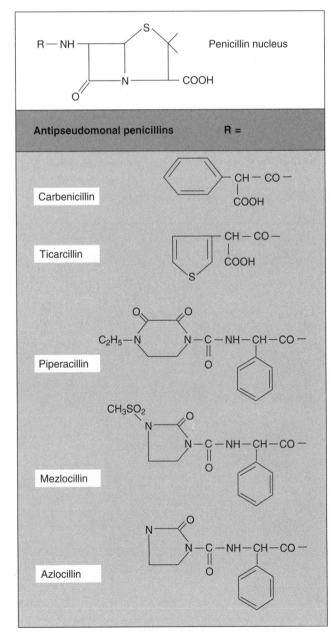

FIGURE 4–6. Structures of antipseudomonal penicillins.

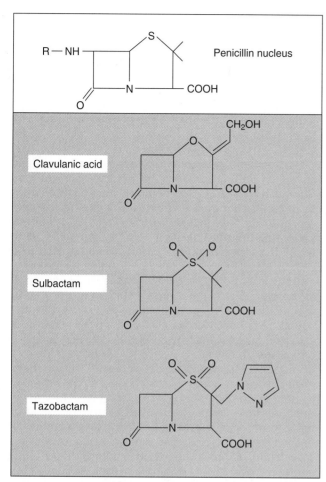

FIGURE 4–7. Structures of clavulanic acid, sulbactam, and tazobactam. These penicillin analogues have poor antibacterial activity but are excellent competitive inhibitors of most beta-lactamases. They are given in combination with broad-spectrum penicillins to treat infections caused by penicillinase-producing bacteria.

lactamases. It appears that the beta-lactamase cleaves the beta-lactam ring of the penicillin analogue but then forms a stable but inactive complex with the cleaved beta-lactam ring—a mechanism known as suicide inactivation. Three **penicillin analogues** are commercially available: **clavulanic acid, sulbactam,** and **tazobactam** (Fig. 4–7). Clavulanic acid is excreted by *Streptomyces clavuligerus,* and sulbactam is synthesized from 6-aminopenicillanic acid. Currently available combinations of penicillin and analogue include ampicillin/sulbactam, amoxicillin/clavulanate, ticarcillin/clavulanate, and piperacillin/tazobactam. The ampicillin/sulbactam and amoxicillin/clavulanate combinations, for example, each extend the spectrum of action to include beta-lactamase–producing strains of *Bacteroides fragilis, Enterobacter, E. coli, Haemophilus ducreyi, H. influenzae, Klebsiella, Moraxella catarrhalis, N. gonorrhoeae, Proteus, Providencia, Staphylococcus epidermidis,* and methicillin-sensitive *S. aureus.*

Other Penicillinlike Antibiotics. Two newer classes of penicillinlike antibiotics were developed by investigators using radically different approaches to create antibiotics that retained the beta-lactam

ring but looked very different from standard penicillins. These antibiotics are known as carbapenems and monobactams.

(1) Carbapenems. Carbapenems are derived synthetically from thienamycin, an antibiotic that is produced by the bacterium *Streptomyces cattleya.* Although thienamycin is not itself suitable for human use, one of its formimidoyl derivatives, known as **imipenem,** has proved to be the broadest-spectrum beta-lactam antibiotic now available. Carbapenems have a double-ring structure that includes a beta-lactam ring, but the five-membered ring retains a C instead of an S at position 1, and the ring is unsaturated (Fig. 4–8). Imipenem inhibits transpeptidation by binding tightly to PBP-1 and PBP-2. It is stable in the presence of most beta-lactamases, including chromosomal class I beta-lactamases that degrade third-generation cephalosporins.

Imipenem penetrates well into gram-negative bacteria and is active against anaerobes. Thus, it is active against beta-lactamase–producing strains of *Acinetobacter, Listeria, N. gonorrhoeae, N. meningitidis, P. aeruginosa, Streptococcus pneumoniae,* gram-negative enteric rods, and a variety of strict anaerobes. It is not effective, however, against *Burkholderia (Pseudomonas) cepacia, Enterococcus faecium, Stenotrophomonas (Xanthomonas) maltophilia,* or obligately intracellular bacteria. It appears that the resistance of *Stenotrophomonas* to imipenem is due to the production of a unique beta-lactamase. Although often not effective as a cidal agent against *Enterococcus faecalis,* imipenem acts as a static agent against this organism.

Imipenem induces the expression of chromosomal class I beta-lactamases. This is not a problem

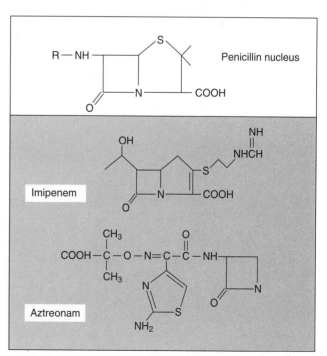

FIGURE 4–8. Structures of imipenem and aztreonam, two penicillinlike antibiotics.

when imipenem is administered alone, because it is not degraded by these enzymes. There can be a problem, however, when it is administered with a cephalosporin, because class I beta-lactamases can inactivate all cephalosporins and are not themselves inactivated by clavulanate or sulbactam.

The spectrum of imipenem can be augmented by administering it in combination with an aminoglycoside. Imipenem is inactivated in the brush border of the proximal renal tubular cells by dehydropeptidase-1. Cilastatin, a specific inhibitor of dehydropeptidase-1, is administered with imipenem at a 1 : 1 ratio to block inactivation of imipenem and to decrease the risk of renal tubular necrosis. Imipenem/cilastatin should not be administered to individuals who have central nervous system lesions (such as strokes or head injuries), a history of convulsions, or renal insufficiency, since reports indicate that 12–32% of these patients develop convulsions as a consequence of receiving this form of treatment. Because of its propensity for eliciting seizures in these patients and because of its cost, imipenem is generally reserved for use in patients who are gravely ill with nosocomial infections caused by multiple pathogens.

Meropenem, another carbapenem, has recently been approved for use in the USA. Although it is similar to imipenem in its spectrum of activity, it can be administered without cilastatin and carries a lower risk of causing seizures.

(2) Monobactams. The first monobactam antibiotic is **aztreonam** (see Fig. 4–8). Monobactams are so named because they have only a single ring, with the central nucleus being the totally synthetic 3-aminobactamic acid. In contrast to imipenem, aztreonam is a narrow-spectrum antibiotic. It inhibits cell division by binding to PBP-3, and it binds poorly or not at all to the PBPs of gram-positive bacteria and anaerobes. In the presence of aztreonam, gram-negative bacteria first grow as elongated filaments and later die. Aztreonam is stable in the presence of many gram-negative beta-lactamases, but it is inactivated by plasmid-encoded beta-lactamases that inactivate the third-generation cephalosporins cefotaxime and ceftazidime—namely, the TEM-3, TEM-5, TEM-7, and SHV-2 beta-lactamases.

The spectrum of aztreonam is sometimes effectively expanded by combining it with a gram-positive penicillin (such as nafcillin or cloxacillin) or with an aminoglycoside. Aztreonam is effective against *N. gonorrhoeae, N. meningitidis, P. aeruginosa,* and most gram-negative enteric bacteria. It appears that patients allergic to penicillins are not allergic to aztreonam.

Cephalosporins, Cephamycins, and Related Antibiotics. The cephalosporins and their relatives, the cephamycins, constitute the largest group of beta-lactam antibiotics. Cephalosporins are semisynthetic derivatives of 7-aminocephalosporanic acid, which contains a beta-lactam ring and a six-membered dihydrothiazine ring (Fig. 4–9).

Up to three R groups are attached to each cephalosporin. The R_1 group is attached at the same site as the R group of penicillins, and variations in this group affect the antibacterial activity of the antibiotic as well as its stability in the presence of specific beta-lactamases. The R_2 group, which is attached to position 3 of the dihydrothiazine ring, influences the metabolism and pharmacokinetic properties of the drug. A few cephalosporins and all cephamycins have a third R group attached to the beta-lactam ring. This R_3 group makes the antibiotic more resistant to the action of most beta-lactamases.

The cephalosporin nucleus, 7-aminocephalosporanic acid, is excreted by the mold *Cephalosporium acremonium.* The cephamycins, which differ from cephalosporins by having a 7α-methoxy group, are each derived semisynthetically from a different source. **Cefoxitin** is derived from cephamycin C, **cefotetan** from organomycin G, and **cefmetazole** from 7-aminocephalosporanic acid. Cephalosporins are resistant to the action of penicillinases, and some cephalosporins (third-generation cephalosporins) resist inactivation by all beta-lactamases except chromosomal class I beta-lactamases and a newly described class of plasmid-encoded beta-lactamases found in only a few bacteria.

Cephalosporins are divided into three major groups (or "generations") according to their efficacy against gram-negative bacteria. Some recently developed cephalosporins have been touted as constituting a fourth major group, but this classification has not yet gained widespread acceptance. Examples of the structural variations that produce the different cephalosporin generations are presented in Fig. 4–9, and the members of each cephalosporin generation are listed in Table 4–1.

(1) First-Generation Cephalosporins. The earliest cephalosporins developed were the first-generation cephalosporins. These antibiotics are effective primarily against a group of gram-positive bacteria that includes pneumococci, streptococci, *Clostridium perfringens, Corynebacterium diphtheriae, S. epidermidis,* and methicillin-sensitive *S. aureus.* They are not effective against another group of gram-positive bacteria that resist the actions of all generations of cephalosporins and that include *E. faecalis, Listeria monocytogenes,* and methicillin-resistant *S. aureus.* First-generation cephalosporins are also ineffective against beta-lactamase–producing strains of *S. pneumoniae.* The clinically relevant spectrum of activity of first-generation cephalosporins against gram-negative bacteria is limited to the enteric rods *E. coli, Klebsiella,* and *Proteus mirabilis.* Most orally administered cephalosporins are from the first-generation group.

(2) Second-Generation Cephalosporins. The second-generation cephalosporins are more extensively modified than are the first-generation cephalosporins. Additionally, most cephamycins are considered to be analogous to second-generation cephalosporins. The second-generation cephalosporins are more active against gram-negative bacteria, and their efficacy against gram-positive bacteria is comparable to or only slightly less than that of the

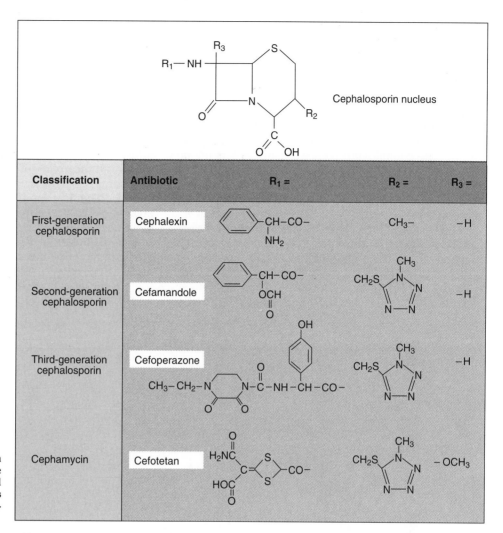

FIGURE 4–9. The cephalosporin nucleus and examples of the structures of first-, second-, and third-generation cephalosporins and the structure of a cephamycin.

first-generation cephalosporins. **Cefuroxime** has proved to be highly effective against beta-lactamase–producing strains of *H. influenzae* and *N. meningitidis,* two important causes of meningitis in children. Additionally, **cefotetan** and **cefoxitin** are effective against *N. gonorrhoeae,* including penicillinase-producing strains. The cephamycin cefotetan has proved to be so effective against gram-negative enteric rods (such as *E. coli, Klebsiella,* and *Proteus*) that many consider it to be a third-generation antibiotic. Second-generation cephalosporins are not, however, generally recommended for use in treating infections caused by gram-positive bacteria, because they are more expensive than first-generation cephalosporins, most of them have to be administered parenterally, and they offer no clinical advantage over first-generation cephalosporins. Second-generation cephalosporins are not effective against *P. aeruginosa.*

(3) Third-Generation Cephalosporins. Third-generation cephalosporins are highly resistant to the actions of beta-lactamases because of their large and unusual R groups (see Fig. 4–9 for an example). Although third-generation cephalosporins have the widest spectrum of activity of all cephalosporins against gram-negative bacteria, they have the poor-

est coverage against gram-positive bacteria. In general, third-generation cephalosporins are highly effective agents against the following gram-negative organisms: *N. gonorrhoeae* (including penicillinase-producing strains), *N. meningitidis, H. influenzae, M. catarrhalis,* and most enteric bacteria (including many *Citrobacter* strains, *E. coli, Klebsiella, Morganella, Proteus, Providencia, Salmonella,* and *Shigella*). Their excellent efficacy against these organisms is due to their strong affinity for gram-negative PBPs and to their unusual resistance to inactivation by beta-lactamases. Third-generation cephalosporins are inactivated by chromosomal class I beta-lactamases (produced by some *Citrobacter, Enterobacter,* and *Pseudomonas* strains), but they resist inactivation by most other beta-lactamases. **Ceftazidime** has the strongest activity against *P. aeruginosa,* with **cefoperazone** also having moderate antipseudomonal activity.

(4) "Fourth-Generation" Cephalosporins. The most recently developed group of cephalosporins includes **cefepime** and **cefpirome.** Although these drugs are similar to the third-generation cephalosporins in activity against gram-negative bacteria, they are roughly similar to the first-generation

cephalosporins in efficacy against some of the gram-positive bacteria. Some clinicians and pharmaceutical firms have dubbed the newest antibiotics "fourth-generation" cephalosporins, but others consider them to be third-generation cephalosporins with extended gram-positive coverage. The newest antibiotics also have lower affinity for class I beta-lactamases than do the third-generation cephalosporins.

(5) Moxalactam and Loracarbef. Closely related to the cephalosporins are the antibiotics moxalactam and loracarbef (Fig. 4–10). Moxalactam differs from the cephalosporins by having an oxygen at position 1 of the six-membered ring, while loracarbef has a carbon at the same site. Thus, moxalactam is an **oxacepham,** and loracarbef is a **carbacepham.** Moxalactam is similar to third-generation cephalosporins in its spectrum of activity, but it is rarely chosen for treatment because its use has been associated with bleeding abnormalities. Moreover, it is no longer available in the USA. Loracarbef is an oral antibiotic that is similar to some oral first- and second-generation cephalosporins in its spectrum of activity. It is used mainly to treat acute otitis media in pediatric patients.

Bacterial Resistance to Beta-Lactam Antibiotics. Bacterial resistance to beta-lactam antibiotics may be acquired via mutation of a chromosomal gene or transfer of a plasmid. Chromosomally mediated changes in sensitivity to beta-lactam antibiotics generally involve alterations in permeability to the antibiotics or in the ability of PBPs to recognize antibiotics, but some beta-lactamases are chromosomally encoded. Plasmid-encoded resistance to beta-lactams always involves the introduction of a beta-lactamase gene.

(1) Changes in Permeability of the Bacterium. Bacteria may become less permeable to beta-lactam antibiotics as a consequence of changes in outer membrane porins or lipopolysaccharide. The gram-negative outer membrane is asymmetric, with porins

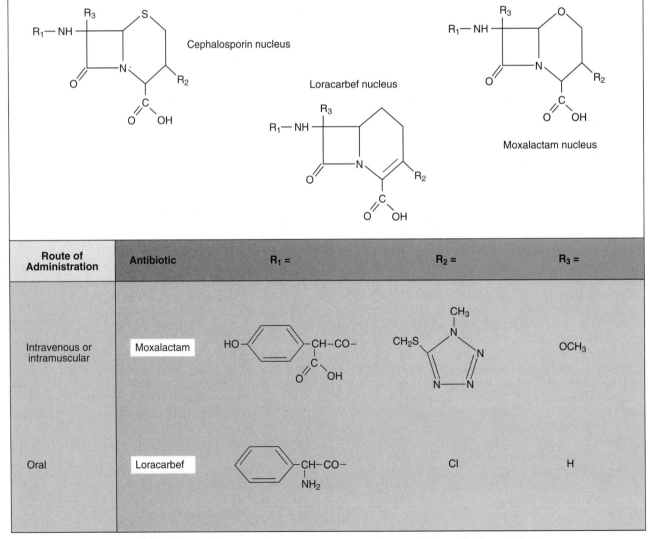

FIGURE 4–10. Structures of moxalactam and loracarbef, two cephalosporinlike antibiotics.

Route of Administration	Antibiotic	R₁ =	R₂ =	R₃ =
Intravenous or intramuscular	Moxalactam			OCH₃
Oral	Loracarbef		Cl	H

and lipopolysaccharide inserted in the outer leaflet. *E. coli* has about 1×10^5 porin molecules per cell, and these can exist as either large (OmpF) or small (OmpC) channels. When an *E. coli* outer membrane is populated primarily with OmpC channels, carbenicillin and other drugs that usually penetrate slowly will be essentially unable to enter the bacterium. In contrast to *E. coli* isolates, *Enterobacter cloacae* and *P. aeruginosa* isolates vary significantly in their susceptibility to penicillins following changes in their lipopolysaccharide composition.

(2) Effects of Beta-Lactamases. The single most troublesome antibiotic resistance mechanism has been that of beta-lactamases. A beta-lactamase is an enzyme that binds to a beta-lactam antibiotic noncovalently, forms a covalent bond, hydrolyzes the cyclic amide bond of the lactam ring, and then releases the altered (inactive) antibiotic. The beta-lactamases compete with PBPs for beta-lactam antibiotics. To date, more than 80 beta-lactamases have been described, each with its own patterns of specificity, affinity, and so forth. Although the beta-lactamases are widely distributed among gram-negative and gram-positive bacteria, their distribution seems to fall into several large categories. Two widely used classification systems have been developed for beta-lactamases.

The first system divides the beta-lactamases into three large categories (types A, B, and C), based on molecular size and homology. This system has been largely supplanted by the system of M. H. Richmond and R. B. Sykes, with some modifications.

The **Richmond-Sykes system** sorts beta-lactamases by substrate profiles and inhibition studies. The **gram-positive beta-lactamases,** which are placed within a **single class** in this system, are enzymes that are produced in large amounts and are secreted into the environment, where they can inactivate beta-lactam antibiotics outside the cell. In so doing, they protect bacteria that do not produce beta-lactamases themselves. This phenomenon is called the **inoculum effect** and is associated with any antibiotic-inactivating enzyme that is secreted into the environment by resistant bacteria. The **gram-negative beta-lactamases** are divided into **six major classes.** Possibly the most important of the beta-lactamases under the Richmond-Sykes system are those in class I. The **class I beta-lactamases** are not inhibited by clavulanate or sulbactam, and some of them can hydrolyze third-generation cephalosporins. Most beta-lactamases are constitutive, but staphylococcal and class I beta-lactamases are induced by cefamandole, cefoxitin, and imipenem. The **class II through class VI beta-lactamases** are all inhibited by clavulanate or sulbactam. These beta-lactamases are produced in small amounts and are restricted to the periplasmic space. Thus, outer membrane permeability greatly influences their efficacy, and there is no inoculum effect. If there is a porin change that results in some loss of permeability, the efficacy of the beta-lactamases may increase greatly.

(3) Changes in Target Affinity. The third major mechanism of resistance to beta-lactam antibiotics involves changing the affinity of PBPs for beta-lactam antibiotics. The greatest clinical impact from this mechanism has been the emergence of methicillin-resistant *S. aureus.* Other bacteria with altered PBP-mediated resistance to beta-lactams include *C. perfringens* (resistant to all penicillins); *H. influenzae* and *Serratia* (resistant to third-generation cephalosporins and some penicillins); and *N. gonorrhoeae* and *S. pneumoniae* (resistant to penicillin G).

(4) Failure to Induce Autolysis. Some bacteria are considered to be tolerant of beta-lactam antibiotics. Beta-lactam antibiotics fail to induce autolysis in these organisms, and the ratio of the minimum bactericidal concentration (MBC) to the minimum inhibitory concentration (MIC) is 32 or greater. This means that the penicillin or cephalosporin is bacteriostatic rather than bactericidal unless extremely high antibiotic levels are achieved. This can be a therapeutic problem in immunosuppressed or neutropenic patients. Bacteria that occasionally exhibit **beta-lactam tolerance** include *L. monocytogenes, S. aureus, S. epidermidis, Streptococcus agalactiae, Streptococcus mutans, S. pneumoniae,* and *Streptococcus sanguis;* all of these bacteria are gram-positive.

Vancomycin and Other Glycopeptide Antibiotics

Characteristics. The first glycopeptide antibiotic, vancomycin, was introduced during the late 1950s as an alternative to penicillin G in treating staphylococcal infections. Because the early vancomycin preparations were relatively impure, physicians found the antibiotic to be unacceptably toxic for routine use. Vancomycin was soon replaced by beta-lactamase–resistant penicillins and by cephalosporins. With the emergence of methicillin-resistant *S. aureus* and other highly resistant gram-positive cocci, vancomycin has returned as an important antibiotic.

In addition to vancomycin, the glycopeptide family now includes teicoplanin, ristocetin, and ramoplanin. While **vancomycin** and **teicoplanin** are commercially available for human use, **ramoplanin** is only available as an investigational drug. **Ristocetin** is too toxic to be used clinically but is often employed in hematology laboratories and serves as an in vitro platelet aggregation agent.

The glycopeptide antibiotics are large, complex antibiotics produced by *Actinoplanes* and *Streptomyces* species. Each has a domain of seven amino acids at its core, with five of these amino acids being identical in all glycopeptide antibiotics. The structure of teicoplanin is depicted in Fig. 4–11.

Mechanisms of Action. Because the glycopeptides are large molecules, they cannot penetrate either the outer membrane of gram-negative bacteria or the cytoplasmic membrane of gram-positive bacteria. Thus, their activity is restricted to events happening outside the cytoplasmic membrane of gram-positive bacteria. Each glycopeptide antibiotic forms a braceletlike configuration with a cleft that binds tightly

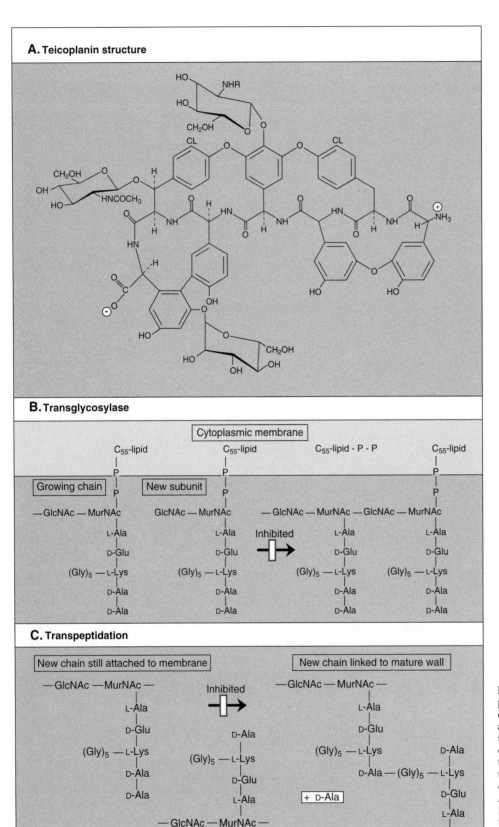

FIGURE 4–11. **Structure and primary mechanism of action of teicoplanin, a glycopeptide antibiotic.** Diagram **A** shows the chemical structure of teicoplanin. Diagram **B** shows that the primary mechanism of action involves inhibition of the donation of *N*-acetylglucosamine-*N*-acetylmuramic acid (GlcNAc-MurNAc) to the murein (peptidoglycan) growth point by bactoprenyl diphosphate. Diagram **C** shows that glycopeptides also sterically inhibit the transpeptidation reaction.

to the target of the antibiotic. The active sites of vancomycin and teicoplanin have been shown to recognize tripeptides with a stereochemical configuration of L-D-D. This configuration is found only within the MurNAc pentapeptide, where an L-amino acid at position 3 is followed by consecutive D-alanines.

When vancomycin is administered to susceptible gram-positive bacteria, it first binds (via hydrogen bonding) to all available acyl-D-alanine-D-alanine residues in the cell wall. Once these are saturated, it binds to the acyl-D-alanine-D-alanine of GlcNAc-MurNAc moieties that are attached to bactoprenyl diphosphate (P-P-bactoprenol) and are at the outer face of the cytoplasmic membrane. In doing so, it exerts its actions at two sites. First, vancomycin bound to GlcNAc-MurNAc-P-P-bactoprenol acts as a space-occupying mass that blocks the ability of peptidoglycan transglycosidase to get close enough to the complex to transfer the disaccharide unit to the murein (peptidoglycan) growth point. Second, attachment of vancomycin to the acyl-D-alanine-D-alanine of non–cross-linked dipeptides already within the cell wall blocks their ability to be cross-linked. In each case, the antibiotic's action is due to its ability to make the substrate unavailable to an enzyme. It is generally believed that the critical step in the efficacy of vancomycin is its ability to block donation of disaccharide units to the murein growth point.

Uses and Adverse Reactions.   Vancomycin and teicoplanin are used to treat severe infections caused by *Clostridium difficile,* by multiply resistant strains of *S. aureus* (including methicillin-resistant strains) and coagulase-negative staphylococci, and by penicillinase-producing strains of *S. pneumoniae* and *Streptococcus pyogenes.* A glycopeptide may also be combined with an aminoglycoside to treat infections caused by the highly resistant *E. faecalis.*

Although the use of vancomycin has occasionally been associated with ototoxicity, nephrotoxicity, and a nonimmune histamine release reaction, the highly purified preparations of vancomycin now available are generally considered safe for most patients when properly administered.

Bacterial Resistance to Glycopeptide Antibiotics.   Resistance to glycopeptide antibiotics has occurred mainly among the *Enterococcus* species and has been due primarily to production of a cytoplasmic membrane–bound protein known as VanA. VanA is a D-alanine-D-alanine ligase, and it synthesizes other mixed dipeptides that can replace D-alanine-D-alanine within MurNAc. VanA-containing enterococci are resistant to glycopeptides because they no longer express an L-D-D target that binds the antibiotic. VanA has been transferred to other bacteria via conjugation. Less common are VanB and VanC, proteins whose modes of action are probably similar to that of VanA but which have not been transferred via conjugation.

Bacitracin and Cycloserine

Characteristics and Mechanisms of Action. Bacitracin and cycloserine (Fig. 4–12) are cell wall

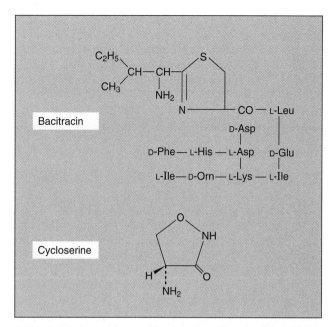

FIGURE 4–12. Structures of bacitracin and cycloserine. These antibiotics inhibit cell wall synthesis.

synthesis inhibitors that are fairly toxic when administered systemically. Bacitracin is a mixture of polypeptide antibiotics produced by the gram-positive bacterium *Bacillus subtilis.* It is a bactericidal antibiotic that blocks dephosphorylation of the bactoprenyl diphosphate carrier molecule after it has donated its GlcNAc-MurNAc to the murein growth point. As a result, no bactoprenyl phosphate is available to receive new cell wall units, and cell wall synthesis is halted. Because it blocks regeneration of the lipid carrier, bacitracin halts the synthesis of all molecules that depend on the availability of bactoprenol, including peptidoglycan, teichoic acid, lipopolysaccharide, and capsules.

Cycloserine is an analogue of D-alanine-D-alanine. As such, it inhibits the formation of the peptidoglycan cross-link by acting as a competitive inhibitor of transpeptidase enzymes.

Uses and Adverse Reactions.   Bacitracin is extremely toxic when administered parenterally. Therefore, it is restricted to topical and oral use. It is found in topical creams for treating eye and skin infections caused by staphylococci and streptococci, as well as in oral preparations for the treatment of pseudomembranous colitis caused by *C. difficile,* a gram-positive anaerobe. Bacitracin is not absorbed when taken orally.

Cycloserine is indicated primarily as a second-line treatment for tuberculosis. Its use has been associated with a high risk of convulsions.

Agents That Disturb Cell Membrane Integrity

Polymyxin antibiotics are large polypeptide antibiotics that contain fatty acids, multiple positive charges, and a long alkyl side chain (Fig. 4–13). Polymyxins act as cationic detergents, binding avidly to lipopolysaccharide and phosphatidylethanolamine in gram-negative outer membranes but poorly to phosphatidylcholine (a constituent of human cell but not bacterial cell membranes). Thus, polymyxins are effective against gram-negative bacteria. Because they disrupt the integrity of the outer membrane, polymyxins are bactericidal and do not require that their target bacteria be multiplying.

Two polymyxins are marketed in the USA: **polymyxin B** and **polymyxin E.** Because of their toxicity, polymyxins are not the drug of choice for treating any bacterial infection. They are used as secondary drugs to treat severe or life-threatening infections caused by *P. aeruginosa* or other gram-negative rods when such infections have not responded to standard therapies.

ANTIBIOTICS THAT INHIBIT PROTEIN SYNTHESIS
General Principles

Unlike human cells, which contain 80S ribosomes, bacteria carry out their protein synthesis through the use of 70S ribosomes. Bacterial ribosomes contain 30S and 50S fragments, which are complexed around polycistronic mRNA transcribed from the chromosome.

A number of antibiotics target specific steps of bacterial protein synthesis that depend on either the 30S or the 50S ribosomal fragment. Because the protein synthesis machinery in bacteria differs appreciably from that in human cells, these antibiotics are selectively toxic for bacteria. However, at high concentrations, antibiotics that inhibit bacterial protein synthesis may interfere with eukaryotic protein synthesis. Furthermore, mitochondria contain 70S ribosomes. Some antibiotics that accumulate well within host cells can damage tissues (such as bone marrow) that are rich in mitochondria. Most antibiotics that inhibit protein synthesis are bacteriostatic, although the aminoglycosides are bactericidal against the majority of susceptible bacteria at physiologic concentrations.

Agents That Affect the 50S Ribosomal Fragment

Chloramphenicol, macrolides, and lincosamides affect the 50S ribosomal fragment.

Chloramphenicol

Characteristics and Mechanisms of Action. Chloramphenicol (Fig. 4–14) is a bacteriostatic antibiotic that inhibits the action of peptidyl transferase and does not allow a peptide bond to form. Because of the drug's bacteriostatic action, it is generally not administered in combination with a bactericidal antibiotic (such as a beta-lactam or an aminoglycoside).

Uses and Adverse Reactions. Chloramphenicol was one of the earliest discovered antimicrobial agents that inhibit protein synthesis. Because chloramphenicol is a broad-spectrum antibiotic and it accumulates well within host cells, many believed at first that it might be the elusive "silver bullet" capable of killing all pathogens. Chloramphenicol also penetrates well into the central nervous system and accumulates within the cerebrospinal fluid.

During the first years after its introduction, chloramphenicol was used almost indiscriminately, but when some patients developed aplastic anemia, it became evident that the drug was often not being used properly. It is now known that this drug's excellent ability to penetrate into host cells is simultaneously advantageous and detrimental. Unlike the beta-lactam antibiotics, which penetrate poorly into host cells, chloramphenicol accumulates in the cytoplasm. Here, it can both kill intracellular bacteria and interfere with mitochondrial protein synthesis. This is likely responsible for the ability of chloramphenicol to depress bone marrow activity and cause aplastic anemia. Chloramphenicol is also toxic to premature infants, who may develop a condition known as gray baby syndrome. For these reasons, clinicians in the USA have shied away from treating patients with chloramphenicol. Used properly, however, it is effective in treating infections caused by *Chlamydia psittaci* (psittacosis), *Haemophilus influenzae* (meningitis), *Rickettsia* species (Rocky Mountain spotted fever, typhus, and other rickettsial diseases), *Salmonella* serotype *typhi* (typhoid), *Yersinia enterocolitica* (enterocolitis), and *Yersinia pestis* (plague). All of these pathogens except *Haemophilus* are facultatively or obligately intracellular pathogens. The use-

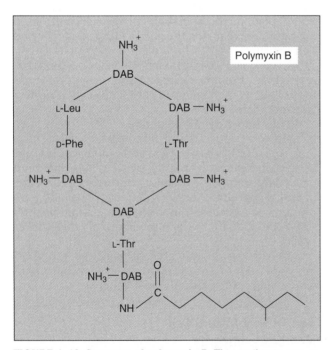

FIGURE 4–13. Structure of polymyxin B. This antibiotic acts as a cationic detergent, dissolving the outer membranes of gram-negative bacteria. DAB = α,γ-diaminobutyric acid.

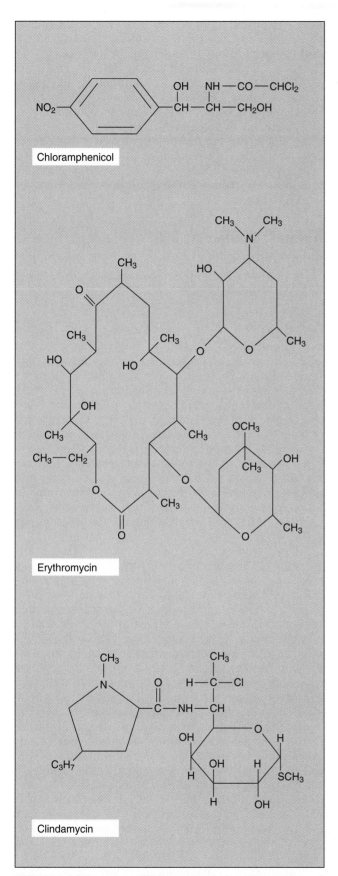

fulness of chloramphenicol in the treatment of meningitis caused by *H. influenzae* is related largely to the ability of the drug to accumulate within the cerebrospinal fluid. Worldwide, chloramphenicol is one of the most widely used antibiotics.

Bacterial Resistance to Chloramphenicol. The enteric bacteria are the organisms in which resistance to chloramphenicol occurs most frequently. In this case, the resistance is usually caused by an R factor containing resistance genes to both chloramphenicol and the tetracyclines and encoding an enzyme that inactivates chloramphenicol by acetylation. This mechanism of resistance occurs commonly, especially in *Salmonella* serotype *typhi* and *Shigella* species. Chloramphenicol acetylase is released into the environment, where it produces an inoculum effect.

Two other mechanisms of resistance to chloramphenicol have been reported. Enteric bacteria and *Pseudomonas* occasionally possess an R factor that encodes reduced permeability of the drug into the bacterium. Other bacteria sometimes experience a mutation of a chromosomal gene for a portion of the 50S subunit, and this results in the antibiotic being poorly recognized by its target.

Erythromycin and Other Macrolides

Characteristics and Mechanisms of Action. The macrolide antibiotics are large cyclic molecules that contain a lactone ring. For many years, **erythromycin** (see Fig. 4–14) was the only macrolide available, but the increasing level of antibiotic resistance among bacteria has led to the development of the new macrolides **azithromycin, clarithromycin, dirithromycin,** and **troleandomycin.** The macrolide antibiotics are bacteriostatic at low concentrations and bactericidal at high concentrations.

Most studies concerning the mechanisms of action of the macrolides have focused on erythromycin. Erythromycin binds reversibly to free ribosomes but does not bind to polysomes (multiple ribosomes reading a single piece of polycistronic mRNA in tandem). It remains bound to the ribosome during initiation and allows a short peptide to be formed, but then it blocks any further synthesis. Both translocation and elongation are blocked. The blocked complex is unstable, so the ribosomal fragments are released from the mRNA. These fragments can reassemble on new mRNA, but their function will once again be blocked.

Uses and Adverse Reactions. Erythromycin has been a popular antibiotic because it has an antimicrobial spectrum similar to that of penicillin G, is not susceptible to inactivation by beta-lactamases, can be administered orally, and is not very toxic when used appropriately. Most adverse reactions to erythromycin consist of gastrointestinal upset. Erythromy-

FIGURE 4–14. Structures of chloramphenicol, erythromycin, and clindamycin. These antibiotics affect the function of the 50S ribosomal fragment. Erythromycin is a macrolide antibiotic and contains a lactone group. Clindamycin is structurally unrelated to the

macrolides but has a similar spectrum of activity and is inactivated by the same resistance mechanisms.

cin is used in the treatment of legionnaires' disease, diphtheria, pertussis, and atypical pneumonia caused by *Mycoplasma* or *Chlamydia.*

The newer macrolides broaden the macrolide spectrum of action slightly and tend to be tolerated by the gastrointestinal tract somewhat better than erythromycin. Azithromycin has been shown to also be effective against *Borrelia burgdorferi* (the agent responsible for Lyme disease), *H. influenzae,* and the parasite *Toxoplasma gondii.* Clarithromycin is unusual in that it is also effective against *Mycobacterium avium-intracellulare* and several so-called atypical mycobacteria. Troleandomycin is used to treat pneumococcal pneumonia and to eradicate carriage of *Streptococcus pyogenes* from the pharynx. Roxithromycin, an investigational drug, has been shown to be effective against *Helicobacter pylori, Moraxella catarrhalis,* some staphylococcal species, and many streptococcal species, in addition to having the usual macrolide spectrum of activity.

Bacterial Resistance to Macrolides. Bacteria resist the action of macrolides by two mechanisms. First, many bacteria experience a mutation of a chromosomal gene encoding the L4 or the L12 protein in the 50S ribosomal fragment. Second, some bacteria carry an R factor that encodes an enzyme which dimethylates 23S rRNA in the 50S ribosomal fragment. As a result of either of these mechanisms, the 50S fragment fails to avidly recognize the antibiotic. When the mechanism is due to an R factor, the bacterium is resistant to all macrolides and lincosamides.

Lincomycin, Clindamycin, and Other Lincosamides

Characteristics and Mechanisms of Action. Lincosamides are traditionally grouped with the macrolides because of their similar spectrum of activity and mechanisms of action, but the macrolides and lincosamides are chemically unrelated. The lincosamides include the antibiotics lincomycin and clindamycin (see Fig. 4–14). Clindamycin differs from lincomycin in having a chlorine rather than a hydroxyl group at position 7. This change makes clindamycin more easily absorbed and more active against anaerobic bacteria.

The lincosamides bind to the same receptor on the 50S ribosomal fragment as does chloramphenicol. Here, they block the formation of the peptide bond. Unlike chloramphenicol, the lincosamides cause the ribosomes to dissociate rapidly into their constituent 50S and 30S subunits. The precise mechanism of action of the lincosamides is not well understood but is believed to involve interference with the relative positions of the aminoacyl-tRNA and peptidyl-tRNA within the assembled ribosome.

Uses and Adverse Reactions. The spectrum of action of clindamycin is similar to that of penicillin G and erythromycin, but clindamycin is used primarily in treating infections caused by the strict anaerobe *Bacteroides fragilis,* especially in penicillin-allergic patients. It is sometimes used to treat abscesses or sepsis due to other *Bacteroides* species, *Actinobacillus, Actinomyces, Capnocytophaga, Clostridium, Flavobacterium, Fusobacterium,* or *Peptostreptococcus.* Most of these organisms are anaerobic or microaerophilic bacteria. Clindamycin can also be used to treat deep staphylococcal infections. In combination with gentamicin (an aminoglycoside), clindamycin is used to treat complicated pelvic inflammatory disease.

Bacterial Resistance to Lincosamides. Bacterial resistance to lincosamides is linked to and occurs concomitantly with resistance to macrolides. When resistance to the lincosamides occurs, it is generally due to the erythromycin-induced RNA methylase described above.

Agents That Affect the 30S Ribosomal Fragment

The aminoglycosides and the tetracyclines affect the 30S ribosomal fragment.

Aminoglycosides

Characteristics. The aminoglycosides consist of a large group of bactericidal antibiotics that contain an aminocyclitol nucleus. The aminocyclitol nucleus is a cyclic molecule, such as inositol or an inositol-derived sugar, in which at least some hydroxyl groups have been replaced with amino groups or substituted amino groups. **Kasugamycin** (which is not used clinically in the USA) is the simplest aminoglycoside and contains a substituted inositol; **streptomycin** contains the amino sugar streptamine; and **amikacin, gentamicin, kanamycin,** and **tobramycin** contain 2-deoxystreptamine. The structures of some representative aminoglycosides are depicted in Fig. 4–15.

Aminoglycosides generally have the suffix "mycin" if they are produced by *Streptomyces* species, and "micin" if they are produced by a *Micromonospora.* There are exceptions to this pattern, however, because some aminoglycosides were named before adoption of this convention for their nomenclature. New aminoglycosides are now being developed by mutasynthesis, a process in which mutants are blocked at various stages and moieties are synthetically attached to the incomplete antibiotic.

Mechanisms of Action. The oldest and best-studied aminoglycoside is **streptomycin.** At low concentrations, streptomycin binds to the S12 protein in the 30S ribosomal subunit. Streptomycin causes misreading by distorting the conformation of the mRNA so that the wrong aminoacyl-tRNA binds to the codon. The ability of an aminoglycoside to cause misreading and the ability to kill bacteria both apparently depend on the presence of the streptamine or 2-deoxystreptamine nucleus; **spectinomycin,** which has a non–streptamine-derived aminocyclitol nucleus, does not cause misreading and is bacteriostatic.

At higher concentrations, streptomycin fixes to the ribosome and complexes with the mRNA. F-met-tRNA initiates protein synthesis under these circumstances, but protein synthesis does not continue

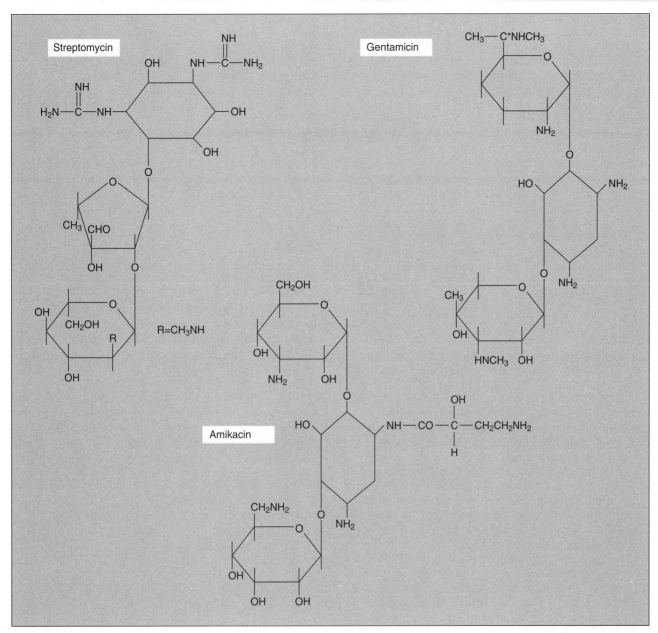

FIGURE 4–15. Structures of streptomycin, gentamicin, and amikacin. These aminoglycoside antibiotics affect the function of the 30S ribosomal fragment.

beyond initiation. After about 5 minutes, the permanently altered ribosome falls off the mRNA. If the altered ribosome complexes with a new piece of mRNA, it will block reading of the message by any other ribosome that subsequently attaches to the mRNA. This polysomal blockade completely halts protein synthesis.

Uses and Adverse Reactions. Aminoglycosides have a broad spectrum and are bactericidal. They are subject, however, to several limiting factors. First, the bactericidal activity of aminoglycosides requires that at least some protein synthesis be occurring. Thus, starvation or reversible inhibition of protein synthesis interferes with aminoglycoside activity. It is for this reason that aminoglycosides are not bacte-

ricidal in the presence of chloramphenicol. Second, the rate of bactericidal killing by aminoglycosides increases with drug concentration, and the amount of antibiotic that enters the bacterium is the rate-limiting factor in the efficacy of aminoglycosides. Third, aminoglycosides are ineffective under anaerobic conditions. Thus, they are ineffective against obligate anaerobes. When facultative bacteria shift to an anaerobic environment, there is a tenfold drop in aminoglycoside efficacy against these organisms. Fourth, aminoglycosides are ineffective against bacteria located in sites where acid and salt concentrations are high. Fifth, because aminoglycosides penetrate poorly into host cells, they are not effective against intracellular bacteria. Finally, aminoglycosides are relatively toxic and exhibit a narrow therapeutic margin. Their use is associated with damage to the eighth cranial nerve (ototoxicity) and to the kidneys.

Aminoglycosides are effective primarily against aerobic or facultatively anaerobic gram-negative rods and are ineffective in treating infections caused by obligately anaerobic organisms. Clinicians have learned to deal with the toxicity of aminoglycosides by administering them with a beta-lactam antibiotic. As discussed above, beta-lactam antibiotics and aminoglycosides act synergistically against many gram-negative rods, possibly because the penicillin or cephalosporin increases the amount of aminoglycoside that enters the target bacterium. Combination therapy greatly increases the therapeutic margin of the aminoglycosides as well as their antimicrobial spectrum.

Today, almost all aminoglycoside use in the USA is in combination therapy against gram-negative rods, including *Pseudomonas*. For example, **gentamicin** is often used in combination with carbenicillin, while **tobramycin** is used with piperacillin or ticarcillin. Because of their antipseudomonal activity, **amikacin, gentamicin, netilmicin,** and **tobramycin** are known as antipseudomonal aminoglycosides; of these, amikacin has the greatest antipseudomonal activity.

Spectinomycin is an unusual aminoglycoside. Reserved primarily for use against *Neisseria gonorrhoeae,* it is bacteriostatic. Its lack of bactericidal activity seems to be due to its lack of an amino sugar as its aminocyclitol nucleus.

Bacterial Resistance to Aminoglycosides. The efficacy of an aminoglycoside is directly related to the amount of the antibiotic that is able to accumulate within the bacterium. This separates aminoglycosides from beta-lactam antibiotics whose effectiveness is related mainly to the growth rate of the bacterium. The aminoglycosides are transported across the cytoplasmic membrane by a specific carrier that is driven by proton motive force (PMF). Bacteria that generate weak PMF or no PMF are intrinsically resistant. Because anaerobes typically generate weak PMF and because strict fermenters (such as streptococci) generate no PMF, these bacteria do not transport aminoglycosides and are aminoglycoside-resistant. Thus, anaerobic or streptococcal infections cannot be treated effectively with aminoglycosides.

Acquired aminoglycoside resistance is most commonly due to the presence of a plasmid (R factor) that encodes an enzyme which inactivates aminoglycosides by attaching an acetyl, phosphate, or adenyl group to them. The modifying enzyme is located in the cytoplasmic membrane. Here, the enzyme attaches a group to the aminoglycoside during transport, and the inactivated antibiotic is released into the cytoplasm. This has a secondary effect of slowing antibiotic transport. In the absence of the modifying enzyme, aminoglycosides interact with ribosomes immediately after entering the bacterium. Binding of aminoglycosides to ribosomes lowers the apparent concentration of free aminoglycoside within the bacterium, and this accelerates aminoglycoside

transport. In the presence of the modifying enzyme, however, aminoglycosides do not interact with ribosomes, so there is no acceleration of transport.

Two other less common modes of resistance to aminoglycosides have been described. In the first mode, *Pseudomonas aeruginosa* and, occasionally, enteric bacteria undergo a smooth to rough lipopolysaccharide transition that greatly reduces the ability of aminoglycosides to pass through the outer membrane. In the second mode, *Enterococcus* (a gram-positive coccus related to *Streptococcus*) and *Pseudomonas* experience a mutation in the S12 protein gene, causing the gene to lose its ability to recognize and avidly bind streptomycin.

Tetracyclines

Characteristics and Mechanisms of Action. Tetracyclines are broad-spectrum bacteriostatic antibiotics that penetrate well into host cells. They are effective only against rapidly multiplying bacteria. The tetracycline group (Fig. 4–16) includes **tetracycline, chlortetracycline, demeclocycline, oxytetracycline, doxycycline,** and **minocycline,** all of which vary according to their R group substitutions at four sites along the central tetracycline nucleus.

Tetracyclines bind to the 30S ribosomal fragment and allow an aminoacyl-tRNA to come into the A site. The aminoacyl-tRNA is not able to bind stably to the A site, and elongation of the peptide is blocked.

Uses and Adverse Reactions. The early oral tetracyclines have a tendency to kill much of the resident gastrointestinal flora, leaving a bacterial vacuum in the gut that can be filled by pathogens. Thus, tetra-

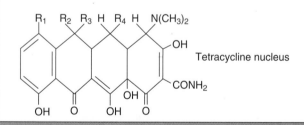

Natural tetracyclines	$R_1 =$	$R_2 =$	$R_3 =$	$R_4 =$
Tetracycline	H	OH	CH_3	H
Chlortetracycline	Cl	OH	CH_3	H
Demeclocycline	Cl	OH	H	H
Oxytetracycline	H	OH	CH_3	OH
Semisynthetic tetracyclines	$R_1 =$	$R_2 =$	$R_3 =$	$R_4 =$
Doxycycline	H	H	CH_3	OH
Minocycline	$N(CH_3)_2$	H	H	H

FIGURE 4–16. Structure of the tetracyclines. There are four natural tetracyclines and two semisynthetic tetracyclines, each differentiated by key R group substitutions at four sites.

cycline use has been associated with the development of colitis. The semisynthetic tetracyclines (doxycycline and minocycline) are more lipophilic, however, and their greater intestinal absorption has made tetracycline-associated colitis less of a problem. Tetracyclines are bone-seeking drugs, and their use in children under 12 years of age can impair bone development and stain the teeth. Intravenous administration of tetracyclines in pregnant women can result in liver necrosis.

Tetracyclines are used primarily to treat infections caused by intracellular bacteria such as *Chlamydia* or *Rickettsia,* pneumonia caused by *Mycoplasma pneumoniae,* and urinary tract infections caused by sensitive gram-negative rods. Doxycycline can be combined with other antibiotics to treat urethritis, which is often a mixed infection caused by *Chlamydia trachomatis* and *N. gonorrhoeae.* Because tetracyclines are readily absorbed from the gastrointestinal tract, they can be administered orally. They do not cross the blood-brain barrier, however, so they are not used to treat meningitis.

Bacterial Resistance to Tetracyclines. Acquired resistance to multiple tetracyclines, including minocycline and doxycycline, has been reported in gram-negative bacteria and usually occurs when a bacterium gains a plasmid that encodes an inducible active efflux system. This system does not affect entry of the tetracyclines. Instead, the tetracyclines are transported normally and are then rapidly pumped back out of the bacterium. In the enteric bacteria, five genes that do this have been described. Although the standard mode of tetracycline resistance is plasmid-mediated efflux, some strains of *B. fragilis, N. gonorrhoeae,* and *Streptococcus pyogenes* exhibit a reduction in tetracycline transport that is due to a mutation of a chromosomal gene.

Other Agents That Inhibit Protein Synthesis

Mupirocin is a pseudomonic acid antibiotic that inhibits protein synthesis by inhibiting the activity of isoleucyl-tRNA synthetase in susceptible bacteria. Thus, when protein synthesis calls for an isoleucyl-tRNA, none is available, and protein synthesis stops. Mupirocin is bactericidal, but because it is so rapidly metabolized when administered systemically, it is useful only in topical preparations. Mupirocin is effective against most staphylococci and streptococci, *Escherichia coli, H. influenzae,* and *Neisseria.* It is used topically to treat impetigo (which is usually due to streptococci or staphylococci) and is administered intranasally to eliminate nasal carriage of *Staphylococcus aureus.*

ANTIBIOTICS THAT AFFECT NUCLEIC ACID SYNTHESIS AND STRUCTURE
General Principles

An important target of antibiotic action is the machinery that maintains and copies bacterial nucleic acids. Unlike eukaryotic cells, bacteria are hap-

loid, have no nucleus, and have a chromosome that is a supercoiled molecule which lies in the cytoplasm of the cell. Because the enzymes responsible for maintaining the supercoiled nature of the chromosome, copying the chromosome, and synthesizing RNA differ from those found in eukaryotic cells, these enzymes serve as good targets for antibiotic action. Most antibiotics that interfere with the function or synthesis of bacterial nucleic acids are bactericidal.

Specific Nucleic Acid Synthesis Inhibitors

Five specific antibiotics or antibiotic groups are discussed: rifampin and other rifamycins; nalidixic acid and the fluoroquinolones; novobiocin; metronidazole; and clofazimine.

Rifampin and Other Rifamycins

Characteristics and Mechanisms of Action. Rifampin (Fig. 4–17) is a semisynthetic derivative of rifamycin B. The rifamycins are ansa compounds, characterized by an aromatic ring system that contains a long aliphatic chain. Rifampin is a bactericidal antibiotic and has a wide spectrum of activity.

Rifampin is a transcriptional inhibitor. It binds to the β subunit of DNA-dependent RNA polymerase, allows an initial phosphodiester bond to form, and then blocks the formation of subsequent phosphodiester bonds. Thus, it is considered to block chain initiation during RNA synthesis.

Uses, Adverse Reactions, and Resistance. Resistance to **rifampin** is usually due to a mutation of the gene for the β subunit of the RNA polymerase. As a result of the mutation, rifampin is no longer recognized by the polymerase. Because bacteria of-

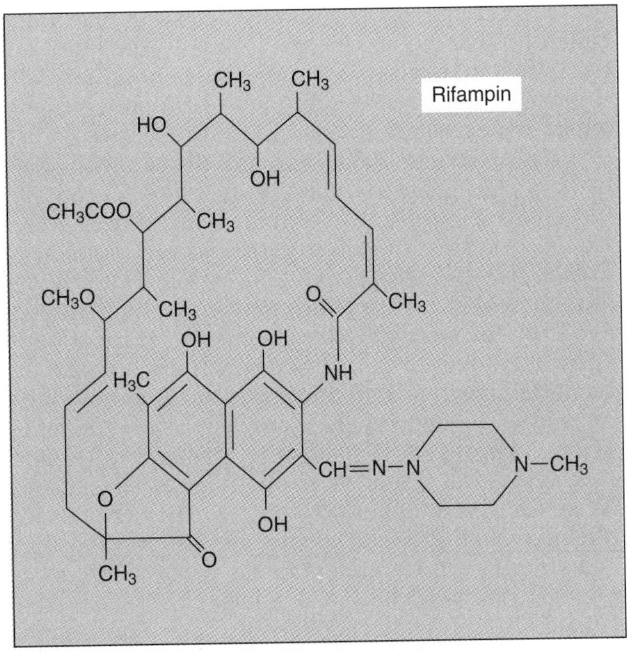

FIGURE 4–17. Structure of rifampin. This antibiotic is a nucleic acid synthesis inhibitor.

ten mutate to resistance during rifampin therapy, the use of rifampin has been restricted to (1) long-term treatment of tuberculosis and leprosy; (2) chemoprophylaxis for individuals exposed to patients with meningitis caused by *Haemophilus influenzae* type b or by *Neisseria meningitidis;* and (3) combination therapy (with vancomycin or nafcillin) in the treatment of endocarditis or osteomyelitis caused by *Staphylococcus aureus* or *Staphylococcus epidermidis.*

Rifabutin, another ansa-type antibiotic, has been reported to have the same mechanism of action as rifampin but to exhibit greater activity against the *Mycobacterium avium-intracellulare* complex. Rifabutin is currently used primarily in the treatment or prevention of infection caused by this complex in patients who have acquired immunodeficiency syndrome (AIDS).

Nalidixic Acid and the Fluoroquinolones

Characteristics and Mechanisms of Action. Nalidixic acid (Fig. 4–18) is an older antibiotic whose primary use is in the treatment of urinary tract infections. Because bacteria exposed to nalidixic acid rapidly become resistant, its use has diminished as better antibiotics have become available. Recently, however, a group of synthetic quinolone derivatives called fluoroquinolones have been developed (see Fig. 4–18). Unlike their predecessor, the fluoroquinolones are broad-spectrum antibiotics that are effective against most gram-negative and some gram-positive bacteria. The commercially available fluoroquinolones include **ciprofloxacin, enoxacin, lomefloxacin, norfloxacin,** and **ofloxacin.** Two other fluoroquinolones, **pefloxacin** and **rufloxacin,** are investigational drugs. All fluoroquinolones are bactericidal antibiotics.

Nalidixic acid and the fluoroquinolones are reported to bind the A subunit of DNA gyrase (also called topoisomerase II) and to inhibit the ability of the gyrase to form phosphodiester bonds. This kills the bacterium by interfering with DNA supercoiling, which is necessary for DNA to be replicated.

Uses, Adverse Reactions, and Resistance. Nalidixic acid is relatively inactive as administered, but it is cleaved to its active form in the urine. It is active primarily against the urinary pathogens *Enterobacter, Escherichia coli, Klebsiella,* and *Proteus.* The fluoroquinolones, in contrast, are active as administered, and they can be used to treat infections in most body sites, including urinary tract infections, gonorrhea, bacterial diarrhea, and infections of the skin, bones, or joints. The fluoroquinolones vary in their efficacy against different pathogens: they are generally effective against all urinary tract pathogens and against *Neisseria gonorrhoeae* and *S. aureus;* they are usually effective against *Pseudomonas aeruginosa;* and they are unique in their ability to kill chronic strains of *Coxiella burnetii,* an intracellular bacterium that causes Q fever and endocarditis. The fluoroquinolones have not shown good activity against streptococci, pneumococci, and *Listeria,* so this limits their

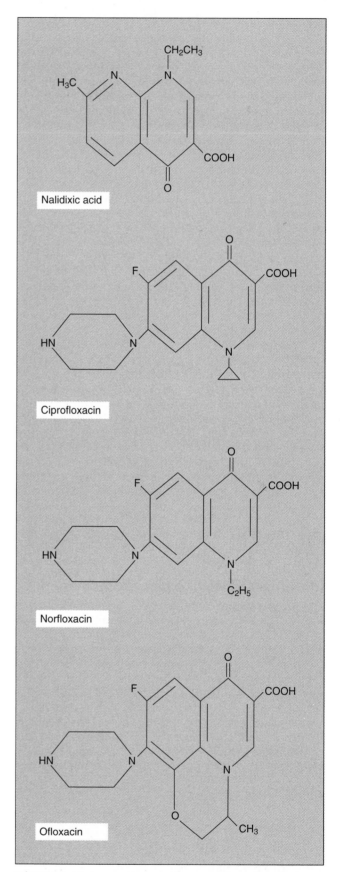

FIGURE 4–18. Structures of nalidixic acid and of three related fluoroquinolones (ciprofloxacin, norfloxacin, and ofloxacin).

usefulness in treating infections of the lower respiratory tract.

Resistance to quinolone antibiotics is generally due to mutation of the gyrA gene. During the course of treatment with nalidixic acid, 2–14% of patients develop bacterial resistance to the drug. Studies are being undertaken to assess the prevalence of resistance to the fluoroquinolones.

Some patients receiving nalidixic acid experience nausea, vomiting, and urticaria, while others have reported photosensitivity. In general, however, nalidixic acid and the fluoroquinolones are well tolerated.

Novobiocin

Novobiocin is a bacteriostatic antibiotic that competes with adenosine triphosphate for the B subunit of DNA gyrase and inhibits both DNA and teichoic acid synthesis. Resistance occurs frequently as a result of a mutation of the gyrB gene of DNA gyrase. Novobiocin is fairly toxic and is used primarily as a secondary antibiotic for treatment of infections caused by S. aureus.

Metronidazole

Metronidazole, a bactericidal antibiotic, has a nitro group that is reduced under anaerobic conditions by bacteria that have a proper nitro reductase. Short-lived, highly cytotoxic intermediates develop and disrupt the bacterial chromosome.

Metronidazole is used most often to treat protozoal infections (especially those caused by amebas, Giardia, and Trichomonas), but it has also become the mainstay of therapy against Bacteroides fragilis, a bacterium that is a strict anaerobe. The efficacy of metronidazole in the treatment of vaginitis associated with Gardnerella vaginalis has been attributed to the ability of the drug to eliminate anaerobes that contribute to what is probably a mixed bacterial infection. Metronidazole is not effective in the treatment of infections caused by nonsporulating grampositive anaerobes.

Gastrointestinal upset is the most common side effect of treatment with metronidazole. The drug has been shown to be carcinogenic in laboratory rodents and mutagenic in bacteria, but its mutagenic capability in eukaryotic cells is not known. It is generally recommended that metronidazole not be given during the first trimester of pregnancy.

Clofazimine

Clofazimine is a slowly bactericidal antibiotic. It is primarily used in combination therapy for leprosy but is sometimes used in the treatment of infections caused by M. avium-intracellulare. Its precise mode of action is uncertain, but death of mycobacteria has been associated with binding of clofazimine to mycobacterial DNA. Clofazimine is a red-colored compound, and most patients being treated with it experience a reddening of the skin, conjunctivas, urine, sweat, and tears. When therapy is discontinued, the discoloration fades and disappears. About half of patients receiving high-dose clofazimine therapy also experience some nausea and vomiting.

ANTIMETABOLITE ANTIBIOTICS
General Principles

Although bacteria use many of the same metabolic cycles as do eukaryotic cells, some of the compounds that human cells obtain from the environment must be synthesized de novo by bacteria, and unusual substrates must be metabolized by bacteria to make energy. Microbiologists and pharmacologists have capitalized on these unique bacterial pathways by producing antibiotics that are analogues of substrates needed by bacteria but not by human cells. Many of these antimetabolite antibiotics are analogues of p-aminobenzoic acid (PABA), which is used by bacteria to synthesize tetrahydrofolate. In general, the antimetabolites competitively inhibit key bacterial enzymes by mimicking the substrate of those enzymes, and their activity can be diminished by increasing the concentration of available genuine substrate.

Specific Antimetabolite Antibiotics

Examples of specific antimetabolite antibiotics are the sulfonamides, trimethoprim, aminosalicylate sodium, dapsone, isoniazid, ethionamide, and ethambutol.

Sulfonamides

The development of Prontosil, or **sulfanilamide,** in the early 1930s heralded the antibiotic era. This antibiotic was not active in vitro but was converted to its active form within the body. Since that time, many sulfonamides have been developed. Those available in the USA include **sulfacytine, sulfadiazine, sulfamerazine, sulfamethazine, sulfamethizole, sulfamethoxazole, sulfasalazine,** and **sulfisoxazole.**

The sulfonamides are bacteriostatic antibiotics that inhibit the formation of folic acid in susceptible bacteria by acting as competitive inhibitors of dihydropteroate synthetase (Fig. 4–19). The synthesis of folic acid in many bacteria begins with the fusion of pteridine (as 2-amino-4-hydroxy-6-dihydropteridinylmethyl pyrophosphate) with PABA to form dihydropteroic acid. The sulfonamides, which are analogues of PABA (Fig. 4–20), competitively inhibit this reaction by serving as an alternative substrate for dihydropteroate synthetase. When resistance occurs, it is due to (1) a chromosomal mutation that results in an enzyme with a poor affinity for sulfonamides, (2) the introduction of an R factor that encodes a new dihydropteroate synthetase, or (3) the

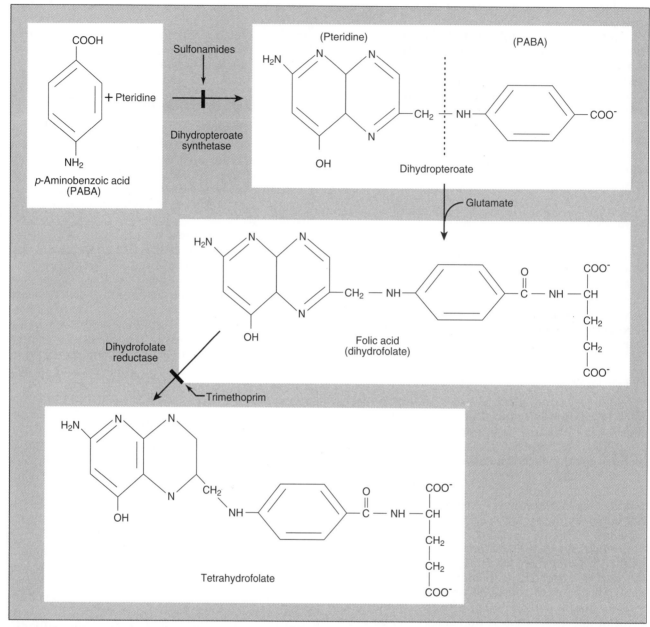

FIGURE 4–19. The pathway used by bacteria to synthesize tetrahydrofolate from *p*-aminobenzoic acid (PABA), pteridine, and glutamate. The sulfonamides inhibit the activity of dihydropteroate synthetase, while trimethoprim blocks the action of dihydrofolate reductase.

introduction of an R factor that encodes an enzyme which inactivates the sulfonamide.

Sulfonamides are used alone in the treatment of uncomplicated urinary tract infections caused by *Escherichia coli* or *Proteus mirabilis,* as an alternative therapy for recurrent acute otitis media, in chemoprophylaxis against sulfonamide-sensitive strains of *Neisseria meningitidis,* and in the treatment of abscesses caused by *Nocardia asteroides.* Because bacteria use folic acid to synthesize purine, glycine, methionine, and thymine, the sulfonamides are ineffective when these substrates are readily available. Thus, sulfonamides are contraindicated in the treatment of infections that involve extensive tissue dam-

age (wounds or burns) or purulent exudates. The greatest use of sulfonamides is in combination with trimethoprim, as discussed below.

Trimethoprim

Dihydropteroic acid synthesized from pteridine and PABA is converted to dihydrofolic acid by the addition of glutamic acid, and the molecule is converted to tetrahydrofolate by the action of dihydrofolate reductase (see Fig. 4–19). Trimethoprim (Fig. 4–21), which is a structural analogue of the pteridine portion of dihydrofolate, blocks this reaction. Resistance occurs when an R factor introduces a gene for a new dihydrofolate reductase.

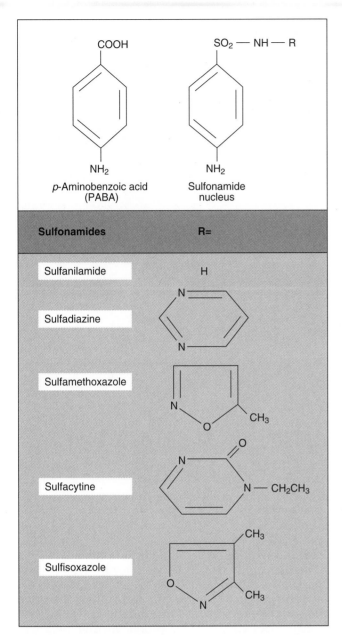

FIGURE 4–20. Structures of sulfonamides, which are analogues of *p*-aminobenzoic acid (PABA).

Listeria monocytogenes, Moraxella catarrhalis, N. asteroides, P. mirabilis, Providencia, Salmonella serotype *typhi, Shigella, Stenotrophomonas (Xanthomonas) maltophilia, Vibrio cholerae,* and *Yersinia enterocolitica,* as well as protozoal infections due to *Isospora belli* and *Pneumocystis carinii.* Since TMP/SMX is fairly inexpensive, is tolerated well by most patients, and has such an amazing spectrum of activity, it is in many ways a "wonder drug."

Other Antimetabolites

Aminosalicylate Sodium. Aminosalicylate sodium, or ***p*-aminosalicylate** (PAS), is a structural analogue of PABA (see Fig. 4–21). Its mode of action is the same as that of the sulfonamides, and it is bacteriostatic. PAS penetrates well into host cells and is sometimes used in combination therapy in the treatment of tuberculosis.

Dapsone. Dapsone is a sulfone antibiotic (see Fig. 4–21) and is identical to the sulfonamides in its mode of action. For many years, dapsone was the treatment of choice against *Mycobacterium leprae.* With the rise in dapsone resistance among leprosy bacilli during the past few years, standard treatment against leprosy now combines dapsone with other antimycobacterial drugs. Dapsone is bacteriostatic.

Isoniazid and Ethionamide. Isoniazid, which is also called **isonicotinic acid hydrazide** (INH), is a bactericidal antibiotic that is an analogue of both nicotinamide and pyridoxamine (see Fig. 4–21). Isoniazid interferes with the synthesis of mycolic acid, an essential component of the cell wall complex of *Mycobacterium tuberculosis.* It is used in combination therapy in the treatment of tuberculosis. Another antimycobacterial drug, ethionamide, is closely related to isoniazid and has the same mode of action.

Ethambutol. Ethambutol is a bactericidal antibiotic that inhibits the synthesis of cell metabolites in an unknown fashion. In combination with other drugs, it is used in the short-term treatment of tuberculosis. Ethambutol causes optic neuritis in about 0.8% of patients, but optic neuritis rarely occurs in patients with normal renal function.

OTHER ANTIBACTERIAL AGENTS
General Principles

Most antibiotics are metabolic analogues or are agents that target the bacterial cell envelope, protein synthesis machinery, or DNA structure or function. There are a small number of antibiotics, however, whose mode of action falls outside these categories or is unknown. These include methenamine, nitrofurantoin, and pyrazinamide.

Specific Antibiotics
Methenamine

Methenamine (Fig. 4–22) is a cyclic condensation of formaldehyde and ammonia. It is inactive in vitro, but when administered orally, its active form accumu-

Trimethoprim (TMP) is occasionally used alone to treat urinary tract infections, but its greatest usefulness is in combination therapy with a sulfonamide, usually sulfamethoxazole (SMX). Because TMP and SMX block separate steps of tetrahydrofolate synthesis, they act synergistically against susceptible bacteria, as well as against some parasites.

TMP/SMX is used to treat acute otitis media, uncomplicated urinary tract infections (cystitis and pyelonephritis), diarrhea, pneumonia in cystic fibrosis patients, bronchitis, and acute sinusitis. It is effective in the treatment of bacterial infections due to *Aeromonas hydrophila, Bordetella pertussis, Brucella, Burkholderia (Pseudomonas) cepacia, Burkholderia (Pseudomonas) pseudomallei, Flavobacterium, Haemophilus ducreyi, Haemophilus influenzae,*

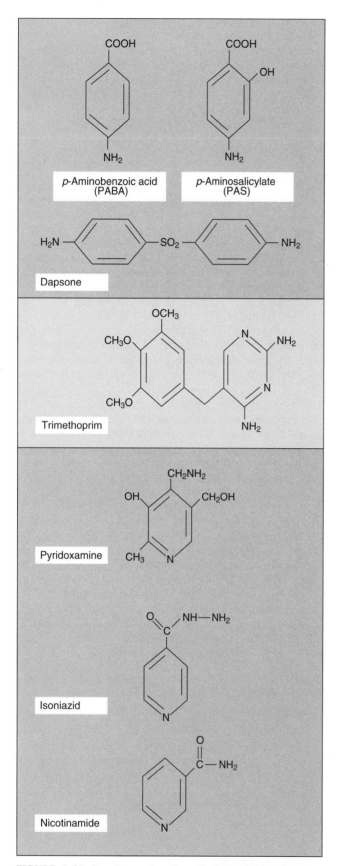

FIGURE 4–21. Structures of aminosalicylate sodium, dapsone, trimethoprim, and isoniazid. These four antibiotics are antimetabolites. Aminosalicylate sodium (*p*-aminosalicylate, or PAS) and dapsone are analogues of *p*-aminobenzoic acid (PABA); trimetho-

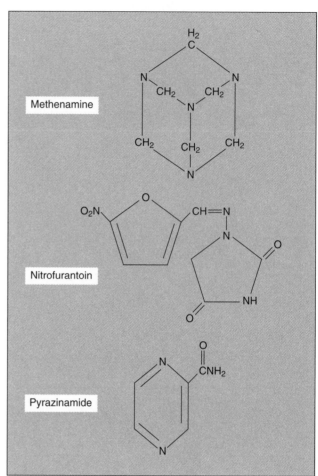

FIGURE 4–22. Structures of methenamine, nitrofurantoin, and pyrazinamide.

lates in the urine. When the pH of urine is less than 5, methenamine is split to yield formaldehyde, and this kills bacteria in the urine. Methenamine is administered with mandelic acid to ensure that the urine pH is acidic enough to activate the antibiotic. Because it alkalinizes the urine by producing ammonia and carbon dioxide, the important urinary pathogen *Proteus* is resistant to the action of methenamine.

Nitrofurantoin

Nitrofurantoin (see Fig. 4–22) and other nitrofurans inhibit the metabolism of susceptible bacteria by an unknown mechanism. Various hypotheses concerning the mode of action of these antibiotics include inhibition of the activity of tricarboxylic acid enzymes and inhibition of translation of inducible enzymes involved in carbohydrate metabolism. The nitrofurans have a broad spectrum and are bacterio-

prim is an analogue of pteridine; and isoniazid (isonicotinic acid hydrazide, or INH) is an analogue of pyridoxamine and nicotinamide.

static. Because they accumulate in the urine, nitrofurans are used primarily to treat uncomplicated urinary tract infections.

Pyrazinamide

Pyrazinamide (see Fig. 4–22) is an antimycobacterial agent whose mode of action is not well understood. The drug is not active as administered but is converted to its active form, pyrazinoic acid, by mycobacteria that have pyrazinamidase activity. Early studies suggested that this took place within the acidic environment of macrophage phagolysosomes, but recent studies have placed this hypothesis in doubt. Pyrazinamide is used in combination therapy of tuberculosis.

Selected Readings

Barradell, L. B., G. L. Plosker, and D. McTavish. Clarithromycin: a review of its pharmacologic properties and therapeutic use in *Mycobacterium avium-intracellulare* complex infection in patients with acquired immunodeficiency syndrome. Drugs 46:289–312, 1993.

Bennett, D. R., ed. Drug Evaluations Annual. Chicago, American Medical Association, 1996. [Updated annually.]

Bennett, P. M., and P. M. Hawkey. The future contribution of transposition to antibiotic resistance. J Hosp Infect 18(supplement A):211–221, 1991.

Bugg, T. D., and C. T. Walsh. Intracellular steps of bacterial cell wall peptidoglycan synthesis: enzymology, antibiotics, and antibiotic resistance. Nat Prod Rep 9:199–215, 1992.

Jacoby, G. A., and G. L. Archer. New mechanisms of bacterial resistance to antimicrobial agents. N Engl J Med 324:601–612, 1991.

Lehrer, R. I., and T. Ganz. Defensins: endogenous antibiotic peptides from human leukocytes. Ciba Found Symp 171:276–293, 1992.

Murray, B. E. Problems and dilemmas of antimicrobial resistance. Pharmacotherapy 12:86S–93S, 1992.

Okamoto, M. P., et al. Cefepime: a new fourth-generation cephalosporin. Am J Hosp Pharm 51:463–477, 1994.

Rakel, R. E., ed. Conn's Current Therapy. Philadelphia, W. B. Saunders Company, 1996. [Updated annually.]

Reynolds, P. E. Structure, biochemistry, and mechanism of action of glycopeptide antibiotics. Eur J Clin Microbiol Infect Dis 8:943–950, 1989.

Sanford, J. Guide to Antimicrobial Therapy. Dallas, Antimicrobial Therapy, Inc., 1996. [Updated annually.]

Smith, J. T., and C. S. Lewin. Mechanisms of antimicrobial resistance and implications for epidemiology. Vet Microbiol 35:233–242, 1993.

Speer, B. S., N. B. Shoemaker, and A. A. Salyers. Bacterial resistance to tetracycline: mechanisms, transfer, and clinical significance. Clin Microbiol Rev 5:387–399, 1992.

Stratton, C. W. Activity of beta-lactamases against beta-lactams. J Antimicrob Chemother 22(supplement A):23–35, 1988.

Tierney, L. M., Jr., S. J. McPhee, and M. A. Papadakis, eds. Current Medical Diagnosis and Treatment. Norwalk, Conn., Appleton and Lange, 1996. [Updated annually.]

Wagenvoort, J. H. The value of new antimicrobial agents. Eur J Clin Microbiol Infect Dis 12(supplement 1):49S–54S, 1993.

Wiseman, L. R., et al. Meropenem: a review of its antibacterial activity, pharmacokinetic properties, and clinical efficacy. Drugs 50:73–101, 1995.

Woodley, M., and A. Whelan. Manual of Medical Therapeutics, 27th ed. Boston, Little, Brown, and Company, 1992.

CHAPTER FIVE

GRAM-POSITIVE

PYOGENIC COCCI

Enterococcus, Staphylococcus, and *Streptococcus*

Based on the general models of infection and disease that are caused by the pathogenic bacteria, these bacteria can be grouped into three categories: extracellular invasive pathogens, intracellular pathogens, and toxigenic pathogens. This chapter focuses on the first category of organisms.

EXTRACELLULAR INVASIVE PATHOGENS

Some extracellular invasive pathogens produce toxins, but the diseases that these pathogens cause are primarily due to their invasion and growth within tissue, rather than to their production and dissemination of a toxin.

Extracellular invasive bacteria typically cause acute infections that involve the formation of a purulent exudate and are accompanied by fever. Some diseases occur when the bacteria elicit an inflammatory response as they grow on a mucosal surface. Other diseases are due to pathogenic events (such as cytokine production) that occur when the bacteria disseminate in the blood or grow within a target organ. In the case of gram-negative infections, septic shock can be a dangerous complication of entry of the bacteria into the blood. Late manifestations of infection with extracellular invasive bacteria may involve immune-mediated phenomena, such as antigenic mimicry, immune complex disease, or hyperimmune responses to bacterial superantigens.

The most important extracellular invasive bacteria are (1) the pyogenic cocci (*Enterococcus, Staphylococcus, Streptococcus, Neisseria,* and some *Moraxella* species); (2) the pyogenic coccobacilli (*Bordetella, Haemophilus,* and other *Moraxella* species); (3) the enteric organisms (*Campylobacter, Enterobacter, Escherichia, Helicobacter, Klebsiella, Proteus, Salmonella, Serratia, Shigella,* and *Yersinia*); and (4) the pseudomonads (*Pseudomonas aeruginosa* and other *Pseu-*

domonas species). Enterococci, staphylococci, and streptococci are discussed in this chapter, while the other organisms are discussed in subsequent chapters.

STREPTOCOCCI

The streptococci are a large group of gram-positive cocci that grow in pairs or in chains. Streptococci grow as pairs in extremely rich media, but they grow in progressively longer chains as they are cultured in simpler media. The streptococci in the chains are connected by intercellular bridges through which the cytoplasm of adjacent bacteria can pass. As a result, when streptococci are serially diluted and plated on a solid medium, colonies originate not from individual bacteria but instead from groups of tightly connected bacteria that are referred to as streptococcal units. Most streptococci are facultative anaerobes, but some are obligate anaerobes. Streptococci are grouped among the lactic acid bacteria because they ferment glucose to produce lactose.

Clinical laboratory technicians are frequently called upon to distinguish pathogenic streptococci from nonpathogenic streptococci and staphylococci that can also be found on the skin and oropharyngeal mucosa. Streptococci and staphylococci can be quickly differentiated by performing a **catalase test.** A portion of a bacterial colony is smeared onto filter paper, and a drop of hydrogen peroxide is placed on the smear. Staphylococci have a catalase enzyme that rapidly breaks down hydrogen peroxide, causing the peroxide drop to bubble vigorously, but little or no effervescence will be seen in a drop of peroxide placed on streptococci. This test should not be performed directly on colonies that are on blood agar, since blood contains catalase.

Table 5–1 presents a list of the clinically impor-

TABLE 5–1. Characteristics and Clinical Significance of the Major Streptococci and Enterococci

Species	Lancefield Group and Hemolytic Classification	Natural Habitat	Associated Diseases
Streptococcus pyogenes	Group A; β-hemolytic.	Upper respiratory tract of 5–20% of general population.	Pharyngitis, scarlet fever, pyoderma, erysipelas, necrotizing fasciitis, toxic streptococcal syndrome, rheumatic fever, rheumatic heart disease, and glomerulonephritis.
Streptococcus agalactiae	Group B; β-hemolytic.	Gastrointestinal tract, vagina, and some animal sources (such as raw milk).	Early-onset and delayed-onset neonatal disease (meningitis, respiratory distress, and sepsis), puerperal sepsis, and pharyngitis.
Streptococcus pneumoniae	No Lancefield antigens; α-hemolytic.	Upper respiratory tract of 5–70% of general population.	Pneumonia, meningitis, otitis media, sinusitis, and conjunctivitis.
Streptococcus mutans	No Lancefield antigens; viridans streptococci; α-hemolytic.	Mouth.	Dental caries and endocarditis.
Streptococcus mitis, Streptococcus salivarius, and *Streptococcus sanguis*	Wide variety of Lancefield antigens; viridans streptococci; α-hemolytic.	Mouth (commensals).	Endocarditis.
Streptococcus intermedius group	Groups A, C, F, and G; variable hemolysis.	Mouth, gastrointestinal tract, and vagina.	Sinusitis, endocarditis, and brain and liver abscesses.
Streptococcus dysgalactiae and *Streptococcus equi*	Groups C and G; β-hemolytic.	Skin and mucosae.	Pharyngitis, erysipelas, impetigo, neonatal meningitis, endocarditis, septic arthritis, and wound infections.
Streptococcus bovis	Group D; α-hemolytic or nonhemolytic.	Gastrointestinal tract.	Endocarditis in patients with gastrointestinal tumors.
Enterococcus faecalis	Group D; variable hemolysis.	Gastrointestinal tract, oral cavity, gallbladder, urethra, and vagina.	Endocarditis, bacteremia, urinary tract infections, abdominal infections, neonatal sepsis, and soft tissue infections. Nosocomial infections in patients with catheters and other indwelling devices.
Enterococcus faecium	Group D; α-hemolytic or nonhemolytic.	Gastrointestinal tract.	Neonatal meningitis.

tant streptococci and enterococci. Because *Enterococcus faecalis* was, until recently, classified as a group D streptococcus and because it shares many characteristics with the genus *Streptococcus,* it is included in this list. The most important pathogens among the group shown are *Streptococcus pyogenes, Streptococcus agalactiae, Streptococcus pneumoniae,* and *E. faecalis.*

Classification of Streptococci

The earliest systems used to classify streptococci were based on the abilities of organisms to lyse erythrocytes when grown on a solid medium. Investigators noted that when different colonies of streptococci were grown on blood agar, they produced different patterns in the agar: some produced a surrounding zone of clearing and were termed **β-hemolytic streptococci;** others produced a surrounding zone of greenish discoloration and were termed **α-hemolytic streptococci;** and still others grew without changing the appearance of the agar and were termed **nonhemolytic or γ-hemolytic streptococci.** While β hemolysis occurs when extracellular streptococcal enzymes known as streptolysins destroy erythro-

cytes, α hemolysis occurs when streptococcal H_2O_2 reduces erythrocyte hemoglobin.

Most streptococcal pathogens are β-hemolytic, as are *S. pyogenes* and *S. agalactiae.* However, *S. pneumoniae* is α-hemolytic, and *E. faecalis,* which is only now becoming appreciated as a pathogen, is variable in its hemolytic activity. Thus, further streptococcal characteristics needed to be identified to differentiate these pathogens from one another and from nonpathogenic streptococci. This was most important for the pneumococcus, which shares α hemolysis with many nonpathogenic "viridans" (green) streptococci that are oral commensals.

A major breakthrough in streptococcal classification and identification came from Rebecca Lancefield, who discovered in 1933 that streptococci could be differentiated by carbohydrate antigens found within their cell walls. These **C carbohydrates,** many of which are teichoic acids, could be identified using type-specific antibody. Twenty-one groups of C carbohydrates were identified and assigned letter designations from A to U. Based on the **Lancefield classification system,** most human streptococcal disease is caused by group A β-hemolytic streptococci (*S. pyogenes*), while group B streptococci (*S. agalactiae*) and group D organisms (such as *E. faecalis*) are also important pathogens. *S. pneumoniae* does not exhibit Lancefield antigens.

Group A Streptococci: *Streptococcus pyogenes*

The clinically significant streptococcus in group A is *Streptococcus pyogenes*. Clinical samples containing this organism are reported by the laboratory as containing group A β-hemolytic streptococci, sometimes shortened to GABHS or GAS.

Characteristics of Group A Streptococci

General Features

(1) Activities, Structures, and Antigens. The group A antigen is a polymer of *N*-acetylglucosamine and rhamnose at a ratio of 1:2 and is located within the cell wall. GABHS are isolated on blood agar as small, β-hemolytic colonies of gram-positive cocci.

Three tests can be used to subsequently identify the organisms as group A streptococci. First, because most group A streptococci are sensitive to bacitracin, a filter paper disk impregnated with bacitracin can be placed on a blood agar plate that has been streaked with suspected GABHS; if the streptococci are group A, their growth will be inhibited around the disk. Unfortunately, because some GABHS are bacitracin-resistant and because a few group B streptococci are bacitracin-sensitive, this **bacitracin test** is not completely reliable. Second, group A streptococci can be reliably distinguished from other β-hemolytic streptococci by a colorimetric test that identifies the presence of L-pyrrolidonyl-β-naphthylamide aminopeptidase activity and is referred to as the **PYR test.** Finally, streptococcal samples can be extracted and tested for the presence of group A antigen by a **rapid agglutination test.** This last test is highly specific and is advantageous because it can also be used to identify other streptococcal groups and can be performed within only a few hours.

Group A streptococci can be further differentiated into about 100 serogroups by their M proteins. **M protein serotype identification** is not done routinely, but it serves as an important epidemiologic tool when there are outbreaks of severe streptococcal diseases (such as rheumatic fever, scarlet fever, glomerulonephritis, toxic streptococcal syndrome, and necrotizing fasciitis) that are associated with a restricted number of streptococcal strains. Investigators have subdivided M proteins into two groups. Those in group I have a particular set of repeating sequences and are associated with streptococci that cause acute rheumatic fever (rheumatogenic strains). Those in group II produce opacity factor, do not have the same set of repeating sequences, and do not cause rheumatic fever.

The synthesis of M protein is controlled by the so-called virulence regulon that encodes M protein, streptococcal C5a peptidase, and opacity factor. As

Fig. 5–1 shows, the M protein layer that covers the surface of the streptococcus appears as a fringed border of fibrils (fimbriae). With rare exceptions, each streptococcus expresses a single type of M protein. M proteins are dimeric proteins (Fig. 5–2) with a seven-residue periodicity that allows them to form an α-helical coil. M proteins can be cleaved about midway along their length with pepsin to yield a hypervariable amino terminus that extends into the environment and a highly conserved carboxy terminus that is embedded in the cytoplasmic membrane.

Studies using cleavage products of M-5 have shown that the pepsin-derived amino terminus (so-called *pep*M5) contains a random coil at its tip and that this randomly coiled section comprises most of the segment which elicits the formation of antibodies that opsonize streptococci. The *pep*M region of at least some M proteins also has epitopes that mimic antigens found in heart valve tissue and elicit autoantibodies in patients. However, the most important function of M protein is to allow the streptococcus to resist phagocytosis by polymorphonuclear leukocytes (PMNs). The mechanism by which this occurs is not certain, but it has been shown that epitopes in the *pep*M segment prevent nonimmune opsonization by binding fibrinogen and complement control factor H. It is believed that bound fibrinogen masks C3b-binding sites on the streptococcus and that binding of factor H inhibits both alternative complement pathway C3 convertase and classic pathway C5 convertase. Yet M protein–mediated resistance to phagocytosis may involve more than inhibition of complement deposition, since early studies showed that M protein protected streptococci from phagocytosis in the absence of serum.

M protein and the streptococcal capsule are the two key streptococcal antiphagocytic structures. Antibodies to M protein are opsonic and will protect the patient from developing disease caused by a GABHS strain. The antibodies will not, however, prevent the patient from carrying that GABHS strain asymptomat-

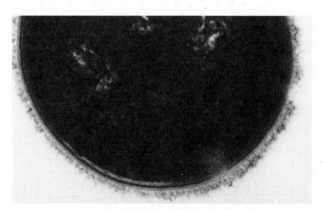

FIGURE 5–1. Negatively stained *Streptococcus pyogenes.* The M protein layer that covers the streptococcal surface appears as a fringed border of fibrils. (Reproduced, with permission, from Dale, J. B., et al. Hyaluronate capsule and surface M protein in resistance to opsonization of group A streptococci. Infect Immun 64:1495–1501, 1996.)

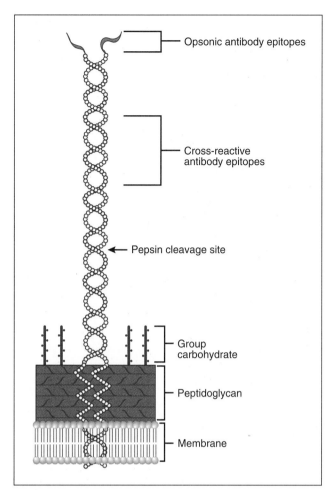

- Opsonic antibody epitopes
- Cross-reactive antibody epitopes
- Pepsin cleavage site
- Group carbohydrate
- Peptidoglycan
- Membrane

FIGURE 5–2. The dimeric coiled structure of streptococcal M protein. Cleavage studies using M-5 have located distinct epitopes that elicit opsonic antibody or elicit antibody that cross-reacts with host tissues. (Redrawn and reproduced, with permission, from Robinson, J. H., and M. A. Kehoe. Group A streptococcal M proteins: virulence factors and protective antigens. Immunol Today 13:362–367, 1992.)

ically in his or her oropharynx. The antiphagocytic capsule of GABHS is constructed of hydrated hyaluronic acid, which is indistinguishable from the ground substance in joints. It has long been believed that the GABHS capsule is nonantigenic, but recent studies have shown that animals used as models of streptococcal disease will form antibodies to the capsule, and other studies are under way to determine if human infections elicit similar antibodies.

In the 1950s, investigators showed that the GABHS capsule worked in concert with M protein to block phagocytosis of streptococci. Fully encapsulated streptococci coated with M protein were phagocytosed by 3% of the PMNs in a suspension. The rate of phagocytosis increased to 41% when the capsule alone was removed, 49% when the M protein alone was removed, and 64% when both the capsule and the M protein were digested away. Thus, the capsule and M protein acted cooperatively to protect the streptococcus. This phenomenon is indirectly evidenced by recent observations that streptococcal

strains which are highly virulent will form mucoid colonies (because they have unusually large capsules) and are of a restricted number of M serotypes.

Streptococci have teichoic acids, some of which are **lipoteichoic acids** (LTAs) that coat streptococcal surface fimbriae. It is believed that streptococci adhere to **fibronectin** in a two-step process that involves initial loose binding with LTA, followed by tighter binding involving M protein or one of several putative streptococcal surface **fibronectin-binding proteins** (Fig. 5–3).

GABHS also exhibit cell wall proteins known as **T antigens.** The functions of these proteins are not known, but antibody directed against T antigens is used by reference laboratories as a secondary means of typing streptococci. Typing systems that use T antigens tend to be less specific than typing systems that use M proteins.

(2) Streptococcal Exoenzymes and Toxins. Group A streptococci hemolyze blood agar because they produce lytic molecules known as streptolysins. **Streptolysin O** (SLO) is a protein that is active only under anaerobic conditions; the O in SLO stands for oxygen-labile. SLO binds to cholesterol-containing sites on the erythrocyte membrane, and the destabilized membrane lyses as a result of osmotic pressure. SLO may damage cardiac cells, and it also has been shown to destroy PMNs by causing their lysosomes to spill into the cytoplasm. SLO is antigenic, and antibody to SLO—known as **antistreptolysin O** (ASO)—can be detected in the sera of patients suffering from streptococcal diseases.

Streptococci are hemolytic when grown aerobically, a property that is due to production of an oxygen-stable streptolysin known as **streptolysin S** (SLS); the second S in SLS stands for oxygen-stable. SLS binds to erythrocyte membrane phospholipids, destabilizes the membrane, and induces osmotic lysis. SLS is nonantigenic.

Some group A streptococci produce one of a group of exotoxins known variously as **erythrogenic toxins, scarlet fever toxins,** and **streptococcal pyrogenic exotoxins** (SPEs). There are four SPEs, called SPE-A, SPE-B, SPE-C, and SPE-F. The genes for SPE-A and SPE-C are introduced into streptococci via phage conversion, while the genes for SPE-B and SPE-F appear to be present in all strains of *S. pyogenes.* SPE-A, the best-studied streptococcal toxin, is synthesized and secreted as a 251-amino-acid precursor, and a 30-amino-acid signal peptide is cleaved to yield the active form of the toxin. SPE-C is believed to be similar to SPE-A. SPE-B is now thought to be identical to an enzyme previously identified as streptococcal cysteine protease and as streptococcal proteinase precursor (SPP). SPE-B is synthesized in an extremely narrow pH range and is activated by cleavage. Once converted to extracellular cysteine protease, SPE-B damages host cells in synergy with streptococcal cell wall antigens and streptolysin O.

The SPEs are responsible for the rash and toxicity of scarlet fever and are thought to be responsible for the manifestations of toxic streptococcal syn-

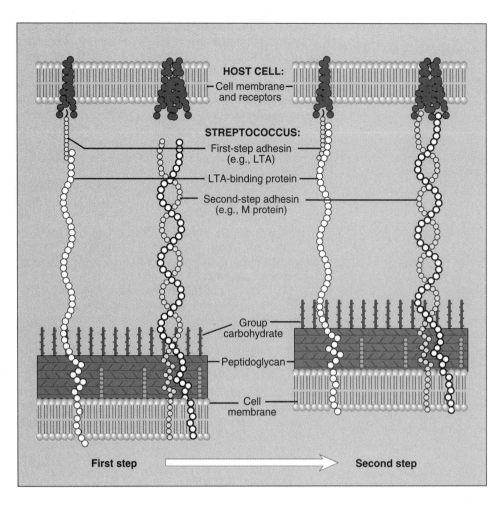

HOST CELL:
— Cell membrane and receptors

STREPTOCOCCUS:
First-step adhesin (e.g., LTA)

LTA-binding protein

Second-step adhesin (e.g., M protein)

Group carbohydrate

Peptidoglycan

Cell membrane

First step ⟶ **Second step**

FIGURE 5–3. Hypothesized two-step process by which group A streptococci bind to host cells. A first-step adhesin, such as lipoteichoic acid (LTA), binds loosely to cell membrane receptors. This brings a second-step adhesin, such as a fibronectin-binding protein or M protein, close to the cellular receptors, and tight binding between the streptococcus and host cell ensues. (Redrawn and reproduced, with permission, from Hasty, D. L., et al. Multiple adhesins of streptococci. Infect Immun 60:2147–2152, 1992.)

drome (also known as toxic shock–like syndrome). The SPEs belong to a family of pyrogenic exotoxins that include the staphylococcal toxins: toxic shock syndrome toxin 1 (TSST-1) and staphylococcal enterotoxin B. These toxins share the characteristic of being polyclonal T cell activators known as **superantigens.** Fig. 5–4 shows how superantigens are believed to function. Most antigens are presented to T cells by antigen-presenting cells (APCs) within a three-dimensional antigen-binding groove in the major histocompatibility complex (MHC) class II molecule. The α and β chains of the T cell receptor (TCR) recognize the combination of antigen and MHC, and the T cell is activated. The combined requirement for antigen and MHC compatibility restricts the response to clones of T cells specific for that antigen. Superantigens bypass this mechanism and act as an external "staple" that links the MHC class II antigen to any of a large group of T cells bearing certain TCR variable region alloantigens. SPE-B activates T cells in the Th2 subclass, while the other SPEs activate T cells in both the Th1 and Th2 subclasses. In contrast to conventional antigens, which activate about 0.001% of available T cells, each SPE can activate between 5% and 40% of the T cell population.

Recent studies have shown that different superantigens recognize different sites on the receptors and that each superantigen recognizes its own set of V_β and V_γ TCR regions. Superantigens activate T cells of varying specificities to release cytokines and monokines and to initiate an immune response that can be either amplified or suppressed. Because T cells activated by superantigens release large amounts of inflammatory mediators and because these mediators elicit the release of other mediators from monocytes, macrophages, PMNs, platelets, and endothelial cells, the presence of a superantigen is often accompanied by signs and symptoms of systemic toxicity, including peripheral vascular collapse. These are the dominant signs and symptoms of severe scarlet fever, toxic shock syndrome, and toxic streptococcal syndrome (toxic shock–like syndrome). Nevertheless, the systemic effects of SPE-B may be mostly due to the direct toxic effects rather than the superantigenicity of SPE-B.

GABHS release a number of enzymes into their environment. These exoenzymes are believed to help the streptococci survive and spread within various body niches. Most helpful to microbiologists is that these exoenzymes elicit an antibody response. Thus, the presence of antibodies can be used as evidence of a current or recent streptococcal infection. The six key exoenzymes are DNAase, NADase, streptokinase, C5a peptidase, IgAase, and hyaluronidase.

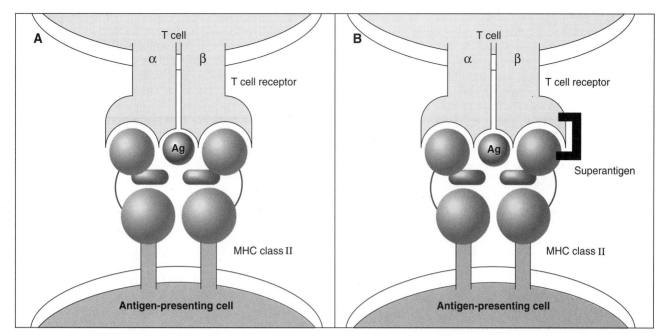

FIGURE 5–4. Hypothesized mechanism by which superantigens elicit massive T cell responses. Diagram **A** shows the normal T cell response to antigens. When the antigen (Ag) is presented to a T cell within an antigen-binding groove in the major histocompatibility complex (MHC) class II receptor, the antigen interacts directly with both the α chain and the β chain of the T cell receptor. As shown in diagram **B**, the superantigen binds to MHC class II regions outside the antigen-binding groove, and it acts as a "staple" to connect the antigen-MHC complex to the V_β chain of the T cell receptor. This allows the superantigen to turn on T cells of a variety of specificities that share specific V_β sequences. (Source: Zumla, A. Superantigens, T cells, and microbes. Clin Infect Dis 15:313–320, 1992. Redrawn and reproduced, with permission, from the University of Chicago Press.)

GABHS produce four serologic types of **streptococcal DNAase,** or **streptodornase.** These types of enzyme degrade DNA, and they are believed to be synthesized to degrade the DNA that is released into boils when there is extensive host cell damage. Antibody titers to DNAase B are helpful in diagnosing streptococcal pyoderma and poststreptococcal glomerulonephritis (which most often follows pyoderma), because these diseases are often not accompanied by elevated ASO titers.

Streptococcal strains that cause glomerulonephritis (the so-called nephritogenic strains) are also good producers of **NADase,** and anti-NADase titers can be used to establish these strains as etiologic agents in suspected cases of streptococcal pyoderma and glomerulonephritis.

Group A and group C β-hemolytic streptococci produce **streptokinase.** Streptokinase cleaves plasminogen to form plasmin, which subsequently hydrolyzes fibrin in blood clots. For this reason, streptokinase is used clinically to dissolve clots in the hearts of patients suffering from myocardial infarction.

Finally, GABHS release C5a peptidase, IgAase, and hyaluronidase. **C5a peptidase** protects streptococci by degrading C5a produced by either the alternative or classic complement pathway. **IgAase** splits secretory IgA (sIgA) and may protect streptococci from the antiadherence properties of sIgA. **Hyaluronidase,** which is also called spreading factor, may promote streptococcal spread into the tissue when causing pyoderma.

Mechanisms of Pathogenicity

(1) Acute Localized Disease. The most commonly seen acute localized streptococcal disease is streptococcal pharyngitis, known commonly as "strep throat." GABHS are often carried in the oropharynx without disease, but some people who are infected develop an exudative pharyngitis accompanied by constitutional symptoms such as fever and abdominal pain. Streptococci adhere to the oral mucosa via LTA and fibronectin-binding proteins and elicit a vigorous neutrophilic response. Because GABHS have M protein and a capsule, they resist phagocytosis until specific anti–M protein antibody appears. Some localized damage may result from the activities of streptolysins and various extracellular streptococcal enzymes, but much localized inflammation is likely to be due to PMN-mediated damage of the infected mucosa. During frustrated phagocytosis, PMNs release hydrolytic enzymes, as well as oxidative free radicals, and mediators such as leukotrienes contribute to the mucosal inflammation. In studies of GABHS pharyngitis and scarlet fever, only 0.3% of patients were found to be bacteremic. Thus, the combination of antibody, complement activation, and phagocytosis restricts the streptococci to the mucosa. When dissemination occurs, it is usually because the strain is one of a small number of M serotypes that are serum-resistant, lack opacity factor, and have extremely large capsules.

Streptococcal pyoderma, also called impetigo, occurs most often in young children living in warm climates, although it is also seen during warm weather months in colder climates. Infection is promoted by poor hygiene and crowded living conditions. Streptococci enter through insect bites, abrasions, eczema, or areas of scabies infestation, and then they multiply within the epidermis. The inflammatory processes are similar to those seen in pharyngitis, but extracellular enzymes such as streptodornase, NADase, and hyaluronidase are believed to play a greater role in the persistence of the streptococci in the area of infection. There seems to be a propensity for a restricted number of "skin" strains of GABHS to cause streptococcal pyoderma. Impetigo can also be caused by *Staphylococcus aureus* or by a mixed infection with GABHS and *S. aureus.*

Erysipelas is an infection of the soft tissues and lymphatics. It occurs most often in young children when GABHS are introduced into the skin via a puncture, laceration, or abrasion. The streptococci multiply within the soft tissues and lymphatics, and they may spread rapidly into the blood. The danger of erysipelas is not the very evident localized inflammation and lymphangitis (usually seen on the face or lower leg) but the possibility that sepsis will develop.

GABHS can also cause purulent pneumonia, meningitis, fasciitis, myositis, and puerperal sepsis. In each case, localized multiplication of streptococci elicits a vigorous neutrophilic response, and the patient can develop septicemia.

(2) Toxigenic Disease. Most diseases caused by GABHS are due to the combined effects of streptococcal multiplication and inflammatory damage, but streptococci can also cause systemic disease that is due primarily to the effects of one or more toxins.

Although rare in the USA today, scarlet fever was once a common complication of streptococcal pharyngitis. The reduced incidence of scarlet fever was initially attributed to a combination of factors, including a reduction in the incidence of streptococcal pharyngitis; an improvement in socioeconomic conditions, with a concomitant reduction in person-to-person transmission of streptococci; and the early treatment of pharyngitis with penicillin. Subsequent surveys have shown that the incidence of streptococcal pharyngitis has not changed with the introduction of penicillin but that the prevalence of certain M serotypes has varied considerably.

Scarlet fever and toxic streptococcal syndrome are caused by SPEs. During the early part of the century, SPE-A–producing strains (such as M-1, M-5, and M-18) were common, and severe scarlet fever was frequently seen. In 1921–1922 in one district in China, for example, about 200,000 people had scarlet fever, and 50,000 died. As M-12 became the prevalent pharyngitis strain, fewer people were infected with the SPE-A–producing strains, and severe scarlet fever became rare. Recently, these strains have become common again in selected locales, and their appearance has been accompanied by outbreaks of scarlet fever and of toxic streptococcal syndrome. Because most of these strains are also rheumatogenic, some of the

affected areas have also experienced a dramatic rise in the incidence of rheumatic fever.

Scarlet fever occurs when SPE-producing streptococci infect the oral mucosa, while toxic streptococcal syndrome occurs when these streptococci cause cellulitis or fasciitis. The streptococci multiply locally and may or may not cause bacteremia. The diseases result primarily from hematogenous dissemination of the SPE. Diseases associated with SPE-A are reported most often in the USA, while those associated with SPE-B are reported most often in Europe.

As discussed above, SPE-A is a superantigen. When superantigens are produced, they connect MHC class II molecules and TCRs outside the antigen-binding regions and cause entire subsets of T cells to be activated. The systemic signs of these processes, which may include organ failure, immunosuppression, and shock, are due to the elicitation of a variety of monokines, cytokines, prostanoids, and other inflammatory and vascular mediators from T cells, endothelial cells, platelets, macrophages, and monocytes. Among the mediators that have been associated with SPE superantigen activity are interleukin-1 (IL-1), interleukin-6 (IL-6), tumor necrosis factor alpha (TNF-α), and a variety of arachidonate-derived products. It is uncertain whether SPE-B is a superantigen, and the mechanisms by which SPE-B causes systemic effects are less clear.

(3) Nonsuppurative Disease. When primary acute streptococcal infections are not treated with antibiotics, some patients develop late sequelae that are immunologically mediated. The two most important late sequelae are acute rheumatic fever (ARF) and acute glomerulonephritis (AGN). In each case, disease is associated with a specific subset of GABHS strains, as identified by their M protein profiles.

The oropharynx is always the initial infection site in patients with ARF. ARF occurs in about 3% of patients who have suffered from streptococcal pharyngitis, but ARF can also follow an asymptomatic pharyngeal infection. ARF occurs in patients infected with rheumatogenic M serotypes 1, 3, 5, 6, 14, 18, 19, 24, 27, and 29. All of these strains have a long terminal antigenic domain on their M protein, have M protein epitopes that are shared with sarcolemmal membrane proteins and cardiac myosin, are heavily encapsulated (form mucoid colonies), are highly resistant to phagocytosis, elicit a strong antibody response during pharyngeal infection, and do not produce opacity factor. (Opacity factor is a streptococcal product that cleaves lipids from serum α_1-lipoprotein, an activity that causes the serum to become opaque. The relevance of opacity factor to streptococcal survival is not understood.) Fortunately, in the USA, most streptococcal pharyngitis is caused by the nonrheumatogenic M serotypes 2, 4, and 12.

ARF is believed to result from **antigenic mimicry.** When patients are infected with rheumatogenic streptococci, antibodies made against the M protein cross-react with sarcolemmal membrane proteins and cardiac myosin. It is the antibodies to myosin that are believed to play a key role in the cardiac damage seen during ARF. Antigens found in the cytoplasmic membrane and cell wall have also been shown to mimic antigens found in the synovium, kidney, and brain, and they may play a role in the development of Sydenham's chorea (also called St. Vitus' dance) in some patients with ARF and in the characteristic arthritis of ARF. For example, antibodies to several streptococcal membrane antigens have been shown to bind to the cytoplasm of subthalamic and caudate nuclei of the brain, and high titers of these antibodies have been identified in patients with Sydenham's chorea.

There is some evidence that the M proteins of rheumatogenic streptococcal strains act as superantigens. Thus, some investigators have suggested that the superantigenic M proteins cause an exaggeration of the antibody response to streptococcal antigens that mimic host antigens. However, there is no definitive proof that the carditis, polyarthritis, or chorea of ARF is directly due to autoantibodies. Other investigators have proposed a role for SLO toxicity in the generation of carditis, but this hypothesis also remains largely unconfirmed.

The possible immune etiology of ARF is supported by the following observations: ARF typically develops 1–3 weeks (mean of 19 days) after streptococcal pharyngitis begins; there are no streptococci on the valvular lesions; and the course of the disease is often mirrored by the titer of heart-reactive antibody. Moreover, studies have shown that patients who have suffered from previous bouts of ARF are at high risk of developing subsequent ARF attacks when reinfected with rheumatogenic strains of GABHS. In patients with untreated streptococcal pharyngitis, the ARF attack rate is 40–50% among those with previous ARF, in contrast to about 3% among those without previous ARF.

Poststreptococcal AGN occurs about 10 days after pharyngitis or 21 days after pyoderma caused by a nephritogenic strain of GABHS. AGN most often follows pharyngitis caused by M serotype 1, 4, or 12 or pyoderma caused by M serotype 49, 55, 57, or 60. Thus, only a single M strain (M-1) is both nephritogenic and rheumatogenic, but two of the three most common causes of streptococcal pharyngitis in the USA (M-4 and M-12) are nephritogenic strains. Although some investigators have suggested that autoantibodies play a role in the pathogenesis of AGN, it appears that AGN is primarily an immune complex disease that occurs when soluble complexes of antibody and streptococcal antigens deposit in the renal basement membrane and elicit a destructive inflammatory response. The presence of immune complexes in the basement membrane is evidenced by a "lumpy-bumpy" pattern of immunofluorescence when fluorescein isothiocyanate (FITC) conjugated anti-immunoglobulin antibodies are used. Both PMN damage and complement-mediated damage occur.

Unlike ARF, AGN does not predispose its victims to increased susceptibility to further attacks when they are later infected with GABHS.

Acute Primary Diseases Due to Group A Streptococci

Diagnosis

(1) Pharyngitis and Scarlet Fever. In the USA, pharyngitis generates over 40 million office calls per year and is the third to seventh most common reason for emergency room visits.

GABHS can be cultured from about 10% of adults and 25–35% of children with pharyngitis. However, because GABHS are carried at least transiently by 5–20% of the general population, it has been estimated that up to half of patients with pharyngitis who are culture-positive for GABHS are suffering from viral, mycoplasmal, or chlamydial disease and are simply carrying GABHS. It might be argued that because most patients with pharyngitis recover spontaneously, there is no need to scrupulously diagnose and treat pharyngitis. However, primary streptococcal diseases, particularly streptococcal pharyngitis, can follow a biphasic clinical course (Fig. 5–5) in which the primary suppurative disease lasts 4–10 days, remits spontaneously, and is then followed several weeks later by a nonsuppurative sequela such as ARF, AGN, or erythema nodosum. Because the incidence of ARF became quite low during the past few years, some clinicians began to question the need to treat streptococcal pharyngitis with antibiotics to prevent the occurrence of ARF. However, with the recent resurgence of ARF in the USA and elsewhere—a resurgence due to the return of several key rheumatogenic streptococcal strains—the diagnosis and treatment of streptococcal pharyngitis has once more become important.

Most nonexudative pharyngitis is caused by viruses, but GABHS can also be responsible for this condition. GABHS are most commonly associated with exudative pharyngitis. Groups B, C, F, and G streptococci also cause pharyngitis but much less

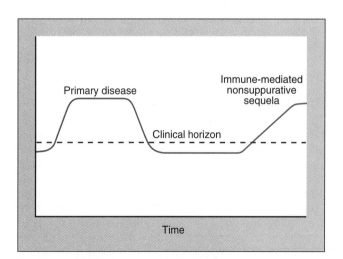

FIGURE 5–5. The biphasic course of streptococcal diseases. A primary streptococcal disease (such as pharyngitis or impetigo) may spontaneously remit, go through an asymptomatic period of several weeks, and then recur as an immune-mediated nonsuppurative sequela (such as acute rheumatic fever, acute glomerulonephritis, or erythema nodosum).

commonly than group A. Unlike the pharyngitis caused by group A, that caused by other groups is never followed by ARF, although it has occasionally been reported to be followed by AGN.

The following are other fairly common causes of pharyngitis and associated problems: (1) up to 200 different viruses, including adenoviruses (responsible for 42% of pediatric cases of exudative pharyngitis in one study), coxsackieviruses (responsible for herpangina, lymphonodular pharyngitis, and hand-foot-and-mouth disease), Epstein-Barr virus (infectious mononucleosis), parainfluenza virus, and influenza virus; (2) numerous bacteria, including *Neisseria gonorrhoea* (sexually transmitted exudative pharyngitis), *Francisella tularensis* (tularemia), the fusobacteria and *Treponema vincentii* (Vincent's angina), *Chlamydia pneumoniae, Mycoplasma pneumoniae,* and *Arcanobacterium haemolyticum;* and (3) the yeast *Candida albicans.* Pharyngitis may also occur as a symptom of more severe systemic disease, such as botulism, toxic shock syndrome, or toxic streptococcal syndrome. Finally, patients may suffer from pharyngitis that is autoimmune or immune complex–mediated (such as erythema multiforme) or allergic in its etiology. Thus, the diagnosis of pharyngitis presents a bewildering array of possibilities.

Streptococcal pharyngitis occurs 48–72 hours after a susceptible individual is exposed to GABHS or, less frequently, to group B, C, F, or G streptococci. GABHS is carried asymptomatically by many people, and nasal carriers are the most frequent source of GABHS infection. The infection is usually acquired by touching bits of infected mucus on the hands of carriers and on fomites, but food-borne epidemics sometimes occur. Most outbreaks of pharyngitis due to streptococci other than group A are food-borne.

Streptococcal pharyngitis has its peak incidence from January to May and during the month of September, the latter possibly related to the return of children to school. About 50% of the cases of streptococcal pharyngitis occur in patients who are 5–15 years old, but 25% of all cases of pharyngitis in children under 3 years old are due to GABHS.

Patients suffer from sore throat, fever, nausea, malaise, and tender cervical lymphadenopathy. Abdominal pain may also be present. Examination of the throat usually reveals that the throat and soft palate are edematous and inflamed. Adenitis, if present, is accompanied by a yellowish exudate that is composed of PMNs and is characteristic of streptococcal pharyngitis. This contrasts with the exudate seen in viral pharyngitis, which is more likely to contain macrophages and lymphocytes. Since many patients with streptococcal pharyngitis do not exhibit exudate, this makes clinical differentiation of GABHS and viral pharyngitis difficult. Patients with pharyngitis and no accompanying illness typically recover in 4–10 days without treatment. Some patients also suffer from otitis media, and rare patients develop pneumonia or meningitis.

If the patient is infected with a GABHS strain that produces an SPE, scarlet fever will develop. Scarlet fever begins as a rash on the neck, usually 24–48 hours after the onset of streptococcal pharyngitis. The rash, which is a diffuse erythema with punctate red spots, spreads to the trunk, abdomen, and extremities. The rash is most intense in the groin and axillas. The face is flushed except around the mouth (circumoral pallor), and the patient's tongue is coated and has large papillae, giving the appearance of a "strawberry tongue." The rash fades in 2–5 days, leaving a fine desquamation.

Scarlet fever can be fairly mild, but it may be life-threatening, with signs of systemic toxicity and shock. In 1895, Sir William Osler described three forms of malignant (severe) scarlet fever: the anginose form, which involved localized necrosis of the soft tissues of the oropharynx; the hemorrhagic form, which extended the hemorrhaging to the skin and was accompanied by hematuria and epistaxis; and the atactic form, which was characterized by fulminating acute systemic toxicity. Twenty years later, G. H. Weaver divided scarlet fever into four modes: mild, moderate, toxic, and septic. Mild and moderate scarlet fever corresponded to what Osler characterized as benign scarlet fever. Toxic scarlet fever was accompanied by a severely sore throat, high temperature (41–42 °C, or 107–108 °F), delirium, skin rash, and cervical adenopathy, with some patients dying within 24 hours. Although most cases of scarlet fever in the USA today correspond with Weaver's classification of mild or moderate disease, the return of dangerous strains of GABHS that produce SPE-A suggests that malignant scarlet fever may return.

While the rash of scarlet fever is fairly characteristic, similar rashes can be seen in several viral diseases as well as during toxic shock syndrome and toxic streptococcal syndrome. The gold standard for diagnosis of both streptococcal pharyngitis and scarlet fever is to obtain a positive throat culture. The sample should be swabbed onto two plates, one a plain blood agar plate and the other a trimethoprim-sulfamethoxazole blood agar plate. Use of two plates increases the sensitivity of culture from about 80% to nearly 100%.

Although some streptococcal experts insist that throat cultures are the only consistently reliable and cost-effective means of diagnosing GABHS pharyngitis, rapid streptococcal diagnostic tests have become the usual means of diagnosis. These are usually based on enzyme-linked immunosorbent assay or agglutination technology, and they can be performed within minutes of obtaining a sample from a patient. Their advantage is that a positive diagnosis can be made while the patient is still in the office, allowing treatment to be initiated immediately. This may reduce the spread of GABHS to the patient's contacts and may offer early relief from the symptoms of pharyngitis. There are disadvantages, however, to this procedure. Although the specificity of rapid streptococcal antigen tests is high (about 95%), the sensitivity of such tests varies widely (from more than 90% to less than 50%), owing not only to an innate problem with rapid diagnostic tests but also to variations in factors such as technician skill, storage conditions, and sample conditions.

The current recommendation is that outpatients with pharyngitis be tested with a rapid diagnostic test. Those who test positive for the presence of streptococcal antigen should receive antibiotics. Those who test negative but have a clinical presentation consistent with streptococcal pharyngitis should have a throat culture performed and should be treated if the culture is positive for GABHS. When the diagnosis is uncertain, it may be helpful to test for antibodies to SLO (the ASO test) or antibodies to DNAase B or NADase. The delay in treating patients should not be of concern. In fact, studies have shown that patients whose treatment is delayed for 48 hours have a significantly lower rate of recurrence than patients who are treated immediately. This is because the delay allows time for specific antistreptococcal antibody to form and because some who receive early treatment fail to develop protective immunity.

Diagnosing strictly on clinical grounds is not recommended, since research has shown that physicians tend to grossly overestimate the number of patients with GABHS pharyngitis. In one major study, only 8 of 104 patients clinically defined as having GABHS pharyngitis had positive cultures. In another study, physicians could predict culture positivity at a 35% rate.

(2) Pyoderma. Streptococcal pyoderma, commonly known as impetigo, is caused primarily by so-called skin strains of GABHS, although isolated cases of impetigo due to group B, C, or G streptococci have been identified. M serotypes of GABHS associated with impetigo include types 2, 33, 39, 41, 43, 49, 52–58, 60, 61, 63, 66, and 68. Of these, types 49, 55, 57, and 60 are known to be nephritogenic strains, with type 49 being the classic "Red Lake strain" that is a worldwide cause of impetigo followed by AGN. Only one skin strain (M serotype 2) is also a common cause of GABHS pharyngitis. Impetigo is also commonly caused by *S. aureus.*

Impetigo is a disease of hot, humid weather and is spread by contact with infected material. It is not unusual for impetigo to spread rapidly among siblings in a family or through children in a day-care center, probably because infants and toddlers touch one another extensively. The streptococci grow on the skin surface and enter the skin through breaks such as abrasions and insect bites. The lesions, which are often on the face or other exposed areas of skin, begin as vesicles but rapidly become pustules, characterized by a thick yellowish crust forming over a layer of thin pus. The lesions itch, and scratching them can cause satellite lesions to develop along the scratch lines. In addition to containing streptococci, the late lesions may contain staphylococci, but their presence in the lesions is probably not significant.

Most patients develop palpable regional lymphadenopathy. Uncomplicated cases of streptococcal pyoderma are not dangerous, but some patients may develop scarlet fever or erysipelas. Occasional patients develop allergic reactions such as urticaria (hives) or erythema multiforme. Most important, patients may develop AGN as a delayed sequela of impetigo.

The diagnosis of pyoderma is based largely on a combination of the clinical appearance of the lesions and the results of cultures. The diagnosis can be confirmed by determining the titer of antibody to DNAase B or NADase, but pyoderma is not generally accompanied by an elevated ASO titer.

(3) Erysipelas. Erysipelas, an acute lymphangitis of the skin, primarily affects children and elderly individuals. In the preantibiotic era, erysipelas occurred as a fulminating and rapidly fatal complication of streptococcal pyoderma. In the UK, it became known as St. Anthony's fire because prayers were offered for its victims in the Chapel of St. Anthony outside Edinburgh and because the disease was characterized by a painful, hot, rapidly spreading, inflamed area of swelling with an advancing bright red margin.

Erysipelas is most often seen on the face and lower extremities and is typically accompanied by regional lymphadenopathy and signs of systemic toxicity. The disease begins with fever, headache, chills, vomiting, and mental confusion. The characteristic bright red lesion is evident by the second day, and it spreads rapidly and irregularly. As the lesion spreads, it tends to clear in the middle, but bullae and vesicles may appear. The advancing margin of the lesion is sharply defined and is slightly raised. Patients may become bacteremic and may develop life-threatening sepsis or pneumonia.

The diagnosis of erysipelas is made primarily on clinical grounds and can be confirmed by positive cultures in only about 25% of patients. Erysipelas can also be caused by *Haemophilus influenzae* and *S. aureus.*

(4) Necrotizing Fasciitis. The 1990s were heralded by tabloid headlines that shrieked "Patient's leg dissolved by flesh-eating bacteria!" In the USA and UK, there were isolated cases of patients with rapidly progressive necrotizing fasciitis, and the public was fascinated and horrified. But necrotizing fasciitis is not a new disease. It was first described during the American Civil War as "hospital gangrene" in which "the skin of the affected part melts away." It was referred to as "hemolytic streptococcus gangrene" in the 1920s and began to be called necrotizing fasciitis in 1952. The disease can be caused by a variety of bacteria, including streptococci, staphylococci, and mixtures of enteric rods and strict anaerobes. However, in the USA, it is most often caused by GABHS.

Necrotizing fasciitis usually occurs in an area that has suffered from minor trauma. In some cases, the precipitating trauma has penetrated the skin (as with insect bites, surgery, abrasions, varicella lesions, and lacerations). In other cases, necrotizing fasciitis has developed following a deep bruise or pulled muscle with no break in the skin. Historically, necrotizing fasciitis has occurred in individuals with an underlying predisposing condition that compromises immune function. Examples are patients with diabetes mellitus, peripheral vascular disease, cancer, or alcoholism; intravenous drug users; women during the postpartum period; and newborn infants. A number of recent cases have, however, occurred in patients with no known predisposing condition. These patients have been infected with a small number of GABHS isolates, particularly M serotypes 1, 3, 12, and 28, all of which have been shown to produce SPEs. Many patients have subsequently developed toxic streptococcal syndrome, although this syndrome does not always occur concurrently with necrotizing fasciitis.

Necrotizing fasciitis progressively destroys the fascia and fat, but the overlying skin may be spared. From 1 to 4 days after the initial traumatic event, necrotizing fasciitis begins with swelling, heat, erythema, and tenderness in the traumatized region. The lesion progresses with alarming speed, changing color from red to purple and, finally, to blue. Bullae appear within 24–48 hours and are filled with clear liquid. By the fourth or fifth day, the affected area is frankly gangrenous. Between the seventh and tenth day, the skin separates to reveal that the underlying tissue is necrotic. Because the nerves passing through the superficial fascia are destroyed, the wound is anesthetic. If a blunt instrument can be passed without resistance between subcutaneous tissues and fascia, this indicates that necrosis is occurring along fascial planes.

Patients with necrotizing fasciitis are febrile from the time of presentation and become increasingly more prostrate and mentally cloudy as the disease progresses. About half of the patients develop bacteremia, which can result not only in sepsis but also in the development of ectopic foci, with further thrombosis and gangrene. Some patients develop myositis. Studies before the late 1980s indicate that 20–30% of patients who developed myositis died and that death occurred in 12–14 days. However, recent reports of necrotizing fasciitis in previously healthy individuals have described a more fulminating course. According to these reports, about 60% of patients infected with streptococcal strains that produce SPE-A or SPE-B have died, and death has occurred as soon as 17.5 hours after the onset of symptoms. This higher fatality rate may reflect the concurrent occurrence of toxic streptococcal syndrome in many of these patients.

The diagnosis of necrotizing fasciitis is based largely on the clinical presentation, but laboratory studies are helpful. Material from the lesion can be Gram-stained. Pus, biopsy material from the center of the lesion, fluid from bullae, and blood samples should be cultured. Serum should be tested for antibodies to DNAase B and hyaluronidase, but ASO titers are not considered to be helpful. Microscopic examination of sections taken from the lesion should reveal an intense PMN exudate, focal necrosis, microabscesses, hemorrhage, and fibrosis of the subcutaneous tissues and fascia. Necrotizing fasciitis must be differentiated from clostridial gas gangrene, erysipelas, myositis, and progressive synergistic gangrene.

(5) Toxic Streptococcal Syndrome. This toxic shock–like syndrome came to the attention of the public when it led to the death of puppeteer Jim Henson in 1990. Toxic streptococcal syndrome and necrotizing fasciitis are remarkable for their similarities to the forms of scarlet fever that were characterized by Osler as hemorrhagic and atactic forms and by Weaver as septic and toxic forms of the disease (see Pharyngitis and Scarlet Fever, above). These may be good analogies, because the streptococcal strains responsible for toxic streptococcal syndrome and necrotizing fasciitis appear to be the same as those responsible for the malignant forms of scarlet fever. In the USA, most cases of toxic streptococcal syndrome have been caused by M serotypes 1, 3, and 18. In Europe, most have been caused by serotypes 1, 3, and 28. These serotypes are all mucoid and produce SPE-A. Outbreaks due to serotypes that produce SPE-B have also been reported in Europe.

The hallmarks of toxic streptococcal syndrome are bacteremia, soft tissue infection, shock, and multiorgan failure. Whereas the fatality rate for toxic shock syndrome (the staphylococcal syndrome) is about 5–10%, the fatality rate for toxic streptococcal syndrome is 30%. The two syndromes have the same mechanisms of pathogenicity, but toxic shock syndrome is caused by the superantigenic activities of staphylococcal enterotoxin B and of TSST-1, while toxic streptococcal syndrome is caused by the superantigenic activities of the SPEs. The two syndromes differ in several other ways: (1) bacteremia accompanies streptococcal but not staphylococcal disease; (2) a significant number of staphylococcal cases are vaginal in origin; and (3) a rash is prominent in patients with staphylococcal disease but is not always present in patients with streptococcal disease (some studies of the streptococcal syndrome have reported no rash in patients, while others have reported a rash in up to 81% of patients).

Toxic streptococcal syndrome occurs most often in patients who are 20–50 years of age and have no predisposing underlying illness. In 45% of patients, no definitive initial infection portal can be identified. The most frequently identified portal of entry for the streptococci is through a break in the skin or through the mucous membranes, although patients have been reported to have developed toxic streptococcal syndrome after liposuction, hysterectomy, vaginal birth, bunion removal, bone pinning, varicella, hematomas, deep bruises, muscle strain during exercise, and pharyngeal infection. About 20% of patients have a prodrome that consists of fever, chills, myalgia, and diarrhea and is so suggestive of influenza that some have been treated initially with amantadine.

The acute syndrome begins abruptly with intense limb or abdominal pain. The patient rapidly develops fever or hypothermia, shock, confusion (55% of patients), tachycardia (80%), and evidence of soft tissue swelling and edema (80%). Of the 80% with soft tissue swelling, 70% develop necrotizing fasciitis, myositis, or both. Some patients develop a scarlet fever–like rash, which may later desquamate.

About 55% of patients rapidly develop adult respiratory distress syndrome.

Laboratory tests show evidence of multiorgan dysfunction. Serum creatinine levels are extremely high, and hemoglobin is found in the urine. Patients typically are hypoalbuminemic, and they have leukocytosis with a profound left shift. Definitive diagnosis is based on the finding of GABHS in cultures. Blood cultures are positive in about 60% of patients, while cultures of material from affected soft tissues are positive in 95%.

The fatality rate in patients with toxic streptococcal syndrome is about 30%, and death is usually due to refractory hypotension and multiorgan failure.

(6) Other Acute Infections Due to Group A Streptococci.   In Europe during the 1800s, puerperal sepsis killed one out of every five women during the postpartum period. In fact, during one year in the 1860s, it was reported that not one woman who gave birth in a hospital in Normandy survived. Ignaz Semmelweis, who showed that physicians were spreading the contagion on their hands to women during delivery, instituted the practice of decontaminating the physicians' hands before any obstetric procedures were begun. Although the first year of this practice saw the antepartum fatality rate drop from about 26% to less than 1%, Semmelweis's colleagues were largely unimpressed, and the practice eventually cost him his job, his sanity, and his life. He was lionized in the UK and the USA, however, where Joseph Lister and Oliver Wendell Holmes followed his lead in introducing the use of sterile techniques during parturition and surgery.

In most cases of puerperal sepsis, acute endometritis occurs 24–48 hours after vaginal delivery. The patient is gravely ill with bacteremia and may have peritonitis. The diagnosis involves recognizing the clinical presentation and culturing streptococci from the blood and from the infected tissues. Puerperal sepsis can also occur as a consequence of abortion, the premature rupture of membranes, or the use of instrumentation to aid in delivery. Although puerperal sepsis is most often caused by GABHS, it can be caused by a wide variety of aerobic and anaerobic bacteria.

GABHS is occasionally the cause of pneumonia and of otitis media.

Treatment and Prognosis

(1) Pharyngitis and Scarlet Fever.   There are four goals of treating streptococcal pharyngitis: to block the occurrence of ARF, to stop the dissemination of streptococci to friends and family, to preclude the development of severe suppurative complications, and to hasten recovery from immediate symptoms. Appropriate antibiotic therapy accomplishes the first three goals, but studies of the effects of antibiotics on the symptoms of "strep throat" have produced contradictory results. Interestingly, although antibiotics can completely block the development of ARF if administered during the first 9 days after the onset of pharyngitis, the use of antibiotics seems to have no significant effect on the development of AGN as a sequela of infection.

In most cases, streptococcal pharyngitis should be treated with a 10-day oral course of penicillin V potassium or with a single intramuscular injection of penicillin G benzathine. At least one major study showed that the failure rate for oral antibiotics (38%) was much higher than that for parenteral antibiotics (8%). This finding was probably related to poor patient compliance. When penicillin is taken orally for only 7 days, its effectiveness is greatly diminished. Yet 71% of patients in one study stopped taking their medicine by day 6, and 82% stopped by day 9. Because they "felt better," they believed that they no longer needed the medication.

Patients with pharyngitis and otitis media can be given amoxicillin. Penicillin-allergic patients can usually be treated with a cephalosporin or with erythromycin. However, in some countries, such as Japan, resistance to erythromycin is common. Tetracyclines, sulfonamides, and trimethoprim-sulfamethoxazole are not reliably effective. Tonsillectomy may be indicated for patients who have recurrent peritonsillar abscesses or other forms of refractory tonsillitis.

Some investigators have explored the issue of whether all patients with pharyngitis should be treated. Microbiologic questions aside, cost analyses have shown that when more than 20% of cases of pharyngitis are due to GABHS, it is most cost-effective to treat all of the patients with antibiotics. But when the rate is lower, it is most cost-effective to treat only those who are culture-positive for GABHS. In the USA, the overall rate of cases due to GABHS is below 20%. Once treatment is complete, the patient should not be retested for GABHS, since up to 30% of patients continue to carry GABHS oropharyngeally following treatment. The presence of these streptococci in the oropharynx is no cause for concern.

(2) Pyoderma.   Impetigo can be caused by either GABHS or staphylococci. It is currently recommended that patients receive oral treatment with a first-generation cephalosporin (but not cefixime) or with erythromycin. Alternatives are topical mupirocin, oral amoxicillin with potassium clavulanate, or an oral second-generation cephalosporin. Appropriate treatment should speed recovery but will not prevent the development of AGN. Because children with impetigo are highly contagious, they should not be put in nurseries or day-care facilities until the lesions have healed.

(3) Erysipelas.   Although erysipelas is most often caused by GABHS, a significant number of cases are due to *S. aureus,* so empiric therapy must cover both possibilities. The affected area is immobilized and elevated, and moist heat is applied. If the agent is not known, dicloxacillin or erythromycin is given. If the patient is acutely ill, penicillin is administered with dicloxacillin intravenously. If the agent is known to be GABHS, penicillin G can be administered.

(4) Necrotizing Fasciitis.   Since necrotizing fasciitis progresses rapidly, treatment must be initiated immediately on the basis of clinical manifestations. The affected area must be thoroughly debrided and surgically explored. Parenteral antibiotics should be given without delay. Because necrotizing fasciitis can be caused by a variety of organisms, combination therapy with ampicillin, gentamicin, and clindamycin or metronidazole is recommended for empiric therapy. If a diagnosis of GABHS is confirmed, penicillin G can be administered. Supportive measures should be given as needed. The overall fatality rate is probably above 50%, with peripheral vascular disease, diabetes mellitus, age greater than 50 years, delay in treatment, extensive disease at time of initiation of treatment, and malnutrition predisposing patients to higher fatality rates.

(5) Toxic Streptococcal Syndrome. Treatment of toxic streptococcal syndrome is similar to that of necrotizing fasciitis. Critical factors for survival are early recognition, treatment with penicillin, and extensive debridement to remove the focus of infection.

Secondary (Immune-Mediated) Diseases Due to Group A Streptococci

Diagnosis

(1) Acute Rheumatic Fever and Rheumatic Heart Disease. Worldwide, rheumatic heart disease is the most common cause of cardiovascular death in children and young adults, with about 30 million children suffering from the disease in developing countries. In India alone, about 6 million children and young adults suffer from rheumatic heart disease, and at least 250,000 new pediatric cases of acute rheumatic fever (ARF) are reported annually. This contrasts with conditions in the USA, where it has become fashionable to believe that ARF has disappeared. Yet an outbreak of 74 cases of ARF in Salt Lake City, Utah, in 1985 was a signal that ARF is, in fact, making a comeback.

Since 1985, there have been clusters of ARF cases in about half of the states in the USA. Two significant observations have come out of these miniepidemics. First, the return of ARF has been paralleled by a rise in the prevalence of rheumatogenic GABHS strains. It is likely that the waning of ARF for a number of years in the USA was related primarily to variations in the distribution of rheumatogenic GABHS, rather than to changes in socioeconomic conditions or to improved recognition and treatment of GABHS pharyngitis. The rheumatogenic GABHS strains are believed to be M serotypes 1, 3, 5, 6, 14, 18, 19, 24, 27, and 29. The lack of a relationship to early treatment of pharyngitis is highlighted by the observation that in eight of the outbreaks, the percentage of patients who had an antecedent sore throat varied from 24% to 74%, with a median of 55%. Thus, in some cases, three-fourths of the patients had no reason to believe that they had a streptococcal infection until they were stricken with ARF. Second, although ARF was traditionally considered to be a disease of poor (usually black) children who live in the inner city and do not have easy access to health care, most of the children in the recent outbreaks were from white, middle-class, suburban or rural families with good access to health care. Thus, there has been a radical shift in the demographics of ARF.

ARF occurs as a sequela of streptococcal pharyngitis in about 3% of untreated patients who have never previously suffered from ARF and in about 40–50% of those who have. The criteria for diagnosing ARF, as originally set forth by T. Duckett Jones in 1944 and periodically updated, are summarized in Table 5–2. ARF typically begins 1–3 weeks (mean is 19 days) after an attack of GABHS pharyngitis. The primary infection site for ARF is always the oropharynx. Patients develop a fever, migratory polyarthritis (about 50% of patients), and carditis (78% of patients). There is no joint damage caused by the arthritis, but if the valvular lesions fail to heal, the patient will develop rheumatic heart disease. About 5% develop Sydenham's chorea, 2% exhibit erythema marginatum, and 5% suffer from erythema nodosum. Sydenham's chorea is the transient development of involuntary, semipurposeful, ineffective movements of the face, neck, and limbs. The chorea is accentuated by voluntary movements and disappears during sleep. Erythema marginatum is a blotchy, red, flat (macular) rash that is of short duration. Erythema nodosum is characterized by painful subcutaneous nodules and is usually seen on the lower legs.

Although throat cultures can be done to establish the presence of GABHS in the oropharynx, antecedent streptococcal infection is best established by showing that the patient has elevated titers of antibody to SLO. When results are equivocal, tests can be performed to demonstrate antibodies to DNAase B, NADase, or hyaluronidase. There are no streptococci in the blood, valvular lesions, or the synovium of arthritic joints.

(2) Acute Glomerulonephritis. Acute glomerulonephritis (AGN) is usually a fairly benign disease that follows streptococcal pyoderma or pharyngitis.

TABLE 5–2. The Modified Jones Criteria for Diagnosis of Acute Rheumatic Fever*

Major Manifestations	Minor Manifestations	
	Clinical Evidence	Laboratory Evidence
Carditis	Arthralgia	Elevated C-reactive
Erythema	Fever	protein
marginatum	Previous rheumatic	Elevated erythrocyte
Polyarthritis	fever or	sedimentation rate
Subcutaneous	rheumatic heart	Leukocytosis
nodules	disease	Prolonged P-R interval
Sydenham's chorea		

*Diagnosis of acute rheumatic fever requires that two major manifestations or one major plus two minor manifestations be documented. It also requires that there be evidence of an antecedent group A β-hemolytic streptococcal infection, which can be established by a positive throat culture, evidence of increased antibody titers to streptococcal antigens (antistreptolysin O, antihyaluronidase, anti-DNAase B, and anti-NADase titers), or evidence that the patient has recently suffered from scarlet fever.

AGN most often occurs about 21 days after GABHS pyoderma, although it may also occur about 10 days after GABHS pharyngitis. When it follows pyoderma, AGN is usually due to M serotype 49, 55, 57, or 60. When it follows pharyngitis, it is most often associated with M serotype 1, 4, or 12. These serotypes are all characterized as nephritogenic strains.

In patients with AGN, signs of impaired renal function begin abruptly and include edema of the face and legs, proteinuria, hematuria, azotemia, and hypertension. Serum complement levels are low. Titers of antibody to DNAase B, hyaluronidase, and NADase are typically high, but ASO titers are often normal.

Treatment and Prognosis

(1) Acute Rheumatic Fever and Rheumatic Heart Disease. When streptococcal pharyngitis is diagnosed and treated appropriately, ARF should not occur as a sequela. Unfortunately, this will not prevent ARF following asymptomatic pharyngeal streptococcal infections. Effective treatment of ARF involves elimination of the infective focus of GABHS in the oropharynx. Patients are usually treated with parenteral penicillin G benzathine, but penicillin V or erythromycin is a suitable alternative in the USA. Salicylates are administered to relieve inflammation.

Once treatment is complete, patients should receive long-term chemoprophylaxis to prevent the recurrence of ARF and the development of rheumatic heart disease. They can be given penicillin G benzathine as monthly injections or can take oral penicillin V twice daily. Chemoprophylaxis is usually continued into the third decade of life, but many physicians recommend that patients with rheumatic heart disease receive chemoprophylaxis for the rest of their lives.

(2) Acute Glomerulonephritis. Antibiotic treatment of streptococcal pharyngitis or pyoderma does not halt the development of AGN, and antibiotics do not seem to abate renal damage once AGN has begun. Patients may need to be treated for uremia and hypertension. For 95% of patients, AGN is a self-limiting disease. Unfortunately, about 5% of patients develop chronic or fatal AGN.

Group B Streptococci: *Streptococcus agalactiae*

The Lancefield group B streptococci (GBS) are strains of *Streptococcus agalactiae.* GBS were first recognized as human pathogens in 1935, when they were reported to be the cause of three cases of fatal puerperal sepsis. Since that time, they have been found to cause meningitis, bacteremia, pneumonia, arthritis, and osteomyelitis both in newborns and in adults, as well as causing cellulitis, puerperal sepsis, and endocarditis in adults. GBS also occasionally have been reported to cause pharyngitis, but they do not cause rheumatic fever. Their greatest clinical significance lies in their ability to cause neonatal and peripartum infections.

Characteristics of Group B Streptococci

General Features. GBS are normal inhabitants of the gastrointestinal and lower genital tracts. The group B antigen is a combination of D-galactose, D-glucosamine, D-rhamnose, and D-glucitol. GBS are encapsulated, and three major capsule types have been identified: types I, II, and III. The type I capsule has been further divided into subtypes Ia, Ib, and Ic. Type III GBS are the cause of 80% of the cases of early-onset neonatal GBS meningitis and 93% of all cases of delayed-onset neonatal disease, but most adult meningitis is caused by type II GBS.

On blood agar, GBS grow as opaque, grayish-white colonies that are surrounded by a narrow band of β hemolysis. The zone of hemolysis is so small for some strains that the colony must be lifted from the agar to see the hemolysis, and 5–10% of GBS strains are nonhemolytic. GBS are differentiated from GABHS by their resistance to bacitracin (although some investigators have reported that up to 10% of GBS are bacitracin-sensitive), by their ability to hydrolyze sodium hippurate to benzoic acid and glycine, and by their reaction in the **Christie, Atkins, Munch-Petersen (CAMP) test.** The CAMP test capitalizes on the synergistic hemolytic action of GBS hemolysin and staphylococcal β-lysin (sphingomyelinase C). A single streak of suspected GBS is made perpendicular to but not touching a single streak of β-lysin–producing *Staphylococcus aureus.* If the organism in question is GBS, there will be an arrowhead-shaped zone of synergistic hemolysis where the two streaks join. GBS are also commonly identified by means of immunologic tests that use specific anti–group B antibody (such as the latex agglutination test and staphylococcal coagglutination test) or that directly identify the presence of GBS in urine and cerebrospinal fluid (CSF) samples.

Mechanisms of Pathogenicity. Each year in the USA, there are about 48,000 cases of maternal postpartum febrile GBS disease, many of which involve puerperal sepsis. Moreover, there are 12,000–15,000 cases of GBS infection in infants, about 2000 of which are fatal. Newborn disease is defined as early-onset GBS disease if it occurs during the first 5 days of life (mean onset is 20 hours postpartum) and is acquired vertically from the mother. It is defined as delayed-onset disease if it begins between the 6th and 90th day of life (mean onset is 24 days postpartum) and is acquired horizontally from a care-giver or from another infant.

Between 8% and 40% of mothers are vaginally or rectally infected with GBS during late pregnancy. Of the infants born to these women, only 1–2% become ill with GBS disease. Why more infants do not develop acute GBS disease is largely unknown. Studies have shown, however, that infants are most likely to develop early-onset GBS disease if any of the following risk factors are present: the maternal amniotic membranes rupture before 37 weeks of gestation or rupture 18 or more hours before delivery; the mother has a fever during labor; the mother is carrying more than one child; the mother has previously delivered an infant with early-onset disease; or the mother is heavily colonized with GBS or has low levels of anti-GBS antibody. Many women whose infants develop early-onset disease suffer from maternal complications during delivery.

Premature rupture of amniotic membranes places infants at risk because it prolongs exposure to GBS: infants born 6 hours after membrane rupture are twice as likely as other infants to develop early-onset disease, and those born more than 18 hours after membrane rupture are seven times as likely. Although most early-onset disease occurs in full-term infants, infants born at less than 37 months of gestation are at a 15-fold increased risk of developing early-onset disease. Some of the risk attributed to prematurity may be related to the fact that preterm infants receive less maternal antibody than do full-term infants. In addition, studies in newborn animals have shown that the age of the newborn affects the proliferative rate of granulocytic stem cells and that the myeloid storage pools of newborns could be rapidly overcome by GBS infection, with fatal results. Thus, premature infants may be at increased risk of GBS disease because they do not have enough maternal anti-GBS antibody and the protective capacity of their neutrophil supply is rapidly overcome during infection.

The development of delayed-onset disease in an infant is not associated with maternal childbirth complications. Type III GBS are most often the cause of severe delayed-onset disease and are considered to be more virulent than the other types. The reason for the increased invasiveness of type III GBS is not well understood. Some investigators have reported that type III GBS produce greater amounts of neuraminidase than do other types and that type III capsules, which have a high sialic acid content, are unusually effective in inactivating the alternative complement pathway.

Diseases Due to Group B Streptococci

Diagnosis

(1) Early-Onset Neonatal Disease. The three most common forms of early-onset GBS disease are pneumonia, meningitis, and bacteremia with no identifiable focus of infection. Because the fetus usually acquires GBS infection by swallowing or aspirating GBS-contaminated amniotic fluid, most infants with early-onset GBS disease have at least some pulmonary symptoms. In addition, infants with early-onset disease typically are pale, do not eat well, and have an unstable body temperature, lethargy, jaundice, and grunting respirations. About 25% are hypotensive. If pneumonia is present, the infants will suffer from tachypnea, apnea, and cyanosis, and most will have a pulmonary x-ray pattern that is indistinguishable from hyaline membrane disease. Almost all with pneumonia will have signs of acute respiratory distress within hours of being born. Infants with meningitis suffer from respiratory distress and from seizures,

which begin during the first day of life in about half of the cases.

Results of laboratory studies show that affected infants are hypoxic, have respiratory or metabolic acidosis, are neutropenic (with an absolute neutrophil count under $1500/\mu L$), and have a disproportionate percentage of immature cells among the neutrophils (a left shift). Rapid diagnostic tests that identify group B antigen can be used to test body fluids, including CSF and urine. Latex agglutination and staphylococcal coagglutination tests are the most widely used rapid tests, but the enzyme-linked immunosorbent assay or counterimmunoelectrophoresis can also be used. Results must be interpreted cautiously, however, since studies have shown that currently available rapid tests are of questionable sensitivity and specificity. Many laboratories first test body fluids and culture samples by a rapid diagnostic method. If the results are positive, the patient is treated. If the results are negative, the culture sample is further grown and is retested 18 hours later for GBS using an agglutination method.

Definitive diagnosis is based on culturing GBS from the blood or CSF. It is of no significance if GBS are isolated from mucosae. Fluid samples should be placed first in a selective enrichment medium such as Todd-Hewitt broth to enhance GBS growth while suppressing the growth of other organisms.

(2) Delayed-Onset Neonatal Disease. Delayed-onset disease often occurs as a nosocomial infection, and 93% of cases are due to type III GBS. Factors that promote the spread of organisms to infants include being in a crowded nursery where sanitary procedures are not strictly followed and being exposed to mothers with a high endogenous GBS carrier rate.

Although some infants have bacteremia without meningitis, a combination of bacteremia and meningitis is the most common form of the disease and is usually accompanied by fever, lethargy, and neurologic abnormalities. Some infants also develop osteomyelitis, septic arthritis, cellulitis, or a combination of these. The disease progresses rapidly to septic shock and seizures. The mainstays of laboratory diagnosis are the same as for early-onset disease and include blood cultures, CSF cultures, and antigen testing of urine and CSF. When the CSF is Gram-stained, sheets of gram-positive cocci and PMNs may be seen. Patients with prolonged seizures, neutropenia, and high amounts of type III GBS polysaccharide in their CSF are in grave danger.

(3) Other Diseases Due to Group B Streptococci. GBS can cause a wide variety of diseases, including postpartum infections, meningitis, pneumonia, endocarditis, arthritis, osteomyelitis, and skin and soft tissue infections. GBS are opportunistic pathogens that frequently infect immunocompromised patients.

The most common GBS infections in adults are those which occur in postpartum women. Although the afterbirth (lochia) of affected women appears normal, signs of endometritis usually develop within 48 hours of delivery and include fever, chills, malaise, and abdominal and uterine tenderness. About 2% of patients subsequently develop pelvic abscess or sepsis. Some patients develop GBS urinary tract infections. The diagnosis is based on clinical manifestations and positive cultures of GBS from the affected areas.

Treatment and Prognosis. Penicillin G and ampicillin are the antibiotics of choice in the treatment of neonatal and adult GBS infections. Vancomycin, macrolides, and cephalosporins may be suitable alternatives. The use of tetracyclines, aminoglycosides, fluoroquinolones, metronidazole, or aztreonam is ineffective.

Early-onset neonatal GBS disease has a fatality rate of 13–37%, while delayed-onset disease has a fatality rate of 10–15%. Between 25% and 50% of infants who survive GBS meningitis (whether early-onset or delayed-onset) have permanent neurologic sequelae, such as blindness, mental retardation, and global developmental delay. The prognosis in adults with GBS infection varies, depending on the type of illness.

Prevention. To prevent the occurrence of early-onset GBS disease, the American Academy of Pediatrics (AAP) has recommended that all pregnant women be tested for GBS rectovaginal infection at 26–28 weeks of gestation and that all culture-positive women with one of several risk factors be treated during parturition with ampicillin, penicillin G, cephalothin, or erythromycin. Risk factors for chemoprophylaxis include preterm labor (less than 37 weeks), premature rupture of membranes (less than 37 weeks), prolonged rupture of membranes (longer than 18 hours), maternal intrapartum temperature higher than 38.4 °C (101.1 °F), previous delivery of an infected infant, and multiple gestation.

In a recent study, investigators examined the AAP recommendation and 18 other options by meta-analysis to determine the chemoprophylactic regimens that offered the least risk to mother and child, the greatest efficacy in preventing early-onset GBS disease, and the lowest total cost. They concluded that the AAP-recommended procedure was among the least effective and most costly options. They found that three regimens were by far superior to the others: (1) treating all pregnant women with antibiotics throughout labor, (2) testing no one but giving antibiotics throughout labor to all women with risk factors, and (3) testing all women for rectovaginal GBS at 36 weeks and treating all women whose deliveries occur preterm and those women who are culture-positive. The last choice was the one favored by the authors of the study.

Viridans Streptococci

The viridans streptococci derive their name from the fact that they are α-hemolytic and produce a greenish zone of discoloration when grown on blood agar. *Streptococcus mutans, Streptococcus sanguis,* and other viridans species are not inhibited by optochin (ethylhydrocupreine hydrochloride) and can thus be distinguished from *Streptococcus pneumoniae* (which is also α-hemolytic but is inhibited by optochin and is not a member of the viridans group). The viridans streptococci are not easily antigenically classified. Many are nontypeable, while others exhibit antigens that agglutinate with sera directed against serotypes F, G, H, K, M, and O. The viridans streptococci comprise 30–60% of the normal oral flora, and some researchers suspect that they also grow on the urogenital and gastrointestinal mucosae.

Two clinically important phenomena are associated with viridans streptococci. First, *S. mutans* is the principal cause of **dental caries** (tooth decay). *S. mutans* adheres to dental surfaces via extracellular carbohydrates (dextran) and erodes the teeth by converting sucrose to acetic acid and lactate. Second, viridans streptococci are responsible for about half of all cases of **infective endocarditis,** which makes them the most common cause of this disease. About two-thirds of the viridans-associated cases are due to *S. sanguis* and *S. mutans.* Another group of viridans streptococci known as nutritionally variant streptococci account for 6–7% of endocarditis cases. Most patients have underlying valvular heart disease, and the course of the endocarditis is generally subacute. Dental procedures, vigorous tooth brushing or chewing, and use of a water pick to clean teeth can cause a transient bacteremia that is enough to initiate valvular infection in a person with damaged valvular tissue.

Endocarditis of natural valves is usually treated with penicillin plus gentamicin, while endocarditis of prosthetic valves may require a combination of vancomycin, gentamicin, and rifampin, sometimes with prosthetic valve replacement.

Group D Streptococci

For a discussion of recent changes in the classification of group D organisms, see Classification of Enterococci and Group D Streptococci, below.

Streptococcus pneumoniae

Streptococcus pneumoniae is known simply as the pneumococcus. Once called the "captain of the men of death," *S. pneumoniae* is today the fifth leading cause of death in the USA, with pneumococcal pneumonia that follows influenza being the only infectious disease among the top ten. From 150,000 to 270,000 cases of pneumococcal pneumonia and from 2600 to 6200 cases of pneumococcal meningitis are estimated to occur each year in the USA. *S. pneumoniae* also causes about half the cases of acute otitis media and is the most common cause of conjunctivitis, sinusitis, and community-acquired pneumonia.

Pneumococcal diseases are **endogenous diseases**—that is, they are not acquired de novo from other patients with active disease but occur when a patient's own pneumococci turn on him or her. Pneumococci are carried asymptomatically in the upper respiratory tract by 5–70% of the general population, depending on several factors. The carriage rate is lowest in adults living with no children in the house;

highest among children and among people in closed populations (such as orphanages and military units); and highest when the weather is cold. Disease usually is the result of a breakdown of the defense systems that keep pneumococci out of the lungs, subarachnoid space, and blood. Thus, predisposing factors for pneumococcal disease include respiratory tract infection, splenic dysfunction or splenectomy, epiglottal dysfunction (due to alcoholism or anesthesia), old age, head trauma, and congestive heart disease.

Characteristics of *S. pneumoniae*

General Features. The pneumococci were once known as *Diplococcus pneumoniae* because they typically appear as diplococci rather than as chains of bacteria. They have no Lancefield antigens, so they cannot be typed by their C carbohydrates.

Pneumococci are α-hemolytic streptococci and are differentiated from viridans streptococci on the basis of three criteria: (1) pneumococcal growth on blood agar is inhibited around a disk that is impregnated with a dye known as optochin (ethylhydrocupreine hydrochloride); (2) pneumococci rapidly kill mice when the bacteria are injected into the mice intraperitoneally; and (3) pneumococci are bile-soluble—that is, they lyse rapidly when placed in a broth that contains 10% deoxycholate. Bile solubility is due to activation of an amidase that splits the bond between alanine and muramic acid in pneumococcal peptidoglycan. The activity of pneumococcal amidase can be seen in older cultures, where prolonged growth on agar results in lysis of the bacteria in the center of the colony. This makes the older colonies look like doughnuts.

Since pneumococci are resistant to gentamicin, gentamicin is placed in selective media used to isolate pneumococci from respiratory samples.

When incubated anaerobically, pneumococci produce β hemolysis on blood agar, owing to the production of a 63-kD protein known as **pneumolysin O.** Pneumolysin O is active only under anaerobic conditions and has been shown to damage leukocytes. It is related to streptolysin O and is released by pneumococci during autolysis. Pneumolysin has two components. One is a hemolysin that acts on host cells, including erythrocytes, and the other is a complement-activating region. In animal models of pneumonia, the hemolysin activity has been shown to cause acute lung injury and to promote pneumococcal growth during the first 3–6 hours of infection. The complement-activating region, in comparison, appears to promote bacterial growth and the generation of bacteremia after 24 hours.

Streptococcal **neuraminidase** may promote pneumococcal access to the lungs by thinning mucinous secretions. Pneumococci secrete an **IgA protease** that cleaves sIgA, IgA, IgG, and IgM. This protease may protect pneumococci from sIgA that can block pneumococcal adherence to mucosal surfaces. Although pneumococci have an **M protein,** it is not a significant factor in protecting pneumococci from phagocytosis, and antibody to pneumococcal M protein does not protect patients from infection. Pneumococci also produce an extracellular cysteine protease that rapidly converts plasma kininogens to kinins. Kinins cause hypotension, increase vascular permeability, contract smooth muscles, and induce the expression of fever and pain.

Pneumococci have a choline-substituted ribitol teichoic acid called **C substance.** C substance is best known for its ability to combine with a nonspecific β-globulin that appears in the serum during certain infections. This C-reactive substance (CRS) is precipitated by C substance in the presence of calcium. CRS was once used in the diagnosis of pneumococcal pneumonia and acute rheumatic fever because it is elevated in the sera of affected patients. Pneumococci also have a lipoteichoic acid that is called **F substance** because it cross-reacts with a mammalian cell surface antigen known as the Forssman antigen. F substance is believed to regulate pneumococcal autolytic amidase activity.

The key pneumococcal antigen is its typespecific capsule. Almost 90 **capsule serotypes** have been described, but most disease is caused by types 1 through 9. Two systems are used to type pneumococci and are referred to as the American and Danish typing systems. The first 25 serotypes of each are essentially the same, but because the two systems view partially cross-reacting strains in a different manner, the systems differ with respect to the higher-numbered strains.

Capsules can be serotyped on the basis of a capsular swelling reaction known as the **Neufeld reaction,** or **quellung reaction.** Culture suspensions, spinal fluid, sputum, or exudate can be placed on a slide and air-dried. After a loopful of antipneumococcal antiserum that contains methylene blue is added, the slide is incubated and the sample examined microscopically. If the sample contains pneumococci that react with the type-specific antiserum, they will appear as diplococci surrounded by a large clear zone that contains the capsule, but nonreactive bacteria will not be surrounded by such a zone. The ability of specific antibody to cause the capsule to appear to swell is probably related to an increase in the effective size of the capsule owing to the binding of antibody to the capsule and to increased refraction.

The pneumococcal capsule protects the pneumococci from being phagocytosed by PMNs. Pneumococci do not have cytochromes, so respiration involves a flavoprotein system that converts O_2 to H_2O_2. This is toxic to pneumococci because they have no external catalase or peroxidase enzymes. When pneumococci are phagocytosed, they are rapidly destroyed by their own H_2O_2 within the phagocytic vacuole. As a result, pneumococci are readily killed when phagocytosis occurs, even when the PMNs are from children who have chronic granulomatous disease, a familial leukocytic disorder in which PMNs are unable to form oxidative free radicals during phagocytosis. Because pneumococci are so susceptible to intraleukocytic killing, they must avoid PMNs if they are to survive. In the absence of specific antibody, encapsulated pneumococci resist phagocytosis. The mechanism by which this occurs is not fully understood, but it may involve inhibition of deposition of opsonic C3b on the bacterial surface. Immunity to pneumococci and recovery from infection depend on the formation of capsule-specific antibody that facilitates phagocytosis of pneumococci by PMNs. Encapsulated (smooth) pneumococci are virulent, but nonencapsulated (rough) pneumococci do not cause disease in humans or in animal models of infection.

Pneumococcal capsules are composed of repeating polysaccharide units. Their effectiveness in protecting pneumococci against phagocytosis is not strictly related to capsule size, but strains with the largest capsules are responsible for the most severe disease. Type 3 pneumococci are the most dangerous of the pneumococci, exhibit the largest capsule, and cause most pneumococcal pulmonary abscesses. The type 3 capsule is composed of repeating units of D-glucuronic β1,4-D-glucose. Pneumococci produce the greatest amount of capsule during log phase, and they have the least amount during the stationary phase of growth. Some pneumococcal capsules cross-react with the capsules of other bacteria (such as those of *Escherichia coli, Klebsiella pneumoniae,* and *Salmonella* species), while others with terminal *N*-acetylglucosamine residues cross-react with ABO blood alloantigens (A, B, H, and Le[a]).

Mechanisms of Pathogenicity

(1) Pneumococcal Pneumonia. Pneumococci are the most common cause of community-acquired pneumonia. Pneumococcal pneumonia is not an epidemic disease but results when a patient's own pneumococci enter the lungs and multiply within the alveoli. This occurs when patients with impaired immune systems aspirate upper respiratory tract secretions. Thus, any condition that diminishes antibody responses or PMN function or increases the aspiration of respiratory secretions will increase the incidence and severity of pneumococcal pneumonia. Some factors that promote infection and disease include alcoholism, anesthesia, upper respiratory tract infections, sickle cell disease, splenectomy, immunosuppression, cancer, and congestive heart failure. Pneumococcal pneumonia can be rapidly fatal in patients who have been splenectomized or have sickle cell disease.

Because infection is initiated by aspirating upper respiratory tract secretions, disease usually begins in the lower lobe or the lower middle lobe. Young adults generally develop lobar pneumonia, while children and the elderly are more likely to develop bronchopneumonia. If there is fluid in the alveoli (such as during congestive heart failure), the pneumococci will multiply rapidly. Before antibody appears, some of the pneumococci will be phagocytosed when they are trapped by PMNs or alveolar macrophages against lung fibrils. This process of surface phagocytosis is fairly inefficient, however, and little phagocytosis occurs until anticapsular antibody appears.

As the lesion of pneumococcal pneumonia spreads and heals centrally, four histologic zones are noted. In the outer zone, the pneumococci multiply rapidly in the serous fluid because there are no phagocytes present. As PMNs are called into the area, they gradually congest the lesion and then clear it of pneumococci. Finally, the lesion begins to heal without scarring. On a larger scale, these processes are reflected in the four phases of gross pathologic findings in the lung—phases known as congestion, red hepatization, gray hepatization, and resolution. Initially, the lung shows edema. By days 2 and 3, it becomes red and undergoes a threefold or fourfold increase in weight owing to the accumulation of red cells, bacteria, and PMNs. By days 4 and 5, as further PMNs and fibrin accumulate, the lung becomes grayish-white, and the alveoli contain PMNs but no detectable pneumococci. This vigorous PMN movement into the lungs can overwhelm the ability of severely ill patients to summon more PMNs from the bone marrow. Thus, when severe pneumococcal disease results in neutropenia, the patient is in grave danger.

About 25% of patients develop pleural effusions, and 25–30% become bacteremic. Bacteremia is dangerous because it may lead to sepsis, endocarditis, or meningitis. Endocarditis occurs in about 10% of patients with untreated pneumococcal pneumonia. Unlike endocarditis caused by viridans streptococci or enterococci, endocarditis caused by pneumococci is acute and can result in damage to the aortic valve. Empyema (the presence of intrapleural abscesses) occurs primarily in patients infected with pneumococcal serotype 3 but occasionally occurs in those infected with serotype 2.

(2) Pneumococcal Meningitis. Pneumococci are the second most prevalent cause of meningitis in the USA. Patients usually acquire pneumococcal meningitis following bacteremia associated with another primary focus of infection (such as the lung) or following an injury or malformation that allows bacteria from the respiratory tract to gain access to the subarachnoid space. About 25% of patients with pneumococcal meningitis also have pneumococcal pneumonia, and many others have suffered from skull fractures. Pneumococcal meningitis is a purulent form of meningitis. Like meningitis due to *Neisseria meningitidis* (see Chapter 6), meningitis due to pneumococci is influenced by the production of cytokines, monokines, and autacoids by host inflammatory cells.

(3) Otitis Media. Most cases of otitis media are due to pneumococci, although *Streptococcus pyogenes* and *Haemophilus influenzae* also commonly cause acute infection of the middle ear. In order of frequency, the pneumococcal serotypes that are usually responsible are types 19, 6, 23, and 3. The first three of these are the three serotypes most commonly carried asymptomatically in the upper respiratory tract. Upper respiratory tract infections and allergies congest the respiratory tract and promote the development of otitis media.

Diseases Due to *S. pneumoniae*

Diagnosis

(1) Pneumococcal Pneumonia. In about 75% of patients, pneumococcal pneumonia begins 1–3 days after the onset of an upper respiratory tract infection and is heralded by a single shaking chill and temperature that rapidly rises to 38.8–41.4 °C (102–106 °F). The chills begin so dramatically that many patients can pinpoint the time that the bout began. Patients typically suffer from pleurisy (inflammation of the pleura); develop a rusty-colored sputum that contains blood; and experience chest pain (pleuritic pain), which is often so severe that pneumococcal pneumonia is called the stabbing disease in some African countries. Other typical manifestations include weakness, anorexia, rapid but shallow breathing, and rapid heart rate. Patients may lie on the affected side to splint the infected lung. Some patients with lower lobe pneumonia experience severe abdominal pain that may be mistaken for an acute abdomen.

X-rays should be taken to determine the nature of the pulmonary disease. Laboratory analyses may reveal hypoxia, increased P_{CO_2}, and leukocytosis (70–90% PMNs) with a profound left shift (many immature leukocytes). From 25% to 30% of patients are bacteremic, placing them at risk for developing endocarditis, septic arthritis, or meningitis. The presence of pneumococci in the blood is considered definitive proof of pneumococcal disease.

Sputum and blood samples should be cultured to determine if *S. pneumoniae* is present. Care should be taken to collect sputum samples that contain no epithelial cells and are really sputum, rather than merely being upper respiratory tract secretions. If the patient is unable to expectorate, samples can be taken by percutaneous transtracheal aspiration. Samples should be examined for a quellung reaction and a response to Gram's staining, and they should also be cultured under CO_2 on blood agar that contains gentamicin. Counterimmunoelectrophoresis, enzyme-linked immunosorbent assay, or an agglutination test can be used to detect the presence of pneumococcal antigens in blood and urine (blood is positive in 45–80% of patients with pneumococcal disease, while urine is positive in 50–65%).

(2) Pneumococcal Meningitis. Pneumococcal meningitis may occur as a primary disease or as a complication of pneumonia. About one-fourth of patients suffer from both pneumococcal pneumonia and meningitis. Head trauma, such as that which occurs during an automobile accident, is also a risk factor for pneumococcal meningitis. Clinical manifestations of meningitis may include a stiff neck (nuchal rigidity), severe headache, somnolence, seizures, and other signs of neurologic abnormalities. Neurologic examination and laboratory testing of patients with meningitis are described in detail in Chapter 6 (see the discussion of meningococcal meningitis under *Neisseria meningitis*).

(3) Otitis Media. Infants and young children are particularly susceptible to developing otitis media for several reasons: their auditory tubes (eustachian tubes) are almost horizontal and are easily plugged; they tend to suffer from many viral infections of the upper respiratory tract, and this contributes to blockage of the auditory tubes; and they lack antibody to the common causative agents of otitis media. The practice of allowing an infant to lie supine and suck from a bottle placed in the crib (bottle propping) predisposes the infant to recurrent otitis media because the liquid tends to jet from the nasopharynx into the auditory tubes when the infant drinks. Otitis media almost always follows a viral infection of the upper respiratory tract, and about 10% of children with measles will also develop bacterial otitis media. Otitis media is sometimes followed by meningitis, particularly in patients under 5 years of age.

Acute bacterial otitis media involves swelling of the soft tissues in the ear and collection of pus behind the tympanic membrane. This may cause a feeling of pressure, sometimes accompanied by temporary loss of hearing or by extreme pain. On otoscopic examination, the tympanic membrane will appear fiery red and bulging. The agent responsible may be identified by culturing a sample of pus that has drained into the ear canal or a sample that has been taken by myringotomy (an incision made in the tympanic membrane) or needle biopsy. Myringotomy is often performed to relieve pressure and pain, but a needle biopsy provides a cleaner sample for culture.

Three bacterial agents are responsible for most *acute* middle ear infections: *S. pneumoniae* (more than one-half of all cases); *H. influenzae* (about one-third of cases, most during infancy); and *S. pyogenes* (10–15% of cases). *Moraxella catarrhalis* is an occasional cause. In infants under 6 weeks of age, coliforms (*E. coli* and closely related bacteria) and staphylococci are common causes of acute otitis media. In older infants and children, if chronic otitis media develops, there is a shift in the bacterial population to gram-negative rods—particularly *Proteus*, *Klebsiella*, *Enterobacter*, and *Pseudomonas*.

(4) Other Diseases Due to S. pneumoniae. Conjunctivitis (pinkeye) is characterized by conjunctival hyperemia and mucoid secretions that cause the eyelids to stick together. The infection makes the eye feel scratchy and appear pink, and it may cause blurred vision. Conjunctivitis may be due to *Neisseria gonorrhoeae*, *Haemophilus*, an allergic reaction, or adenovirus, but it is most commonly due to *S. pneumoniae* and is generally diagnosed on clinical grounds alone. Although conjunctivitis sometimes resolves spontaneously in about a week, it usually needs to be treated.

Sinusitis is an extremely common problem in cold, damp environments and is caused by *S. pneumoniae* (30–40% of cases), *H. influenzae* (about 20%), *M. catarrhalis* (about 20%), and *Staphylococcus aureus* (less than 20%). Sinusitis usually follows an upper respiratory tract infection that blocks the paranasal sinuses and is characterized by pain and tenderness over the sinus and by a purulent discharge. The patient may experience fever with chills and headaches. The diagnosis is usually made on the basis of clinical signs and symptoms. However, refractile sinusitis sometimes requires a precise microbiologic identification, in which case the patient may need to be sedated or anesthetized so that a transnasal sinus aspirate can be obtained and cultured.

Treatment and Prognosis.   In the past, pneumococci were uniformly sensitive to penicillin G, so all pneumococcal diseases were treated with penicillin. Today, "relative" penicillin resistance (minimum inhibitory concentration, or MIC, of 0.1–0.9 μg/mL) is seen frequently in the USA, while high-level resistance (MIC ≥ 1.0 μg/mL) is seen occasionally. Penicillin G is still the recommended treatment, but cefotaxime, ceftriaxone, imipenem, or vancomycin can be substituted as indicated by sensitivity testing. Tetracyclines should not be used, because many pneumococci are tetracycline-resistant.

Five factors affect the outcome of pneumococcal pneumonia: patient age, presence of underlying disease, severity of disease, pneumococcal serotype, and delay of therapy. Patients over age 40 are at greatly increased risk of death, and the treated mortality rate is about 25% among the elderly. Pneumococcal pneumonia can be rapidly fatal in patients with sickle cell disease, splenectomy, multiple myeloma, emphysema, congestive heart failure, or other underlying disease or immunologic defect. Patients with severe disease characterized by multilobar involvement are at greatly increased risk. Disease caused by type 3 or type 2 pneumococci is the most dangerous. The later that antibiotic treatment begins during the first 4 days of disease, the worse the prognosis is.

Otitis media, conjunctivitis, and sinusitis are generally treated empirically with regimens designed to provide coverage against the prevalent causes of each disease. Otitis media in patients 4 years or younger is treated with a mixture of erythromycin and sulfonamide, while that in patients over 4 years old is treated with trimethoprim-sulfamethoxazole or with cefuroxime. Conjunctivitis is generally treated with an ointment or drops that contain either sulfacetamide or a combination of neomycin and polymyxin. Sinusitis is treated with measures to relieve congestion (water-saturated air and decongestants) and with antibiotics (ampicillin, amoxicillin, trimethoprim-sulfamethoxazole, or a second-generation cephalosporin). Patients with chronic sinusitis may require surgical treatment.

Prevention.   A patient at high risk for pneumococcal disease should not be hospitalized in the same room as a patient who is suffering from pneumococcal pneumonia. Individuals at risk should be immunized periodically with a pneumococcal vaccine. The one that is currently available is a killed vaccine that contains material from the 23 most prevalent serotypes of pneumococcal disease. While reimmunization is recommended every 6 years for adults, it is recommended every 3–6 years for children with specific risk factors.

Other Streptococci

Group C streptococci, group G streptococci, and members of the *Streptococcus intermedius* group (*Streptococcus anginosus, Streptococcus constellatus,*

and *Streptococcus* MG) are occasional causes of human disease, as described in Table 5–1. The *S. intermedius* group is also called the *Streptococcus milleri* or *Streptococcus anginosus-milleri* group.

ENTEROCOCCI
Classification of Enterococci and Group D Streptococci

Until recently, Lancefield group D streptococci were divided into two classes: the enterococci and the nonenterococcal group D streptococci. During the 1980s, the genus *Streptococcus* was divided into three genera, and the enterococci were placed within the genus *Enterococcus*. Although there are currently 12 *Enterococcus* species, between 80% and 90% of all enterococcal disease is caused by *Enterococcus faecalis,* with most of the rest caused by *Enterococcus faecium*. The most important of the nonenterococcal group D streptococci is *Streptococcus bovis,* which is most often the cause of endocarditis in patients with gastrointestinal tumors.

Enterococcus faecalis and *Enterococcus faecium*

While *Enterococcus faecalis* and *Enterococcus faecium* both cause disease in humans, the discussion here focuses on the first of these, since it is the key enterococcal pathogen. *E. faecalis* is carried in the gastrointestinal tract, oral cavity, gallbladder, urethra, and vagina. It is spread to new hosts on the hands and can persist for some time on fomites. For this reason, *E. faecalis* is an important cause of nosocomial disease. While *E. faecalis* used to be the fourth most prevalent nosocomial pathogen, in less than a decade it became the second most prevalent, with *Escherichia coli* currently being first on the list. Enterococci are opportunistic pathogens that often colonize patients via indwelling catheters, and they preferentially cause disease in patients who are debilitated or immunocompromised. Other risk factors are major surgery, wounds, cystoscopy, and intravenous drug use. Enterococcal infections can result in development of endocarditis, bacteremia, urinary tract infections, intra-abdominal abscesses, soft tissue infections, and neonatal sepsis.

Characteristics of *E. faecalis* and *E. faecium*

General Features.   When cultivated on blood agar, enterococci are variable in their hemolysis, causing either α hemolysis or no hemolysis. They are distinguished from other gram-positive cocci on the basis of the ability of enterococci to (1) grow at a wide temperature range (10–45 °C), (2) grow in a medium that contains 6.5% sodium chloride, (3) hydrolyze esculin in 40% bile, and (4) hydrolyze L-pyrrolidonyl-β-naphthylamide.

Mechanisms of Pathogenicity.   If there is a single outstanding characteristic of enterococci that allows them to cause disease, it is their unusual resistance to antibiotics. Some enterococci are reported to be resistant to every known antibiotic, while others are reported to be impervious to all antibiotics except glycopeptides (vancomycin and teicoplanin) or imipenem. *E. faecium* tends to be more antibiotic-resistant than is *E. faecalis.*

Both *E. faecalis* and *E. faecium* harbor plasmids that encode resistance to a wide variety of antibiotics, including tetracyclines, penicillins, cephalosporins, macrolides, chloramphenicol, and aminoglycosides. The enterococci are naturally tolerant to beta-lactam antibiotics, ostensibly because their penicillin-binding proteins have relatively low affinities for most beta-lactam drugs. Additionally, some enterococci demonstrate a curious response to beta-lactam antibiotics known as the **eagle effect.** Eagle effect–positive enterococci exhibit their greatest bactericidal response to penicillins at a concentration just above the MIC of the antibiotic; as the concentration of penicillin is increased above this value, the bactericidal effect against the enterococci is decreased. The molecular basis of the eagle effect is not known.

While some enterococci are sensitive to gentamicin, others exhibit either high-level resistance (MIC $\geq$2000 μg/mL) or low-level resistance (MIC <2000 μg/mL) to this drug. Aminoglycosides work synergistically with penicillins or vancomycin when gentamicin resistance is low but not when it is high.

Diseases Due to *E. faecalis* and *E. faecium*

Diagnosis. Among the diseases caused by enterococci, the five most important are endocarditis, primary bacteremia, urinary tract infections, abdominal infections, and neonatal meningitis.

(1) Endocarditis. Infective endocarditis can be caused by a wide variety of organisms, including streptococci, which account for about 70% of cases. The viridans streptococci that are oral commensals are the most prevalent cause of infective endocarditis; staphylococci are the second most prevalent; *E. faecalis* has been reported to cause 5–20% of cases; and *Streptococcus bovis,* a nonenterococcal group D streptococcus, is also responsible for cases of infective endocarditis.

Enterococcal endocarditis is often subacute, rather than acute, and occurs most frequently in elderly men, young women, and intravenous drug users. Elderly men are at risk because they often undergo genitourinary tract procedures, such as cystoscopy and catheterization. Two-thirds of patients with enterococcal endocarditis have preexisting valvular abnormalities.

Patients with endocarditis show signs of general systemic infection, such as fever, weakness, anorexia, myalgia, arthralgia, weight loss, and leukocytosis. The combination of fever and heart murmur suggests the presence of infectious endocarditis. Patients often develop manifestations whose origins are from emboli precipitated by cardiac vegetations. Some of these are splenomegaly with upper left abdominal quadrant pain, strokes and toxic encephalopathy, petechiae, splinter hemorrhages under the fingernails

and on the conjunctivas, Osler's nodes (raised reddish-blue nodules, usually on the fingertips), Janeway's spots (flat red macules on the extremities), and focal embolic nephritis. Clubbing of the fingers is associated with the development of chronic endocarditis.

The keystone to diagnosis of infective endocarditis is blood culture. Venous blood samples are taken at intervals of 6–8 hours for 3–5 days before antibiotic therapy is instituted. Once isolated, enterococci must be differentiated from viridans streptococci and *S. bovis.* If the organism is identified as *S. bovis,* the patient should be further examined for the presence of a gastrointestinal tumor. In cases of endocarditis due to *E. faecalis,* the fatality rate is about 70% for patients with natural valves but only 10–15% for those with prosthetic valves.

(2) Bacteremia. Primary enterococcal bacteremia occurs most often in men who are older than 50 years and have a preexisting medical condition, such as recent major surgery, severe burns, or multiple trauma. In about 80% of cases, the infection is nosocomial. Other major risk factors are bladder catheterization and cephalosporin use. According to one study, 98% of bacteremic patients received cephalosporins or other broad-spectrum antibiotics before the onset of their bacteremia.

Patients with bacteremia exhibit signs of generalized systemic disease and may also suffer from endocarditis. The diagnosis is confirmed by blood culture.

(3) Urinary Tract Infections. *E. faecalis* causes about 10% of urinary tract infections in the general population and is the second most prevalent cause of these infections in hospitalized patients. Risk factors include impaired host defense and urinary catheterization. Enterococci can cause pyelonephritis or cystitis. While either of these infections may be characterized by urgent, frequent, and painful urination, pyelonephritis is also associated with fever, chills, and flank pain and is sometimes accompanied by nausea and diarrhea. Cystitis is associated with suprapubic discomfort and is not accompanied by fever. In each case, bacteria can be isolated from midstream urine, but absolute bacterial counts are considerably higher in patients with pyelonephritis. Unlike patients with cystitis, those with pyelonephritis have leukocytosis with a left shift and also have urinary bacteria that are coated with antibody.

(4) Abdominal Infections. *E. faecalis* is occasionally the cause of intra-abdominal infections, usually as part of a mixed infection with *E. coli, Staphylococcus aureus,* and *Staphylococcus epidermidis.* The case fatality rate is high when the infection contains both enterococci and *E. coli.*

(5) Neonatal Meningitis. *E. faecium* has caused sporadic epidemics of enterococcal neonatal meningitis. The affected infants were of low birth weight, were premature (mean gestational age of 29 weeks), were under 16 days old, had received penicillin G or ampicillin previously, and had either an intravenous catheter or nasogastric tube. The infection was thought to have been transmitted to the infants from the hands of attending health care workers.

Treatment. Because enterococci have a high frequency of antibiotic resistance, the selection of antibiotics is difficult. Generally, the recommendation for treatment of enterococcal infections outside the bladder is combination therapy with penicillin or a glycopeptide (vancomycin or teicoplanin) plus an aminoglycoside. For treatment of cystitis, the recommendation is to use penicillin, ampicillin, or a glycopeptide. Cephalosporins are not indicated, because they predispose patients to enterococcal superinfections.

Before treatment is begun, enterococci should be tested for penicillin and gentamicin sensitivity. If the patient is not allergic to penicillin and the enterococcus is penicillin-sensitive, the infection should be treated with penicillin or ampicillin plus an aminoglycoside; otherwise, vancomycin plus an aminoglycoside should be used. If the enterococcus exhibits high-level gentamicin resistance, sensitivity to streptomycin should be tested. Whereas streptomycin-sensitive bacteria should be treated with streptomycin plus a penicillin, streptomycin-resistant bacteria should be treated with a prolonged course of either penicillin or a glycopeptide. If the patient suffers from endocarditis, combination treatment is with intravenous antibiotics.

STAPHYLOCOCCI

The staphylococci are the quintessential pyogenic cocci. Infection with staphylococci is almost always accompanied by the accumulation of large amounts of pus. In fact, staphylococci are responsible for more than 80% of all suppurative infections and are capable of causing such diverse conditions as boils (furuncles and carbuncles), folliculitis, impetigo, pneumonia, endocarditis, pyoarthrosis, burn infections with bacteremia, acute enteritis, food poisoning, scalded skin syndrome, and toxic shock syndrome.

Classification of Staphylococci

Staphylococci appear as masses of gram-positive cocci and derive their name from the Greek *staphylē,* which means "a cluster of grapes." Unlike streptococci, which are catalase-negative, staphylococci are catalase-positive (for a description of the catalase test, see the earlier discussion of streptococci).

There are more than 20 species of staphylococci, but only 3 are associated with human disease: *Staphylococcus aureus, Staphylococcus epidermidis,* and *Staphylococcus saprophyticus.* Of these, only *S. aureus*

is considered to be frankly pathogenic and only *S. aureus* is coagulase-positive. **Coagulase** is a staphylococcal enzyme that complexes with prothrombin in serum to split fibrinogen to fibrin. Thus, when *S. aureus* is placed into a tube of serum that contains prothrombin and fibrinogen, the serum becomes gelatinous. *S. epidermidis* and *S. saprophyticus* are coagulase-negative. Although *Staphylococcus hyicus* and *Staphylococcus intermedius* also produce coagulase, they are not isolated from human sources. Many laboratories merely report staphylococci as being either *S. aureus* or coagulase-negative staphylococci.

As Table 5–3 shows, *S. aureus* grows as β-hemolytic colonies on blood agar. The name "aureus" was given to this organism because many strains have yellowish (or golden) colonies, but not all *S. aureus* strains have this characteristic.

Staphylococci can be isolated on mannitol salt agar, which is a medium that is high in salt (7.5% NaCl) and contains mannitol as a source of carbon and energy. *S. aureus* ferments the mannitol and causes the medium to turn yellow. While other staphylococci grow on the medium, they are variable in their ability to ferment mannitol. The staphylococci vary in the sugars they ferment, but when cultured in fermentation tubes, each species produces acid but no gas from sugars. *S. epidermidis* can be differentiated from *S. aureus* and *S. saprophyticus* by its requirement for biotin for growth, while *S. saprophyticus* can be identified by its novobiocin resistance. Among the findings that allow staphylococcal species to be identified are that *S. saprophyticus* does not reduce nitrate or utilize arginine and that *S. epidermidis* does not ferment D-trehalose.

S. aureus is unique in that it has a surface structure known as **protein A,** which is an Fc receptor for IgG1, IgG2, and IgG4. The presence of protein A can be detected by using a **latex agglutination test** in which the latex beads are coated with plasma that contains clumping factor (discussed below) and antibody to protein A. A sample of a colony suspected of being *S. aureus* is mixed with saline and latex bead reagent on a card, and the presence of *S. aureus* is evidenced by a visible clumping reaction. For purposes of epidemiologic studies, reference laboratories are able to divide *S. aureus* strains into four groups, based on their patterns of sensitivity to various lysogenic phages.

Staphylococcus aureus

Staphylococcus aureus is consistently one of the top four causes of nosocomial infections, along with

TABLE 5–3.   A Comparison of the Characteristics of Three Important Staphylococci and *Streptococcus pyogenes*

Species	Hemolysis	Catalase	Coagulase	Protein A	Biotin	Novobiocin
Staphylococcus aureus	Beta	Positive	Positive	Present	Not required for growth	Sensitive
Staphylococcus epidermidis	Variable	Positive	Negative	Absent	Required	Sensitive
Staphylococcus saprophyticus	Variable	Positive	Negative	Absent	Not required	Resistant
Streptococcus pyogenes	Beta	Negative	Negative	Absent	Not required	Sensitive

Escherichia coli, Enterococcus faecalis, and *Pseudomonas aeruginosa.*

Although *S. aureus* is a normal resident of the nares and bowel of 30–50% of the general population, the organism is carried by about 90% of the hospital clinical staff. It is unusually resistant to drying, so it is rapidly and easily spread to patients from the hands of the clinical staff and from fomites such as clothes, sheets, and equipment. *S. aureus* strains typically are resistant to many drugs and are able to avoid being killed by most disinfectants. Thus, they are able to persist and thrive in the hospital environment, where they can be passed to individuals who are highly susceptible to staphylococcal infection, including newborns, immunosuppressed patients, burn victims, and patients with indwelling devices such as catheters.

Characteristics of *S. aureus*

General Features. *S. aureus* is a β-hemolytic, gram-positive coccus that is catalase-positive, is coagulase-positive, and ferments mannitol.

(1) Cell Surface Antigens. Staphylococci have a variety of cell surface antigens, and some staphylococcal strains have a weakly antiphagocytic capsule. This **capsule** is lost when the strain is subcultured, and its significance in pathogenesis is not known.

Covalently linked to the peptidoglycan of *S. aureus* is **protein A,** a 42-kD protein that binds the Fc region of IgG1, IgG2, and IgG4, as well as some IgM and IgA. About one-third of the protein A produced is also released into the environment, where it binds IgG and elicits a cell-mediated immune response (CMIR). Each molecule of protein A expressed on the cell surface can bind up to four molecules of IgG. If a staphylococcal boil is present, binding of IgG to the bacterial surface via the Fc region will not only interfere with phagocytosis of the staphylococci but will also elicit a CMIR that may be responsible for much of the cytolysis and necrolysis seen within the boil.

S. aureus expresses a substituted ribitol phosphate **teichoic acid** that is sometimes identified as **polysaccharide A.** Teichoic acid–peptidoglycan complexes are released into the environment, where they activate complement away from the bacterium. This protects the organism from opsonization by depleting complement, but it attracts PMNs into the lesion when chemotactic peptides are generated. Polysaccharide A that is not released also elicits a CMIR, and the combined effects of complement activation, PMN accumulation, and CMIR contribute to the festering of staphylococcal boils.

S. aureus has a cell wall component known as **clumping factor,** which aggregates staphylococci by binding fibrinogen. Aggregated staphylococci are difficult to phagocytose.

The **cell wall peptidoglycan** of staphylococci is highly cross-linked with pentaglycine bridges. Patients with staphylococcal infections form antibodies to this peptidoglycan, probably because of its high peptide content. These antibodies can form damaging immune complexes with peptidoglycan monomers released by staphylococci during growth.

Staphylococci exhibit **binding sites** for a number of serum proteins, including **fibronectin, C1q, lamanin,** and **collagen.** The binding sites may allow staphylococci to persist in areas where these substances abound. For example, wounds contain much fibronectin, and the persistence of staphylococci in wounds may be related to the ability of the organisms to attach to cells via fibronectin. Lamanin is the major glycoprotein in mammalian basement membranes, so staphylococci with lamanin receptors may have increased ability to colonize basement membranes.

(2) Extracellular Enzymes. Of the staphylococci that colonize humans, *S. aureus* is the only one that produces **coagulase,** as discussed above. *S. aureus* also releases several hydrolases into the environment. Staphylococcal **lipases** digest fats and are believed to be important in the pathogenesis of boils. **Staphylokinase,** which is encoded by a temperate phage, is similar to streptokinase; both convert plasminogen to fibrinolytic plasmin. Staphylococci also produce **hyaluronidase,** several **proteases,** and a **nuclease** that cleaves both RNA and DNA.

S. aureus produces four hemolysins that differ in structure, specificity, and mechanism of action. The **α-hemolysin (alpha toxin)** is a 34-kD protein that lyses cells by forming transmembrane channels. Some investigators have noted that these channels resemble the terminal transmembrane attack complex formed by activated complement components. Encoded on a transposon, alpha toxin lyses rabbit erythrocytes (but not human erythrocytes) and produces β hemolysis on agar containing rabbit blood. Alpha toxin has been shown to damage a variety of cells, including human platelets and many types of cultured cells. Its dermonecrotic action seems to come from its spastic effects on vascular smooth muscle. The **β-hemolysin** is a "hot-cold" hemolysin produced by 10–20% of human *S. aureus* isolates. A sphingomyelinase, it lyses erythrocytes (including human erythrocytes) when they are incubated at 37 °C and then shifted to cold temperatures. The β-hemolysin is toxic for a wide variety of cultured cells. The **γ-hemolysin** is a combination of two proteins that lyse human, sheep, and rabbit erythrocytes. The function of γ-hemolysin in infection is not understood. The **δ-hemolysin** is a detergentlike toxin that damages many types of cells and may elicit the formation of platelet-activating factor.

Most *S. aureus* strains produce **Panton-Valentine leukocidin.** This toxin has two components, known as S and F. The S component binds to GM_1 gangliosides and phosphatidylcholine, making phospholipid-derived products available when it activates a membrane-bound phospholipase A_2. The cell is lysed when F binds to these products and forms a K^+-specific ion channel.

(3) Staphylococcal Exotoxins. Staphylococci may produce three types of exotoxins: staphylococcal enterotoxin, exfoliative toxin, and toxic shock syndrome toxin 1.

Staphylococcal enterotoxins (SEs) derive their name from the fact that they affect the functions of the gastrointestinal tract. The SE genes are carried by a limited number of bacteriophages and are introduced into staphylococci via phage conversion. The SEs are produced only by phage group III *S. aureus,* and their production occurs when the bacteria are multiplying logarithmically. SEs are resistant to the action of proteolytic enzymes and are not inactivated when exposed to a temperature of 100 °C for 30 minutes. Thus, cooking food suspected of containing an SE will not reliably inactivate the toxin. There are seven SEs, designated as SE-A, SE-B, SE-C1, SE-C2, SE-D, SE-E, and SE-F. While SE-A is the enterotoxin most often encountered, SE-B plays a role in toxic shock syndrome. In the gut, the SEs stimulate local neural receptors that travel to the vomiting center. Thus, an individual who eats food that contains an SE will experience explosive vomiting and may suffer from diarrhea. It is believed that SE-B is a **superantigen** and that its participation in the generation of toxic shock syndrome is due to its superantigenic properties.

Exfoliative toxins (ETs) are produced by about 5% of *S. aureus* isolates, most of which are in phage group II. ETs, which are sometimes called epidermolytic toxins, are responsible for staphylococcal scalded skin syndrome (toxic epidermal necrolysis) and for bullous impetigo. They cause intraepidermal separation by splitting and disrupting desmosomes at the intercellular contact sites in the granular layer of the epidermis. When the affected skin is stroked lightly, it will peel and wrinkle (a positive Nikolsky sign). Skin affected by ETs heals without scarring. There are two ETs, designated as ETA and ETB. ETB is more commonly seen, is encoded on a plasmid, and is produced by staphylococci in phage group II. ETA is chromosomally encoded, and its production is not restricted to a particular phage group.

Toxic shock syndrome toxin 1 (TSST-1) is a 24-kD protein produced primarily by staphylococci that are sensitive to one or two specific bacteriophages (bacteriophage 29, 52, or both) and exhibit chromosomally encoded resistance to cadmium, arsenate, and penicillin G. Like SE-B and like streptococcal pyrogenic exotoxins A and C (SPE-A and SPE-C), TSST-1 is a **superantigen** that causes selective expression of T cell subsets with concomitant hyperproduction of cytokines, monokines, and autacoids. This process is discussed at length in the section concerning SPEs (see Group A Streptococci, above). TSST-1 also causes extensive capillary leakage that results in hypovolemia and is directly toxic to the myocardium, kidneys, liver, lungs, lymphoid tissues, central nervous system, and peripheral nerves.

Mechanisms of Pathogenicity. The ability of staphylococci to cause disease is influenced by the ability to freely exchange genetic information. Many characteristics are transferred by bacteriophages, either via generalized transduction or via phage conversion, but a process akin to conjugation has also been described among the staphylococci. Certain diseases correspond to specific phage groups. For example, phage group II staphylococci most often cause skin infections, while phage group III staphylococci most often cause gastrointestinal infections. Staphylococci carry many plasmids that encode antibiotic resistance, and these plasmids have been shown to be transmitted efficiently among staphylococci by both transduction and conjugation. Thus, staphylococci are often antibiotic-resistant, making antibiotic selection a problem.

Although SEs, ETs, and TSST-1 can be identified as the proximal causes of staphylococcal food poisoning, scalded skin syndrome, and toxic shock syndrome, respectively, most staphylococcal diseases are pyogenic infections in which no single pathogenic attribute of staphylococci can be said to be critical. Rather, it is the aggregate pyogenic and necrotic activities of staphylococci that make them successful pathogens. These include the activities of invasive factors (lipases, nuclease, coagulase, staphylokinase, hyaluronidase, and proteases), local toxins (α-, β-, γ-, and δ-hemolysins), and cell surface antigens (capsule, protein A, polysaccharide A, clumping factor, peptidoglycan, and binding sites for host receptors). The impact of these substances is accentuated by antibody and cellular immune responses that contribute to the formation of pus and local necrosis. Because staphylococci resist phagocytosis, they are able to persist long enough to elicit a vigorous pyogenic response. The result is usually the formation of a suppurative (pus-producing) lesion.

Suppurative Infections Due to *S. aureus*

Diagnosis

(1) Folliculitis, Furuncles, and Carbuncles. Staphylococci are the main cause of suppurative skin and tissue infections, including folliculitis, furuncles, and carbuncles. Staphylococci commonly enter the skin via an insect bite or hair follicle and form a pus-filled lesion (pustule). **Folliculitis** occurs when the lesion is restricted to the hair follicle, and it is often seen as aggregates of pustules on the bearded area of the face or as areas of the scalp where there is a pustule at the base of each hair. The lesion can become a **furuncle** (boil) when the pustule spreads into the subcutaneous tissues. Furuncles are hot, can be exquisitely tender, and may be accompanied by low-grade fever. Furuncles may spread beneath the skin and form interconnecting channels to construct a complex lesion known as a **carbuncle.** Carbuncles are most often seen on the neck or upper back. Some patients with carbuncles develop staphylococcal cellulitis, and immunosuppressed patients are at risk of becoming bacteremic. Patients infected with staphylococcal strains that produce TSST-1, SE-B, or both of these toxins are at risk of developing toxic shock syndrome. Patients who are nasal carriers of *S. aureus* may suffer from recurrent folliculitis or furuncles.

Material from staphylococcal pyoderma can be examined by Gram's stain for the presence of clumps of gram-positive cocci, but the results are only suggestive. Definitive diagnosis involves culturing material on blood agar (rabbit blood is best) and demonstrating the presence of β-hemolytic, catalase-positive, coagulase-positive, gram-positive cocci.

(2) Impetigo. *S. aureus* is now the most common cause of impetigo in children. Staphylococcal impetigo occurs most often around the nose and is most likely spread from the nares to the face by runny noses and nose picking. Diagnosis of staphylococcal impetigo involves culturing the organisms from the superficial lesions. The crusts can be moistened and dissolved to facilitate isolation of the staphylococci.

(3) Pneumonia. *S. aureus* is responsible for 1–5% of all cases of pneumonia in the USA. Staphylococcal pneumonia most often occurs as a sequela of influenza, and 75% of affected patients in the USA are under 1 year of age. At risk are patients with impaired immune or pulmonary function, including those with cystic fibrosis, measles, or emphysema and those receiving chemotherapy. Staphylococcal pneumonia is an acute pneumonia and is often accompanied by empyema (intrapleural abscesses). The signs and symptoms of staphylococcal pneumonia are similar to those of pneumococcal pneumonia, and definitive diagnosis requires that the organisms be cultured from sputum, blood, or transtracheal aspirates.

(4) Other Suppurative Infections Due to *S. aureus*. Patients who have had orthopedic surgery are at risk of developing staphylococcal **pyoarthrosis** or **osteomyelitis.** Patients with third-degree burns (burns that destroy the full thickness of the skin) are at risk of developing suppurative **infections of the burned area** and **bacteremia.** In each case, bacteremia resulting from the primary infection can lead to staphylococcal **endocarditis.** Staphylococcal endocarditis is an acute, rapidly progressive endocarditis that can destroy natural valves within days and has a fatality rate of 40–80% with appropriate treatment. Finally, patients who have received large doses of broad-spectrum antibiotics may develop a bacterial vacuum in the gut. When the depopulated intestinal mucosa is repopulated with drug-resistant staphylococci, the patient will develop **acute staphylococcal enteritis.** Staphylococci may necrose the bowel wall, resulting in bacteremia and endocarditis. Each of these diseases is definitively diagnosed by culturing staphylococci from lesion exudate and from the blood.

Treatment
(1) Folliculitis, Furuncles, and Carbuncles. Folliculitis is treated with mupirocin, which is applied directly to the affected area and to the nostrils to keep patients from reinfecting themselves. A systemic antibiotic, such as dicloxacillin or erythromycin, may also be required. The prevalence of methicillin resistance in many vicinities has made treatment of staphylococcal infections more difficult. Carbuncles and furuncles should be "ripened" by the application of heat and then incised and drained. If the patient is febrile, dicloxacillin or erythromycin should be administered. Again, staphylococcal carriage should be eliminated by intranasal mupirocin.

(2) Impetigo. Patients with impetigo should be treated with topical mupirocin and systemic dicloxacillin or erythromycin.

(3) Pneumonia and Other Suppurative Infections. Systemic suppurative infections, such as pneumonia, are treated with systemic antibiotics. Systemic infections caused by methicillin-sensitive staphylococci are usually treated with a penicillinase-resistant penicillin (nafcillin, oxacillin, or methicillin). Alternatively, vancomycin, clindamycin, or a first-generation cephalosporin can be used. Pneumonia caused by methicillin-resistant staphylococci is treated with vancomycin.

Nonsuppurative Infections Due to *S. aureus*

Diagnosis
(1) Staphylococcal Scalded Skin Syndrome. Scalded skin syndrome is a disease found in young children, usually under 2 years of age but occasionally as old as 4 years. Affected children are usually nonimmune children whose umbilical stump, conjunctiva, or external ear canal has been colonized with a strain of *S. aureus* that produces ET. ET-producing staphylococci are in phage group II, and most are susceptible to phage 71. The ET is disseminated hematogenously, and cultures of the affected skin do not yield toxigenic *S. aureus*.

There are two forms of scalded skin syndrome. Patients who develop **bullous impetigo** break out in clusters of large blisters (bullae) that occur most often on intertriginous surfaces and rupture to become moist red or crusted lesions. Others develop **generalized scalded skin syndrome,** which begins on the face and neck, under the arms, and in the groin and then spreads over the body during the next 24–48 hours, causing generalized reddening of the skin. The skin is loose and wrinkled, can be sloughed off with gentle pressure (a positive Nikolsky sign), and looks as if it has been scalded with boiling water. In addition to skin involvement, patients may have a low-grade fever and be irritable. Although the skin peels in sheets, only the granular layer is involved. Thus, scalded skin syndrome and bullous impetigo lesions heal without scarring in 7–10 days.

The diagnosis rests heavily on clinical findings, because the area of skin that looks scalded is not infected. Skin and mucosal areas usually colonized by *S. aureus* can be cultured to determine if the patient is harboring phage group II staphylococci. Scalded skin syndrome must be differentiated from drug-induced toxic epidermal necrolysis and from erythema multiforme.

(2) Toxic Shock Syndrome. Toxic shock syndrome (TSS) was first described in 1978 in a group of seven children and adolescents (three boys and four girls) between the ages of 8 and 17 years. During the early 1980s, there was an explosion of TSS cases, most of which occurred in menstruating women who were using superabsorbent tampons. Because of the dramatic association of TSS with tampons, many have forgotten that TSS is not a disease only of women.

TSS may also occur in individuals who have a boil or other focus of staphylococcal infection. TSS is caused by *S. aureus* strains that produce either TSST-1 or SE-B.

Patients with TSS develop a generalized pruritic maculopapular rash similar to that seen during scarlet fever. The rash desquamates on the fingers, toes, palms, and soles. Patients may suffer hair and nail loss and feel extreme fatigue. Systemic signs of toxicity and multiorgan involvement will be present and may consist of adult respiratory distress syndrome, hyponatremia, acidosis, acute renal failure, thrombocytopenia, disseminated intravascular coagulation, pericardial and pleural edema, hepatic dysfunction, central nervous system dysfunction (including irrational behavior or seizures), or a combination of these findings. The mucous membranes of the mouth and gastrointestinal tract often desquamate, and the patient suffers from prolonged myalgia and muscle weakness. There may also be neuropathies and peripheral gangrene. From 5% to 10% of patients die, usually from noncardiogenic shock.

The clinical diagnosis may be supported by cultivation of staphylococci from a boil or from tampons. TSS must be differentiated from the more dangerous toxic streptococcal syndrome.

(3) Kawasaki Disease. Kawasaki disease is an acute disease of childhood and early infancy and is the main cause of acquired heart disease among children in the USA. Its etiology is unknown, but recent studies have shown that most children with Kawasaki disease carry TSST-1–producing strains of *S. aureus*, and those who are negative for these staphylococci carry *Streptococcus pyogenes* strains that produce SPE-B or SPE-C. Thus, Kawasaki disease may be the result of the superantigenic activity of staphylococcal and streptococcal toxins, with selective expansion of $V\beta2^+$ T cells.

Kawasaki disease is a multisystem disease that includes a rash and lymphadenopathy. It results in coronary artery abnormalities in 15–25% of patients. The diagnosis is made on clinical grounds. In addition to having a temperature that spikes to over 39.4 °C (over 103 °F) for at least 5 days, patients have at least four of the following five criteria: (1) the conjunctivas are injected; (2) the lips are fissured, the throat is injected, or there is a strawberry tongue; (3) the palms and soles are red, the hands and feet are swollen, or the skin on the hands and feet desquamates; (4) a generalized scarlet fever–like rash is present; and (5) cervical lymphadenopathy is present. Patients often have sore joints, and heart sounds may indicate that there is cardiac involvement.

(4) Staphylococcal Food Poisoning. The most common form of food poisoning in the USA is staphylococcal food poisoning, which is not an infection but is an intoxication with staphylococcal enterotoxin. The signs of food poisoning begin 1–6 hours after the patient has eaten a protein-rich food (such as pastry fillings, ham salad, chicken salad, cottage cheese, or lunch meat) that is infected with an enterotoxin-producing *S. aureus* strain. Food can be easily contam-

inated when it is handled by individuals who carry *S. aureus* on their hands or in their nose. If the food is not stored properly (is kept too long, for example, in a picnic basket on a warm day or under a warming light in a restaurant), the staphylococci multiply and produce enterotoxin. It is important to remember that staphylococcal enterotoxins are heat-stable and cannot be destroyed by warming the food. Furthermore, foods containing staphylococcal enterotoxins typically do not appear to be spoiled. Thus, if there is reason to suspect that food is contaminated with staphylococci, the food should be thrown away.

Patients suffer from vomiting and diarrhea that are severe and may last between 6 and 48 hours. Staphylococcal food poisoning can be life-threatening in the elderly and in infants because they are easily imperiled by changes in hydration. The diagnosis of staphylococcal food poisoning is made on clinical grounds alone.

Treatment
(1) Staphylococcal Scalded Skin Syndrome. A penicillinase-resistant penicillin is usually used. However, if methicillin-resistant *S. aureus* (MRSA) is isolated, vancomycin is used.

(2) Toxic Shock Syndrome. Because this syndrome is so often caused by MRSA, patients receive vancomycin and supportive measures for shock.

(3) Kawasaki Disease. Since the etiology of Kawasaki disease is usually uncertain, therapeutic approaches have centered on giving adequate supportive measures. The possibility that the disease is caused by staphylococci and streptococci may alter the way that affected patients are treated.

(4) Staphylococcal Food Poisoning. No antibiotic therapy is required, because the condition is an intoxication rather than an infection. Patients should be adequately hydrated, and their electrolyte status should be monitored and corrected as needed.

Staphylococcus epidermidis

Staphylococcus epidermidis is a ubiquitous inhabitant of human skin surfaces. *S. epidermidis* may be α-hemolytic or nonhemolytic and can be differentiated from *Staphylococcus aureus* by its requirement for biotin for growth and its lack of coagulase activity. *S. epidermidis* has a glycerol teichoic acid and has no protein A.

Most diseases caused by *S. epidermidis* involve infection of an implanted device such as a heart valve, hip prosthesis, pacemaker, vascular graft, or intravenous catheter. *S. epidermidis* also causes urinary tract infections in elderly hospitalized men and causes natural valve endocarditis in intravenous drug users. Treatment of *S. epidermidis* infections is problematic because the organism is usually resistant to many drugs. Penicillins and cephalosporins are often ineffective, so vancomycin has become the drug of choice. Even with appropriate antibiotic therapy, eradication of the organism is difficult because it often grows in an implanted device, where it is relatively inaccessible to the circulation, and because patients are so often debilitated.

Staphylococcus saprophyticus

Staphylococcus saprophyticus tends to be only a transient part of the normal flora, usually on the skin or in and around the urethra. *S. saprophyticus* is coagulase-negative and has no protein A. It can be differentiated from *Staphylococcus epidermidis* by its inability to ferment glucose and by its unusual resistance to novobiocin.

S. saprophyticus is the second most frequent cause of urinary tract infections in sexually active young women. Patients may suffer from cystitis (infection of the bladder) or pyelonephritis (inflammation of the renal parenchyma and pelvis). In men, urinary tract infections caused by this organism are uncommon and usually occur after age 50.

Trimethoprim-sulfamethoxazole is the treatment of choice for *S. saprophyticus* infections. Ampicillin, amoxicillin, or a fluoroquinolone can be used as an alternative.

Selected Readings

Bisno, A. L. Group A streptococcal infections and rheumatic fever. N Engl J Med 325:783–793, 1991.

Cunningham, R., et al. Clinical and molecular aspects of the pathogenesis of *Staphylococcus aureus* bone and joint infections. J Med Microbiol 44:157–164, 1996.

Daly, J. A. Rapid diagnostic tests in microbiology in the 1990s. Am J Clin Pathol 101(supplement 4):S22–S26, 1994.

Edmond, M. B., et al. Vancomycin-resistant *Staphylococcus aureus:* perspectives on measures needed for control. Ann Intern Med 124:329–334, 1996.

Froude, J., et al. Cross-reactivity between streptococci and human tissue: a model of molecular mimicry and autoimmunity. Curr Top Microbiol Immunol 145:5–26, 1989.

Hasty, D. L., et al. Multiple adhesins of streptococci. Infect Immun 60:2147–2152, 1992.

Herwald, H., et al. Streptococcal cysteine protease releases kinins: a virulence mechanism. J Exp Med 184:665–673, 1996.

Johnson, H. E., et al. Superantigens: structure and relevance to human disease. Proc Soc Exp Biol Med 212:99–109, 1996.

Kim, Y. S., and M. G. Tauber. Neurotoxicity of glia activated by gram-positive bacterial products depends on nitric oxide production. Infect Immun 64:3148–3153, 1996.

Pichichera, M. E., et al. Comparative reliability of clinical, culture, and antigen detection methods for the diagnosis of group A beta-hemolytic streptococcal tonsillopharyngitis. Pediatr Ann 21:798–805, 1992.

Rink, L., et al. Induction of a cytokine network by superantigens with parallel Th1 and Th2 stimulation. J Interferon Cytokine Res 16:41–47, 1996.

Robinson, J. H., and M. A. Kehoe. Group A streptococcal M proteins: virulence factors and protective antigens. Immunol Today 13:362–367, 1992.

Rouse, D. J., et al. Strategies for the prevention of early-onset neonatal group B streptococcal sepsis: a decision analysis. Obstet Gynecol 83:483–494, 1994.

Rubins, J. B., et al. Distinct roles for pneumolysin's cytotoxic and complement activities in the pathogenesis of pneumococcal pneumonia. Am J Respir Crit Care Med 153:1339–1346, 1996.

Shanley, T. P., et al. Streptococcal cysteine protease augments lung injury produced by products of group A streptococci. Infect Immun 64:870–877, 1996.

Stevens, D. L. Invasive group A streptococcal infections. Clin Infect Dis 14:2–13, 1992.

Stollerman, G. H. Rheumatogenic group A streptococci and the return of rheumatic fever. Adv Intern Med 35:1–26, 1990.

Strausbaugh, L. J. Toxic shock syndrome: are you recognizing its changing presentations? Postgrad Med 94:107–118, 1993.

Wood, T. F., M. A. Potter, and O. Jonasson. Streptococcal toxic shock–like syndrome: the importance of surgical intervention. Ann Surg 217:109–114, 1993.

Zumla, A. Superantigens, T cells, and microbes. Clin Infect Dis 15:313–320, 1992.

CHAPTER SIX

GRAM-NEGATIVE

PYOGENIC BACTERIA

Bordetella, Haemophilus, Moraxella, and *Neisseria*

While Chapter 5 discussed the gram-positive pyogenic cocci, Chapter 6 discusses the gram-negative pyogenic bacteria and focuses on four genera that are important human pathogens: *Bordetella, Haemophilus, Moraxella,* and *Neisseria.*

The gram-negative pyogenic bacteria are cocci or coccobacilli whose associated diseases usually involve the accumulation of copious amounts of pus and frequently affect the genital or respiratory tract. These diseases include purulent urethritis (gonorrhea), meningitis, pneumonia, bronchitis, sinusitis, otitis media, conjunctivitis, epiglottitis, and whooping cough (pertussis).

NEISSERIA SPECIES
General Characteristics and Classification

The neisseriae are diplococci that are shaped like kidney beans. Many of the organisms are encapsulated, and some are heavily piliated (Fig. 6–1). Neisseriae are distinguished from other mucosal cocci by their nutritional fastidiousness, their Gram-staining characteristics (see Chapter 1), and their reaction in the oxidase test.

In the **oxidase test,** dimethyl or trimethyl paraphenylenediamine is used as an oxidase reagent. A drop of the reagent is placed directly on a bacterial colony or on several colonies that have been smeared on filter paper. If the bacteria in the colony have a terminal cytochrome oxidase, they will turn black or purple within seconds. A disk oxidase test is also available. Neisseriae are oxidase-positive.

There are two pathogenic species of *Neisseria: Neisseria gonorrhoeae* and *Neisseria meningitidis.* Table 6–1 compares the characteristics of pathogenic and commensal neisseriae with other organisms that are commonly isolated from mucosal surfaces. Commensal neisseriae and *N. meningitidis* can be cultivated either on blood agar or on chocolate agar

(a chocolate-colored medium that contains heated blood). Because *N. gonorrhoeae* is so nutritionally fastidious, it cannot be cultivated on blood agar. Instead, it must be cultivated either on chocolate agar or on selective media that are nutritionally supplemented and contain antibiotics that inhibit the growth of competing organisms from mucosal surfaces. Examples of selective media are modified Thayer-Martin agar, Martin-Lewis agar, and New York City medium. The neisseriae are aerobes, but pathogenic neisseriae require increased CO_2 tension for growth. Therefore, primary isolates are cultured in an incubator or candle jar containing 5% CO_2. Some commensal neisseriae are β-hemolytic, but the pathogenic neisseriae are not. Additionally, some commensal neisseriae can be cultured at 22 °C.

Once an isolate has been identified as a neisserial organism, its species must be determined. *Neisseria* species can be differentiated by their ability to convert four carbohydrates (glucose, maltose, sucrose, and lactose) to acetate via the Entner-Doudoroff pathway (see Chapter 2 and Fig. 2–5). In the **cystine trypticase agar (CTA) test,** neisserial organisms are placed in four tubes of CTA, each containing one of the carbohydrates. If the organisms convert the carbohydrate to acetate, the color of the tube will change from red to yellow. Table 6–2 compares the reactions elicited by *N. gonorrhoeae, N. meningitidis,* and several other species of *Neisseria.* A rapid **colorimetric test for carbohydrate utilization** (API QuadFERM+) is also available.

The **superoxol test** can be used to differentiate *N. gonorrhoeae* from *N. meningitidis* and *Neisseria lactamica.* The superoxol test is similar to the peroxidase test, except that 30% rather than 3% hydrogen peroxide is used. When organisms are mixed with 30% hydrogen peroxide and placed on a glass slide, the emulsion will immediately begin to bubble briskly if the organisms are *N. gonorrhoeae* but will produce

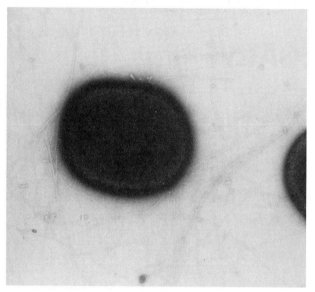

FIGURE 6–1. *Neisseria subflava,* **an example of a** *Neisseria* **species that exhibits numerous pili.**

little or no bubbling if the organisms are *N. meningitidis* or *N. lactamica.*

Neisseria gonorrhoeae

Humans are the only known host of *Neisseria gonorrhoeae,* an organism that is commonly called the **gonococcus** and is the cause of gonorrhea and other types of disease. Although gonococci are not part of the normal flora, they can cause asymptomatic infections, usually in women.

Characteristics of *N. gonorrhoeae*

General Features. As discussed above, gonococci must be cultivated on special media. The organisms grow best at 35 °C in an atmosphere of 5% CO_2. When exposed to room air, gonococci rapidly autolyze. Gonococci can be differentiated from other *Neisseria* species by their ability to convert glucose (but not maltose, sucrose, and lactose) to acid in the CTA test (see Table 6–2) and by their positive response in the oxidase and superoxol tests.

Gonococci are usually visualized within purulent exudates as intracellular gram-negative diplococci. When initially isolated, gonococci grow as tiny colonies with a circumscribed edge. When these colonies are viewed under a dissecting microscope and the ground glass reflector is used to illuminate the colonies from below, each colony appears to be surrounded by a halo. If the organisms are subcultured indiscriminately, however, the gonococci will revert to one of several other **colony types** that are large, flattened, and have no halo.

Mechanisms of Pathogenicity. Early studies of the pathogenicity of gonorrhea failed to recognize changes in colony types, and investigators were frustrated in their attempts to elicit gonorrhea in subjects exposed to serially subcultured gonococci. During the late 1960s, Douglas Kellogg discovered that gonococci undergo **phase variation** during subculture. Fred Sparling later showed that the initial **small-colony gonococci** were piliated and virulent but that subcultured **large-colony gonococci** were unpiliated and avirulent. The small-colony types were named T1 and T2 gonococci, and the large-colony types were named T3, T4, and T5. Scientists now know that gonococcal phase variation occurs as a result of chromosomal rearrangement.

(1) Gonococcal Antigens and Virulence Determinants. Gonococci are mucosal pathogens. As such, they must persist in an environment where they risk being eliminated by desquamation and fluid flow, are exposed to the actions of antibodies (particularly sIgA and IgG), and must resist being destroyed by polymorphonuclear leukocytes (PMNs). In addition, gonococci move from the mucosal lumen to the submucosa during infection, and some strains invade the blood. These activities require the concerted participation of pili, outer membrane proteins, lipooligosaccharide, peptidoglycan, and other surface structures and virulence determinants.

(a) Pili. Gonococcal phase variation during subculture results in the concomitant loss of pili and loss of virulence. T1 and T2 gonococci are heavily piliated, and their pili mediate two processes: adherence to mucosal epithelial cells and resistance to phagocytosis by PMNs.

Clinical studies have shown that only piliated gonococci initiate urethral disease in human subjects. Antipilus antibody is opsonic and protects subjects from infection. Pilus vaccines have been tested, but they have been unsuccessful because there are many antigenic types of gonococcal pili and gonococci change their pilin antigens.

TABLE 6–1. **Characteristics of Neisseriae and Other Bacteria Commonly Isolated From Mucosal Surfaces**

Organisms	Gram's Stain Reaction	Type of Hemolysis	Growth on Blood Agar	Growth on Chocolate Agar	Oxidase Test Results	Catalase Test Results
Commensal neisseriae	Gram-negative diplococci	Variable	+	+	+	+
Pathogenic neisseriae	Gram-negative diplococci	Gamma	Variable*	+	+	+
Group A streptococci	Gram-positive cocci (chains)	Beta	+	+	–	–
Viridans streptococci	Gram-positive cocci (chains)	Alpha	+	+	–	–
Pneumococci	Gram-positive diplococci	Alpha	+	+	–	–
Staphylococcus aureus	Gram-positive cocci (clumps)	Beta	+	+	–	+

Neisseria meningitidis can be cultured on blood agar, but *Neisseria gonorrhoeae* cannot.

TABLE 6–2.   Ability of *Neisseria* Species to Convert Four Carbohydrates to Acetate in the Cystine Trypticase Agar (CTA) Test

Species	Pathogenic	Glucose Conversion	Maltose Conversion	Sucrose Conversion	Lactose Conversion
Neisseria gonorrhoeae	Yes	+	−	−	−
Neisseria meningitidis	Yes	+	+	−	−
Neisseria flavescens	No	−	−	−	−
Neisseria lactamica	No	+	+	−	+
Neisseria sicca	No	+	+	+	−

Gonococcal pili are constructed largely of repeating units of a pilin that contains 159 amino acids and can be divided into three major regions by cyanogen bromide digestion. Region 2 and region 3 of gonococcal pilin are believed to be the receptor-binding region and the type-specific region, respectively. Region 2 recognizes cellular receptors and elicits antibody that is opsonic and protective. Because this region is constant in its amino acid sequence, it would be a good candidate for a pilus vaccine. Unfortunately, it is overshadowed immunologically by region 3. This type-specific region contains a hypervariable loop that dominates the immune response to gonococcal pili. Each pilus serotype elicits a strong response against the hypervariable loop and protects the patient from the serotype that is present but not from the dozens of other pilus serotypes.

Changes in gonococcal pilin antigens occur as a result of chromosomal rearrangement and introduction of new genes via transformation. Gonococci can be transformed only when piliated. The hypervariability in pilin antigens and the specificity of the immune response make reinfection with gonococci possible. Indeed, **recidivism** (repeat infection) is a common occurrence.

(b) Outer Membrane Proteins.   Although gonococcal outer membrane proteins are known to be an important determinant of virulence, their precise roles have been difficult to elucidate because of the lack of a satisfactory animal model for gonococcal urethritis. There are three membrane proteins. **Protein I** (PI) is the principal outer membrane protein (POMP) of the gonococcus. This protein is antigenically variable and occurs in high- and low-molecular-weight forms. **Protein II** (PII) was first discovered in opaque-colony gonococcal variants and is also called opacity protein (Opa) or opacity-associated protein. **Protein III** (PIII), which complexes with PI to form gonococcal porin molecules, is reported to be the major binding site for IgG antibody. This so-called blocking antibody interferes with complement-mediated killing.

When gonococci with low-molecular-weight PI are in the patient's serum, they resist elimination by bactericidal agents (serum killing). Most patients with disseminated gonococcal disease are infected with organisms that have this form of PI. Gonococcal strains with low-molecular-weight PI are auxotrophs that require arginine, hypoxanthine, and uracil for growth. Gonococcal strains with high-molecular-

weight PI are not resistant to serum killing and are usually found only in the urethra. The serum bactericidal activity that restricts these strains to the urethra is believed to be complement-dependent killing of gonococci. Supporting this notion is the observation that patients who are deficient in late complement components can develop disseminated disease when infected with any gonococcal strain.

PII (or Opa) is subject to phase variation, so there are several variants of this protein. In some cases, a gonococcus expresses no PII. In other cases, a single gonococcus can express up to three PII variants simultaneously. Gonococcal strains that cause disseminated disease are usually PII-negative, whereas strains that cause urethritis are generally PII-positive. Under certain circumstances, PII-positive gonococci will autoagglutinate and adhere to epithelial cells and PMNs. The PII-positive organisms have been shown to invade epithelial cells via a process that resembles phagocytosis in that it involves polymerization of F-actin and is blocked in the presence of cytochalasin D.

(c) Lipooligosaccharide.   Like other gram-negative bacteria, gonococci have an outer membrane whose outer leaflet is filled with lipopolysaccharide (LPS). Gonococcal LPS is unusual, however, in that it has no O antigen and is therefore considered to be naturally rough. Rough LPS is called lipooligosaccharide (LOS) to differentiate it from O antigen–containing LPS. The LOS of gonococci is more antigenically complex than the LPS of bacteria such as *Escherichia coli* and *Salmonella* species.

Multiplying gonococci release blebs of outer membrane. These blebs are heavily impregnated with LOS and are toxic for ciliated epithelial cells. Cilia exposed to LOS stop beating, and then the ciliated cells are sloughed from the epithelium. Thus, LOS protects gonococci from being eliminated from the mucosa via ciliary activity.

Recent studies of gonococcal LOS have focused on similarities between human glycosphingolipids and gonococcal LOS, and investigators have identified LOS of varying molecular weights. One study showed that urethritis developed in human subjects who were infected with gonococci that exhibited low-molecular-weight LOS; however, when gonococci were isolated from the urethral exudate of these subjects, they uniformly exhibited high-molecular-weight LOS. This change in LOS molecular weight was accompanied by sialylation of the LOS terminal galactose. Other studies have shown that gonococci with sialylated LOS are resistant to antibody-mediated serum bactericidal activity. Thus, the addition of sialic acid to gonococcal LOS may protect the organisms from antibody-mediated defense processes. *Neisseria meningitidis* and *Haemophilus influenzae* also express LOS, and their LOS can bind sialic acid.

(d) Peptidoglycan. Gonococci have been found to shed peptidoglycan fragments during in vitro growth and are thought to shed these fragments in vivo. *N. gonorrhoeae* is one of 11 bacterial species that are known to acetylate the C-6 hydroxyl group of *N*-acetylmuramic acid. Various investigators have reported that between 34% and 52% of the gonococcal muramyl residues are *O*-acetylated. *O*-acetylated peptidoglycan is resistant to the lytic action of lysozyme, and *O*-acetylated peptidoglycan fragments have been reported to be arthritogenic and to induce slow-wave sleep, activate complement, induce fever, and damage ciliated epithelium. Because these fragments are quite stable and tend to persist, their influence on the pathogenesis of gonorrhea may be significant.

(e) Other Characteristics. Gonococci secrete an **IgAase** that cleaves the Fc region from sIgA1. It is unclear how this helps the gonococcus, since IgA is not directly opsonic and does not activate complement via the classic pathway. Some investigators believe that IgAase diminishes the adherence-blocking activity of IgA and makes agglutinated IgA unable to activate complement via the alternative pathway. Additionally, some have suggested that binding of IgA Fab fragments to the gonococcus may protect the organism from IgG by masking key surface antigens.

Gonococci require iron to maintain their virulence. They do not express siderophores but acquire iron via a receptor-mediated, high-affinity iron-binding system, possibly involving **ferric iron–binding protein**.

Using electron microscopes, investigators have taken photomicrographs in which gonococci appear to be in tissue surrounded by a **capsule**. It is not clear whether a capsule actually exists and has an effect on gonococcal virulence.

Finally, gonococci were recently found to secrete a protein called **alpha protein** or **alpha factor.** This protein is secreted concomitantly with IgA protease and is found in culture supernatants either free or attached to IgA protease. Sequence analysis of alpha protein suggests that it is a hormone-like substance. Its activities and possible effects on virulence are currently being studied.

(2) Pathogenic Processes. The absence of a suitable animal model for gonorrhea has made it difficult to assess the role of various virulence determinants in the pathogenesis of disease. The strong host specificity of gonococci is believed to be due at least in part to the specificity of gonococcal adherence to epithelial cells. Piliated gonococci adhere poorly to epithelial cells from every nonhuman species that has been tested. Several investigators have, however, used human fallopian tube organ cultures to investigate the pathogenesis of gonorrhea, and studies using human volunteers have been helpful. What follows

is a hypothetical model of what happens during a gonococcal infection of the urethra. This model has been pieced together from in vivo and in vitro studies.

Gonococci are introduced into the urogenital mucosa during intercourse. Piliated gonococci adhere via their pili to squamous epithelium but not columnar epithelium. As the gonococci multiply, they release peptidoglycan fragments and LOS, each of which elicits an inflammatory response. These bacterial products may also cause the ciliated epithelium first to stop beating and then to slough. Complement activation attracts PMNs to the vicinity, producing a purulent exudate. Meanwhile, adherent gonococci are phagocytosed by epithelial cells, are transported across the cytoplasm in vesicles, and are released via exocytosis into the submucosa.

In the submucosa, the gonococci multiply and spread, eroding the epithelium above. PII probably facilitates epithelial invasion. Antibody and complement restrict the gonococci to the mucosa via complement-mediated lysis. T1 and T2 gonococci resist phagocytosis until specific antigonococcal antibody is available, but naturally arising T3, T4, and T5 gonococci are rapidly phagocytosed and eliminated. Eventually, the antibody and PMN response will eliminate the gonococci.

If a patient suffers from repeated bouts of gonorrhea, there may be considerable scarring, which can block the urethra or fallopian tubes. Blockage of the urethra may cause urination to be painful (dysuria), and blockage of the fallopian tubes may cause sterility.

Diseases Due to *N. gonorrhoeae*

Epidemiology. Gonorrhea is one of the most common bacterial infectious diseases. In the USA, the incidence of gonorrhea peaked at about 450 cases per 100,000 people in 1975. Since that time, the incidence has gradually declined to just under 300 per 100,000. This represents between 600,000 and 1.2 million cases of gonorrhea per year. In addition, there are more than 500,000 cases of pelvic inflammatory disease annually in the USA, with about half of the cases caused by *N. gonorrhoeae* and the remainder caused by *Chlamydia trachomatis, Mycoplasma hominis,* or *Ureaplasma urealyticum.*

Gonorrhea is primarily a disease of youth, with more than 80% of cases occurring between the ages of 15 and 29 years, when people tend to be most sexually active and have the greatest number of partners. Although more than 90% of men suffer from painful urethritis when infected by gonococci, fewer than 30% of women are symptomatic. Thus, most men seek urgent treatment to ease their pain, whereas most women go untreated and can continue to spread the infection. In men who have unprotected intercourse with an infected partner, there is a 1 in 5 chance of contracting gonorrhea. For this reason, it is critical that all sexual contacts of a patient with gonorrhea be identified and treated.

Diagnosis. Patients with gonococcal infection

may present with urethritis, pelvic inflammatory disease, disseminated disease, or other forms of infection.

(1) History and Physical Examination

(a) Urethritis (Gonorrhea). In men, gonorrhea begins from 2 to 8 days (mean of 4 days) after unprotected intercourse with an infected partner. Manifestations include a copious yellow-green discharge that can block the urethra, causing dysuria and increased urinary urgency and frequency. Although most infected men seek treatment, gonorrhea usually resolves spontaneously but painfully in about 1 month. Nevertheless, serious complications occur in about 1% of untreated men and include epididymitis, prostatitis, and blockage of the urethra by scar tissue.

Many infected women are asymptomatic and therefore do not know that they have gonorrhea. Those with symptoms experience dysuria, frequent and urgent urination, vaginal discharge, and abdominal pain. When urethral symptoms do not occur and no treatment is sought, the patient may develop pelvic inflammatory disease (PID).

(b) Pelvic Inflammatory Disease. PID occurs when gonococci spread from the endocervix to the fallopian tubes and cause salpingitis. The fallopian tubes can become blocked by scar tissue, trapping discharge material. The surrounding pelvic tissues can become involved, and the exudate may spill into the peritoneum. Thus, some patients develop gonococcal perihepatitis (Fitz-Hugh–Curtis syndrome) or peritonitis.

PID is often first suspected because the patient has an unusually severe and prolonged menstrual period. Other clinical manifestations include fever, lower abdominal pain and tenderness, and leukocytosis. When the cervix is moved during pelvic examination, the patient suffers from bilateral pain.

PID caused by *N. gonorrhoeae* is usually acute, whereas PID caused by nongonococcal organisms is more often chronic.

(c) Disseminated Gonococcal Infection. About 1% of men and 3% of women who are infected with *N. gonorrhoeae* develop disseminated gonococcal infection. In individuals who are deficient in late complement components, any gonococcal strain can cause disseminated infection. In the vast majority of cases, however, the disseminated disease is caused by unusual gonococcal strains that preferentially activate complement via the alternative pathway and are exquisitely sensitive to penicillin treatment. Activation of the alternative complement pathway causes chemotactic factors to be generated slowly. As a result, patients rarely experience an attack of gonococcal urethritis before dissemination occurs.

Common manifestations of disseminated disease include skin lesions, fever, polyarthritis, and bacteremia. Rarely, patients also suffer from endocarditis or meningitis.

In most patients, skin lesions erupt 7–30 days after the initial infection with gonococci. The lesions usually begin as hemorrhagic macules but then become hemorrhagic pustules within 24–48 hours. Typically, between 3 and 20 lesions are found on the distal extremities. In some cases, however, lesions are found on the hands and the soles. Two-thirds of the lesions contain gonococci. Gonococcal arthritis is often asymmetric, and many patients have arthritis in only one knee.

Patients with inflammation of the tendon and its enveloping sheath usually develop **gonococcal arthritis-dermatitis syndrome** (GADS), characterized by fever, tenosynovitis, acute arthritis in one or more joints, and the presence of a few distal pustular or hemorrhagic skin lesions. GADS is the most common form of septic arthritis in patients between the ages of 16 and 50 years, and about 75% of patients with GADS are women.

(d) Ophthalmia Neonatorum. The eyes of an infant who passes through the birth canal of a woman with active gonorrhea may become infected, resulting in ophthalmia neonatorum. The longer the gap between the time of membrane rupture and the birth of the infant, the greater the risk that an infected mother will pass gonococci to her child. About 2–3 days postpartum, the infected infant develops redness and swelling of both eyelids, and a purulent discharge is noted. In some cases, the infant may develop corneal ulceration and perforation, and the lens may be extruded. If not treated immediately, ophthalmia neonatorum results in blindness.

(e) Other Gonococcal Infections. Infants, women, and homosexual men may present with anorectal gonorrhea, characterized by rectal pain, tenesmus, rectal bleeding, and a mucopurulent rectal discharge.

(2) Laboratory Analysis. Laboratory diagnosis of gonorrhea involves examining the purulent exudate and culturing the organisms. Laboratory diagnosis of disseminated gonococcal infection involves culturing the organisms from blood, skin lesions, and joints. Although ophthalmia neonatorum can be diagnosed by examining exudate and culturing gonococci from ophthalmologic samples, treatment is urgent and is therefore initiated primarily on the basis of clinical manifestations.

If gonorrhea is suspected, samples of purulent exudate should be collected using Dacron or rayon swabs, because calcium alginate and cotton swabs may contain materials toxic for gonococci. Exudate from patients with gonorrhea contains many PMNs with intracellular gram-negative diplococci. Gonococci grow on chocolate agar as gram-negative, oxidase-positive diplococci that ferment only glucose in the CTA test. If a sample cannot be cultured immediately, it can be transported using one of several nonnutritive swab transport systems or a culture medium transport system.

Many laboratories use a nucleic acid probe to test samples directly for the presence of gonococci. A chemiluminescence-enhanced probe assay called PACE detects gonococcal rRNA and has been reported to be 90% sensitive and 99.4% specific for *N. gonorrhoea*. This assay can be performed on samples from genital lesions in about 2 hours, but it does have three major limitations. First, extragenital samples (for example, from the rectum or blood) cannot be tested by this method. Second, the method is less sensitive than culturing the organisms. Third, results from samples tested by this method cannot be confirmed by culture, because the method makes the sample unusable for other tests.

Another rRNA probe system called Accuprobe has been shown to be a highly reliable means of identifying gonococci once they are isolated on a selective medium. Suspected gonococci grown in pure culture can also be speciated using fluorescent antigonococcal antiserum.

Treatment and Prognosis. Gonococci were once quite susceptible to penicillin G, and treatment involved the administration of penicillin alone. Over time, gonococci became less permeable to penicillin, so penicillin was given in combination with probenecid to keep the blood levels of penicillin adequately elevated. This regimen became obsolete when **penicillinase-producing _N. gonorrhoeae_** (PPNG) appeared during the 1970s. Today, because of the prevalence of PPNG, penicillinase-resistant cephalosporins must be used to treat gonorrhea.

Another therapeutic problem has arisen from the fact that approximately half of the patients with **gonococcal urethritis** (gonorrhea) are also infected with one or more agents of **nongonococcal urethritis** (NGU). NGU is most often caused by _C. trachomatis_ but can also be caused by _M. hominis_ or _U. urealyticum_. Patients who suffer from concomitant gonorrhea and NGU will experience gonorrhea that is followed 2–3 weeks later by NGU. For this reason, most physicians now treat patients for both diseases. In some cases, a two-drug combination consisting of ceftriaxone plus doxycycline, tetracycline, or azithromycin is used. The ceftriaxone kills gonococci, and the other agents kill nongonococcal organisms. If PPNG organisms are not prevalent, a three-drug combination consisting of amoxicillin, probenecid, and doxycycline may be used.

Patients with disseminated gonococcal infection are usually treated with ceftriaxone, cefotaxime, or ceftizoxime. Ophthalmia neonatorum is treated with ceftriaxone.

In general, patients with gonococcal infections respond well to treatment. Failure to treat GADS may result in destructive arthritis, and failure to provide immediate treatment for ophthalmia neonatorum will result in blindness. Repeated bouts of gonococcal urethritis can cause scarring and stricture of the urethra. Repeated bouts of PID pose a significant risk of sterility, with one study reporting a 21% risk of sterility after one bout of PID, a 35% risk after two bouts, and a 75% risk after three bouts.

Prevention. There is no vaccine against gonococcal infection. Individuals who do not use condoms and who have multiple sexual partners are at increased risk of infection. Therefore, condom use and monogamy seem to be the best solutions to slowing the spread of gonorrhea.

To prevent ophthalmia neonatorum, hospital personnel instill a 1% silver nitrate solution in the eyes of infants immediately after their birth.

Neisseria meningitidis

Neisseria meningitidis is commonly called the **meningococcus.** It can be carried asymptomatically and is isolated in 5–20% of healthy individuals.

Characteristics of _N. meningitidis_

General Features. Meningococci are superoxol-negative and can be identified by their ability to convert glucose and maltose to acid in the CTA test (see Table 6–2). When cultivated at 35 °C on blood agar or chocolate agar, meningococci usually form gray colonies. In some cases, however, the organisms form yellowish colonies on blood agar. Meningococci cannot be cultured on these media at 22 °C. Primary cultures are usually obtained using a selective medium, such as modified Thayer-Martin agar. Blood, urine, or cerebrospinal fluid (CSF) samples from patients should not be refrigerated before being cultured, because refrigeration kills meningococci.

Mechanisms of Pathogenicity. The virulence of meningococci appears to depend primarily on the ability of the organisms to invade the blood and meninges and to survive in the face of a brisk PMN response.

(1) Meningococcal Antigens and Virulence Determinants. Although the capsule is the key virulence determinant of the meningococcus, other determinants include pili, LOS, outer membrane proteins, and IgAase.

(a) Capsule. Thirteen capsule serotypes of _N. meningitidis_ have now been identified and designated as types A, B, C, D, H, I, K, L, X, Y, Z, W-135, and 29E. Worldwide, types A and B are the most prevalent causes of meningitis. On the African continent, type A is the cause of widespread multiyear epidemics of meningitis. In the USA, type A is responsible for fewer than 1% of cases of meningococcal disease, and the most prevalent meningococcal pathogens are type B (responsible for 46% of cases), type C (48%), and types W-135 and Y (5%).

Most meningococcal capsules are polysaccharide homopolymers or contain repeating polysaccharide units. The primary function of the meningococcal capsule is to prevent meningococci from being phagocytosed by PMNs. The capsules of types A, C, W-135, and Y meningococci have been shown to be antiphagocytic. Although the capsule of type B meningococci may protect the organisms from complement-mediated lysis, it may not be an effective antiphagocytic device.

Antimeningococcal antibody activates complement to lyse the meningococci. However, immunity to meningococci depends on the development of type-specific anticapsular antibody. This antibody opsonizes meningococci, and then the meningococci can be phagocytosed and rapidly killed. Because the structures of the meningococcal capsules are known, it has been possible to prepare effective antimeningococcal vaccines. Three vaccines are currently licensed: a univalent vaccine directed against type A, another univalent vaccine directed against type C, and a polyvalent vaccine directed against types A, C, W-135, and Y. The capsule of type B meningococci is a poor immunogen in adults and appears to be completely nonimmunogenic in children.

(b) Pili. Some strains of *N. meningitidis* are not piliated, but most strains of newly isolated meningococci possess pili. Although several investigators have shown that these pili can mediate adherence to host cells, the role played by *N. meningitidis* pili in the pathogenesis of disease may be less prominent than the role played by *Neisseria gonorrhoeae* pili.

(c) Lipooligosaccharide. Like gonococci, meningococci have a rough form of lipopolysaccharide that is referred to as lipooligosaccharide (LOS) and is able to be sialylated. Meningococcal LOS is highly endotoxic, making meningococcal septicemia extremely dangerous.

(d) Other Characteristics. *N. meningitidis* is able to obtain iron from transferrin and produces an **IgAase** that cleaves IgA1. *N. meningitidis* also has at least five classes of **outer membrane proteins,** which may help meningococci to survive and cause disease. Class 5 proteins are similar to gonococcal protein II and include the Opa and Opc proteins. Class 5 proteins are involved in attachment to and invasion of epithelial cells. Because class 2 and class 3 proteins are the major outer membrane proteins, some laboratories have developed a system that classifies meningococci on the basis of proteins from these two classes. Classification schemes that combine capsule serotype, LOS determinants, and class 2 and 3 protein serotypes are used as epidemiologic tools.

(2) Pathogenic Processes. Meningococcal meningitis is frequently preceded by an upper respiratory tract infection and almost always occurs soon after the patient has become newly infected with *N. meningitidis*. The initial site of infection appears to be the nasopharynx, where the meningococci adhere via pili to squamous epithelial cells and then enter the blood. Investigators believe that most meningococci cross the mucosa when they are phagocytosed and that the organisms are then exocytosed at the basement membrane. Some meningococci, however, may pass through intercellular junctions. The ability to invade the epithelium has been associated with meningococci that possess Opc protein, lack capsule, lack pili, have nonsialylated LOS, and express a 28-kD opacity outer membrane protein.

Several studies have shown that meningococcemia does not occur in individuals with preexisting specific anticapsular antibody and that complement-mediated lysis restricts meningococci to the mucosa in most cases. Moreover, at least some meningococcal capsules inhibit the activity of the alternative pathway of complement activation by promoting the binding of factor H to C3b on the capsule surface. This blocks the ability of C3b to bind factor B.

Once in the blood, meningococci may cross the blood-brain barrier and infect the leptomeninges, or they may remain in the blood, where they multiply to enormous numbers. Unlike gonococci, which are difficult to locate in patients with gonococcemia, meningococci can be readily seen in Giemsa-stained blood smears from patients with meningococcemia.

Meningococcemia is dangerous because meningococci release highly endotoxic LOS as they multiply. Some patients with fulminating meningococcemia develop purpura fulminans. This disorder is characterized by fever and ecchymoses and is sometimes accompanied by shock secondary to peripheral vascular collapse. Others develop disseminated intravascular coagulation (DIC). Patients with Waterhouse-Friderichsen syndrome have reduced adrenal activity because there is hemorrhaging into the adrenal glands. Many patients develop only meningococcemia and do not develop meningitis.

Peptidoglycan and LOS fragments released by meningococci elicit the production of interleukin-1 and tumor necrosis factor (TNF). These substances increase the permeability of the vessels and the blood-brain barrier, and they also cause endothelial cells to express two cellular receptors for PMNs (CD62 and ELAM-1). PMNs initially bind loosely to the endothelium, and interleukin-8 then causes the endothelial cells and the PMNs to express new receptors (ICAM-1 and CD18 integrins, respectively). When the PMNs cross into the subarachnoid space, they phagocytose antibody-coated meningococci.

The combination of PMN activation and endothelial cell activation results in the production of a wide variety of effectors, including TNF, interleukin-1, interleukin-6, interleukin-8, various prostaglandins and leukotrienes, platelet-activating factor, superoxide, H_2O_2, hydroxyl radical, and singlet-excited oxygen. Together, these products cause a diffuse granulocytic inflammation of the leptomeninges, alter the general metabolism of the brain to produce excess lactic acid, cause vasogenic edema, decrease the cerebral perfusion pressure, cause cerebral ischemia, and increase the intracranial pressure. To reverse these processes, it may be necessary to kill the bacteria with bactericidal antibiotics and also to halt the production of inflammatory cytokines, monokines, and autacoids.

Diseases Due to *N. meningitidis*

Epidemiology. In the USA, meningococcal meningitis is a sporadic disease. There are, however, localized outbreaks in closed populations, such as populations of military recruits. While the carriage rate in the general US population is in the 5–20% range, carriage rates of higher than 90% have been reported in military recruits. Attack rates of meningococcal meningitis are between 1 and 3 cases per 100,000 people in the general US population but are from 500 to 800 times higher in household contacts of patients with meningitis. This is because meningococcal meningitis usually occurs when a person is newly infected with meningococci. Even though the patient may have been carrying a strain of *N. meningitidis,* the disease has its onset after the patient is infected with a different strain.

The Inuit in Canada have experienced attack rates higher than 200 cases per 100,000 people. Moreover, attack rates as high as 1700 cases per 100,000 have been reported in sub-Saharan Africa, which is often called the meningitis belt.

The most important risk factor for meningitis is age. Under the age of 1 year, the incidence rate for meningococcal disease ranges from 10 to 100 per 100,000 children. Other risk factors are deficiencies in late complement components (C5–C9) and crowded living conditions.

Diagnosis

(1) History and Physical Examination. The onset of **meningococcal meningitis** may be acute or gradual. Patients initially complain of chills, malaise, fever, lethargy, and a severe headache that may be diffuse or frontal. In many cases, the pain radiates from the head down the spine.

At least one-third of patients with meningococcal disease develop a petechial rash during the first 3 days of disease. This rash is seen most prominently in areas subject to pressure, such as along the belt line. The petechiae rapidly progress to ecchymoses and purpura. Patients may also develop maculopapular nodules up to 2 cm in diameter on the trunk and arms. Children with Waterhouse-Friderichsen syndrome develop extensive purpura.

Nuchal rigidity (stiff neck) and other signs of increased cranial pressure are the hallmark of meningitis but are difficult to recognize in an infant. Infants with meningitis often cry a lot, vomit, and refuse food. The crying increases when they are picked up, because this bends the neck and spine. The vomiting begins early in the disease and may be severe enough to cause dehydration.

Patients should be examined closely for signs of meningeal irritation. As meningococcal disease progresses, the patient may progressively develop twitching, signs of cranial nerve dysfunction, exaggerated reflexes, photophobia, seizures, opisthotonos (characterized by a rigid and bowed back), and coma.

(2) Laboratory Analysis. CSF samples are taken via lumbar puncture. Blood samples should be obtained before antibiotics are initiated. The samples can be stained and examined for the presence of PMNs and meningococci, tested for protein and glucose levels, cultured on modified Thayer-Martin agar, and tested immunologically for the presence of meningococcal capsular material.

In patients with meningococcal meningitis, the CSF is usually turbid and has a PMN count of 400–20,000/μL. Gram-negative diplococci can be readily seen in centrifuged CSF. CSF protein levels are elevated (80–500 mg per 100 mL), and glucose levels are depressed (less than 35 mg per 100 mL).

A rapid preliminary diagnosis can be made on the basis of immunologic methods to detect the presence of meningococcal capsule. Agglutination tests can detect the presence of several encapsulated organisms, including meningococci, pneumococci, and *Haemophilus influenzae* type b, in samples of blood, CSF, and urine. Counterimmunoelectrophoresis can also be used but is less sensitive.

Treatment and Prognosis. Meningitis is a medical emergency, and treatment is usually initiated before a definitive diagnosis is made. Therefore, the antibiotics given initially are chosen on the basis of their effectiveness against all the likely causes of meningitis in the patient's risk group. Bactericidal antibiotics must be used because immune function in the subarachnoid space is less than optimal. Fortunately, inflammation of the meninges allows some antibiotics that normally do not cross the blood-brain barrier to enter the subarachnoid space fairly well.

If a diagnosis of meningococcal meningitis is certain, penicillin G or ceftriaxone is usually administered. Otherwise, empiric therapy is based on the age of the patient: infants between the ages of 1 and 3 months are given a two-drug combination of ampicillin plus cefotaxime or ceftriaxone; infants and children between the ages of 3 months and 7 years are treated with ceftriaxone or cefotaxime; and older children and adults are given a two-drug combination of ampicillin or penicillin G plus ceftriaxone or cefotaxime. Recent studies have suggested that dexamethasone reduces morbidity and mortality rates if it is administered before antibiotics are begun. Therefore, many clinicians recommend that this drug be given 15 minutes before antibiotics are started.

Untreated meningococcal meningitis is fatal in 70% of patients. Antibiotic treatment reduces the mortality rate to 8–13%. Many patients who recover, however, suffer from residual neurologic defects, including hearing loss, speech deficits, mental retardation, motor abnormalities, and visual impairment.

Prevention. The spread of meningococcal meningitis can be prevented by chemoprophylaxis and by immunization.

Household and other close contacts of patients with meningococcal meningitis are usually treated with rifampin for 2 days.

US military personnel are routinely immunized with a tetravalent **meningococcal meningitis vaccine** against types A, C, W-135, and Y meningococci. Unfortunately, no vaccine is available against type B, which is a prevalent cause of meningococcal meningitis in the USA.

MORAXELLA SPECIES
General Characteristics and Classification

Members of the genus *Moraxella* are closely related to the neisseriae. In fact, *Moraxella catarrhalis,* the key human pathogen in the genus, was for many years classified as *Neisseria catarrhalis* because it is a gram-negative, oxidase-positive diplococcus and is a mucosal inhabitant. Later, when its guanine plus cytosine (G+C) ratio was found to differ so much from that of the neisseriae, the organism was reclassified first as *Branhamella catarrhalis* and next as *M. catarrhalis*.

Moraxella catarrhalis
Characteristics of M. catarrhalis

M. catarrhalis can be cultured on blood agar, chocolate agar, or modified Martin-Thayer agar. The organism utilizes no sugars in the CTA test and may cause the CTA medium to become alkaline. *M. catarrhalis* is also identified by its ability to reduce nitrite and nitrate, its DNAase activity, and its ability to hydrolyze ester-linked butyrate groups (butyrate esterase).

Many *M. catarrhalis* strains produce an inducible beta-lactamase that cannot be detected by rapid penicillinase tests that measure the conversion of penicillin to penicilloic acid, so *M. catarrhalis* should be tested for beta-lactamase production using an iodometric method or a chromogenic cephalosporinase test.

Diseases Due to M. catarrhalis

Epidemiology. *M. catarrhalis* is found in the respiratory tracts of 1.5–5.4% of healthy young and middle-aged adults, 26.5% of healthy elderly people, and 50.8% of healthy children. It is therefore recognized as a significant potential pathogen of the respiratory tract, including the sinuses, bronchi, and larynx.

Diagnosis. **Sinusitis** usually follows an upper respiratory tract infection and is characterized by fever, sinus pain, and a purulent discharge. The diagnosis is generally made on clinical grounds alone; however, when necessary, sinus exudate can be collected by needle puncture and cultured. While 20% of the cases of sinusitis are due to *M. catarrhalis*, other common causes include *Haemophilus influenzae*, *Streptococcus pneumoniae*, and *Streptococcus pyogenes*.

Chronic **bronchitis** among smokers is often caused by *M. catarrhalis*. Although **laryngitis** is occasionally caused by this organism, about 90% of cases are due to viruses.

Treatment. Disease known to be due to *M. catarrhalis* can be treated with one of the following: amoxicillin plus clavulanate; an oral second- or third-generation cephalosporin; an extended-spectrum macrolide, such as azithromycin; or trimethoprim-sulfamethoxazole (TMP/SMX). Although these treatment regimens can be used empirically to treat sinusitis or bronchitis, TMP/SMX is ineffective against many strains of *S. pyogenes* and is therefore not the first choice for empiric therapy of sinusitis.

HAEMOPHILUS SPECIES
General Characteristics and Classification

The term *Haemophilus* is derived from the Greek and means "blood-loving." *Haemophilus* species are small gram-negative rods that require one or two specific growth factors present in blood. Some require X factor, consisting of heme, hematin, or other tetrapyrroles. Others require V factor, consisting of nicotinamide adenine dinucleotide (NAD) or NAD phosphate (NADP). *Haemophilus* species that require V factor cannot be cultured on sheep blood agar, because sheep blood contains enzymes that hydrolyze V factor. These species must be grown on blood agar made from horse or rabbit blood or on chocolate agar. The heating process used to make chocolate agar inactivates the enzymes that degrade V factor.

More than 15 *Haemophilus* species have been identified, and about 10 of these are known to cause disease in humans. *Haemophilus influenzae* is the most important human pathogen, while *Haemophilus aegyptius*, *Haemophilus ducreyi*, and *Haemophilus parainfluenzae* are also significant causes of human disease. Table 6–3 lists the diseases associated with *Haemophilus* infection.

Haemophilus influenzae

Haemophilus influenzae is a major pathogen that is best known for its ability to cause life-threatening diseases, including meningitis and epiglottitis, in young children.

Characteristics of H. influenzae

General Features. *H. influenzae* is a small gram-negative rod (a coccobacillus) that requires both X and V factors for growth. As such, it can be cultivated on chocolate agar, selective *Haemophilus* media, and blood agar that contains either horse or rabbit blood. *H. influenzae* is nonhemolytic.

X and V factor requirements can be determined by a variety of means, including the satellite test and filter paper strip test. If the **satellite test** is used, suspected *H. influenzae* organisms are spread across a sheep blood agar plate. A single streak of *Staphylococcus aureus* is made across the agar. Because *S. aureus* will provide the V factor absent in sheep blood agar, *H. influenzae* will grow as tiny colonies in the vicinity of the *S. aureus* streak. If a **filter paper strip test** is used, the suspected *H. influenzae* organisms are spread across an agar that is deficient in both X and V factor. Two strips of filter paper—one impregnated with X factor and the other impregnated with V factor—are placed about 2 cm apart on the agar. *H. influenzae* will grow only in the areas where there is convergence of X and V diffusing from the two strips of paper.

H. influenzae is also differentiated from other *Haemophilus* species by its inability to synthesize protoporphyrin from delta-aminolevulinic acid (ALA). Several rapid ALA-porphyrin tests are available. Unlike *H. influenzae*, *Haemophilus parainfluenzae* is ALA-positive and requires only V factor. Unlike *Haemophilus haemolyticus*, *H. influenzae* is nonhemolytic and is unable to ferment fructose. Unlike *Haemophilus aegyptius*, most strains of *H. influenzae* are indole-positive and ornithine decarboxylase–positive.

Eight biotypes of *H. influenzae* have been established on the basis of fermentation reactions and on the basis of indole, urease, and ornithine decarboxylase activities. These biotypes are used by reference

TABLE 6–3. Diseases Commonly Caused by *Haemophilus* Species

Disease	Species	Clinical Manifestations
Brazilian purpuric fever	*Haemophilus aegyptius* (BPF strain).	Fever, abdominal pain, vomiting, petechiae, and conjunctivitis. Clinical picture similar to that of meningococcemia.
Bronchitis	*Haemophilus influenzae* (usually nontypeable strains).	Wheezing and nonproductive cough. Tends to come and go.
Cellulitis	*H. influenzae* type b.	Infection of buccal mucosa that spreads to the face and neck, causing swelling with bluish-red discoloration of the skin. Sometimes accompanied by epiglottitis or sepsis. Clinical picture similar to that of erysipelas.
Chancroid	*Haemophilus ducreyi*.	Sexually transmitted disease characterized by painful ulcerative genital lesions and inguinal buboes.
Conjunctivitis	*H. aegyptius*.	Mucopurulent conjunctival discharge.
Endocarditis	*Haemophilus aphrophilus, Haemophilus paraphrophilus, Haemophilus parainfluenzae,* and *H. influenzae*.	Infection of mitral or aortic valve, accompanied by spiking fever, leukocytosis, weight loss, anemia, and embolization.
Epiglottitis	*H. influenzae* type b.	Fulminating airway obstruction due to swollen and stiff epiglottis. May lead to sepsis.
Laryngotracheobronchitis and acute pharyngitis	*H. influenzae* type b.	Sore throat with crouplike cough, exudate, and stridor.
Meningitis	*H. influenzae* type b and *H. parainfluenzae*.	Stiff neck (nuchal rigidity), vomiting, fever, headache, seizures, and cranial nerve involvement, usually in an infant or young child.
Otitis media	*H. influenzae* (usually nontypeable strains).	Fever, irritability, and pain, usually in an infant or young child. Exudate in the ear causes the tympanic membrane to bulge. May accompany or precede meningitis.
Pneumonia	*H. influenzae* (often type b, but nontypeable strains may infect older patients).	Lobar or segmental pneumonia with cough, pleuritic pain, and sputum production. Similar to pneumococcal pneumonia. Bacteremia may develop.
Puerperal sepsis	*H. influenzae* (nontypeable strains) and *H. parainfluenzae*.	Urethritis or endometritis, accompanied by abdominal pain, fever, and sepsis.
Sinusitis (acute)	*H. influenzae* (nontypeable strains) and *H. parainfluenzae*.	Frontal headaches with fever, sinus swelling, and sinus exudate.

laboratories as an epidemiologic tool. Most cases of *H. influenzae* meningitis are due to biotype I.

Mechanisms of Pathogenicity

(1) *H. influenzae* Antigens and Virulence Determinants. The key virulence determinant of *H. influenzae* is the antiphagocytic capsule. Other determinants include lipooligosaccharide, pili, blastogenic factor, and IgA protease.

(a) Capsule. There are six capsule types, designated as types a through f. Almost all systemic childhood disease is due to organisms that express capsule type b. These organisms are referred to as ***H. influenzae* type b** (Hib). The type b capsule is the only capsule that contains a pentose sugar. It is composed of polyribose and ribitol phosphate chains and is usually designated simply as PRP (polyribose phosphate). The type b capsule is similar to teichoic acids in its structure. Many *H. influenzae* strains associated with localized infections have no capsule and are referred to as nontypeable strains. Because of the importance of the capsule to systemic *Haemophilus* disease, tests are available to identify the serotype of each *H. influenzae* isolate. Additionally, agglutination tests can be used to detect the presence of free capsule in blood, urine, and CSF samples from patients.

(b) Lipooligosaccharide. Like the outer membrane of pathogenic neisseriae, the outer membrane of *H. influenzae* contains a naturally rough lipopolysaccharide (LPS) called lipooligosaccharide (LOS). Unlike the LPS of enteric bacilli, the core polysaccha-

rides found in the LOS of *Haemophilus* are highly variable and are subject to phase variation. LOS is released in outer membrane blebs by multiplying Hib and is also released when the bacteria lyse. LOS acts as a ciliostatic factor, damaging the ciliated epithelium and causing the epithelial cells to slough. In experimental studies of meningitis, LOS has been reported to increase the permeability of the blood-brain barrier. Because LOS contains a high percentage of lipid A, patients with bacteremia are at risk for sepsis.

(c) Other Antigens and Cell Products. *H. influenzae* organisms express several types of **pili** that mediate adherence to epithelial cells and erythrocytes. These pili are subject to phase variation, and loss of pili promotes invasion of the epithelium. *H. influenzae* organisms appear to be piliated when in the nasopharynx, but when they reach the blood and begin to multiply rapidly, strains that cause systemic disease stop expressing pili on their surfaces.

In addition to releasing a lymphocyte mitogen called **blastogenic factor**, *H. influenzae* releases an **IgA protease.** At least one group has reported that *H. influenzae* produces **histamine.** Finally, like the pathogenic neisseriae, *H. influenzae* can derive iron directly from human transferrin.

(2) Pathogenic Processes. *H. influenzae* adheres to the nasal mucosa via pili and possibly via other outer membrane proteins. Unlike meningococci, which are phagocytosed and transported through the epithelium to the basement membrane,

H. influenzae organisms adhere tightly to areas of mucosal damage, where they pass to the subendothelium between epithelial cells. If the infective agent has a type b capsule, dissemination will occur.

The key to the ability of Hib to cause systemic disease is its antiphagocytic capsule. Hib releases about half of the capsular material it synthesizes into the environment, where it may act as a decoy for anti-PRP antibody. Binding of anti-PRP antibody to capsular material not located on the bacterial surface may tie up needed opsonic antibody and deplete activated complement components. Thus, the capsule is believed to protect Hib both from opsonization and from immune-mediated lysis.

The type b capsule is a poor immunogen in children with developing immune systems. Before the age of 1 year, little if any antibody is elicited by purified PRP. Thus, until children are able to mount an effective immune response against the type b capsule, they are susceptible to Hib systemic diseases, such as meningitis and epiglottitis. During the first few months of life, infants are at least partially protected by maternal antibody. For this reason, Hib rarely causes neonatal meningitis. Protection against Hib meningitis is not absolute, however, so Hib meningitis begins to appear among infants starting at about 2 months of age. Maternal antibody seems to offer better protection against epiglottitis, because most epiglottitis cases occur in children who are 6 months or older. Once the titer of maternal antibody begins to wane, children become susceptible to Hib and remain so until they begin to make their own anti-PRP antibody.

Dissemination of *H. influenzae* organisms seems to follow the same general pattern as dissemination of pathogenic neisseriae. In the case of *H. influenzae,* dissemination in immunocompetent individuals occurs only when the type b capsule is present to block the opsonic and lytic actions of complement, and antibody directed against the type b capsule is protective. Investigators have hypothesized that complement acts as an opsonin and thereby contains the dissemination of organisms. Two types of evidence support this hypothesis. First, patients deficient in C3 are highly susceptible to disseminated Hib disease, but those deficient in late complement components are not; this points to the critical nature of the opsonic function of C3b. Second, the importance of phagocytosis in preventing dissemination of *H. influenzae* organisms is supported by the observation that splenectomized patients are highly susceptible to disseminated disease.

Meningitis and other systemic Hib diseases occur only in the presence of marked bacteremia. Apparently, the presence of a large number of Hib organisms in the blood allows efficient seeding of the meninges, joints, heart, and other tissues. In the case of meningitis, Hib organisms cross the endothelium into the subarachnoid space via phagocytosis and are transported to the inner aspect of the endothelium. Once in the subarachnoid space, the organisms infect the leptomeninges.

Diseases Due to *H. influenzae*

Epidemiology. Although 35–85% of adults carry *H. influenzae* in the upper respiratory tract (nasopharynx and oropharynx), only about 0.4% carry Hib. An estimated 60–90% of children carry *H. influenzae.* About 5% of all children and as many as 60% of children in day-care centers are Hib carriers. *H. influenzae* is disseminated via respiratory secretions.

Meningitis and epiglottitis are severe diseases that occur primarily in infants and young children. In the USA, the annual number of cases of meningitis ranges from 10,000 to 12,000. Hib is the most common cause of meningitis in children between the ages of 2 months and 5 years. The peak occurrence of meningitis is between 6 and 8 months of age, while the peak occurrence of epiglottitis is at about 9 months of age.

Diagnosis. In addition to meningitis and epiglottitis, *H. influenzae* can cause cellulitis, otitis media, bronchitis, sinusitis, pneumonia, bacteremia, endometritis, salpingitis, sepsis, pericarditis, and endocarditis.

(1) History and Physical Examination

(a) Meningitis. Almost all cases of *H. influenzae* meningitis in children are caused by Hib. Meningitis is usually preceded by a respiratory infection or otitis media. The organisms spread into the blood from the nasopharynx or middle ear and then enter the central nervous system at the highly vascularized choroid plexus. Once in the subarachnoid space, they are largely isolated from the immune system and are able to multiply rapidly. Eventually, antibody and PMN enter the CSF, but by this time many bacteria are present and therapeutic intervention is needed.

H. influenzae meningitis occurs occasionally in older children and adults and can be caused by typeable or nontypeable strains. The significant pathogenetic factor in these cases is not the presence of capsule but, instead, the predisposing condition of the patient. About 50% of adults with *H. influenzae* meningitis have recently experienced head trauma (for example, a concussion or fractured skull), and another 25% suffer from chronic *H. influenzae* otitis media. In these patients, meningitis is thought to result from the spread of organisms from the pharynx or middle ear without the occurrence of bacteremia.

In patients with meningitis due to any cause, clinical findings may include a high fever, stiff neck, vomiting, twitching, cranial nerve palsies, seizures, and other abnormal neurologic signs. Infants with meningitis cry when picked up, because being held bends the back and neck and causes pain.

(b) Cellulitis and Epiglottitis. Cellulitis and epiglottitis are life-threatening pediatric infections that are almost always due to Hib.

Hib cellulitis begins as an infection of the buccal mucosa and spreads to the face and neck, where it causes swelling, bluish-red discoloration of the skin, and fever. The infection is similar in appearance to erysipelas and is sometimes classified as a form of erysipelas. Spread of Hib from the tissues to the blood may cause rapid sepsis and death.

Epiglottitis, often called **croup,** is a specialized form of cellulitis that affects the loose tissues of the epiglottis. Most cases of epiglottitis occur between the ages of 6 months and 2 years. Epiglottitis begins as a sore throat accompanied by fever, hoarseness, and a barking cough. Within hours, prostration, dyspnea, and cyanosis occur. Acutely ill patients gasp for breath because the epiglottis is inflamed, swollen, and stiff. Each breath requires tremendous effort and is accompanied by stridor and marked retraction of the suprasternal notch. Examination reveals that the epiglottis is beefy red and swollen, and leukocytosis and bacteremia are found. Although a sample of epiglottal exudate can be sent for culture, treatment is urgent and is initiated on clinical grounds alone.

(c) Otitis Media. While *Streptococcus pneumoniae* is the most common cause of otitis media (see Chapter 5), *H. influenzae* is the second most common cause, responsible for 21% of cases. At least 90% of *H. influenzae* strains isolated from patients with otitis media are nontypeable.

(d) Respiratory Infections. *H. influenzae* is the second most common cause of acute purulent sinusitis and of community-acquired pneumonia, trailing only *S. pneumoniae* as a cause of these two conditions. *H. influenzae* has also been associated with the occurrence of purulent bronchitis, and it may exacerbate chronic bronchitis in patients with chronic obstructive pulmonary disease (COPD) or emphysema.

In adults, respiratory infections may be caused by nontypeable *H. influenza* strains, Hib, or a combination of both. In infants and toddlers, the strains that disseminate and cause life-threatening infections are almost always Hib.

H. influenzae pneumonia commonly occurs in children under 5 years of age and in elderly patients with COPD. Other significant risk factors are alcoholism, malnutrition, cancer, and diabetes mellitus. Manifestations of pneumonia include fever, pleuritic pain, and productive cough. Although pneumonia caused by nontypeable strains of *H. influenzae* is rarely accompanied by bacteremia, 30% of patients with pneumonia caused by Hib show signs of bacteremia. This is dangerous because bacteremia can lead to meningitis, endocarditis, hepatomegaly, jaundice, arthritis, or septic shock.

(e) Other Infections. *H. influenzae* causes about 20% of the acute febrile cases of primary bacteremia in pediatric patients. A primary bacteremia is a bacteremia in which there is no obvious nonvascular focus of infection. Primary *H. influenzae* bacteremia occurs mainly in children who have sickle cell disease or have undergone splenectomy. Almost all cases of primary *H. influenzae* bacteremia are due to Hib.

Nontypeable strains of biotype IV *H. influenzae* preferentially colonize the female genital tract and cause acute endometritis, salpingitis, puerperal sepsis, and sepsis in newborns. These diseases have also been associated with biotypes I and II *H. parainfluenzae.*

H. influenzae has been identified as a cause of purulent pericarditis. It is also an occasional cause of endocarditis, but *Haemophilus aphrophilus, Haemophilus paraphrophilus,* and *H. parainfluenzae* are more commonly implicated.

(2) Laboratory Analysis. Laboratory diagnosis of Hib meningitis is based on direct visualization of PMNs and gram-negative coccobacilli in CSF samples; demonstration of low glucose and high protein levels in CSF samples; immunologic demonstration of Hib capsular material in blood, CSF, or urine samples; and the culture of Hib organisms from CSF samples.

Several immunologic tests are available for detecting the presence of capsular material. Most laboratories use either a latex agglutination (LA) test or a staphylococcal protein A coagglutination (COA) test. These tests involve the use of anti-PRP antibodies, which are attached to latex beads in the LA test and are attached to staphylococci in the COA test. A small sample of blood, CSF, or urine is added to the conjugate, and if PRP is present, the beads or staphylococci will agglutinate within seconds or minutes. The LA test appears to be the most sensitive immunologic test available. However, an enzyme immunoassay that was developed more recently than the LA or COA test has been shown to be more specific for the detection of Hib capsular antigen.

Immunologic tests are not useful in the diagnosis of meningitis that is due to nontypeable strains of *H. influenzae.* While positive results in immunologic tests lend support to the diagnosis of meningitis due to Hib, negative results cannot rule out this diagnosis. The definitive diagnosis of meningitis due to Hib or other strains of *H. influenzae* requires that the organisms be cultured from CSF samples. The definitive diagnosis of other diseases due to *H. influenzae* also requires culturing of organisms.

Because *H. influenzae* organisms are extremely sensitive to changes in their environment, clinical samples to be cultured should be collected before antibiotics are administered, should be transported to the laboratory as quickly as possible, and should not be refrigerated. Specimens of blood, CSF, and exudate can be cultured on chocolate agar or on one of the many selective *H. influenzae* media that are commercially available. Each selective medium includes defibrinated horse blood, which contains both X and V factors. Bacitracin is added to most of the selective media to inhibit the growth of other organisms likely to be found on the oropharyngeal and nasopharyngeal mucosae.

After a *Haemophilus* isolate is cultured, a panel of biochemical tests can be used to speciate and biotype the organisms. A slide agglutination test using specific anticapsular antibodies can then be used to determine the capsule type expressed by *H. influenzae* isolates.

Treatment and Prognosis. Until recently, patients with life-threatening epiglottitis or meningitis due to *H. influenzae* were treated with ampicillin plus chloramphenicol. This practice has changed because 25–35% of Hib isolates in the USA are ampicillin-resistant and because drugs that are less toxic than chloramphenicol are now available.

Life-threatening epiglottitis is now usually treated with ceftriaxone or cefotaxime. Patients may also need to have an airway established via tracheostomy or cricothyrotomy.

If the cause of meningitis is unknown but Hib is suspected, patients are treated empirically with ampicillin plus ceftriaxone or cefotaxime. Many physicians also administer dexamethasone 15 minutes before administration of antibiotics, since dexamethasone is thought to reduce the severity of the acute phase of meningitis and to lower the risk of developing neurologic sequelae. Dexamethasone use is controversial, however, because it has been associated with gastrointestinal bleeding in some patients.

Most non–life threatening illnesses due to *H. influenzae* are treated with one of the following: amoxicillin plus clavulanate; an oral second- or third-generation cephalosporin; an extended-spectrum macrolide; or ampicillin plus sulbactam.

The fatality rate associated with Hib meningitis in treated patients has been reported to be as low as 3% and as high as 17.5%. Children at increased risk of death from Hib meningitis include those who have sickle cell anemia, are asplenic, are receiving immunotherapy, have hypogammaglobulinemia, or lack the KM(1) immunoglobulin allotype.

Long-term sequelae to Hib meningitis include hearing deficits, seizures, motor abnormalities, mental retardation, language disorders, visual impairments, hydrocephalus, and isolated cranial nerve palsies.

Prevention. The spread of meningitis and other systemic diseases that are due to Hib can be prevented by immunization and by chemoprophylaxis.

Three ***H. influenzae* type b (HIB) vaccines** are now available: (1) the PRP-D vaccine, in which Hib PRP capsular material is conjugated to diphtheria toxoid; (2) the HbOC vaccine, in which PRP is conjugated to CRM_{197}, a nontoxic fragment of diphtheria toxin; and (3) the PRP-OMP vaccine, in which PRP is conjugated to an outer membrane protein of *Neisseria meningitidis*. While the first of these vaccines is licensed for use in children at the age of 15 months, the other two vaccines are licensed for use as early as 2 months of age. Infants should be immunized against Hib using HbOC or PRP-OMP at 2, 4, and 6 months of age.

Rifampin can be used to prevent Hib infection in immune and nonimmune household members who have been exposed to a child with Hib meningitis. Some experts recommend that rifampin be given for 4 days to all household members if the index case has any siblings under the age of 48 months. Chemoprophylaxis is about 95% effective in eliminating the carriage of Hib.

Other *Haemophilus* Species

Diseases caused by other *Haemophilus* species are summarized in Table 6–3. *Haemophilus aegyptius,* also known as the Koch-Weeks bacillus, is sometimes classified as a biotype III *Haemophilus influenzae.* It is a common cause of conjunctivitis, and the so-called BPF strains of this organism are responsible for a life-threatening disease called Brazilian purpuric fever. *Haemophilus ducreyi* is rare in the USA and causes a sexually transmitted disease known as chancroid. *Haemophilus parainfluenzae* is an uncommon cause of endocarditis and meningitis.

BORDETELLA SPECIES
General Characteristics and Classification

Three species of *Bordetella* infect humans: *Bordetella pertussis, Bordetella bronchiseptica,* and *Bordetella parapertussis.* A fourth species, *Bordetella avium,* infects birds. Because genetic studies have shown that the four species are so closely related, some investigators believe that they are actually four subspecies of a single *Bordetella* species.

Bordetellae are fastidious and grow quite slowly. *B. pertussis* must be cultivated on a special medium that contains starch, charcoal, or resin beads to remove fatty acids and other toxic substances that are released by the organism as it grows. Examples of these media are Bordet-Gengou agar (which contains potato starch) and Regan-Lowe agar (which contains charcoal). Other *Bordetella* species can be cultivated on chocolate agar. After 2–7 days of growth, bordetellae appear as tiny translucent colonies.

Bordetella pertussis

Bordetella pertussis is the most common pathogenic species and is the cause of whooping cough (pertussis).

Characteristics of *B. pertussis*

General Features. *B. pertussis* is a tiny gram-negative rod that grows on the ciliated epithelium of the human nasopharyngeal mucosa and trachea. Like *Bordetella parapertussis* but unlike the other *Bordetella* species, *B. pertussis* is nonmotile and unable to reduce nitrate. Unlike any other *Bordetella* species, *B. pertussis* has no urease activity, cannot be cultured on chocolate agar, and cannot be grown on citrate. The most important difference is that, unlike other species, *B. pertussis* produces **pertussis toxin.** This toxin is responsible for many of the symptoms and pathologic findings associated with whooping cough.

Mechanisms of Pathogenicity. Primary isolates of *B. pertussis* produce toxins and are highly virulent, but nonselective serial subculture results in the appearance of new colony types of bordetellae that have varying degrees of virulence. These changes in virulence are due to phase variation. There are four *B. pertussis* phases or colony types. Phase I isolates (fresh isolates) are encapsulated, piliated, toxic, and virulent. Subculturing results in the gradual appearance of phase II, III, and IV organisms, with the concomitant loss of virulence characteristics. Phase IV isolates are unencapsulated, unpiliated, and avirulent.

(1) *B. pertussis* Antigens and Virulence Determinants. At least four types of adhesins are found on the surface of *B. pertussis,* and the organism produces four key toxins.

(a) Adhesins. Pertactin, pili, filamentous hemagglutinin, and pertussis toxin–hemagglutinin are found on the surface of each organism and are needed to initiate and establish nasopharyngeal colonization.

Pertactin is a 69-kD protein that is synthesized as a 93-kD precursor, processed, and expressed on the bacterial surface. Pertactin has been shown to facilitate the adherence of *B. pertussis* to cultured Chinese hamster ovary cells and to HeLa cells. Pertactin contains an Arg-Gly-Asp sequence (also known as an RGD sequence) in its binding site, and it has multiple repeating units of Gly-Gly-Xaa-Xaa-Pro and Pro-Gln-Pro in its structural regions. The Arg-Gly-Asp sequence facilitates entry of *B. pertussis* into the cytoplasm of cultured cells.

Phase I bordetellae express several types of **pili.** At least two serotypes of *B. pertussis* pili have been described and are called pili or fimbriae 2 and 3. Investigators sometimes refer to these serotypes as agglutinogens. Pili are probably not the key adhesin of *B. pertussis,* but they have been shown to mediate adherence to human erythrocytes and to ciliated epithelial cells in tracheal ring cultures. Results of experiments in mice suggest that *B. pertussis* pili play an important role in the ability of *B. pertussis* to persist in the trachea but may not be a significant adhesin in the nasopharynx.

Filamentous hemagglutinin (FHA) is thought to be the key *B. pertussis* adhesin. FHA is synthesized as a 370-kD precursor and is then processed to yield the active 220-kD FHA adhesin. FHA mediates adherence to a variety of cultured cells, including ciliated epithelial cells in tracheal ring cultures. Results of experiments in mice suggest that FHA is a significant adhesin in both the nasopharynx and the trachea. Like the binding site of pertactin, the binding site of FHA contains an Arg-Gly-Asp sequence (RGD sequence). Unlike the sequence in pertactin, however, the sequence in FHA does not appear to promote cellular invasion.

FHA has three separate binding regions: the Arg-Gly-Asp region binds to lactosylceramide, and two yet-undefined regions bind separately to heparin and to the leukocyte integrin complement receptor 3 (CR3). FHA has been reported to bind to CR3 by mimicking the endothelial receptor for CR3. Antibody to FHA binds to endothelial cells, interferes with leukocyte recruitment, and increases the permeability of the endothelium. *B. pertussis* enters macrophages by binding to CR3 on the macrophage surface. Because the organisms are not killed within macrophages, they are able to persist within the lungs.

Some studies have shown that respiratory and oral immunization of mice with purified FHA protects them against tracheal and lung infection with *B. pertussis.* Other studies have shown that mice immunized intraperitoneally or intramuscularly with purified FHA were protected against lung and trachea

colonization with *B. pertussis* and that this protective effect was due to production of IgG and IgM (rather than IgA) antibodies to FHA.

Pertussis toxin–hemagglutinin (TOX-HA) is a hemagglutinin that has about 5% the adhesive capacity of FHA and is released from *B. pertussis* organisms into the environment. Some investigators have speculated that TOX-HA promotes secondary infection in *B. pertussis*–infected sites by adhering to other mucosal pathogens, such as *Haemophilus influenzae* and *Streptococcus pneumoniae.*

(b) Toxins. *B. pertussis* produces four important toxins: pertussis toxin, pertussis adenylate cyclase, dermonecrotic toxin, and tracheal cytotoxin.

Pertussis toxin is the key to the ability of *B. pertussis* to cause whooping cough. In fact, it is probably the lack of pertussis toxin production by other *Bordetella* species that makes them so rarely the cause of pertussislike disease in humans.

Pertussis toxin is a type A-B toxin. Its A (toxic) region consists of a single S1 subunit, while its B (receptor-binding) region contains two dimers. One of the two dimers consists of subunits S2–S3, and the other contains the subunit complex S2–S4. The two dimers are joined by a single S5. The A-B model is a common one for bacterial exotoxins.

Fig. 6–2 shows the putative mechanism of pertussis toxin. *B. pertussis* releases pertussis toxin into the environment. The B region binds to cellular receptors, and the A region enters the affected cell. Inside the cell, the toxin splits nicotinamide adenine dinucleotide (NAD) and then attaches adenosine diphosphate plus ribose (ADP-R) to the α subunit of a membrane-bound G_i protein. (Proteins that have guanosine triphosphatase activity are called G proteins, and the function of a G_i protein is to inhibit, or down-regulate, the activity of an adenylate cyclase to which it is coupled.)

ADP-ribosylation inactivates the G_i protein, uncoupling it from the adenylate cyclase. Because there is now no mechanism to halt adenylate cyclase activity, the affected cell accumulates huge amounts of cyclic adenosine monophosphate (cAMP) in response to any effector that activates adenylate cyclase. Chloride excretion is stimulated by the excess cAMP, and changes in ion flux cause the affected cells to secrete massive amounts of fluids and electrolytes. Although the mechanism is different, the net effect of this pertussis toxin activity is the same as that of cholera toxin activity (see Chapter 14).

Pertussis toxin is a lymphocytosis-promoting factor and histamine-sensitizing factor. Investigators believe that the toxin promotes lymphocytosis by inducing the synthesis of interleukin-1 and that it potentiates the effects of histamine in a variety of cells. The toxin causes the respiratory tract to produce massive amounts of mucoid secretions and to be exquisitely sensitive to irritants. Slight irritations of the upper respiratory tract can cause the patient to suffer from violent fits of coughing.

B. pertussis produces two adenylate cyclases. One of these remains within the bacterium, and the

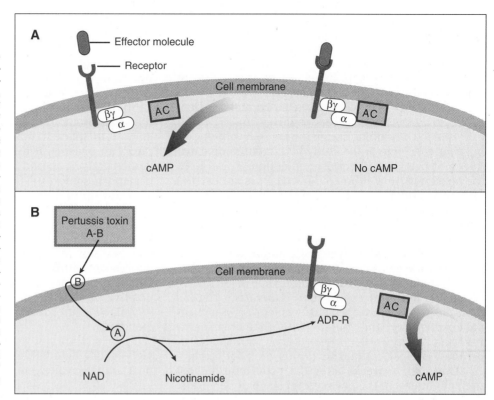

FIGURE 6–2. The putative mechanisms of pertussis toxin. Diagram **A** shows the normal function of the α subunit of the G_i protein. This subunit normally responds to external stimuli by associating with a coupled membrane-bound adenylate cyclase (AC). The association halts the activity of AC. Diagram **B** shows that when pertussis toxin is present, the B region of the toxin binds to cell surface receptors and facilitates the entry of the A region into the cell. The A region splits nicotinamide adenine dinucleotide (NAD), and adenosine diphosphate plus ribose (ADP-R) becomes attached to the α subunit of the G_i protein. The ADP-ribosylated G_i protein is permanently uncoupled from its corresponding AC, and massive amounts of cyclic adenosine monophosphate (cAMP) are synthesized by the now unregulated AC. Accumulation of cAMP causes hypersecretion of fluids and electrolytes.

other is secreted. **Pertussis adenylate cyclase** enters host cells either alone or in conjunction with the entry of *B. pertussis* organisms into the cell cytoplasm. Inside the host cell, the adenylate cyclase is activated by calmodulin. The activated pertussis adenylate cyclase in turn activates dermonecrotic toxin. Although the role of adenylate cyclase in disease is not well understood, experimental studies have shown that *B. pertussis* strains which do not produce adenylate cyclase are avirulent.

Dermonecrotic toxin, also called **heat-labile toxin,** is released when phase I *B. pertussis* organisms lyse. Its contribution to the pathogenesis of pertussis remains largely speculative, but it has been shown to be ciliostatic and cytotoxic, to cause tissue necrosis ("dermonecrosis"), and to be unstable at 56 °C ("heat-labile"). Dermonecrotic toxin is lethal when injected intraperitoneally into mice.

Tracheal cytotoxin (TCT) is a 921-dalton peptidoglycan fragment that is released by growing *B. pertussis.* Another name for TCT is *N*-acetylglucosaminyl-1,6-anhydromuramylalanyl-γ-glutamyldiaminopimelylalanine. This is the same molecule released by growing gonococci and is identical to a molecule that is known as FS_u or factor S and appears in the CSF of sleep-deprived animals. TCT and related muramyl peptides have been shown to have immunomodulating activity, to be ciliostatic or ciliocidal, and to block adherence of 5-hydroxytryptamine to cellular receptors.

(2) Pathogenic Processes. *B. pertussis* is an exquisitely viscerotropic bacterium that has a strict affinity for ciliated epithelial cells. The pertactin, FHA,

and pili of *B. pertussis* promote the adherence of organisms to these cells in the nasopharynx and trachea. The organisms also spread into the bronchi, where they may be phagocytosed by macrophages. Some organisms multiply within macrophages and epithelial cells, but most pathologic changes are caused by extracellular organisms that adhere to the ciliated epithelium.

The toxins produced by *B. pertussis* are responsible for the clinical manifestations of pertussis. Pertussis toxin causes massive hypersecretion and also causes the mucosa to become hypersensitive to histamine. Dermonecrotic toxin and TCT damage the ciliated epithelium and reduce the ability of cilia to clear bacteria and secretions from the mucociliary tree. Damage to the nasopharynx acts as an irritant and causes the patient to sneeze frequently. Histamine hypersensitivity elicits more hypersecretion and causes spasms when any histamine-inducing agent (such as an allergen or viral infection) is present. Eventually, the ciliated epithelium of the trachea and nasopharynx becomes covered with a massive purulent exudate. The combined effects of hypersecretion, purulent exudation, histamine sensitivity, and necrosis cause the patient to suffer from terrible paroxysms (fits) of coughing.

Diseases Due to *B. pertussis*

Epidemiology. In the USA, pertussis primarily affects young children, with most cases reported in those under 1 year of age. During the late 1950s, the incidence of pertussis was about 23 per 100,000 people. With widespread use of pertussis vaccine, the incidence has dropped to under 2 cases per 100,000.

In unvaccinated individuals who are exposed to active *B. pertussis* organisms, the rate of disease is reported to be 90–95%. Extensive efforts to locate asymptomatic carriers of *B. pertussis* have been fruitless. In a study of unvaccinated individuals in Denmark, however, investigators reported that 61% had experienced whooping cough during their childhood but that everyone in the study had immunologic evidence of previous *B. pertussis* infection. This raises the possibility that although *B. pertussis* is not carried asymptomatically, some patients develop a very mild respiratory disease that is not recognized as whooping cough.

Diagnosis

(1) History and Physical Examination. There are three stages of pertussis, or whooping cough.

The **catarrhal stage** is the prodrome of pertussis. About 10 days after exposure to *B. pertussis,* the patient has a runny nose, extensive sneezing, a nocturnal cough, fever, and conjunctivitis. Like measles virus and many other respiratory pathogens, *B. pertussis* is most contagious during the prodrome.

One or two weeks after the prodrome begins, the patient enters the **paroxysmal stage** of pertussis. During each coughing paroxysm, which lasts 30 seconds or more, the patient coughs violently 5–20 times without taking intervening breaths, and mucinous secretions may bubble in massive amounts from the nose and mouth. By the end of a paroxysm, the patient may become anoxic and turn blue. Then as air rushes back into the air-depleted lungs, there is a loud "whooping" or "crowing" sound. Other manifestations of disease in the paroxysmal stage are vomiting, epistaxis (bloody nose), periorbital edema, and conjunctival hemorrhage. Fever is present only if the patient is secondarily infected with another bacterial agent. Secondary infection with group A streptococci is not unusual. Lymphocytic leukocytosis is seen in about 25% of patients under 6 months of age and in 75% of patients 6 months or older. The average duration of the paroxysmal stage is 2 weeks, but some patients suffer from paroxysms for up to 6 weeks.

Pertussis gradually resolves during the **convalescent stage.** This stage usually lasts 2 weeks. However, for the next few months, the patient is unusually susceptible to life-threatening pneumonia and other respiratory tract infections caused by pathogens such as group A streptococci, pneumococci, and *H. influenzae.* This is because the patient's respiratory ciliated epithelium has been severely damaged, removing an important obstacle to pulmonary infections.

(2) Laboratory Analysis. Because *B. pertussis* is rarely recovered from patients who have been infected more than 4 weeks, cultures should be attempted as early in the disease as possible. Cotton is toxic to *B. pertussis,* so cotton swabs should not be used to collect specimens for culture. Instead, a calcium alginate or Dacron swab should be used. The swab is passed to the posterior pharyngeal wall,

where it is left for a moment to allow it to become soaked with exudate. The specimen is then used to inoculate a plate of selective *Bordetella* agar.

Among the selective media most often used are Bordet-Gengou agar, Stanier-Scholte agar, and Regan-Lowe agar. If the medium to be used does not contain antibiotics, as is the case with Bordet-Gengou agar, the swab should be passed through a drop of penicillin G on the plate to inhibit the growth of other respiratory organisms. If the sample cannot be cultured immediately, it should be transported in Regan-Lowe transport medium. The samples are incubated at 35 °C for up to 7 days in 5–7% CO_2.

A direct fluorescent antibody test can be used to examine exudate samples for *B. pertussis.* This test is rapid, but it is significantly less sensitive than are cultures. For example, one group reported that the fluorescent antibody test yielded positive results in only 6 of 20 specimens from patients with culture-positive pertussis. Thus, until the sensitivity of this technique is improved, its use is not generally recommended.

Patients are not tested for antibody to *B. pertussis,* because detectable levels of antibody do not appear until convalescence. Blood cultures are not useful, because pertussis has no bacteremic phase. Efforts are under way to produce a reliable test using polymerase chain reaction technology.

Treatment and Prognosis. Erythromycin is the treatment of choice for patients with pertussis. Alternatively, ampicillin or trimethoprim-sulfamethoxazole (TMP/SMX) can be used. Antibiotic therapy does not appear to change the course of the disease unless administered early during the prodrome. In later stages, inexorable mucosal damage has already occurred, and elimination of the organisms will not reverse this damage significantly. Nevertheless, because *B. pertussis* is so contagious, all patients should be treated with antibiotics and placed under respiratory isolation. In addition, proper acid-base balance must be maintained, and the patient must have adequate oxygen support available during and immediately after paroxysms.

The fatality rate associated with untreated pertussis is about 1%.

Prevention. The spread of pertussis can be prevented by immunization and by chemoprophylaxis.

The currently used **pertussis vaccine** contains killed phase I organisms and is generally administered in combination with diphtheria and tetanus toxoids (as DTP or DPT vaccine). The rate of neurologic sequelae in vaccine recipients is about 0.00032% (1 in every 310,000 vaccinated people), whereas the rate of neurologic sequelae in hospitalized patients with pertussis is between 1.5% and 14%. For this reason, all children should be immunized.

To prevent infection in nonimmune children and adults who have been exposed to *B. pertussis,* a 10-day course of erythromycin should be given. A booster of pertussis vaccine should also be given to exposed children under 4 years old.

Because of the fear of neurologic sequelae in

recipients of whole-cell pertussis vaccines, investigators have developed several acellular vaccines. In clinical trials, acellular vaccines that contain pertussis toxin, filamentous hemagglutinin, or pertactin have been shown to be safe and about as effective as whole-cell vaccines.

Selected Readings

Burroughs, M., et al. Bacterial components and the pathophysiology of injury to the blood-brain barrier: does cell wall add to the effects of endotoxin in gram-negative meningitis? J Infect Dis 165(supplement 1):S82–S85, 1992.

Cookson, B. T., et al. Primary structure of the peptidoglycan-derived tracheal cytotoxin of *Bordetella pertussis.* Biochemistry 28:1744–1749, 1989.

Cuevas, L. E., and C. A. Hart. Chemoprophylaxis of bacterial meningitis. J Antimicrob Chemother 31(supplement B):79–91, 1993.

DeVries, F. P., et al. Invasion of primary nasopharyngeal epithelial cells by *Neisseria meningitidis* is controlled by phase variation of multiple surface antigens. Infect Immun 64:2998–3006, 1996.

Edwards, K. M., and M. D. Decker. Acellular pertussis vaccines for infants. N Engl J Med 334:391–392, 1996.

Gorby, G. L., and G. B. Schaefer. Effect of attachment factors (pili plus Opa) on *Neisseria gonorrhoeae* invasion of human fallopian tube tissue in vitro: quantitation by computerized image analysis. Microb Pathog 13:93–108, 1992.

Gray, L. D., and D. P. Fedorko. Laboratory diagnosis of bacterial meningitis. Clin Microbiol 5:130–145, 1992.

Heike, U., et al. Gonococcal opacity protein promotes bacterial entry-associated rearrangements of the epithelial cell actin cytoskeleton. Infect Immun 64:1621–1630, 1996.

Heininger, U., et al. Clinical characteristics of illness caused by *Bordetella parapertussis* compared with illness caused by *Bordetella pertussis.* Pediatr Infect Dis J 13:306–309, 1994.

Kellogg, D. S., Jr., et al. *Neisseria gonorrhoeae.* 1. Virulence genetically linked to clonal variation. J Bacteriol 85:1274–1279, 1963.

Kellogg, D. S., Jr., et al. *Neisseria gonorrhoeae.* 2. Clonal variation and pathogenicity during 35 months in vitro. J Bacteriol 96:596–605, 1968.

Kilian, M., et al. Biological significance of IgA1 proteases in bacterial colonization and pathogenesis: critical evaluation of experimental evidence. APMIS 104:321–338, 1996.

Kimura, A., et al. *Bordetella pertussis* filamentous hemagglutinin: evaluation as a protective antigen and colonization factor in a mouse respiratory infection model. Infect Immun 58:7–16, 1990.

Lagergard, T., et al. Evidence of *Haemophilus ducreyi* adherence to and cytotoxin destruction of human epithelial cells. Microb Pathog 14:417–431, 1993.

Leininger, E., et al. Pertactin, an Arg-Gly-Asp-containing *Bordetella pertussis* surface protein that promotes adherence of mammalian cells. Proc Natl Acad Sci USA 88:345–349, 1991.

Madore, D. V. Impact of immunization on *Haemophilus influenzae* type b disease. Infect Agents Dis 5:8–20, 1996.

Mandrell, R. E., and M. A. Apicella. Lipooligosaccharides (LOS) of mucosal pathogens: molecular mimicry and host modification of LOS. Immunobiology 187:382–402, 1993.

Punsalang, A. P., and W. D. Sawyer. Role of pili in the virulence of *Neisseria gonorrhoeae.* Infect Immun 8:255–263, 1973.

Quagliarello, V. M., and W. M. Scheld. Bacterial meningitis: pathogenesis, pathophysiology, and progress. N Engl J Med 327:864–869, 1992.

Sarosi, G. A. Bacterial pneumonia: *Streptococcus pneumoniae* and *Haemophilus influenzae* are the villains. Postgrad Med 93:43–50, 1993.

Saukkonen, K., et al. Integrin-mediated localization of *Bordetella pertussis* within macrophages: role in pulmonary colonization. J Exp Med 173:1143–1149, 1991.

Stephens, D. S., and M. M. Farley. Pathogenetic events during infection of the human nasopharynx with *Neisseria meningitidis* and *Haemophilus influenzae.* Rev Infect Dis 13:22–33, 1991.

Tarlow, M. J. Should we use dexamethasone in meningitis? Arch Dis Child 67:1398–1401, 1992.

Thongthai, C. F., and W. D. Sawyer. Studies on the virulence of *Neisseria gonorrhoeae.* 1. Relation of colonial morphology and resistance to phagocytosis by polymorphonuclear leukocytes. Infect Immun 7:373–379, 1973.

Verheul, A. F., et al. Meningococcal lipopolysaccharides: virulence factor and potential vaccine component. Microbiol Rev 57:34–49, 1993.

CHAPTER SEVEN

ENTEROBACTERIACEAE

AND ASSOCIATED BACTERIA

Campylobacter, Citrobacter, Edwardsiella, Enterobacter, Escherichia, Hafnia, Helicobacter, Klebsiella, Morganella, Pantoea, Proteus, Providencia, Salmonella, Serratia, Shigella, and *Yersinia*

Chapter 7 focuses on members of the family Enterobacteriaceae and members of the genera *Campylobacter* and *Helicobacter*.

Members of the family Enterobacteriaceae are called **enteric organisms** because they so often reside in the gastrointestinal tract of animals and humans, although many species are also found in water and soil. Among the medically important genera in this family are *Enterobacter, Escherichia, Klebsiella, Proteus, Salmonella, Serratia, Shigella,* and *Yersinia*.

Except for the genera *Salmonella, Shigella,* and *Yersinia,* Enterobacteriaceae are seen primarily as normal flora or environmental bacteria. When the organisms are introduced into a body site that is usually sterile, however, they can cause diseases such as pneumonia, urinary tract infections, septicemia, neonatal infections, wound infections, and postoperative infections. Enteric organisms are generally opportunistic and cause disease mainly in patients who are immunosuppressed, catheterized, or debilitated. As such, the organisms are common causes of nosocomial disease. The greatest danger posed by opportunistic enteric infections is the development of sepsis. The frankly pathogenic enteric organisms cause gastrointestinal infections that may become systemic.

Like members of the family Enterobacteriaceae, members of the genera *Campylobacter* and *Helicobacter* are gram-negative rods that cause gastrointestinal disease.

ENTEROBACTERIACEAE
General Characteristics and Classification

The family Enterobacteriaceae consists of organisms that are gram-negative rods; are about 0.5–2.0 μm wide by 2–4 μm long; are facultative anaerobes that ferment glucose when grown anaerobically; are cytochrome oxidase–negative; are capable of reducing nitrate to nitrite; and are peritrichous when motile.

Much of what is known about bacteria has come from studies involving *Escherichia coli, Salmonella* species, and other Enterobacteriaceae. Indeed, data presented in the early chapters of this book were derived largely from studies of *E. coli,* and *Salmonella* species have been used extensively to study the structure and expression of lipopolysaccharide molecules. Although the enteric organisms are the best-studied bacteria and have become the standard against which all other gram-negative bacteria are judged, the taxonomy of the family Enterobacteriaceae remains confusing and controversial.

The 1984 edition of *Bergey's Manual of Determinative Bacteriology* proposed 20 enteric genera based largely on "DNA findings." This scheme moved *Shigella* into the tribe Escherichieae and divided *Salmonella* into various subgenera. In 1986, W. H. Ewing proposed a new scheme that kept *Shigella* within the tribe Escherichieae (Table 7–1) but recognized only a single *Salmonella* species, which was known as *Salmonella enterica* and had five subspecies. In 1989, the Centers for Disease Control (CDC) established a classification scheme that was similar to the previous two, but it placed *Escherichia* and *Shigella* into a single genus known as *Escherichia-Shigella* and grouped the salmonellae as many serotypes within a single genus, *Salmonella*. Today, the CDC and state laboratories use the 1989 CDC taxonomic scheme in their reporting, but many investigators, hospitals, clinicians, and journals use variations of the other taxonomic schemes.

TABLE 7–1. Tribes and Genera in the Family Enterobacteriaceae*

Tribe I: Escherichieae
*Escherichia**
*Shigella**

Tribe II: Edwardsielleae
Edwardsiella

Tribe III: Salmonelleae
Salmonella

Tribe IV: Citrobactereae
Citrobacter

Tribe V: Klebsielleae
Enterobacter
Hafnia
Klebsiella
Pantoea
Serratia

Tribe VI: Proteeae
Morganella
Proteus
Providencia

Tribe VII: Yersinieae
Yersinia

Tribe VIII: Erwinieae
Erwinia

*The classification scheme proposed by the Centers for Disease Control in 1989 combines *Escherichia* and *Shigella* into one genus called *Escherichia-Shigella.*

In the classification of enteric organisms, the relative significance of biochemical tests versus nucleic acid homologies is a subject of considerable disagreement. Although nucleic acid homology would seem to be the most pertinent taxonomic characteristic, the clinical laboratory relies primarily on biochemical and immunologic tests to identify bacterial species. These biochemical identification schemes do not always seem to coincide with nucleic acid–based taxonomic divisions. For example, the ability to ferment lactose is considered to be a key characteristic in any taxonomic identification pathway. *E. coli* is a motile, lactose-positive, opportunistic pathogen. Yet recent taxonomic schemes have allied it closely with *Shigella,* an organism previously considered to be distinct from *E. coli* because it is a nonmotile, lactose-negative, invasive organism. These types of disputes have kept the problem of classifying the enteric organisms unresolved.

Culture and Identification of Enteric Organisms

Opportunistic enteric organisms are often present as normal flora, so isolating them from gastrointestinal specimens (such as fecal samples or rectal swabs) is not considered to be of significance. However, when invasive enteric organisms—namely, *Sal-* monella, Shigella, and Yersinia—are present in these samples, it is likely that they are a cause of disease.

Culture Media

Selective culture media have been developed to inhibit the growth of gram-positive bacteria and opportunistic enteric bacteria but allow invasive enteric organisms to multiply freely. These media take advantage of the fact that *Salmonella* grows well in the presence of bile salts, but *E. coli* does not. Most of these media contain lactose as an energy source and include indicators that change color when lactose is fermented. Some media contain multiple sugars. The selective media used most often are eosin–methylene blue (EMB) agar, Hektoen enteric (HE) agar, MacConkey (MC) agar, Salmonella-Shigella (SS) agar, and xylose-lysine-deoxycholate (XLD) agar. Table 7–2 outlines the characteristics of lactose fermenters and nonfermenters on these agars.

When infections due to salmonellae or shigellae involve small numbers of bacteria, **enrichment media** may be used as the primary culture media. Each enrichment medium contains chemicals that inhibit the growth of coliforms (opportunistic enteric organisms similar to and including *E. coli*), holding them in a prolonged lag phase. After an enrichment medium is inoculated with a specimen drawn from the patient, it is incubated 4–12 hours to allow salmonellae or shigellae to grow. Then a sample of the medium is used to inoculate HE agar. The most commonly used enrichment media are selenite broth and gram-negative (GN) broth.

Culture Techniques

The correct culture technique depends on the type of samples taken.

Blood, wound exudate, or other specimens that are not taken from the gastrointestinal tract may contain opportunistic enteric organisms that are responsible for the patient's infection. These samples should be streaked on two plates of agar: blood agar and either MC agar or EMB agar.

Fecal samples or rectal swabs are more likely to contain *Salmonella, Shigella,* or *Yersinia,* so they must be tested on media that will selectively culture these organisms. The samples should be streaked on two plates of agar, the first containing either MC agar or EMB agar to identify all enteric organisms present and the second containing either XLD agar or HE agar to selectively culture salmonellae or shigellae. A small sample should also be enriched in selenite broth for 8–12 hours or in GN broth for 4 hours, and then the enriched broth is used to inoculate HE agar.

After these initial steps are followed, all specimens are treated in the same manner. The plates are incubated for 24–48 hours. Then each colony type is Gram-stained, streaked for isolation as needed, and characterized by a series of biochemical tests. The biochemical tests are almost always performed using commercially available kits to identify characteristics such as carbohydrate fermentation; citrate utiliza-

TABLE 7–2. Characteristics of Selective Media for the Culture of Enterobacteriaceae

Medium	Sugars in Medium	Rapid Lactose Fermenters	Slow Lactose Fermenters	Nonfermenters
Eosin–methylene blue (EMB) agar	Lactose and sucrose.	Green-black colonies with green sheen.	Purple colonies in 24–48 hours.	Transparent colonies.
Hektoen enteric (HE) agar	Lactose, sucrose, and salicin.	Growth partially inhibited; bright orange to salmon-colored colonies.	Growth partially inhibited; bright orange to salmon-colored colonies.	Green (*Shigella*); blue-green with black centers (*Salmonella*).
MacConkey (MC) agar	Lactose.	Red colonies.	Pink colonies surrounded by bile precipitate.	Transparent after 24–48 hours.
Salmonella-Shigella (SS) agar	Lactose.	Red colonies.	Red colonies.	Transparent (*Shigella*); transparent with black centers (*Salmonella*).
Xylose-lysine-deoxycholate (XLD) agar	Lactose, xylose, and sucrose.	Bright yellow colonies.	Bright yellow colonies.	Translucent (*Shigella*); red with black centers (*Salmonella*).

tion; decarboxylation of lysine, ornithine, and arginine; hydrogen sulfide production; indole production from tryptophan; motility; orthonitrophenyl-β-D-galactopyranoside (ONPG) utilization; phenylalanine deaminase production; and Voges-Proskauer activity (production of acetoin).

Surface Antigens of Enteric Organisms

Three types of surface antigens are widely used to serotype enteric organisms: O antigens, H antigens, and K antigens.

O antigens are the O antigenic carbohydrates of bacteria that have a "smooth" or complete lipopolysaccharide molecule. The enteric organisms have a powerful endotoxic activity that is due to the lipid A portion of their lipopolysaccharide. Thus, enteric infections carry the threat of sepsis, a condition associated with a high fatality rate. O antigen typing is a key step in serotyping enteric strains. Because bacteriophages may carry O antigen genes, some enteric organisms express more than one O antigen specificity at a time.

H antigens are flagellar antigens. Enteric rods that are motile exhibit peritrichous flagellation. By use of special media, motile enteric rods can be induced to express either phase I or phase II H antigens. The pattern of expression is then used to serotype the organisms. *Shigella* species are not motile and do not express H antigens.

K antigens are usually capsular antigens, but a few are now known to be pili (fimbriae). These antigens are found on all encapsulated enteric organisms. In most cases, they are referred to as K antigens. By convention, however, they are called **Vi antigens** when they are found on salmonellae. K comes from the German word *Kapsel,* and Vi is the shortened form of the word *virulence.*

When outbreaks of uncommon enteric diseases occur, epidemiologists use these antigens as a tool to determine if the outbreak is due to a single strain and to trace the source of origin of the outbreak. For example, strains of *E. coli* that have been responsible for outbreaks of bloody diarrhea and hemolytic-uremic syndrome in the northwestern USA have almost always been identified as O157:H7.

Escherichia and *Shigella* Species

Until recently, the tribe **Escherichieae** contained only a single species, *Escherichia coli.* During the past few years, two changes have come to this tribe. First, new species of *Escherichia* were discovered. (Because these species are rarely pathogenic for humans, they will not be discussed in this chapter.) Second, the genus *Shigella* was moved into the tribe Escherichieae on the basis of studies in which nucleic acid homology was used as an indicator of genetic relatedness.

The two genera in the tribe—*Escherichia* and *Shigella*—seem to be strange bedfellows. *E. coli* is a motile lactose fermenter, and most strains of this organism are considered to be opportunistic pathogens at best. *E. coli* usually causes kidney and bladder infections, respiratory infections, neonatal meningitis, pulmonary disease in debilitated and catheterized patients, and sepsis. In contrast, *Shigella* is nonmotile, does not ferment lactose, and is a frank pathogen. It causes bacillary dysentery, characterized by massive invasion and erosion of the colonic mucosa and by bloody, mucoid diarrhea.

Characteristics of *Escherichia*

General Features. *E. coli* is a facultative anaerobe and is part of the normal gut flora of animals and humans. Each gram of human feces contains up to 10^8 *E. coli* organisms. *E. coli* grows well on very simple media; is motile and has peritrichous flagella; ferments lactose and forms a green sheen on eosin–methylene blue agar; has lysine decarboxylase activity; can utilize acetate as its sole carbon source; and hydrolyzes tryptophan to form indole.

Reference laboratories identify individual *E. coli* strains by their O, H, and K antigen serotypes. Hundreds of O antigens and dozens of H and K antigens have been identified, and K antigens have been subdivided into three groups (L, A, and B). A typical *E. coli* strain designation is *E. coli* O26:K60(B6):H11.

Mechanisms of Pathogenicity. Most *E. coli* infections are opportunistic infections of the kidney, bladder, wounds, lungs, or meninges, and each may lead to life-threatening sepsis. As such, *E. coli* is one of the key nosocomial pathogens. But *E. coli* also causes community-acquired urinary tract infections, and special *E. coli* strains cause diarrhea. These special strains are classified as **enterotoxigenic** (ETEC), **enteropathogenic** (EPEC), **enteroinvasive** (EIEC), and **enterohemorrhagic** (EHEC). In addition, because EHEC strains produce verotoxin (described below), they are sometimes classified as **verotoxigenic** (VTEC) strains.

(1) Bacterial Products Involved in Virulence

(a) Adhesins. Pili, or fimbriae, are important *E. coli* virulence factors because they allow *E. coli* to adhere to mucosa.

More than 80% of *E. coli* strains known to cause pyelonephritis exhibit **P fimbriae** that bind to glycolipids containing galactose disaccharide units. P fimbriae bind avidly to mucosal and renal cells and seem to inhibit the ability of *E. coli* to be phagocytosed by polymorphonuclear leukocytes (PMNs).

EPEC strains of *E. coli,* which cause diarrhea in infants, are believed to adhere to intestinal mucosa via **type IV pili.** These pili are also known as bundle-forming pili and are similar to the pili of *Vibrio cholerae* and *Neisseria gonorrhoeae.* Other diarrhea-inducing strains of *E. coli* have been reported to express pili known as **colonization factor antigens** (CFA). There are two types of CFA. While the adherence of CFA/I is inhibited by mannose, that of CFA/II is unaffected by mannose.

(b) Endotoxin. *E. coli* is a major cause of sepsis. The endotoxicity associated with *E. coli* sepsis is due to the lipid A portion of lipopolysaccharide. *E. coli* sepsis may occur in patients with community-acquired urinary tract infections, but it is most often seen when debilitated patients develop nosocomial *E. coli* infections. The pathogenesis of sepsis is discussed fully in Chapter 1.

(c) Enterotoxins. Enterotoxins are protein toxins that affect the function of the gastrointestinal tract. Two *E. coli* enterotoxins have been described: **heat-stable enterotoxin** (ST) and **heat-labile enterotoxin** (LT). Patients infected with *E. coli* strains that produce ST or LT suffer from profuse, watery, cholera-like diarrhea. *E. coli* enterotoxins are plasmid-encoded.

ST is an nonantigenic enterotoxin that is produced by ETEC strains of *E. coli.* Two forms of the toxin, STa and STb, may be produced. STa causes hypersecretion by stimulating the activity of guanylate cyclase. The mechanism of STb is not well understood.

LT is an antigenic enterotoxin that binds to GM_1 gangliosides on the surface of intestinal epithelial cells. LT stimulates adenylate cyclase activity by activating a G protein in the cell membrane. Its mode of action is identical to that of cholera toxin (see Chapter 14). Like cholera toxin, LT causes hypersecretion of fluids and electrolytes without affecting fluid resorption. Thus, patients with diarrhea caused by LT or cholera toxin can be rehydrated orally. Although their mechanisms of action are similar, LT and cholera toxin are structurally unrelated.

(d) Verotoxin. EHEC (VTEC) strains of *E. coli* produce a toxin that is called verotoxin (because of its ability to kill cultured Vero cells) or Shiga-like toxin (because of its similarity to the Shiga neurotoxin produced by *Shigella dysenteriae*). Verotoxin is encoded on the genome of a bacteriophage, and the gene enters the *E. coli* via phage conversion. Two forms of verotoxin are found: verotoxin-1 and verotoxin-2.

Verotoxin-1 is identical to Shiga toxin. It has one A subunit (the active component) and multiple B subunits (receptor-binding components). The entire toxin is transcribed as an operon. The B subunits bind to globotriaosylceramide (Gb3), and this allows the A subunit to enter the target cell. The A subunit cleaves an *N*-glycosidic bond in 28S rRNA, thereby releasing adenosine from position 4324. As a result, elongation factor 1 (EF-1) is no longer able to facilitate the binding of aminoacyl tRNA to ribosome. Protein synthesis is blocked, and the cell dies.

Verotoxin-2 has a similar mode of action, but it is structurally different from Shiga toxin. Antibody directed against Shiga toxin neutralizes verotoxin-1 but not verotoxin-2.

Verotoxin activity causes bloody diarrhea, hemolytic-uremic syndrome, or both. The means by which this occurs is not certain, but investigators believe that verotoxin damages endothelial cells, causing a decrease in the production of prostaglandin I_2 (PGI_2 or prostacyclin) and an increase in the release of von Willebrand factor multimers. The combined effects of these agents may cause platelet aggregation and thrombocytopenia, the suspected precursors of hemolytic-uremic syndrome. Hemolytic-uremic syndrome consists of a triad of microangiopathic hemolytic anemia, acute renal failure, and thrombocytopenia.

(e) Other Pathogenetic Products. *E. coli* strains that are commonly associated with pyelonephritis often produce a **hemolysin** that lyses erythrocytes and damages a variety of host cells. The hemolysin damages cell membranes by inserting itself into the membrane to form cation-selective channels. The presence of hemolysin seems to increase the nephropathogenicity of *E. coli.*

An iron-chelating siderophore known as **aerobactin** has been described, but its relationship to disease is not known.

(2) Pathogenesis of Opportunistic Infections. *E. coli* organisms are found in large numbers in the intestine of every human and are spread by fecal contamination. In hospitalized patients, studies have shown that as the frequency of invasive procedures increases, the incidence of *E. coli* infections also increases. For example, debilitated patients are routinely infected when hands contaminated with

E. coli touch indwelling devices such as catheters. Among the risk factors for the development of *E. coli* meningitis in neonates are traumatic delivery, premature birth, low birth weight, and use of *E. coli*–contaminated instruments to assist delivery.

(3) Pathogenesis of Urinary Tract Infections. Community-acquired *E. coli* urinary tract infections are generally caused by self-infection and occur most often in women. Because the female urethra is short and the vagina can be colonized by coliforms, *E. coli* can readily ascend the urethra to the bladder and kidney. Intercourse is often the precipitating event for urinary tract infections in women, and cystitis is a common occurrence in newly married women ("honeymoon cystitis"). In men over the age of 45, prostatic hypertrophy is a risk factor for urinary tract infection. Other risk factors in men and women include diabetes and the presence of kidney stones.

(4) Pathogenesis of Diarrheal Disease. Diarrhea is caused by a limited number of *E. coli* strains. Although diarrhea is little more than a nuisance to most people in the USA, it is a major killer of infants and toddlers in developing countries. Fig. 7–1 shows how ETEC, EPEC, EHEC, and EIEC strains of *E. coli* cause diarrhea, and Table 7–3 lists the common serogroups.

(a) Enterotoxigenic *E. coli*. ETEC is a common cause of watery diarrhea in malnourished infants and is the major cause of traveler's diarrhea. Infection is acquired by ingesting feces-contaminated food or water. The ETEC organisms colonize the proximal small intestine, where they adhere to the mucosa via pili and release ST or LT. The ST or LT causes hypersecretion of fluids and electrolytes, and this leads to watery diarrhea.

(b) Enteropathogenic *E. coli*. EPEC has been implicated in epidemics of diarrhea among infants, particularly those living in urban areas and those who are hospitalized. EPEC rarely causes disease after 1 year of age, and almost all patients are 6 months of age or younger. EPEC outbreaks have occurred occasionally in child-care settings in the USA and are sometimes the cause of prolonged diarrhea.

EPEC organisms adhere closely to enterocyte membranes through a process known as localized adherence. Rather than covering the cells uniformly, the bacteria adhere via type IV pili to the epithelium in distinct microcolonies. In a process controlled in concert by chromosomal and plasmid genes, the bacteria cause calcium levels inside the target cell to rise and the microvilli to efface. A second adhesin known as intimin then promotes tight adherence to the enterocyte, and this results in proliferation of filamentous actin under each adherent bacterium.

Some cell invasion occurs with EPEC, but invasion is not as extensive as that seen with EIEC. The effacement of microvilli in this process may cause some malabsorption to occur, but the precise source of diarrhea seen with EPEC infections is not known. The diarrhea caused by EPEC is copious, watery, and mucoid, but the stools contain no blood.

(c) Enterohemorrhagic *E. coli*. Cattle serve as the primary reservoir for EHEC, and EHEC diarrhea can result from ingesting undercooked hamburger that contains unacceptably high levels of bovine feces. EHEC diarrhea in the USA occurs most often in the Pacific Northwest and is caused by *E. coli* O157:H7, while diarrhea in Canada is most often caused by *E. coli* O26:H11 strain 30. Sporadic outbreaks have been reported among nursing home patients and children in day-care facilities. EHEC organisms cause diarrhea by adhering to the colonic mucosa and producing verotoxins. The diarrhea is copious and bloody but can be distinguished from dysentery by the absence of PMNs in the stool. EHEC diarrhea is dangerous in itself, but it is doubly dangerous because 2–11% of patients develop hemolytic-uremic syndrome.

(d) Enteroinvasive *E. coli*. EIEC organisms are found primarily in developing countries and are rarely seen in the USA. When EIEC organisms are ingested in feces-contaminated food or water, they attach to the colonic mucosa and then invade the mucosa and lamina propria. Although this initially causes watery diarrhea, the diarrhea soon becomes similar to that seen in patients with bacillary dysentery, and blood and mucus are found in the stool.

(e) Enteroaggregative *E. coli*. Investigators have discovered an *E. coli* strain that is able to adhere in clumps to HEp-2 cells in vitro. This enteroaggregative strain also adheres to the colonic mucosa via bundle-forming pili and causes watery diarrhea by producing a low-molecular-weight heat-stable enterotoxin that is distinct from ST and LT. Most cases of diarrhea caused by this strain have occurred in Southeast Asia.

(f) Other Strains of *E. coli*. Nontoxigenic *E. coli* organisms that have mannose-resistant pili (CFA/II) will adhere to the small intestine and cause prolonged diarrhea in malnourished patients. The mechanism of action in this type of diarrhea is unknown.

Diseases Due to *Escherichia*

Epidemiology. Table 7–3 shows the *E. coli* serogroups most often associated with opportunistic infections, urinary tract infections, and diarrhea.

Diagnosis

(1) Opportunistic Infections. Debilitated patients, particularly those who have indwelling catheters or undergo invasive procedures, are at risk of acquiring *E. coli* infections. Nosocomial infection with *E. coli* is a common cause of **pneumonia,** especially in patients who are over 50 years of age and have a chronic underlying disease. *E. coli* pneumonia is often complicated by **empyema** and **sepsis** and is usually acquired by aspirating oral secretions.

E. coli is a frequent cause of **wound and postoperative infections,** particularly if the wound or surgery involves the bowel. Abdominal infections may lead to peritonitis and sepsis. *E. coli* may also cause sepsis with no obvious point of origin.

E. coli strains that have K1 antigen can cause **meningitis** in neonates. The antigen protects the or-

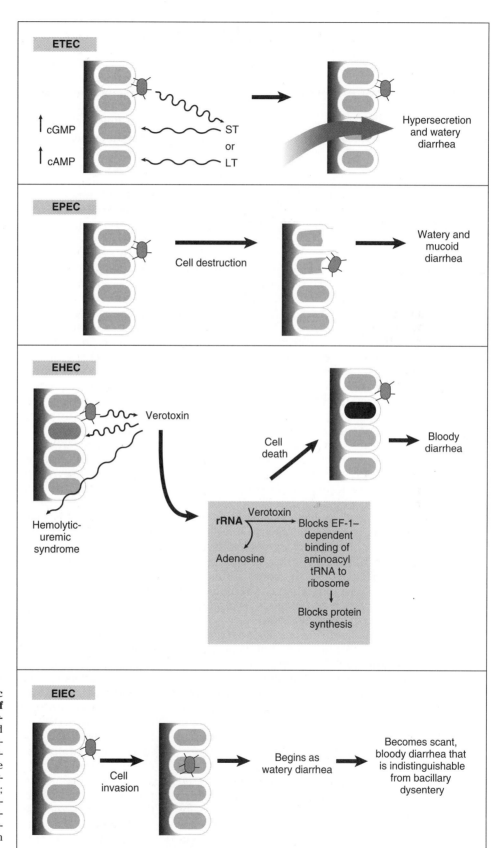

FIGURE 7–1. The pathogenetic mechanisms of four strains of *Escherichia coli* that cause diarrhea. ETEC, EPEC, EHEC, and EIEC are the enterotoxigenic, enteropathogenic, enterohemorrhagic, and enteroinvasive strains, respectively. cGMP = cyclic guanosine monophosphate; cAMP = cyclic adenosine monophosphate; ST = heat-stable enterotoxin; LT = heat-labile enterotoxin; and EF-1 = elongation factor 1.

TABLE 7–3. Categorization of _Escherichia coli_ Serogroups

Category	O Antigen Serogroups
Normal enteric flora	1, 2, 4, 6, 7, 8, 18, 25, 45, 75, and 81
Causes of opportunistic infections	1, 2, 4, 6, 7, 8, 9, 11, 18, 22, 25, 62, and 75
Causes of urinary tract infections	1, 4, 6, 18, and 75
Causes of diarrhea	
Enterotoxigenic (ETEC) strains	6, 8, 15, 20, 25, 27, 63, 78, 80, 85, 115, 128ac, 139, 148, 153, 159, and 167
Enteropathogenic (EPEC) strains	18, 44, 55, 86, 111, 112, 114, 119, 125, 126, 127, 128ab, and 142
Enterohemorrhagic (EHEC) strains	26, 111, and 157
Enteroinvasive (EIEC) strains	29, 124, 136, 143, 144, 152, 164, and 167

ganisms from phagocytosis by PMNs and serum killing. Thus, the organisms are not restricted to the mucosa by the immune system. _E. coli_ meningitis has a high fatality rate, and most survivors suffer from neurologic sequelae.

Opportunistic infections are diagnosed by culturing blood or samples of infected tissue, and _E. coli_ is identified by use of a battery of biochemical tests, as described earlier.

(2) Urinary Tract Infections. Patients with _E. coli_ infection of the urinary tract may present with cystitis, pyelonephritis, or sepsis.

Cystitis is an infection of the urinary bladder. Although it is accompanied by urinary frequency and dysuria, fever is rarely present and flank pain is always absent. In contrast, **pyelonephritis** is an infection of the renal parenchyma and pelvis. It is usually accompanied by fever, flank pain, urinary frequency, and dysuria. In some cases, patients also have chills, nausea, vomiting, diarrhea, leukocytosis with a left shift, and bacteremia. Pyelonephritis is a significant risk factor for **sepsis,** particularly among elderly patients. Sepsis, which develops when _E. coli_ organisms spill from the urinary tract to the blood, is a medical emergency with a high mortality rate.

Cystitis and pyelonephritis are diagnosed definitively by obtaining, testing, and culturing a midstream urine sample (a "clean catch" sample). The urine of patients with cystitis contains erythrocytes, leukocytes, and bacteria, and fluorescent antibody testing shows that the bacteria are not coated with antibody. In contrast, the urine of patients with pyelonephritis contains erythrocytes, casts, and bacteria, and the bacteria are antibody-coated.

In the majority of patients with cystitis and in as many as 80–90% of patients with uncomplicated pyelonephritis, _E. coli_ is found to be the cause. Other causes of cystitis include _Staphylococcus saprophyticus_ and _Enterococcus faecalis,_ while other causes of pyelonephritis include _Proteus mirabilis, Proteus vulgaris,_ and _Enterococcus._

Enteric bacteria isolated from the urine should be tested for antibiotic sensitivity.

(3) Diarrheal Disease. In about 90% of cases of diarrheal disease, patients have **watery diarrhea.** In the USA and other industrialized nations, watery diarrhea is generally viral in origin. In developing countries, however, watery diarrhea is usually caused by an ETEC, EPEC, or enteroaggregative strain of _E. coli;_ by rotavirus; or by _Campylobacter jejuni._ In the remaining 10% of cases, patients have **bloody diarrhea,** and this may be due to EIEC or EHEC.

Clinical manifestations are as follows: (a) **ETEC infection** causes watery diarrhea, nausea, abdominal cramps, and a low-grade fever. (b) **EPEC infection** causes watery diarrhea that is copious and is accompanied by fever, malaise, and vomiting. The stools are filled with mucus, but there is no grossly observable blood. (c) **Enteroaggregative _E. coli_ infection** causes watery diarrhea that may be prolonged. (d) **EIEC infection** causes watery diarrhea that progresses to **dysentery.** Stools are scanty and contain blood and mucus. Other manifestations include fever, abdominal cramps, malaise, and toxemia. (e) **EHEC infection** causes watery diarrhea and abdominal cramps 4 days after the patient ingests EHEC organisms. On the fifth day, about 40% of patients develop copious bloody diarrhea. This diarrhea, known as **hemorrhagic colitis,** is typically accompanied by intense abdominal pain, but most patients are afebrile. Up to 11% of patients with hemorrhagic colitis soon develop **hemolytic-uremic syndrome.**

Stool cultures are expensive and laborious, and their results are not likely to alter the choice of a treatment regimen. For this reason, they should not be performed routinely. However, if a patient has unexplained severe or prolonged diarrhea, a stool sample should be collected in a cup, examined, and cultured. The gross appearance of the stool should be noted, as this may suggest the site, mechanism, and type of infection. The stool should be examined microscopically for PMNs, erythrocytes, and parasites. Specimens of stool should be cultured on selective media as soon as possible. If the culture cannot be initiated within 4 hours of collecting the stool sample, the sample should be refrigerated.

After _E. coli_ has been cultured, individual _E. coli_ strains can be identified in a variety of ways: (a) **ETEC organisms** can be identified by looking for ST and LT. Gene probes and bioassays are available for each of these toxins and can be performed by reference laboratories. (b) **EPEC organisms** are identified by serotyping. (c) **Enteroaggregative organisms** can be identified by a DNA probe. (d) **EIEC organisms** can be identified by use of the Sereny test. In this test, fluid that contains organisms is instilled in the eye of a guinea pig, and if keratoconjunctivitis is elicited, the results are considered positive. Like shigellae, EIEC organisms yield positive results in the Sereny test. The enteroinvasiveness of the EIEC strain can be demonstrated by the ability of EIEC organisms to invade HeLa cells in vitro. Moreover, if a drop of fecal material is placed on a slide and stained with methylene blue, sheets of PMNs can be easily seen. (e) **EHEC organisms** are identified by two techniques.

Most *E. coli* strains ferment sorbitol when grown on MacConkey agar supplemented with sorbitol, but EHEC does not. Thus, EHEC can be identified as sorbitol-negative *E. coli* and then serotyped. Moreover, EHEC organisms produce verotoxin, so they can be identified by a bioassay using Vero cells.

Treatment. As shown in Table 7–4, various antibiotics can be used in the treatment of *E. coli* infections. The precise selection of antibiotics depends on the type of infection and the antibiotic sensitivity of the *E. coli* strain isolated.

In the treatment of diarrhea, regardless of the causative *E. coli* strain, adequate rehydration is imperative to replenish fluids and electrolytes. The World Health Organization has developed a standard rehydration formula that can be given orally, and many other oral rehydration solutions are available commercially. Because antimotility agents increase the duration and severity of *E. coli* diarrhea, they should not be used.

Prevention. The prevalence of opportunistic *E. coli* infections can be reduced by observing strict aseptic techniques in clinical settings and by avoiding the unnecessary use of invasive procedures such as catheterization.

Maintenance of a potable water supply, thorough cooking of meats, breast-feeding of infants, and pasteurization of milk should reduce the frequency of *E. coli* diarrhea. When travelers visit developing countries, they should avoid eating anything that is not thoroughly cooked and should avoid drinking anything that is not commercially bottled or boiled. Chemoprophylaxis is not generally recommended for travelers, but use of a fluoroquinolone (such as ciprofloxacin, norfloxacin, or ofloxacin) may be indicated for some high-risk individuals.

Characteristics of *Shigella*

Shigella has traditionally been grouped with *Salmonella* and *Yersinia* because these three genera are invasive organisms that do not ferment lactose. However, recent taxonomic studies that have focused on DNA homology have shown that *Shigella* is closely related to *Escherichia*, and some researchers believe that it is a subspecies of *Escherichia coli*.

Shigella species can be distinguished from *E. coli* by their inability to ferment lactose, their lack of motility, their lack of lysine decarboxylase activity, and their failure to produce gas from any carbohydrate.

TABLE 7–4. Recommended Antibiotics for the Treatment of Diseases Caused by Common Gram-Negative Enteric Rods

Organism	Disease	Effective Antibiotic Treatments*
Enterobacter species	All types.	Imipenem; or antipseudomonal penicillin plus antipseudomonal aminoglycoside.
Escherichia coli	Cystitis.	TMP/SMX; cephalexin; or fluoroquinolone.
	EHEC diarrhea.[†]	TMP/SMX plus rehydration.
	EIEC diarrhea.[†]	TMP/SMX plus rehydration; or fluoroquinolone plus rehydration.
	EPEC diarrhea.[†]	TMP/SMX plus rehydration; gentamicin plus rehydration; or colistin plus rehydration.
	ETEC diarrhea.[†]	TMP/SMX plus rehydration; or fluoroquinolone plus rehydration.
	Pyelonephritis.	If acute and uncomplicated: ampicillin plus gentamicin; TMP/SMX; or ciprofloxacin. If complicated or nosocomial: third-generation cephalosporin; ticarcillin plus clavulanate; antipseudomonal penicillin plus antipseudomonal aminoglycoside; or ciprofloxacin.
Klebsiella oxytoca	All types.	Antipseudomonal third-generation cephalosporin; or ciprofloxacin.
Klebsiella ozaenae	Atrophic rhinitis and ozena.	Ciprofloxacin; or rifampin plus TMP/SMX.
Klebsiella pneumoniae	All types.	Antipseudomonal third-generation cephalosporin; or ciprofloxacin.
Klebsiella rhinoscleromatis	Rhinoscleroma.	Ciprofloxacin; or rifampin plus TMP/SMX.
Proteus mirabilis	All types.	Ampicillin; or TMP/SMX.
Proteus vulgaris	All types.	Antipseudomonal third-generation cephalosporin; or fluoroquinolone.
Salmonella non-*typhi* serotypes	Enteritis.	No antibiotics.
	Primary septicemia.	Ciprofloxacin; ceftriaxone; cefoperazone; or TMP/SMX.
Salmonella serotype *typhi*	Typhoid.	In Mexico or Southeast Asia: amoxicillin; or TMP/SMX. In other areas: chloramphenicol; ciprofloxacin; ceftriaxone; cefoperazone; or TMP/SMX.
Serratia species	All types.	Gentamicin; antipseudomonal third-generation cephalosporin; imipenem; or fluoroquinolone.
Shigella species	Shigellosis.	For adults: rehydration if necessary; no antibiotics; norfloxacin; or ciprofloxacin. For children in Latin America and the Middle East: TMP/SMX plus rehydration. For children in other areas: TMP/SMX plus rehydration; or ampicillin plus rehydration.
Yersinia enterocolitica	All types.	Antipseudomonal third-generation cephalosporin plus antipseudomonal aminoglycoside; doxycycline; or TMP/SMX.
Yersinia pseudotuberculosis	All types.	Antipseudomonal third-generation cephalosporin plus antipseudomonal aminoglycoside; doxycycline; or TMP/SMX.

*Antibiotics are listed in their general order of recommended use, with the drug or drug combination used most often listed first. TMP = trimethoprim; and SMX = sulfamethoxazole.
†Diarrhea is caused by the following strains of *E. coli:* enterohemorrhagic (EHEC), enteroinvasive (EIEC), enteropathogenic (EPEC), and enterotoxigenic (ETEC).

Shigella species are differentiated from *Salmonella* species by their lack of motility and their failure to produce H₂S.

General Features. Four species (groups) of *Shigella* have been identified: *Shigella dysenteriae* (group A), *Shigella flexneri* (group B), *Shigella boydii* (group C), and *Shigella sonnei* (group D).

Under the CDC classification scheme, the first three *Shigella* species are lumped together as "*Shigella*-serogroups A,B,C" because they are biochemically similar. *S. sonnei*, which is responsible for most cases of *Shigella* infection in the USA, can be easily distinguished from the first three because it has ornithine decarboxylase and β-galactosidase activities. *S. dysenteriae*, which causes the most severe disease but is rare in the USA, is distinguished from the other species by its inability to ferment mannitol and by its production of Shiga neurotoxin. The *Shigella* species can also be differentiated by their O antigenic specificities.

Mechanisms of Pathogenicity. *Shigella* species are the cause of bacillary dysentery, and they owe their pathogenicity primarily to their ability to invade the colonic mucosa. The ability of *S. dysenteriae* to cause more severe disease than its cohorts has been attributed to its production of Shiga neurotoxin. Investigators have studied the effects of shigellae on monkeys, cultured human colonic and noncolonic cell lines, and ligated rabbit ileal loops and are beginning to put together a picture of how shigellae cause dysentery.

(1) Bacterial Products Involved in Virulence. The ability of shigellae to invade host cells depends on the presence of a 220-kb plasmid that encodes for a set of proteins known as **invasion plasmid antigens** (Ipa). One of these antigens, **IpaD**, is believed to be an adhesin that allows the bacterium to be phagocytosed. The host cell receptor for IpaD is not known, but it is expressed only on the basolateral pole of enterocytes.

Once the shigella is inside the host phagosome, a cell-associated **hemolysin** lyses the phagosome, and the bacterium multiplies within the cell cytoplasm. Within 2 hours of entry, the shigella is coated with gelatinized **actin.** This coat is soon converted to a "tail" of polymerized actin that streams away from the bacterium. Actin polymerization is caused by a 120-kD **outer membrane protein.** This polymerization allows the shigella to move directly from cell to cell in a process that is similar to the intercellular and intracellular movement of *Listeria monocytogenes* (see Chapter 10).

S. dysenteriae produces **Shiga neurotoxin.** This toxin is identical to the verotoxin-1 produced by enterohemorrhagic strains of *E. coli*, and it has a mode of action that is identical to that of ricin, a plant lectin. Shiga toxin production is not needed to kill host colonic epithelial cells. In fact, invasion seems to be the critical event in cell death and kills host cells faster than does Shiga toxin. Nevertheless, shigellae that produce Shiga toxin cause more severe disease, possibly because the toxin damages the capillaries of the lamina propria of the colonic villi, causing ischemia and hemorrhagic colitis.

(2) The *Shigella* Infection Cycle. The infection cycle is depicted in Fig. 7–2. Shigellae transiently infect the small intestine during the first few days of disease, and dysentery occurs when the colon is infected. Invasion of the colon is probably initiated through colonic lymphoid follicles that are rich in M cells and are analogous to Peyer's patches found in the small intestine. The shigellae adhere, undergo parasite-directed phagocytosis, and escape the phagosome.

Inside the cytoplasm, the shigellae multiply once every 40 minutes and fill the parasitized cell. The bacteria are apparently propelled by actin filaments and stress fibers, and they move directly from cell to cell without passing into the extracellular space. Some shigellae subsequently invade the connective tissue (the lamina propria), elicit an inflammatory response, and cause ulceration at the invasion site. The inflammatory response involves PMNs, and a fibrin pseudomembrane typically forms over the ulcer.

Shiga toxin may exacerbate the inflammation by causing ischemia and hemorrhage. Shiga toxin that enters the circulation may also cause hemolytic-uremic syndrome. Unlike salmonellae, shigellae are restricted to the mucosa and submucosa and rarely cause bacteremia or sepsis.

Diseases Due to *Shigella*

Epidemiology. Each year, about 25,000 cases of shigellosis are reported in the USA, and millions of cases occur worldwide.

Shigella is one of the most infectious of bacteria, and ingestion of as few as 100–200 organisms will cause disease. This low ID₅₀ makes *Shigella* species dangerous organisms in the laboratory, and labora-

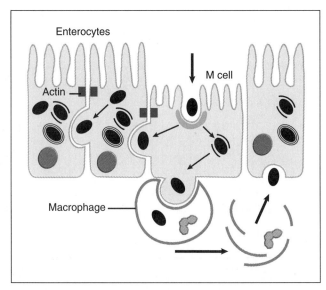

FIGURE 7–2. Invasion of the intestinal epithelium by *Shigella* species and formation of mucosal abscesses.

tory workers are often infected when they handle clinical samples containing shigellae.

Most individuals are infected with shigellae when they ingest food or water contaminated with human fecal material. Shigellae can survive up to 30 days in milk, eggs, cheese, or shrimp. Spread is always from a human source and generally involves one of the five f's: food, fingers, feces, flies, or fomites. This is in contrast to salmonellae, which are often spread to humans from infected animals.

Infants and toddlers are most susceptible to shigellosis. About 60% of infants younger than 1 year of age develop dysentery when exposed to shigellae, but the infection rate drops to about 20% after the age of 1 year. Most disease worldwide occurs in children under the age of 10 years, and shigellosis is responsible for about 15% of pediatric cases of diarrhea in the USA.

Dysentery outbreaks are usually associated with closed populations, such as families, cruise ships, mental hospitals, children in day-care facilities, and prisoners. Bacillary dysentery has also been a major force during wars, often rendering complete armies temporarily unfit for battle.

Diagnosis. Two to three days after exposure to shigellae, the symptoms of **shigellosis** begin. There is a sudden onset of fever, abdominal cramping and tenderness, and diarrhea. During the first 2–3 days, fluid loss may be extensive and may endanger the lives of children and others who tolerate fluid and electrolyte loss poorly. The onset of tenesmus (straining at stool) is usually accompanied by a decrease in the number and volume of stools.

Sigmoidoscopy reveals that the mucosa is hyperemic and hemorrhagic and demonstrates the presence of ulcerations covered with a fibrin pseudomembrane. The finding of mucus, PMNs, and blood in the stool is the hallmark of **dysentery** and indicates that the bowel wall has been invaded.

To identify the causative agent, stool samples can be cultured. The best sample for culture, however, consists of a rectal swab of an ulcer and is obtained during sigmoidoscopy. Dysentery due to *Shigella* must be differentiated from dysenterylike diseases caused by enteroinvasive *E. coli, Campylobacter jejuni,* and the parasites *Entamoeba histolytica* and *Balantidium coli.*

Treatment. Table 7–4 summarizes the recommended antibiotic therapies for shigellosis. Adults often recover without antibiotic treatment but should be adequately rehydrated. Antidiarrheal agents should not be administered, because they tend to prolong the disease.

Prevention. No vaccine is currently available, so preventive measures focus on breaking the transmission cycle. Adequate water supplies should be maintained, sewage should be cared for properly, human carriers should be identified and treated, and the frequent washing of hands with soap should be encouraged. In developing countries, mothers should be encouraged to breast-feed their infants, rather than using formulas mixed with potentially contaminated water.

Salmonella Species

The tribe **Salmonelleae** consists of a single genus, *Salmonella.* The genus *Salmonella* contains the organisms known previously as *Salmonella* and *Arizona.* The taxonomy of the salmonellae has been in flux for many years, and taxonomists have devised widely divergent classification schemes that have utilized both biochemical and immunologic techniques.

Characteristics of Salmonella

General Features. The salmonellae are an enormous group of enteric organisms, consisting of some 2200 serotypes. The organisms do not ferment lactose, are negative for indole and ONPG, and are positive for hydrogen sulfide production, citrate utilization, and motility.

Under the current CDC classification scheme, there is only a single *Salmonella* species, and this species is divided into 7 subgroups (subgroups 1, 2, 3a, 3b, 4, 5, and 6). Serogrouping is based on reactions of isolates with antibody directed against specific O, H, and Vi antigens. Clinical laboratories generally do not report the *Salmonella* subgroups. Instead, they report isolates as genus-serotype. For example, instead of reporting *Salmonella* subgroup 1 serotype *typhi,* the clinical laboratory will report *Salmonella* serotype *typhi* or *Salmonella typhi.*

Earlier classification systems included (1) the Kauffman-White system, which identified each serotype as an individual *Salmonella* species; (2) the Edwards-Ewing system, which divided the salmonellae into three species *(Salmonella choleraesuis, Salmonella enteritidis,* and *Salmonella typhi)* and hundreds of serotypes; and (3) a DNA hybridization scheme that lumped the salmonellae into a single species known as *Salmonella enteritidis* and then subdivided this species into the subspecies *arizonae, bongori, diarizonae, enterica, houtenae,* and *salamae.* This last scheme is the one that the CDC modified for current use.

Although the classification of salmonellae relies primarily on serotyping of surface antigens, the *typhi* serotype can be differentiated from the other serotypes on the basis of its relatively inert biochemical behavior. The *typhi* serotype is negative for Simmons' citrate; ornithine decarboxylase; gas from glucose; fermentation of dulcitol, arabinose, rhamnose, and mucinate; and acetate utilization. This distinction is important because the *typhi* serotype is responsible for most cases of enteric fever (typhoid). Other serotypes generally cause enteritis.

Mechanisms of Pathogenicity

(1) Bacterial Products Involved in Virulence. Salmonellae owe their pathogenicity largely to their ability to invade tissue and to survive within macrophages. The **Vi antigen** is a capsule that affords salmonellae some protection from phagocytosis. Once phagocytosed, *S. typhi* inhibits generation of oxidative free radicals and intraphagosomal killing. Additionally, salmonellae have endotoxic **lipopolysaccharide,** which is responsible for septic shock in patients with bacteremia.

Salmonellae that cause enteritis produce at least two **enterotoxins** that are responsible for many of the clinical signs of enteritis. The first of these is a small (25–30 kD) protein that binds to GM_1 gangliosides and causes hypersecretion of fluids and electrolytes by elevating levels of cyclic adenosine monophosphate (cAMP). It appears that both protein kinase C and prostaglandin E_2 are involved in this process. The second enterotoxin is larger (about 100 kD) and is unrelated in structure and mechanism of activity to the first enterotoxin.

Salmonella strains that produce enterotoxins have been reported to invade the intestinal wall more effectively and to be more virulent than their nontoxigenic counterparts. Between two-thirds and three-fourths of *Salmonella* strains isolated from patients with enteritis produce enterotoxins.

(2) The *Salmonella* Infection Cycle.   Intestinal infection with salmonellae can follow one of two infection cycles, as depicted in Fig. 7–3. One cycle causes enteritis, and the other causes typhoid.

(a) Enteritis.   Most serotypes cause enteritis, an infection that is limited to the terminal ileum. The salmonellae invade the intestinal wall and produce enterotoxins that cause nausea, vomiting, and diarrhea. Tissue invasion is evidenced by the presence of PMNs in the stool, but the bacteria rarely spread beyond the gastrointestinal tract.

(b) Enteric Fever (Typhoid).   Two serotypes—*typhi* and *paratyphi*—can cause typhoid. The salmonellae invade the wall of the terminal ileum and then spread to the intestinal lymphatics, where they are phagocytosed by PMNs and cells of the macrophage-monocyte series. Salmonellae phagocytosed by PMNs are killed, but those phagocytosed by macrophages survive and multiply within phagocytic vacuoles. Wandering macrophages that contain salmonellae act as "taxicabs" that deliver salmonellae to various reticuloendothelial tissues. Infected macrophages are eventually destroyed, and salmonellae released from lysed macrophages cause septicemia.

Some salmonellae begin to disseminate hematogenously to a variety of ectopic sites, including the bones, kidneys, lungs, liver, and brain, where they cause osteomyelitis, pyelonephritis, empyema, hepatic necrosis, and meningitis, respectively. Other

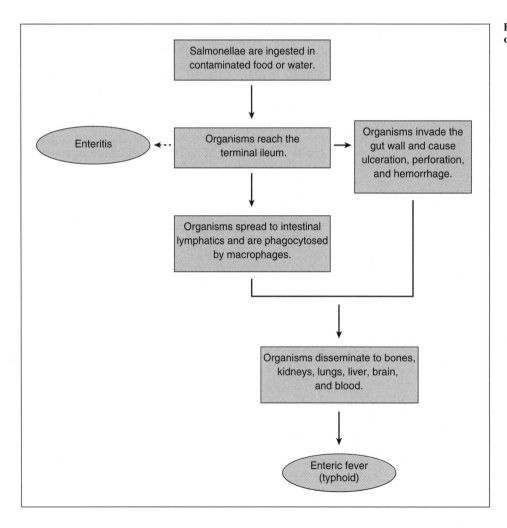

FIGURE 7–3. Infection patterns of *Salmonella*.

salmonellae remain in the intestine, where they invade the gut wall and may cause ulceration, perforation, and hemorrhage. Salmonellae multiply avidly in the gallbladder and bile, and the infected bile continues to circulate salmonellae to the intestine. Salmonellae also multiply well in gut-associated lymphoid tissue and may ulcerate Peyer's patches.

Diseases Due to *Salmonella*

Epidemiology. In the USA, *Salmonella* enteritis is the third most commonly reported form of "food poisoning." About 50,000 cases of *Salmonella* enteritis are reported each year, and most are caused by *Salmonella* serotype *typhimurium.* The infection is zoonotic, and poultry is the source of infection in about half of the cases. Salmonellae are spread from the poultry carcasses to humans when the poultry is eaten undercooked or when meat handlers fail to wash their hands or utensils properly. Other common sources of *Salmonella* enteritis include milk products, food, and water contaminated with animal feces or urine.

The largest documented outbreak of *Salmonella* enteritis in the USA occurred in 1985, when a faulty valve allowed milk marketed by a major grocer in the Midwest to become contaminated with salmonellae. Although only about 16,000 cases were confirmed by culture, estimates of the total number of cases ranged from 150,000 to 200,000.

In the past, pet turtles were a major source of *Salmonella* enteritis in children. Small turtles sold in pet stores were raised in turtle farms that were merely an area of a pond or bayou that was enclosed by a steel mesh curtain. The turtles were infected with salmonellae when raw sewage contaminated the water in their pens. Children became infected when they handled the turtles and then ate without washing their hands.

Typhoid is usually caused by *S. typhi* and is always acquired from a human source. In most cases, *S. typhi* is acquired when people consume food or water contaminated with human feces or urine. Unlike shigellae, salmonellae are sensitive to stomach acid, so a dose of 10^6–10^7 organisms must be ingested to reliably establish infection. Thus, people who take antacids or other drugs that lower the acidity of the stomach are usually susceptible to a lower infective dose of salmonellae.

S. typhi tends to localize in the gallbladder, and some people carry salmonellae in their gallbladder without suffering from disease. These carriers may shed salmonellae for many years. The archetypical *Salmonella* carrier was "typhoid Mary" (Mary Mallon), who worked in restaurants in New York City at the beginning of the 20th century and was implicated as the source of an outbreak of typhoid that involved 1300 reported cases. Because she continued to seek jobs in restaurants (under assumed names), she was placed under detention from 1915 until her death in 1938.

In the USA, the usual number of cases of typhoid is about 400 per year, but large outbreaks have occurred. In an outbreak in Florida, 225 residents of a community developed typhoid when a water chlorinator malfunctioned. In an outbreak in San Antonio, Texas, 80 cases of typhoid were traced to a carrier of *S. typhi* who worked as a food preparer in a restaurant.

Ingestion of food contaminated with *S. choleraesuis* has been reported to cause primary septicemia in people with sickle cell anemia or malaria.

Diagnosis

(1) Enteritis. Nausea, vomiting, abdominal pain, and diarrhea begin 8–24 hours after the ingestion of food or drink contaminated with *Salmonella.* In some cases, manifestations include a low-grade fever, headache, and chills. *Salmonella* enteritis is a self-limiting disease that usually lasts about 5 days, but severe loss of fluids and electrolytes may be life-threatening in infants and elderly patients.

The feces of patients with enteritis can be Gram-stained for the presence of PMNs. Stool cultures will reveal the presence of *Salmonella,* and antibody can be used to serotype the organisms.

Recovery from enteritis does not confer immunity against reinfection.

(2) Enteric Fever (Typhoid). About 7–14 days after ingesting salmonellae, patients begin to develop symptoms and signs of typhoid, including anorexia, lethargy, a dull frontal headache, a nonproductive cough, constipation, abdominal pain, and a temperature that increases steadily and reaches 40 °C (104 °F). At this time, there are no salmonellae detected in the blood, and leukocyte counts are normal.

By the second or third week of disease, salmonellae have escaped macrophages and the patient is severely ill. Rose spots that are 2–5 mm in diameter may appear on the trunk, and these maculopapular lesions contain salmonellae. Weakness and confusion are accompanied by a dull and expressionless look. In some cases, patients suffer from delirium.

If Peyer's patches become perforated, peritonitis may develop. Dissemination of salmonellae to ectopic foci may result in liver necrosis, empyema, meningitis, osteomyelitis, endocarditis, or pyelonephritis. The fatality rate is 2–10%.

In patients with *S. typhi* infection, the organisms can be cultured from samples of blood, feces, urine, bone marrow, and exudate from rose spots. Although the organisms can be cultured in 80% of blood samples and 20% of stool samples during the first week of clinical disease, this rate shifts to 25% of blood samples and 85% of stool samples during the fourth week. In many patients, the urine remains culture-positive throughout the course of typhoid. In addition to positive culture results, patients with typhoid exhibit a fourfold or greater rise in serum antibody to *S. typhi.*

Recovery from typhoid is a prolonged process that lasts a month or longer, and about 5–20% of patients suffer a relapse during the first month of convalescence. Recovery confers lifelong immunity against typhoid.

(3) Primary Septicemia. Patients with anemia

may develop septicemia after asymptomatic ileal infection with *S. choleraesuis.* Manifestations include spiking fever, weight loss, anorexia, anemia, bacteremia, and hepatosplenomegaly. Bacteremia may lead to sepsis or cause seeding of organs and ectopic infection. Blood cultures should be obtained from patients with septicemia.

Treatment.   Specific treatments for diseases caused by *Salmonella* are summarized in Table 7–4.

About 3% of patients who recover from typhoid become carriers of *S. typhi.* Older women with gallbladder disease or gallstones are at highest risk of becoming carriers. Carriage of *S. typhi* can be eliminated by administering antibiotics and performing cholecystectomy.

In patients with *Salmonella* enteritis, treatment with antibiotics has not proved effective in reducing the severity or duration of disease, and it promotes carriage of organisms in the gallbladder. For these reasons, clinicians do not recommend antibiotic treatment. Instead, patients should be kept adequately hydrated, and electrolytes should be replenished as needed.

Prevention.   Attenuated oral and killed parenteral **typhoid vaccines** are available. Prevention also rests on effective public health measures, including the following: sewage must be properly disposed of and treated; an unpolluted water supply must be maintained; milk must be pasteurized to kill *S. typhi* and other pathogens; and carriers must be identified, excluded from food handling, and treated to eliminate carriage of salmonellae.

Klebsiella, Enterobacter, and Serratia Species

Klebsiella, Enterobacter, and *Serratia* are three members of the tribe **Klebsielleae** and are often known as the **KES group.** The organisms in this group are opportunistic pathogens and are common causes of nosocomial infections.

Characteristics of Klebsiella

General Features.   The genus *Klebsiella* contains two pathogenic species: *Klebsiella pneumoniae* and *Klebsiella oxytoca.* Although *Klebsiella ozaenae* and *Klebsiella rhinoscleromatis* are subspecies of *K. pneumoniae,* they are considered separately from *K. pneumoniae* by clinicians and clinical laboratories because of the unique diseases they cause.

The members of the genus *Klebsiella* are nonmotile enteric organisms that ferment lactose, decarboxylate lysine but not ornithine, and hydrolyze urea slowly. *K. pneumoniae,* once known as Friedländer's bacillus, is notable for its large mucoid colonies, which are moist because of the presence of capsular material. Table 7–5 shows other key features used to differentiate among the klebsiellae.

Mechanisms of Pathogenicity.   *K. pneumoniae* owes its pathogenicity to the presence of an antiphagocytic **capsule** (K antigen). About 80 different **K antigens** of *K. pneumoniae* have been described, and some infections caused by *K. pneumoniae* are restricted to specific serotypes. The *Klebsiella* capsule allows the organism to persist in the face of a mounting immune response, and dissemination of *Klebsiella* may result in septic shock.

Diseases Due to Klebsiella

K. pneumoniae causes pneumonia and urinary tract infections, usually in debilitated or catheterized patients. *K. ozaenae* causes atrophic rhinitis and ozena, and *K. rhinoscleromatis* causes rhinoscleroma.

Epidemiology.   *K. pneumoniae* can be isolated from the upper respiratory tract or gastrointestinal tract of about 5% of the general population. Thus, the origin of infection is generally via aspiration of respiratory secretions or contamination of catheters with organisms from the gastrointestinal tract. *Klebsiella* pneumonia occurs mainly in hospitalized patients who have impaired mucociliary function. Other high-risk individuals are nonhospitalized patients with chronic obstructive pulmonary disease (COPD), diabetes, or alcoholism. Strains of *K. pneumoniae* that cause pneumonia are usually capsule serotypes 1 and 2. Strains that cause urinary tract infections are capsule serotypes 8, 9, 19, and 24.

The origin of rhinoscleroma is unknown, but it is endemic in Latin America, the Near East, and the republics of the former Soviet Union.

Diagnosis

(1) Urinary Tract Infections.   Although *K. pneumoniae* may cause **pyelonephritis** and **cystitis** in catheterized patients, it rarely causes these infections in others. Urine samples should be collected and cultured, as described in the earlier section on *Escherichia coli.*

(2) Pneumonia.   In debilitated patients with *K. pneumoniae* infection, pneumonia begins insidiously and is usually accompanied by pleuritic pain. The

TABLE 7–5.   Key Characteristics of Four Species of *Klebsiella*

Species	Methyl Red Reaction	Voges-Proskauer Activity	Urease Activity	Malonate Production	Indole Production
Klebsiella oxytoca	+	−	−	−	−
Klebsiella ozaenae	Variable	+	+	+	+
Klebsiella pneumoniae	−	+	+	+	−
Klebsiella rhinoscleromatis	+	−	−	+	−

sputum may be thick and bloody, or it may be thin and have the consistency of currant jelly. Weakened patients eventually develop abscesses, necrosis, and septicemia.

Samples of sputum, blood, or transtracheal aspirate should be collected, stained, examined directly for gram-negative rods, and cultured on appropriate media. It is critical to differentiate *K. pneumoniae* pneumonia from pneumococcal pneumonia. *K. pneumoniae* strains are typically resistant to many drugs and generally cause more severe disease. Even with appropriate therapy, the fatality rate of pneumonia due to *K. pneumoniae* is 40–60%.

(3) Rhinitis. Infection of the nasal epithelium with *K. ozaenae* can lead to **atrophic rhinitis.** This chronic form of rhinitis is characterized by focal areas of squamous metaplasia, wasting of the mucous glands, and impairment of mucus secretion. In affected patients, the nasal mucosa looks dry, glazed, and shiny. Infection with *K. ozaenae* can also cause **ozena,** a rare form of suppurative rhinitis in which a foul-smelling greenish exudate obstructs the nasal passages. The diagnosis is confirmed by culturing the exudate.

(4) Rhinoscleroma. Rhinoscleroma that is caused by *K. rhinoscleromatis* begins with symptoms resembling those of an ordinary cold. Granulomatous inflammation of the nasal airway leads to development of tumorlike submucosal masses. The masses can become quite large and may close the nares and cause the face to swell. If the masses extend into the larynx and adjacent airways, they may suffocate the patient.

The diagnosis of rhinoscleroma is based on direct microscopic examination, which reveals that lesions contain many foamy macrophages, giant cells, and encapsulated bacilli.

Treatment.   Specific antibiotic therapies for diseases caused by klebsiellae are summarized in Table 7–4.

Characteristics of *Enterobacter*

Enterobacter is part of the commensal enteric flora, but it is also found in water, sewage, soil, and plants. It was once called *Aerobacter* because so much gas is produced by the organism when carbohydrates are fermented. Unlike *Klebsiella, Enterobacter* is a motile, ornithine decarboxylase–positive organism. *Enterobacter* colonies are moist, owing to the presence of capsular material, but they are not as moist as *Klebsiella* colonies.

Eleven *Enterobacter* species have been described, but most human disease is caused by *Enterobacter aerogenes* and *Enterobacter cloacae. Enterobacter* isolates can be serotyped on the basis of O, H, and K antigens.

Diseases Due to *Enterobacter*

Enterobacter species cause opportunistic infections. Most often, they cause **urinary tract infections** in debilitated or catheterized patients. Occasionally, they cause **pneumonia, wound infections,** and **sepsis** in hospitalized patients.

Like many enteric organisms, *Enterobacter* species are often resistant to numerous drugs, and specific therapy requires determination of antibiotic sensitivities. For example, some *E. cloacae* isolates produce class I beta-lactamases that cannot be inhibited by clavulanate or sulbactam, and others are capable of degrading third-generation cephalosporins.

Table 7–4 lists specific antibiotic therapies for diseases caused by *Enterobacter.*

Characteristics of *Serratia*

Nine species of *Serratia* have been described, but most human disease is due to a single species, *Serratia marcescens.* Organisms in this species are slow lactose fermenters, are motile, and are positive for lipase, gelatinase, ornithine decarboxylase, and DNAase activities.

Serratia isolates can be typed by their O and H antigens. Many strains of *Serratia* are easily recognized in culture because they produce an orange-red pigment known as prodigiosin. At one time, *S. marcescens* was believed to be a harmless environmental bacterium, and laboratory workers used the organism's brightly colored colonies for various diversions and experiments. For example, during the Christmas holidays, workers decorated "agar cakes" with green *Pseudomonas* and red *Serratia* colonies. Some researchers are reported to have studied air currents by dispersing *Serratia* from airplanes and then cultivating environmental samples to identify the easily recognized red colonies of *Serratia.* Today, *S. marcescens* is known to be a pathogen, and experiments such as this are no longer performed.

Diseases Due to *Serratia*

Between 75% and 90% of all *Serratia* infections are nosocomial. *Serratia* causes **pneumonia** and **sepsis,** particularly in patients who have reticuloendothelial cancer and are receiving chemotherapy. It also occasionally causes **urinary tract infections** and **wound infections** in hospitalized patients.

Table 7–4 summarizes recommended treatments for *Serratia* infections.

Proteus Species

Proteus species, which are members of the tribe **Proteeae,** are part of the normal human gastrointestinal flora and exist in water and soil as saprophytic organisms.

Characteristics of *Proteus*

General Features.   Members of the genus *Proteus* exhibit strong urease activity, produce hydrogen sulfide, are motile, are positive for phenylalanine deaminase activity, and are negative for lactose fermentation. Although four *Proteus* species have been identified, only two cause human disease: *Proteus mirabilis* and *Proteus vulgaris.*

P. mirabilis is the more common of the two pathogens and is distinguished from *P. vulgaris* by its failure to convert tryptophan to indole. Many isolates of *P. mirabilis* and *P. vulgaris* are extremely motile and exhibit "swarming motility" on blood agar plates. Swarming *Proteus* isolates spread in waves across the agar surface and sometimes make isolation of other organisms on the plate extremely difficult.

Proteus isolates can be serotyped by O, H, and K antigens. Antibodies to three *Proteus* O antigens are used in the Weil-Felix test to diagnose certain rickettsial diseases.

Mechanisms of Pathogenicity. The principal virulence determinants of *Proteus* species are lipopolysaccharide, pili, urease activity, and capsule.

The **lipopolysaccharide** of *Proteus,* like that of other enteric organisms, exhibits endotoxic activity. The *Proteus* **pili** promote colonization of the kidney, and the *Proteus* **urease** converts urea to NH_4 and CO_2. These products of urea hydrolysis alkalinize the urine, and this precipitates Mg^{2+} and Ca^{2+} and leads to the formation of renal calculi (kidney stones). NH_4 also protects *Proteus* in the kidney from the classic complement pathway by splitting C4. Studies have shown that the *Proteus* **capsule** not only protects the organisms from phagocytosis but also precipitates $MgNH_4PO_4 \cdot 6H_2O$ (struvite). Struvite calculi are a frequent complication of *P. mirabilis* urinary tract infections.

Diseases Due to *Proteus*

P. mirabilis is a common cause of nosocomial and community-acquired **urinary tract infections,** including **pyelonephritis** and **cystitis.** As with pyelonephritis due to *Escherichia coli,* pyelonephritis due to *P. mirabilis* may lead to **sepsis.** Because *Proteus* infection alkalinizes the urine, patients with repeated infections may develop **renal calculi.** In hospitalized patients with indwelling urinary catheters, *P. mirabilis* can cause **bladder infections** that sometimes lead to sepsis. Other *Proteus* infections include **wound infections** and **pneumonia.**

P. mirabilis is responsible for most *Proteus* infections. *P. vulgaris* is isolated primarily from immunosuppressed patients.

Specific antibiotic treatments for diseases caused by *P. mirabilis* and *P. vulgaris* are summarized in Table 7–4.

Yersinia Species

The tribe **Yersinieae** consists of a single genus, *Yersinia.* Eleven *Yersinia* species have been described, but only three have been reported to be frankly pathogenic in humans. One of these, *Yersinia pestis,* is the cause of the plague. Because of its epidemiologic position as a zoonotic disease, *Y. pestis* is discussed in Chapter 10, with other zoonoses. The other two pathogenic species, *Yersinia pseudotuberculosis* and *Yersinia enterocolitica,* are discussed in this section.

Characteristics of *Yersinia*

General Features. The yersiniae are coccobacilli that grow as small lactose-negative colonies on MacConkey agar or Salmonella-Shigella agar after 48 hours of incubation at room temperature. The optimal growth temperature for yersiniae, unlike that of other enteric organisms, is 25–32 °C.

Y. pseudotuberculosis and *Y. enterocolitica* differ from *Y. pestis* in that they are motile and have either polar or peritrichous flagella. *Y. pseudotuberculosis* ferments rhamnose and melibiose, while *Y. enterocolitica* decarboxylates ornithine and ferments sucrose, cellobiose, and sorbitol.

The yersiniae are serotyped by O and H antigenic specificities. *Y. pseudotuberculosis* has 6 serotypes, and *Y. enterocolitica* has 27. *Y. enterocolitica* O:9 reacts to antibody directed against *Brucella* antigens, so patients with elevated titers of *Brucella* antibody may actually be suffering from a *Yersinia* infection.

Mechanisms of Pathogenicity. The yersiniae are facultatively intracellular pathogens that invade macrophages and epithelial cells. The best-studied *Yersinia* virulence factors are several proteins that mediate attachment and entry into these cells.

(1) Bacterial Products Involved in Virulence. The expression of many of the proteins involved in virulence is regulated by Ca^{2+} concentrations and temperature, and several of the proteins are encoded on a 70- to 75-kb virulence plasmid.

Both *Y. pseudotuberculosis* and *Y. enterocolitica* express **Inv proteins,** which are 108-kD "invasion" proteins that bind to β_1 integrins and promote the ability of yersiniae to invade host cells. The Inv proteins are expressed maximally at 28 °C and are probably most important in invasion of Peyer's patches soon after the yersiniae are ingested. *Y. enterocolitica* expresses **Ail proteins,** which are 15-kD "invasion-attachment locus" proteins that promote entry into host cells. It also expresses **YadA proteins,** which are plasmid-encoded fibrillar adhesins that bind to fibronectin and collagen and allow yersiniae to invade the ileal epithelium. *Y. pseudotuberculosis,* like *Y. pestis,* produces the **pH 6 adhesin,** a substance that allows the bacteria to bind to epithelial cells.

Other *Yersinia* virulence factors include **Yops surface proteins,** some of which are antiphagocytic proteins; the **V and W antigens** (discussed fully with plague); and an endotoxic **lipopolysaccharide.**

Y. pseudotuberculosis produces an **exotoxin** that is identical to the murine toxin of *Y. pestis.* This toxin inhibits mitochondrial respiration by splitting nicotinamide adenine dinucleotide (NAD) to yield adenosine diphosphate and ribose (ADP-ribose) and nicotinamide.

(2) The *Yersinia* Infection Cycle. Humans are infected with gastrointestinal yersiniae when they ingest food or water contaminated with the feces of infected animals or humans. The organisms initially invade the intestinal epithelium and Peyer's patches. Yersiniae that invade lymphoid tissue multiply within the phagocytic vacuoles of macrophages. Invasion of the intestinal wall produces ulceration of the mucosa, and lymphoid invasion causes the nodes to become enlarged and firm. The mesenteric nodes are most prominently affected.

In most cases, the infection is restricted to the intestinal mucosa and mesenteric nodes, but a few individuals develop bacteremia, sepsis, and disseminated disease. The organisms may grow in the liver, where their presence results in the development of liver abscesses. Individuals at risk of disseminated disease include those with preexisting liver disease, infants under 1 year of age, patients with hemoglobinopathies or diabetes, and patients receiving large doses of corticosteroids.

Diseases Due to *Yersinia*

Epidemiology.   *Y. pseudotuberculosis* and *Y. enterocolitica* infect a wide variety of wild and domestic animals, and humans are often infected when they ingest food or water contaminated with the feces of infected animals. *Y. pseudotuberculosis* infections are most often acquired from wild animal sources, while *Y. enterocolitica* infections are frequently acquired from pigs or dogs.

Cases of *Yersinia* infection often occur in clusters. After a single person has been infected, it is not uncommon for close contacts to be secondarily infected, especially if the person handles or prepares food for others. In Japan, for example, a single patient was the source case for an outbreak that infected 20% of the children in a school. In New York, 218 children in a school developed disease after drinking contaminated milk. Outbreaks of diarrhea caused by *Yersinia* have often originated from contaminated water supplies. Most types of water-borne diarrhea, including those caused by other enteric rods, viruses, and *Giardia,* are prevalent during the summer because the organisms "bloom" in the warm water. The pattern of water-borne diarrhea caused by *Yersinia* is the opposite. Because yersiniae survive longest in cold water, most cases of diarrhea caused by these organisms occur during the winter or early spring.

Diagnosis.   About 24 hours after exposure to *Yersinia,* patients begin to develop symptoms. The infection follows one of four patterns. (1) Children under 5 years old usually develop acute **enteritis** with prolonged diarrhea. (2) Older children and adults are more likely to develop **gastroenteritis, terminal ileitis, mesenteric lymphadenitis,** or a combination of these. Affected patients suffer from diarrhea, mesenteric lymph node enlargement, headache, malaise, fever, and severe abdominal pain. Patients with high fever may convulse. The combination of mesenteric lymph node enlargement and severe abdominal pain may cause clinicians to mistake the disease for acute appendicitis. (3) Women between the ages of 15 and 45 may develop **diarrhea** that is accompanied by **arthritis** and **erythema nodosum.** (4) Individuals with preexisting liver disease, infants, patients with hemoglobinopathies or diabetes, and patients receiving

high-dose corticosteroid therapy may develop **liver abscesses** that are accompanied by **sepsis.**

Yersiniosis must be differentiated from appendicitis, cat-scratch disease, salmonellosis, and tularemia.

The diagnosis of yersiniosis can be confirmed by culturing the organisms in stool samples, blood samples (if sepsis is present), biopsies of mesenteric lymph nodes, or specimens from other infected sites. The organisms can be selectively enriched by placing the samples in isotonic saline and refrigerating them up to 3 weeks. An agglutination test is also available to detect the presence of antibody to *Yersinia.*

Treatment.   Specific antibiotic treatments for diseases caused by *Yersinia* species are summarized in Table 7–4. Patients who become dehydrated should have fluids and electrolytes replenished as needed.

Other Enterobacteriaceae

Table 7–6 presents information about *Citrobacter, Edwardsiella, Hafnia, Morganella, Pantoea,* and *Providencia.* These Enterobacteriaceae are infrequent causes of disease.

OTHER BACTERIA THAT CAUSE GASTROINTESTINAL DISEASE
Campylobacter Species

Members of the genus *Campylobacter* are curved gram-negative rods whose characteristics are similar to those of the genera *Arcobacter, Flexispira, Helicobacter,* and *Wolinella.* The *Campylobacter* species and subspecies most commonly associated with human disease are *Campylobacter jejuni* subspecies *jejuni; Campylobacter coli; Campylobacter fetus* subspecies *fetus;* and *Campylobacter lari* (formerly called *Campylobacter laridis*).

Characteristics of *Campylobacter*

General Features.   *Campylobacter* species are microaerophilic, and each organism has a single polar flagellum. The organisms can be cultured on special media at 42 °C under an atmosphere of 5% O_2, 10% CO_2, and 85% N_2. The most commonly used specialized medium is called Campy BAP. This medium contains Brucella agar base supplemented with 10% sheep blood, as well as a variety of antibiotics (vancomycin, trimethoprim, polymyxin B, cephalothin, and amphotericin B). *Campylobacter* species also grow on media containing 0.5% glycine. They reduce nitrate but do not hydrolyze urea.

Individual *Campylobacter* species are distinguished by their catalase activity, hydrogen sulfide production, indoxyl acetate hydrolysis, nalidixic acid and cephalothin susceptibility, hippurate hydrolysis, and resistance to triphenyltetrazolium chloride.

Mechanisms of Pathogenicity.   *C. fetus* is unusual among the *Campylobacter* species in its ability to cause disseminated infection. *C. fetus* exhibits para-

TABLE 7–6. Characteristics of Uncommon Gram-Negative Enteric Rods

Organism	Tribe	Distinguishing Characteristics*	Sources of Infection	Diseases	Effective Antibiotic Treatments†
Citrobacter species	Citrobactereae	Lactose-negative; H$_2$S-positive; lysine decarboxylase–negative; ONPG-positive; and grows on potassium cyanide (KCN) medium.	Environment and contaminated infant formula.	Diarrhea, neonatal meningitis, and brain abscesses.	Imipenem; antipseudomonal third-generation cephalosporin; or fluoroquinolone.
Edwardsiella tarda	Edwardsielleae	Lactose-negative; H$_2$S-positive; and motile.	Water.	Wound infections; primary bacteremia in individuals with sickle cell anemia; and primary liver abscess.	Ampicillin.
Hafnia alvei	Klebsielleae	Lactose-negative; ferments arabinose; lysine decarboxylase–positive; ornithine decarboxylase–positive; DNAase-negative; and lipase-negative.	Human feces.	Wound infections.	Antipseudomonal aminoglycoside; or imipenem.
Morganella morganii	Proteeae	Lactose-negative; H$_2$S-negative; ornithine decarboxylase–negative; and urease-positive.	Soil, water, and feces.	Diarrhea, urinary tract infections, and wound infections.	Imipenem; antipseudomonal aminoglycoside; or fluoroquinolone.
Pantoea agglomerans	Klebsielleae	Lactose-variant; lysine decarboxylase–negative; and ornithine decarboxylase–negative.	Environment and contaminated intravenous fluids.	Primary sepsis.	Imipenem; or antipseudomonal penicillin plus antipseudomonal aminoglycoside.
Providencia species	Proteeae	Lactose-negative; H$_2$S-negative; and phenylalanine deaminase–positive.	Human feces.	Nosocomial urinary tract infections.	Amikacin; fluoroquinolone; or TMP/SMX.

* ONPG = orthonitrophenyl-β-D-galactopyranoside.
† Antibiotics are listed in their general order of recommended use, with the drug or drug combination used most often listed first. TMP = trimethoprim; and SMX = sulfamethoxazole.

crystalline surface layers called **S-layers.** These layers are composed of acidic high-molecular-weight proteins and show great antigenic diversity among isolates. The S-layers protect *C. fetus* from opsonization and phagocytosis by inhibiting the binding of C3b to the bacterial surface. Thus, *C. fetus* resists serum bactericidal activity and is unusually suited to grow in the blood.

C. jejuni causes diarrhea that may be either watery or bloody. Various strains of *C. jejuni* have been reported to produce a heat-labile **enterotoxin** similar to the toxins produced by *Shigella dysenteriae* and enterotoxigenic strains of *Escherichia coli.* The diarrheogenic strains of *C. jejuni* invade the intestinal epithelium in a manner similar to that seen in *Shigella* infections. The *Campylobacter* organisms invade the lamina propria of both the large and small intestines and cause crypt abscesses. Unlike *C. fetus, C. jejuni* is extremely sensitive to the lytic and opsonic activities of antibody and complement.

Diseases Due to *Campylobacter*

Epidemiology. Most *Campylobacter* infections are acquired from ingesting raw milk, poultry products, and contaminated water. In addition, pets—

especially dogs with diarrhea—can infect humans via the fecal-oral route. Although raw milk is a common source of *C. jejuni* and *Salmonella* infections, the *Campylobacter* organisms, unlike the *Salmonella* organisms, do not multiply in milk. Surveys of chicken carcasses in stores have shown that about 33% are infected with *Campylobacter* and only about 3.5% are infected with *Salmonella.* Beef and pork are not infected with *Campylobacter,* probably because the organisms grow best at the high body temperatures typically found in birds.

Humans with active *Campylobacter* infection can serve as a source of infection. In the USA, carriers are rare. However, in some developing countries, up to 40% of children sampled have been shown to carry *C. jejuni* without symptoms of diarrhea.

The ID$_{50}$ of *C. jejuni* is low, and infection in humans can result from ingestion of only 500–1000 organisms. In the USA, diarrhea due to *Campylobacter* has the highest rate of infection in people from 10 to 29 years old and occurs most frequently during the summer months. Various studies have estimated that *Campylobacter* is the cause of between 3% and 14% of all cases of diarrhea. This means that *Campylobacter* causes more cases of diarrhea than *Salmonella* and *Shigella* together cause in the USA. In some countries, up to 35% of the cases of acute diarrhea have been attributed to *Campylobacter* infection.

Diagnosis.   The disease most commonly associated with *Campylobacter* infection is **acute enteritis.** From 3 to 5 days after infection, the disease begins with profuse **diarrhea** that may be watery or bloody. The diarrhea is typically accompanied by fever and abdominal pain. In some cases, abdominal pain is so severe that it mimics the pain of appendicitis or acute ulcerative colitis. The stools contain many vibrio-like bacteria and may contain blood and sheets of PMNs. *Campylobacter* enteritis is a self-limiting disease that generally lasts 1–7 days.

C. fetus can cause **acute, febrile primary bacteremia,** particularly in older men with cancer, cirrhosis, or some other debilitating disease. This organism has also been implicated as a cause of **meningitis** in neonates and of **respiratory disease** in pregnant women.

Campylobacter species can be cultured from fecal samples or rectal swabs. Campy BAP or another special medium is used, and the organisms are incubated under microaerophilic conditions at 42 °C. Gas-liquid chromatography can also be used to identify unique 19-cyclopropane fatty acids formed by *Campylobacter* species.

Treatment.   Diarrhea caused by *C. jejuni* is treated with a fluoroquinolone or with erythromycin, and patients are rehydrated as needed. Systemic disease caused by *C. fetus* is treated with imipenem plus cilastatin or with gentamicin.

Helicobacter Species

In 1983, B. J. Marshall and J. R. Warren reported that they had isolated a spiral microaerophilic bacterium from human gastric mucosa, and they demonstrated that the presence of this bacterium was associated with the presence of gastric inflammation. The organism was originally named *Campylobacter pylori,* but rRNA gene sequence analysis and ultrastructural studies led to the creation of a new genus, *Helicobacter,* and the renaming of this organism as *Helicobacter pylori.* Today, about a dozen species of *Helicobacter* have been described.

Helicobacter species are found in a variety of animals. Most species of organisms reside in the stomach; however, some species are isolated from both the liver and stomach, and several urease-negative species are residents of the intestine alone. *H. pylori* is the cause of active chronic gastritis in humans, is the major cause of duodenal and gastric ulcers, and is a significant risk factor for the development of gastric adenocarcinoma and low-grade B cell lymphomas of gastric mucosa–associated lymphoid tissue.

Characteristics of Helicobacter

General Features.   *H. pylori* is a slightly curved microaerophilic rod that has multiple polar flagella. Although the organism was once classified as a species of *Campylobacter,* it cannot be cultured on Campy BAP agar, because it is susceptible to cephalothin. *H. pylori* can be cultured on Brucella agar, brain-heart infusion medium, or trypticase soy agar that contains 5% defibrinated sheep or horse blood. Colonies will appear on each medium in 3–5 days when incubated at 37 °C in a Campy GasPak Jar. *H. pylori* will grow in an atmosphere that contains 10% CO_2, 5% O_2, and 85% N_2, or it will grow in air that contains 10% CO_2.

H. pylori is weakly hemolytic, is oxidase-positive and catalase-positive, and exhibits intense urease activity. It differs from *Campylobacter* species in its fatty acid profile, with a high percentage of 14:0 fatty acid, little 16:0, and the presence of a 3-OH-18:0 fatty acid.

Mechanisms of Pathogenicity

(1) Bacterial Products Involved in Virulence. The key bacterial products involved in the pathogenesis of *H. pylori* infections are believed to be adhesins, urease, flagella, vacuolating cytotoxin, CagA protein, superoxide dismutase, catalase, and phospholipases.

(a) Adhesins.   At least two *H. pylori* adhesins have been described. One is a fibrillar hemagglutinin that binds to *N*-acetylneuraminyl lactose, while the other is an adhesive pilus that binds to phosphatidylethanolamine and laminin.

(b) Urease.   The *H. pylori* urease is believed to help the organism survive in an acidic environment. The production of ammonia by urease provides a microhaven that is less acidic than the general environment. Urease may promote inflammation of the gastric mucosa by recruiting and activating PMNs and monocytes. In addition, urease may play a role in eliciting the excess gastrin and acid production that occurs during *H. pylori* infection. The importance of urease to *H. pylori* is underscored by two findings: urease-deficient *H. pylori* organisms are unable to survive in the stomach, and urease-negative *Helicobacter* species can be found only in the intestine.

(c) Flagella.   Flagella are thought to promote the survival of *Helicobacter* by allowing the organism to move efficiently through mucus.

(d) Vacuolating Cytotoxin.   In studies of *Helicobacter* organisms, investigators have described a vacuolating cytotoxin that causes cultured cells to develop many cytoplasmic vacuoles. The role of this toxin in disease is in dispute. On the one hand, vacuolated cells are rarely seen in sites of *Helicobacter* colonization of the gastric mucosa. On the other hand, studies have shown that 60% of *H. pylori* strains produce the cytotoxin, most patients with duodenal ulcers carry toxin-producing strains, most patients with long-term nonulcerative gastritis carry strains that produce no toxin, and most patients with duodenal ulcers exhibit antitoxin antibodies.

(e) Other Pathogenetic Products.   The function of the **CagA protein** is unknown, but its expression has been reported to accentuate the activity of the vacuolating cytotoxin. **Superoxide dismutase** and **catalase** probably allow *H. pylori* to survive within PMNs and monocytes when phagocytosed. Investigators have shown that *H. pylori* exhibits **phospholipase A1, A2, and C activity** and that samples from infected patients contain lysophosphatides released by this activity. The phospholipases may contribute to damage of the gastric and duodenal mucosa. Studies have shown that *H. pylori* **lipopolysaccharide** (LPS) mimics Lewis blood groups in structure. Because Lewis blood group antigens are present in the gastric mucosa, some investigators believe that *H. pylori* LPS camouflages the organisms and protects them from elimination by the immune system. *H. pylori* LPS may also contribute to the loss of mucosal integrity by interfering with interactions between laminin and gastric cell receptors.

(2) The *Helicobacter* Infection Cycle. *H. pylori* organisms occupy an unusual niche in the gastric mucosa. Their most common site of infection is the antrum (the non–acid-secreting area close to the pyloric sphincter), where the organisms persist for many years (usually 30 years or more). As shown in Fig. 7–4, *H. pylori* infection predisposes patients to a variety of diseases.

Helicobacter does not invade the mucosa but apparently produces substances that erode the mucosa. This initially causes chronic superficial gastritis, a condition that usually produces no noticeable symptoms. It later causes ulcers in some patients. Scientists have found that cells in the vicinity of *H. pylori* infection express class II major histocompatibility complex (MHC) gene products. Moreover, they have noted that tumor necrosis factor alpha, interleukin-6, and interleukin-8 can be readily found in in-fected areas. These substances may play a role in the localized inflammation that leads to ulcers. In combination with cytotoxin and urease activity, these substances may also cause chronic inflammation of the gastric mucosa.

Investigators have reported that *H. pylori* heat-shock proteins share antigens with host tissues. These cross-reactive antigens are believed to elicit autoimmunity in the form of an antibody or cell-mediated response, and this may result in a low-level inflammation that lasts for decades. *H. pylori* infection is similar to leprosy in that the infectious agent elicits a moderate immune response that causes a persistent low-grade inflammation but fails to eradicate the microbe.

H. pylori infection has been shown to increase the secretion of gastrin and gastric acid. This increased acid load causes gastric metaplasia, and this in turn promotes colonization of the duodenum by *H. pylori*. Once the organisms are growing at sites of epithelial metaplasia, the various *H. pylori* products act in combination with gastric acid and the immune responses to damage the mucosa and cause inflammation.

Diseases Due to *Helicobacter*

Epidemiology. *H. pylori* has been found within feces, oral secretions, and dental plaque. For this

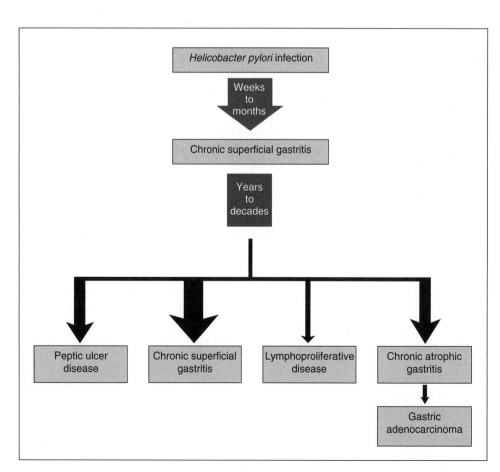

FIGURE 7–4. The relative distribution of the various outcomes of infection with *Helicobacter pylori*. (Source: Blaser, M. J., and J. Parsonnet. Parasitism by the "slow" bacterium *Helicobacter pylori* leads to altered gastric homeostasis and neoplasia. Redrawn and reproduced from The Journal of Clinical Investigation, 1994, vol. 94, pp. 4–8, by copyright permission of The American Society for Clinical Investigation.)

reason, investigators have hypothesized that the organism is transmitted by either an oral-oral route or a fecal-oral route. About 40% of adults in industrialized countries and about 80% of adults in developing countries are infected with *H. pylori*.

Diagnosis. Most *H. pylori* infections cause **active chronic gastritis.** Affected individuals are usually asymptomatic, but some develop **chronic superficial gastritis,** a condition that is associated with aging and predisposes individuals to a variety of disorders, including ulcers. *H. pylori* infection is believed to be the cause of most **gastric ulcers** and of essentially all **duodenal ulcers** that are not caused by nonsteroidal anti-inflammatory drugs. These ulcers, known as **peptic ulcers,** cause epigastric pain that is more intense when the stomach is empty.

H. pylori infection is a significant risk factor for the development of **gastric adenocarcinoma.** For example, in one study, 89.2% of individuals with epidemic-type gastric cancer were found to be culture-positive for *H. pylori*. Worldwide, gastric adenocarcinoma is one of the most common and most deadly neoplasms. Manifestations may include epigastric pain, unexplained weight loss, nausea, and vomiting. Patients often present with cancer that is well advanced. About 50% of them have a palpable epigastric mass, and about one-third have metastases.

Gastric infection with *H. pylori* can be diagnosed by a variety of means, the most common of which are biopsy, culture, antibody determination, and urea breath test. Gene probes, immunofluorescence techniques, and polymerase chain reaction systems are used in some laboratories but are not yet generally available.

Endoscopic biopsy sections can be cultured on Brucella or trypticase soy agar containing 5% sheep blood and incubated under microaerophilic conditions. The organism can be identified by its biochemical characteristics. Biopsy samples can also be stained and examined directly for the presence of *H. pylori*.

Several antibody tests have been developed for detecting the presence of antibodies to *H. pylori* in serum samples. In one study, an enzyme-linked immunosorbent assay was shown to be 93% sensitive and 81% specific for *H. pylori* infection. In contrast, a microhemagglutination test was 87% sensitive and 69% specific, and a latex agglutination test was 71% sensitive and 74% specific.

A urea breath test can be used to detect the presence of *H. pylori* in the stomach without performing an invasive procedure. The patient ingests ^{13}C- or ^{14}C-labeled urea, and if *H. pylori* is present, it converts the urea to CO_2 in the stomach. This test has a reported sensitivity and specificity of 95–100%.

Treatment. The key to effective treatment of *H. pylori* infection is the use of combination therapy. Treatment of this infection is analogous to treatment of bacterial meningitis or endocarditis. The organisms are in a protected site, so bactericidal antibiotics must be used and every bacterium must be eliminated. *H. pylori* infection is usually treated with the combination of bismuth subsalicylate, metronidazole, and either amoxicillin or tetracycline. Patients should take these drugs for 2 weeks and should be tested for *H. pylori* reinfection weeks or months later to ensure that the treatment was effective. Alternatively, the combination of ranitidine, bismuth citrate, and clarithromycin or the combination of a proton pump inhibitor and either amoxicillin or clarithromycin can be used.

Studies have shown that H_2-receptor antagonists, often given to treat ulcers, reduce the pain associated with ulcers but do not completely heal the ulcers themselves. When acid-reducing drugs are used alone to treat peptic ulcers, about 70% recur within 1 year. In contrast, when ulcers are treated as an *H. pylori* infection, fewer than 5% recur within a year, whether or not the antibiotics were administered with an acid-reducing drug.

A recent study has indicated that treatment of chronic gastritis with only a proton pump inhibitor (omeprazole) placed those infected with *H. pylori* at greatly increased risk of developing atrophic gastritis.

Selected Readings

Ashkenazi, S. Role of bacterial cytotoxins in hemolytic-uremic syndrome and thrombotic thrombocytopenic purpura. Annu Rev Med 44:11–18, 1993.

Cover, T. L., and M. J. Blaser. *Helicobacter pylori:* a bacterial cause of gastritis, peptic ulcer disease, and gastric cancer. ASM News 61:21–26, 1995.

Donnenberg, M. S., and J. B. Kaper. Enteropathogenic *Escherichia coli.* Infect Immun 60:3953–3961, 1992.

Dumanski, A. J., et al. Unique ability of the *Proteus mirabilis* capsule to enhance mineral growth in infectious urinary calculi. Infect Immun 62:2998–3003, 1994.

Galan, J. E., C. Ginocchio, and P. Costeas. Molecular and functional characterization of the *Salmonella* invasion gene *invA*: homology of InvA to members of a new protein family. J Bacteriol 174:4338–4349, 1992.

Goldberg, M. B., and P. J. Sansonetti. *Shigella* subversion of the cellular cytoskeleton: a strategy for epithelial colonization. Infect Immun 61:4941–4946, 1993.

High, N., et al. IpaB of *Shigella flexneri* causes entry into epithelial cells and escape from the phagocytic vacuole. EMBO J 11:1991–1999, 1992.

Hunt, R. H. Eradication of *Helicobacter pylori* infection. Am J Med 100:42S–50S, 1996.

Kuipers, E. J., et al. Atrophic gastritis and *Helicobacter pylori* infection in patients with reflux esophagitis treated with omeprazole or fundoplication. N Engl J Med 334:1018–1022, 1996.

Lee, A., J. Fox, and S. Hazell. Pathogenicity of *Helicobacter pylori:* a perspective. Infect Immun 61:1601–1610, 1993.

Moran, A. P. The role of lipopolysaccharide in *Helicobacter pylori* pathogenesis. Aliment Pharmacol Ther 10(supplement 1):39–50, 1996.

Neild, G. H. Haemolytic-uraemic syndrome in practice. Lancet 343:398–401, 1994.

Phadnis, S. H., et al. Pathological significance and molecular characterization of the vacuolating toxin gene of *Helicobacter pylori*. Infect Immun 62:1557–1565, 1994.

Prevost, M. C., et al. Unipolar reorganization of F-actin layer at bacterial division and bundling of actin filaments by plastin correlate with movement of *Shigella flexneri* within HeLa cells. Infect Immun 60:4088–4099, 1992.

Sansonetti, P. J. Molecular and cellular biology of *Shigella flexneri* invasiveness: from cell assay systems to shigellosis. Curr Top Microbiol Immunol 180:1–19, 1992.

Straley, S. C., et al. Yops of *Yersinia* species pathogenic for humans. Infect Immun 61:3105–3110, 1993.

Tewari, R., et al. The *pap*G tip adhesin of P fimbriae protects

Escherichia coli from neutrophil bactericidal activity. Infect Immun 62:5296–5304, 1994.

Zeitlyn, S., and F. Islam. The use of soap and water in two Bangladeshi communities: implications for the transmission of diarrhea. Rev Infect Dis 13(supplement 4):S259–S264, 1991.

PSEUDOMONADACEAE

Burkholderia, Pseudomonas, and *Stenotrophomonas (Xanthomonas)*

General Characteristics and Classification

Like the family Enterobacteriaceae, the family Pseudomonadaceae consists of a large group of gram-negative rods. Unlike the Enterobacteriaceae, however, the Pseudomonadaceae have one or more polar flagella, are usually oxidase-positive, and can be grown on very simple media.

The Pseudomonadaceae have been divided into five groups on the basis of ribosomal RNA (rRNA) homologies, but only three of these groups—groups I, II, and V—contain organisms that are human pathogens. **Groups I and II** consist of members of the genus *Pseudomonas* (pseudomonads), as shown in Table 8–1. **Group V** consists of a single species, *Stenotrophomonas (Xanthomonas) maltophilia.*

Pseudomonas aeruginosa and *Burkholderia (Pseudomonas) pseudomallei,* two common causes of disease, are discussed below. The characteristics and associated diseases of *Burkholderia (Pseudomonas) cepacia, Pseudomonas stutzeri,* and *S. maltophilia* are summarized in Table 8–2.

Pseudomonas aeruginosa

Pseudomonas aeruginosa, the best-known pseudomonad, is the most frequent cause of nosocomial infections in patients hospitalized for 10 days or longer. The organism is in the fluorescent subgroup of rRNA group I Pseudomonadaceae. Like all of the organisms in the subgroup, it produces **pyoverdin,** a pigment that fluoresces white to blue-green when illuminated under a Wood's lamp (400 nm). However, *P. aeruginosa* is unique in that more than half of the clinical strains of this organism produce a water-soluble pigment known as **pyocyanin.** When this pigment is present, exudates containing *P. aeruginosa* appear blue-green. Some strains also produce the fluorescent dye **fluorescein.** Because the organisms fluoresce, patients with burns can be monitored for *P. aeruginosa* infections by passing a Wood's lamp over the burned skin to look for fluorescent patches.

Characteristics of *P. aeruginosa*

General Features. *P. aeruginosa* is an oxidase-positive, motile, gram-negative rod that is 0.5–0.8 μm wide by 1.5–3.0 μm long and has one to three polar flagella. It is an obligate aerobe except when grown in the presence of nitrate, which it can reduce to nitrite. *P. aeruginosa* does not ferment carbohydrates, but it is nutritionally adaptable, able to metabolize more than 80 organic compounds yet be cultivated on simple media. These metabolic characteristics reflect the role of *P. aeruginosa* in nature. The organisms are found in water and soil and are involved in the decomposition of organic substances.

P. aeruginosa is Simmons' citrate–positive, arginine dihydrolase–positive, lysine decarboxylase–negative, and ornithine decarboxylase–negative. It does not produce H_2S in Kligler iron agar. Because it produces trimethylamine, cultures of *P. aeruginosa* typically have a characteristic fruity odor.

Mechanisms of Pathogenicity. *P. aeruginosa* is an opportunistic pathogen that causes disease primarily in patients with catheters and in patients with immune defects, such as neutropenia. Pseudomonads are often hard to eradicate because the patients are immunologically unable to deal with the infection and because the isolates are typically resistant to multiple drugs, sometimes producing beta-lactamases capable of degrading or inactivating third-generation cephalosporins.

(1) Bacterial Factors in the Pathogenesis of *Pseudomonas* Infections. *P. aeruginosa* expresses a wide variety of structures and cell products that contribute to its ability to cause disease by serving as adhesins, protecting from phagocytosis, altering the immune response, or damaging host tissues.

(a) Lipopolysaccharide. Most strains of *P. aeruginosa* have lipopolysaccharide inserted in their outer membrane, although mucoid strains are rough. More than one antigenic type of O antigen may be expressed simultaneously, and growth conditions can affect the expression of O antigens. The lipid A portion of *P. aeruginosa* lipopolysaccharide is similar to that of the enteric organisms in its endotoxic activity, but it differs structurally in that it has more phosphate groups and lacks β-hydroxymyristic acid. A scheme that utilizes lipopolysaccharide antigenicity is used to type *P. aeruginosa* and is known as the **international antigenic typing system** (IATS).

TABLE 8–1.   Group I and Group II Pseudomonads

Ribosomal RNA Group and Subgroup	Organisms
Group I	
Alcaligenes subgroup	*Pseudomonas alcaligenes, Pseudomonas pseudoalcaligenes,* and *Pseudomonas* species group 1.
Fluorescent subgroup	*Pseudomonas aeruginosa, Pseudomonas fluorescens,* and *Pseudomonas putida.*
Stutzeri subgroup	*Pseudomonas mendocina, Pseudomonas stutzeri,* and CDC group Vb-3.
Group II	*Burkholderia (Pseudomonas) cepacia, Burkholderia (Pseudomonas) pseudomallei, Pseudomonas gladioli, Pseudomonas mallei,* and *Pseudomonas pickettii.*

Pseudomonads with smooth lipopolysaccharide are resistant to the bactericidal activity of serum, but those with rough lipopolysaccharide are sensitive. The production of alginate (discussed below) and expression of O antigen are coupled, so that strains producing alginate stop expressing O antigen on their outer membrane surface. Endotoxic shock occurs in patients with *Pseudomonas* bacteremia.

(b) Extracellular Proteases.   At least three key extracellular proteases are produced by *P. aeruginosa:* elastase, alkaline protease, and protease IV.

Pseudomonas **elastase** activates an enzyme that is called **matrix metalloproteinase 2** (MMP-2) and is produced by corneal cells. This enzyme damages the eye and causes keratitis by degrading type IV, V, and VII collagens, which are part of the structure of the corneal basement membrane and stroma. Elastase also plays a key role in the pathogenesis of tissue necrosis in patients with burns and of pulmonary disease in patients with cystic fibrosis. Its role in these diseases has been attributed to its abilities to do the following: degrade complement components, particularly C3b; degrade IgG and IgA; break down other serum proteins, including α_1-antichymotrypsin,

α_1-proteinase inhibitor, and C1 inhibitor; inhibit polymorphonuclear leukocyte (PMN) chemotaxis and chemiluminescence; cleave CD4 and interleukin-2; and inhibit natural killer cell activity by cleaving CD16. Under some environmental conditions, elastase may assist in the acquisition of iron by degrading host transferrin. Elastase may also contribute to lung damage and bacterial invasion of lung tissue by damaging tight junction–associated proteins.

Less is known about *Pseudomonas* **alkaline protease.** This 57-kD protein is believed to contribute to immunosuppression and necrosis by cleaving a wide variety of host proteins, including interleukin-2 and several leukocyte adhesion molecules.

Protease IV remains largely uncharacterized, but studies in rabbits have shown that protease IV activity damages the eye and can contribute to the development of keratitis.

(c) ADP-Ribosyl Transferase Exotoxins.   *P. aeruginosa* produces at least three adenosine diphosphate–ribosyl (ADP-ribosyl) transferases: exotoxin A, exoenzyme S, and high-molecular-weight leukocidin.

About 90% of *P. aeruginosa* strains produce **exotoxin A** (ETA), a substance that blocks protein synthesis and kills cells by inactivating elongation factor 2 (EF-2). ETA works by utilizing nicotinamide adenine dinucleotide (NAD) to ADP-ribosylate EF-2. Although the mechanisms of diphtheria toxin (see Chapter 14) and ETA are identical, the structures of these toxins are unrelated. ETA has three domains. Domain I binds to host cell receptors and initiates endocytosis. When the endosome is acidified, domain II promotes movement of the toxin into the cell cytoplasm, and domain III catalyzes the ADP-ribosylation of EF-2.

About 40% of *P. aeruginosa* strains produce **exoenzyme S** (ExoS). ExoS ADP-ribosylates host cell proteins other than EF-2. Among its targets are vimentin and several proteins that bind guanosine triphosphate (GTP). Because these GTP-binding proteins are involved in the movement of lysosomes, ExoS may protect *P. aeruginosa* from being killed by PMNs and macrophages. ExoS seems to be a critical component in the development of *P. aeruginosa* infections in patients with burns.

TABLE 8–2.   Uncommon Members of the Pseudomonadaceae Family and Their Associated Diseases

Organism	Source of Infection	Diseases	Treatment*
Burkholderia (Pseudomonas) cepacia	Fluids containing nitrogen, including water, detergents, disinfectants, and irrigation solutions.	Cepacia syndrome in patients with cystic fibrosis; conjunctivitis; endocarditis; jungle rot (foot infection); neonatal meningitis; and nosocomial urinary tract infections.	TMP/SMX; ceftazidime; or ciprofloxacin.
Pseudomonas stutzeri	Cosmetics; soil; and infant formula, water, and other environmental fluids.	Conjunctivitis; otitis media; pneumonia; and septic arthritis.	Broad-spectrum antibiotics.
Stenotrophomonas (Xanthomonas) maltophilia	Disinfectants and water.	Nosocomial infections, including pneumonia, primary bacteremia, sepsis, and urinary tract infections.	Chloramphenicol; TMP/SMX; or ticarcillin plus clavulanate.

*TMP/SMX = trimethoprim-sulfamethoxazole. Many broad-spectrum antibiotics are effective in the treatment of *P. stutzeri* infection, but antibiotics are generally not very effective in the treatment of *S. maltophilia* infection.

High-molecular-weight leukocidin has been reported to initiate ADP-ribosylation and is thought to activate protein kinase C.

(d) Siderophores.   There is little free iron in the body fluids. Instead, extracellular iron is complexed with transferrin and lactoferrin. Because bacteria need iron, organisms that cannot scavenge iron cannot invade host tissues. *P. aeruginosa* utilizes two siderophores, known as **pyoverdin** and **pyochelin,** to obtain Fe^{3+} from transferrin. The precise role of siderophores in virulence is not fully understood, but pyoverdin-deficient isolates of *P. aeruginosa* are unable to cause disease in mice that have sustained burns.

(e) Pili.   Many isolates of *P. aeruginosa* have numerous type IV pili extending from their surface. These pili, which are similar to the pili of *Bacteroides nodosus, Moraxella bovis, Neisseria gonorrhoeae,* and *Vibrio cholerae,* mediate adherence to mucins and epithelial cells. Mucins are high-molecular-weight O-linked glycoproteins secreted by the goblet cells and mucous glands of the respiratory mucosa, and patients with cystic fibrosis produce excess mucins. The pili of *P. aeruginosa* bind to oligosaccharide moieties of the glycosphingolipids asialo-GM_1 and asialo-GM_2. These receptors are revealed when epithelial cells are stripped of fibronectin by proteases.

Two interesting observations have been made about the relationship between the pili of *P. aeruginosa* and pulmonary infections in patients with cystic fibrosis. First, *P. aeruginosa* strains isolated during the earliest phases of *Pseudomonas* pulmonary infection are piliated, have smooth lipopolysaccharide, and are nonmucoid, but strains isolated during later phases are nonpiliated, have rough lipopolysaccharide, and are mucoid. Second, epithelial cells from patients who have cystic fibrosis exhibit about twice as many receptors for pili as do the epithelial cells from individuals who do not have cystic fibrosis. In patients with cystic fibrosis, it appears that *Pseudomonas* infections are established in the lungs by piliated bacteria that adhere preferentially to the respiratory epithelium and abundant mucins. Once the infection has become established and the bacteria need to resist phagocytosis, pili and O antigen are no longer expressed and the bacterial colony becomes coated with an antiphagocytic alginate gel.

(f) Rhamnolipids.   *P. aeruginosa* produces two detergentlike glycolipids that are rhamnolipids. **Monorhamnolipid** is rhamnose linked to a dimer of β-hydroxydecanoic acid, and **dirhamnolipid** is a rhamnose dimer linked to a dimer of β-hydroxydecanoic acid. Rhamnolipids are believed to contribute to the ability of *P. aeruginosa* to cause lung infections. They have been shown to inhibit the activity of respiratory cilia, stimulate mucin secretion, kill monocyte-derived macrophages, inhibit macrophage phagocytosis, and alter epithelial ion transport.

(g) Phospholipase C.   Two forms of phospholipase C (PLC) are produced by *P. aeruginosa*. High-molecular-weight PLC is hemolytic (PLC-H), while low-molecular-weight PLC is nonhemolytic (PLC-N).

When environmental carbohydrate levels are elevated and inorganic phosphate (Pi) levels are low, the synthesis of PLC-H and PLC-N is stimulated 8-fold and 30-fold, respectively. These proteins are part of a large group of genes under coordinate control within the Pi regulon.

PLC-H and PLC-N degrade phosphorylcholine, the principal constituent of lung surfactant. Degradation of phosphorylcholine liberates diacylglycerol and choline, leads to atelectasis, stimulates further PLC-H synthesis, and results in the formation of prostaglandins, thromboxanes, and leukotrienes. These products of arachidonate metabolism may contribute to pathologic changes that occur in the lungs of patients who have cystic fibrosis and chronic *P. aeruginosa* pulmonary infections. The major products of PLC activity are also osmoprotectors, and they may protect the bacteria from the high osmotic pressure present in the lungs of these patients.

(h) Cytotoxin.   Cytotoxin (CTX) was originally known as **leukocidin** because of its ability to kill PMNs. CTX is a 29-kD protein encoded on the genome of phage ϕCTX, and the gene is introduced into *P. aeruginosa* via **phage conversion.** CTX is synthesized as a prototoxin, is released by bacteriolysis, and is converted to its active form when cleaved by extracellular proteases. CTX binds to host cell membranes, forms 1-nm holes in the membrane, and destabilizes membrane integrity.

(i) Alginate.   Alginate is the substance that makes up the gelatinous slime layer on *P. aeruginosa* strains that cause chronic pulmonary infections in patients with cystic fibrosis. Alginate is composed of D-mannuronic acid and its 5′ epimer, L-guluronic acid (Fig. 8–1).

Alginate is believed to be necessary for the persistence of *P. aeruginosa* within the lungs of patients with cystic fibrosis. Although only 0.8–2.0% of all *Pseudomonas* infections are caused by mucoid *P. aeruginosa* strains, 80–90% of patients with cystic fibro-

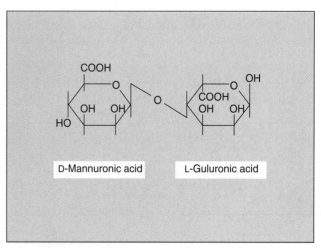

FIGURE 8–1. The structure of the disaccharide subunit of alginate. Alginate contains D-mannuronic acid and L-guluronic acid linked by β1,4 bonds. The ratio of D-mannuronic acid to L-guluronic acid ranges from 4:1 to 1:1.

sis develop pulmonary infections caused by alginate-producing *P. aeruginosa* strains. *Pseudomonas* strains that initiate infection in the tracheobronchial tree are not mucoid, but growth in the lungs of patients with cystic fibrosis initiates a phenotypic change that causes the organisms to stop expressing pili and O antigen and to begin synthesizing alginate.

The key regulatory signals for alginate synthesis are NaCl, KCl, and desiccants, each of which activates the *algD* promoter. The AlgD protein is GDP-mannose dehydrogenase, a key enzyme in the synthesis of alginate. The lungs of patients with cystic fibrosis are an ideal site for activation of alginate synthesis because they contain high concentrations of Na^+, Cl^-, Ca^{2+}, and K^+; are desiccated; and allow the organisms to grow as gelatinous microcolonies surrounded by alginate. According to one study, the concentration of alginate in sputum samples of patients with pulmonary disease ranges from 4 to 100 $\mu g/mL$, with a median concentration of 35.5 $\mu g/mL$.

A wide variety of properties have been attributed to alginate (Table 8–3), probably the most important of which is its ability to prevent pseudomonads from being phagocytosed and killed by PMNs and alveolar macrophages.

(j) Other Virulence Factors. A lectinlike substance known as **PA-I lectin** has been shown to kill or inhibit the growth of respiratory epithelial cells in a concentration-dependent manner. Several **outer membrane proteins** have been shown to adhere to mucins from patients with cystic fibrosis. **Phenazine pigments** such as **pyocyanin** have been reported to be ciliostatic agents, to help pseudomonads compete for iron by reducing Fe^{3+} to the more soluble Fe^{2+} form, and to inhibit the blastogenic response of T cells to mitogens and specific antigens.

(2) Host Factors in the Pathogenesis of *Pseudomonas* Infections. Host factors also play a key role in the development of disease due to *P. aeruginosa*. These factors are most clearly demonstrated in the development of keratitis, pulmonary infections in patients with cystic fibrosis, and tissue necrosis in patients with burns.

(a) Keratitis. Keratitis occurs when *P. aeruginosa* colonizes an eye damaged by trauma, by herpes simplex infection, or by prolonged use of soft contact lenses. The bacteria may be introduced via contaminated wash solutions, and their initial persistence may be related to the patient's immune status. Once established within a corneal ulceration, the bacteria spread and necrose the cornea as they produce ETA, ExoS, proteases, and other cytotoxic products.

(b) Pulmonary Infections in Patients With Cystic Fibrosis. *P. aeruginosa* is not a primary pathogen in patients with cystic fibrosis. Young patients typically suffer from repeated *Staphylococcus aureus* and *Haemophilus influenzae* infections that damage the lungs. Patients who have suffered from decreased lung function for 3 years or longer develop intermittent *P. aeruginosa* infections over 6 months to 2 years, and these lead to a chronic pulmonary infection with mucoid strains of *P. aeruginosa*.

Investigators believe that the pulmonary damage caused by *S. aureus* and *H. influenzae* infections and by excess proteases in the mucin strips fibronectin from the surfaces of epithelial cells and exposes ganglioside receptors for *Pseudomonas* adhesins. This allows piliated nonmucoid strains to adhere to the respiratory epithelium, and the bacteria eventually migrate into the lungs, where they begin to produce alginate. Alginate protects the organisms from destruction by phagocytic cells and thereby allows them to establish chronic infection. The lungs are damaged not only by *P. aeruginosa* products but also by host cell factors. Type III hypersensitivity reactions seem to be at the center of the generation of lung damage. PMNs unable to phagocytose microcolonies of organisms damage the lung by releasing oxygen-derived free radicals and hydrolytic enzymes, such as elastase.

(c) Tissue Necrosis and Sepsis in Patients With Burns. Patients with severe burns have high levels of endogenous proteolytic activity in the affected tissues. Studies suggest that the presence of protease-producing *P. aeruginosa* pushes the total proteolytic load in the tissues beyond the inhibitory capacity of available serum protease inhibitors. The excess load activates Hageman factor, which begins a cascade of events that lead to the generation of fibrin, activated complement components, kinin, and eicosanoids. Patients suffer from excess clotting, depressed opsonic activity, increased activity of suppressor T cells, decreased activity of helper T cells and natural killer cells, decreased antigen presentation, and generalized immunosuppression. The importance of protease activity is illustrated by the fact that *P. aeruginosa* infections in patients with burns are fatal only if the infecting strain produces abundant proteases. ExoS is also believed to participate in the development of burn infections, but its precise role is not understood.

TABLE 8–3. Virulence Properties Attributed to the Alginate Slime Layer of Mucoid Strains of *Pseudomonas aeruginosa*

Inhibits leukocyte chemotaxis.
Directly interferes with phagocytosis.
Inhibits phagocytosis by chelating divalent cations.
Inhibits phagocytosis by providing a hydrophilic surface.
Potentiates antibody production by acting as an adjuvant.
Intensifies polymorphonuclear leukocyte production of superoxide in response to *N*-formyl-methionyl-leucyl-phenylalanine (FMLP).
Scavenges toxic free radicals.
Acts as a nonactivator surface for complement activation.
Provides biofilm to allow pseudomonads to enter the human body via catheters.
Adheres to mucins.

Diseases Due to *P. aeruginosa*

Epidemiology. *P. aeruginosa* is a ubiquitous organism, found in water, soil, and vegetation. It is carried on the skin and in the gastrointestinal tract and throat of about 3% of the general population, but carriage rates among hospital personnel may exceed 20%. *P. aeruginosa* tends to persist in the hospital environment because of its ability to resist the activities of so many antibiotics.

P. aeruginosa is a true opportunistic pathogen, causing nosocomial disease in patients who are debilitated or immunosuppressed. The organisms are sensitive to drying, so they are not easily spread on fomites. Instead, they are often spread via water used to cleanse respirators, nebulizers, other equipment, and wounds; flowers brought to the patient; and green salads fed to the patient. Infections commonly begin at sites where moisture accumulates, such as in tracheostomies, indwelling catheters, burned skin, the external ear, and weeping cutaneous wounds.

Patients at highest risk are those with diminished numbers of PMNs (particularly cancer patients receiving cytotoxic drugs), depressed PMN function, or a condition that makes a body surface suitable for pseudomonads to adhere and grow. Among those at risk are individuals who have received intravenous broad-spectrum antibiotics and those who have diabetes mellitus, leukemia, neutropenia, cystic fibrosis, third-degree burns, eye ulcers, traumatic wounds, or an indwelling catheter.

Diagnosis

(1) History and Physical Examination. *P. aeruginosa* is associated with a wide variety of opportunistic infections.

(a) Bacteremia. While *Escherichia coli, Klebsiella,* and *Enterobacter* are the three leading causes of primary hospital-acquired bacteremia, *P. aeruginosa* is fourth. Patients at risk for primary bacteremia are usually debilitated or immunosuppressed, as discussed above. Bacteremia may also be secondary, occurring as an extension of pneumonia, pyelonephritis, or gastrointestinal infections.

Patients with bacteremia due to *Pseudomonas* suffer from typical gram-negative sepsis. They generally exhibit fever, tachycardia, tachypnea, respiratory distress, hypotension, and azotemia. Sepsis may lead to refractory shock and renal failure.

Bacteremia may be accompanied by erythematous skin lesions known as **ecthyma gangrenosum.** These lesions begin as vesicles that hemorrhage, necrose, and ulcerate as they become indurated nodules. Ecthyma gangrenosum is seen most often as patches of lesions in the perineal area, in the axillas, or on the extremities, but lesions may occur anywhere, including on the mucous membranes. The ulcerated lesions contain *P. aeruginosa* organisms but little or no pus.

As with any gram-negative sepsis, *Pseudomonas* sepsis is rapidly fulminating, and death occurs in 33–38% of patients.

(b) Bone and Joint Infections. The bones and joints of patients may become infected with *P. aeruginosa* either by hematogenous spread of organisms from a primary infection site or by direct extension of infection from a contiguous site. Those at greatest risk for hematogenous spread are intravenous drug users and patients with urinary tract or pelvic infections. Those at risk for direct extension of infection include patients with penetrating wounds and patients with cellulitis. Pain in the affected area is sometimes accompanied by fever and loss of range of motion.

(c) Central Nervous System Infections. *P. aeruginosa* causes **meningitis** and **brain abscesses** in patients with preexisting immunologic defects or head trauma. The organisms may be introduced into the central nervous system by trauma, hematogenous spread, or direct extension from a chronic ear or sinus infection. Meningitis due to *P. aeruginosa* often occurs in cancer patients and is usually accompanied by fever, headache, nuchal rigidity (stiff neck), confusion, and other neurologic signs of meningitis. In the absence of bacteremia, the disease tends to be subacute. Patients with bacteremia may suffer from fulminating disease accompanied by septic shock.

(d) Ear Infections. *P. aeruginosa* can cause **otitis externa,** a rather benign but extremely painful infection that is also called **swimmer's ear** because it most often affects individuals who have been swimming in a body of warm water, such as a pond or gravel pit. The ear canal, which swells tremendously and contains debris, itches at first and then begins to ache.

Elderly diabetic patients and infants may develop a more dangerous infection that is called **malignant otitis externa.** This condition is characterized by invasion of the soft tissues, sometimes leading to necrosis, cranial nerve damage, bacteremia, and sepsis. Typical manifestations include a tender and swollen ear canal, purulent discharge, and granulation in the posteroinferior canal wall. Cranial nerve involvement may be heralded by facial palsies, but any of the cranial nerves may become involved. Patients sometimes complain of trismus and hearing loss, and sepsis may occur. Fatality rates of 15–20% in treated patients have been reported.

P. aeruginosa may cause **otitis media** in newborns and is the most common cause of **chronic suppurative otitis media** in children and adults. Diabetic patients may develop **mastoiditis,** often secondary to malignant otitis externa or to otitis media.

(e) Eye Infections. *P. aeruginosa* causes a fulminating ulceration of the cornea that is known as **keratitis.** As mentioned above, risk factors include damage of the conjunctiva by herpes simplex infection, trauma, or use of soft contact lenses. The infection begins as a small corneal ulcer that rapidly spreads concentrically, causing pain and swelling of the eyelid. The epidermis and stroma become necrotic, and exudate collects in the ulcer. The eye may fill with pus (hypopyon), and ocular function is rapidly lost. *Pseudomonas* keratitis is a medical emergency because patients with penetrating injuries may develop panophthalmitis that destroys the eye within hours or days.

(f) Gastrointestinal Tract Infections. *Pseudomonas* infections of the gastrointestinal tract occur primarily in newborn infants and immunocompromised patients. Some newborn infants develop life-threatening **enterocolitis.** In neutropenic cancer patients, asymptomatic infections of the intestine sometimes progress to sepsis or disseminated ectopic infections, but frank enterocolitis also occurs. Neutropenic patients with enterocolitis develop hemorrhagic and necrotic lesions of the intestinal mucosa. Like the skin lesions of ecthyma gangrenosum, these lesions contain organisms but few inflammatory cells.

A pediatric disease that is called **Shanghai fever** and is similar to typhoid fever is also believed to be caused by *P. aeruginosa.*

(g) Infective Endocarditis.   *P. aeruginosa* is responsible for nearly two-thirds of all cases of infective endocarditis in intravenous drug users, with almost 90% of affected individuals being black males under the age of 30 years. Although people with prosthetic valves are occasionally infected, *P. aeruginosa* endocarditis occurs almost exclusively in drug users. *P. aeruginosa* is believed to be in the water or paraphernalia used to prepare drugs, rather than in the drugs themselves. The organisms adhere well to native valves, which in some cases may have been slightly damaged by impurities in the drug mixture.

Patients with subacute endocarditis of the tricuspid valve suffer from fever, murmurs, and septic pulmonary emboli. These emboli are typically accompanied by a productive cough, pleuritic chest pain, pleural effusions, and pulmonary infiltrates. Patients with acute endocarditis of the mitral or aortic valve may suffer from congestive heart failure and systemic arterial emboli.

(h) Respiratory Tract Infections.   *P. aeruginosa* infections of the respiratory tract occur in a variety of forms.

Primary nonbacteremic pneumonia is usually acquired when patients with chronic lung disease or congestive heart failure receive respiratory therapy using contaminated ventilator equipment or nebulizers. The patients suffer from a fulminating bronchopneumonia with fever, dyspnea, copious purulent sputum, cyanosis, pleural effusions, microabscesses, and focal hemorrhaging. The disease is similar to staphylococcal pneumonia in its clinical presentation and is often fatal.

Primary bacteremic pneumonia is seen most often in patients with cancer and neutropenia. In these patients, the necrotic lesions that develop in the lung are similar to the skin lesions of ecthyma gangrenosum. The disease characteristically progresses rapidly from pulmonary vascular congestion to pulmonary edema to necrotizing bronchopneumonia. Patients often suffer from sepsis, and death may occur in 3–4 days.

Chronic pulmonary infections occur in older patients with cystic fibrosis. As described earlier, the respiratory epithelium in these patients is prepared for *Pseudomonas* infection by years of intermittent infections with *H. influenzae* and *S. aureus* and by the presence of excess mucins. Patients develop chronic suppuration, mucus plugging of the airways, bronchi-

ectasis, atelectasis, and fibrosis. As a result, they suffer from rapid breathing, wheezing, productive cough, and loss of appetite and weight. The disease tends to wax and wane, with lingering chronic disease interrupted by acute exacerbations. Some patients also become infected with *Burkholderia* (*Pseudomonas*) *cepacia* and develop an acute pulmonary disease that is known as **cepacia syndrome** and may lead to death within 1 year.

(i) Skin and Soft Tissue Infections.   Staphylococci were once the major cause of death in patients with severe burns. With improvement in the management of severe burns, patients more often survive early staphylococcal infections, only to develop *Pseudomonas* infections that cause **tissue necrosis** and **sepsis** and can be rapidly fatal. Pseudomonads colonize the burn eschar and grow to densities of greater than 10^5 bacteria per gram of tissue. The infected burn becomes discolored and dark, and the skin adjacent to the burn becomes edematous and hemorrhagic. The patient exhibits disorientation, fever or hypothermia, abdominal pain with vomiting and diarrhea (ileus), and leukopenia. Once a necrotic infection is established, the pseudomonads can spread rapidly into the blood and cause fulminating sepsis. In patients with burns, isolation has been an effective tool in delaying the onset of *Pseudomonas* infection (from 19 days to 41 days following the burn) and reducing the number of deaths due to *Pseudomonas* infection (from 77% to 21% of infected patients).

P. aeruginosa can cause **hot tub dermatitis** in people who use hot tubs contaminated with the organism. *P. aeruginosa* can also cause **tropical immersion foot** in patients with athlete's foot. This condition is characterized by an infection of the toe webs following exposure of the feet to high temperature, humidity, and stress. **Green nail syndrome** is a form of paronychia caused by *P. aeruginosa.* The characteristic green hue of the nail bed is due to the production of pyocyanin by the organisms.

(j) Urinary Tract Infections.   *E. coli, Enterococcus* species, and *P. aeruginosa* are the three most common causes of hospital-acquired urinary tract infections. The patients most frequently affected are those with indwelling urinary catheters, chronic prostatitis, or kidney stones. Like other gram-negative organisms (see Chapter 7), *P. aeruginosa* is also responsible for some cases of community-acquired pyelonephritis in women.

(2) Laboratory Analysis.   *P. aeruginosa* infections are often suspected when blue-green pus is present in lesions. Sputum, pus, and biopsy material from burns, keratitis, and ecthyma gangrenosum can be stained and examined directly for the presence of gram-negative rods. The diagnosis can be confirmed by cultivating the organisms on standard bacteriologic media and performing biochemical tests.

Treatment.   Treatment of infections caused by *P. aeruginosa* is difficult because the organisms are typically resistant to numerous drugs and because some isolates produce cephalosporinases that inactivate or degrade third-generation cephalosporins. Antibiotic therapy and other treatment measures used for bacteremia and infections of various organ systems are listed in Table 8–4.

Burkholderia (Pseudomonas) pseudomallei

Burkholderia (Pseudomonas) pseudomallei is a free-living bacterium found in warm water and wet soil, primarily in Southeast Asia. It is particularly common in southern Thailand and in Vietnam, where it grows abundantly in flooded rice paddies and causes a disease called melioidosis.

Characteristics of B. pseudomallei

General Features. *B. pseudomallei* is classified as a member of rRNA group II Pseudomonadaceae (the pseudomallei group). It grows well on many standard microbiologic media, producing characteristic wrinkled colonies. *B. pseudomallei* exhibits bipolar staining that gives it the appearance of a safety pin when examined microscopically. The organism is oxidase-positive and reduces nitrate to nitrite. In triple sugar iron (TSI) agar, it produces an acid slant that has a neutral butt after 24 hours but changes to an acid butt after 72 hours of incubation. Antisera can be used to definitively identify isolates of *B. pseudomallei*.

Mechanisms of Pathogenicity. Human infections with *B. pseudomallei* usually begin when the organisms enter through abrasions, cuts, or ulcers. In some cases, however, infections begin when healthy individuals inhale the organisms; when hospitalized patients are exposed to contaminated antiseptics, bronchoscopy equipment, or urinary catheters; or when laboratory workers are exposed while culturing *B. pseudomallei*.

The means by which *B. pseudomallei* causes meli-

TABLE 8–4. Recommended Treatment for Diseases Caused by *Pseudomonas aeruginosa*

Disease	Recommended Treatment
Bacteremia	Aggressive antibiotic therapy (antipseudomonal aminoglycoside alone or in combination with antipseudomonal penicillin) and supportive care for sepsis.
Bone and joint infections	Surgery, drainage of pus, and antibiotics (antipseudomonal aminoglycoside alone or in combination with antipseudomonal penicillin).
Central nervous system infections	
Brain abscess	Surgical drainage and antibiotics.
Meningitis	Ceftazidime.
Ear infections	
Chronic suppurative otitis media	Tympanomastoid surgery and parenteral antibiotics.
Malignant otitis externa	Surgery and beta-lactam aminoglycosides plus antipseudomonal aminoglycosides.
Mastoiditis in patients with diabetes	Surgery and antibiotics as indicated by susceptibility testing.
Otitis externa	Topical antibiotics and corticosteroids, 2% acetic acid, and drying agents.
Otitis media	Third-generation antipseudomonal cephalosporin.
Eye infections	High-dose topical gentamicin.
Gastrointestinal tract infections	Antibiotics as indicated by susceptibility testing.
Infective endocarditis	
Mitral or aortic valve disease	Immediate valve replacement and high-dose parenteral antibiotics (antipseudomonal penicillin plus antipseudomonal aminoglycoside); splenectomy if splenic abscesses are present.
Tricuspid valve disease	High-dose parenteral antibiotics (antipseudomonal penicillin plus antipseudomonal aminoglycoside); valve replacement if bacteremia persists.
Respiratory tract infections	
Chronic pulmonary infections in patients with cystic fibrosis	High-dose parenteral antibiotics (usually antipseudomonal aminoglycoside in combination with a third-generation antipseudomonal cephalosporin or antipseudomonal penicillin).
Primary bacteremic pneumonia	High-dose parenteral antibiotics (usually antipseudomonal penicillin; ticarcillin plus clavulanate; or imipenem).
Primary nonbacteremic pneumonia	High-dose parenteral antibiotics (usually antipseudomonal penicillin; ticarcillin plus clavulanate; or imipenem).
Skin and soft tissue infections	
Green nail syndrome	A solution of 3% thymol in absolute alcohol.
Hot tub dermatitis	No specific treatment. Clean hot tub.
Tissue necrosis and sepsis in patients with burns	Isolation and antipseudomonal aminoglycoside plus antipseudomonal penicillin.
Tropical immersion foot	General measures (drying and resting the feet) and antibiotics as needed.
Urinary tract infections	Parenteral third-generation antipseudomonal cephalosporin; ticarcillin plus clavulanate; or antipseudomonal penicillin plus antipseudomonal aminoglycoside.

oidosis are not well described. *B. pseudomallei* has an endotoxic **lipopolysaccharide** and produces an extracellular **protease.** Its most unusual property is its ability to survive quietly within the liver and spleen for many years and then to be reactivated and cause rapidly fulminating, life-threatening infection.

Diseases Due to *B. pseudomallei*

Epidemiology.   *B. pseudomallei* is found primarily in Southeast Asia, but cases of melioidosis that are believed to be indigenous have been reported in 31 countries, including those as geographically diverse as the USA, Australia, Burma, India, Russia, Chad, Burkina Faso, England, and Ecuador.

In Australia, serologic surveys using an indirect hemagglutination test in northern Queensland showed that 5.7% of all residents living in this area and 29.1% of Vietnamese refugees living in this area had antibody to *B. pseudomallei.* In the USA, similar serologic surveys have suggested that as many as 225,000 members of the military who served during the Vietnam War were infected with this organism and may carry it in their reticuloendothelial system.

The worldwide prevalence of melioidosis is difficult to determine for two reasons: most cases occur in countries without adequate systems to survey and report infectious diseases, and most patients are thought to be asymptomatic.

Diagnosis

(1) History and Physical Examination.   Most patients infected with *B. pseudomallei* do not develop disease. Those who develop **melioidosis** have one of three basic disease patterns: localized infection that can be suppurative and acute or can be granulomatous and chronic; septicemia that begins abruptly and rapidly disseminates to ectopic foci; or prolonged fever that may not be accompanied by signs of localized infection.

Infection often begins as acute pneumonitis, a chronic tuberculosislike syndrome, or localized cellulitis at the site of entry. Acute *B. pseudomallei* infection is often confused with *Staphylococcus aureus* infection, and chronic melioidosis has been mistaken for deep fungal infections, tuberculosis, and anaerobic infections. Melioidosis is sometimes called the "great imitator" because of its propensity for dissemination and ectopic infection in a variety of sites (Table 8–5). It is also called the "Vietnamese time bomb" because individuals suffering from chronic pulmonary infections or asymptomatic infections have developed rapidly fatal septicemia years after acquiring *B. pseudomallei* infection in Vietnam. In each case, an immunosuppressive or debilitating condition, such as diabetes mellitus, cirrhosis, or cancer, has precipitated the fatal attack of acute melioidosis.

(2) Laboratory Analysis.   A diagnosis of melioidosis is suspected when patients with appropriate symptoms and history exhibit antibodies to *B. pseudomallei* in the indirect hemagglutination test. Exudate or granuloma samples can be stained and exam-

TABLE 8–5.   Major Ectopic Infections Caused by *Burkholderia (Pseudomonas) pseudomallei*

Organ or System	Types of Infection
Cardiovascular system	Pericarditis and pericardial effusion.
Genitourinary system	Pyelonephritis, prostatitis, and prostatic abscess.
Liver	Liver abscess.
Lymphatic system	Lymphadenitis and lymph node abscess.
Respiratory system	Pneumonitis, lung abscess, empyema, pleural effusion, and miliary granuloma.
Skeletal system	Septic arthritis and osteomyelitis.
Skin and soft tissue	Cellulitis, subcutaneous abscess, and granuloma.
Spleen	Splenic abscess.

ined for the presence of gram-negative rods that are shaped like safety pins. Unlike in *Pseudomonas aeruginosa* infections, in *B. pseudomallei* infections few organisms are found in exudate samples. Definitive diagnosis of melioidosis requires that the organisms be cultured from infection sites.

Treatment.   Without treatment, about 95% of patients with acute melioidosis die. Although disseminated melioidosis does not respond well to antibiotic therapy, ceftazidime has been shown to reduce the mortality rate by about 50%. The following treatment regimens have also been used with some success: chloramphenicol; doxycycline; tetracycline; kanamycin; trimethoprim-sulfamethoxazole (TMP/SMX); piperacillin; amoxicillin plus clavulanate; and imipenem plus cilastatin. Nondisseminated melioidosis has a lower fatality rate (about 20%) and responds well to antibiotic treatment. Surgical drainage of abscesses should not be performed until antibiotics have been initiated, because drainage of abscesses in untreated patients has resulted in rapid dissemination of the organisms and early death.

Selected Readings

Azghani, A. D. *Pseudomonas aeruginosa* and epithelial permeability: role of virulence factors elastase and exotoxin A. Am J Respir Cell Mol Biol 15:132–140, 1996.

Carrell, D. T., M. E. Hammond, and W. D. Odell. Evidence for an autocrine/paracrine function of chorionic gonadotropin in *Xanthomonas maltophilia.* Endocrinology 132:1085–1089, 1993.

Coburn, J., and D. M. Gill. ADP-ribosylation of p21[ras] and related proteins by *Pseudomonas aeruginosa* exoenzyme S. Infect Immun 59:4259–4262, 1991.

Dance, D. A. Melioidosis: the tip of the iceberg? Clin Microbiol Rev 4:52–60, 1991.

Dart, J. K., and D. V. Seal. Pathogenesis and therapy of *Pseudomonas aeruginosa* keratitis. Eye 2(supplement):S46–S55, 1988.

Fleiszig, S. M., et al. Relationship between cytotoxicity and corneal epithelial cell invasion by clinical isolates of *Pseudomonas aeruginosa.* Infect Immun 64:2288–2294, 1996.

Gilligan, P. H. Microbiology of airway disease in patients with cystic fibrosis. Clin Microbiol Rev 4:35–51, 1991.

Holder, I. A., and A. N. Neely. The role of proteases in *Pseudomonas* infections in burns: a current hypothesis. Antibiot Chemother 44:99–105, 1991.

Leelarasamee, A., and S. Bovornkitti. Melioidosis: review and update. Rev Infect Dis 11:413–425, 1989.

Matsumoto, K., et al. Proteolytic activation of corneal metalloprotease by *Pseudomonas aeruginosa.* Curr Eye Res 11:1105–1109, 1992.

McClure, C. D., and N. L. Schiller. Effects of *Pseudomonas aeruginosa* rhamnolipids on human monocyte-derived macrophages. J Leukoc Biol 51:97–102, 1992.

McClure, C. D., and N. L. Schiller. Inhibition of macrophage phagocytosis by *Pseudomonas aeruginosa* rhamnolipids in vitro and in vivo. Curr Microbiol 33:109–117, 1996.

Pedersen, S. S., et al. *Pseudomonas aeruginosa* alginate in cystic fibrosis sputum and the inflammatory response. Infect Immun 58:3363–3368, 1990.

Prince, A. Adhesins and receptors of *Pseudomonas aeruginosa* associated with infection of the respiratory tract. Microb Pathog 13:251–260, 1992.

Roilides, E., et al. *Pseudomonas* infections in children with human immunodeficiency virus infection. Pediatr Infect Dis J 11:547–553, 1992.

Roychoudhury, S., et al. *Pseudomonas aeruginosa* infection in cystic fibrosis: biosynthesis of alginate as a virulence factor. Antibiot Chemother 44:63–67, 1991.

Sajjan, U. S., et al. Binding of *Pseudomonas cepacia* to normal human intestinal mucin and respiratory mucin from patients with cystic fibrosis. J Clin Invest 89:648–656, 1992.

Villarno, M. E., et al. Risk factors for epidemic *Xanthomonas maltophilia* infection and colonization in intensive care unit patients. Infect Control Hosp Epidemiol 13:201–206, 1992.

Whitchurch, C. B., et al. The alginate regulator AlgR and an associated sensor FimS are required for twitching motility in *Pseudomonas aeruginosa.* Proc Natl Acad Sci USA 93:9839–9843, 1996.

Wick, M. J., et al. Structure, function, and regulation of *Pseudomonas aeruginosa* exotoxin A. Annu Rev Microbiol 44:335–363, 1990.

CHAPTER NINE

FUNGUSLIKE BACTERIA

Actinomadura, Actinomyces, Mycobacterium, Nocardia, Streptomyces, and *Tropheryma*

The *Actinomadura, Actinomyces, Mycobacterium, Nocardia, Streptomyces,* and *Tropheryma* species discussed in this chapter are grouped together as funguslike bacteria. These bacteria resemble fungi in that most are found throughout the environment, most grow slowly, and many grow as long filaments that look like fungal hyphae. Moreover, the effective immune response to them is largely a cell-mediated response. However, all these bacteria are prokaryotes, whereas all fungi are eukaryotes. Thus, similarities between these bacteria and the fungi are largely superficial and analogical.

MYCOBACTERIA

The mycobacteria are acid-fast, gram-positive bacilli that are highly resistant to environmental conditions. Their unusual resistance comes from their complex cell envelopes, which contain waxes, glycoproteins, and glycolipids. Many of the mycobacteria are found throughout the environment, but *Mycobacterium tuberculosis* and *Mycobacterium leprae* are strictly parasitic. The mycobacteria are facultatively intracellular bacteria that multiply within cells of the reticuloendothelial system, particularly macrophages and monocytes. Mycobacteria typically cause chronic diseases, often characterized by a prolonged latent period. The host develops a vigorous antibody response, but recovery from mycobacterial diseases depends on the development of a cell-mediated immune response. Once macrophages are activated by cytokines, mycobacteria are killed and the disease is arrested.

Mycobacterium tuberculosis

Among the earlier names for the mycobacterial disease now known as tuberculosis were phthisis and consumption. Around 1000 B.C., Hippocrates described phthisis, a term that meant "to waste away." During the 17th and 18th centuries, phthisis was reported to cause 20–30% of all deaths in London. The propensity of tuberculosis to chronically sap the strength of the patient and cause prolonged weight loss was recognized in its subsequent name, consumption. The disease became known as tuberculosis in 1834, and Robert Koch isolated *Mycobacterium tuberculosis* in 1882. *M. tuberculosis* is the major agent of tuberculosis, but tuberculosis due to *Mycobacterium bovis* sometimes occurs, usually as a result of drinking raw milk obtained from infected cattle.

The World Health Organization has estimated that perhaps up to half of the world's population is infected with *M. tuberculosis* and that 3 million or more die each year from tuberculosis. Since 1990, the number of cases in the USA has been increasing, with between 20,000 and 30,000 new tuberculosis cases identified each year.

Characteristics of *M. tuberculosis*

General Features. *M. tuberculosis* is a facultatively intracellular bacterium that is resistant to acids and alkalies because of its multilayered and hydrophobic cell wall complex. The organisms stain faintly gram-positive, appearing as straight to slightly curved bacilli that are 1–10 μm long and 0.2–0.6 μm wide. Specimens from patients are usually cleared of debris using the *N*-acetyl-L-cysteine procedure and are then tested using one of the following three acid-fast procedures for identification of *Mycobacterium* species: Ziehl-Neelsen staining, Kinyoun staining, or the auramine fluorochrome procedure. The mycobacteria are acid-fast, so they resist decolorization by the acid-alcohol mixtures used in these procedures.

Because of the lengthy period needed to produce visible growth, the media used to culture *M. tuberculosis* contain malachite green or antibiotics to inhibit the growth of other bacteria. The organisms are routinely cultivated on media that contain whole eggs and potato flour, but media that contain no eggs have also been developed. Examples of mycobacterial media are listed in Table 9–1. Isolation from clinical samples can be facilitated using special BACTEC rapid culture systems, and nucleic acid probes can be used to identify the cultured organism as *M. tuberculosis.*

Mechanisms of Pathogenicity. The structural components and products of the cell wall complex

TABLE 9–1.   Characteristics of
Mycobacterium tuberculosis

Optimal conditions for culture
3–11% CO_2 level
37 °C (does not grow at 30 °C or 42–45 °C)

Growth media
American Thoracic Society medium
Löwenstein-Jensen culture medium
Middlebrook 7H10 agar
Middlebrook 7H11 agar
Middlebrook 7H12 agar or broth
Petragnani culture medium

Tests and results
Arylsulfatase activity	Negative
Catalase activity	Negative
Niacin accumulation	Positive
Nitrate reduction	Positive
Pyrazinamidase activity	Positive
Thiopene 2-carboxylic acid	Inhibits growth
Urease activity	Positive

of *M. tuberculosis* are responsible for the organism's virulence and ability to survive harsh environmental conditions.

(1) Components of the Cell Wall Complex. As shown in Fig. 9–1, the cell wall complex consists of an inner cytoplasmic membrane surrounded by a typical gram-positive cell wall (peptidoglycan). The cell wall is attached via disaccharide bridges to a layer of arabinogalactan. Mycolic acids and mycocerosic acids are attached to arabinogalactan, and the outermost layer of the complex is composed of sulfated glycolipids known as sulfatides. This phalanx of macromolecules makes the mycobacterial wall complex fairly impenetrable. The peptidoglycan and arabinogalactan layers are similar in all species of *Mycobacterium,* but the lipoarabinomannan, mycolic acids, mycocerosic acids, and other attached macromolecules vary among the species.

(a) Cytoplasmic Membrane. The cytoplasmic membrane of *M. tuberculosis* is a typical trilaminar membrane consisting of phospholipids and proteins. It contains phosphatidylinositol, which serves as an anchor for the mannophosphoinositides and lipoarabinomannan. Lipoarabinomannan is analogous to the lipopolysaccharide of gram-negative bacteria. The phosphoinositol units are substituted with palmitate and 10-methyloctadecanoate (tuberculostearate).

(b) Peptidoglycan-Arabinogalactan Complex. The peptidoglycan of *M. tuberculosis* is very much like that of *Escherichia coli,* consisting of N-acetylglucosamine-N-acetylmuramic acid. However, it is linked via a rhamnose-N-acetylglucosamine disaccharide bridge to arabinogalactan, which in turn is linked to the mycolic acids and mycocerosic acids. The mycolic acids are of particular importance because they are believed to be crucial factors in the virulence of *M. tuberculosis.* Mycolic acids are α-substituted β-hydroxy fatty acids that are esterified to cell wall polysaccharides (Fig. 9–2). The length of the associated hydrocarbon chains is a species-specific characteristic within the mycobacteria. The complex of mycolic acid and arabinogalactan forms the mycolylarabinogalactan cell wall complex, which may comprise up to 35% of the cell wall complex mass.

(c) Other Cell Surface Structures. *M. tuberculosis* has an outer layer of sulfated glycolipids, or sulfatides, that are involved in virulence. Other species of *Mycobacterium,* such as *Mycobacterium avium-intracellulare, Mycobacterium chelonae, Mycobacterium lepraemurium,* and *Mycobacterium scrofulaceum,* exhibit peptide-containing glycolipids that serve as a highly antigenic capsular structure and were initially known as C-mycosides or Schaefer antigens. In *M. bovis, Mycobacterium kansasii, Mycobacterium leprae,* and *Mycobacterium marinum,* the cell surface is surrounded by a layer of phenolated glycolipids.

(2) Products Related to Virulence.   Table 9–2

FIGURE 9–1. The cell envelope complex of *Mycobacterium tuberculosis.* (Source: Gaylord, H., and P. J. Brennan. Leprosy and the leprosy bacillus: recent developments in characterization of antigens and immunology of the disease. Ann Rev Microbiol 41:645–675, 1987. Redrawn and reproduced, with permission, from the Annual Review of Microbiology, Volume 41, © 1987, by Annual Reviews Inc.)

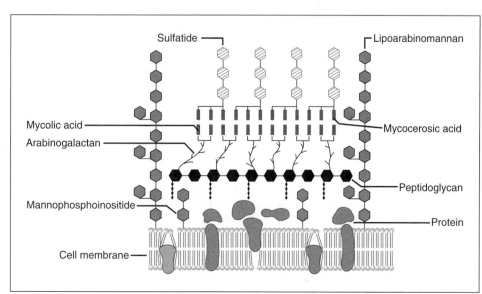

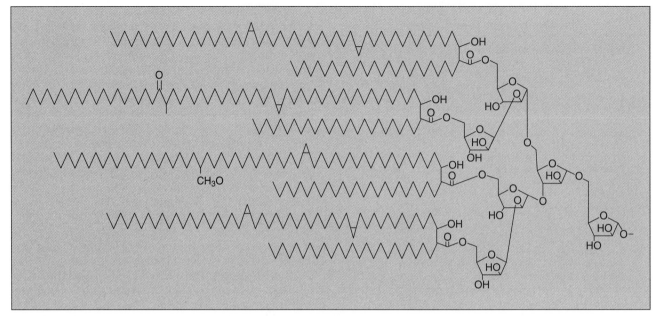

FIGURE 9–2. The general structure of mycolic acids.

lists numerous mycobacterial virulence determinants and outlines their activities.

(a) Cord Factor. Cord factor is produced by members of the genera *Corynebacterium, Mycobacterium, Nocardia,* and *Rhodococcus.* It is the most important mycoside produced by *M. tuberculosis,* and it is called cord factor because it causes the organism to grow as rope-like lateral aggregates. Cord factor consists of trehalose 6-6'-dimycolate (Fig. 9–3), and trehalose is glucose α-1-1'-D-glucoside. Studies have shown that mycobacterial organisms lacking cord factor are unable to cause disease. When injected into mice, 10 μg of cord factor in oil causes hemorrhagic pneumonitis, and three such doses are fatal. Cord factor causes the mice to develop granulomas and lung procoagulant activity. Perhaps most important, cord factor inhibits fusion of macrophage lysosomes with phagosomes, a phenomenon that is believed to be key in the ability of *M. tuberculosis* to survive within macrophages.

(b) Sulfatides. The sulfatides, which are anionic trehalose sulfate derivatives that contain long-chain fatty acids, are located on the outermost surface of mycobacteria. Studies of the most abundant of the *M. tuberculosis* sulfatides, SL-1, have shown that this sulfatide can block or reverse the priming of monocytes by lipopolysaccharide or interferon-gamma. This causes the monocytes to produce little superoxide radical, and it may protect phagocytosed *M. tuberculosis* from intracellular killing. Monocytes exposed to SL-1 have limited protein kinase C activity, but they produce high amounts of interleukin-1β and tumor necrosis factor alpha (TNF-α).

(c) Arabinogalactan and Lipoarabinomannan. In conjunction with arabinogalactan, lipoarabinomannan elicits a strong but ineffective antibody response. Lipoarabinomannan works in concert with cord factor to produce tuberculous granulomas and tissue necrosis.

(d) Tuberculoproteins. The proteins of *M. tu-*

TABLE 9–2. Mycobacterial Virulence Determinants and Their Activities

Virulence Determinant	Activities
Adenylate cyclase	Inhibits macrophage degranulation.
Arabinogalactan	Elicits futile antibody response.
Lipoarabinomannan	Elicits futile antibody response; suppresses T cell activity; inhibits antigenic responsiveness of peripheral blood lymphocytes; inhibits antigen presentation; induces production of tumor necrosis factor alpha (TNF-α); and inhibits interferon-gamma–mediated macrophage activation.
Mycolic acids	Confer acid-fastness and protect against acids and alkalies.
Mycosides (such as cord factor)	Inhibit leukocyte migration; stimulate granuloma formation; destroy mitochondrial membranes; inhibit cellular response; inhibit monocyte release of interleukin-6 (IL-6); and inhibit fusion of macrophage lysosomes with phagosomes.
Sulfatides	Potentiate cord factor effects; immobilize or inactivate macrophage hydrolytic enzymes; block macrophage degranulation; and cause virulent *Mycobacterium tuberculosis* strains to stain with neutral red.
Tuberculoproteins	Interfere with immune response; promote cellular invasion; and elicit delayed-type hypersensitivity.
Wax D	Acts as an adjuvant.

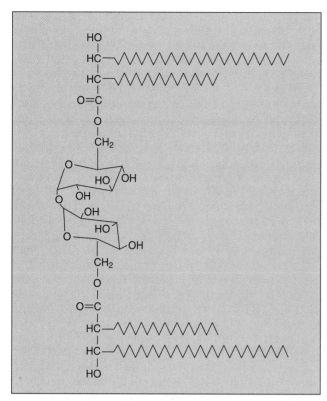

FIGURE 9–3. The structure of cord factor.

berculosis have drawn considerable interest since the early discovery that proteins extracted by boiling culture filtrates of the organism could elicit a cutaneous reaction when injected intradermally into individuals infected with *M. tuberculosis.* The fairly raw protein preparation used for skin testing became known as **old tuberculin** (OT). OT can be precipitated with ammonium sulfate to produce **purified protein derivative** (PPD), which is the antigenic mixture used today for tuberculosis skin testing. When PPD is injected intradermally into a person infected with *M. tuberculosis,* there is an initial nonspecific wheal that quickly disappears. From 48 to 72 hours later, the infected patient develops an indurated lump that is due to delayed-type hypersensitivity to PPD. This procedure, which is used to diagnose tuberculosis, is known as the **Mantoux test** and is discussed more fully below.

(3) Host Response to Infection. The survival of *M. tuberculosis* within the host depends on the organism's ability to multiply within macrophages and monocytes. The host's immunity to *M. tuberculosis* depends on the development of a vigorous antimycobacterial cellular response that activates macrophages to kill or restrict the growth of intracellular organisms. Investigators who work with tuberculosis differentiate between the regenerative and destructive aspects of the cellular response, referring to effective cellular immunity as the **cell-mediated immune response** (CMIR) and referring to cellular damage to tissues as **delayed-type hypersensitivity** (DTH).

The pathologic hallmark of tuberculosis is the formation of granulomas around the foci of infection. When mycobacteria enter the lung, they are phagocytosed by macrophages that vary in their abilities to kill the organisms. Patients with acquired immunodeficiency syndrome (AIDS) are uniquely susceptible to tuberculosis, and the reason for this may be that their macrophages are naturally deficient in tuberculocidal activity even before cell activation occurs. Investigators believe that a key step in halting infection with *M. tuberculosis* is the initial interaction between quiescent macrophages and the organism. They also believe that a monocyte chemotactic protein (MCP-1), three interleukins (IL-1, IL-2, and IL-8), TNF-α, and interferon-gamma play key roles in the development of granulomas and the control of infections with *M. tuberculosis.*

Early in the infection, macrophages are attracted to each infection site by generation of the chemotactic factors C5a and MCP-1. T cells are attracted by IL-8. Unstimulated macrophages phagocytose the mycobacteria but do not control the infection until a specific CMIR first appears during weeks 3–10. Macrophages attracted by MCP-1 may be better suited to control the mycobacteria than are the initial macrophages that encounter the mycobacteria, since MCP-1 stimulates the macrophage respiratory burst.

The lipoarabinomannan of *M. tuberculosis* stimulates monocytes and macrophages to secrete TNF-α. This substance acts synergistically with interferon-gamma to cause macrophages to kill the mycobacteria. It also activates nitric oxide–dependent killing of intracellular bacteria and induces granuloma formation. In fact, studies have shown that animals depleted of TNF activity are unable to control the multiplication of mycobacteria or form granulomas.

CD4$^+$ T lymphocytes have been divided into Th1 and Th2 phenotypes. Th1 cells secrete interferon-gamma and IL-2 in response to specific antigenic stimuli, while Th2 cells secrete IL-4, IL-5, IL-6, and IL-10. Animals infected with *M. tuberculosis* preferentially expand Th1 T cell clones, and the expansion of these clones has been related to their ability to recover from infection. Additionally, at least two populations of T cell receptors (TCRs) exist. Most T cells express alpha/beta TCR, but a small proportion of T cells express gamma/delta TCR. Most gamma/delta T cells are CD4$^-$/CD8$^-$, and they seem to be important to recovery from intracellular infections. Patients who are infected with *M. tuberculosis* and do not develop disease appear to preferentially expand gamma/delta T cell clones, although the bulk of the T cell response consists of alpha/beta T cells.

Finally, cytotoxic T lymphocytes (CTLs) and natural killer cells are believed to be important to recovery from infection with *M. tuberculosis,* because they kill the organism-infected macrophages and monocytes.

(4) Dynamics of Infection. In a 1948 study of patients with tuberculosis, E. M. Medlar showed that primary lesions were located throughout the lungs

(Fig. 9–4A) and that 85% of the lesions were within 1 cm of the pleural surface.

Studies using animal models have shown that *M. tuberculosis* initially infects the parenchyma throughout the lungs, causing damage particularly within the lower lung fields. When infectious droplets that are 5 μm or smaller and contain 1–10 organisms are inhaled into the lower lung fields, infection is initiated and leads to the formation of a primary lesion.

Mycobacteria are quickly phagocytosed by alveolar macrophages when the complement component C3bi deposits on the surface of the organisms and interacts with the macrophage complement receptor 3 (CR3). Mycobacteria multiply within these macrophages by blocking degranulation of primary and secondary lysosomes into the phagocytic vacuole and by blocking acidification of phagosomes. The virulence of *M. tuberculosis* isolates varies, as does the antimycobacterial activity of macrophages.

Investigators believe that infection begins when a highly virulent isolate of *M. tuberculosis* infects a weak macrophage. Initially, the mycobacteria grow symbiotically within the macrophage, but infected macrophages are eventually destroyed by the multiplying mycobacteria. When the organisms enter the extracellular space, they are again phagocytosed. As this cycle is repeated, some organisms migrate to the draining lymphatic vessels, where they multiply intracellularly and cause the lymph node to swell. The hilar and mediastinal lymph nodes are most commonly affected, and lymphadenopathy is most prominent in children. When organisms escape the node

and enter the blood, they are disseminated to ectopic sites such as the bone marrow, kidneys, meninges, and the lung apex.

The granulomas of tuberculosis are called **tubercles.** The center of each tubercle contains Langhans' giant cells. A zone of epithelioid cells surrounds the giant cells, and a zone containing fibroblasts and lymphocytes forms the outermost layer of the tubercle. The generation of a CMIR causes the center of the tubercle to become crumbly and cheese-like, a condition known as caseation. The CMIR develops within 3–10 weeks of the initiation of infection, causing caseation and sterilizing most of the primary and metastatic foci. Mycobacterial growth is restricted within activated macrophages, and CTLs kill the mycobacteria-infected macrophages. At this time, most lesions are microscopic or barely visible, and patients generally recover with no radiographic or clinical evidence of disease. However, mycobacteria that have migrated to the lung apex survive in a dormant state. In about 95% of cases, these bacteria remain dormant for the life of the patient. In the other 5% of cases, the bacteria later reactivate to cause clinically apparent tuberculosis.

About 5% of patients develop progressive primary tuberculosis at the time of initial infection, with exudative or granulomatous lesions at each ectopic focus, and some develop numerous small lesions throughout both lungs. These small lesions are known as **miliary lesions** because they look somewhat like a millet seed.

M. tuberculosis is an aerobe, and the well-aerated

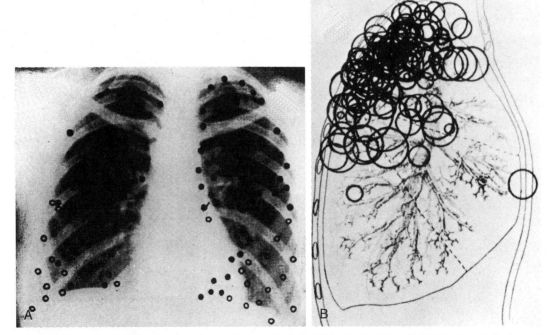

FIGURE 9–4. Distribution of calcified primary lesions of tuberculosis in 105 patients (A) and distribution of single cavitary lesions of tuberculosis in 204 patients (B). (Sources: Medlar, E. M. The pathogenesis of minimal pulmonary tuberculosis: a study of 1225 necropsies in cases of sudden and unexpected death. Am Rev Tuberc 58:583–611, 1948. Sweany, H. C., et al. A study of the position of primary cavities in pulmonary tuberculosis. Am Rev Tuberc 24:558–582, 1931. Reproduced, with permission, from American Journal of Respiratory and Critical Care Medicine.)

lung apex provides it with a hospitable environment (Fig. 9–4B). Investigators believe that part of the reason mycobacteria persist in the lung apex is that the CMIR is unable to sterilize a caseous apical lesion. The caseous lesion is avascular, and adjacent blood vessels are thrombosed, making it difficult for macrophages to reach mycobacteria in the center of the lesion. Despite the relatively good aeration of the lung apex, growth of mycobacteria within the apical caseous lesion is slow or nonexistent. This may be because toxic fatty acids accumulate in the lesion, the lesion is relatively anoxic, and the pH of the lesion is low. Small foci are eventually eliminated by macrophages, but larger lesions (5–20 mm) persist indefinitely.

In the USA, many cases of active tuberculosis in adults are cases of **reactivation tuberculosis** that occur with the waning and waxing of the CMIR to mycobacteria. The mycobacteria multiply in the apical focus, and the newly reinvigorated CMIR causes intense necrosis, liquefaction of tissue, and the formation of tissue cavities. Liquefaction is thought to be the result of tissue damage caused by macrophage hydrolytic enzymes released when macrophages are unable to cope with a concentrated nidus of mycobacteria. When the organisms are released from the cells, they multiply to great numbers, allowing toxic mycobacterial products to accumulate. In the presence of these products, DTH results in necrosis and rupture of the bronchial wall and the formation of a cavity. This process is critical to the development of active tuberculosis in at least two ways. First, cavity formation allows the mycobacteria to enter the airways, and the patient now sheds organisms in each respiratory droplet as he or she coughs. Second, the accumulation of huge numbers of mycobacteria within the lesion favors the development of antibiotic resistance. Lesions may become encapsulated within fibrous material or may be exudative. If a cavity forms near a blood vessel, the mycobacteria may disseminate to ectopic sites and granulomas will form wherever the mycobacteria grow.

(5) Transmission of Infection. *M. tuberculosis* is spread from person to person via **droplet nuclei,** which are respiratory droplets shed when patients with active tuberculosis cough, talk, or sing. About half of the droplets spread by coughing remain airborne and infectious for 30 minutes, but only 6% of those aerosolized during talking remain airborne for the same duration. Because of their small size (1–5 μm), droplet nuclei are able to travel down the bronchi to the alveolus, where infection begins.

Patients with cavitary pulmonary or laryngeal tuberculosis are most likely to spread mycobacteria if they have a chronic cough, have acid-fast bacilli in their sputum, fail to cover their face when they cough, and are not being treated with antibiotics or have been taking antibiotics for only a short time. Patients with laryngeal tuberculosis are particularly dangerous. Individuals who are exposed to these patients in areas of inadequate ventilation are at high risk of being infected. Patients shedding mycobacteria infect about 29% of their close contacts (family members and coworkers who share restricted air spaces with a patient for substantial periods of time) and about 15% of semiclose contacts.

About 5% of patients who are infected with *M. tuberculosis* will develop disease within 2 years. Although some will develop clinical manifestations of disease much later, most will never develop symptoms. Among the groups with a high risk of developing tuberculosis following infection are the following: members of medically underserved minority populations; homeless people; intravenous drug users; people born in countries where *M. tuberculosis* is prevalent; people who are 10% or more below ideal body weight; individuals recently infected with *M. tuberculosis;* children 5 years of age or younger; patients who have silicosis or have had a gastrectomy or jejunoileal bypass; patients with chronic renal failure; patients with diabetes; patients with old fibrotic lung lesions that can be seen radiographically; and immunocompromised individuals, including those with human immunodeficiency virus (HIV) infection or AIDS.

Infections in children are considered to be primary tuberculosis. In developing countries, where *M. tuberculosis* is prevalent, tuberculosis in adults is often primary tuberculosis. In countries where *M. tuberculosis* is not prevalent, such as the USA, most cases of tuberculosis in adults were thought to be due to reactivation of latent infection. However, recent studies in San Francisco and New York have shown that about one-third of the observed cases of adult tuberculosis were due to primary infection. This epidemiologic shift may be related to the emergence of HIV-infected individuals as a population unusually susceptible to tuberculosis.

Tuberculosis has been reported to occur before an AIDS-defining illness in 50–75% of HIV-infected people. Moreover, people who are infected with both HIV and *M. tuberculosis* are estimated to have an 8–10% risk of developing active tuberculosis each year, as compared to a 10% risk over the lifetime of people with normal immune systems and *M. tuberculosis* infection. This unusual susceptibility to mycobacterial infection has been attributed to two factors. One is that unstimulated macrophages from HIV-infected people appear too weak to restrict the growth of mycobacteria. The other is that the interferon-gamma response of HIV-infected people appears inadequate to initiate a vigorous CMIR to the mycobacteria.

Not only is the HIV-infected group unusually susceptible to tuberculosis, but *M. tuberculosis* may actually hasten the onset of AIDS in this group. Mycobacterial infection causes macrophages and T cells to secrete increased amounts of TNF-α, which in turn causes HIV in latent infected cells to be expressed. Expression of HIV increases TNF production, which accelerates further HIV production, and so on. The loss of CD4$^+$ T cell activity that accompanies AIDS makes the body further unable to control the mycobacterial infection, and the patient develops both active tuberculosis and AIDS.

About 21% of HIV-infected people who develop

tuberculosis die within 1 year, but only 13% of these deaths are directly due to tuberculosis. Instead, most deaths are attributable to other AIDS-related diseases, such as pneumonia or pneumonitis due to *Pneumocystis carinii* or various bacteria.

Diseases Due to *M. tuberculosis*

Diagnosis

(1) History and Physical Examination. The clinical manifestations of tuberculosis occur late during the disease and include inexplicable weight loss, constant fatigue, temperature that may reach 40 °C (104 °F), night sweats, shortness of breath, and chest pain. The cough is productive of mucopurulent sputum that is often tinged with blood. Cavitation leads to development of frankly purulent sputum. Patients with pleural effusions typically suffer from pleuritic pain and dyspnea. When dissemination occurs, the symptoms reflect the presence of a granuloma in the affected tissues.

(a) Primary Progressive Tuberculosis. This form of tuberculosis is seen most often in children and immunodeficient adults. Children typically develop prominent hilar lymphadenopathy but rarely develop cavitary lesions. In children, the lesions may be found anywhere in the lungs. The organisms are disseminated in the blood, and ectopic foci of infection may be established. Although the pulmonary and lymph node lesions usually heal spontaneously, some children develop rapidly progressive miliary tuberculosis, which is fatal within a year if untreated. Adults with primary progressive tuberculosis have little lymph node involvement, but they frequently develop cavitary lesions in the lung apex. Unless the patient is severely immunocompromised, *M. tuberculosis* disseminates less frequently in adults than in children.

(b) Reactivation Tuberculosis. Reactivation tuberculosis usually occurs in older patients and is accompanied by the formation of cavitary lesions in the lung apex. The cavities progress slowly, and mycobacteria may spread into the bronchi.

(2) Tuberculin Skin Test. Individuals who have been exposed to active tuberculosis or have clinical signs of tuberculosis should be skin-tested for evidence of a DTH reaction to *M. tuberculosis*. The intradermal **Mantoux test** should be used, rather than the tine test or other multiple-puncture tests. In the Mantoux test, the volar or dorsal surface of the forearm is injected intradermally with 0.1 mL of a solution containing 5 tuberculin units (TU) of PPD. A wheal 6–10 mm in diameter is formed immediately, but this wheal quickly dissipates. The reaction to the test is read 48–72 hours later by measuring the area of induration seen on the forearm. Positive reactions fall into three major categories, as described in Table 9–3.

The results of skin testing must be interpreted cautiously. A single, isolated positive result in the Mantoux test means only that the patient has, at some time, been exposed to an immunogenic dose of *M. tuberculosis*. Patients previously infected with *M. tu-*

TABLE 9–3. Results Considered Positive in the Mantoux Tuberculin Skin Test

Risk Category	Result in Mantoux Test	Presence of Other Risk Factor
Group 1	Induration ≥5 mm	Infected with human immunodeficiency virus (HIV). Recently exposed to active tuberculosis. Healed tuberculosis lesion found on x-ray.
Group 2	Induration ≥10 mm	Born in a country where tuberculosis is common. Intravenous drug user. Member of a medically underserved group. Member of a low-income group. Patient with diabetes, gastrectomy, leukemia, or silicosis. Resident of a long-term care facility (such as a nursing home or prison).
Group 3	Induration ≥15 mm	None of the above risk factors.

berculosis will be PPD-positive for years, and patients infected with "atypical" mycobacteria (discussed below) exhibit varying degrees of cross-reactivity to skin testing. For these reasons, it is important to determine the size of the indurated region and to know the size of induration when the patient was last tested.

Results of skin testing may be falsely negative in patients with very recent infection (infection occurring 3–10 weeks before testing). Results obtained from older patients (55 years or older) may also be misleading, but in this case it is because of the **booster phenomenon.** DTH wanes over time. Thus, older patients may initially test PPD-negative, but when retested months later may have a positive reaction that is due to reactivation of their preexisting DTH. For this reason, some physicians use a two-step test for older patients. The patient is administered PPD, the first test is not read, and then a second Mantoux test is performed within the next few weeks. The result of the second test is usually considered positive if the area of induration is greater than 15 mm. If the result is positive or borderline, subsequent tests must yield an increase of 15 mm or more in the area of induration to be considered positive.

(3) Chest X-Rays. Patients with active pulmonary tuberculosis should be examined for radiographic evidence of primary lesions, pleural effusions, or upper lobe cavity formation. Healed primary complexes often calcify, leaving a scar called a **Ghon complex** that can be seen by radiograph as a spot on the lung. Ghon complexes can also be caused by fungal pulmonary infections, such as histoplasmosis. Some patients develop large calcified masses known as **tuberculomas.** In patients with reactivation tuberculosis, radiographs may show a single large, air-containing space in the lung or may reveal a small cavity encapsulated by fibrous material.

(4) Laboratory Analysis. Confirmation of the diagnosis of tuberculosis rests on the results of skin testing and chest x-rays, the examination of sputum smears, and the culture and identification of organisms.

(a) Sputum Smears. Sputum samples should be collected from patients and examined directly for the presence of acid-fast bacilli. It is important that the samples collected are sputum and not respiratory secretions. Sputum comes from the lungs and contains no epithelial cells. If the patient cannot cough up sputum, he or she can be placed in a respiratory isolation site (in a special cubicle or under a hood) where an aerosol of hypertonic saline can be inhaled to facilitate sputum collection. Alternatively, sputum can be obtained from early-morning gastric aspiration samples collected after an 8- to 10-hour fast.

Sputum samples should be cleared of debris using the N-acetyl-L-cysteine procedure and stained by the Ziehl-Neelsen, Kinyoun, or auramine fluorochrome procedure. If acid-fast bacilli are present, they can usually be detected within 24 hours of sample collection. The number of acid-fast bacilli per milliliter of sputum should be estimated to determine the extent of infection. The results of sputum smear examination are positive in 50–80% of patients with pulmonary tuberculosis.

(b) Culture and Identification of the Organisms. The most popular of the rapid culture systems for *M. tuberculosis* is a BACTEC system that uses Middlebrook 7H12 agar containing a ^{14}C-labeled palmitic acid substrate. *M. tuberculosis* can grow in this system in 10–14 days, and samples can then be used to inoculate a BACTEC-NAP medium that confirms the presence of *M. tuberculosis* in another 7 days (for a total of 17–21 days) by specifically inhibiting the growth of the organism in the presence of p-nitro-α-acetylamino-β-hydroxypropiophenone (NAP). Alternatively, samples from the BACTEC medium can be tested by a rapid DNA probe that identifies *M. tuberculosis* within 2–8 hours after isolation (for a total of 10–15 days). The BACTEC systems have reduced the time needed to culture and identify *M. tuberculosis* from the 3–5 weeks needed when a conventional medium (such as Löwenstein-Jensen medium) is used.

Treatment. At one time, patients with tuberculosis were isolated in sanatoriums to restrict the spread of the disease. Tuberculosis was treated by collapsing the lung, a procedure that was effective because mycobacteria are so strictly aerobic.

Today, antibiotics are the capstone of tuberculosis treatment, but several problems must be addressed when designing a course of antibiotic therapy for a patient with tuberculosis. First, mycobacteria are intracellular bacteria, so the antibiotics utilized must be able to accumulate within host cells, including within macrophage phagosomes. Second, mycobacteria grow slowly, so antibiotics that are effective only against rapidly growing bacteria are not useful. Because slow growth and the high culture densities within liquefied lesions are conditions that allow resistant mutants to appear, the treatment must involve multiple antibiotics. Third, the antibiotics used must be well tolerated when given over a prolonged period of time and should be able to be administered infrequently enough to make patient compliance a reasonable expectation. If the cost of the antibiotics is too great or the dosing is too frequent, many patients will not complete their treatments.

The approach to treatment of suspected or confirmed infection with *M. tuberculosis* is based on a variety of factors. Table 9–4 shows the currently recommended regimens for three groups: exposed individuals with negative results in the Mantoux test; exposed individuals with positive results in the Mantoux test but no other signs of infection; and patients with clinical manifestations of tuberculosis. Mitigating factors include age, country of origin, infection with drug-resistant strains of *M. tuberculosis,* site of infection, pregnancy, intensity of disease, and immune status.

The various antibiotics currently used can be divided into two groups. The first-line antimycobacterial drugs include ethambutol, isoniazid (INH), pyrazinamide, rifampin, and streptomycin. The second-line drugs, which are either less effective or more difficult to use, include amikacin, aminosalicylate sodium, capreomycin, ciprofloxacin, clofazimine, dapsone, ethionamide, ofloxacin, and rifabutin.

Prevention. Patients with active pulmonary tuberculosis should be isolated during the first few weeks of treatment until acid-fast bacilli are no longer seen in sputum samples. Patients with extrapulmonary tuberculosis are not infectious to others and need not be isolated.

Community prevention of tuberculosis is carried out by one of two methods. In countries where tuberculosis is relatively infrequent, members of the general population may be routinely tested for tuberculosis by the Mantoux skin test. Children with positive skin test results and adults whose results have recently converted from negative to positive may be treated with INH as described in Table 9–4. In countries where tuberculosis is common, individuals are immunized with **bacillus Calmette-Guérin vaccine (BCG vaccine),** which consists of a live, attenuated strain of *M. bovis.*

BCG immunization is believed to act as a primary infection. When BCG-immunized persons are infected with *M. tuberculosis,* a vigorous CMIR response ensues and controls the infection. Thus, the purpose of BCG immunization is not to prevent infection but to ensure that any *M. tuberculosis* infection remains localized. This should reduce spread to others by preventing cavity formation and should protect the patient from developing disseminated disease.

Unfortunately, BCG immunization is not as effective as investigators hoped. Studies have shown that there is a wide variability in the protective efficacy of BCG, with efficacy rates ranging from 0% to about 80%. This variation is likely related to differences

TABLE 9–4.   Recommended Steps in the Management of Suspected or Confirmed Infection With *Mycobacterium tuberculosis*

Diagnosis Group	Management
Exposed individuals with negative results in the Mantoux test	For newborns, give isoniazid for 3 months. Repeat Mantoux test. If positive, give isoniazid plus rifampin for 3 more months.
	For children under 5 years of age, give isoniazid for 3 months. Repeat Mantoux test. If positive, give isoniazid for 3 more months.
	For older children or adults, repeat Mantoux test in 3 months. If positive, give isoniazid for 9 months.
Exposed individuals with positive results in the Mantoux test but no other signs of infection	For patients of all ages, give isoniazid for 6–12 months. If organisms are resistant to isoniazid or rifampin, give pyrazinamide plus ethambutol and monitor for retrobulbar neuritis.
Patients with clinical manifestations of tuberculosis	For patients with pulmonary tuberculosis, give a combination of three drugs—isoniazid, rifampin, and pyrazinamide—for 2 months, followed by isoniazid plus pyrazinamide for 4 months. Alternatively, give a combination of four drugs—isoniazid, rifampin, pyrazinamide, and either streptomycin or ethambutol—for 2 months by daily observed therapy, followed by isoniazid plus rifampin for 4 months.
	For patients with extrapulmonary tuberculosis, give the same treatment as for pulmonary tuberculosis but continue it for 9 months.
	For patients with meningitis, give a combination of four drugs—isoniazid, rifampin, pyrazinamide, and ethambutol—for 9 months.
	For patients with human immunodeficiency virus (HIV) infection or acquired immunodeficiency syndrome (AIDS), give a combination of three drugs—isoniazid, rifampin, and pyrazinamide—for 9 months or for 6 months beyond the point at which cultures become negative for *M. tuberculosis*.
	For patients with suspected or proved multidrug-resistant disease, give a combination of four drugs: (1) ethambutol; (2) pyrazinamide; (3) either amikacin, capreomycin, or kanamycin; and (4) either ciprofloxacin or ofloxacin.
	For patients who are pregnant, give a combination of three drugs—isoniazid, rifampin, and ethambutol—for 9 months. Do not give pyrazinamide or streptomycin.
	For patients with a relapse of tuberculosis, change the regimen to include at least two drugs not previously used.

both in BCG strains and in the virulence of *M. tuberculosis* strains that are prevalent in different locales. Efforts have been made to develop a killed vaccine. To date, however, BCG has proved to be more effective than killed vaccines, possibly for two reasons. First, BCG grows within the host, producing a larger dose of immunogen than the dose originally injected into the host. Second, as BCG grows, it releases multiple proteins, each of which elicits an immune response. Thus, the BCG vaccine is an expanding complex pool of antigens.

Some AIDS patients who were immunized with BCG subsequently developed disseminated BCG infection. For this reason, BCG should not be administered to immunocompromised patients.

Mycobacterium leprae

Mycobacterium leprae causes leprosy, a disease sometimes called **Hansen's disease** in the USA. The earliest description of leprosy originated in India around 600 B.C. Whether the Old Testament references to "leprosy" actually refer to the disease now known to be caused by *M. leprae* or instead refer to various forms of eczema is a point of controversy. The Hebrew word *tsara-ath,* which was translated as "leprosy" in English versions of the Bible, may be better translated as "ceremonial uncleanness."

Soldiers of Alexander the Great are believed to have carried leprosy back to Greece, and Straton (about 300–250 B.C.) described a new disease that he called elephantiasis Graecorum and is thought to have been leprosy. The term "lepra" was introduced in the 9th century by Johannes Damascenes, and leprosy became a common disease in Europe during the so-called Dark Ages. In 1873, the leprosy bacillus was first observed in tissues from leprosy patients, but it was not until 1971 that *M. leprae* was cultivated in nine-banded armadillos, an event that ushered in the modern era of leprosy research.

Today, leprosy is found worldwide and affects from 12 million to 13 million individuals. The disease is most commonly seen in sub-Saharan Africa, India, South America, the Philippines, Southeast Asia, and the South Pacific. In the USA, leprosy is endemic in California, Florida, Hawaii, Louisiana, and Texas. Leprosy in the USA has an incidence of about 100–150 new cases per year and a prevalence of about 6000 cases, but the infection in about 90% of these cases originates outside the country.

Characteristics of *M. leprae*

General Features. *M. leprae* is an acid-fast gram-positive bacillus that measures 0.3–0.5 μm by 4–7 μm. Unlike the acid-fastness of other mycobacteria, that of *M. leprae* can be extracted with pyridine. *M. leprae* is an intracellular bacterium that grows within macrophages, Schwann cells, endothelial cells, and epithelial cells. It has the longest generation time of any known human pathogen, doubling once every 11–13 days. *M. leprae* is thought to have a propensity for growing in cool tissues. It has never been cultivated in an artificial medium or cell culture. Instead, it is grown in animals, particularly mice (in mouse footpads) and nine-banded armadillos.

Mechanisms of Pathogenicity

(1) Components of the Cell Wall Complex.   The cell envelope structure of *M. leprae* is similar to that of the other mycobacteria, but the outermost layer of the complex is composed of phenolic glycolipids. The cell wall contains various virulence determinants (including arabinogalactan, lipoarabinomannan, and mycolic acids) and peptidoglycan, but *M. leprae* peptidoglycan contains glycine instead of alanine within its tetrapeptide.

(2) Host Response to Infection.   *M. leprae* grows well within macrophages. Its phagocytosis is accelerated when complement is activated, because entry into macrophages involves interactions between C3bi and CR3 on the macrophage surface. Once inside a macrophage, *M. leprae* blocks degranulation, and the macrophage becomes impervious to activation by interferon-gamma. A vigorous antibody response is generated and may contribute to pathogenicity by causing Arthus-type reactions in infected tissues. Recovery depends on development of a CMIR. When an inadequate CMIR develops, the clinical signs of disease appear.

Five major forms of the disease, each related to a different level of CMIR, have been identified (Table 9–5). Patients with a good CMIR develop the least severe form, which is called tuberculoid leprosy and is characterized by the formation of granulomas, the presence of few *M. leprae* bacilli in the body fluids, and the development of extensive nerve damage caused by CMIR efforts to eliminate the bacteria. Patients with a poor CMIR develop the most severe form, which is called lepromatous leprosy and is characterized by the absence of granulomas, the presence of huge numbers of bacilli in the body fluids, and the progressive development of disfiguring lesions.

The cellular response of patients with tuberculoid leprosy involves CD4$^+$ T cells of the Th1 subclass, while that of patients with lepromatous leprosy involves CD8$^+$ T cells of the Th2 subclass. Th1 T cells are the most effective in initiating an effective CMIR, and they produce the cytokines interleukin-2 (IL-2) and interferon-gamma. Skin lesions of patients with lepromatous leprosy contain elevated levels of type 2 cytokines, including IL-4 and IL-10. It appears that *M. leprae* causes macrophages in patients who develop lepromatous leprosy to release IL-10, which in turn causes CD4$^+$ T cells to become unresponsive.

The **Mitsuda skin test** may be administered to determine the immune status of patients and assess the form of leprosy present. This test uses an antigen preparation that is called **lepromin** and is obtained from infected armadillos. Patients with a positive reaction develop an area of red induration at the site of intradermal injection of lepromin after 24–48 hours (the Fernandez reaction), followed 3–4 weeks later by an epithelioid granuloma that is greater than 5 mm in diameter (the Mitsuda reaction). A positive Mitsuda reaction indicates that the patient is able to develop a CMIR to *M. leprae* antigens. About 90% of infected *and* uninfected individuals have a positive reaction in the Mitsuda test.

(3) Transmission of Infection.   Leprosy probably is spread from person to person via the respiratory secretions of patients with lepromatous leprosy or other forms of leprosy characterized by the presence of many bacilli. Children are thought to be most susceptible to infection. The usual incubation period is 2–5 years, but latent periods of up to 26 years have been described. Placental transmission may occur, and some believe that the bacilli may be disseminated to infants via breast milk.

In populations where leprosy is common, some individuals carry the bacilli transiently in the nasopharynx, and the organisms can survive weeks to months in wet or shaded soil. Thus, asymptomatic carriers and environmental samples are potential sources of infection.

About 95% of humans are naturally resistant to infection with *M. leprae,* and the outcome of infection is an HLA-linked phenomenon. Lymphocyte transformation studies have shown that about half of the close contacts of leprosy patients develop active cellular immunity against *M. leprae.* Thus, many close contacts are probably transiently infected with *M.*

TABLE 9–5.   Classification of Leprosy by the Ridley-Jopling System

Characteristic	Tuberculoid Leprosy (TT)	Borderline-Tuberculoid Leprosy (BT)	Borderline Leprosy (BB)	Borderline-Lepromatous Leprosy (BL)	Lepromatous Leprosy (LL)
Lesion type	Few and well-defined macules and plaques	More lesions than TT but less defined	More lesions than BT and borders are vague	Many lesions	Many macules and nodules
Nerve involvement	Early nerve damage and anesthesia	Damage common	Damage common but nerves not destroyed	Some nerve damage	Some late nerve damage
Grenz zone	No	Yes	Yes	Yes	Yes
Granulomas	Yes	Yes	Some	No	No
Foamy histiocytes	No	No	Some	Yes	Yes
Epithelioid cells	Many	Some	Some	No	No
Bacilli in lesions	Not seen	Rare	Some	Yes	Many
Bacilli in nerves	Rare	Some	Yes	Yes	Yes

leprae but are naturally resistant to developing disease. As many as 50% of some Asian populations develop lepromatous leprosy when infected, but only 5–10% of patients in Africa develop the lepromatous form of the disease. This variability in the course of the disease may also be an HLA-linked phenomenon.

Leprosy may be a zoonotic disease. Naturally occurring lepromatous leprosy has been described in nine-banded armadillos, chimpanzees, and sooty mangabey monkeys. One report has placed the incidence of leprosy in armadillos in Louisiana at about 10%, and there have been at least two reports of possible leprosy transmission from armadillos to humans.

Diseases Due to *M. leprae*

Classification of Disease. In 1966, D. S. Ridley and W. H. Jopling divided leprosy into five major forms, reflecting the immunologic status of patients and histologic presentation of disease. As Table 9–5 shows, the five forms of leprosy in this classification system are tuberculoid (TT), borderline-tuberculoid (BT), borderline (BB), borderline-lepromatous (BL), and lepromatous (LL).

At least four other forms of leprosy are reported in the medical literature, and these are known as indeterminate leprosy, Lucio's leprosy (spotted leprosy), neural leprosy, and histoid leprosy.

The World Health Organization has constructed a two-category system, based on the extent of infection. Patients are considered to have multibacillary infection (MB) if their skin smears reveal the presence of *M. leprae.* They are considered to have paucibacillary infection (PB) if their skin smears are negative or if they have three or fewer skin lesions and have no erythema, induration, or neuritis.

Diagnosis. Leprosy usually begins as indeterminate leprosy, with a hypopigmented or red lesion that is slightly hypoesthetic and appears on the trunk or a limb. What happens next depends on the immune response that is mounted. The three most recognizable forms of leprosy are lepromatous, tuberculoid, and borderline leprosy. The diagnosis of each of these is based on the history and physical examination and is confirmed by microscopic examination of samples taken from lesions. A small incision is made at the edge of an earlobe or along the margin of a lesion; the area is scraped; and the sample is smeared on a slide, stained by the Ziehl-Neelsen or Kinyoun method, and then examined for the presence of acid-fast rods. The number of bacteria per microscopic field is determined, along with the morphology and extent of staining of the individual organisms. Nasal secretions and punch biopsy samples of lesions can also be examined. Biopsy samples are best stained by the Fite-Ferraco method, rather than by acid-fast stains. Although a Mitsuda skin test may be administered to determine the immune status of the patient, the test is not used for the diagnosis of disease.

(1) Lepromatous Leprosy. Lepromatous leprosy is characterized by severe, progressive, disfiguring lesions that may affect the face and ears, as well as the exterior surface of the extremities. Patients commonly lose their eyebrows. Invasion of the larynx may cause the voice to change; testicular invasion may cause sterility; and invasion of the nasal mucosa causes the nose to become "stuffy." Early lesions are slightly hypoesthetic, and the lesions may become anesthetic. As the nerve trunks become more heavily infected, there is sensory loss that tends to be bilateral and relatively symmetric. The degree of sensory loss is much less in lepromatous leprosy than in tuberculoid leprosy.

The peripheral nerve trunks, skin, nasal secretions, larynx, eyes, testes, and blood contain many leprosy bacilli. Nasal secretions may contain up to 10^7 bacilli per milliliter. The lesions also contain many histiocytes filled with lipids (foamy histiocytes), but there are few lymphocytes (Fig. 9–5). The usual type of lesion is surrounded by a layer of collagen known as the grenz zone. However, patients in Mexico may develop diffuse cutaneous infiltrations rather than discrete lesions. The affected areas contain infected endothelial cells and exhibit punched-out ulcerations (Lucio's phenomenon). The condition characterized by these ulcerations is called **Lucio's leprosy,** or **spotted leprosy.**

About 50% of patients with lepromatous leprosy experience hypersensitivity reactions. These so-called **reversal reactions,** which are most common in patients with borderline disease, are believed to be a cellular response to previously masked *M. leprae* antigens. Lesions intensify and become edematous as lymphocytes and giant cells collect within them. After a period of intense neuritis, the lesions return to the form that preceded the reaction.

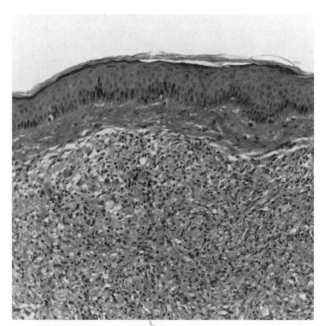

FIGURE 9–5. A cross-section of a dermal lesion of lepromatous leprosy. Note the predominance of histiocytes. (Courtesy of Armed Forces Institute of Pathology. AFIP photo 65-1653.)

Erythema nodosum leprosum is an immune complex reaction that occurs in patients with lepromatous or borderline-lepromatous leprosy. The reaction is similar to the erythema nodosum seen in streptococcal and coccidioidal infections, with development of tender subcutaneous nodules on extensor surfaces of the legs or arms (Fig. 9–6). Nodule formation is often accompanied by constitutional symptoms, including malaise, fever, and inflammation of the iris and ciliary body (iridocyclitis).

Patients with lepromatous leprosy have extremely high levels of antibody to *M. leprae,* but this immune response is ineffective, since recovery from leprosy requires development of an effective CMIR. Patients with lepromatous leprosy show negative results in the Mitsuda skin test. They also generate a serum factor that inactivates the complement components C3 and C5.

Untreated patients may develop waxy deposits of immunoglobulin light chains in the viscera. This condition, known as amyloidosis, is sometimes fatal.

(2) Tuberculoid Leprosy.   Patients with tuberculoid leprosy have mounted an active CMIR to *M. leprae.* As a result, they show positive results in the Mitsuda skin test, and *M. leprae* is difficult to locate in lesions or body fluids. Unlike lepromatous leprosy, tuberculoid leprosy is accompanied by a modest rise or no rise in the titer of antibodies to *M. leprae.* The disease is referred to as tuberculoid leprosy because patients develop red cutaneous nodules that resemble tubercles (are "tuberculoid") and contain granulomas (Figs. 9–7 and 9–8). Most patients have only one nodule or a small number of them.

As bacteria invade nerves, the CMIR attacks the infected nerves and causes considerable damage. Thus, nerve damage and anesthesia are prominent features of tuberculoid leprosy. Sensory nerves are usually the first and most severely affected, but motor and autonomic nerves may also be damaged. Some of the effects of nerve damage include tissue necrosis, loss of sweating, loss of vasomotor functions, and

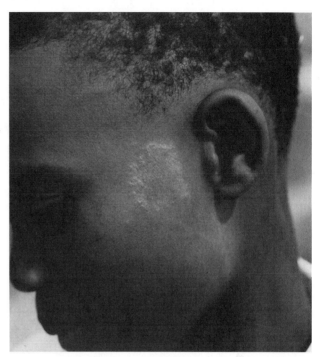

FIGURE 9–7. A single lesion in tuberculoid leprosy. (Courtesy of Armed Forces Institute of Pathology. AFIP photo 75-15598.)

development of secondary bacterial infections such as osteomyelitis and cellulitis.

(3) Borderline Leprosy.   Borderline leprosy is characterized by flat lesions that are white or red. Patients with borderline leprosy have bacteria within lesions and nerves and show equivocal or positive results in the Mitsuda skin test. Nerve damage and anesthesia occur, but lesions contain few granulomas and foamy histiocytes. Patients with borderline leprosy often suffer from clawing of the hands, footdrop, or facial palsy.

Treatment.   Effective treatment of leprosy re-

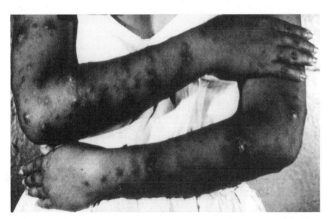

FIGURE 9–6. Clinical manifestations of erythema nodosum leprosum. (Courtesy of Armed Forces Institute of Pathology. AFIP photo 74-9029-7.)

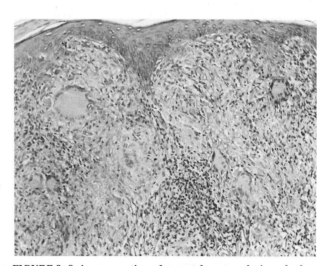

FIGURE 9–8. A cross-section of a granulomatous lesion of tuberculoid leprosy. The lesion is filled with epithelioid cells, Langhans' giant cells, and lymphocytes. (Courtesy of Armed Forces Institute of Pathology. AFIP photo 72-12465.)

quires combination drug therapy that usually involves two or more of the following: dapsone, clofazimine, rifampin, and ethionamide. Dapsone and clofazimine are both bacteriostatic, whereas the other two drugs are bactericidal.

Paucibacillary forms of leprosy are commonly treated with dapsone plus rifampin for 6 months. Multibacillary forms are generally treated with a combination of dapsone, clofazimine, and rifampin for at least 2 years. Ethionamide may be substituted for clofazimine. Attacks of erythema nodosum leprosum may be treated with prednisone or thalidomide.

Prevention. Efforts are under way to develop a leprosy vaccine, but none now exists. BCG has been used as a vaccine against leprosy with some success. Currently, most efforts are directed toward identifying patients with leprosy and ensuring that they receive adequate treatment. Family members and close contacts are identified and treated in the same manner as patients with paucibacillary leprosy. Patients with multibacillary leprosy are separated from prolonged contact with children until the disease enters remission.

"ATYPICAL" MYCOBACTERIA

Early studies of mycobacteria focused on *Mycobacterium tuberculosis* and its common manifestations of disease. When other bacteria were occasionally identified as causes of a tuberculosislike illness that was atypical in its course and caused atypical results in the tuberculin skin test, these bacteria were called atypical mycobacteria. They are members of a large group of mycobacteria that are found in soil and water and have gained increasing recognition as important opportunistic environmental agents. Along with this increased recognition has been a movement to assign the atypical mycobacteria a designation that better typifies them. Some investigators commonly refer to them as **mycobacteria other than tubercle bacilli** (MOTT bacilli), while others prefer to call them **potentially pathogenic environmental mycobacteria** (PPEM). The discussion that follows uses the designation PPEM to emphasize that these organisms are important opportunistic environmental bacteria.

Based on the classification system of E. H. Runyon, the PPEM are divided into four large groups: photochromogens (group I), scotochromogens (group II), nonphotochromogens (group III), and rapid-growing mycobacteria (group IV). In contrast to the **rapid-growing mycobacteria,** which form colonies on agar within 7 days, the other three groups require more than 7 days to form colonies. **Photochromogens** produce pigments after exposure to light; **scotochromogens** produce pigments in the dark; and **nonphotochromogens** fail to produce pigments. Some PPEM are not categorized within the four Runyon groups.

PPEM are similar to the pathogenic mycobacteria in having complex cell walls that contain mycolic acids, arabinomannan, and peptides, and they survive within unstimulated macrophages. Infections may be evidenced by borderline or false-positive results in the tuberculin skin test.

At least a dozen species of PPEM have been identified as significant causes of human disease (Table 9–6). The most important of these are the *Mycobacterium avium-intracellulare* complex, *Mycobacterium kansasii, Mycobacterium marinum,* and *Mycobacterium scrofulaceum.*

The *Mycobacterium avium-intracellulare* Complex

The *Mycobacterium avium-intracellulare* complex (MAC), once known as the Battey bacillus, is a complex of mycobacteria that are ubiquitous in nature and are commonly found in soil and water samples. The organisms rarely cause disease in immunocompetent individuals but are important opportunistic pathogens with a special predilection for causing disease in patients with AIDS.

Characteristics of the *M. avium-intracellulare* Complex

General Features. MAC is a complex of 28 serovars of two mycobacterial species, *Mycobacterium avium* and *Mycobacterium intracellulare*. The first of these can be divided into three subspecies, known as *Mycobacterium avium avium, Mycobacterium avium paratuberculosis,* and *Mycobacterium avium silvaticum.* Although three colony types of MAC are seen, it is the smooth transparent colonies that are usually isolated from diseased patients, and various studies have shown that the bacteria in these colonies are more resistant to antibiotics and more virulent than the bacteria in the other two colony types.

Mechanisms of Pathogenicity

(1) Components of the Cell Wall Complex. MAC is similar to *Mycobacterium tuberculosis* in that is has a complex cell envelope containing arabinogalactan, peptidoglycan, lipoarabinomannan, and mycolic acids. Thus, MAC is fairly impermeable to antibiotics and resists being killed by acids and alkalies. Polar and apolar glycopeptidolipids serve as key surface antigens for MAC.

(2) Dynamics of Infection. MAC is an opportunistic pathogen that is believed to enter immunocompromised patients through the gastrointestinal tract, and studies have shown that the organisms invade intestinal epithelial cells in vitro. A 27-kD protein has been tentatively identified as the MAC adhesin for fibroblasts and epithelial cells. MAC organisms also multiply within unstimulated macrophages. It appears that they enter macrophages via parasite-directed phagocytosis and that entry involves either the macrophage CR3 receptor or the integrin-fibronectin receptor. Like *M. tuberculosis,* MAC inhibits lysosomal fusion with the phagosome, and both superoxide dismutase and heat shock proteins allow the phagocytosed MAC to resist intraphagosomal killing.

MAC organisms in the intestine multiply in the gut-associated lymphoid tissue for 4–5 months, after

TABLE 9–6. Atypical *Mycobacterium* Species Associated With Human Disease

Runyon Classification	Species	Disease	Treatment
Group I	*Mycobacterium asiatica*	Chronic pulmonary disease.	No general recommendation.
	Mycobacterium kansasii	Chronic pulmonary disease or osteomyelitis.	Rifampin plus isoniazid plus ethambutol.
		Cervical or cutaneous lymphadenopathy, soft tissue infection, or granulomatous tenosynovitis.	Surgery.
	Mycobacterium marinum	Swimming pool granuloma.	Rifampin plus ethambutol plus surgery.
	Mycobacterium simiae	Chronic pulmonary disease.	No general recommendation.
Group II	*Mycobacterium gordonae*	Pulmonary, bone, or skin infection.	Rifampin plus isoniazid plus ethambutol.
	Mycobacterium scrofulaceum	Cervical lymphadenopathy.	Surgery; or rifampin plus cycloserine plus either isoniazid or streptomycin.
	Mycobacterium szulgai	Chronic pulmonary disease.	No general recommendation.
	Mycobacterium xenopi	Chronic pulmonary disease.	No general recommendation.
Group III	*Mycobacterium avium-intracellulare* complex	Pulmonary disease.	Clarithromycin in combination with ethambutol, clofazimine, or ciprofloxacin.
		Subacute lymphadenitis.	Surgery.
		Disseminated disease.	Either a combination of rifabutin plus ethambutol or a combination of clarithromycin plus clofazimine.
	Mycobacterium haemophilum	Disseminated granulomas.	No general recommendation.
Group IV	*Mycobacterium fortuitum-chelonae* complex	Skin, soft tissue, pulmonary, bone, or intestinal infection; hepatitis; keratitis; endocarditis after heart surgery; or prosthetic valve infection.	A combination of amikacin plus cefoxitin plus probenecid; followed by trimethoprim plus sulfamethoxazole for *M. fortuitum* or by clarithromycin for *M. chelonae*.
No group	*Mycobacterium ulcerans*	Buruli ulcer.	Ethambutol plus trimethoprim plus sulfamethoxazole plus surgery.

which they enter the blood. During the early phase of infection, the mesenteric lymph nodes and Peyer's patches become heavily infected, and the intestinal epithelium may be substantially eroded. Intestinal erosion causes the patient to suffer from chronic diarrhea. Mycobacteremia is seen in 75–85% of patients during the first year of infection and is the route by which organisms spread to ectopic sites. This differs from *M. tuberculosis* infections, in which mycobacteremia is rarely seen. MAC may disseminate to various organs, with pulmonary, gastrointestinal, liver, spleen, lymphatic, bone marrow, and skin infections most commonly seen.

(3) Host Response to Infection. Recovery from MAC infection involves generation of an effective CMIR. The stimulation of T cells elicits cytokine production and macrophage activation that result in intraleukocytic killing of MAC. Interferon-gamma potentiates the ability of macrophages to kill some MAC strains, and both granulocyte-macrophage colony-stimulating factor (GM-CSF) and TNF increase the killing of phagocytosed MAC. Although the bulk of the T cell response involves expansion of alpha/beta TCR-bearing CD4+ T cell clones, there seems to be selective expansion of gamma/delta T cells, particularly V-delta-9 and V-delta-2 T cells. It is also believed that effective immunity involves the killing of infected macrophages by natural killer cells.

(4) Transmission of Infection. Although MAC organisms are found worldwide, disease is most prevalent in northern regions, particularly in the USA, Canada, Europe, and Japan. MAC infections are rare

in individuals with normal immune systems. About 98% of MAC infections in AIDS patients and 60% of MAC infections in non-AIDS patients are due to *M. avium*. Fresh water and salt water constitute the greatest single source of human infections, but poultry-associated *M. avium* infections have been documented. Most patients are infected by ingesting the organisms, which then attach to and multiply in the gut-associated lymphoid tissue.

One study showed that the risk of MAC infection in AIDS patients was 21% at 1 year after the AIDS diagnosis and 43% at 2 years. At 1 year after the AIDS diagnosis, 39% of patients with CD4+ cell counts under 10/μL were infected with MAC but only 3% of patients with CD4+ counts of 100–200/μL were infected. This makes MAC quite different from *M. tuberculosis*, whose infection rates have not been observed to vary in this manner with CD4+ cell counts. In fact, a diagnosis of tuberculosis precedes the AIDS diagnosis in 50–75% of AIDS patients, but most MAC infections in AIDS patients occur late in the course of AIDS, when CD4+ counts are under 100/μL.

Diseases Due to the
M. avium-intracellulare Complex

Diagnosis. The three forms of MAC disease most often diagnosed are pulmonary disease, subacute lymphadenitis, and disseminated disease. The form found most often in immunocompetent patients is pulmonary disease, while that in immunocompromised patients is disseminated disease. Confirmation of the diagnosis of MAC disease depends on cultivating the organisms from sputum, blood, stool, or biopsy samples. Sputum samples are usually culture-negative, but about 75–85% of patients with MAC disease have bacteremia, and about half have MAC in their stools.

At least two culture systems should be used. One sample should be used to inoculate a radioactive BACTEC culture system, such as the BACTEC TB system or BACTEC 13A medium. A second sample should be used to inoculate a standard agar or egg-based medium such as Middlebrook 7H11 or Löwenstein-Jensen medium. Because the MAC organisms are primarily within macrophages, isolation is potentiated by using a commercial lysis-centrifugation technique to liberate the intracellular organisms. Cultures may yield positive results in 7–14 days with the BACTEC system and in 21 days or longer with the conventional medium. DNA probes can then be used to confirm the identity of the sample growth as MAC.

(1) Pulmonary Disease. MAC pulmonary disease is seen most often in white men who are 45–65 years old and have a preexisting pulmonary disease, such as inactive or active tuberculosis, cystic fibrosis, bronchiectasis, chronic obstructive pulmonary disease, emphysema, chronic or recurrent pneumonia, pneumoconiosis, or bronchogenic carcinoma. Clinical manifestations of MAC pulmonary disease are similar to those of pulmonary tuberculosis and include chronic productive cough (sometimes accompanied by hemoptysis), dyspnea, fever, night sweats, malaise, and fatigue. About 75% of immunocompetent patients have radiographic evidence of thin-walled infiltrated cavities, usually in the apex and anterior segments of the upper lobes. The lesions of MAC pulmonary disease are granulomas, and they may be caseating or noncaseating. Many patients experience granulomatous vasculitis or nonspecific interstitial pneumonitis. Patients with AIDS are more likely to exhibit diffuse interstitial or reticulonodular infiltrates without forming cavities, and granulomas that form are poorly organized.

Fairly mild pulmonary MAC disease of the middle lobe or the lingula pulmonis sinistri has also been reported among elderly women. This disease is called Lady Windermere's disease, named for a character in an Oscar Wilde play who had a fastidious habit of suppressing her cough—a habit that may predispose elderly women to MAC infection.

(2) Subacute Lymphadenitis. MAC is the most common cause of subacute lymphadenitis in children under 5 years of age. The lymph nodes involved are most often those in the neck and face. Cervical, submandibular, submaxillary, or preauricular lymphadenopathy may be caused by MAC (63–80% of cases); *Mycobacterium scrofulaceum* (10–20% of cases); *M. tuberculosis;* or *Bartonella (Rochalimaea) henselae,* the agent of cat-scratch disease. Usually, several nodes on one side of the body are involved and are swollen but not painful. Subacute lymphadenitis rarely occurs among MAC-infected patients with AIDS.

(3) Disseminated Disease. More than 90% of individuals with disseminated MAC disease are AIDS patients. When first seen by a physician, many patients report that they have suffered for 2 weeks with diarrhea, vomiting, abdominal pain, and weight loss. When MAC disease progresses, it is associated with intermittent fever, night sweats, anorexia, and weakness, in addition to symptoms and signs reflecting the presence of inflammation in involved organs. Almost any organ system may be infected, including the skin, brain, adrenal glands, testes, large airways, gastrointestinal tract, bones, joints, eyes, and thyroid.

Differential Diagnosis. Because tuberculosis in AIDS patients follows a fulminating course but MAC disease follows a much milder course, it is important to differentiate between tuberculosis and MAC disease. A comparison of findings is presented in Table 9–7.

Treatment. MAC infections fail to respond to most antibiotics used routinely to treat other mycobacterial infections. Immunocompetent patients with chronic pulmonary MAC disease or disseminated MAC disease are usually treated with clarithromycin plus one of the following: ethambutol, clofazimine, or ciprofloxacin. Immunocompromised patients with disseminated disease may be treated either with a combination of rifabutin plus ethambutol or with a combination of clarithromycin plus clofazimine. Children with subacute lymphadenitis can usually be cured by surgically removing infected lymph nodes.

Mycobacterium kansasii

Although infections caused by *Mycobacterium kansasii* are similar to those caused by the *Mycobacterium avium-intracellulare* complex (MAC), *M. kansasii* is responsible for more severe disease in normal hosts. This may be because *M. kansasii* elicits the

TABLE 9–7. A Comparison of Tuberculosis and Disseminated Disease Caused by the *Mycobacterium avium-intracellulare* Complex (MAC)

Characteristic	Tuberculosis	Disseminated Disease Caused by MAC
Staining of sputum sample yields positive results	60% of cases	16% of cases
Culture of sputum sample yields positive results	50–80% of cases	25% of cases
Mantoux test yields positive results	Yes	No
Bacteremia is present	2–12% of cases	75–85% of cases
Chest x-ray yields abnormal results	80–90% of cases	25% of cases
Hilar lymphadenopathy is present	25% of cases	Rarely
Acquired immunodeficiency syndrome (AIDS) is present	<30% of cases	>90% of cases
Immune status of patient	Competent or compromised	Compromised; CD4$^+$ cells <100/μL

release of significantly less TNF-α and IL-6 from macrophages than MAC elicits.

Characteristics of *M. kansasii*

M. kansasii is an environmental mycobacterium that stains unevenly with the Ziehl-Neelsen (acid-fast) stain, giving it a barred or beaded appearance. When *M. kansasii* is cultivated on a standard medium and placed in the dark, it grows as smooth, ivory-colored colonies after 1–2 weeks. When cultivated in the light, its colonies are initially lemon-yellow but gradually turn orange or reddish-orange owing to the accumulation of beta-carotene crystals. As a result, *M. kansasii* was initially known as "the yellow bacillus." *M. kansasii* cross-reacts immunologically with *Mycobacterium tuberculosis,* and infection produces cross-reactive results in the tuberculin skin test.

Diseases Due to *M. kansasii*

Infections caused by *M. kansasii* occur most often in Texas, Louisiana, Florida, Illinois, and California. Men with disease outnumber women 3:1, and most infections occur in people living in large urban areas. Disease occurs most often in middle-aged white men who either have preexisting lung disease or are immunocompromised. A single large study reported that 0.2% of patients with AIDS were infected with *M. kansasii.* However, a study of AIDS patients in Louisiana, where *M. kansasii* infections are prevalent, showed that 31.9% of AIDS patients were infected with *M. kansasii.*

M. kansasii most often causes chronic pulmonary disease that looks much like classic pulmonary tuberculosis. The disease progresses slowly over many years, with multiple thin-walled cavities forming in the upper lobe of the lung. The disease is generally milder than the pulmonary disease caused by *M. tuberculosis.* AIDS patients, however, may develop disseminated disease that can be rapidly fatal.

M. kansasii infections are usually treated with a combination of rifampin, isoniazid (INH), and ethambutol. For patients with HIV infection, treatment is commonly continued for a minimum of 15 months. If cervical or cutaneous lymphadenitis is present, the nodes should be surgically excised.

Mycobacterium scrofulaceum

Mycobacterium scrofulaceum is a slow-growing mycobacterium that takes 4–6 weeks to form colonies. It grows as smooth, buttery colonies that are light yellow to deep orange.

M. scrofulaceum causes **cervical lymphadenitis,** a disease that was formerly called **scrofula** and generally affects young children. Investigators believe that cervical lymphadenitis originates endogenously from the mycobacteria in the throat and mouth, and some think that the infection spreads when new teeth erupt and the tooth eruption disturbs the gums. Affected patients are usually between 18 months and 4 years of age. Lymph nodes high in the neck area near the mandible swell, and some nodes may suppurate and drain. The nodes are not painful, and most patients are otherwise healthy, with no constitutional symptoms.

Cervical lymphadenitis can also be caused by other mycobacteria, including *Mycobacterium tuberculosis* and the *Mycobacterium avium-intracellulare* complex.

Most patients recover completely from lymphadenitis if the infected nodes are surgically removed. Antibiotics are rarely indicated. When they are indicated, isoniazid (INH) or streptomycin can be combined with rifampin and cycloserine.

Mycobacterium marinum

Mycobacterium marinum is commonly found in unchlorinated fresh or salt water. It grows optimally at 30–32 °C and grows poorly or not at all at 37 °C. Deep yellow colonies appear in 8–14 days when the organism is cultivated on a standard mycobacterial medium.

M. marinum causes a noncaseating granulomatous infection known commonly as **swimming pool granuloma.** Patients become infected when minor skin abrasions are exposed to inadequately chlorinated fresh or salt water, such as in swimming pools, tropical fish aquariums, and water cooling towers. A small papule forms in 2–3 weeks, gradually increases in size, and becomes a suppurative ulcer. The subcutaneous lesions are tender and red or reddish-blue, and they are most often located on the knee, elbow, toe, or finger. The lesions of swimming pool granuloma generally heal in several months, but occasionally a patient has a lesion that persists for 2 years or longer. Some patients develop chronic lesions that spread to the lymphatic system.

The diagnosis of *M. marinum* infection is confirmed by examining ulcer exudates or biopsy specimens for the microscopic presence of acid-fast bacilli. Samples can also be cultured and identified.

Treatment usually consists of surgical removal of the granulomas and administration of rifampin plus ethambutol. Minocycline or trimethoprim-sulfamethoxazole may also be useful.

NOCARDIA SPECIES

Nocardia species are nonsporulating gram-positive bacteria that are partially acid-fast. Partial acid-fastness is the ability to avoid decolorization when treated with 1% sulfuric acid or 3% hydrochloric acid. Nocardiae are decolorized in the Ziehl-Neelsen or Kinyoun stains when acid-alcohol is used as the decolorizing agent. The nocardiae appear as branching filaments that tend to fragment into rods and cocci. They are considered to be aerobic actinomycetes and are similar to *Rhodococcus* and *Oerskovia.*

Nocardia species are found in mud, peat, muddy water, compost, and rotting vegetables. It is believed that nocardiae may also grow as saprophytic pathogens in respiratory lesions. When grown on a standard medium, they can be cultivated at temperatures as high as 45 °C. They grow as tough, adherent colonies in 3 days to 2 weeks and emit an odor reminiscent of freshly turned soil or a musty basement.

Nocardia species have complex cell walls, containing *meso*-diaminopimelic acid, arabinose, and galactose. Like the mycobacteria, the nocardiae have mycolic acids. Nocardiae survive within macrophages, possibly by inhibiting lysosome fusion and by using external catalase and superoxide dismutase to detoxify oxygen-derived products.

Nocardia asteroides

Nocardia asteroides is primarily an opportunistic pathogen that causes **nocardiosis** in patients with underlying immunodeficiencies. Patients inhale airborne spores, and the nocardiae multiply in the lungs, where they cause primary pneumonitis and resist being destroyed by nonactivated macrophages. Patients suffer from fever and a cough that produces mucopurulent sputum. The infection may follow a wide variety of courses, with some patients developing pleural effusions, others developing lobar pneumonia or bronchopneumonia with extensive consolidation, and still others developing sinus tracts that connect a lung abscess to the chest wall.

Between 50% and 70% of patients with pulmonary disease develop ectopic foci of infection as a consequence of the nocardiae traveling through the blood. Almost any organ may become infected, but brain abscesses are reported in about 30% of patients and kidney infections are also common. Ectopic nocardial abscesses tend to become necrotic and contain many polymorphonuclear leukocytes.

Nocardiosis is confirmed by visualizing the organisms in exudate samples and by culture. Exudates often contain yellow, red, brown, black, or white granules that represent aggregated colonies of *Nocardia* and are known as sulfur granules. These granules can be crushed, stained, and examined microscopically. Visualization of *Nocardia* in biopsy specimens can be aided by first digesting the material with *N*-acetyl-L-cysteine. Nocardiae will appear as partially acid-fast, gram-positive, branching filaments that form no endospores. *Nocardia* can be cultivated on a wide variety of media, including media used for mycobacteria or fungi.

Patients with milder forms of pulmonary nocardiosis are usually treated with trimethoprim-sulfamethoxazole (TMP/SMX) or a sulfonamide. Patients with brain abscesses or overwhelming disease are treated with sulfamethoxazole or TMP/SMX plus ceftriaxone plus amikacin. Ectopic nocardiosis does not respond well to treatment and is associated with a 45% mortality rate in treated patients.

Nocardia brasiliensis

Introduction of *Nocardia brasiliensis* into a foot wound can result in the formation of a granulomatous abscess known as **Madura foot.** This disease is frequently caused by other actinomycetes or by fungi

and is discussed below (see *Actinomadura* Species). Nocardiae introduced into a wound can also cause a lymphocutaneous disease that is similar in appearance to a fungal disease known as sporotrichosis. Laboratory diagnosis is as described for *Nocardia asteroides*.

Infections caused by *N. brasiliensis* may be treated with amoxicillin plus clavulanate or with amikacin plus ceftriaxone.

ACTINOMYCES AND ACTINOMADURA SPECIES

Actinomyces and *Actinomadura* are normal residents of the human oropharynx and may be facultative anaerobes, obligate anaerobes, or microaerophilic bacteria. They are grouped with *Bifidobacterium, Eubacterium,* and *Propionibacterium* as anaerobic, non–spore-forming, gram-positive bacilli that are not acid-fast. *Actinomyces* and *Actinomadura* appear microscopically as club-shaped or branched rods. When they are seen in oral samples, they are referred to as "diphtheroids" because of their general morphologic resemblance to the agent of diphtheria, *Corynebacterium diphtheriae.*

Actinomyces Species

Actinomyces species are cultivated anaerobically or microaerophilically on blood agar. They are identified by their microscopic morphology (branching filaments), by their relative requirement for oxygen, and by their production of acetic acid, lactic acid, and succinic acid when cultivated in peptone–yeast extract–glucose medium. The most important actinomycotic pathogen, *Actinomyces israelii,* is identified by its rough growth on agar, its slow growth, its ability to hydrolyze esculin but be inhibited by bile, and its ability to ferment glucose, mannitol, and rhamnose.

Human infections are most often caused by *A. israelii* organisms that are residents of the oropharynx. It is believed that trauma or surgery, including dental work, is usually the event that precipitates infection. *Actinomyces* species are also found in the soil, and some infections may occur as a consequence of soil entering a deep wound.

Actinomyces causes destructive abscesses of the connective tissues. The abscesses tend to expand into adjacent tissues and form burrowing sinus tracts that extend to the skin. The lesions may become walled off by granulomatous material, and a purulent exudate may drain from open skin lesions. Abscesses due to *Actinomyces* occur most often in the cecum and appendix (up to 50% of cases), the face and neck (30–60% of cases), and the lungs and chest wall (up to 20% of cases).

Laboratory diagnosis involves identifying sulfur granules in purulent exudates. These granules are clusters of *Actinomyces* colonies and may be several millimeters in diameter. The colonies are crushed, stained, and examined for the presence of the typical gram-positive diphtheroid rods or branched filaments. Samples from lesions are cultured anaerobically, and organisms are identified by their cultural and biochemical characteristics. Immunofluorescence can be used to speciate *Actinomyces* isolates.

Most *Actinomyces* infections are treated with penicillin G or ampicillin, and the lesions are drained or excised surgically. Cervicofacial lesions respond well to treatment, with about 90% of patients recovering, but other abscesses do not reliably respond well. Doxycycline or ceftriaxone can be used as an alternative treatment.

Actinomadura Species

Actinomadura species are aerobic actinomycetes that are found in the soil. They form tough, membranous colonies of branched filaments that bear short chains of conidia. *Actinomadura* species are not acid-fast. They hydrolyze casein, tyrosine, and hypoxanthine but do not hydrolyze xanthine.

Actinomadura madurae or *Actinomadura pelletieri* is sometimes the cause of a suppurative foot infection known as **Madura foot.** Soil organisms are introduced into a foot wound, and a purulent lesion with interconnecting sinuses develops. Worldwide, about 50% of Madura foot lesions are caused by *Actinomadura* species, with most of the rest due to fungi or *Nocardia brasiliensis.* The fungus *Pseudoallescheria boydii* is the most common cause of Madura foot in the USA, whereas nocardiae predominate in Mexico and *Actinomadura* species are prevalent causes in Africa and Asia.

Madura foot is sometimes referred to as **actinomycotic mycetoma.** It was first described in 1842 by Dr. Gill, who was a member of the Madras Medical Service of the British Army and offered the following report about a patient from the Madurai region of India: "When the leg has been amputated, the foot has been found to be one mass of fibrocartilaginous nature, with entire destruction of joints, cartilages, and ligaments; it has neither shape nor feature and is covered with large fungoid excrescences discharging an offensive ichorous fluid." As Fig. 9–9 shows,

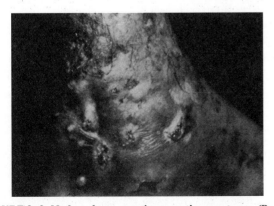

FIGURE 9–9. Madura foot, or actinomycotic mycetoma. (Reproduced, with permission, from Rippon, J. W. Medical Mycology: The Pathogenic Fungi and the Pathogenic Actinomycetes, 3rd ed. Philadelphia, W. B. Saunders Company, 1988.)

Dr. Gill's description was particularly apt. The diagnosis of *Actinomadura* infection is confirmed by examination of sulfur granules and by culture.

Patients with Madura foot are treated with streptomycin sulfate in combination with either trimethoprim-sulfamethoxazole or dapsone. In addition, the abscessed area of the foot is surgically resected.

OTHER FUNGUSLIKE BACTERIA
Streptomyces Species

Members of the genus *Streptomyces* are soil organisms that are valuable to the pharmaceutical industry because some species produce antibiotics. For example, *Streptomyces aureofaciens* synthesizes tetracycline and chlortetracycline; *Streptomyces erythreus* produces erythromycin; *Streptomyces niveus* produces novobiocin; and *Streptomyces venezuelae* produces chloramphenicol.

Streptomyces species are gram-positive bacteria that grow as branching filaments with aerial hyphae that bear conidia. They differ from *Nocardia* in that they are sensitive to lysozyme and are not partially acid-fast. *Streptomyces* species hydrolyze casein, xanthine, and tyrosine.

Streptomyces species only rarely cause human infections. Like the nocardiae, *Streptomyces somaliensis* can cause **mycetomas** when soil is introduced into a wound. These mycetomas occur in eastern Africa, India, and Mexico. The conidia of *Streptomyces* species can also cause **farmer's lung** in allergic patients. This pulmonary allergic response is described more fully in the discussion of *Aspergillus* in Chapter 18.

Streptomyces infections are not responsive to antibiotic therapy. Mycetomas caused by *Streptomyces* species are treated by surgery.

Tropheryma whippelii

In 1907, the *Bulletin of Johns Hopkins Hospital* carried a clinical report of a 36-year-old medical missionary who suffered from migratory polyarthritis, diarrhea, malabsorption syndrome, weight loss, cough, and mesenteric lymphadenitis. The writer of the report, George Whipple, indicated that he found "great numbers of a rod-shaped organism" within silver-stained lymph node sections, but he was unable to culture organisms from any clinical sample. Almost 90 years have passed since Whipple's original description of the disease, and many clinicians have confirmed the presence of what appear to be gram-positive bacteria within macrophages of patients who suffer from **Whipple's disease.** Yet the responsible organism remains uncultured.

In 1961, two groups reported that electron microscopy showed that the intracellular rods were indeed bacteria and were probably gram-positive bacteria. Others had long noted that curative antibiotic therapy caused the rods to break up and disappear, suggesting that they were bacteria. Several groups claimed to have cultivated the rods, but they were unable to repeat their results or to fulfill Koch's postulates with their sample outgrowth.

In 1992, two groups used polymerase chain reaction (PCR) technology to amplify 16S rRNA segments from samples taken from several patients with Whipple's disease, and they identified the putative agent as an actinomycete. K. H. Wilson and colleagues believed that the rRNA sequence was most like that of *Rhodococcus, Arthrobacter,* and *Streptomyces,* and they assigned it a place within the genus *Rhodococcus.* D. A. Relman and colleagues disagreed, presenting evidence that there was some distance between the sequences of *Rhodococcus* and those of the putative agent; they named the agent *Tropheryma whippelii.* Until the responsible organism is cultured and Koch's postulates are fulfilled, this controversy will continue.

Whipple's disease usually affects the central nervous system, mesentery, and heart but can affect almost any organ system. More than 90% of patients with Whipple's disease are white men between the ages of 20 and 67 years. The typical patient is a middle-aged man who has had arthritis, arthralgia, or both for 10–30 years and seeks medical assistance because of diarrhea, abdominal pain, and weight loss. Some patients exhibit lymphadenopathy, fever, and increased skin pigmentation. Depending on the organ system involved, dementia, ataxia, paresis, hearing loss, visual impairment, pericarditis, or other manifestations may also be noted.

Patients who present with the combination of diarrhea, abdominal pain, steatorrhea, weight loss due to fat malabsorption, and long-standing arthralgia should be examined by bowel or lymph node biopsy. Lymph node samples from patients with Whipple's disease contain numerous foamy macrophages bearing diastase-resistant inclusions that stain with periodic acid–Schiff (PAS) stain. These PAS-positive macrophages are often abundant in the lamina propria of the small bowel of patients suffering from steatorrhea. The inclusions are the rod-shaped or sickle-shaped bacteria of Whipple's disease.

Accurate diagnosis of Whipple's disease is critical, because untreated patients invariably die of malabsorption syndrome—that is, they starve to death.

Patients are usually treated with penicillin G plus streptomycin for 10–14 days, followed by a 1-year regimen of tetracycline, chloramphenicol, or trimethoprim-sulfamethoxazole. Patient compliance is critical, because most patients who fail to complete their treatment regimen have a relapse of disease.

Selected Readings

Balusbramanian, V., et al. Pathogenesis of tuberculosis: pathway to apical localization. Tuber Lung Dis 75:168–178, 1994.

Behling, C. A., et al. Development of a trehalose 6,6'-dimycolate model which explains cord formation by *Mycobacterium tuberculosis.* Infect Immun 61:2296–2303, 1993.

Boom, W. H., et al. Characterization of a 10- to 14-kilodalton protease-sensitive *Mycobacterium tuberculosis* H37Ra antigen that stimulates human T cells. Infect Immun 62:5511–5518, 1994.

Brennan, P. J. Structure of mycobacteria: recent developments in defining cell wall carbohydrates and proteins. Rev Infect Dis 11(supplement 2):S420–S430, 1989.

Brozna, J. P., et al. Monocyte response to sulfatide of *Mycobacterium tuberculosis:* inhibition of priming for enhanced release of superoxide, associated with increased secretion of interleukin-1 and tumor necrosis factor alpha, and altered protein phosphorylation. Infect Immun 59:2542–2548, 1991.

Crowle, A. J., et al. Evidence that vesicles containing living, virulent *Mycobacterium tuberculosis* or *Mycobacterium avium* in cultured human macrophages are not acidic. Infect Immun 59:1823–1831, 1991.

Dannenberg, A. M., Jr. Immune mechanisms in the pathogenesis of pulmonary tuberculosis. Rev Infect Dis 11(supplement 2):S369–S378, 1989.

DeSikan, K. V. Extended studies on the viability of *Mycobacterium leprae* outside the human body. Lepr Rev 66:287–295, 1995.

Fagan, M. J., and G. A. Poland. Tuberculin skin testing in medical students: a survey of U.S. medical schools. Ann Intern Med 120:930–931, 1994.

Fenton, M. J., and M. W. Vermeulen. Immunopathology of tuberculosis: roles of macrophages and monocytes. Infect Immun 64:683–690, 1996.

Friedland, J. S. Cytokines, phagocytosis, and *Mycobacterium tuberculosis.* Lymphokine Cytokine Res 12:127–133, 1993.

Gaylord, H., and P. J. Brennan. Leprosy and the leprosy bacillus: recent developments in characterization of antigens and immunology of the disease. Ann Rev Microbiol 41:645–675, 1987.

Houston, S., and A. Fanning. Current and potential treatment of tuberculosis. Drugs 48:689–708, 1994.

Inderlied, C. B., C. A. Kemper, and L. E. Bermudez. The *Mycobacterium avium* complex. Clin Microbiol Rev 6:266–310, 1993.

McNeil, M. R., and P. J. Brennan. Structure, function, and biogenesis of the cell envelope of mycobacteria in relation to bacterial physiology, pathogenesis, and drug resistance: some thoughts and possibilities arising from recent structural information. Res Microbiol 142:451–463, 1991.

Meyers, W. M., and A. M. Marty. Current concepts in the pathogenesis of leprosy: clinical, pathological, immunological, and chemotherapeutic aspects. Drugs 41:832–856, 1991.

Misra, N., et al. Cytokine profile of circulating T cells of leprosy patients reflects both indiscriminate and polarized T helper subsets: T helper phenotype is stable and uninfluenced by related antigens of *Mycobacterium leprae.* Immunology 86:97–103, 1995.

Modlin, R. L. Th1-Th2 paradigm: insights from leprosy. J Invest Dermatol 102:828–832, 1994.

Orme, I. M., P. Andersen, and W. H. Boom. T cell response to *Mycobacterium tuberculosis.* J Infect Dis 167:1481–1497, 1993.

Relman, D. A., et al. Identification of the uncultured bacillus of Whipple's disease. N Engl J Med 327:293–301, 1992.

Smith, D. W., and E. H. Wiegeshaus. What animal models can teach us about the pathogenesis of tuberculosis in humans. Rev Infect Dis 11(supplement 2):S385–S393, 1989.

Spargo, B. J., et al. Cord factor (α,α-trehalose 6,6'-dimycolate) inhibits fusion between phospholipid vesicles. Proc Natl Acad Sci USA 88:737–740, 1991.

Stauffer, F., et al. Release of TNF-α and IL-6 from human monocytes infected with *Mycobacterium kansasii:* a comparison to *Mycobacterium avium.* Infection 22:326–329, 1994.

Wallis, R. S., and J. J. Ellner. Cytokines and tuberculosis. J Leukoc Biol 55:676–681, 1994.

Wayne, L. G., and H. A. Sramek. Agents of newly recognized or infrequently encountered mycobacterial diseases. Clin Microbiol Rev 5:1–25, 1992.

Wiker, H. G., and M. Harboe. The antigen 85 complex: a major secretion product of *Mycobacterium tuberculosis.* Microbiol Rev 56:648–661, 1992.

Wilson, K. H., et al. Phylogeny of the Whipple's disease–associated bacterium. Lancet 338:474–475, 1991.

CHAPTER TEN

ZOONOTIC BACTERIA

Brucella, Capnocytophaga, Erysipelothrix, Francisella, Listeria, Pasteurella, Spirillum, Streptobacillus, and *Yersinia*

The bacteria discussed in detail in this chapter—*Francisella tularensis, Listeria monocytogenes, Yersinia pestis,* and *Brucella* species—have two features in common. First, they are **zoonotic bacteria.** This type of organism most often infects animals and is only occasionally spread to humans. Infection results when humans ingest contaminated food or drink, handle infected animal products, or are bitten by a vector that brings the bacterium from an animal host to a human host. Second, they are **facultatively intracellular bacteria.** This means that although they can multiply in a cell-free environment, their ability to multiply within host cells is critical to their survival within the human body.

Overview of Intracellular Parasitism
Classification of Intracellular Bacteria

Intracellular bacteria can be lumped into two large groups. The first consists of the **facultatively intracellular bacteria,** which spend only part of their lives inside cells and can be cultivated on cell-free media. The second consists of the **obligately intracellular bacteria,** which can multiply only when they are inside host cells. Because they cannot be cultivated on artificial media, obligately intracellular bacteria must be cultivated in animals, eggs, or tissue culture. Table 10–1 presents information about the bacteria in these two groups and their associated diseases.

Obligately intracellular bacteria have sometimes been described as "viruslike bacteria" because, like viruses, they are small, multiply within cells, and cannot be grown on agar. However, to think of them in this way is misleading. The obligately intracellular bacteria are true bacteria, and they typically have DNA and RNA, energy-generating biochemical pathways, biosynthetic pathways, protein synthesis, a cell wall, typical cell membranes, electron transport systems, lipopolysaccharide or lipoteichoic acid, and active transport mechanisms. They do not uncoat, nor do they utilize the replicative machinery of the host cell to duplicate themselves or their nucleic acids.

Moreover, they are susceptible to many antibiotics. For all of these reasons, it is best to think of them as bacteria that occupy an unusual niche—the inside of a host cell—rather than as viruslike organisms.

Requirements of Intracellular Bacteria

Intracellular parasitism provides the bacterium with two basic requirements.

First, the inside of a host cell provides a rich store of nutrients not available outside the cell. For example, rickettsiae and chlamydiae are obligately intracellular parasites that transport adenosine triphosphate (ATP), and rickettsiae also transport a reduced form of nicotinamide adenine dinucleotide (NADH) and nucleoside diphosphate sugars. Many investigators believe that the obligately intracellular bacteria cannot be cultivated outside cells because they need energy products or biosynthetic precursors available only inside cells. The facultatively intracellular bacteria, in contrast, are more self-sufficient and can survive outside the cell, where these substances are not available.

Second, an intracellular bacterium is protected from the immune system of the host. Outside the cell lie antibodies, polymorphonuclear leukocytes (PMNs), complement, macrophages, natural killer cells, and a variety of other host factors that pose a danger to the bacterium. The intracellular bacterium is sequestered from these. Unlike viruses, intracellular bacteria do not place their proteins in host cell membranes. Thus, an infected cell is difficult for the immune system to distinguish from an uninfected cell. Many intracellular bacteria parasitize macrophages and are able to multiply within macrophages that have not been activated. However, intracellular bacteria usually move to new cells through the body fluids, and this movement makes them vulnerable to antibodies, opsonization, and complement-mediated lysis.

Dynamics of Intracellular Infection and Immunity

In general, effective immunity to intracellular bacteria involves generation of an effective **cell-**

TABLE 10–1. Significant Intracellular Pathogens and Their Associated Diseases

Site of Infection	Pathogen	Type of Intracellular Organism	Associated Disease
Endothelia	*Bartonella (Rochalimaea) henselae*	Facultative	Bacillary angiomatosis and peliosis hepatis.
	Bartonella (Rochalimaea) quintana	Facultative	Trench fever.
	Rickettsia prowazekii	Obligate	Typhus.
	Rickettsia rickettsii	Obligate	Rocky Mountain spotted fever.
	Rickettsia tsutsugamushi	Obligate	Scrub typhus.
Erythrocytes	*Bartonella bacilliformis*	Facultative	Carrión's disease.
Eyes	*Chlamydia trachomatis*	Obligate	Keratoconjunctivitis and trachoma.
	Francisella tularensis	Facultative	Oculoglandular tularemia.
Gastrointestinal tract	*Brucella* species	Facultative	Cholecystitis.
	F. tularensis	Facultative	Typhoidal tularemia.
	Listeria monocytogenes	Facultative	Gastroenteritis.
	Salmonella serotype *typhi*	Facultative	Typhoid fever.
Genitourinary tract	*Calymmatobacterium granulomatis*	Facultative	Granuloma inguinale.
	C. trachomatis	Obligate	Lymphogranuloma venereum and nongonococcal urethritis.
	L. monocytogenes	Facultative	Uterine and placental infections.
Lungs	*Chlamydia pneumoniae*	Obligate	Atypical pneumonia.
	Chlamydia psittaci	Obligate	Psittacosis.
	Coxiella burnetii	Obligate	Pneumonitis.
	Mycobacterium tuberculosis	Facultative	Pulmonary tuberculosis.
	Yersinia pestis	Facultative	Pneumonic plaque (bloody pneumonia).
Meninges	*Brucella* species	Facultative	Meningitis.
	L. monocytogenes	Facultative	Meningitis in newborn infants and immunocompromised patients.
Nerves	*Mycobacterium leprae*	Facultative	Leprosy.
Reticuloendothelial system	*Brucella* species	Facultative	Brucellosis, with granulomas and abscesses in various lymphoid tissues.
	F. tularensis	Facultative	Tularemia.
	M. leprae	Facultative	Leprosy.
	M. tuberculosis	Facultative	Tuberculosis.
	Salmonella serotype *typhi*	Facultative	Typhoid fever.
	Y. pestis	Facultative	Plague.

mediated immune response (CMIR), and the bacteria are killed when they are phagocytosed by activated macrophages. In some cases, killing is potentiated by **antibody.**

If the CMIR is vigorous enough, it will rapidly eliminate the organisms by destroying infected cells, sometimes with the formation of caseation necrosis. If the CMIR does not eliminate the infection rapidly, a **granuloma** is formed. A granuloma consists of a focus of macrophages and other immune cells surrounding a nidus of infected cells. Tissue damage accompanies granuloma formation, and the granuloma acts as a space-occupying lesion that may disrupt the functions of the organ or tissue in which it is formed. When intracellular bacteria infect cells that produce chemical mediators, infection may severely disrupt the balance of cytokines, monokines, autacoids, and other cell products. The resulting chemical messenger imbalance can severely disrupt the body's homeostasis.

General Approach to Treatment of Intracellular Infection

Antibiotic treatment of intracellular infection poses some special problems. If the infection is a chronic one, treatment must be with an agent that is effective against slow-growing bacteria and can be tolerated (and afforded) by the patient when administered over several months. Beta-lactam antibiotics cannot be used, because they are effective only against bacteria that grow rapidly. In some cases, combination therapy is used to counteract the possible appearance of resistant strains over a prolonged course of treatment.

Most antibiotics penetrate the host cell, but many do not reach therapeutically significant concentrations inside it. Because the tetracyclines and chloramphenicol can reach appropriate concentrations inside infected host cells, they have become the antibiotics used most often in treating diseases caused by intracellular bacteria. Some facultatively intracellular bacteria spend a significant portion of their growth cycle outside host cells and can be treated with a wider range of antibiotics.

Francisella tularensis

The genus *Francisella* was named after Nobel prize winner Edward Francis, who demonstrated that the organism responsible for a plague-like disease in rodents was also the cause of deerfly fever. Because the early cases of human disease caused by this organism occurred in Tulare County in California, the disease became known as tularemia, and the organism was named *Francisella tularensis*. This is the only species of *Francisella* that causes disease in humans.

Characteristics of *F. tularensis*

General Features. *F. tularensis,* a facultatively intracellular bacterium, is a gram-negative pleomorphic rod that is 0.2 μm wide by 0.2–0.7 μm long. Isolates of *F. tularensis* have been divided into three biogroups: tularensis, palearctica, and novicida. Acute arthropod-borne and animal-borne tularemia is caused by organisms in biogroup tularensis (also called Jellison biogroup A), and mild water-borne disease is caused by biogroup palearctica (Jellison biogroup B). Organisms in biogroup novicida cause human disease rarely and only in children with chronic granulomatous disease and in victims of near-drowning.

Francisella is a dangerous organism to culture because it has an ID_{50} of about 50 organisms and can enter the body through mucosal surfaces (including the conjunctiva) and through breaks in the skin. Thus, samples suspected of containing *Francisella* should be handled only within a certified biohazard hood. *Francisella* can be cultivated on media that contain cysteine or cystine. Conventional chocolate agar is supplemented with an additive that contains cysteine, so it can be used for culture. Alternatively, the organisms can be cultured on cysteine-blood agar or on the charcoal–yeast extract (CYE) agar that is used to cultivate *Legionella.*

Some *F. tularensis* strains ferment glycerol, and all strains ferment glucose. The organisms are non-motile, are oxidase-negative and urease-negative, produce no H_2S on triple sugar iron (TSI) agar, and do not reduce nitrate. Agglutination tests that use specific anti-*Francisella* antisera are used to confirm the identity of cultured *F. tularensis.*

Mechanisms of Pathogenicity. Little is known about the ability of *F. tularensis* to cause disease. *F. tularensis* has **lipopolysaccharide,** but limulus lysate tests have shown that it has little endotoxic activity. *F. tularensis* has a **capsule,** but resistance to phagocytosis is not believed to play an important role in tularemia. Rather, *Francisella* organisms owe much of their pathogenicity to their ability to survive within unstimulated macrophages. The organisms are phagocytosed easily by macrophages, but they resist being killed by oxygen-derived free radicals. This resistance to intracellular killing may be due to an external superoxide dismutase activity. Once macrophages are activated, the organisms are killed by intraleukocytic nitrous oxide.

Infection with *F. tularensis* is countered initially by a localized neutrophilic response, but this response fails to contain the infection. The neutrophilic response forms a localized cutaneous ulcer that later becomes a scarring lesion when the neutrophils are replaced by macrophages. Eventually, the organisms spread to distal sites, where granulomas form. The organisms tend to accumulate in lymphoid tissue, and patients may develop splenomegaly and buboes. When buboes occur, tularemia may be mistaken for plague.

Diseases Due to *F. tularensis*

Epidemiology. *F. tularensis* biogroup tularensis is the cause of most cases of tularemia in the USA. Infection with this biogroup can be acquired by four principal routes: by skinning an infected animal; by being bitten by an infected deerfly, tick, or mosquito; by eating undercooked meat from a diseased animal; and by handling contaminated fomites.

Tularemia is commonly known as "rabbit fever" because it is often associated with skinning *Francisella*-infected rabbits. However, *F. tularensis* has been isolated from hundreds of animal species, so there is a risk associated with skinning, handling, or eating any small wild animal. The organism is so contagious that tularemia can be easily acquired via contact with a tiny amount of contaminated material. For example, a single drop of blood from an infected animal can initiate human infection if it comes in contact with the conjunctiva, the oral mucosa, or a cut or abrasion. *F. tularensis* is passed transovarially in ticks, but deerfly and mosquito transmission is believed to be a mechanical transmission that occurs when the insect feeds on an infected animal and then immediately feeds on a person. *F. tularensis* has been isolated from a variety of ticks, including *Amblyomma, Dermacentor,* and *Ixodes* ticks.

F. tularensis biogroup palearctica is isolated occasionally in the USA and is the principal agent of tularemia in Europe. This biogroup, which causes a mild form of tularemia, is shed by aquatic mammals such as beavers and muskrats. Humans generally are infected when they drink water contaminated by the feces of infected animals.

There are about 300 cases of tularemia each year in the USA, and the disease is most common in Arkansas, Missouri, Montana, Oklahoma, Tennessee, Texas, Utah, and Wyoming. Men are affected more often than women, largely because the disease is associated with eating and handling wild animals.

Diagnosis

(1) History and Physical Examination. Tularemia can occur in any of five forms: ulceroglandular, typhoidal, oculoglandular, oropharyngeal, and pulmonic tularemia. The form exhibited by a patient usually depends on the route by which the patient was infected, although pulmonic tularemia can occur as an extension of any of the other forms.

(a) Ulceroglandular Tularemia. In the USA, the ulceroglandular form is the most common form, occurring in 70–80% of patients with tularemia. About 48 hours after exposure, patients develop a papule at the site where the organism entered the body (for example, the site of a cut, abrasion, or insect bite). The papule itches, swells, and becomes an ulcer with sharply demarcated edges after about 2 days. At this time, patients become acutely ill, with fever, rigors, headache, myalgia, and splenomegaly. They may develop a rash, and the draining lymph nodes may swell and become buboes. If untreated, nonfatal cases of disease may last 3–6 months, and relapses may occur over several years.

(b) Typhoidal Tularemia. The typhoidal form of tularemia is the second most common form in the USA, affecting 7–14% of patients with tularemia. After eating undercooked infected meat, these patients experience symptoms similar to those of typhoid. The disease begins abruptly with back pain, fever, anorexia, and chills. Patients soon develop a nonproductive cough and maculopapular rash, accompanied by nausea, vomiting, and abdominal pain. Some patients also develop septicemia, which can lead to a rapidly fatal form of pneumonia or meningitis.

(c) Oculoglandular, Oropharyngeal, or Pulmonic Tularemia. Patients who are inoculated in the eye with infectious droplets develop oculoglandular tularemia. The infection begins as a conjunctival papule and subsequently develops into a granuloma. Patients who have been splattered by contaminated droplets from infected animals or have inhaled aerosols of *F. tularensis* may develop oropharyngeal tularemia or pulmonic tularemia. The latter is a fulminating pneumonia with a high fatality rate.

(2) Laboratory Analysis. Because of the extreme infectivity of *F. tularensis,* the laboratory should be warned that samples are from patients suspected of having tularemia.

F. tularensis can be cultured from primary ulcers, lymph node aspirates, sputum, and biopsy samples from the spleen, bone marrow, and other infected tissues. Blood cultures are usually not successful but should be attempted. Samples cultured on chocolate agar under increased CO_2 will produce visible colonies in 3–5 days. An agglutination test is used to confirm the presence of *F. tularensis.*

Patients with tularemia often have antibodies to *F. tularensis* and can be tested for these by means of a tube agglutination test or a microagglutination test.

Treatment and Prognosis. Tularemia responds well to treatment with aminoglycoside antibiotics. Streptomycin is the antibiotic of choice, but gentamicin is an acceptable alternative. Chloramphenicol and tetracyclines should not be used to treat tularemia. Their use is often associated with clinical relapses in treated patients.

The fatality rates for untreated cases of ulceroglandular tularemia and pulmonic tularemia are about 5% and 30%, respectively.

Prevention. Hunters, veterinarians, naturalists, and other people who handle small animals should avoid the contamination of cuts, abrasions, and mucosae with the blood of these animals. When in the woods, they should use insecticides containing permethrin; wear long pants tucked into boots; routinely search for and remove ticks; and avoid drinking water from streams and ponds, which may be contaminated in areas where tularemia is endemic.

A **vaccine** against *F. tularensis* is available and is administered by multiple skin punctures (scarification). This vaccine, the oral typhoid vaccine, and the bacillus Calmette-Guérin (BCG) vaccine for tuberculosis are the only live attenuated bacterial vaccines available in the USA.

Listeria monocytogenes

There are eight species of Listeria, but only two—*Listeria monocytogenes* and *Listeria ivanovii*—cause disease in humans. Because *L. ivanovii* is rarely encountered, this discussion focuses on *L. monocytogenes.*

L. monocytogenes is a normal resident of the gastrointestinal tract of many animals. The organism was named *L. monocytogenes* because infection in some animals is accompanied by a striking monocytic response and the organism was once thought to be the cause of infectious monocytosis. Infection in humans is accompanied by neutrophilic leukocytosis.

In immunocompetent individuals, *L. monocytogenes* causes gastrointestinal and uterine infections. In infected pregnant women, it causes premature delivery of an infected infant. In newborns and in immunocompromised patients, the organism also causes meningitis and systemic disease.

Characteristics of *L. monocytogenes*

General Features. *L. monocytogenes* is a gram-positive bacillus that is 0.4–0.5 μm wide by 1–2 μm long. The organism can be cultured on chocolate agar and blood agar in temperatures ranging from −0.4 °C to 50 °C. Colonies of organisms exhibit a green sheen when examined under obliquely transmitted light. When grown between 20 °C and 25 °C, the organisms have many flagella and exhibit an unusual tumbling motility. At other temperatures, they have few flagella and no tumbling motility.

On blood agar, *L. monocytogenes* exhibits a narrow band of β hemolysis that is due to the production of at least two hemolysins. One of these hemolysins is called CAMP hemolysin because it demonstrates positive results in the Christie, Atkins, Munch-Peterson (CAMP) test when cultured at right angles to *Staphylococcus aureus*. Although it is similar to the hemolysin of group B streptococci, the CAMP hemolysin of *L. monocytogenes* produces a square zone of synergistic hemolysis in this test.

L. monocytogenes can be further distinguished from streptococci and from other *Listeria* species by the fact that it is catalase-positive; is optimally motile at 25 °C; is able to ferment glucose, trehalose, α-methyl-D-mannoside, and salicin; is able to hydrolyze esculin; and is virulent in mice. *L. monocytogenes* can be tested for virulence by injecting the organisms intraperitoneally into mice or by performing a conjunctival test known as the Anton test. This test requires that a sample from a 24-hour culture of *Listeria* be dropped into the conjunctival sac of a young rabbit or guinea pig. Virulent *L. monocytogenes* will produce severe, purulent conjunctivitis in the infected eye in 24–36 hours.

Mechanisms of Pathogenicity

(1) *Listeria* Antigens and Virulence Determinants. *L. monocytogenes* has two types of **teichoic acids.** One is a polyribitol phosphate teichoic acid that is attached to the cell wall, while the other is a **lipoteichoic acid** (LTA) that is linked to the cytoplasmic membrane by a glycolipid moiety. *L. monocytogenes* organisms have been divided into 13 serovars, based on the antigenic specificities of their surface LTA. Investigators refer to these as O (somatic) antigen specificities. Unfortunately, this practice often causes confusion between the lipopolysaccharide of gram-negative bacteria and the LTA of *Listeria,* a gram-positive bacterium. Serovar 4b is considered to be the **epidemic strain** of *L. monocytogenes* and has been associated with large outbreaks of foodborne listeriosis. Serotype 1/2b is also commonly isolated from patients.

Virulent *L. monocytogenes* strains produce a protein that allows them to mobilize iron from human transferrin. The ability to acquire iron when in the tissues or blood is a common theme among pathogens that are able to cause disseminated disease.

L. monocytogenes must invade host cells during human infection. A 60-kD extracellular protein that facilitates entry into host cells is produced only by virulent strains of *L. monocytogenes,* but its precise role in the infection cycle is not known. The organisms adhere to a **galactose receptor** on the surface of target cells as a prelude to entry, but the listerial adhesin has not been fully characterized.

The key virulence determinant of *L. monocytogenes* is believed to be the **listeriolysin O** hemolysin. Listeriolysin O is a 58-kD protein that lyses a variety of erythrocytes. It is believed to lyse the phagocytic vacuole, allowing endocytosed organisms to escape into the cytoplasm of their target cells, where they multiply. Strains that lack listeriolysin O remain within phagosomes after being phagocytosed and do not multiply intracellularly.

At least three other listerial antigens may contribute to virulence: **glyceride A,** a wall component that elicits the strong monocytic response associated with listeriosis in animals; **ActA protein,** a surface protein that mobilizes and polymerizes actin filaments; and **phospholipase C,** a substance that promotes survival of organisms within phagosomes in a yet-undefined manner.

(2) The *Listeria* **Infection Cycle.** Fig. 10–1 shows the infection cycle of *L. monocytogenes.* The key to the pathogenicity of the organism is its ability to multiply within unstimulated macrophages.

Listeria organisms adhere to the galactose receptor on the surface of macrophages and other cells. During parasite-directed endocytosis, adherent bacteria are phagocytosed and then quickly escape the phagocytic vacuole, probably by utilizing listeriolysin O to lyse the vacuole membrane. The bacteria now multiply within the host cell cytoplasm. As new bacteria are formed, they are encapsulated by host cell–derived actin filaments. The polymerized actin filaments, which form a long tail that extends from one end of each organism (Fig. 10–2), eventually propel the bacterium through the host cell cytoplasm to the cell membrane. The encapsulated bacterium pushes against the cell membrane to form a pseudopod that extends into an adjacent cell. The membranes of the two cells eventually fuse, and the bacterium in the

pseudopod is introduced into a new host cell. The bacterium will escape this vacuole, and the cell cycle will be restarted.

In this manner, *Listeria* organisms can move directly from cell to cell without passing through the extracellular space. This protects the bacteria from antibody and complement. Thus, effective immunity to *L. monocytogenes* requires that specifically sensitized lymphocytes be elicited and that macrophages be activated.

Diseases Due to *L. monocytogenes*

Epidemiology. In the USA, about 1700 cases of listeriosis are reported each year. The annual incidence rates are 0.7 cases per 100,000 in the general population, 12.7 per 100,000 in newborn infants and pregnant women, and 90 per 100,000 in patients with acquired immunodeficiency syndrome (AIDS). A recent survey from 16 countries revealed that 31% of patients with listeriosis were over 60 years old and that 22% were under 1 month old. A survey of listeriosis from 20 countries showed that 43% of the cases were maternal and neonatal infections, 29% involved septicemia, and 24% were infections of the central nervous system. Patients with deficiencies in T cell immunity are at greatest risk for listeriosis.

Adults acquire listeriosis when they eat foods that are contaminated with the feces of animals infected with *L. monocytogenes.* Between 5% and 10% of people carry *L. monocytogenes* in their gastrointestinal tract, but carriage seems to be transitory rather than permanent. In general, strains that are carried by humans are deemed nonpathogenic on the basis of results in the Anton test. If a woman is already carrying *L. monocytogenes* in her gastrointestinal tract before she becomes pregnant, her infant will not be infected. However, if she acquires infection during pregnancy, the infection may be transmitted to the infant in utero or during passage from the birth canal.

Listeriosis usually occurs as a sporadic disease, but large food-borne outbreaks have been reported. One survey showed that 2–3% of dairy products, 8% of shrimp and cooked crab meat, up to 20% of ground beef, and 90% of poultry available in the supermarket are contaminated with *L. monocytogenes.* Other foods that are frequently contaminated are vegetables, cheese rinds, and salads, especially salads containing cabbage or lettuce that was fertilized with manure. With the current emphasis on organic foods, listeriosis may become more prevalent.

One famous outbreak of listeriosis occurred in the maritime provinces of Canada in 1981. The disease was reported in 41 people who ate contaminated coleslaw. In this group, 34 were pregnant women, who later gave birth to 23 infected infants (6 of whom died), 9 stillbirths, and 2 healthy infants. The coleslaw contained cabbage grown by a farmer who fertilized with composted sheep manure. Two of his sheep had died from listeriosis (one in 1979 and one in 1981), and the cabbage had been harvested and stored in

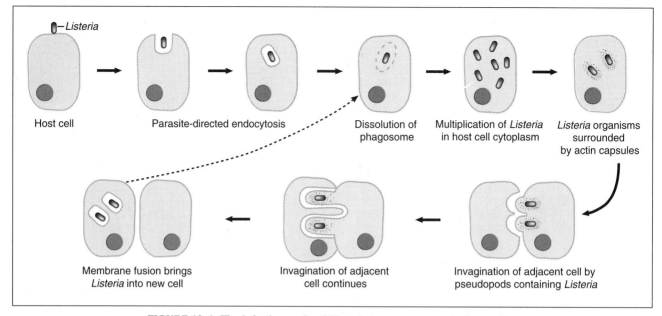

FIGURE 10–1. The infection cycle of *Listeria monocytogenes* in host cells.

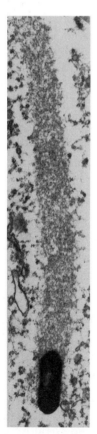

FIGURE 10–2. Intracellular *Listeria monocytogenes.* Note the long tail of polymerized actin extending from one end of the bacterium. (Reproduced, with permission, from Kocks, C., et al. *Listeria monocytogenes*–induced actin assembly requires the ActA gene product, a surface protein. Cell 68:521–531, 1992. © Cell Press.)

a cold-storage shed. Apparently, *L. monocytogenes* grew on the cabbage in the cold temperatures of the shed and persisted on the cabbage throughout the preparation of the slaw.

Outbreaks have also been associated with eating whey cheese, Mexican-style soft cheese, hot dogs, celery, tomatoes, and pasteurized milk. There is some evidence that pasteurization does not reliably kill *L. monocytogenes*. The use of antacids and agents that reduce stomach acid production lower the dose of organisms required to initiate infection.

Diagnosis

(1) History and Physical Examination. In adults, the pattern of **listeriosis** depends on the age and immune status of the infected individual. Elderly individuals and patients with diabetes, cancer, renal transplants, and deficiencies in T cell function usually develop fulminating systemic disease that results in **meningitis.** Renal transplant recipients and patients with leukemia may also develop **brain abscesses.** Listeriosis in elderly and immunocompromised patients begins with a headache, vomiting, fever, and malaise. Focal signs of acute meningitis soon follow, sometimes accompanied by symptoms and signs of sepsis or endocarditis.

Pregnant women and other immunocompetent adults who have eaten food contaminated with *L. monocytogenes* develop a **mild influenza-like illness** whose manifestations may include fever, headache, vomiting, abdominal pain, and cramps in the lower back. The disease is self-limited in these adults. However, an infected pregnant woman may transmit the infection to her infant, especially if the woman is in her third trimester of pregnancy, and this may result in stillbirth, premature delivery, or neonatal infection.

Infants infected transplacentally develop **early-onset listeriosis** (granulomatous disease with pneumonia), and those infected by coming into contact with contaminated body fluids during delivery develop **late-onset listeriosis** (meningitis). Table 10–2 compares these infections.

(2) Laboratory Analysis.   Meningitis caused by *L. monocytogenes* must be distinguished from meningitis caused by *Neisseria meningitidis* or *Streptococcus pneumoniae* in adults and from meningitis and similar diseases caused by group B streptococci or enteric bacilli in newborn infants.

Appropriate clinical specimens, such as stool, blood, cerebrospinal fluid, meconium, amniotic fluid, and placental samples, should be cultured on sheep blood agar or on Columbia colistin–nalidixic acid (CNA) agar. Because many *L. monocytogenes* organisms are inside cells, portions of each clinical sample should be diluted (one part specimen to nine parts broth) in tryptose broth or trypticase soy broth and held for up to 2 months at 4 °C. At various intervals, an aliquot from each sample should be used to inoculate a solid medium. Cold storage is believed to enhance isolation of *L. monocytogenes* by lysing host cells that contain the organisms. The organisms should grow as short, β-hemolytic, gram-positive rods and can be speciated as described previously.

Although serodiagnosis of listeriosis is not effective, centrifuged samples of cerebrospinal fluid can be Gram-stained and examined for the presence of organisms.

Treatment and Prognosis.   The treatment of choice for listeriosis in elderly individuals, immunocompromised patients, and infants is ampicillin. Alternatively, trimethoprim-sulfamethoxazole can be used. Untreated listeriosis in these groups of patients is almost always fatal. Even with appropriate treatment, death occurs in 13–34% of adults with acute systemic listeriosis, 15–50% of infants with early-onset listeriosis, and 10–20% of infants with late-onset listeriosis.

Infection in immunocompetent adults is usually mild and self-limited and therefore requires no treatment.

Yersinia pestis

Although there are 11 species of *Yersinia,* only 3 species are significant causes of human disease.

Yersinia enterocolitica and *Yersinia pseudotuberculosis* cause food-borne diseases and are discussed with the enteric rods in Chapter 7. *Yersinia pestis* causes plague, a disease whose very name evokes fear and stirs the imagination—and not inappropriately so, given its impact on literature and history.

The earliest likely reference to plague was in the Old Testament, which described an epidemic that was characterized by inguinal buboes and affected the Philistines after they took the Ark of the Covenant from the Israelites. The first plague pandemic began in northern Africa in 542 A.D., during the reign of Roman Emperor Justinian I, and quickly spread across Europe. It continued to rage for 60 years, killing over 100 million people and completely depopulating some regions. The second pandemic began in Asia and spread like wildfire across Asia and Europe during the 14th century. In Europe alone, it killed 25 million, or roughly one-fourth of the population. The third pandemic began in Burma in 1894, spread to China and Hong Kong, and was then transported to ports around the world on rat-infested ships. This was the first of the pandemics to reach the shores of North America, and many died in port cities such as San Francisco. India was hardest hit by this pandemic, with an estimated 10 million deaths.

Plague has been memorialized in the nursery rhyme "Ring Around a Rosie" and in Edgar Allen Poe's story "The Masque of the Red Death." This disease, along with typhus, led to the malthusian hypothesis that whenever the population reaches an unmanageable size, it is pared back by pestilence or war.

Today, plague is spread sporadically from infected rodents to humans through the bites of fleas. Worldwide, about 1000 cases are confirmed each year, and 90% of them occur in eastern Asia. In the USA, the annual rate is about 10–20 cases, most of which occur in the southwestern states, where small rodents such as field mice or prairie dogs sometimes harbor the bacilli. Often, dogs or cats help spread the disease by bringing infected rodents to humans. Native American populations in these states are at greatest risk because of their contact with feral rodents.

Characteristics of Y. pestis

General Features.   *Y. pestis* is a pleomorphic gram-negative rod. When stained with Wayson stain

TABLE 10–2.   A Comparison of Early-Onset and Late-Onset Listeriosis in Newborn Infants

Characteristic	Early-Onset Listeriosis	Late-Onset Listeriosis
Route of infection	Transplacental.	Contact with contaminated body fluids during delivery or postpartum.
Usual onset of symptoms and signs	Two days postpartum.	One to two weeks postpartum.
Major clinical manifestations	Granulomatosis infantiseptica: disseminated granulomas and abscesses, with respiratory distress, cyanosis, apnea, and pneumonia.	Meningitis.
Fatality rate in treated patients	15–50%.	10–20%.
Percentage of mothers with identifiable listeriosis	50%.	<5%.

or Giemsa stain, it looks much like a safety pin because the organism stains bipolarly. *Y. pestis* is a member of the family Enterobacteriaceae and can be cultured on standard media selective for enteric rods, including MacConkey (MC) agar and Salmonella-Shigella (SS) agar. Virulent isolates of *Y. pestis* produce colored colonies when grown on media that contain hemin or Congo red.

The yersiniae were originally classified as members of the genus *Pasteurella,* and they exhibit reactions on triple sugar iron (TSI) agar that are similar to those of *Pasteurella* species. Unlike *Pasteurella* species, however, yersiniae demonstrate β-galactosidase activity.

Although *Y. enterocolitica* and *Y. pseudotuberculosis* are motile at 25 °C, *Y. pestis* is not. Unlike *Y. enterocolitica, Y. pestis* is ornithine decarboxylase–negative and does not ferment sucrose, cellobiose, or sorbitol. Unlike *Y. pseudotuberculosis, Y. pestis* does not ferment rhamnose.

Mechanisms of Pathogenicity

(1) *Yersinia* Antigens and Virulence Determinants. The virulence of *Y. pestis* is a complex process, involving a large number of factors encoded on three virulence plasmids (Pst, Lcr, and Tox) and the chromosome.

(a) Factors Encoded on the Pesticin (Pst) Plasmid. The Pst plasmid is a 10-kb plasmid that encodes the synthesis of three factors: an enzyme that serves as a posttranslational modifier of *Yersinia* outer membrane proteins; **pesticin,** a bacteriocinlike protein that has no relevance to virulence; and *Yersinia* **plasminogen activator,** a substance required for the yersiniae to disseminate from the original infection site. The fibrinolytic activity of plasminogen activator is thought to be the key factor in dissemination. The coagulase activity of the plasminogen activator may also clot blood in the stomach of infected fleas, causing the fleas to regurgitate yersiniae when they feed on mammalian hosts.

(b) Factors Encoded on the Low-Calcium-Response (Lcr) Plasmid. The Lcr plasmid, which is activated when calcium levels are low, is the only one of the three plasmids that is found in *Yersinia* species other that *Y. pestis.*

The Lcr plasmid is a 70-kb plasmid that encodes a series of *Yersinia* **outer membrane proteins** (Yops). YopE, YopK, YopL, and YopM are involved in rapid growth of yersiniae in tissues, and YopN is a temperature sensor. YopM is immunologically similar to the platelet antigen GPIba and inhibits platelet aggregation. YopK and YopL are believed to interfere with the development of a CMIR to *Y. pestis.* YopH is a protein tyrosine kinase that protects the yersiniae from being phagocytosed by leukocytes. It is believed that many copies of the Yops are shed by yersiniae and that their primary effects may be at sites away from the bacteria.

The Lcr plasmid also encodes **V and W antigens.** V is a 38-kD monomer that tends to aggregate, and W is a 140-kD protein. V and W are believed to be secreted as a complex with the chaperon protein GroEL. V and W have variously been reported to be immunosuppressive, antiphagocytic, protective antigens and to be promoters of Ca^{2+} dependence.

When Ca^{2+} levels are above 2.5 mmol and the temperature is 37 °C, yersiniae multiply rapidly and produce no V and W. When Ca^{2+} levels are below 2.5 mmol, as occurs within host cells, yersiniae stop multiplying, the adenylate energy charge drops, and the products of the Lcr plasmid (V, W, and Yops) are synthesized maximally.

(c) Factors Encoded on the Exotoxin (Tox) Plasmid. The Tox plasmid is a 100-kb plasmid that is incompletely characterized. Its most important products are believed to be the *Y. pestis* capsule and the *Y. pestis* murine exotoxin. The **capsule,** called fraction 1 (Fx1), is an antiphagocytic glycoprotein capsule that is not produced at low temperatures. The exotoxin is called **murine exotoxin** because its injection into mice is rapidly lethal. Murine exotoxin has been reported to deplete NAD by splitting it to ADP-ribose and nicotinamide. It has also been reported to block beta receptors for catecholamines. This is believed to interfere with the ability of the sympathetic nervous system to regulate body temperature and may cause the patient to suffer from a fatal form of hypothermia.

(d) Chromosomal Products. Numerous chromosomal products contribute to virulence. The **lipopolysaccharide** of *Yersinia* is similar to that of other Enterobacteriaceae and has potent endotoxic activity. **Pigmentation peptide F** is a hemin storage protein that allows yersiniae to obtain iron. **Inv and Ail proteins** are substances that promote the invasion of "nonprofessional" phagocytes (cells other than leukocytes) by yersiniae. The **pH 6 antigen,** also called **antigen 4,** is a fibrillar protein that may form a layer of adhesive fimbriae on the surface of yersiniae. **Antigen 5** is a catalase that promotes the survival of yersiniae within phagocytic vacuoles.

(2) The *Yersinia* Infection Cycle. *Y. pestis* is a facultatively intracellular pathogen that survives within macrophages and neutrophils but multiplies well in the extracellular space. In fact, some investigators prefer to think of yersiniae as extracellular pathogens that can invade host cells. Yersiniae must contend with three different environments: the gastrointestinal tract of the flea, the interior of mammalian host cells, and the blood and tissues of the mammalian host.

When yersiniae are inside the flea, many of their virulence factors are not expressed, because of the cool temperatures and the lack of Ca^{2+} in this environment. The coagulase activity of the yersiniae coagulates blood and blocks the flea's proventriculus. As a result, when the flea feeds on a new host, it regurgitates yersiniae into the bite. Because the yersiniae that are introduced into the mammalian host lack Fx1, V, W, and other key virulence determinants, they are phagocytosed by macrophages.

In the low-calcium environment of the macrophage at 37 °C, the yersiniae stop multiplying but continue to synthesize Lcr plasmid products. The macrophage is killed, and fully virulent yersiniae are released into the circulation. These yersiniae resist phagocytosis, multiply rapidly in blood and tissues, invade nonprofessional phagocytes, and produce toxins that damage host tissues.

Plasminogen activator potentiates the dissemination of yersiniae throughout the body. Sepsis and disseminated intravascular coagulation (DIC) can cause the fingers, toes, nose, and ears to necrose and turn black—the classic signs of the "black death." Spread of organisms to the lungs causes fulminating pneumonia. The septicemic form of plague is spread from person to person via *Pulex irritans,* a flea that bites humans. The pneumonic form is spread via infectious aerosols.

Diseases Due to *Y. pestis*

Epidemiology. About 200 species of small animals have been found to carry plague. Some species are rapidly killed, but others suffer little or no ill effects. The yersiniae can be spread from animal to animal through flea bites or by direct contact. This completely zootic cycle of spread is called **sylvatic plague** (literally, plague of the woods). Sometimes the first sign of plague is the death of numerous rats. If rats contract the disease from sylvatic rodents and then spread the disease via fleas to humans, the cycle of spread is called **urban plague.**

As shown in Fig. 10–3, humans enter the cycle when they come in contact with infected animals or their fleas. In the USA, the animals most often associated with spread to humans are ground squirrels, prairie dogs, marmots, chipmunks, rabbits, hares, wood rats, and deer mice. Because men and children are more likely to come in contact with these animals, about two-thirds of infected patients are males and about three-fourths are under 25 years old.

Person-to-person spread of plague, either via human fleas or via infectious respiratory droplets, is called **demic plague.**

Diagnosis

(1) History and Physical Examination. Plague has three major clinical presentations, known as bubonic plague, septicemic plague, and pneumonic plague.

(a) Bubonic Plague. The triad of high fever, buboes, and conjunctivitis strongly suggests bubonic plague. From 2 to 6 days after an individual is bitten by an infected flea, a vesicular lesion develops at the site of the bite. Before buboes appear, most patients develop systemic signs of disease, such as fever, chills, confusion, malaise, nausea, and pain in the back and legs. The yersiniae quickly spread to the draining lymph nodes, where they cause swelling and the formation of exquisitely tender buboes. Congestion of blood vessels in the eye causes conjunctivitis.

Most buboes are inguinal, but some are axillary or cervical. It is unusual for buboes to occur at more than one site. The skin around buboes becomes reddened and may ulcerate. At this time, blood cultures reveal the presence of yersiniae. If treatment is not initiated, the bacteremia may lead to overwhelming sepsis, hemorrhagic pneumonia, or meningitis.

(b) Septicemic Plague. Although septicemic plague usually occurs as an extension of bubonic plague, about 20% of *Y. pestis* infections in the USA begin as septicemic plague with little or no evidence of buboes. This form of plague, which can be easily spread to others via fleas, is a rapidly fulminating disease, with early DIC and vascular collapse.

(c) Pneumonic Plague. Patients with pneumonic plague have hemorrhagic pneumonia accompanied by respiratory distress. In some patients, this

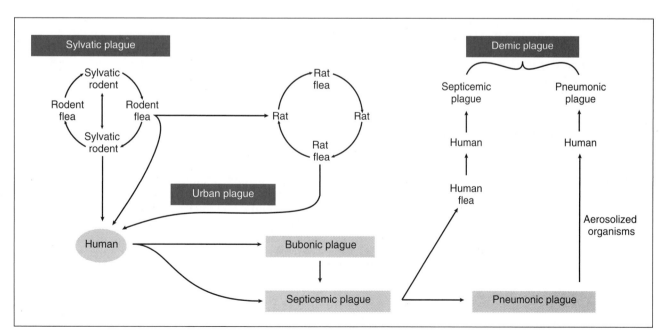

FIGURE 10–3. The transmission of *Yersinia pestis,* the cause of plague in animals and humans.

form of plague occurs as an extension of septicemic plague. In others, *Yersinia* infection begins as pneumonic plague and is the result of breathing infectious droplets shed by another patient with pneumonic plague. Plague acquired via the respiratory route has an incubation period of 2–3 days before symptoms begin. The average time from the first clinical manifestations to death is 2 days, and many die within 24 hours of their first symptoms.

(2) Laboratory Analysis. Because *Y. pestis* is highly contagious, laboratory workers must be warned when clinical samples are suspected of containing this organism. Sputum samples from patients with pneumonia or aspirate from fluctuant buboes in other patients should be stained and examined directly for the presence of organisms that show bipolar staining. Reference laboratories can perform fluorescent antibody tests to make a preliminary identification of *Y. pestis*. When blood, bubo aspirates, and other appropriate body fluids are cultured on MC and SS agar, yersiniae will usually appear in 48 hours as small lactose-negative colonies.

Treatment and Prognosis. Antibiotic treatment should be started as soon as possible—optimally, within 12–15 hours of the first symptoms of plague. Streptomycin or gentamicin is the antibiotic of choice, but patients have also been treated successfully with chloramphenicol or tetracycline. Neither ampicillin nor doxycycline is recommended, since these antibiotics are not uniformly effective. Because plague is often accompanied by DIC, good supportive care is critical, and arm boards or restraints should not be used.

In some patients, a transient intensification of the symptoms of plague is noted during treatment. This reaction, called the **Jarisch-Herxheimer reaction,** is believed to be due to the rapid killing of large numbers of bacteria and the concomitant release of toxic intracellular materials during bacterial lysis. Some clinicians administer corticosteroids with streptomycin to ameliorate the reaction.

Bubonic plague is fatal in 50–80% of patients who are not treated with antibiotics and in 18–19% of patients who are treated. All patients with septicemic plague or pneumonic plague die unless they receive appropriate and timely antibiotic therapy.

Prevention. Plague is an internationally quarantined disease, and patients must be strictly isolated. Contacts of patients should be treated prophylactically with tetracycline.

An inactivated **vaccine** that contains formalinized Fx1 fragments has been administered widely to US soldiers. Although the vaccine sometimes causes a transient fever and nausea, its use is recommended for people who will travel to areas where plague is endemic. The vaccine is about 90% effective in preventing bubonic plague, but its efficacy against pneumonic plague is not known. Booster injections of plague vaccine are administered annually.

Brucella Species

Brucella was named after Sir David Bruce, a physician who established the etiology of what was known at the time as Malta fever or melitosis. Bruce was a British army physician who insisted on studying the diseases he found in the exotic sites where he was stationed. In the late 1880s, he was sent to Malta (or Melita), where he discovered that people with undulant fever were infected with a bacterium that was spread to humans from goats. This organism was later named *Brucella melitensis*. The British army did not appreciate Bruce's meddling with indigenous diseases or his research efforts, so they shipped him to Tanganyika. As soon as Bruce arrived in eastern Africa, he set to work on a new disease, sleeping sickness, and found the etiologic agent, which is now called *Trypanosoma brucei*.

Characteristics of *Brucella*

There are six *Brucella* species, and each species is strongly associated with a particular host. *Brucella abortus* most often causes disease in cattle; *Brucella canis* causes disease in dogs; *B. melitensis* infects goats and sheep; *Brucella neotomae* usually causes disease in wood rats; *Brucella ovis* infects sheep; and *Brucella suis* infects pigs, horses, reindeer, and rodents.

General Features. Brucellae are gram-negative coccobacilli that are typically 0.5–0.7 μm wide by 0.6–1.5 μm long, but some are even smaller. Primary cultures are isolated on specialized media using biphasic culture systems. Clinical isolates grow slowly, often producing colonies in 5–10 days but sometimes requiring as long as 4–6 weeks to produce visible growth. Brucellae can also be grown on blood, chocolate, trypticase soy, Brucella, and serum dextrose agars. Brucellae are strict aerobes, do not form spores, and lack capsules.

Individual species of *Brucella* are identified by fermentation reactions, urease and H_2S production, CO_2 requirements for growth, ability to grow on media containing thionine and basic fuchsin dyes, and agglutination with specific antisera. These characteristics have also been used to divide the brucellae into biovars. *B. melitensis* and *B. suis* each have four biovars, and *B. abortus* has eight.

Mechanisms of Pathogenicity. Brucellae cause acute and chronic infections of the reticuloendothelial system. The key pathogenic characteristic of the organisms is their ability to survive within unstimulated macrophages.

(1) *Brucella* Antigens and Virulence Determinants. Primary isolates of *Brucella* are said to exhibit a smooth (S) morphology, but subcultured isolates become rough (R). Although the terms smooth and rough are used to describe changes in encapsulation in other bacteria, the brucellae have no capsule. Instead, the changes in brucellae reflect changes in the **outer membrane.** The transition from the S form to the R form appears to be a response to the accumulation of D-alanine excreted by S forms and to the lowering of the Po_2 level of the medium during the growth of brucellae. S forms seem better able than R forms to survive within phagocytes.

Three surface antigens have been identified on brucellae, two of which are expressed by S forms and one of which is expressed by R forms. The antigens of S forms are more specific than those of R forms, and their presence varies among the individual species. *B. melitensis* primarily expresses **M antigen** (for melitensis), while *B. abortus* and *B. suis* express large amounts of **A antigen** (for abortus) and small amounts of M antigen. Primary isolates of *B. canis* and *B. ovis* express **R antigen** (for rough).

(2) The *Brucella* Infection Cycle. Humans acquire brucellosis by one of three routes: via ingestion of contaminated undercooked meat or unpasteurized milk; via contact with the tissues, blood, or other body fluids of infected animals and subsequent entry of organisms through mucous membranes, cuts, or abrasions; or via inhalation of organisms when working with them in the laboratory.

Inside the human body, brucellae are phagocytosed by PMNs. The brucellae survive within these cells and use the leukocytes as "taxicabs" to transport them to various lymphatic tissues, such as the liver, spleen, and bone marrow, as well as to other selected sites.

The hallmark of acute brucellosis is the formation of granulomas within lymphatic tissues. Multiplication of brucellae within macrophages fills and destroys the cells, and patients develop bacteremia. If the CMIR that develops during this phase is insufficient to control the brucellae, the liver, spleen, bone marrow, and lymph nodes may become extensively infected. Granulomas form around infection foci, and the sinusoids of the liver may become filled with parasitized macrophages. If the patient is infected with *B. suis,* granulomas may lead to caseation necrosis. In patients with chronic brucellosis, granulomas form in the kidneys, central nervous system, subcutaneous tissues, and testes or ovaries.

Studies indicate that brucellae inhibit granulocyte degranulation by producing 5'-guanosine monophosphate (GMP) and adenosine. In addition, some investigators have reported that brucellae inhibit the oxygen burst that generates toxic free radicals within phagosomes. Thus, brucellae avoid being killed by the myeloperoxidase–halide–free radical bactericidal system of phagocytic cells.

Brucellosis is most often a disease of grazing animals. Ruminants infected with brucellae often develop placental infections that cause septic abortions, yet this never happens during human infections. This is because the placental fluid of ruminants contains erythritol, a carbon and energy source that promotes rapid multiplication of brucellae. In contrast, the placental fluid of humans contains erythrose, which does not support the growth of brucellae.

Diseases Due to *Brucella*

Epidemiology. *B. melitensis* infections are acquired most often from goats and tend to be acute infections with disabling complications. *B. abortus* infections are acquired from cattle and are generally less severe than *B. melitensis* infections. *B. suis* infections are acquired from swine and are often characterized by the formation of caseation necrosis and abscesses in lymphoid tissues. Milk, cheese, and meat are the usual sources of infection. Brucellae infect the mammary glands of ruminants and then appear in their milk.

According to the World Health Organization, about 500,000 confirmed cases of brucellosis are reported worldwide each year, but possibly millions of cases are unrecognized and unreported. In the USA, 100–200 cases are reported annually and an estimated 25 cases go unrecognized. Slaughterhouse workers, veterinarians, and hospital laboratory technicians are at highest risk of contracting brucellosis because they are most likely to come into contact with infected animal tissues.

Diagnosis

(1) History and Physical Examination. There are five forms of human brucellosis: subclinical, bacteremic, serologic, localized, and chronic forms. Although the actual course of disease varies with the infecting *Brucella* species, up to 85% of all patients with brucellosis develop osteoarticular manifestations, such as arthralgia, arthritis, bursitis, osteomyelitis, spondylitis, tenosynovitis, and sacroiliitis.

(a) Subclinical Brucellosis. Patients with subclinical brucellosis have only vague symptoms and signs of disease. They complain of fatigue and headaches and have a history of contact with raw animal products or with grazing animals.

(b) Bacteremic Brucellosis. Bacteremic brucellosis is an acute systemic form of disease and is most often due to *B. melitensis.* Patients develop a fever 2–3 weeks after exposure to infected animals or their products. Because the fever tends to wax and wane, this form of brucellosis is also called **undulant fever.** Other manifestations may include intense headaches, vomiting, weakness, severe muscle and joint pain, anorexia, depression, and enlargement of the spleen, liver, and lymph nodes. Dissemination of the organisms may lead to meningitis, endocarditis, suppurative joint infections, or renal damage. Bacteremic brucellosis may become chronic.

(c) Serologic Brucellosis. Affected patients have mild systemic signs of brucellosis and a history of drinking raw milk or eating cheese made from unpasteurized milk. The diagnosis of serologic brucellosis is usually established by demonstrating the presence of antibody to *Brucella* species.

(d) Localized Brucellosis. Most often caused by *B. melitensis* or *B. suis,* this form of brucellosis is characterized by the gradual onset of systemic signs of brucellosis, including headache, fever, and arthritis. Granulomas form in the liver, bone marrow, spleen, and other lymphoid tissues. The clinical course and symptoms depend on the site, size, and number of granulomas. Patients may develop chronic brucellosis.

(e) Chronic Brucellosis. Bacteremic or localized brucellosis may become chronic, with numerous exacerbations and remissions occurring over months

TABLE 10–3.   Uncommon Zoonotic Bacteria and Their Associated Diseases

Organism	Characteristics*	Source of Infection	Disease	Treatment
Capnocytophaga canimorsus and *Capnocytophaga cynodegmi*	Thin, fusiform gram-negative rods; are catalase-positive, arginine dihydrolase–positive, and ONPG-positive.	Bite of dog or cat.	Localized and painful cellulitis in otherwise healthy people. Patients with alcoholism, asplenia, or leukemia may develop overwhelming sepsis. Fatality rate is 25%.	Amoxicillin; cefoxitin; clindamycin; erythromycin; or penicillin G.
Erysipelothrix rhusiopathiae	Gram-positive rod; is α-hemolytic or nonhemolytic; ferments glucose; is catalase-negative, H$_2$S-positive, and esculin-negative.	Usually, contact of skin abrasion with pig feces.	Erysipeloid, characterized by a hard, swollen, burning, itching, purplish swelling on the hand, with no pus in the lesion. Patients with alcoholism may develop septicemia, arthritis, or endocarditis.	Ampicillin; penicillin G; or first-generation cephalosporin.
Pasteurella multocida	Gram-negative rod with bipolar staining; is nonhemolytic; grows on enteric media; is oxidase-positive, catalase-positive, ornithine decarboxylase–positive, indole-positive, and urease-negative.	Scratch or bite of dog or cat.	Localized, discolored, swollen, and painful bite infection in otherwise healthy people. Draining lymph nodes swell, and infection may spread to adjacent tissues, causing polyarthritis, synovitis, or osteomyelitis. Patients with chronic lung disease may develop a suppurative respiratory tract infection. Patients with liver disease or cancer may develop sepsis.	Penicillin G; doxycycline; or amoxicillin plus clavulanate.
Spirillum minus	Helical gram-negative rod; cannot be cultured on artificial media.	Bite of cat, ferret, rat, or weasel.	Rat-bite fever, or sodoku, with swelling of the bitten area 5–14 days after bite, lymphadenopathy, and eschar formation. Fever appears for 1–2 days, remits for 3–9 days, recurs repeatedly, and is accompanied by a purplish maculopapular rash. Some patients develop endocarditis or secondary pyogenic infections. Fatality rate is 10%.	Ampicillin; penicillin G; or streptomycin.
Streptobacillus moniliformis	Pleomorphic gram-negative rod; has many L phase variants; cannot be cultured on standard media; requires special biphasic serum agar.	Bite of rat; contact with dogs, cats, mice, or pigs; ingestion of contaminated milk.	Rat-bite fever, or Haverhill fever, with onset of fever, chills, headache, and vomiting 1–5 days after exposure. Within 48 hours of onset, patients develop swelling of one or more joints, accompanied by an extensive rash on the extremities, including the palms and soles. Some patients develop arthritis, pneumonia, or abscesses in multiple organ systems. Fatality rate is 10%.	Ampicillin; penicillin G; chloramphenicol; streptomycin; or tetracycline.

* ONPG = orthonitrophenyl-β-D-galactopyranoside.

or years. Patients have been reported to suffer exacerbations of bacteremic brucellosis for as long as 20 years. Chronic complications of localized or bacteremic brucellosis include meningitis, granulomatous hepatitis, abscesses of the liver and spleen, cholecystitis, endocarditis, erythema nodosum, and chronic skin ulcers.

(2) Laboratory Analysis. *Brucella* species are highly infectious, and laboratory workers should be warned when clinical samples are believed to contain brucellae. All patients with subclinical, bacteremic, and serologic brucellosis and most patients with localized brucellosis will have antibodies to *Brucella* species that can be detected by a tube agglutination method. Brucellae can be cultured from the blood and bone marrow of patients with bacteremic brucellosis, and they can be cultured from the tissue of infected organs of patients with localized brucellosis. Cultures are usually unsuccessful, however, when performed on materials taken from patients with subclinical, serologic, or chronic brucellosis.

Treatment and Prognosis. The management of brucellosis is somewhat controversial, because treatment is long-term and patients often suffer from relapses. One major problem has been the failure of many clinicians to recognize that antibiotics used to treat brucellosis must accumulate within host cells at therapeutically effective concentrations. Because of the duration of treatment, effective management of brucellosis involves combination therapy, usually with tetracycline for 3 weeks and streptomycin for 2 weeks. Up to 10% of patients using this treatment regimen relapse. Alternatively, patients may be treated with the combination of streptomycin plus doxycycline or minocycline; the combination of doxycycline plus rifampin; or the combination of ceftriaxone plus rifampin.

Prevention. In the USA, there is no vaccine for use in humans. There is, however, a live attenuated vaccine for immunizing cattle against *B. abortus*. The pasteurization of milk and the immunization of cattle have helped control the occurrence of human brucellosis.

Other Zoonotic Bacteria

Table 10-3 summarizes information concerning six other zoonotic agents.

Capnocytophaga canimorsus and *Capnocytophaga cynodegmi* are found in the mouths of dogs and cats. The organisms can cause localized and painful **cellulitis** in otherwise healthy people who are bitten by these animals. In patients with alcoholism, asplenia, or leukemia, infection may lead to overwhelming sepsis.

Erysipelothrix rhusiopathiae is usually acquired when a skin abrasion comes into contact with pig feces containing this organism. Infection causes **erysipeloid,** characterized by a large, purplish swelling on the hand, with no pus in the lesion. In patients with a history of alcohol abuse, the infection may disseminate and cause septicemia, arthritis, and endocarditis.

Pasteurella multocida is carried in the mouths of most dogs and cats, where it plays the role that viridans streptococci do in the mouths of humans. *P. multocida* causes localized **bite infections** in otherwise healthy people and causes a **suppurative respiratory tract infection** in patients with chronic lung disease.

Spirillum minus causes a severe form of **rat-bite fever** and may be acquired from the bites of cats, ferrets, rats, and weasels. The disease is also called **sodoku** and is characterized by a fever that appears for 1–2 days, remits for 3–9 days, and then recurs. Death occurs in about 10% of patients.

Streptobacillus moniliformis causes a systemic disease with fever, rash, and arthritis. The disease is called **rat-bite fever** in those who acquire it from a rodent bite and is called **Haverhill fever** in those who acquire it from contaminated milk.

Selected Readings

Anthony, L. S., P. J. Morrisey, and F. E. Nano. Growth inhibition of *Francisella tularensis* live vaccine strain by interferon-gamma–activated macrophages is mediated by reactive nitrogen intermediates derived from L-arginine metabolism. J Immunol 148:1829–1834, 1992.

Brubaker, R. R. Factors promoting acute and chronic diseases caused by yersiniae. Clin Microbiol Rev 4:309–324, 1991.

Evans, M. E., et al. Tularemia: a 30-year experience with 88 cases. Medicine (Baltimore) 64:251–269, 1985.

Farber, J. M., and P. I. Peterkin. *Listeria monocytogenes,* a foodborne pathogen. Microbiol Rev 55:476–511, 1991.

Kocks, C., et al. *Listeria monocytogenes*–induced actin assembly requires the ActA gene product, a surface protein. Cell 68:521–531, 1992.

Leung, K. Y., and S. C. Straley. The *yop*M gene of *Yersinia pestis* encodes a released protein having homology with the human platelet surface protein GPIba. J Bacteriol 171:4623–4632, 1989.

Lindler, L. E., and B. D. Tall. *Yersinia pestis* pH 6 antigen forms fimbriae and is induced by intracellular association with macrophages. Mol Microbiol 8:311–324, 1993.

Polsinelli, T., M. S. Meltzer, and A. H. Fortier. Nitric oxide–independent killing of *Francisella tularensis* by interferon-gamma–stimulated murine alveolar macrophages. J Immunol 153:1238–1245, 1994.

Schwan, W. R., et al. Phosphoinositol-specific phospholipase C from *Listeria monocytogenes* contributes to the intracellular survival of *Listeria* inocula. Infect Immun 62:4795–4803, 1994.

Southworth, F. S., and D. L. Purich. Intracellular pathogenesis of listeriosis. N Engl J Med 334:770–776, 1996.

Straley, S. C. The plasmid-encoded outer membrane proteins of *Yersinia pestis.* Rev Infect Dis 10(supplement 2):S323–S326, 1988.

Straley, S. C., and M. L. Cibull. Differential clearance and host-pathogen interactions of YopE⁻ and YopK⁻ *Yersinia pestis* in BALB/c mice. Infect Immun 57:1200–1210, 1989.

Tilney, L. G., and D. A. Portnoy. Actin filaments and the growth, movement, and spread of the intracellular bacterial parasite *Listeria monocytogenes.* J Cell Biol 109:1597–1608, 1989.

Zhan, Y., et al. Tumor necrosis factor alpha and interleukin-12 contribute to resistance to the intracellular bacterium *Brucella abortus* by different mechanisms. Infect Immun 64:2782–2786, 1996.

CHAPTER ELEVEN

MYCOPLASMAS, RICKETTSIAE, AND OTHER UNUSUAL BACTERIA

Bartonella, Chlamydia, Coxiella, Ehrlichia, Mycoplasma, Rickettsia, and *Ureaplasma*

MYCOPLASMAS
Classification

The earliest mycoplasmas described were the agents of bovine pleuropneumonia. These agents, which were thought to be viruses because they could pass through the pores of a Berkefeld filter, were known as pleuropneumonia organisms (PPO). As new mycoplasmas were discovered, they were referred to as pleuropneumonia-like organisms (PPLO). During World War II, a mycoplasma known as the Eaton agent was found to be responsible for primary atypical pneumonia, which was common among the Allied soldiers. Eventually, the Eaton agent was named *Mycoplasma pneumoniae.*

Mycoplasmas are the smallest type of bacteria. They are wall-less and are members of the class Mollicutes (meaning "soft skin"), the order Mycoplasmatales, and the family Mycoplasmataceae. Two genera in this family have been cultured from humans: *Mycoplasma* and *Ureaplasma.*

Mollicutes contains three orders: Mycoplasmatales, which are facultative mycoplasmas that require cholesterol for growth; Anaeroplasmatales, which are anaerobic organisms that require cholesterol; and Acholeplasmatales, which are facultative organisms that do not require cholesterol. One member of the order Acholeplasmatales (*Acholeplasma laidlawii*) is a commensal of the human mouth.

M. pneumoniae, which causes primary atypical pneumonia and tracheobronchitis, is the sole mycoplasma that has been definitively shown to be a human pathogen. Studies have indicated that *Mycoplasma genitalium, Mycoplasma hominis,* and *Ureaplasma urealyticum* are strongly associated with the occurrence of nongonococcal urethritis and have suggested that several newly discovered mycoplasmas are cofactors in the development of acquired immunodeficiency syndrome (AIDS) in individuals infected with the human immunodeficiency virus (HIV).

Structure, Metabolism, and Culture

The mycoplasmas have an average diameter of 0.2–0.3 μm. Their genome is only one-third to one-fifth the size of the *Escherichia coli* genome, with the *Ureaplasma* chromosome consisting of fewer than 10^6 base pairs. Mycoplasmas contain cholesterol in their cell membranes. Because they lack a rigid cell wall, they are extremely pleomorphic. Although *M. pneumoniae* moves by gliding motility, some other mycoplasmas (for example, *Spiroplasma*) utilize a spiraling motility that looks like the movement of spirochetes.

The mycoplasmas multiply by binary fission, but their division is not well coordinated with DNA replication. Thus, many small buds that contain no DNA are produced during mycoplasmal growth. The organisms are fastidious bacteria and can be isolated on media that contain a source of preformed protein and nucleic acid precursors (provided by peptone base and yeast extract) and cholesterol (provided by serum). Depending on the mycoplasma that is expected, the medium is supplemented with glucose, arginine, or urea. Phenol red is added to the medium as an indicator of relative pH, and thallium acetate and penicillin can be added to prevent the growth of organisms other than mycoplasmas.

If the diagnosis of *Mycoplasma* or *Ureaplasma* infection is suspected, clinical samples are collected for culture. One sample is used to inoculate an agar medium described above and is incubated in an atmosphere of 5% CO_2 and 95% air for *Mycoplasma* species or in an atmosphere of 10–20% CO_2 and 80–90% N_2 for *Ureaplasma.* A second sample is used to inoculate a biphasic enrichment medium, which is later used to inoculate a plate of agar medium.

The growth of *Mycoplasma* or *Ureaplasma* is evidenced by the acidification of glucose-containing agar or the alkalinization of media that contain arginine or urea. The tiny colonies of organisms erode the medium. While the colonies of most mycoplasmas

medium. While the colonies of most mycoplasmas take on the appearance of a fried egg, those of *M. pneumoniae* do not.

Mycoplasma pneumoniae

As mentioned above, *Mycoplasma pneumoniae* is the only mycoplasma definitively shown to be a human pathogen. In addition to causing primary atypical pneumonia, the organism is a common cause of acute tracheobronchitis in children and young adults.

Characteristics of *M. pneumoniae*

General Features.   *M. pneumoniae* is identified by its ability to convert glucose to acid; its relatively slow growth (8–15 days) in biphasic media; its production of β hemolysis on appropriate media; and its ability to reduce triphenyl tetrazolium to a red compound, formazan. *M. pneumoniae* colonies are able to adsorb erythrocytes when the agar plate is flooded with guinea pig erythrocytes. Moreover, colonies suspected of being *M. pneumoniae* can be identified by flooding the plate with fluorescein-tagged antibodies to *Mycoplasma* and then examining the washed colonies by epifluorescence microscopy.

Mechanisms of Pathogenicity.   *M. pneumoniae* is a strictly extracellular pathogen and does not invade the respiratory epithelium. Instead, it attaches to host cells in the epithelium via a specialized tip. This tip contains P1, a protein adhesin that adheres to neuraminic acid residues and is responsible for the ability of virulent *M. pneumoniae* isolates to adsorb guinea pig erythrocytes. After the filamentous organisms attach to the host cells, they damage the mucosa by producing copious amounts of H_2O_2.

Some investigators believe that the systemic symptoms associated with *M. pneumoniae* infection are related to the ability of some mycoplasmal antigens to act as superantigens. Variations in the immune response to mycoplasmal antigens may be responsible for variations in disease severity. The disease tends to be most severe in patients who are older and have a more vigorous immune response. The bronchiolar walls of lungs infected with *M. pneumoniae* are infiltrated with lymphocytes, monocytes, and macrophages, and the alveoli are infiltrated with lymphocytes. When the bronchiolar walls become thickened, a pneumonic lesion develops, and this lesion contains clear serous fluid.

Diseases Due to *M. pneumoniae*

Epidemiology.   In the USA, *M. pneumoniae* infects an estimated 12 million people each year but causes symptomatic disease in only 5–10% of those infected. Of those with disease, most develop tracheobronchitis only, but 30–40% also develop primary atypical pneumonia. Thus, there are between 250,000 and 500,000 cases of mycoplasmal pneumonia each year, representing about 15% of all cases of pneumonia.

Investigators believe that *M. pneumoniae* is

spread directly from person to person via respiratory droplets. Disease occurs most commonly in people who are between the ages of 5 and 25 years. Although *M. pneumoniae* is endemic worldwide, epidemics occur at intervals of 4–6 years in some locales. Cases are often clustered among close contacts, such as family members, schoolmates, or soldiers housed in a single barracks.

Diagnosis

(1) History and Physical Examination.   About 2–3 weeks after exposure to *M. pneumoniae*, patients gradually develop symptoms and signs of **tracheobronchitis,** including fever (temperature up to 39.5 °C or 103 °F), chills, malaise, a sore throat, nasal congestion, headache, and a hacking, nonproductive cough. Some patients complain of an earache caused by myringitis. If the disease progresses from tracheobronchitis to **pneumonia,** the cough becomes productive with sputum that is mucoid or mucopurulent, and some patients develop nonpleuritic chest pain. Auscultation reveals rales, rhonchi, or both. Radiographs show a diffuse bronchopneumonia that involves several lobes, but there is no consolidation.

Mycoplasmal pneumonia is known as primary atypical pneumonia for two reasons. First, unlike pneumonias caused by gram-negative rods and anaerobes, it is not secondary to another disease. Second, its course and characteristics are more like those of viral pneumonia than those of bacterial pneumonia. Patients with mycoplasmal pneumonia are usually not severely ill. Although fatigue and malaise may result in their absence from work or school, they are often said to be suffering from "walking pneumonia." Table 11–1 compares some of the key characteristics of mycoplasmal pneumonia with those of pneumo-

TABLE 11–1.   A Comparison of Key Characteristics of Mycoplasmal Pneumonia and Pneumococcal Pneumonia

Mycoplasmal Pneumonia	Pneumococcal Pneumonia
Pneumonia may be preceded by pharyngitis.	Pneumonia is not preceded by pharyngitis.
Disease has a gradual onset.	Disease has a rapid onset with chills.
Bacteremia is rare.	Bacteremia is common.
Chest pain is nonpleuritic.	Chest pain is pleuritic and may be severe.
Sputum is usually clear.	Sputum is rust-colored and purulent and contains polymorphonuclear leukocytes, red blood cells, and cocci.
Leukocytosis is absent.	Leukocytosis is usually present, but neutropenia is seen in those who are critically ill.
Empyema is absent.	Empyema is sometimes present.
Disease is treated with a macrolide antibiotic or tetracycline; beta-lactam antibiotics are ineffective.	Disease is treated with penicillin G or vancomycin.
Disease causes few deaths.	Disease causes death in 20–30% of patients.

coccal pneumonia, the archetypal bacterial pneumonia.

Complications of mycoplasmal pneumonia are rare but may include diarrhea, erythema multiforme, intravascular coagulopathy, hepatitis, pericarditis, myocarditis, meningoencephalitis, Guillain-Barré syndrome, and a variety of neuropathies. Fatal hemolytic anemia due to either complement-mediated lysis (intravascular hemolysis) or splenic erythrophagocytosis (extravascular hemolysis) has been reported. Patients with extremely high antibody levels and patients with hypogammaglobulinemia tend to develop more severe pneumonia.

(2) Laboratory Analysis. Early diagnosis of mycoplasmal disease is made primarily on clinical grounds. The organisms can be cultivated from sputum samples and throat swabs, but this often takes 2 weeks or longer.

Some patients with mycoplasmal pneumonia develop antibodies against the human erythrocyte I antigen. The antibodies are called cold agglutinins because they agglutinate human O erythrocytes at 4 °C but not at 37 °C. The usefulness of cold agglutinins as a diagnostic aid is limited because many patients do not develop these agglutinins and because some false-positive results occur in antigen testing. Patients with mycoplasmal pneumonia may also develop antibodies that agglutinate *Streptococcus* MG.

Treatment and Prognosis. Mycoplasmal tracheobronchitis and pneumonia are generally self-limiting, with overt disease lasting 3–10 days and radiographic abnormalities persisting for 10 days to 6 weeks. Although treatment with antibiotics does not eradicate the organisms, it does reduce the duration of the clinical disease. For this reason, most clinicians recommend antibiotic treatment. The drug of choice is a macrolide antibiotic such as erythromycin, azithromycin, or clarithromycin. An effective alternative is doxycycline. Because mycoplasmas have no cell wall, treatment with cell wall–reactive agents (such as penicillins, cephalosporins, monobactams, imipenem, and vancomycin) is ineffective.

Other Mycoplasmas

The cause of 50–70% of cases of nongonococcal urethritis (NGU) in the USA is not known, but circumstantial evidence suggests that *Mycoplasma hominis* and *Ureaplasma urealyticum* may be common agents of urethritis. *M. hominis* and *U. urealyticum* have also been implicated as causes of pelvic inflammatory disease, endometritis, infertility, chorioamnionitis, premature delivery, postpartum fever, and neonatal infection. These organisms have been found in the genitourinary and respiratory tracts of 18–45% of infants born to women infected with *M. hominis* or *U. urealyticum*. About 30% of infants infected with *U. urealyticum* develop chronic lung disease, and *M. hominis* and *U. urealyticum* are sporadic causes of neonatal meningitis.

At least one new *Mycoplasma* species, *Mycoplasma penetrans,* has been closely associated with

the development of AIDS in HIV-positive individuals. Although other *Mycoplasma* species have also been found in AIDS patients, those who have Kaposi's sarcoma are 11.7-fold more likely than other AIDS patients to have antibody to *M. penetrans.* In HIV-positive individuals, 40% with AIDS and 0.3% without AIDS have antibody to *M. penetrans.* In contrast, fewer than 0.5% of individuals who are immunocompetent or have immunosuppressive diseases other than AIDS have antibody to this organism.

Some investigators believe that *M. penetrans* acts as a cofactor in AIDS and may accelerate the rate at which HIV-positive individuals develop AIDS. Mycoplasmas have been shown to potentiate HIV-induced cytopathic effects by acting synergistically with HIV to kill host cells. It appears that *Mycoplasma* infection may also trigger HIV-infected cells to rapidly produce viral progeny. Mycoplasmas can induce the production of substances such as tumor necrosis factor alpha and interleukin-1, which activate viral replication in HIV-infected host cells.

CHLAMYDIAE
Classification

Early investigators were unsure where to place chlamydiae. Because of the small size and intracellular location of the organisms, many thought they were viruses or viruslike organisms. It is clear now that the organisms are gram-negative bacteria that occupy an unusual niche—the inside of a cell. They have all the parts native to bacteria, have their own metabolism, do not uncoat, and replicate themselves by transverse binary fission. They differ from most bacteria, however, in that they have a complex life cycle and exist in two morphologic forms.

Chlamydiae are members of the order Chlamydiales and the family Chlamydiaceae. Although there are several genera in this family, members of the genus *Chlamydia* are the only ones that cause human disease. There are three *Chlamydia* species: *Chlamydia pneumoniae, Chlamydia psittaci,* and *Chlamydia trachomatis.* The diseases associated with each of the chlamydiae are listed in Table 11–2.

Structure, Metabolism, and Life Cycle

Chlamydiae have the smallest bacterial genome, containing only about 600 kb. This is about one-fourth

TABLE 11–2. The Clinically Important Chlamydiae and Their Associated Diseases

Organism	Associated Diseases
Chlamydia pneumoniae	Atypical pneumonia, bronchitis, pharyngitis, and sinusitis.
Chlamydia psittaci	Psittacosis.
Chlamydia trachomatis	
Serovars A, B1, B2, and C	Trachoma.
Serovars D through K	Inclusion conjunctivitis, neonatal pneumonia, Reiter's syndrome, and urethritis.
Serovars L1, L2, and L3	Lymphogranuloma venereum.

the size of the chromosome of *Escherichia coli.* Additionally, two plasmids have been described in chlamydiae, one in *C. trachomatis* and the other in *C. psittaci.*

The two morphologic forms of chlamydiae are known as elementary bodies and reticulate bodies and are shown in Fig. 11–1.

Elementary bodies are the extracellular form. They are electron-dense structures that are 0.2–0.4 μm in diameter and are metabolically inert. Although their cell wall contains no detectable muramic acid, it contains D-alanine and carbohydrates, as well as peptides that are linked by sulfhydryl groups. Lipopolysaccharide on the outer membrane contains no O antigen and is structurally similar to severe-rough (Re) lipopolysaccharide found in some enteric organisms. Elementary bodies are released from host cells at the end of the infection cycle and invade target cells.

Once inside the target cells, chlamydiae become **reticulate bodies,** which are 0.6–1.0 μm in diameter, are metabolically active, and multiply within host vacuoles. Chlamydiae are energy parasites. Their reticulate bodies have no tricarboxylic acid cycle and must obtain adenosine triphosphate (ATP) directly from the host cell. Rickettsiae (discussed below) and chlamydiae are the only bacteria known to possess an ATP translocase.

The complex life cycle of chlamydiae is depicted in Fig. 11–2. Chlamydial elementary bodies attach to host cells via adhesins that can be digested by trypsin. Two surface proteins with adhesin activity have been described in *C. trachomatis,* and the major outer membrane protein (MOMP) is also thought to act as an adhesin. The host cell receptor has not been identified, but adherence of chlamydiae to host cells is inhibited by heparin, neuraminidase treatment, and addition of wheat germ agglutinin, suggesting that the host receptor for chlamydiae is a sialic acid.

The natural host cells for *C. trachomatis* are ciliated epithelial cells. Chlamydiae attach preferentially to the microvilli of these cells and are endocytosed at the sites of coated pits on the cell surface. The internalized chlamydiae remain within the phagocytic vacuole, where they protect themselves by blocking degranulation (blocking fusion of lysosomes with the phagocytic vacuole). Chlamydiae also are phagocytosed by monocytes and polymorphonuclear leukocytes (PMNs), and they survive within the monocytes by blocking degranulation.

Inside the phagocytic vacuole, elementary bodies are converted to metabolically active reticulate bodies. The reticulate bodies multiply by transverse binary fission, and the phagosome containing these bodies is converted into a large intracellular **inclusion body** that can be seen in stained cells. As the reticulate bodies multiply, mitochondria come close to the parasitized vacuole. Each reticulate body contains about 18 small surface projections that apparently penetrate the vacuolar membrane and move into the adjacent mitochondria. Investigators believe that these surface projections allow ATP and other nutrients to pass from mitochondria to the reticulate bodies.

Eventually, the reticulate bodies differentiate into elementary bodies, and the contents of the intracellular inclusion are released into the extracellular environment. The entry of a single elementary body into a host cell will result in the development of an inclusion body that contains 100–500 elementary bodies.

Culture

Chlamydiae are not routinely cultivated in hospital clinical laboratories. This is because the cultivation of *C. psittaci* and of some strains of *C. trachomatis* is dangerous unless strict containment facilities are available and also because chlamydiae must be grown in eggs or cell culture. Chlamydiae are cultured

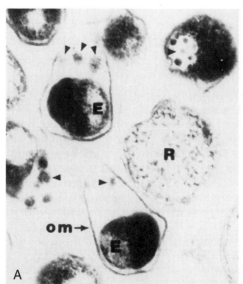
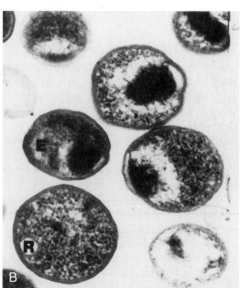

FIGURE 11–1. Chlamydiae have two morphologic forms. Electron micrographs show *Chlamydia pneumoniae* **(A)** and *Chlamydia trachomatis* **(B).** Arrowheads point to miniature bodies. E = elementary body; R = reticulate body; and om = outer membrane. (Reproduced, with permission, from Chi, E. Y., C. C. Kuo, and J. T. Grayston. Unique ultrastructure in the elementary body of *Chlamydia* sp. strain TWAR. J Bacteriol 169:3757–3763, 1987.)

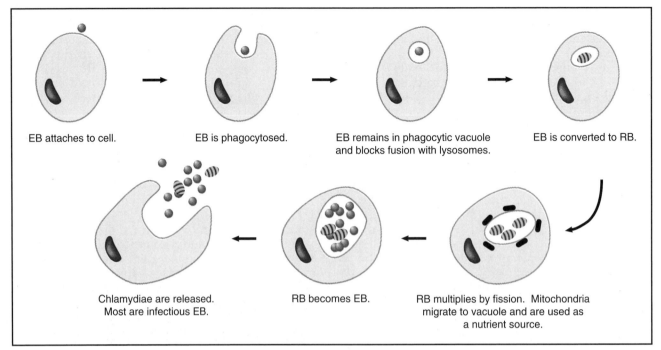

EB attaches to cell.

EB is phagocytosed.

EB remains in phagocytic vacuole and blocks fusion with lysosomes.

EB is converted to RB.

Chlamydiae are released. Most are infectious EB.

RB becomes EB.

RB multiplies by fission. Mitochondria migrate to vacuole and are used as a nutrient source.

FIGURE 11–2. The complex life cycle of *Chlamydia trachomatis.* EB = elementary body; and RB = reticulate body.

most often in McCoy cells that have been irradiated or treated with cycloheximide to prevent further growth of the cell monolayer. The clinical sample suspected of containing chlamydiae is centrifuged onto the monolayer, and the infected flasks are incubated for 48–72 hours. The presence of chlamydiae can be detected with immunofluorescence or by staining the granules (which contain glycogen) with iodine.

Chlamydia trachomatis

About 15 serovars of *Chlamydia trachomatis* have been identified. As shown in Table 11–2, the individual diseases caused by *C. trachomatis* are restricted to specific sets of serovars.

Characteristics of *C. trachomatis*

C. trachomatis is an obligately intracellular bacterium that infects and multiplies within epithelial cells and macrophages. Chlamydiae tend to cause prolonged infections in vivo, and in vitro studies suggest that chlamydial infections are characterized by alternating cycles of cell destruction and host cell proliferation. PMNs are involved in the early response to chlamydiae, but lymphocytes, macrophages, and monocytes eventually predominate.

Ocular infections can develop when organisms are spread from the eyes or genitals to the eyes of others via hands, flies, clothing, or shared towels and washcloths. Repeated infections with *C. trachomatis* cause extensive lymphoid proliferation, with the formation of the characteristic lymphoid follicles of trachoma, an eye infection that can cause blindness.

In patients with lymphogranuloma venereum, a sexually transmitted disease, a prominent granuloma is the characteristic pathologic lesion. Infants born to mothers with genital chlamydial infections may develop ocular or pulmonary *C. trachomatis* infections.

The mechanism of pathogenicity of Reiter's syndrome is poorly understood. Until recently, investigators thought that the arthritis in patients with this syndrome was a sterile immune-mediated phenomenon. Studies using RNA probes and polymerase chain reaction technology have indicated, however, that chlamydial elementary bodies are present in the synovial membrane during the first 4 weeks of the syndrome. Investigators now believe that the expression of HLA-B27 modulates the immune response to chlamydiae, alters susceptibility to dissemination of the organisms, and promotes development of an arthrogenic immune response.

Diseases Due to *C. trachomatis*

Epidemiology. An estimated 20 million people are blind today because of trachoma, the major cause of acquired blindness in the world. Trachoma is primarily a disease of poverty and is prevalent in Asia, the Middle East, and the Pacific islands. In these locations, children are often initially infected as early as 2–3 months of age, and most children are infected at least once with *C. trachomatis* by the age of 7 years.

C. trachomatis is found in association with lymphogranuloma venereum and nongonococcal urethritis, both of which are sexually transmitted. Lymphogranuloma venereum is primarily a disease of developing countries. In the USA, only about 300 cases occur each year, with most being reported in men who are black or homosexual. Nongonococcal urethritis is the most common sexually transmitted disease in the Western nations. *C. trachomatis* has been identified as the causative agent in 30–50% of patients suffering from this form of urethritis. In addition, 20–30% of patients with gonorrhea are concurrently infected with *C. trachomatis.*

Diagnosis

(1) History and Physical Examination

(a) Trachoma and Inclusion Conjunctivitis. Trachoma is more severe than inclusion conjunctivitis and is caused by serovars A through C. Four stages of trachoma are recognized: keratitis with exudate, ingrowth of eyelashes, scarring of the conjunctivas, and ingrowth of new vessels into the cornea (pannus). The undersides of normal eyelids are fairly smooth, but the undersides of the eyelids of patients with trachoma are rough and have the appearance of a cobblestone pavement (Fig. 11–3). This rough appearance is due to the formation of lymphoid follicles in the eyelid epithelium, which occurs as part of the inflammatory response to chlamydiae. The eyelashes grow downward and into the eyes and scratch the conjunctivas. The conjunctivas are further scarred by pannus. Repeated infections produce additional scarring, and the outcome may be blindness.

Inclusion conjunctivitis is caused by serovars D through K. Newborn infants who are infected when passing through the birth canal develop a mucopurulent discharge of the eyes 2–25 days after parturition. The conjunctivas are inflamed and edematous. In adults, the disease is similar, but the corneas are also inflamed (keratitis) and photophobia is present. In most infants, the conjunctivitis resolves spontaneously within several months and has no sequelae. In adults, it resolves in 2 months to 2 years.

(b) Neonatal Pneumonia. Infants born to mothers with genital *C. trachomatis* infections may develop a mild, afebrile form of pneumonia that causes them to cough and wheeze. The pneumonia has its onset

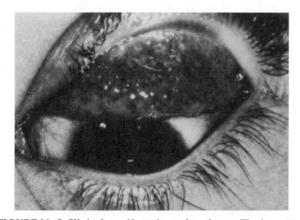

FIGURE 11–3. Clinical manifestations of trachoma. The formation of lymphoid follicles causes the undersides of the eyelids to have a cobblestone appearance, and the conjunctivas are scarred by pannus. (Reproduced, with permission, from Strickland, G. T. Hunter's Tropical Medicine, 7th ed. Philadelphia, W. B. Saunders, 1991.)

4–16 weeks after birth and is generally preceded by inclusion conjunctivitis.

(c) Urethritis. Chlamydial urethritis can lead to pelvic inflammatory disease, sterility, ectopic pregnancy, premature delivery, and perinatal morbidity. Patients often develop gonorrhea 2–7 days after intercourse and then develop chlamydial urethritis 2–3 weeks later. Chlamydial urethritis is similar in its clinical presentation to gonorrhea, but no bacteria are seen in the exudate.

(d) Reiter's Syndrome. Reiter's syndrome was originally characterized by the triad of conjunctivitis, urethritis, and reactive arthritis. The latter is an immune-mediated form of arthritis that occurs at a site distal to a primary focus of infection. Two factors are strongly associated with the development of this syndrome: a genitourinary or gastrointestinal infection with *C. trachomatis* or another organism such as *Campylobacter, Klebsiella, Mycoplasma hominis, Salmonella, Shigella,* or *Yersinia;* and the presence of HLA-B27 (found in about 80% of patients with Reiter's syndrome).

Based on the criteria established by the American Rheumatism Association, Reiter's syndrome is present if the patient has asymmetric polyarthritis that primarily involves the joints of the lower extremities and lasts for at least 1 month and if the patient also has at least one of the following: urethritis; inflammatory eye disease; mouth ulcers; circinate balanitis (glans penis inflammation attributed to spirochetes); keratoderma blennorrhagicum (purulent skin lesions with thick coverings); nail changes; dysentery; heel pain; or radiographic evidence of sacroiliitis, periostitis, or heel spurs.

(e) Lymphogranuloma Venereum. Inguinal and anogenitorectal forms of lymphogranuloma venereum are seen.

The inguinal form occurs 1–4 weeks after sexual intercourse with a partner infected with an L1, L2, or L3 serovar of *C. trachomatis.* Between 10% and 40% of patients develop a small, painless vesicular lesion on or around the genitals. All patients subsequently develop regional lymphadenitis with nodes that are firm and moderately painful. These nodes, known as inguinal buboes, may become abscessed and cause extreme pain. A characteristic cleft can be seen between adjacent buboes, and the buboes contain aggregates of large monocytes and epithelial cells, as well as some giant cells. In some cases, patients develop chronic inguinal buboes.

The anogenitorectal form of lymphogranuloma venereum occurs primarily in women. It is characterized by a bloody mucopurulent rectal discharge, which may be accompanied by tenesmus, abdominal pain, diarrhea, and rectal perforation.

(2) Laboratory Analysis. In patients with eye infections or urethritis, the diagnosis is based on demonstrating that mucosal scrapings contain *C. trachomatis* or that tears or sera contain antibody to *C. trachomatis* in immunofluorescent antibody tests. Cervical samples should be obtained after mucus is carefully removed. Purulent urethral discharge, urine, and semen are not acceptable samples for diagnosis.

The infected mucosa should be scraped with a Dacron or rayon swab, since cotton or calcium alginate may be toxic to the chlamydiae. Mucosal scrapings can be handled in one of several different ways. After the specimen is smeared on a glass slide, it can be examined for the presence of chlamydiae by use of a direct immunofluorescence technique. The smear can be stained by the Gimenez method or with Giemsa stain and examined for the presence of the characteristic inclusion bodies (known as Halberstaedter-Prowazek bodies). An enzyme immunoassay is also available and is 70–100% sensitive. DNA probes are now becoming available, but their reliability as diagnostic aids is still under investigation. The gold standard for chlamydial diagnosis is to culture the organisms in McCoy cell cultures. Cell culture for chlamydiae is not available in many hospitals, but when a definitive diagnosis is necessary (such as in criminal trials), infection should be culture-confirmed.

A diagnosis of lymphogranuloma venereum is supported by detection of antibodies to L1, L2, and L3 serovars of *C. trachomatis* using a complement fixation or microimmunofluorescence test.

In neonates with pneumonia, chlamydiae cannot be found in the blood, but eosinophilia and high titers of antibody to *C. trachomatis* are usually present.

Treatment. Trachoma is usually treated with doxycycline or azithromycin, but a suitable alternative is erythromycin or a fluoroquinolone. In adults, inclusion conjunctivitis and urethritis are treated with doxycycline, and lymphogranuloma venereum is treated with doxycycline, erythromycin, or sulfisoxazole. If urethritis is present in patients with Reiter's syndrome, treatment with tetracycline may be beneficial. In neonates, pneumonia is treated with erythromycin or a sulfonamide.

Chlamydia psittaci

Chlamydia psittaci is the cause of **psittacosis,** a disease also known as **parrot fever** or **ornithosis.** Psittacosis came to public attention during 1929 and 1930, when more than 750 people in 12 countries developed life-threatening pneumonia that was traced to shipments of diseased parrots from South America. The disease was named psittacosis because parrots are psittacine birds. Some experts prefer the name ornithosis because the disease can also be acquired from turkeys, ducks, parakeets, and a variety of small birds.

Patients are infected with *C. psittaci* when they breathe air contaminated with the feces of diseased birds. In many cases, the patient has a parrot or budgerigar that is lethargic and has a cough and diarrhea. When the bird flaps its wings, dried feces in its cage are stirred up and can be inhaled. From 1 to 3 weeks later, the patient develops a fever, nonproductive cough, rales, sore throat, myalgia, and a frontal headache. While some patients have mild pneumonia

or pneumonitis, others become acutely ill with vomiting, cyanosis, and central nervous system symptoms that can include encephalitis, delirium, and coma. About 5–20% of untreated patients die.

Laboratory confirmation of psittacosis is based on demonstrating that macrophages in sputum samples contain inclusion bodies and on identifying antibody to *Chlamydia.* Organisms can be cultured from the sputum and blood, but culture should be performed only if adequate containment facilities are available.

Patients with psittacosis are usually treated with tetracycline and placed in isolation to prevent the disease from spreading to others via respiratory droplets. Because *C. psittaci* is sulfonamide-resistant, sulfonamides should not be used.

Chlamydia pneumoniae

Chlamydia pneumoniae was discovered during the early 1980s. The organism was originally isolated from a Taiwanese child and was designated as the TWAR agent because the laboratory codes for the initial isolates were TW-183 and AR-39. This designation quickly became an acronym for *Tai*wan *a*cute *r*espiratory agent because the organism was most commonly associated with human respiratory tract infection. In 1989, the TWAR agent was named *C. pneumoniae.*

Characteristics of C. pneumoniae

C. pneumoniae was recognized as being distinct from the other chlamydial species on the bases of at least two significant factors: genetics and morphology. First, although the chromosomes of individual *C. pneumoniae* isolates show 94% homology, the DNA of *C. pneumoniae* shows only 5% homology with that of *Chlamydia trachomatis* and 10% homology with that of *Chlamydia psittaci.* Second, the elementary bodies of *C. pneumoniae* are oblong (pear-shaped), have a large periplasmic space, and contain miniature bodies (Fig. 11–4). This contrasts with the dense, round elementary bodies of other chlamydial species.

Investigators believe that only humans are infected with *C. pneumoniae* and that there are no animal reservoirs. Although organisms are probably spread from person to person via respiratory droplets, they are not easily spread to others. Family members of patients are rarely infected, and nosocomial transmission has not been documented. Reinfection of adults is common but seems to be associated with a milder clinical course.

Retrospective serologic surveys indicate that *C. pneumoniae* infections tend to occur in cycles, with the incidence of disease being high for 2–3 years and then low for 4–6 years. Asymptomatic patients may play a major role in the infection cycle. About 90% of those infected with *C. pneumoniae* do not become ill.

Polymerase chain reaction assays and immunofluorescence studies have recently shown that *C. pneumoniae* is present in most atherosclerotic coronary arteries but is only rarely present in nonathero-

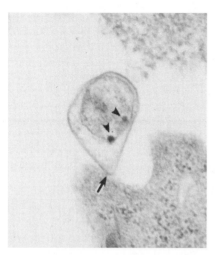

FIGURE 11–4. The distinctive pear-shaped elementary bodies of *Chlamydia pneumoniae*. The arrowheads point to the miniature bodies, and the full arrows point to the usual site of attachment of chlamydiae to host cells. (Reproduced, with permission, from Kuo, C. C., E. Y. Chi, and J. T. Grayston. Ultrastructural study of entry of *Chlamydia* strain TWAR into HeLa cells. Infect Immun 56:1668–1672, 1988.)

sclerotic arteries. This suggests that *C. pneumoniae* may be at least in part responsible for the development of atherosclerosis.

Diseases Due to *C. pneumoniae*

Epidemiology. *C. pneumoniae* is a common cause of adult upper and lower respiratory tract infections in all countries that have been surveyed. In industrialized countries, infection before the age of 5 years is rare, but almost every person is infected at some time during life and adults are commonly reinfected. Infection tends to be most severe in older individuals and in patients with an underlying pulmonary disease, such as chronic obstructive pulmonary disease (COPD) or emphysema.

C. pneumoniae is most often associated with mild upper respiratory tract diseases in young adults, but it causes pneumonia in about 70% of patients over 60 years of age. In contrast, *Mycoplasma pneumoniae* causes the highest rates of pneumonia and tracheobronchitis in children and young adults. Each year in the USA, *C. pneumoniae* is responsible for 200,000 to 300,000 cases of pneumonia (or 6–12% of all cases of pneumonia), while *M. pneumoniae* is responsible for 250,000 to 500,000 cases.

Diagnosis

(1) History and Physical Examination. In addition to causing atypical pneumonia, bronchitis, pharyngitis, and sinusitis, *C. pneumoniae* is thought to be responsible for fever in many cases that were previously diagnosed as fever of unknown origin (FUO). *C. pneumoniae* may also play a role in the development of atherosclerosis.

The incubation period for **pneumonia** is long, with symptoms appearing 30 days or more after exposure to *C. pneumoniae*. Often, the disease follows a biphasic course in which an initial upper respiratory tract illness regresses spontaneously and is followed days to weeks later by pneumonia or bronchitis.

Manifestations of the first phase of disease may include pharyngitis, hoarseness, and fever. Patients often suffer from sinusitis that may persist throughout both phases of the disease. In the second phase, which begins with cough and malaise, fever is uncommon. Most patients are not very ill unless they are elderly or suffer from underlying pulmonary disease. Auscultation reveals rhonchi and rales, even in those with fairly mild disease, and one study showed that 36% of patients with pneumonia also had sinus tenderness to percussion. Chest radiographs usually demonstrate the presence of pneumonitis with a single subsegmental lesion, but bilateral pneumonitis is sometimes seen in severe cases.

A small number of patients with *C. pneumoniae* infections develop myocarditis or endocarditis as a complication of pneumonia.

(2) Laboratory Analysis. A diagnosis of pneumonia due to *C. pneumoniae* is best established by culture. However, many patients are culture-negative, the organisms are difficult to isolate, and many hospitals do not have the facilities to culture *C. pneumoniae*. Therefore, laboratory confirmation of *C. pneumoniae* infection is likely to be based on showing that the patient has antibodies to *Chlamydia*.

If chlamydial culture is available, clinical specimens should be cultured in HL cells. Like the inclusion bodies of *C. psittaci,* those of *C. pneumoniae* contain no glycogen and cannot be stained with iodine.

The most readily available antibody test is the complement fixation (CF) test originally developed to diagnose psittacosis. This test identifies a genus-specific antigen and does not differentiate among chlamydial species. The diagnosis of *C. pneumoniae* infection is made if the patient has pneumonia, positive results in the CF test, and a history inconsistent with psittacosis. Alternatively, a microimmunofluorescence (MIF) test can be used to demonstrate IgG or IgM antibodies to *C. pneumoniae*. This test is specific and sensitive but is available in only a few reference laboratories.

Antibody test results in patients who have primary disease differ from those in patients who have been reinfected with *C. pneumoniae*. In primary infection, CF-demonstrable antibody and MIF-demonstrable IgM antibody appear by weeks 2–4, and MIF-demonstrable IgG antibody appears during weeks 6–8. Reinfected patients may not develop CF or IgM antibodies, or these antibodies may be present at very low titers. IgG, however, rises rapidly to extremely high titers in reinfected patients. Thus, a series of serum samples should be drawn from patients, with the first sample collected as soon as possible after admission, the next one collected 3–4 weeks later, and the third one collected 3–4 weeks after the second sample.

In general, a fourfold or greater rise in antibody titer between sequential serum samples indicates that the patient has an active infection. Mere demonstration of an elevated antibody titer does not confirm the presence of *C. pneumoniae* infection, because elevated titers of IgG antibody may persist for years. IgM and CF antibodies disappear 2–6 months after recovery.

Treatment and Prognosis.   Disease caused by *C. pneumoniae* is best managed with prolonged, high-dose tetracycline or doxycycline treatment. Erythromycin is a suitable alternative but is more often associated with relapse. Sulfonamides should not be used, because *C. pneumoniae* is resistant to these antibiotics. Recovery does not confer lasting immunity, and reinfection is common in adults.

RICKETTSIAE
Classification

Members of the genera *Rickettsia* and *Coxiella* are obligately intracellular bacteria that belong to the order Rickettsiales and the tribe Rickettsieae. One *Coxiella* species and numerous *Rickettsia* species are significant human pathogens. The *Coxiella* species was originally called *Rickettsia burnetii,* but because the agent differs significantly from other *Rickettsia* species in its nucleic acid composition (as reflected in its G+C ratio) and in its physical characteristics, its name was changed to *Coxiella burnetii.*

Rickettsia species differ from chlamydiae and ehrlichiae in that they (1) multiply within the cytoplasm of their target cells, rather than within host phagocytic vacuoles; (2) do not have a complex life cycle; and (3) can be transmitted by arthropod vectors. *Coxiella* organisms are more like the chlamydiae and ehrlichiae in that they have a complex life cycle that is completed within host vacuoles.

Based on clinical, immunologic, and genetic crite-

ria, the rickettsiae can be divided into four groups: typhus rickettsiae, spotted fever rickettsiae, scrub typhus rickettsiae, and coxiellae. Table 11–3 provides information on the most important members of these groups. Because the first three groups have so much in common, this section begins with an overview of their structure, metabolism, and infection cycle. The characteristics of the fourth group are discussed later in the section.

Structure and Metabolism of *Rickettsia* Species

Rickettsia species are in many ways typical gram-negative bacteria, but they multiply only within eukaryotic cells. The organisms are rods measuring 0.3–0.6 μm wide by 0.8–2.0 μm long. They have a standard bacterial life cycle, and they multiply by transverse binary fission. Like other gram-negative bacteria, they have a peptidoglycan cell wall and an outer membrane that contains lipopolysaccharide.

Although *Rickettsia* species actively transport a variety of substrates and metabolize glutamate via the Krebs cycle, they do not possess glycolytic enzymes. For this reason, cell wall precursors (uridine diphosphate sugars) must be obtained from the host cell. At least some species have the unusual ability to transport adenosine diphosphate and triphosphate (ADP and ATP) by an obligate exchange system. The obligate exchange mechanism used to transport ATP allows an organism to equilibrate itself to the energy charge of the host cell when it is intracellular, but it ensures that no ATP is exported when the organism moves into the ATP-poor extracellular environment.

Possibly the most important characteristic of *Rickettsia* species is their hemolytic activity, which

TABLE 11–3.   Classification and Characteristics of the Major Pathogenic Rickettsiae

Rickettsial Group	Disease	Distribution	Vector	Reservoir
Typhus rickettsiae				
Rickettsia prowazekii	Epidemic typhus.	Worldwide.	Body louse.	Humans and flying squirrels.
Rickettsia typhi	Endemic typhus (murine typhus).	Worldwide.	Flea.	Rodents.
Spotted fever rickettsiae				
Rickettsia akari	Rickettsialpox.	Worldwide.	Mite.	Mice.
Rickettsia australis	Australian tick typhus (Queensland tick typhus).	Australia.	Tick.	Rodents and marsupials.
Rickettsia conorii	Boutonneuse fever.	Mediterranean countries, India, and Africa.	Tick.	Rodents and dogs.
Rickettsia rickettsii	Rocky Mountain spotted fever.	North and South America.	Tick.	Rodents and dogs.
Rickettsia siberica	North Asian tick typhus (Siberian tick typhus).	Siberia, Mongolia, and China.	Tick.	Rodents.
Scrub typhus rickettsiae				
Rickettsia tsutsugamushi	Scrub typhus.	Asia and Australia.	Mite.	Many animals.
Coxiellae				
Coxiella burnetii	Q fever.	Worldwide.	Aerosolized coxiellae, meat, milk, and tick.	Many animals.

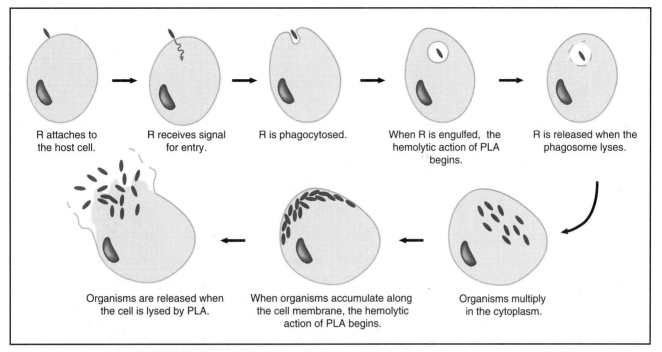

FIGURE 11–5. The typical rickettsial infection cycle. R = rickettsial organism; and PLA = phospholipase A.

is due to a phospholipase A that rapidly destroys host cell membranes. This activity generates arachidonic acid and lysophosphatides that can be converted by the host cell to pharmacologically active products such as prostaglandins and leukotrienes. Phospholipase A is believed to play a critical role in the infection cycle of rickettsiae and in the pathogenesis of rickettsial diseases.

Infection Cycle of *Rickettsia* Species

Rickettsia species are parasites of endothelial cells, and virulent strains can multiply within unstimulated macrophages. Fig. 11–5 shows the typical rickettsial infection cycle. The rickettsial organism enters a host cell when it attaches to a host receptor and is phagocytosed. The precise host receptor has not been identified, but the organism binds to cholesterol palmitate–containing sites on the erythrocyte membranes. Each organism promotes its own entry into host cells via a process requiring the expenditure of energy. Once phagocytosed, the organism rapidly lyses the phagocytic vacuole and escapes into the cytoplasm (Fig. 11–6).

Rickettsiae multiply by transverse binary fission and fill the cytoplasm of the host cell. Both scrub typhus and spotted fever rickettsiae form tails of polymerized actin (Fig. 11–7) that may propel them through the host cell cytoplasm and allow them to pass directly between cells in a manner similar to that seen with *Listeria* and *Shigella* species. Spotted fever rickettsiae are unusual in that they multiply within both the cytoplasm and the nucleus of endothelial cells. After rickettsiae accumulate along the cell membrane, they are released. Scrub typhus rick-

ettsiae are extruded individually from the parasitized endothelial cell, but spotted fever rickettsiae are released in a burst of organisms when the rickettsial phospholipase A lyses the cell.

Diseases caused by *Rickettsia* species are characterized by vasculitis, fever, and rash. The nidus of infection in the endothelium becomes a "vascular nodule" filled with inflammatory cells such as PMNs and macrophages (Fig. 11–8). As the infection spreads within the endothelium, the permeability of

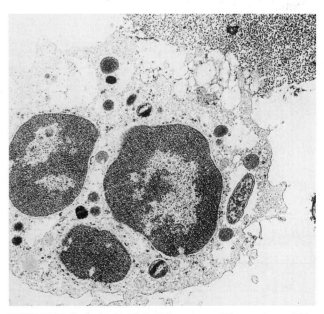

FIGURE 11–6. A single *Rickettsia prowazekii* organism within the cytoplasm of a host cell.

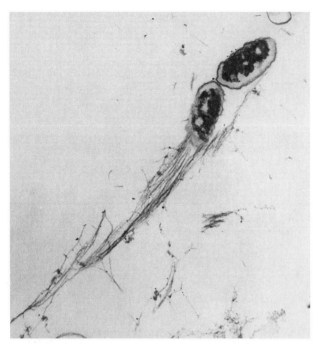

FIGURE 11–7. **Polymerized actin tails produced by intracellular** *Rickettsia rickettsii.* (Reproduced, with permission, from Heinzen, R. A., et al. Directional actin polymerization associated with spotted fever group rickettsial infection of Vero cells. Infect Immun 61:1926–1935, 1993.)

the blood vessels increases. Fluid leaks into the tissues, causing the affected area to become edematous and the blood volume to decrease. Infection of the skin microvasculature causes the eruption of a rash that looks similar to the rash seen in patients with rubeola or meningococcemia. Thrombosis and vascular collapse decrease regional blood supplies, leading to tissue anoxia. Eventually, loss of blood volume causes blood pressure to drop, and moribund patients develop shock secondary to peripheral vascular collapse. The origin of the profound vascular changes that occur during rickettsial disease is not well understood. Early investigators looked for a toxin because blood vessels not infected with rickettsiae showed pathologic changes. The presence of a rickettsial toxin was also inferred from the fact that intravenous injection of living (but not dead) rickettsiae killed mice within a few hours, and their death was due to peripheral vascular collapse secondary to increased vascular permeability. Thus, rickettsiae killed mice without multiplying within the vasculature. Other investigators suggested that the clinical signs of rickettsial disease could be attributed to vascular denudement caused when infected cells were lysed by rickettsiae. Many investigators now believe that the key to the pathogenesis of rickettsial disease lies in the fact that rickettsiae infect endothelial cells and alter their production of a wide variety of effector molecules and cell surface antigens that modulate thrombosis, vascular permeability, and the immune response (Fig. 11–9).

Recovery from a rickettsial disease requires the generation of antibody and activated macrophages.

Rickettsiae are readily killed when phagocytosed by PMNs, but virulent rickettsiae survive within unstimulated macrophages and monocytes in the absence of antibody to *Rickettsia*. Maximal killing of virulent rickettsiae occurs when the organisms are phagocytosed by activated macrophages in the presence of antibody. The antibody may prevent the organisms from utilizing their phospholipase to escape the phagosome. Interferon-gamma may also play a role in restricting the intracellular multiplication of organisms.

Methods of Diagnosing Rickettsial Diseases

Diseases caused by the typhus rickettsiae, spotted fever rickettsiae, and scrub typhus rickettsieae are acute vector-borne exanthematous diseases.

Patients should be questioned about possible exposure to the vectors listed in Table 11–3 and about the spread of rash on the body. The rash caused by typhus rickettsiae begins on the trunk and spreads to the extremities, but the rash caused by spotted fever rickettsiae begins on the extremities and spreads later to the trunk. A history of tick bites may indicate that the patient has a form of spotted fever. If a living tick is still present, the tick can be sent to a reference laboratory to be examined for the presence of pathogenic rickettsiae. Skin scrapings, blood samples, and serum samples should also be collected and sent to an appropriate laboratory for testing.

Skin scrapings can be tested to see if they react with fluorescein-conjugated antibody to *Rickettsia*.

Because rickettsiae are obligately intracellular bacteria, they cannot be cultivated on microbiologic media. Instead, they must be grown in tissue culture cells (such as chick embryo fibroblasts, L929 cells, or endothelial cells) or within the yolk sacs of embryonated chicken eggs. Although they are gram-negative bacteria, rickettsiae are not routinely stained with Gram's stain, because this stain does not stain intracellular bacteria well. Instead, cells in-

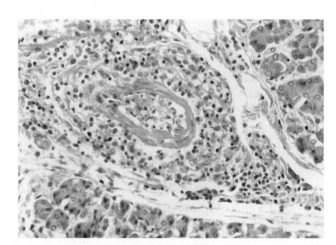

FIGURE 11–8. **Histologic findings in Rocky Mountain spotted fever.** A single blood vessel is surrounded by inflammatory cells. (Reproduced, with permission, from Walker, D. H. *In* Damjanov, I., and J. Linder, eds. Color Atlas of Pathology. St. Louis, Mosby–Year Book, Inc., in press.)

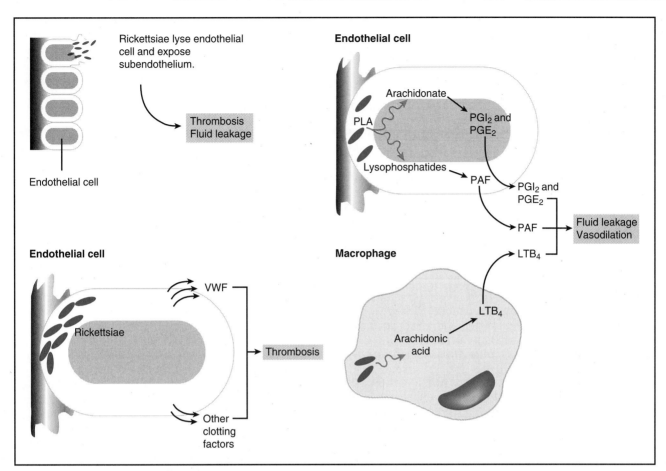

FIGURE 11-9. Processes believed to be involved in the pathogenesis of rickettsial disease. First, rickettsial destruction of endothelial cells exposes the thrombogenic subendothelium and allows leakage of serum into the perivascular space. Second, rickettsial phospholipase A (PLA) releases arachidonate and lysophosphatides from the host cell membrane. In addition, it directly lyses a number of types of cells, including endothelial cells, erythrocytes, and fibroblasts. Third, the endothelial cells convert arachidonate to protaglandin I_2 and E_2 (PGI_2 and PGE_2) and convert lysophosphatides to platelet-activating factor (PAF). PGI_2, a vasodilator and a powerful hypotensive agent, inhibits the adherence of platelets to the endothelium. PGE_2 suppresses the immune response, and PAF increases vascular permeability. Fourth, macrophages and polymorphonuclear leukocytes infected with rickettsiae secrete large amounts of PGE_2 and leukotriene B_4 (LTB_4). These agents act in concert to increase vascular permeability. Fifth, *Rickettsia*-infected endothelial cells produce an excessive number of von Willebrand factor (VWF) monomers. Together these processes lead to vasodilatation, thrombogenesis, peripheral vascular collapse, and noncardiogenic shock.

fected with rickettsiae are stained with Giemsa stain or by the Gimenez method. Host cells stained by the Gimenez method appear blue-green, and intracellular rickettsiae stain bright red.

Serum samples are tested for two types of antirickettsial antibody. An agglutination test called the Weil-Felix test identifies antirickettsial antibodies that agglutinate *Proteus* isolates with particular O antigens. These antibodies often appear first during convalescence, so both acute and convalescent sera should be tested. The Weil-Felix reactions of several rickettsiae are listed in Table 11-4. An indirect fluorescent antibody test can also be used to show that the patient has antibody to group-specific rickettsial antigens. Group-specific antibodies generally appear during the acute phase of disease.

The Typhus Rickettsiae

Throughout history, probably more deaths have been caused by typhus than by any other infectious

TABLE 11-4. The Weil-Felix Reactions of Rickettsiae

Rickettsial Group	Weil-Felix Reactivity to *Proteus* Antigens		
	OX-19	OX-2	OX-K
Typhus rickettsiae			
Epidemic typhus	+++	+	0
Endemic typhus	+++	+	0
Brill-Zinsser disease	0 or +	0	0
Spotted fever rickettsiae			
Rocky Mountain spotted fever	+++	+++	0
Tick typhus	+++	+++	0
Rickettsialpox	0	0	0
Scrub typhus rickettsiae			
Scrub typhus	0	0	+++
Coxiellae			
Q fever	0	0	0

disease except malaria. Epidemic typhus, which is spread by body lice, has long been a specter that haunts the battlefield. During war, soldiers huddle together and rarely bathe, so lice spread rapidly. As a result, typhus has played an important role in a number of historical events. For example, in 1528, the outcome of the siege of Naples was determined when typhus swept through the French camp that surrounded the city. Charles V was at the brink of being deposed, but he had a grisly ally that he never expected. The spread of typhus and rapid deaths of about 30,000 French soldiers brought the siege to a grinding halt, and Charles retained his crown. Soldiers had to contend with typhus in the Spanish wars against the Moors during the 15th century and in the Napoleonic campaign against Russia. In the aftermath of World War I, an estimated 3 million Russians died of typhus.

Characteristics of Typhus Rickettsiae

Typhus is caused by two agents. *Rickettsia prowazekii* causes epidemic typhus and a recrudescent form of typhus known as Brill-Zinsser disease. *Rickettsia typhi,* an agent once known as *Rickettsia mooseri,* causes endemic typhus.

Typhus caused by *R. prowazekii* is called epidemic typhus because it often occurs as massive outbreaks. It is usually spread from person to person via the body louse (*Pediculus humanus corporis*), although the head louse (*Pediculus humanus capitis*) has also been reported to disseminate the infection. Humans are the usual reservoir of rickettsiae, and the louse is infected when it feeds on a person who has typhus. The rickettsiae are spread through the feces of the louse, rather than through the saliva. The louse defecates when it feeds on a person, and the rickettsiae are introduced into the bite when the person scratches the bitten skin. In some case, rickettsiae may be inhaled when a person handles clothes that are heavily infested with lice and the feces of body lice.

Rickettsiae are not spread transovarially to the progeny of lice, so continued spread of typhus requires that the louse-to-human-to-louse cycle continue. This cycle is promoted by the propensity of lice to abandon patients who have high fevers or have died. Infected lice die from the rickettsial infection in 1–3 weeks.

Although flying squirrels have been reported to be the reservoir for some cases of epidemic typhus, the vector has not been found.

Endemic typhus is spread most often via the rat flea (*Xenopsylla cheopis*) and occasionally via the rat louse (*Polyplax spinulosa*). Because of its association with rodents, endemic typhus is also called murine typhus.

The pathogenic mechanisms of disease caused by *R. prowazekii* and *R. typhi* are discussed above (see Infection Cycle of *Rickettsia* Species).

Diseases Due to Typhus Rickettsiae

Epidemiology. Each year in the USA, there are reports of about 10 cases of epidemic typhus and 50 cases of endemic typhus, most of which occur in Texas and some southeastern states. Worldwide, most cases of epidemic typhus are found in Africa, but some cases are reported in Central and South America. Most cases of endemic typhus are found in Mexico and Central America.

Diagnosis. See Methods of Diagnosing Rickettsial Diseases (above).

(1) History and Physical Examination

(a) Epidemic Typhus. The prodrome of typhus, which may last hours or days, begins 8–12 days after the patient is bitten by a *Rickettsia*-infected louse. Manifestations include low-grade fever, headache, and generalized muscle weakness, sometimes accompanied by myalgia in the larger muscles of the back and legs.

The acute phase of typhus begins with high fever (temperature 40–41 °C or 104–106 °F), frontal headaches, and intense myalgia in the back and legs. Between day 4 and day 7 of the acute phase, a rash appears on the shoulders and upper trunk and begins to spread to the periphery. The early rash is macular (flat) but soon becomes maculopapular and may become petechial or hemorrhagic. Patients develop a wide variety of systemic signs of disease, including moist rales, cough, diarrhea, generalized edema, peripheral necrosis, renal failure, and mental changes that may include obstreperousness or stupor. The hazy mental condition of the acutely ill patient is the source of the name "typhus," which is derived from the Greek *typhos,* meaning hazy or smoky.

Complications of typhus are generally related to tissue anoxia secondary to thrombosis and peripheral vascular collapse. Some patients develop gangrene of the extremities and may require amputation of the fingers, toes, or limbs. Patients who recover may suffer for years from the sequelae of tissue anoxia. Death due to typhus may be the result of loss of blood flow to a critical organ, such as the brain; stroke or heart attack secondary to thrombosis; or noncardiogenic shock secondary to peripheral vascular collapse. When death occurs, it is usually between day 9 and day 18 of illness.

(b) Endemic Typhus (Murine Typhus). Endemic typhus is generally milder than epidemic typhus. About 1–2 weeks after being bitten by an infected flea, the patient develops a prodrome similar to that of epidemic typhus. The characteristic rash usually appears between day 3 and day 5, but some patients develop no rash. Typical manifestations include fever, nausea, vomiting, cough, arthralgia, headache, and chills. The disease usually lasts about 2 weeks.

(c) Brill-Zinsser Disease. Brill-Zinsser disease is a recrudescent form of typhus that appears many years after the initial typhus episode. Patients often develop no rash and have a milder course of the symptoms associated with typhus. The most prominent manifestations are headache, myalgia, and malaise.

(2) Laboratory Analysis. As discussed earlier, laboratory confirmation of typhus rests primarily upon demonstrating that the patient has antibodies to typhus rickettsiae. In the Weil-Felix test (see Table 11–4), antibodies to OX-19 tend to have the highest titer. Antibodies to OX-19 and OX-2 do not appear until late in the acute phase or during convalescence. For this reason, a negative result in serum drawn early does not rule out a diagnosis of typhus. Patients with endemic typhus may not develop OX-19 and OX-2 antibodies. In the indirect fluorescent antibody test, specific typhus-group antibodies can be detected during the acute phase in most patients with epidemic or endemic typhus, usually during the second week of disease.

Treatment and Prognosis. Typhus is treated with doxycycline or chloramphenicol. Patients suffering from thrombosis and vascular collapse will need appropriate supportive measures. In untreated patients, the fatality rate of epidemic typhus ranges from 20% to 70% and that of endemic typhus is about 2%. Death due to Brill-Zinsser disease is extremely rare.

The Spotted Fever Rickettsiae

The spotted fever rickettsiae are responsible for Rocky Mountain spotted fever (RMSF), rickettsialpox, boutonneuse fever, Israeli spotted fever, Australian tick typhus (Queensland tick typhus), North Asian tick typhus (Siberian tick typhus), and a growing number of other regional spotted fevers.

Characteristics of Spotted Fever Rickettsiae

RMSF is caused by *Rickettsia rickettsii.* The organism is passed to humans via the bite of ticks, most often the dog tick (*Dermacentor variabilis*) and wood tick (*Dermacentor andersoni*). A third tick, the rabbit tick (*Haemaphysalis leporispalustris*) is believed to participate in the persistence of RMSF among reservoir animals by transmitting *R. rickettsii* among rodents, rabbits, and hares. Dogs, deer, and other animals also serve as reservoirs, but the persistence of *R. rickettsii* is also facilitated by the ability of ticks to transfer the organism to their offspring. Because RMSF is a tick-borne disease, most disease occurs during the months when ticks are feeding—namely, April through August.

As shown in Table 11–3, most other forms of spotted fever are also spread by ticks. The exception is *Rickettsia akari,* the agent of rickettsialpox, which is spread via the bites of mites (*Allodermanyssus sanguineus*). The mite vector is a parasite of house mice and feeds on humans primarily when the rodent population is reduced.

In general, spotted fevers are similar to typhus in their clinical and pathologic presentation (see Infection Cycle of *Rickettsia* Species, above). The notable exceptions are listed in Table 11–5.

Two factors that are thought to play key roles in immunity against spotted fever rickettsiae are interferon-gamma and tumor necrosis factor. In experiments with *Rickettsia conorii,* mice that were depleted of either of these factors developed rapidly fatal disseminated spotted fever. In contrast, mice

TABLE 11–5. A Comparison of Key Characteristics of Spotted Fevers and Typhus

Spotted Fevers	Typhus
Disease vector is the tick; vector passes rickettsiae to progeny.	Disease vector is the body louse; vector does not pass rickettsiae to progeny.
Disease occurs in humans during late spring through early autumn in the USA and is acquired via the bite of an infected tick.	Disease occurs in humans during winter in the USA and is acquired via contact with the feces of infected body lice.
Rickettsiae target the endothelial cells, smooth muscle cells, and fibroblasts.	Rickettsiae target the endothelial cells.
Rickettsiae multiply within the cytoplasm and cell nucleus.	Rickettsiae multiply within the cytoplasm only.
Rash spreads from the periphery to the trunk.	Rash spreads from the trunk to the periphery.
Rash is extensive and hemorrhagic and includes petechiae and purpura.	Rash is characterized by maculopapules and petechiae.
Extensive thrombosis and disseminated intravascular coagulation occur.	Thrombosis occurs but is less prominent.

with both interferon-gamma and tumor necrosis factor recovered completely from disease within 9 days. Results of these and other experiments led investigators to conclude that interferon-gamma and tumor necrosis factor induce host cells to produce nitric oxide, which kills intracellular rickettsiae.

Diseases Due to Spotted Fever Rickettsiae

Epidemiology. RMSF received its name because the early isolates of *R. rickettsii* came from the valley that lies between the Bitterroot and Sapphire ranges of the Rocky Mountains in western Montana. The early cases of spotted fever led the US Department of Agriculture to locate its communicable diseases research center in Hamilton, Montana. Today, RMSF occurs primarily within the southeastern and southern states. For example, during one recent year, the states with the greatest number of cases of RMSF were North Carolina (243 cases), Virginia (90), Georgia (83), South Carolina (80), and Maryland (75). Other states where RMSF is prevalent include Oklahoma, New York, Missouri, Illinois, and Ohio. About 600–1000 cases of RMSF are confirmed each year in the USA.

Rickettsialpox is a sporadic disease of urban areas and has been seen most often in New York City, Russia, and Korea.

Diagnosis. See Methods of Diagnosing Rickettsial Diseases (above).

(1) History and Physical Examination

(a) Rocky Mountain Spotted Fever. From 2 to 12 days after the patient is bitten by an infected tick, the disease begins with headache, fever, chills, malaise, and myalgia. Some patients do not develop a rash. In most cases, however, a maculopapular rash

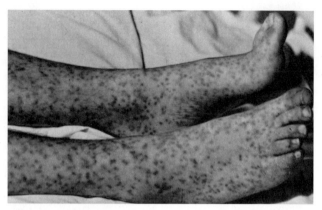

FIGURE 11–10. The rash of Rocky Mountain spotted fever. (Courtesy of Armed Forces Institute of Pathology. AFIP photo 67987-3.)

(Fig. 11–10) appears on the ankles, wrists, and forehead on days 2–4. As the rash spreads to the trunk, it may become petechial or hemorrhagic.

Acutely ill patients may exhibit a wide variety of manifestations, including diarrhea, abdominal pain, stiff neck, renal failure, congestive heart failure, seizures, hyponatremia, and thrombocytopenia. About 25% of patients develop splenomegaly. Patients with signs of disseminated intravascular coagulation suffer from complications related to ischemia of blood vessels that supply various organs. Thrombosis may also lead to loss of blood flow to limbs, and amputation may be necessary.

(b) Rickettsialpox. The first sign of rickettsialpox is a red papule at the site of a mite bite. The papule vesiculates and then becomes a black eschar (an ulcerated lesion covered by a thick, coagulated crust) over the next few days. About 3–7 days after the papule appears, manifestations include fever, chills, lymphadenopathy, and leukopenia. Within 72 hours, the patient develops a maculopapular rash that is similar to chickenpox. Table 11–6 compares the manifestations of rickettsialpox with those of chickenpox.

(2) Laboratory Analysis. If RMSF is suspected on the basis of the patient's history and clinical mani-

festations, treatment is usually begun before laboratory results are available. Confirmation is usually based on the results of antibody tests. Convalescent serum samples from patients with RMSF are strongly positive for OX-19 and OX-2 antibody in the Weil-Felix test (see Table 11–4). Group-specific antibodies to spotted fever rickettsiae are demonstrated in the indirect fluorescent antibody test. Immunofluorescence can be used to show the presence of rickettsiae in skin biopsies, but many patients with RMSF do not test positive.

Patients with rickettsialpox do not show positive results in the Weil-Felix test. Indirect fluorescent antibody testing demonstrates the presence of group-specific antibodies 4–6 weeks after infection begins. Sera can be sent to the Centers for Disease Control and Prevention to be tested for the presence of species-specific antibodies to *R. akari.*

Treatment and Prognosis. RMSF is treated with tetracycline or chloramphenicol. The latter is the antibiotic of choice if the patient is gravely ill. Platelets and supportive care are needed for patients who develop disseminated intravascular coagulation. Rickettsialpox is treated with tetracycline.

Fatality rates associated with RMSF vary from 5% to 90%, depending on the strain of *R. rickettsii* responsible for the disease. Rickettsialpox is a mild disease that rarely causes death.

Prevention. A vaccine consisting of killed bacteria did not prove effective and is no longer available. Tick attachment can be prevented by tucking pants into boots when hiking and by using insect repellents that contain permethrin. Attached ticks should be removed immediately by grasping them with tweezers and pulling firmly until they release their grip.

The Scrub Typhus Rickettsiae

Scrub typhus is caused by *Rickettsia tsutsugamushi.* The disease name stems from the fact that organisms are passed to humans via infected mites that live in isolated patches of scrub vegetation. The species name is derived from the Japanese words *tsutsuga,* which means "something small and dangerous," and *mushi,* which means "creature." During 1995, one group of investigators proposed that the name of this organism be changed to *Orientia tsutsugamushi.*

Characteristics of Scrub Typhus Rickettsiae

Three major antigenic types of *R. tsutsugamushi* have been described and are known as the Karp, Gilliam, and Kato strains.

R. tsutsugamushi is spread by the bites of the larval forms (chiggers) of several species of trombiculid mites. Chiggers are the only stage of the mite that takes a blood meal. The chiggers routinely transmit rickettsiae back and forth from various rodents and only sporadically transmit them to humans. The rickettsiae are passed transovarially to the offspring of the mites, allowing them to act as both vectors and reservoirs of the disease.

TABLE 11–6. A Comparison of the Key Characteristics of Rickettsialpox and Chickenpox

Rickettsialpox	Chickenpox
Fever precedes rash.	Fever follows or accompanies rash.
Fever is remittent.	Fever is nonremittent.
A primary eschar accompanies the rash.	There is no eschar.
Rash is not on palms, soles, or oropharynx.	Rash is everywhere, including palms, soles, and oropharynx.
Lesions are vesicles surrounded by papular rings.	Lesions are vesicles.
Rickettsiae are in vesicular fluid.	Varicella-zoster virus is in vesicular fluid.

The infection cycle of *R. tsutsugamushi* is unusual in that each organism exits the host cell individually rather than being expelled in groups when the cell is lysed. Electron microscopic studies have shown that each organism buds through the cell membrane and coats itself with host membrane material during this process.

Diseases Due to Scrub Typhus Rickettsiae

Epidemiology. Scrub typhus is most prevalent in India, Southeast Asia, Indonesia, Australia, Korea, and Japan. It occurs most often during the rainy season.

Diagnosis

(1) History and Physical Examination. Patients with **scrub typhus,** which is also called **tsutsugamushi disease** or **Japanese river disease,** develop fever, chills, and headache 1–3 weeks after being bitten by an infected chigger. About half of the patients develop a papule at the site of the precipitating mite bite, with the papule becoming first a vesicle and then a black eschar (Fig. 11–11) that leaves a scar when it heals. Lymph nodes that drain the area of the eschar typically are enlarged. During the prodromal phase of disease, patients may also complain of nausea, vomiting, sore muscles, abdominal pain, cough, and sore throat.

The acute phase of scrub typhus is generally heralded by a macular or maculopapular rash that starts on the trunk. The rash appears 5–8 days after the onset of the prodrome, but many patients develop no rash. Splenomegaly and conjunctivitis are common manifestations of acute illness, and some patients develop pneumonia, circulatory failure, delirium, or coma.

(2) Laboratory Analysis. If scrub typhus is suspected on the basis of clinical findings, treatment is usually started without laboratory testing. Because *R.*

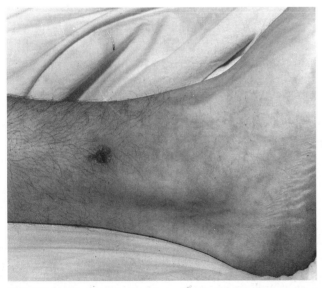

FIGURE 11–11. The black eschar of scrub typhus. (Courtesy of Armed Forces Institute of Pathology. AFIP photo D4451.)

tsutsugamushi strains are antigenically variable, good antibody tests have been difficult to develop. Enzyme-linked immunosorbent assay (ELISA) methods that utilize antigens from the three major *R. tsutsugamushi* strains have recently been developed for field use. Convalescent sera usually contain antibodies to OX-K in the Weil-Felix test (see Table 11–4).

Treatment and Prognosis. Scrub typhus is usually treated with tetracycline or chloramphenicol.

Fatality rates range from 0% to 50%, depending on the particular strain of *R. tsutsugamushi* that caused the disease. Recovery confers only short-term immunity against the other strains, so reinfection is common.

The Coxiellae

In 1935, an outbreak of disease occurred in workers in a meat-packing plant in Brisbane, Australia. Because the etiologic agent was unknown, it was called Q (for query) fever. In 1937, F. M. Burnet and M. Freeman showed that the agent responsible for the initial Q fever outbreak was a rickettsia, and the agent was called *Rickettsia burnetii.* Although the name was later changed to *Coxiella burnetii,* the organism is conventionally grouped with the other major pathogenic rickettsiae, as shown in Table 11–3.

Unlike the other rickettsiae, *C. burnetii* (1) has a complex life cycle with multiple morphologic forms, (2) multiplies within host vacuoles rather than within the cytoplasm, (3) resists harsh environmental conditions, (4) is disseminated to humans primarily via means that do not involve an arthropod vector, and (5) usually causes a mild form of pneumonitis or pneumonia with no accompanying rash.

Characteristics of Coxiellae

General Features. Three morphologic variants of *C. burnetii* can be seen within host cells: small cell variants, large cell variants, and endospores. Of these, small cell variants are the most infectious when used to produce infection in experimental animals. *Coxiella* endospores are so named because of their intracellular location ("endo") and their morphology when viewed by electron microscopy. *Coxiella* endospores should not be confused with the "classic" endospores of gram-positive bacteria such as *Bacillus* and *Clostridium.* While *Coxiella* endospores are not known to be dormant or unusually resistant, classic endospores are dormant and are highly resistant to drying, heat, radiation, and chemicals.

The lipopolysaccharide of coxiellae undergoes phase variation. Phase I organisms are more virulent and more resistant to phagocytosis than are phase II organisms. Most coxiellae isolated from patients are phase I organisms, but the phase II organisms predominate after several rounds of subculture in vitro.

Coxiellae usually infect cattle, sheep, goats, and cats. Infection is spread among these animals by tick bites, contact with infected placentas, ingestion of infected urine or feces, eating the flesh of infected animals, and drinking infected milk. Humans enter the transmission cycle when they breathe aerosols that contain coxiellae, come into contact with infected placentas, or ingest infected meat or milk. Transmission of Q fever to humans via the bites of ticks is unusual.

Mechanisms of Pathogenicity. "Acute" strains of *C. burnetii* cause mild atypical pneumonia, and "chronic" strains cause a persistent form of endocarditis that is accompanied by steady deterioration of the liver or spleen.

Because Q fever pneumonia is rarely fatal, little biopsy material has been available to study the pathogenesis of disease. Severely ill patients exhibit signs of vasculitis, hemorrhage, and necrosis, all of which are probably related to endothelial destruction by coxiellae. The exudative response in pneumonia caused by coxiellae is unusual in that histiocytes, rather than PMNs, predominate.

Q fever endocarditis most often affects the aortic or mitral valve and occurs most frequently in patients with preexisting valvular disease or prosthetic valves. Various investigators have reported that the infected valves show small perforations or brownish-yellow vegetations. The mechanism by which coxiellae damage heart valves is not understood.

Biopsy specimens from patients with liver, spleen, or bone disease have shown the presence of granulomas surrounding the infection foci—a finding that is typical for chronic intracellular infections.

Diseases Due to Coxiellae

Epidemiology. Parturient animals, particularly sheep and cats, play an important role in the dissemination of coxiellae. Latent infection is activated during late pregnancy, and the urine, feces, amniotic fluid, and placentas of these animals are heavily infected. Contact with these infected animal products has often resulted in outbreaks of disease in humans. For example, a large outbreak of Q fever in Nova Scotia occurred when a cat gave birth on the front steps of a boarding house. Those who entered the boarding house through the front door developed Q fever, while those who used the back door did not develop the disease.

Meat-packing houses also are a source of infection. When infected meat is processed, infected particles become airborne, and people who are downwind are at risk of disease. For example, an epidemic of Q fever in Oakland, California, was traced to a rendering plant (slaughterhouse). All those who became ill lived or worked within a triangular area whose tip in the direction of the prevailing wind pointed to the rendering plant. Coxiellae are highly resistant to environmental changes and can remain infectious in particles for years. Moreover, the ID_{50} of coxiellae for humans is extremely low—perhaps as low as a single organism—making *C. burnetii* the most infectious agent known.

Diagnosis

(1) History and Physical Examination. Acute and chronic forms of Q fever have been described. Acute disease is characterized by pneumonia, hepatitis, or both. Chronic disease is characterized by endocarditis and steady deterioration of the liver or spleen.

(a) Acute Q Fever. Acute disease begins 2–6 weeks after exposure to *C. burnetii*. Initial manifestations include high fever, chills, headache, myalgia, retro-orbital pain, and malaise. In some cases, patients also complain of chest pain, cough, nausea, vomiting, and diarrhea. The spleen and liver may be somewhat enlarged, but the disease is primarily a form of pneumonitis or pneumonia and is similar to the pneumonia caused by *Chlamydia pneumoniae* or *Mycoplasma pneumoniae*. Chest films usually reveal infiltrates involving the lower lung fields and sometimes show round, segmented opacities.

Some patients develop hepatitis, with hepatomegaly, liver tenderness, jaundice, and abnormal results in liver function tests. The percentage of patients who have pneumonia, hepatitis, or both varies considerably among geographic locales.

Most patients recover from overt disease in 1–2 weeks without treatment. Rare complications include hemolytic anemia, encephalitis, pericarditis, and myocarditis.

(b) Chronic Q Fever. In individuals infected with "chronic" strains of *C. burnetii*, endocarditis can occur years or even decades after the initial *Coxiella* infection. The aortic tricuspid valve is infected most often, resulting in valve damage and ventricular incompetence. Typical signs include fever, clubbing of the fingers, splinter hemorrhages, hepatomegaly, splenomegaly, thrombocytopenia, and microscopic hematuria. Patients may also suffer from endotoxemia.

(2) Laboratory Analysis. Patients living in areas where Q fever is common are generally treated on the basis of clinical signs alone. Because *C. burnetii* is so highly infectious, it should not be cultivated unless extraordinary containment facilities are available. A complement fixation test is the most widely used diagnostic test. However, ELISA and indirect immunofluorescent antibody tests are also available and are more sensitive than the complement fixation test for detecting antibodies to *Coxiella*. Titers of antibody to phase I antigens and antibody to phase II antigens are measured, and the ratio of the two helps define the stage of disease. In those with acute disease (which is usually pneumonitis), the ratio of phase I to phase II is greater than 1. In those with chronic disease (usually endocarditis), it is less than 1. In those with subacute disease (usually hepatitis), the ratio is greater than or equal to 1.

Treatment and Prognosis. Patients with Q fever pneumonitis should be placed in respiratory isolation. Acute Q fever is treated with doxycycline. Chronic Q fever does not generally respond well to treatment, but some patients have been treated successfully with a fluoroquinolone or with a combination of a fluoroquinolone plus rifampin.

In patients with untreated acute disease, the fatality rate is about 1%. Chronic disease progresses slowly and has a high fatality rate.

Prevention. Individuals at high risk of developing Q fever can be immunized with ***Coxiella* vaccine,** a killed bacteria vaccine that is rather irritating to the injection site. The incidence of Q fever can also be reduced by drinking only pasteurized milk.

EHRLICHIAE
Ehrlichia Species

The ehrlichiae are members of the family Rickettsiaceae and the tribe Ehrlichieae. They are usually veterinary pathogens, but human disease has been attributed to three *Ehrlichia* species: (1) *Ehrlichia chaffeensis,* the agent of human monocytic ehrlichiosis (HME); (2) *Ehrlichia sennetsu,* the agent of a rare disease that is found in Japan and Malaysia and is called Sennetsu fever or Sennetsu mononucleosis; and (3) the yet-unnamed agent of human granulocytic ehrlichiosis (HGE).

Characteristics of Ehrlichiae

Like chlamydiae, ehrlichiae are obligately intracellular bacteria that are gram-negative, are coccoid, have a complex life cycle, and multiply within host cell vacuoles. They survive within phagosomes because lysosomes fail to fuse with vacuoles that contain ehrlichiae. Unlike chlamydiae, ehrlichiae infect mostly monocytes and macrophages, are not energy parasites, and can be transmitted from host to host via arthropod vectors. Ehrlichiae also multiply within platelets and endothelial cells.

The life cycle of ehrlichiae has not been thoroughly described, but two forms of organisms are known to exist: small forms that are called morulae (Fig. 11–12) and larger forms that are tightly wrapped in host membranes. Ehrlichiae metabolize glutamine and glutamate, and they generate ATP from the metabolism of these compounds.

Diseases Due to Ehrlichiae

Epidemiology. In the USA, HME most often is seen south of a line extending from New Jersey to Texas and Oklahoma, but it also is found in Illinois and Missouri. In Georgia, the incidence of HME is nine times that of Rocky Mountain spotted fever (RMSF). In contrast, HGE has been reported primarily in the upper midwestern states. With the public becoming more aware of HGE, cases are now being reported in other areas, including Arkansas, California, Florida, Pennsylvania, New York, and several New England states.

HME and HGE are restricted geographically by the distribution of their vectors. HME is caused by *E. chaffeensis* and is transmitted by *Amblyomma americanum* (the Lone Star tick) and *Dermacentor variabilis* (the American dog tick). HGE is caused by an unnamed *Ehrlichia* that is believed to be a strain of or closely related to *Ehrlichia equi.* HGE is transmitted

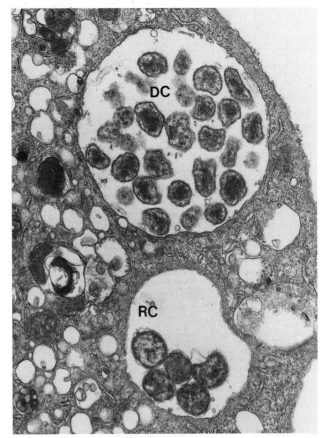

FIGURE 11–12. Two morulae of *Ehrlichia chaffeensis* in a cultured DH82 cell. One morula contains reticulate cells (RC), while the other contains dense-cored cells (DC). (Reproduced, with permission, from Dumler, J. S., et al. Isolation and characterization of a new strain of *Ehrlichia chaffeensis* from a patient with nearly fatal monocytic ehrlichiosis. J Clin Microbiol 33:1704–1711, 1995.)

through the bites of *Ixodes scapularis* (the black-legged or deer tick) and its close relative, *Ixodes pacificus.* These ticks also transmit Lyme disease, and *I. scapularis* is the vector of babesiosis. Indeed, individuals have been shown to suffer concomitantly with Lyme disease and HGE, and some *Ixodes* ticks collected from the wild have been found to harbor the agents of both of these diseases.

Diagnosis
(1) History and Physical Examination. About 3–4 weeks after being bitten by a tick, patients with **human monocytic ehrlichiosis** (HME) develop leukopenia, thrombocytopenia, and abnormal results in liver function tests. Other clinical signs include fever (temperature >38 °C or 100.4 °F), severe headache, vomiting, diarrhea, arthralgia, myalgia, and pneumonia. HME is sometimes diagnosed as rashless RMSF, although about 36% of patients develop a macular rash. The diagnosis is pursued when patients suspected of having RMSF fail to develop OX-19 and OX-2 antibodies detectable by the Weil-Felix test or group-specific antibodies to spotted fever rickettsiae.

About 8 days after exposure to an infected tick, patients with **human granulocytic ehrlichiosis** (HGE) develop fever, chills, headache, malaise, and myalgia.

Many patients also suffer from confusion, coughing, nausea, and vomiting, but only about 2% develop a rash. Patients are acutely ill, and death results in about 5% of cases.

(2) Laboratory Analysis.   Laboratory confirmation of HME depends on demonstrating the presence of characteristic inclusion bodies in macrophages obtained by biopsy of the liver, spleen, or bone marrow and on detecting antibodies to *Ehrlichia* by means of an indirect fluorescent antibody test. Antibodies appear by about the third week of infection. Morulae are rarely seen within circulating monocytes. Diagnostic tests based on polymerase chain reaction technology are under development.

In patients with HGE, peripheral blood smears show PMNs with cytoplasmic vacuoles that contain *Ehrlichia*. During the late acute or early convalescent stage of disease, antibodies are detectable by an indirect fluorescent antibody test that uses *E. equi* as a test antigen.

Treatment.   Patients with HME or HGE generally respond to treatment with doxycycline. When death occurs, it is usually due to pneumonia or to an overwhelming opportunistic infection.

BARTONELLAE

Although bartonellae are members of the family Bartonellaceae and the order Rickettsiales, recent genetic studies suggest that the bartonellae may be more closely related to brucellae than to rickettsiae.

The genus *Bartonella* contains organisms previously classified as *Bartonella* and *Rochalimaea*. Four pathogenic species have been described: *Bartonella bacilliformis,* which causes Carrión's disease; *Bartonella (Rochalimaea) quintana,* which causes trench fever and occasionally causes bacillary angiomatosis; *Bartonella (Rochalimaea) henselae,* which causes cat-scratch disease and is the principal cause of bacillary angiomatosis; and *Bartonella elizabethae,* which has been identified in the lesions of some patients with infective endocarditis.

Bartonella bacilliformis

Bartonellosis is a disease associated with many strange stories, one of which concerns the origin of its name, Carrión's disease. Daniel Carrión was a senior medical student in Lima, Peru, in 1885. For his senior project, he chose to study verruga peruana, a disease characterized by the development of highly endothelialized warts (verrugas). Wishing to chronicle the prodrome of this rather indolent disease, he inoculated himself with verrucous material from a patient. Unfortunately, about 2 weeks later, he developed the acute hemolytic anemia known as Oroya fever. Before his death, he remarked that it was now evident to him that verruga peruana and Oroya fever were two manifestations of the same disease. Daniel Carrión did not graduate from medical school, but there is now a statue in his honor in Lima, and the disease that took his life bears his name.

Characteristics of B. bacilliformis

General Features.   *B. bacilliformis* is a gram-negative rod that is 1–3 μm in length and has tufts of polar flagella. It can be cultured at 29 °C on heart infusion agar that contains rabbit serum and rabbit hemoglobin. Two colony types, T1 and T2, have been described. Although phase variation in organisms has not been shown to correlate with changes in their ability to cause disease, the T2 bacteria are more adherent to erythrocytes. In addition to invading erythrocytes, bartonellae have been reported to invade endothelial cells and macrophages.

Mechanisms of Pathogenicity.   In Oroya fever, there is massive parasitization of mature erythrocytes. In vitro electron microscopic studies suggest that bartonellae adhere to erythrocytes via a flagellum-associated adhesin. In vivo, bartonellae also adhere to human erythrocytes, some of which they apparently enter (Fig. 11–13). The mechanism of entry is uncertain but may involve some sort of forced endocytosis. Patients lose up to 500,000 erythrocytes per microliter per day (equivalent to about 10% of the total erythrocytes of a male adult) and are immunosuppressed. Clinical studies have shown that infected erythrocytes are removed by the spleen, probably via erythrophagocytosis.

In verruga peruana, the warts are the result of massive endothelial proliferation. They are infiltrated with many mast cells and neutrophils, and bartonellae are found in the interstitial spaces. Although some investigators have reported finding bartonellae within endothelial cells, others argue that bartonellae are exclusively extracellular in vivo. Therefore, it remains controversial whether bartonellae invade the endothelium in vivo, even though the organisms have been shown to invade host cells in vitro. As the lesions heal, there is focal necrosis of the endothelium.

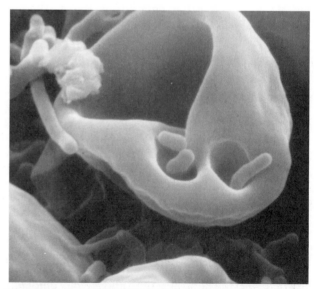

FIGURE 11–13. *Bartonella bacilliformis* **adheres to an erythrocyte and forms deep pits in the cell.** (Reproduced, with permission, from Benson, L. A., et al. Entry of *Bartonella bacilliformis* into erythrocytes. Infect Immun 54:347–353, 1986.)

Diseases Due to *B. bacilliformis*

Epidemiology. Most cases of Carrión's disease are found in the western slopes of the Andes of Peru, Ecuador, Chile, and Colombia. This is because *B. bacilliformis* is spread via the bites of a species of sandfly (*Lutzomyia verrucarum*) that lives at high altitudes in valleys at right angles to the prevailing winds. The sandfly feeds only at dusk, and humans are the only known reservoir. Many asymptomatic individuals in endemic areas have been shown to have low-level *Bartonella* bacteremia.

Diagnosis

(1) History and Physical Examination. People with **Carrión's disease** may have Oroya fever, verruga peruana, or both, but the two manifestations do not occur simultaneously.

Oroya fever is an acute, febrile, hemolytic anemia. About 2–5 weeks after being bitten by an infected sandfly, the patient develops fever, diffuse bone and muscle pain, hepatosplenomegaly, and profound anemia. In some cases, the patient becomes secondarily infected with *Salmonella* serotype *typhi* and develops fatal typhoid.

Verruga peruana, a fairly benign disease, is characterized by the development of bright red angiomatous warts that bleed profusely when touched. The warts are not painful, but they can be quite disfiguring, especially if they appear on the face. The warts may be as large as an egg, but most are much smaller and appear in crops, somewhat like red berries. Patients may experience some fever and malaise while the growths are present. The warts typically last 4–6 months but can persist for up to 2 years.

(2) Laboratory Analysis. Oroya fever is diagnosed by culturing the organisms from the blood and by visualizing parasitized erythrocytes on Giemsa-stained thin blood films. The organisms can be cultured from warts and can be seen in tissue sections. Antibody to *B. bacilliformis* appears during convalescence and is not useful in diagnosing Carrión's disease.

Treatment and Prognosis. Oroya fever has been treated successfully with penicillin, tetracycline, chloramphenicol, or various other antibiotics. The combination of antibiotic treatment and blood transfusion causes dramatic improvement in many patients who have Oroya fever but may not eliminate bacteremia. Verruga peruana does not respond well to antibiotic therapy.

Bartonella (Rochalimaea) quintana

Bartonella quintana is the cause of trench fever, so named because about 1 million German and Allied soldiers suffered from the disease during the trench warfare of World War I. An early investigator of trench fever, Dr. H. da Rocha-Lima, noted that the disease has a fever cycle of roughly 5 days (quintana). For this reason, *B. quintana* was long known as *Rochalimaea quintana*.

Characteristics of *B. quintana*

B. quintana is a coccobacillus that measures 0.2–0.4 μm in length and shows bipolar staining. The organism is an extracellular pathogen that can be cultivated on enriched media containing 5% sheep's blood. Growth becomes confluent after about 7 days of cultivation at 37 °C in an atmosphere of 5% CO_2.

Humans serve as the key reservoir of *B. quintana,* an organism that is transmitted by the body louse (*Pediculus humanus corporis*). The bartonellae grow extracellularly within the louse gut and are not transmitted transovarially to the offspring of the infected louse. Lice have been shown to remain infected with bartonellae for more than a year, and infection does not shorten their life span. As with typhus rickettsiae, with *B. quintana* the organisms are passed in the feces of the louse as it feeds, and the organisms enter the bitten skin when the patient scratches the skin.

Diseases Due to *B. quintana*

Epidemiology. Patients infected with *B. quintana* may develop trench fever, relapsing febrile bacteremia, intraocular inflammation, or bacillary angiomatosis. Serologic studies suggest that many individuals who are infected with *B. quintana* develop mild disease that is not clinically recognized and is sometimes diagnosed as fever of unknown origin (FUO) in Mexico, the USA, and Europe.

Trench fever was seen during both world wars but is now seen only sporadically. Asymptomatic patients have been shown to have *Bartonella* bacteremia that persists for years, resulting in relapse of trench fever as late as 8 years after being initially infected.

Diagnosis. The manifestations of **trench fever** begin 4–35 days after an individual is infected with *B. quintana* and include fever, chills, headache, ocular pain, malaise, and severe pain of the muscles, joints, and bones. Because the shins tend to be extremely painful, the disease is often called **shin bone fever.** A macular rash may appear on the abdomen and look like the rose spots of typhoid. The fever rises steadily for 2–3 days and then subsides over the next 2–3 days, resulting in a typical 5-day or 6-day cycle of trench fever. The disease may follow a relapsing course that lasts several years and may be confused with louse-borne relapsing fever.

Bacillary angiomatosis occurs only among patients who are severely immunosuppressed. Most cases are caused by *Bartonella henselae,* but a few cases have been attributed to *B. quintana.* Both organisms have also been associated with cases of inflammatory **optic neuritis.**

Treatment. *B. quintana* is susceptible in vitro to a wide variety of antibiotics, but patients are treated most often with tetracyclines.

Bartonella (Rochalimaea) henselae

Bartonella (Rochalimaea) henselae was originally identified in clinical samples by the use of polymerase chain reaction technology, which showed it to be closely related to *Bartonella quintana* and *Bartonella vinsonii*. In immunocompetent individuals, infection with *B. henselae* usually results in cat-scratch disease. In immunocompromised patients, particularly those with AIDS, infection results in bacillary angiomatosis, with or without peliosis hepatis. Bacillary angiomatosis is rare in patients with normal immune responses.

Characteristics of *B. henselae*

B. henselae is a gram-negative organism that has been cultivated on enriched blood agar. It takes about 4 days to produce confluent growth at 25 °C.

Little is known of how *B. henselae* produces disease. The organism has been seen within macrophages in patients with cat-scratch disease, but it appears to be primarily an extracellular pathogen in patients with bacillary angiomatosis and peliosis hepatis. Abundant organisms are seen in the interstitium of the angiomatous lesions associated with the latter two diseases. Investigators believe that extracellular bartonellae produce a substance or set of substances that cause endothelial cells to proliferate rapidly. Cat-scratch disease is marked by the formation of granulomas in the lymph nodes that drain the site of a cat bite or scratch.

Diseases Due to *B. henselae*

Epidemiology. Most patients with cat-scratch disease are children, and 87–99% of children and adults with this disease report having been bitten, scratched, or licked by a cat—usually a kitten—prior to its onset. The source of bacillary angiomatosis is less certain. Although one study of 48 patients showed that being bitten or scratched by a cat was the single greatest risk factor for development of bacillary angiomatosis among AIDS patients, about one-third of the patients could recall no such contact. A recent demonstration that cat fleas can be infected with *B. henselae* raises the possibility that the organism may occasionally be transmitted via the bites of fleas.

Some immunocompetent individuals have developed persistent bacteremia with *B. henselae* soon after being bitten by a tick.

Diagnosis
(1) History and Physical Examination
(a) Cat-Scratch Disease. Typical and atypical forms of cat-scratch disease have been described and account for 89% and 11% of cases, respectively.

Patients with **typical cat-scratch disease** develop a macule at the site of entry of the organisms 4–6 days after being bitten or scratched by a cat. The macule quickly becomes a papule or pustule, and the draining lymph nodes gradually swell over the next 7–50 days. Most of the swollen nodes are on the head, neck, or upper extremities and may be confused with the cervical lymphadenopathy of scrofula. The lymphadenopathy of cat-scratch disease is due to the

formation of granulomas and may be accompanied by fever and malaise. Nodes suppurate in about 15% of patients. Typical cat-scratch disease subsides spontaneously in 2–4 months.

Atypical cat-scratch disease has a wide variety of clinical presentations. The most common is **Parinaud's oculoglandular syndrome** (granulomatous conjunctivitis with swelling of the preauricular lymph nodes). Less common are atypical pneumonia, granulomatous hepatitis, encephalitis, tonsillitis, cerebral arteritis, splenitis, and radiculitis. Patients with atypical cat-scratch disease may develop allergic manifestations such as erythema nodosum or erythema annulare or may develop a maculopapular rash. Some suffer from thrombocytopenic purpura.

(b) Bacillary Angiomatosis and Peliosis Hepatis. The proliferation of endothelial cells in patients with angiomatosis may cause dermal nodules, visceral nodules, or both. Dermal nodules most often begin as small red papules. The papules gradually enlarge to a diameter of several centimeters and look like cranberries. Visceral nodules may appear in almost any organ system. If vascular proliferation occurs in the liver, it causes the formation of large blood-filled cysts known as peliosis hepatis.

Patients with angiomatosis may suffer from fever, weight loss, diarrhea, malaise, and signs of dysfunction of organs in which angiomas are located. Patients with peliosis hepatis may have hepatosplenomegaly, a feeling of fullness, and abdominal pain.

(2) Laboratory Analysis. In patients with suspected cat-scratch disease, the diagnosis has long rested on the use of a skin test that utilizes an extract taken from the nodes of patients with confirmed cat-scratch disease. Nodes can be biopsied and cultured for *B. henselae,* and node tissue sections can be stained and examined for evidence of the bacillary forms of *B. henselae* in macrophages. In patients with suspected angiomatosis, *B. henselae* can be cultured from the nodules and can be seen in the interstitial spaces between endothelial cells. An immunofluorescent antibody test can be used to detect antibody to *B. henselae,* and polymerase chain reaction tests have been used at major research and reference laboratories.

Treatment. Cat-scratch disease is usually treated with rifampin, ciprofloxacin, gentamicin, or trimethoprim-sulfamethoxazole. Swollen lymph nodes may be aspirated to relieve pain. Many patients with bacillary angiomatosis are treated with a prolonged course (4–6 weeks) of erythromycin, rifampin, or doxycycline. Alternatively, some have been treated successfully with combined antibiotic therapy (erythromycin plus norfloxacin or chloramphenicol) or sequential antibiotic therapy (ceftriaxone plus gentamicin followed by ciprofloxacin).

Selected Readings

Ativan, W. H., and H. H. Winkler. Permeability of *Rickettsia prowazekii* to nicotinamide adenine dinucleotide. J Bacteriol 171: 761–766, 1989.

Bakken, J. S., et al. Clinical and laboratory characteristics of human granulocytic ehrlichiosis. JAMA 275:199–205, 1996.

Barlough, J. E., et al. Protection against *Ehrlichia equi* is conferred by prior infection with the human granulocytotropic *Ehrlichia* (HGE agent). J Clin Microbiol 33:3333–3334, 1995.

Benson, L. A., et al. Entry of *Bartonella bacilliformis* into erythrocytes. Infect Immun 54:347–353, 1986.

Blanchard, A., and L. Montagnier. AIDS-associated mycoplasmas. Annu Rev Microbiol 48:687–712, 1994.

Dolan, M. J., et al. Syndrome of *Rochalimaea henselae* adenitis suggesting cat-scratch disease. Ann Intern Med 118:331–336, 1993.

Feng, H.-M., V. L. Popov, and D. H. Walker. Depletion of gamma interferon and tumor necrosis factor alpha in mice with *Rickettsia conorii*–infected endothelium: impairment of rickettsicidal nitric oxide production resulting in fatal, overwhelming rickettsial disease. Infect Immun 62:1952–1960, 1994.

Feng, H.-M., J. Wen, and D. H. Walker. *Rickettsia australis* infection: a murine model of highly invasive vasculopathic rickettsiosis. Am J Pathol 142:1471–1482, 1993.

Heinzen, R. A., et al. Differential interactions with endocytic and exocytic pathways distinguish parasitophorous vacuoles of *Coxiella burnetii* and *Chlamydia trachomatis*. Infect Immun 64:796–809, 1996.

Higgins, J. A., et al. Acquisition of the cat-scratch disease agent *Bartonella henselae* by cat fleas. J Med Entomol 33:490–495, 1996.

Hill, E. M., et al. Adhesion to and invasion of cultured human cells by *Bartonella bacilliformis*. Infect Immun 60:4051–4058, 1992.

Igietseme, J. U., et al. Integrin-mediated epithelial–T cell interaction enhances nitric oxide production and increases intracellular inhibition of *Chlamydia*. J Leukoc Biol 59:656–662, 1996.

Kostianovsky, M., Y. Lamy, and M. A. Greco. Immunohistochemical and electron microscopic profiles of cutaneous Kaposi's sarcoma and bacillary angiomatosis. Ultrastruct Pathol 16:629–640, 1992.

Lo, S.-C., et al. Enhancement of HIV-1 cytocidal effects in CD4+ lymphocytes by the AIDS-associated mycoplasma. Science 251:1074–1076, 1991.

Mernaugh, G., and G. M. Ihler. Deformation factor: an extracellular protein synthesized by *Bartonella bacilliformis* that deforms erythrocyte membranes. Infect Immun 60:937–943, 1992.

Moulder, J. W. Interaction of chlamydiae and host cells in vitro. Microbiol Rev 55:143–190, 1991.

Muhlestein, J. B., et al. Increased incidence of *Chlamydia* species within the coronary arteries of patients with symptomatic atherosclerotic versus other forms of cardiovascular disease. J Am Coll Cardiol 27:1555–1561, 1996.

Ong, G., et al. Detection and widespread distribution of *Chlamydia pneumoniae* in the vascular system and its possible implications. J Clin Pathol 49:102–106, 1996.

Raoult, D., et al. Diagnosis of 22 new cases of *Bartonella* endocarditis. Ann Intern Med 125:646–652, 1996.

Slater, L. N., D. F. Welch, and K.-W. Min. *Rochalimaea henselae* causes bacillary angiomatosis and peliosis hepatis. Arch Intern Med 152:602–606, 1992.

Tappero, J. W., et al. The epidemiology of bacillary angiomatosis and bacillary peliosis. JAMA 269:770–775, 1993.

Turco, J., and H. H. Winkler. Relationship of tumor necrosis factor alpha, the nitric oxide synthetase pathway, and lipopolysaccharide to the killing of gamma interferon–treated macrophage-like RAW264.7 cells by *Rickettsia prowazekii*. Infect Immun 62:2568–2574, 1994.

Walker, D. H., and J. S. Dumler. Emergence of the ehrlichioses as human health problems. Emerg Infect Dis 2:18–29, 1996.

Walker, T. S., and C. S. Hoover. Rickettsial effects on leukotriene and prostaglandin secretion by mouse polymorphonuclear leukocytes. Infect Immun 59:351–356, 1991.

Walker, T. S., and G. E. Mellott. Rickettsial stimulation of endothelial platelet-activating factor synthesis. Infect Immun 61:2024–2029, 1993.

Walker, T. S., and D. A. Triplett. Serologic characterization of Rocky Mountain spotted fever: appearance of antibodies reactive with endothelial cells and phospholipids, and factors that alter protein C activation and prostacyclin secretion. Am J Clin Pathol 95:725–732, 1991.

Walker, T. S., et al. Endothelial prostaglandin secretion: effects of typhus rickettsiae. J Infect Dis 162:1136–1144, 1990.

SPIROCHETES

Borrelia, Leptospira, and Treponema

The *borreliae, leptospires, and treponemes* are helical gram-negative bacteria that are members of the order Spirochaetales. There are two families in this order: (1) Spirochaetaceae, which includes the pathogenic genera *Borrelia* and *Treponema;* and (2) Leptospiraceae, which includes the genus *Leptospira.* In general, borreliae are speciated according to their arthropod vectors, treponemal species are determined by the diseases they cause, and leptospiral species reflect the animal that is most often their host.

The spirochetes vary tremendously in length, with some being extremely short and others as long as 250 μm. Each organism is curled helically around one or more axial filaments (Fig. 12–1), and the cell body is surrounded by a sheath composed of the cell wall and outer membrane. Outside the outer membrane is a mucoid layer, which in some cases contains glycosaminoglycan. Spirochetes are motile, and their movement appears to be related to their ability to contract and extend themselves about their axial filaments, the number of which varies with the spirochetal genus. Leptospires have 1 axial filament, virulent treponemes have 3, and borreliae have from 7 to 30. The filaments are attached by knobs to pores at the ends of the spirochetes. Axial filaments are much like the flagella of other bacteria, consisting of a helix made of a simple protein, rather than the 9 + 2 microtubular arrangement seen in eukaryotic fibrils. Spirochetes are slender and are usually visualized in clinical samples by use of darkfield or phase-contrast microscopy.

The spirochetal diseases follow a similar pattern, although each disease has its own idiosyncrasies. First, the spirochetes enter through the skin or mucous membranes, where most cause a primary lesion. Spirochetemia is noted about the time clinical disease begins and the spirochetes disseminate to target organs. Next, the disease typically enters a period of latency, followed by secondary and then tertiary disease. In most spirochetal diseases, the patients can continue to harbor spirochetes for a long period of time, with prolonged infection damaging the central nervous system or heart. Finally, immune-mediated damage plays a key role in producing the secondary or tertiary signs and symptoms associated with most spirochetal diseases.

TREPONEMES

The most important spirochetes from a clinical standpoint are the treponemes. Many treponemes are nonpathogenic and are part of the normal flora of the oral mucosa, but several treponemes cause human disease.

The best-known species of pathogenic treponemes is *Treponema pallidum,* which has three subspecies that are discussed below: (1) *Treponema pallidum* subspecies *pallidum* (previously called *T. pallidum*) causes syphilis; (2) *Treponema pallidum* subspecies *endemicum* (previously called *T. pallidum* II) causes bejel, or endemic syphilis; and (3) *Treponema pallidum* subspecies *pertenue* (previously called *Treponema pertenue*) causes yaws. Another species of pathogenic treponemes, *Treponema carateum,* causes pinta and is also discussed in this chapter.

Treponema pallidum

Treponema pallidum subspecies *pallidum* is the cause of syphilis. This disease burst on the European scene during the Middle Ages, when it was known as the "great pox" (to distinguish it from smallpox). It appears to have been more virulent at that time than it is today, and patients often developed large ulcerative lesions (great pox) and disfiguring granulomas of cartilaginous tissue (gummas). When Shakespeare said, "A pox on you!" he was not speaking of smallpox but of syphilis.

Many of the aristocracy and intelligentsia of Europe suffered from syphilis. For example, the consort of Mary, Queen of Scots, was said to have stopped going out in public because he developed a gumma that eroded his nose. Notable individuals from history and the arts who reportedly succumbed to neurosyphilis (syphilitic insanity) or who had tertiary syphilis and then died of another cause include George Meredith, Baudelaire, Heinrich Heine, Oscar

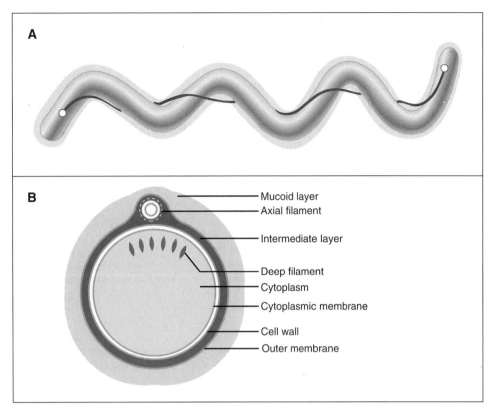

FIGURE 12-1. The structure of spirochetes. The longitudinal view **(A)** shows a helical spirochete with an axial filament inserted at each pole and overlapping in the middle. The cross-sectional view **(B)** depicts a spirochete that has one axial filament.

Wilde, Casanova, Dean Swift, Dostoyevsky, Walt Whitman, Nietzsche, Gaugin, Manet, Schopenhauer, Schumann, Frederick the Great, Ivan the Terrible, Henry VIII, Edward VII, and the popes Alexander VI, Julius II, and Leo X.

Although syphilis was spread to Europe from either the Americas or Africa during the 15th century, it was not until the 18th century that physicians recognized that it was transmitted sexually. Then came a tragic experiment: In 1767, British physician John Hunter inoculated himself with urethral exudate from a patient with gonorrhea. Because Hunter developed a fatal case of syphilis, two generations of physicians believed that syphilis and gonorrhea were the same disease. In 1838, Phillipe Ricord finally convinced the medical community that the diseases were separate; in 1905, *T. pallidum* was discovered to be the causative agent; and within 1 year, August Paul von Wassermann developed his serologic test for syphilis, a test that is used even today.

Syphilis once was believed to be disappearing in the USA, but it has lately made a substantial comeback. By the mid 1980s, the number of syphilis cases in adults (sexually transmitted disease) had become fairly stable, and the number of cases in infants (congenitally acquired disease) had dropped substantially. Subsequently, the number of cases began to rise dramatically, nearly doubling from 1985 to 1989 (25,000 versus 44,000 cases). Epidemiologists have attributed this rise in the incidence of syphilis largely to increased transmission among homosexual men and via prostitutes who are drug users.

Characteristics of *T. pallidum*

General Features.   Considering the clinical impact of syphilis, surprisingly little is known about the organism or its pathogenic properties. This is largely because *T. pallidum* was not able to be cultured in vitro until recently. Even now, culture consists only of transferring the organisms from rabbits to cultured rabbit epithelial cells in which the treponemes multiply for a few generations. Usually, *T. pallidum* is cultured by inoculating the spirochetes into the testes of rabbits. Here they grow very slowly, with a doubling time of about 30 hours.

Mechanisms of Pathogenicity.   *T. pallidum* is a microaerophile. Its virulent strains produce hyaluronidase, an enzyme that may help the treponeme penetrate the glycocalyx surrounding host cells. In vitro studies suggest that virulent treponemes coat themselves with fibronectin, which allows them to bind tightly to endothelial cells. The lesions of *T. pallidum* infections contain treponemes attached to endothelial cells, and the adherent treponemes elicit a cellular inflammatory response that is probably responsible for most of the damage that occurs during syphilis. Primary and secondary lesions also contain activated cytotoxic T cells. Both immune competent cells and antibody participate in producing tissue damage. Syphilis is largely a vasculitis, and *T. pallidum* is an extracellular pathogen. Recent studies have shown that *T. pallidum* has an external layer containing two substances—glycosaminoglycan and sialic acids—and that these substances interfere with the abilities of the classic and alternative complement pathways, respectively, to kill treponemes. Some investigators have also reported that syphilis treponemes secrete prostaglandin E_2 (PGE_2), a potent immunosuppressive chemical that interferes with granulocyte elicitation, migration, and activation.

Diseases Due to *Treponema pallidum* subspecies *pallidum*

Epidemiology. Syphilis can be transmitted sexually to adults or congenitally to fetuses and newborn infants. When a person has sexual intercourse with someone who already has syphilis, the chance of transmitting the infection is 1 in 10 for each incident of sexual contact. The median infective dose (ID_{50}) of *T. p. pallidum* has been estimated to be about 57 organisms. In infected adults, the disease can progress through primary, secondary, latent, and tertiary stages. The risk of transplacental transmission of syphilis from a pregnant woman to her fetus depends on the woman's stage of infection during pregnancy. Primary infection in the pregnant woman carries a 100% risk to the fetus; secondary infection carries a 90% risk; early latent disease carries a 30% risk; and late latent or tertiary disease carries no risk to the fetus.

Diagnosis

(1) History and Physical Examination. The clinical findings of syphilis vary, depending on the stage of disease.

(a) Primary Syphilis. In sexually transmitted disease, the treponemes enter the body through a mucous membrane or an abrasion and rapidly multiply at the site. They then spread through the lymphatics and systemic circulation, and 10–120 days later (mean duration is 3 weeks), an intense inflammatory response develops at the site of entry. The capillary endothelia in the area swell, and plasma cells, monocytes, and lymphocytes infiltrate the region. This process results in the formation of a primary syphilitic lesion called a **chancre** (Fig. 12–2). The chancre is a

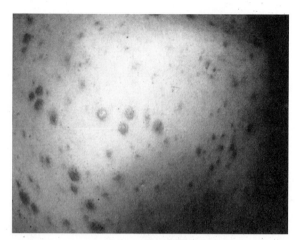

FIGURE 12–3. Lesions of secondary syphilis. The lesions can take many forms and can be found on the skin and mucosae. Secondary lesions contain treponemes and are infectious. (Courtesy of Armed Forces Institute of Pathology. AFIP photo 58-13966-45.)

painless, hard, shallow ulcer that usually occurs on the external genitals but may be oral, anal, or at the site of a previous abrasion. If the chancre becomes secondarily infected, it may become painful. In most cases, there is only one chancre, but some people have multiple chancres. The lymph nodes that drain the area where the chancre occurs swell and are sometimes called satellite buboes, but this lymphadenitis is not painful. The initial syphilitic syndrome is called primary syphilis and is a rather quiescent stage, with the chancre healing spontaneously in 3–6 weeks. Thus, it is not unusual for patients with primary syphilis to discount the danger and fail to seek treatment. Because the chancres are almost always painless, cervical and anal chancres often go unrecognized.

(b) Secondary Syphilis. From 6 to 8 weeks after the appearance of the chancre (but sometimes before the primary lesion heals), the untreated patient develops numerous secondary cutaneous and mucocutaneous lesions, which may be macular, papular, pustular, follicular, or nodular (Fig. 12–3). The secondary lesions are filled with treponemes, are extremely contagious, and are sometimes accompanied by systemic symptoms such as malaise, anorexia, headache, sore throat, generalized lymphadenopathy, and alopecia (hair loss). Some patients develop renal disease or arthritis, which occurs when immune complexes are deposited in the kidneys or joints, while a few develop hepatitis or uveitis. Between 15% and 40% of patients with primary and secondary syphilis have cerebrospinal fluid abnormalities that indicate the presence of transient damage to mesodermally derived structures in the central nervous system, such as the meninges and the blood vessels to the brain. After 2–6 weeks, the secondary disease will wane, and if the patient does not receive antibiotics, the syphilis will become latent.

(c) Latent Syphilis. The disease may remain latent for years. During this time, treponemes grow in ectopic sites, and the immune system tries to elimi-

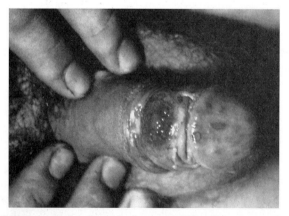

FIGURE 12–2. A lesion of primary syphilis. Chancres, such as the one shown on the penis in this photograph, are usually painless and heal spontaneously in 3–6 weeks. (Courtesy of Armed Forces Institute of Pathology. AFIP photo 82-9103.)

nate them. This causes a chronic vasculitis that produces no symptoms until years later, when treponemes can no longer be found and the damage is substantial. During latency, there are no visible lesions, but results of serologic tests for syphilis remain positive. These tests are discussed in detail below. Briefly, patients with syphilis develop two types of antibodies: nonspecific antibodies against phospholipids, which can be detected by "nontreponemal" serologic tests; and specific antibodies against treponemal surface antigens, which can be detected by "treponemal" serologic tests. During the first 4 years of latency (so-called early latency), infected women can pass syphilis transplacentally to their unborn offspring. While about 25% of infected men and women in early latency have a relapse of symptoms similar to those seen in the secondary stage of disease, relapse after the first 4 years is rare.

(d) Tertiary Syphilis. About one-third of untreated patients develop destructive tertiary syphilis. Patients with this stage of disease are not infectious, and some no longer have serologic evidence of syphilis. Rarely can treponemes be found in the lesions (the organisms were likely to have been eliminated years earlier), but the immune response to the affected tissue continues. There are three major forms of tertiary syphilis: late benign syphilis, cardiovascular syphilis, and neurosyphilis.

Late benign syphilis, or **gumma,** occurs in about 15% of patients with untreated syphilis. Gummas are granulomatous lesions that most frequently affect the skin, cartilage, or bone but sometimes affect the viscera. Gummas begin to appear between 1 and 10 years after primary syphilis.

Cardiovascular syphilis occurs in about 10% of patients with untreated syphilis, usually at least 10 years after primary syphilis. The pathologic hallmark is aortitis. The aortic vasa vasorum is severely damaged, replacing elastic tissue with fibrous tissue. This is occasionally asymptomatic, but it is most often evidenced by aortic regurgitation. The second most frequent cardiac disorder seen is aortic aneurysm, while some patients develop obstruction of the coronary ostia.

Neurosyphilis occurs in about 8% of patients with untreated syphilis, making its first appearance 5–35 years after the primary episode, most often in white males. About one-third of these patients have negative results in the nontreponemal serologic tests, and a few also have negative results in the treponemal serologic tests. Neurosyphilis occurs because the central nervous system (particularly, the brain parenchyma) and its vasculature have been damaged by the chronic immune response to treponemes. The most common sign is **tabes dorsalis,** which is characterized by a chronic, progressive sclerosis of the posterior spinal roots, the posterior columns of the spinal cord, and the peripheral nerves and which results in loss of pain sensation, position recognition, and motion sense. Affected patients at first become extremely uncoordinated in their movements and have lightning pains (sharp, shooting pains). Their mus-

cles atrophy, and sometimes the optic nerve atrophies as well. Because these patients often lack proprioception (a sense of where their extremities are), they may exhibit an odd pattern of walking as they search for the floor with their feet. They may also be impotent or lose bladder function. Eventually, these patients become completely paralyzed and may become blind. Other patients develop **generalized paresis,** a condition that includes increasing muscular weakness, progressive dementia, palsy, and speech disturbances. Many patients with this condition have delusions of grandeur. This is the so-called syphilitic insanity that has left many of its victims spending the last years of their lives incurably insane and paralyzed. A third form of disease affecting the central nervous system is **meningovascular syphilis,** in which damage to the meningeal vasculature results in strokes or seizures. Finally, recent studies have shown that some patients with concurrent syphilis and human immunodeficiency virus (HIV) infection develop neurosyphilis within 6 months of the appearance of a primary chancre. These patients most often suffer from syphilitic meningitis and often exhibit abnormalities of the second and eighth cranial nerves.

(e) Congenital Syphilis. When *T. p. pallidum* is transmitted transplacentally, there is massive treponemal invasion of the fetus. Some offspring of infected women are stillborn or are spontaneously aborted, while others die as neonates, with numerous destructive lesions throughout their bodies. Yet many are born alive and survive the neonatal period.

Infants with congenital syphilis have one or more characteristic clinical signs. The body may be covered with vesicular or bullous eruptions that even affect the palms and soles. The nose may be obstructed with a mucoid or bloody discharge filled with treponemes. This condition is called "snuffles." The nasal secretions are highly infectious, and treponemes may enter the mother or other attendants through an abrasion, mucous membrane, or cut. In some infants, the nasal bones may become inflamed, leading to saddle nose. Treponemal laryngitis may be present, causing infants to have a characteristic weak, forced cry. The long bones may be affected by periostitis or osteochondritis, as seen on x-ray. Treponemal renal disease may also be present.

If infants with congenital disease do not receive appropriate antibiotic therapy, about 25% will die during the first year of life. Of the survivors, most will become serologically positive for syphilis, about 40% will develop the stigmas (permanent defects) of congenital syphilis, and some will develop neurosyphilis. The most prevalent stigmas are Hutchinson's incisors (screwdriver-shaped incisors with notched occlusional surfaces), Moon's teeth (first molars with supernumerary defective cusps), and interstitial keratitis (inflammation of the corneal parenchyma). Other stigmas include saber shins, saddle nose, and Higouménakis's sign (unilateral thickening of the inner third of the clavicle).

(2) Laboratory Tests. Virulent treponemes cannot be routinely cultured, but they can be demonstrated in exudate drawn from lesions and in blood.

(a) Darkfield Microscopy. Primary and secondary syphilitic lesions are filled with treponemes that can be visualized by darkfield microscopy.

(b) Serologic Tests. Two categories of tests—referred to as "nontreponemal" and "treponemal" tests—are used in the diagnosis of syphilis.

The **nontreponemal tests** measure so-called reaginic antibody, which is antibody that recognizes a cardiolipin-lecithin–containing antigen. Syphilis patients produce high levels of antiphospholipid antibodies (APA), and these APA can be detected in a variety of test systems. These APA also appear in people who are being treated with certain drugs or have had certain infections, and they are believed to cause women to miscarry their pregnancies; APA that are not due to treponemal diseases are called lupus anticoagulants. Some of the nontreponemal test systems used in the diagnosis of syphilis are the Venereal Disease Research Laboratory (VDRL) test, the Wassermann test, the automated reagin test (ART), and the rapid plasma reagin (RPR) test. Because the test antigens and concentrations vary among these tests, their results cannot be compared quantitatively. In patients with primary syphilis, results of the VDRL test become positive 1–3 weeks after the chancre appears. All patients with secondary disease have positive results in this test, and the VDRL response begins to fade during latency. Some patients with tertiary syphilis have negative results in the VDRL test. The VDRL and other nontreponemal tests are used to screen people for evidence of syphilis, because they are easy to perform, are inexpensive, and are suitably reliable. At one time, most states in the USA required marriage license applicants to submit to a VDRL test. When the VDRL test yields positive results, the more expensive and difficult—but also more specific—treponemal tests are used to confirm the diagnosis of syphilis.

The **treponemal tests** detect antibody to genuine treponemal antigens. At one time, each serum sample was incubated with living *T. pallidum* on a slide to determine if it contained antibody that would halt the organism's motility. This *T. pallidum* immobilization (TPI) test is difficult to perform correctly and has been replaced in most laboratories by the fluorescent treponemal antibody (FTA) test. The FTA test can be made more specific by first absorbing the patient's serum with a commensal treponeme called Reiter's treponeme to remove less specific antibody that reacts with treponemal group antigens (the FTA-absorption, or FTA-ABS, test). The presence of treponemal infection can also be determined by the treponemal hemagglutination (TPHA) test. Antibody to treponemes (as determined by the FTA test) appears earlier in primary disease than does reaginic antibody. Although some patients will be VDRL-negative at the end of primary disease, essentially all patients are FTA-positive at this time. The relationships between the course of disease and the appearance of FTA and VDRL antibodies are presented in Table 12–1. The FTA test becomes positive much earlier than does the VDRL test, is more specific, and remains positive throughout tertiary syphilis in most patients. Finally, congenital infections should be diagnosed using fluorescein-conjugated anti-IgM (the IgM-FTA-ABS test).

It should be noted that patients with yaws, bejel, and pinta have the same serologic results in all treponemal and nontreponemal tests as do patients with syphilis. The three diseases cannot be differentiated from syphilis on the basis of serologic test results alone. It should also be remembered that because most patients with syphilis become serologically positive for life, the mere presence of a single positive result in the VDRL or FTA test does not warrant a diagnosis of active syphilis.

(3) Laboratory Results. The diagnosis of syphilis rests on a combination of clinical findings and results of the laboratory tests described above.

(a) Primary Syphilis. Antibody to treponemes or to nontreponemal antigens will often appear after the chancre appears, so an early negative serologic test result does not reliably exclude the diagnosis of primary syphilis. If serologic tests yield positive results, however, this strongly supports the diagnosis, especially if the antibody titer is rising. Treponemes can frequently be noted on darkfield examination of exudate from a chancre. If the chancre is on the oral mucosa, however, commensal oral spirochetes will interfere with the darkfield microscopy, since these spirochetes cannot be differentiated from *T. pallidum*. For this reason, it may be necessary to wait for the serologic results to become positive to be sure of the diagnosis.

(b) Secondary Syphilis. This is diagnosed in patients with appropriate clinical signs by using darkfield microscopy to identify treponemes in the exudate of secondary lesions. A positive serologic test result will confirm the diagnosis, because essentially all patients with secondary syphilis have positive results when either treponemal or nontreponemal tests are used.

(c) Latent Syphilis. Patients with latent syphilis are not likely to be routinely identified, since they have no presenting lesions. However, they may be discovered through serologic screening or when they give birth to an infant with congenital syphilis. In a patient with a positive nontreponemal test result, the diagnosis is confirmed by demonstrating the presence of specific antibody to *T. pallidum*.

(d) Tertiary Syphilis. This is diagnosed in patients who have typical signs of cardiovascular syphilis, gummatous lesions, or neurosyphilis and who also have positive results in treponemal or nontreponemal tests. Unfortunately, patients with neurosyphilis are often serologically negative, making diagnosis more difficult.

(e) Congenital Syphilis. In newborn infants with clinical signs such as snuffles, primary lesions, or laryngitis, the diagnosis is made by identifying treponemes in nonoral lesions and by confirming the presence of IgM directed against *T. pallidum*. The IgM-

TABLE 12–1.   Modes of Disease Transmission and Results of Two Serologic Tests—the Venereal Disease Research Laboratory (VDRL) Test and the Fluorescent Treponemal Antibody (FTA) Test—in Various Stages of Syphilis

Stage	Mode of Transmission		Percentage of Patients With Positive Test Results	
	Sexual	Transplacental	VDRL Test	FTA Test
Primary syphilis	Yes	Yes	76	86
Secondary syphilis	Yes	Yes	100	100
Latent syphilis				
Early latency	No	Yes	95	99
Late latency	No	No	72	96
Tertiary syphilis	No	No	70	97

FTA-ABS test is used for this purpose. Remember that the usual serologic tests will identify IgG (rather than IgM) antibody to treponemes and that any IgG found in the newborn is likely to have come across the placenta from the mother.

(f) Syphilis and Acquired Immunodeficiency Syndrome.   AIDS patients who acquire syphilis exhibit a normal serologic response to *T. pallidum,* as evidenced by the time of appearance and peak titers of treponemal and nontreponemal antibodies. Because of the danger of early neurosyphilis in AIDS patients who have serologic evidence of syphilis, some clinicians recommend that their cerebrospinal fluid be examined for evidence of neurologic disease.

Treatment and Prognosis.   In adults, forms of syphilis other than neurosyphilis are treated with benzathine penicillin G. Neurosyphilis and congenital syphilis are treated with a combination of probenecid and aqueous penicillin G; the probenecid keeps serum penicillin levels elevated by slowing excretion of the antibiotic. In some patients, antibiotic therapy causes a **Jarisch-Herxheimer reaction,** characterized by a temporary intensification of fever, chills, and clinical signs. Penicillin halts primary and secondary syphilis, but it is unclear whether antibiotic treatment completely eradicates the treponemes. Gummas remain, but their development is arrested. If penicillin is administered to a pregnant woman during the first trimester, it will prevent congenital syphilis, but this treatment is less successful later during the pregnancy. Treatment of neurosyphilis is of questionable value, but the attempt should be made. If treponemes remain, they will be killed, but the central nervous system damage is irreversible. Doxycycline and ceftriaxone have each been used successfully in treating syphilis when penicillin use was contraindicated.

Most patients who are treated successfully during primary or secondary disease gradually become serologically negative for syphilis within 2 years, but some patients remain seropositive for life. Patients treated appropriately during early primary disease (before antibody appears) may not become serologically positive for syphilis. Reinfection with *T. p. pallidum* is uncommon.

Diseases Due to *Treponema pallidum* subspecies *endemicum*

Treponema pallidum subspecies *endemicum* causes **endemic syphilis,** or **bejel.** This rare form of syphilis occurs mostly in northern Africa (especially Egypt) and in the Middle East and may involve transmission through abrasions. The primary lesions of bejel are usually in the mouth, leading many investigators to believe that the infection is passed via shared eating utensils. Children are often the victims of this infection. The disease is similar to yaws in that the late lesions are gummatous and there is no damage to the heart or central nervous system. Laboratory diagnosis and treatment are the same as for syphilis (see above).

Diseases Due to *Treponema pallidum* subspecies *pertenue*

Treponema pallidum subspecies *pertenue* is the cause of a contagious treponemal disease called **yaws** or **frambesia.** This disease is similar to syphilis except that it is not transmitted sexually and only the late lesions are gummatous. Additionally, many yaws patients but few syphilis patients are children. At one time, there were an estimated 50 million cases of yaws in the world. Today, however, the incidence is greatly reduced, and yaws is endemic only in Africa, India, tropical South America, Indonesia, and the Pacific islands.

Yaws is spread directly by nonsexual contact or indirectly by flies. About 3–4 weeks later, a painless red papule surrounded by erythema develops at the site of treponemal entry; this is the **mother yaw,** or **framboise** (Fig. 12–4). The mother yaw ulcerates, a crust forms, and then the lesion heals in 3–6 months. From 6 to 12 weeks after the appearance of the mother yaw (sometimes before the mother yaw has disappeared), the patient develops crops of papillomatous (wartlike) secondary lesions (Fig. 12–5) that are disfiguring and may later break down and ulcerate. Some patients develop painful secondary lesions on the palms and soles of the feet (Fig. 12–6). These are called **crab yaws** because the lesions make the pa-

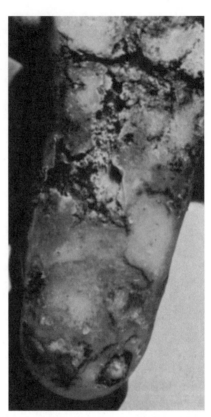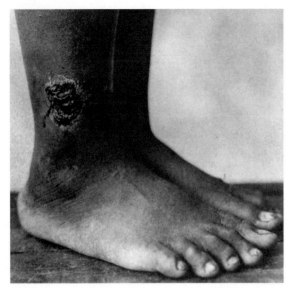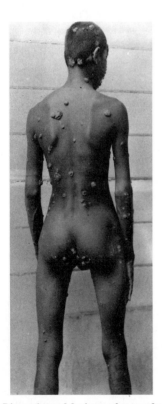

FIGURE 12–4. A lesion of primary yaws. The mother yaw, or framboise, shown here is a hyperkeratotic papilloma that has ulcerated. (Courtesy of Armed Forces Institute of Pathology. AFIP photo 39207.)

tients walk gingerly. The secondary lesions gradually abate, but new crops may appear for up to 5 years. About 10% of untreated patients develop highly destructive granulomatous gummas, some of which are underlaid by periostitis. These lesions may be tremendously disfiguring, and some become secondarily infected and gangrenous. A lesion particularly

FIGURE 12–6. Lesions of crab yaws. These plantar papillomas are painful, causing the patient to walk on the sides of the feet. The odd gait that results gives this form of yaws its name. (Reproduced, with permission, from Strickland, G. T. Hunter's Tropical Medicine, 7th ed. Philadelphia, W. B. Saunders Company, 1991.)

characteristic of yaws is a gumma that ulcerates the nasal area (rhinopharyngitis mutilans).

Laboratory diagnosis of yaws is the same as that of syphilis (see above). Yaws is treated with penicillin G.

Treponema carateum

Treponema carateum is the organism responsible for **pinta,** a disease that occurs in Central and South America and is spread by nonsexual contact. *T. carateum* is less contagious than the three subspecies of *Treponema pallidum* discussed above but has the same mechanisms of pathogenicity. A papule or plaque is seen 2–3 weeks after infection with *T. carateum.* In untreated patients, flat lesions (pintids) develop 3–9 months later and leave the skin depigmented (Fig. 12–7). Repetitive crops of pintids appear for years, making pinta infectious for a far longer time than any of the other treponemal diseases. There are no tertiary cardiac or neurologic lesions, and no destructive gummas occur. Laboratory diagnosis is the same as for syphilis (see above), and pinta is successfully treated with penicillin G.

BORRELIAE
Borrelia recurrentis, Borrelia hermsii, and *Borrelia duttonii*

Epidemic relapsing fever, or louse-borne relapsing fever (LBRF), is caused by *Borrelia recurrentis,* an

FIGURE 12–5. Disseminated lesions of secondary yaws. (Courtesy of Armed Forces Institute of Pathology. AFIP photo 39205.)

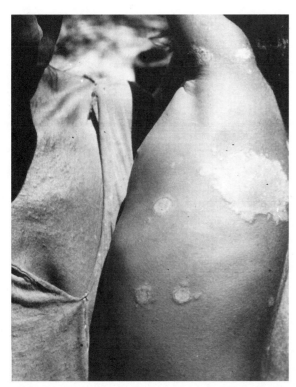

FIGURE 12–7. Lesions of pinta. A large primary lesion and several smaller pintids are shown on the abdomen of an affected child. (Courtesy of Armed Forces Institute of Pathology. AFIP photo 75-5536-2.)

organism that infects body lice. Humans most often acquire LBRF when they squash infected lice with their fingernails. The lice do not pass the infection transovarially to their offspring, so they must continue to feed on infected hosts for the bacteria to persist among a louse population. LBRF was once widespread, but it is now found primarily in eastern Africa. Today, most relapsing fever is of the tick-borne variety.

Endemic relapsing fever, or tick-borne relapsing fever (TBRF), is associated with other borreliae, particularly *Borrelia hermsii* and *Borrelia duttonii.* The fever is acquired via the bite of an infected *Ornithodoros* tick. Infected ticks pass the bacteria to their offspring transovarially, so the infection is able to persist entirely within the vector population. These ticks are soft, feed quickly (in 10–20 minutes), bite primarily during the night, and cause no pain when they bite humans. Thus, many patients with TBRF do not recall having been bitten by a tick. All relapsing fever in the USA is the endemic form. Cases occur primarily in Colorado and Arizona, particularly along the Grand Canyon. Rodents can serve as reservoirs of the infection, and the borreliae are speciated by the vector that passes the infection.

Characteristics of *B. recurrentis, B. hermsii,* and *B. duttonii*

The relapsing fever borreliae are able to change immunodominant proteins called **variable major proteins** (VMPs) on their outer membranes, and this is

what causes the disease to wax and wane. The genes for *Borrelia* VMPs are carried on **linear plasmids,** and each plasmid is present in multiple copies. Only one VMP gene is expressed at a time. This expressed VMP gene is adjacent to the telomere, while the silent genes are located hundreds of nucleotides away from the telomeres of their plasmids (Fig. 12–8). At the beginning of infection, a single VMP is expressed on the surface of each *Borrelia.* When the immune system responds to this VMP, antibody eliminates most of the borreliae through opsonization and complement-mediated lysis. A small number of borreliae persist because they have undergone a transpositional event that resulted in their expressing a new VMP; thus, they are not recognized by the immune response to the first VMP. Soon the borreliae with the new VMP multiply and produce a vigorous bacteremia with its accompanying clinical signs— and the patient relapses.

The mechanism responsible for the gene switch is not fully understood. Investigators believe that a silent gene in the middle of one linear plasmid replaces an expressed gene at the telomere of another plasmid (see Fig. 12–8). The formerly expressed gene is lost, but the newly expressed gene can now be found on both plasmids. The movement of this gene to the telomere results in expression of the gene because it has been moved from a site where there was no upstream promoter to a site where there is a promoter immediately upstream (and the telomere is immediately downstream). With the gene now next to a promoter, it will be read and a new VMP will be produced.

Diseases Due to *B. recurrentis, B. hermsii,* and *B. duttonii*

Diagnosis

(1) History and Physical Examination. From 2 to 15 days after being bitten by an infected tick or after squashing an infected louse, patients with either type of relapsing fever (TBRF or LBRF) experience a sudden onset of fever, chills, headache, lethargy, muscle and joint pain, and extreme weakness. At this time, they may also be photophobic, have a rash on the torso (about one-fourth of cases), and have a tender liver and spleen. These clinical signs last 3–6 days, and then the patients have a rapid drop in temperature, leaving them prostrate and hypotensive. For 5–10 days, they are afebrile and have few borreliae in their blood (in fact, routine blood smears usually will not detect any borreliae at this time). Then a new episode of the acute phase begins. The patients may suffer up to nine such attacks, each less severe than the first. When death occurs, it is usually at the end of the first disease cycle and is due to myocardial collapse. Fatalities have also been attributed to cerebral hemorrhage and to liver failure. TBRF is typically less severe than LBRF.

(2) Laboratory Analysis. The spirochetes can be found on blood films stained with Wright's or Giemsa stain (Fig. 12–9). The organisms can also be cultured on a special medium (Kelly's broth medium),

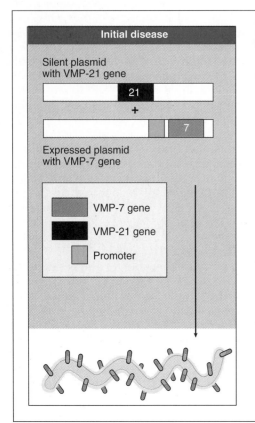
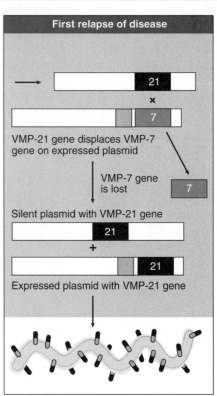

FIGURE 12–8. Genetic control of the antigenic variation responsible for the relapses that occur in patients with relapsing fever. The borreliae that cause the waxing and waning of disease are able to change immunodominant proteins—called variable major proteins (VMPs)—on their outer membranes. During the initial disease (see left side of diagram), the *Borrelia* expresses VMP-7 on its outer membrane because the VMP-7 gene is at the telomere, just downstream from a promoter. The VMP-21 gene is on another plasmid, where it is unexpressed ("silent") because there is no adjacent promoter. An antibody response to VMP-7 develops and removes borreliae from the blood, causing the disease to wane. A transpositional event then occurs in some borreliae and leads to a relapse (see right side of diagram). During the transpositional event, the VMP-7 gene is lost and a copy of the VMP-21 gene takes its place next to the promoter, with the result that the borreliae will now express VMP-21 instead of VMP-7 on their surfaces. Because the immune response does not recognize this new antigen, the borreliae will multiply freely and the disease will relapse.

but the diagnosis most often rests on positive blood smears rather than culture. Patients often are thrombocytopenic and may have elevated serum levels of liver enzymes.

Treatment and Prognosis. Doxycycline is the recommended treatment for either type of relapsing fever, while erythromycin or penicillin G can be used as an acceptable alternative.

Antibiotic treatment of patients with LBRF (and some patients with TBRF) causes a transient but distressing reaction called the **Jarisch-Herxheimer reaction.** This reaction was mentioned previously as occurring occasionally in patients treated for syphilis. Patients typically have rigors (chills) that begin 2–3 hours after antibiotics are initiated. The temperature rises and the blood pressure drops over several hours, causing the patient to feel apprehensive and cold and to complain of head and muscle aches. The signs and symptoms last 12–24 hours and are rarely life-threatening. The molecular cause of the reaction is not understood, but it occurs during the time that the spirochetes disappear from the blood. A Jarisch-Herxheimer reaction is best managed by administering intravenous fluids as needed to control hypotension.

Without antibiotic treatment, about 40% of patients with LBRF die. Untreated TBRF is less severe; its untreated mortality rate is 2–5% overall and 20% in young children.

Borrelia burgdorferi

The history of Lyme disease is an illustration of how physicians sometimes turn a blind eye to patients who present them with something they do not understand. For 10 years, Polly Murray sought help

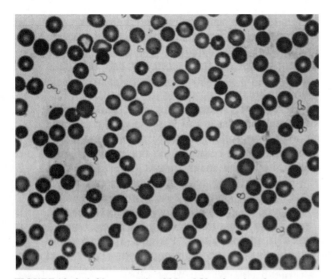

FIGURE 12–9. A Giemsa-stained blood film showing the presence of *Borrelia hermsii*. (Reproduced, with permission, from Strickland, G. T. Hunter's Tropical Medicine, 7th ed. Philadelphia, W. B. Saunders Company, 1991.)

from physicians in Lyme, Connecticut, for her long-standing physical problems, which are now known to have been due to Lyme disease. Before her search was ended, all five members of her family suffered from this disease. Finally, in 1975, a public health physician became interested and invited a rheumatologist, Allen Steere, to investigate. Steere and his associates at Yale University began a process that resulted in the description of a new disease (Lyme disease) and the discovery of its etiologic agent, *Borrelia burgdorferi*. Through the cooperation of mothers, physicians, schools, and local health agencies in the Connecticut towns of Lyme, Old Lyme, and East Haddon (with a combined population of 12,000), Steere's group identified 39 children and 12 adults who had brief recurrent attacks of migratory arthritis affecting the large joints and especially the knees. The attack rate was 12.2 per 1000, at least 100 times greater than that of juvenile rheumatoid arthritis. Thirteen of the patients remembered having had a red papule that became an annular ring, and this reminded Steere's group of a similar disease—erythema chronicum migrans (ECM)—which was discovered in Europe in 1909 and was associated with the bites of *Ixodes ricinus* ticks. In 1983, Willy Burgdorfer and his colleagues at the Rocky Mountain Research Laboratory demonstrated that the disease was due to a *Borrelia,* and the organism was later named *B. burgdorferi.*

B. burgdorferi is now known to be widespread, but most Lyme disease in the USA occurs in three regions: (1) in New England, New York, and Pennsylvania and along the Atlantic seaboard; (2) in Wisconsin, Missouri, and Minnesota; and (3) in western Nevada, California, and Oregon. During the early 1990s, the Centers for Disease Control and Prevention reported that there were between 9000 and 13,000 confirmed cases of Lyme disease in the USA annually, with the number appearing to rise each year. The distribution of Lyme disease is illustrated in Table 12–2, which shows the 11 states in which 94% of the reported cases of Lyme disease occurred during 1994. The restricting factor is the distribution of the vec-

TABLE 12–2. The Distribution of Confirmed Cases of Lyme Disease in the USA

State	Number of Cases of Lyme Disease
New York	5,185
Connecticut	2,013
New Jersey	1,534
Pennsylvania	1,337
Maryland	492
Rhode Island	471
Wisconsin	409
Massachusetts	256
Minnesota	195
Georgia	132
Virginia	131
Total in the above 11 states	12,155*

*This number accounts for 94% of cases in all 50 states in 1994.

tors, which are members of the *I. ricinus* complex of ticks. Lyme disease is the most common vector-borne disease in the USA. As white-tailed deer—the natural hosts of adult *Ixodes* ticks—have increased in number and habitat range, Lyme disease has increased in range as well. Lyme disease also occurs in Europe, where it causes manifestations somewhat different from those seen in the USA, and it is the most common neurologic infection in northern Europe.

Characteristics of *B. burgdorferi*

General Features. *B. burgdorferi* is the longest (20–30 μm) and narrowest (0.2–0.3 μm) of the borreliae. It has the typical corkscrew shape of the spirochetes and has 7–11 axial filaments between the outer envelope and the cytoplasmic membrane. Like the other borreliae, *B. burgdorferi* can be cultured in modified Kelly's medium, where it grows slowly under microaerophilic conditions. Like the borreliae that cause relapsing fever, *B. burgdorferi* has linear plasmids, but the agent of Lyme disease does not undergo waves of antigenic variation within a single host, as do the agents of relapsing fever.

B. burgdorferi grows within ticks of the *I. ricinus* group, including *Ixodes pacificus* in the northwestern USA and *Ixodes scapularis* in the eastern and midwestern USA. (The so-called *Ixodes dammini* tick was considered to be a new species of deer tick that carried both *B. burgdorferi* and the parasite *Babesia microti.* Recently, however, entomologists have become convinced that *I. dammini* is merely a variant of the familiar black-legged deer tick, *I. scapularis,* and have recommended that the name *I. dammini* be abandoned.)

The transmission cycle of *B. burgdorferi* is shown in Fig. 12–10. Ticks of the *I. ricinus* group have a life cycle that carries over 2 calendar years. Lyme disease borreliae are not passed by ticks to their offspring, so when the tick eggs hatch in the late summer, the six-legged larvae are uninfected. That fall, the tick larvae become infected with *B. burgdorferi* when they feed on white-footed field mice. These mice harbor *B. burgdorferi* and develop spirochetemia but do not become ill from the infection. The next spring, the tick larvae molt and become eight-legged nymphs. The nymphs feed on field mice and humans and thereby spread *B. burgdorferi* infection to their hosts. Because the nymphs are tiny (about the size of a pencil point), they are rarely noticed. The nymphs molt in the late summer and become adults, which then feed on white-tailed deer and humans. *I. scapularis* is a small, hard tick (Fig. 12–11). To reliably pass borreliae to a human, the adult tick must engorge itself with blood, a process that takes 48–72 hours and is often long enough for the tick to be noticed and removed. Thus, even though about twice as many adult ticks as nymphs in endemic regions carry *B. burgdorferi* (28% versus 12%), humans more often are infected by the bite of a nymph because the nymphs are so rarely noticed and removed. (In comparison, only 4% of tick larvae in these same areas have detectable borreliae in them.) Two additional *Borrelia* spe-

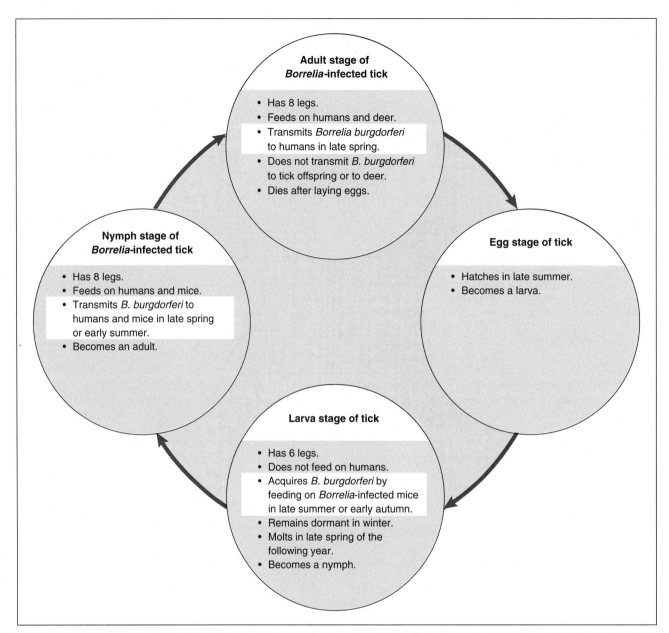

FIGURE 12–10. The infection cycle of *Borrelia burgdorferi* in ticks and humans. Larvae of *Ixodes scapularis* become infected in the late summer or early autumn when they feed on infected white-footed field mice. The following spring, they molt and become nymphs that feed on field mice or humans; both can be infected as a result of hosting infected nymphs. The nymphs molt and become adults that feed on deer and humans, but only humans will become infected.

cies have recently been discovered to cause Lyme disease in Europe. These species, named *Borrelia afzelii* and *Borrelia garinii,* appear to be the agents of a form of Lyme disease that follows an atypical course.

Mechanisms of Pathogenicity. A remarkable feature of *B. burgdorferi* is its ability to cause a wide variety of clinical findings, including skin lesions and flu-like illness (stage 1 disease), neurologic and cardiac abnormalities (stage 2 disease), and persistent arthritis (stage 3 disease). How can a single agent produce so many distinct manifestations? It appears that bacterial products as well as immune-mediated damage are involved.

Borreliae are gram-negative bacteria, albeit rather unusual ones. Several investigators have shown that *B. burgdorferi* has lipopolysaccharide-like (LPS-like) activity as measured by several assays, including the *Limulus* lysate assay. Although *B. burgdorferi* LPS is less potent pharmacologically than *Escherichia coli* LPS, the former has been shown to elicit interleukin-1 (IL-1) production from macrophages and monocytes. This production of IL-1 may be important because IL-1 is chemotactic for leukocytes, causes fever, elicits the release of acute phase proteins, and causes cells to secrete PGE_2 and collagenase. One group of investigators has shown that IL-1 injected into the skin can produce a lesion similar in gross appearance and pattern to ECM (the most common dermatologic manifestation of stage 1 disease), while others have shown that patients with Lyme arthritis (stage 3 dis-

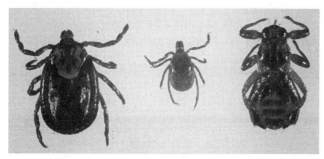

FIGURE 12–11. Magnified view of the black-legged deer tick, *Ixodes scapularis*. The tick in the center is the deer tick. On the left is the dog tick (*Dermacentor variabilis*), which carries the agent of Rocky Mountain spotted fever. On the right is an insect known as a deer ked. (Courtesy of D. J. White, New York State Department of Health.)

ease) have IL-1, PGE$_2$, and collagenase in the synovial fluid of affected joints. Thus, LPS-elicited production of interleukins may play a role in the generation of ECM and arthritis.

Experimental studies have shown that macrophages exposed to *B. burgdorferi* antigens can induce a form of arthritis in hamsters that is indistinguishable from the arthritis seen during Lyme disease. In addition, studies have demonstrated that antibody directed against interleukin-12 (IL-12), which diminishes Th1 immune responses, reduces the severity of Lyme arthritis in mice. Thus, macrophages and Th1 responses may play significant roles in the generation of Lyme arthritis.

The arthritic joints of patients with Lyme disease contain some immune complexes and low levels of borreliae. They also contain T cells and B cell germinal centers that are typical for a chronic hypersensitivity response, and this gives rise to the description of the inflamed joint as an ectopic lymphoid organ. In many ways, the arthritic joint of Lyme disease is similar to the lesions of tertiary syphilis and lepromatous leprosy, in which a tiny number of persistent organisms trigger a chronic plasma cell and T cell response.

In summary, it appears that ECM is the result of borreliae found in the skin, where they elicit inflammatory cells and IL-1 production, while the arthritis of Lyme disease involves the long-term persistence of tiny numbers of borreliae found in the joint, where they cause immune complexes to form, elicit the activation of complement, and stimulate the secretion of IL-1, PGE$_2$, and collagenase—all of which damage the integrity of the joint. Systemic symptoms may be due (at least in part) to LPS-induced production of cytokines. In cases of chronic destructive arthritis that seems to be almost incurable, it appears that the affected patients have a genetic predisposition for this form of disease. At least one major study reported that most of the affected patients expressed alloantigen HLA-DR4, while other studies have made some connection between the occurrence of destructive Lyme arthritis and the expression of HLA-DR2. Affected patients have been shown to have persistently elevated titers of antibody to two *B. burgdorferi*

outer membrane proteins, the so-called outer surface proteins (Osp) OspA and OspB.

At this time, the mechanisms by which *B. burgdorferi* causes neurologic and cardiac abnormalities (stage 2 disease) are poorly understood. However, there have been reports of borreliae in the central nervous system and of the appearance of antibodies to myelin in the cerebrospinal fluid of patients with neurologic damage due to Lyme disease. The significance of these findings is not yet clear, and much work lies ahead in determining the pathogenic events that lead to most of the clinical manifestations of the disease. In the final analysis, it appears that central to the pathogenesis of Lyme disease are (1) the tropism of *B. burgdorferi* for the skin, joints, and central nervous system; (2) the ability of the organisms to persist for years in these areas in small numbers; and (3) the immune response to the persistent organisms.

Experimental and clinical studies indicate that interleukin-4 (IL-4) may play a key role in immunity to *B. burgdorferi*. Administration of recombinant IL-4 to mice infected with borreliae results in rapid control of infection and abrogation of joint swelling. Peripheral blood monocytes from patients with Lyme disease produce significantly less IL-4 than do similar cells from uninfected controls. Thus, lack of IL-4 production in infected patients may lead to persistence of *B. burgdorferi* infection and development of disease.

Diseases Due to *B. burgdorferi*

Manifestations and Terminology. Lyme disease is found in Europe and the USA, although the clinical symptoms and signs vary somewhat in frequency in these two areas.

In Europe, the most prominent components of the disease are two dermatologic manifestations—namely, **erythema chronicum migrans** (ECM) and **acrodermatitis chronica atrophicans** (ACA)—and a neurologic syndrome called the **Garin-Bajadoux-Bannwarth syndrome.** ECM begins as a papule at the site of the tick bite and then spreads peripherally, leaving one or more rings around an area of central clearing. ACA is a reddish symmetric inflammation of the skin that occurs bilaterally on the feet or hands and is usually accompanied by hypertrophy of the horny layer of the skin and by scaling. ACA occurs only in patients infected with *B. afzelii*. The neurologic syndrome, which is often simply called **Bannwarth's syndrome,** is characterized by a triad of diseases: lymphocytic meningitis (inflammation of the meninges with a lymphocytic exudate), cranial neuropathy (often evidenced by bilateral Bell's palsy), and peripheral radiculoneuropathy (inflammation of the spinal root that can be accompanied by pain in the spine or along the sensory nerves).

In the USA, the three most common manifestations of Lyme disease are ECM, a chronic fatigue-like syndrome, and arthritis of the large joints. In addition, 23% of US patients with Lyme disease suffer from cardiac abnormalities (usually atrioventricular block), the neurologic abnormalities listed above, or a combination of these. A small percentage have ACA.

In children and adults, three stages of Lyme disease are recognized. Whether or not *B. burgdorferi* can be passed transplacentally to cause a congenital form of the disease is unknown. There have been anecdotal reports that some women who developed Lyme disease during pregnancy have suffered from miscarriages while others have had infants born prematurely or with birth defects. Yet it has not been established that *B. burgdorferi* was the cause of these events. There has been one report of an infant who died shortly after birth and was found to have *B. burgdorferi* in his brain and liver. That the mother of this infant had been treated successfully for Lyme disease with penicillin during her pregnancy raises concerns about how to approach treatment of Lyme disease in pregnant women. At this time, it is uncertain whether Lyme disease in a pregnant woman is a direct threat to the life of the fetus.

Diagnosis

(1) History and Physical Examination. Table 12–3 lists the clinical manifestations of the three stages of Lyme disease.

(a) Stage 1 Disease. Lyme disease commonly begins as a papule, usually at the site of the tick bite, 3–32 days after the patient is bitten by a tick of the *I. ricinus* group. From this develops an elevated erythematous ring that is warm to the touch and continues growing larger. The advancing border of the lesion is indurated, but the skin inside the ring clears. There may be more than one ring on a patient, and each ring may become as large as 70 cm, although the average size is about 10 cm. Some patients have smaller annular rings within the border of one large ring. These lesions, which are characteristic of ECM,

TABLE 12–3. The Stages of Lyme Disease and the Percentage of Patients Who Suffer From Each Manifestation

Stage of Disease	Manifestation	Percentage of Patients
Stage 1	Erythema chronicum migrans	80–90
Stage 2	Neurologic disorders (lymphocytic meningitis; cranial neuropathy; peripheral radiculoneuropathy)	15
	Cardiac disorders (atrioventricular block with heart palpitations or fainting)	8
	Other disorders (debilitating malaise or fatigue; migratory pain; mild hepatitis; microscopic hematuria or proteinuria)	50
Stage 3	Arthritis (migratory polyarthritis of large joints)	60
	Chronic arthritis with joint damage (HLA-linked disease)	6
	Chronic borreliosis (acrodermatitis chronica atrophicans; encephalopathy; polyneuropathy with spinal or radicular pain)	5

fade in 3–4 weeks. Patients with stage 1 disease may also have myalgia, chills, stiff neck, a low-grade fever, and regional lymphadenopathy. These constitutional symptoms occur because the spirochetes are disseminating. About 17% of patients later develop satellite lesions that are due to dissemination of spirochetes and are similar in appearance to but smaller than the primary lesion. About 10–20% of patients with Lyme disease never suffer from ECM; some in this group are asymptomatic, while others experience flu-like symptoms without ECM. About 20% of patients with stage 1 disease will have no further disease manifestations. Stage 1 usually lasts about 1 month.

(b) Stage 2 Disease. During the next few weeks or months (usually within 1–4 months), about 73% of patients with stage 1 disease progress to stage 2 disease. Some previously asymptomatic patients also develop the clinical signs of stage 2 disease, which are due to disseminated spirochetes. Patients in this stage may have one or more of the following: neurologic abnormalities (such as Bannwarth's syndrome); cardiac disorders (such as atrioventricular block with heart palpitations or fainting spells); migratory pain in the muscles, joints, tendons, or bones; and debilitating malaise and fatigue. Neurologic problems usually resolve spontaneously in 1–9 months, and cardiac problems resolve in 3–6 weeks. However, recovery from the malaise, fatigue, and muscle pain may be prolonged. These manifestations of Lyme disease are hard to differentiate from chronic fatigue syndrome and fibromyalgia. Making this distinction more difficult is the fact that Lyme disease may be one of several events that trigger the onset of fibromyalgia.

(c) Stage 3 Disease. The hallmark of stage 3 disease, which occurs 5–24 months after stage 1 disease, is migratory arthritis. The arthritis usually affects the large joints (most often the knee joints), is sometimes accompanied by swelling, and is present in 60% of patients with untreated Lyme disease. The arthritis gradually resolves over several years in most cases, but about 6% of patients develop a chronic destructive form of arthritis that may not resolve, even with appropriate treatment, and is believed to be an HLA-linked disease. Other manifestations of stage 3 disease include ACA, encephalopathy, and polyneuropathy with spinal or radicular pain.

(2) Laboratory Analysis. The diagnosis of Lyme disease rests on three points: the patient's clinical condition is typical for Lyme disease; the patient has been in an area where Lyme disease is endemic; and antibodies to *B. burgdorferi* are detectable in the patient's serum or cerebrospinal fluid (CSF). Because Lyme disease is spread by the bites of nymphal or adult *Ixodes* ticks, most cases occur during the summer or early fall, but especially during June and July. Diagnosis is never made by culturing the organisms or by demonstrating them in tissues, because the borreliae are typically present in very small numbers and grow too slowly for culture to be of use to the patient. The diagnosis of Lyme disease appears to be quite straightforward, but there are several factors that often make Lyme disease difficult to diagnose.

The first diagnostic problem is that patients with stage 1 disease often have no detectable anti-*Borrelia* antibodies. IgM antibody titers peak between weeks 3 and 6 of disease, but early IgM antibody is often directed against a 41-kD flagellar antigen that is fairly nonspecific, being shared by several spirochetes. IgM directed against the highly specific OspA and OspB antigens often does not appear until late in stage 1 disease. IgG antibody to the borreliae usually appears about 6 weeks after the initiation of ECM and peaks months later. Thus, the standard tests for antibody may not become positive until the patient enters stage 2 Lyme disease, and preliminary diagnosis may have to be made on the presence of ECM alone. Antibodies (both IgG and IgM) are detected by enzyme-linked immunosorbent assay (ELISA), and Western blots can be performed if the ELISA results are equivocal. Patients who are seronegative but have strong clinical evidence of Lyme disease can be tested for a cell-mediated immune response to borreliae by use of a lymphocyte proliferative assay.

The second major diagnostic problem is the lack of standardization of immunologic tests for Lyme disease. Because the tests are not adequately standardized, false-negative results are common and false-positive results are extremely common. This problem is compounded because patients who have stage 1 disease and are treated inadequately may never develop detectable antibody, and patients who become seropositive remain so for years. Thus, patients who have previously had asymptomatic Lyme disease and patients who have recovered from Lyme disease and now have manifestations that mimic Lyme disease may be misdiagnosed. Does this happen often? In one major study of 788 patients diagnosed with Lyme disease and referred to a major Lyme disease referral site, only 23% had active Lyme disease, another 20% had previously had Lyme disease but now suffered from fibromyalgia, and 57% had never suffered from Lyme disease. Thus, 77% of the patients diagnosed with Lyme disease did not have Lyme disease. The similarities between fibromyalgia and the fatigue syndrome of Lyme disease make accurate diagnosis a problem.

Stage 2 disease is particularly difficult to diagnose in patients with neurologic manifestations. Lyme disease must be differentiated from viral meningitis, strokes, multiple sclerosis, Guillain-Barré syndrome, and a host of other neurologic abnormalities. A diagnosis of stage 2 disease is supported by demonstration of lymphocytic pleocytosis in the CSF of patients with clinical signs typical of neurologic Lyme disease and particularly in patients with the triad of meningitis, cranial neuropathy, and radiculoneuropathy. Patients with this triad typically have antibody to borreliae in their CSF and serum. Lyme disease with cardiac manifestations can be distinguished from rheumatic heart disease by the presence of antibody to borreliae in the serum and also by the occurrence of complete heart block, a cardiac problem that

is uncommon in rheumatic heart disease. Remember that ECM does not occur in about 10–20% of patients with Lyme disease, so for many, stage 2 symptoms are the first indication of disease.

Stage 3 disease is confirmed by demonstrating that the serum contains antibodies to borreliae.

Treatment and Prognosis.   Patients with ECM respond well to treatment with oral doxycycline or amoxicillin. Early recognition and treatment of Lyme disease have been highly successful in reducing the occurrence of Lyme arthritis—so much so that *Borrelia*-associated fibromyalgia is now the most commonly seen complication of Lyme disease in the USA. Most patients with neurologic, arthritic, or cardiac manifestations of Lyme disease are treated with ceftriaxone, although some patients with arthritic disease are treated with doxycycline or amoxicillin. Nonchronic arthritis responds to antibiotic treatment, but recovery is slow. Chronic arthritis responds very poorly to antibiotic therapy. Fibromyalgia that occurs as a consequence of Lyme disease does not improve when the borreliae are eliminated.

Prevention.   There is no vaccine against Lyme disease, so prevention involves making certain that infection does not occur. People who hike in areas endemic for Lyme disease can avoid tick bites by wearing long-sleeved shirts, by tucking pants legs into boots, and by coating the clothing with repellents that contain permethrin. Ticks should be removed immediately—not by burning them with a cigarette or yanking them off but instead by grasping the tick's abdomen with tweezers and gently pulling. Usually, after 1–2 minutes, the tick tires and releases its hold on the skin. The tick can then be placed in a small bottle that contains a bit of damp paper towel and be sent to the nearest reference center where ticks are screened for pathogens. The nearest state board of health should be able to give advice about where such testing is performed.

LEPTOSPIRES
Classification

Leptospires are aerobic spirochetes that are 6–20 μm long and have hooked ends and a single axial filament (Fig. 12–12). There is only one pathogenic species of *Leptospira*—namely, *Leptospira interrogans*—but the species includes many serovars (serologic types). Serovars are classified mainly on the basis of the hosts that are typically infected. For example, hosts for the serovar *icterohaemorrhagiae* are rats, while hosts for the serovars *pomona* and *canicola* are dogs and swine, respectively. Disease spreads to humans from these hosts, which serve as reservoirs for the organism.

Leptospira interrogans
Characteristics of *L. interrogans*

Leptospires have the ability to cause hemorrhage, diarrhea, jaundice, severe renal impairment (due to acute tubular necrosis), hypovolemia, and

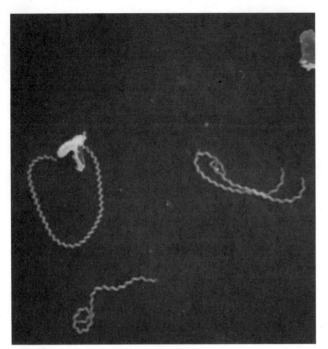

FIGURE 12–12. Darkfield micrograph of *Leptospira interrogans*. (Reproduced, with permission, from Strickland, G. T. Hunter's Tropical Medicine, 7th ed. Philadelphia, W. B. Saunders Company, 1991.)

signs of aseptic meningitis. Yet there is little evidence of direct spirochetal damage to the affected tissues, and many suspect that the leptospires either produce a toxin or elicit toxic substances from host cells. Leptospires enter the cerebrospinal fluid, and signs of meningitis coincide with the appearance of antibody to *Leptospira,* suggesting that this disease may be immune-mediated. Leptospires have endotoxinlike activity (although there is no 2-keto-3-deoxyoctulosonic acid, or KDO), and this activity may be involved in some of their effects on vascular function.

As shown in Fig. 12–13, leptospirosis is a biphasic disease. The first phase is believed to be due to leptospiral invasion and possible toxin production, while the second phase—called the immune phase—is believed to be caused by the immune response to leptospires and their products. At this time, very little is understood of the means by which leptospires produce the pathologic manifestations associated with leptospirosis.

Diseases Due to *L. interrogans*

Epidemiology. All *L. interrogans* serovars can cause leptospirosis in humans, sometimes without jaundice (anicteric disease) and sometimes with jaundice (Weil's disease, the icteric form of the disease). Leptospirosis is spread to humans who come in contact with the urine of infected animals. The contact may be direct, such as in the case of farmers or veterinarians who handle animals, or it may be indirect, such as via contact with contaminated water or mud in flooded streets, rice paddies, and jungle swamps.

Over 150 species of mammals have been shown to harbor and shed leptospires, but rodents (especially the Norway rat) have been found to be key reservoirs. The disease is found worldwide. In the USA, leptospirosis is seen most often in Hawaii among taro farmers who must wade in flooded fields. There are about 100 cases of leptospirosis each year in the USA.

The *autumnalis* serovar of *L. interrogans* causes pretibial fever, a rare disease. In the USA, pretibial fever is also called Fort Bragg fever because an outbreak occurred among soldiers stationed at Fort Bragg in North Carolina. In Europe, the disease is sometimes called pea-picker's disease.

Diagnosis

(1) History and Physical Examination. People are infected with leptospires when the spirochetes in animal urine pass through mucous membranes or abrasions. After an incubation period of 2–20 days, patients are struck abruptly with fever, headache, myalgia, and other flu-like symptoms that are accompanied by a leptospiral septicemia. At this time, the spirochetes can be found in the blood and in various organs, such as the kidneys and the meninges. Some patients have a rash, but there is no consistent pattern to the rash. After 4–7 days of illness, patients undergo rapid improvement and then enter a 1- to 3-day asymptomatic hiatus. The disease disappears at this time because antibody has cleared the spirochetes from the blood and from all tissues except the kidneys and the aqueous humor. When the asymptomatic period ends, one of two very different immune phases begins.

About 90% of leptospirosis patients enter the first type of immune phase and develop a fairly mild disease called **anicteric leptospirosis.** These patients have a low-grade fever, suffer from a mild form of meningitis, and have leptospires in their urine. Occasional patients will experience nerve palsies, myelitis, or encephalitis that lasts several weeks or months, and a few will develop uveitis several months later. Deaths due to anicteric leptospirosis are rare.

The remaining 10% of leptospirosis patients enter the second type of immune phase and develop a dangerous disease called **icteric leptospirosis** or **Weil's disease.** Patients with Weil's disease have jaundice (icterus) and suffer from azotemia, hemorrhagic diathesis, and myocarditis. Azotemia is also called uremia and is an accumulation of nitrogenous waste and urea in the blood, in this case attributable to renal tubular necrosis. Patients with azotemia may suffer from headaches, vomiting, dyspnea, delirium, convulsions, coma, or a combination of these. Hemorrhagic diathesis is a condition in which trivial trauma causes uncontrolled bleeding. In patients with Weil's disease, the skin and mucous membranes are most often affected, but some patients develop massive gastrointestinal bleeding. Myocarditis may lead to cardiogenic shock. Deaths are common (occurring in about 10% of cases) and are most often due to hemorrhage, cardiovascular collapse, or renal failure.

Patients with **pretibial fever** are febrile and have

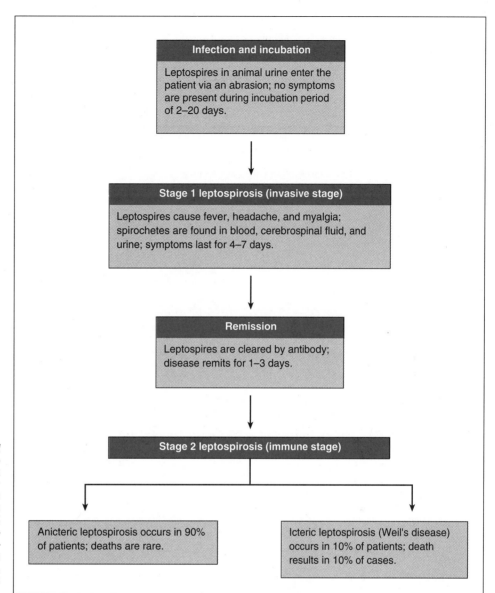

FIGURE 12–13. **The course of untreated leptospirosis in humans.** Liptospirosis begins as an acute disease that remits after 4–7 days. About 90% of patients subsequently develop anicteric leptospirosis, while about 10% develop the more dangerous icteric leptospirosis (Weil's disease). Stage 1 leptospirosis is due to the action of the leptospires, while stage 2 leptospirosis is an immune-mediated disease.

a rash that affects the shins and sometimes appears to be urticarial.

(2) **Laboratory Analysis.** Diagnosis of leptospirosis is based on recognizing the clinical picture and showing that the patient has antibodies to *Leptospira.* A slide agglutination test or an enzyme-linked immunosorbent assay will demonstrate antibodies in serum. Early diagnosis is difficult because the first stage of leptospirosis consists of mundane flu-like symptoms that could be due to almost anything and because there are no antibodies to detect at this stage. Antibodies to *Leptospira* reach detectable levels usually between days 6 and 12 of illness and are maximal during weeks 3 and 4. *L. interrogans* can be cultured on special media, but it may take up to 8 weeks to identify the organisms, and this is too slow for cultures to be of diagnostic value.

Leptospirosis must be differentiated from viral hepatitis, influenza, and appendicitis in the USA and from diseases such as malaria, typhoid, and scrub typhus in the tropics. The difficulty of diagnosing the disease was demonstrated by an epidemiologic survey that found that leptospirosis was considered in the original differential diagnosis of only one-fourth of cases of confirmed leptospirosis.

Treatment. The effectiveness of antibiotic therapy in treating leptospirosis is somewhat controversial, but doxycycline or penicillin G has been used. Pretibial fever is treated with penicillin.

Selected Readings

Anguita, J., et al. Effect of anti–interleukin-12 treatment on murine Lyme borreliosis. J Clin Invest 17:1028–1034, 1996.

Barbour, A. G. Antigenic variation of a relapsing fever *Borrelia* species. Annu Rev Microbiol 44:155–171, 1991.

Barbour, A. G. Molecular biology of antigenic variation in Lyme borreliosis and relapsing fever: a comparative analysis. Scand J Infect Dis Suppl 77:88–93, 1991.

Barbour, A. G., and S. F. Hayes. Biology of *Borrelia* species. Microbiol Rev 50:381–400, 1986.

Barbour, A. G., et al. Variable antigen genes of the relapsing fever agent *Borrelia hermsii* are activated by promoter addition. Mol Microbiol 5:489–493, 1991.

Clark, E. G., and N. Danbolt. The Oslo study of the natural course of untreated syphilis. Med Clin North Am 48:613–623, 1964.

DuChateau, B. K., et al. Macrophages exposed to *Borrelia burgdorferi* induce Lyme arthritis in hamsters. Infect Immun 64:2540–2547, 1996.

Fitzgerald, T. J., and L. A. Repesh. The hyaluronidase associated with *Treponema pallidum* facilitates treponemal dissemination. Infect Immun 55:1023–1028, 1987.

Heath, C. W., A. D. Alexander, and M. M. Galton. Leptospirosis in the United States: analysis of 483 cases in man, 1949–1961. N Engl J Med 273:857–864, 1965.

Keane-Myers, A., et al. Recombinant IL-4 treatment augments resistance to *Borrelia burgdorferi* infections in both normal susceptible and antibody-deficient susceptible mice. J Immunol 156:2488–2494, 1996.

Kitten, T., and A. G. Barbour. The relapsing fever agent *Borrelia hermsii* has multiple copies of its chromosome and linear plasmids. Genetics 132:311–324, 1992.

Musher, D. M., R. T. Hamill, and R. E. Baughn. Effect of human immunodeficiency virus (HIV) infection on the course of syphilis and on the response to treatment. Ann Intern Med 113:872–881, 1990.

Oksi, J., et al. Decreased interleukin-4 and increased gamma interferon production by peripheral blood mononuclear cells of patients with Lyme borreliosis. Infect Immun 64:3620–3623, 1996.

Steere, A. C. Current understanding of Lyme disease. Hosp Pract 28:37–44, 1993.

Steere, A. C. Pathogenesis of Lyme arthritis. Ann NY Acad Sci 539:87–92, 1988.

Steere, A. C., et al. The overdiagnosis of Lyme disease. JAMA 269:1812–1816, 1993.

Steine, B. M., S. Sell, and R. F. Schell. *Treponema pallidum* attachment to surface and matrix proteins of cultured rabbit epithelial cells. J Infect Dis 155:742–748, 1987.

Wang, B., et al. Role of specific antibody in interaction of leptospires with human monocytes and monocyte-derived macrophages. Infect Immun 46:809–813, 1984.

CHAPTER THIRTEEN

LEGIONELLAE

Legionella Species

Investigation of Early Disease Outbreaks

Legionnaires' disease made its dramatic appearance in 1976, when without warning it struck 221 and killed 34 American Legion members who were attending a convention in a Philadelphia hotel. A startled nation watched as television cameras showed patient after patient being wheeled on gurneys from the hotel to awaiting ambulances after being stricken with what appeared to be a modern-day plague. The unknown agent of disease, which caused pneumonia with multisystem effects, was particularly dangerous to people with underlying cardiopulmonary disease, diabetes, or cancer, 29% of whom died. In contrast, its mortality rate was only about 5% in people with previously good health.

Epidemiologists launched a national effort to identify the elusive agent of the deadly pneumonia. After several months, Joe McDade isolated the bacterium on enriched Mueller-Hinton agar after first injecting material from clinical samples into guinea pigs. Because the organism was isolated from legionnaires and because of its propensity for the lungs, it was named *Legionella pneumophila*.

Retrospective investigations have shown that there were earlier cases and outbreaks of *Legionella*. In 1947, Hugh Tatlock isolated a "rickettsia-like" organism from a patient with pneumonia. The so-called Tatlock agent was later identified as *L. pneumophila*. An epidemic that occurred in 1965 in Washington, D.C., and affected 81 psychiatric patients, 15 of whom died, was later attributed to *L. pneumophila*. As a matter of fact, what is now called legionnaires' disease could instead have been called Odd Fellows' disease, since a similar outbreak occurred in 1974 among Odd Fellows who were attending a convention in the same hotel that hosted the organism and its victims in the 1976 outbreak. Because the outbreak at the Odd Fellows convention affected only 11 people, it went unrecognized until several years later.

Human infection most often begins when hot water containing legionellae is aerosolized and breathed. This is a problem in large institutions such as hospitals and hotels, especially when the temperature of hot water supplies is under 57 °C (135 °F), when there are dead ends in hot water systems, when spas and Jacuzzis are used, and when nebulizers and humidifiers are filled with contaminated hot water. The use of silicone-based rubber in hot water supply systems greatly enhances the persistence of legionellae, and vertical evaporation towers that are part of heating and cooling systems may serve as a reservoir for the organisms. If more than 30% of hot water sites in an institution have demonstrable legionellae, there is significant risk that an outbreak of legionnaires' disease will occur.

In Louisiana, an outbreak of legionnaires' disease was traced to an ultrasonic mist machine used to keep vegetables moist in a grocery store display case. This outbreak was of great concern because the mist machine involved was essentially identical to ultrasonic humidifiers that are commonly used in homes.

Today, *Legionella* is a significant cause of hospital-acquired pneumonia and is consistently ranked as one of the three major causes of community-acquired pneumonia in the USA. It is responsible not only for the acute form of pneumonia known as legionnaires' disease but also for a self-limited flu-like illness called Pontiac fever. Legionellae have not been isolated from patients with Pontiac fever, but serum samples from almost all of these patients show high titers of antibody to *Legionella* during convalescence.

Legionella Species

Over 30 *Legionella* species and more than 50 *Legionella* serotypes have been identified. About 85% of cases of legionnaires' disease are caused by *Legionella pneumophila*, with 50% due to serogroup 1 and 10% to serogroup 6. *Legionella micdadei* is the second most common species causing legionnaires' disease. Other *Legionella* species frequently identified by isolation of organisms or by results of serologic testing include *Legionella bozemanii, Legionella dumoffii,* and *Legionella longbeachae*.

Characteristics of *Legionella*

General Features. Most of what is known about legionellae has come from studies of *L. pneumophila* or *L. micdadei*. The legionellae are gram-negative rods

253

that are 0.3–0.9 μm wide by 2–20 μm long and appear as coccobacilli in tissue sections. Although they can be stained with Gram's stain, legionellae are best stained in tissues with the Gimenez method (which is more often used to stain rickettsiae), and paraffin-embedded samples can be stained with Dieterle's stain or Warthin-Starry stain.

Legionellae are fastidious bacteria that are usually isolated on buffered charcoal–yeast extract (CYE) agar. They will not grow in the absence of L-cysteine. For optimal growth, they also need keto acids and iron. *L. pneumophila* reverts rapidly to an attenuated form on some media, apparently in response to the presence of high amounts of NaCl in the agar. Media used to isolate legionellae are made selective by adding an antibiotic (cefamandole, polymyxin B, or vancomycin) or an inhibitor (glycine) to halt the growth of bacteria that reside in the respiratory tract, and dyes are added to better visualize the *Legionella* colonies. Isolation of legionellae from sputum samples is improved when the samples are treated with acid to eliminate respiratory commensals that may be present as contaminants. *L. pneumophila* will multiply between the temperatures of 25 °C and 42 °C, and its colonies will appear after 3–5 days of growth on selective media at 35–37 °C.

Legionellae are relatively chlorine-resistant and are generally present in small numbers in fresh water, including the water in potable water systems and in cooling systems of large buildings. They usually do not grow to great numbers and become a health hazard unless many helper bacteria or protozoa are also present to provide nutrients not normally found in high amounts in fresh water. Some investigators, for example, have reported that certain bacteria and blue-green algae secrete by-products that allow legionellae to grow to high densities in media that previously supported only poor growth of legionellae. But the most compelling evidence for helper activity has been the demonstration that *Legionella* species grow rapidly within free-living amebas (Fig. 13–1) of the genera *Hartmannella* and *Naegleria,* as well as within the ciliated *Tetrahymena.*

Mechanisms of Pathogenicity. In humans, legionellae grow as facultatively intracellular organisms, and their key pathogenic characteristic is their ability to survive within polymorphonuclear leukocytes (PMNs), monocytes, and alveolar macrophages.

(1) *Legionella* Antigens and Virulence Determinants. A number of *Legionella* cell surface antigens and cell products help legionellae survive within phagocytes and cause toxic effects on host cells.

(a) Pili, Outer Membrane Proteins, and Lipopolysaccharide. *L. pneumophila* has a single polar flagellum, and the organisms typically have **pili**. The **major outer membrane protein** (MOMP) is a 24- to 29-kD porin molecule that anchors **lipopolysaccharide** to the outer membrane and facilitates the entry of legionellae into host cells by binding an activated subunit of the complement component C3.

A 24-kD protein called the **macrophage infectivity potentiator** (Mip) is also found on the outer mem-

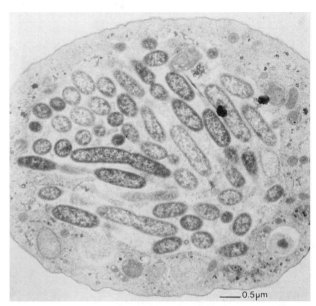

FIGURE 13–1. Phagocytosis of *Legionella pneumophila* by a free-living ameba. The ameba shown here (*Hartmannella vermiformis*) is filled with *L. pneumophila.* Most of the legionellae have left the phagocytic vacuole and are multiplying in the cytoplasm of the ameba. (Courtesy of Barry S. Fields.)

brane and appears to be necessary for legionellae to survive within macrophages. Mip is a peptidyl prolyl *cis-trans* isomerase, an enzyme that is involved in protein folding. Mip promotes intracellular survival of legionellae by an unknown mechanism, and the absence of Mip in mutants results in an 80-fold decrease in the ability of legionellae to survive.

A 58- to 60-kD **heat shock protein** has been found in the periplasmic space of *L. pneumophila.* The function of this protein is unknown, but convalescing patients typically have elevated titers of antibody to it.

(b) Phosphatase. *L. pneumophila* secretes a phosphatase that inhibits superoxide production by reducing the amounts of *sn*-1,2-diacylglycerol (DAG) and *myo*-inositol 1,4,5-triphosphate (IP$_3$) that are available. Fig. 13–2 shows that superoxide production by neutrophils normally involves a reduced form of nicotinamide adenine dinucleotide phosphate oxidase (NADPH oxidase) that is directly or indirectly activated by a protein kinase. The activity of this protein kinase is increased directly by DAG or is increased indirectly when IP$_3$ mobilizes calcium from intracellular stores. IP$_3$ is generated from phosphatidylinositol by the action of phospholipase C, which is itself activated by a G protein that responds to several external stimuli.

(c) Peptide Toxin. Peptide toxin is produced by phagocytosed legionellae and is believed to interfere with early steps in the neutrophil activation series by blocking the action of phospholipase C. Studies have demonstrated that peptide toxin is cytotoxic for host cells, depresses neutrophil hexose monophosphate shunt activity, and greatly inhibits the ability of phagocytes to iodinate and kill bacteria.

(d) Zinc Metalloprotease. A 38-kD zinc metallo-

FIGURE 13–2. The oxidative burst of polymorphonuclear leukocytes (PMNs). Various mechanisms control the expression of the PMN oxidative burst through their effects on the activity of a reduced form of nicotinamide adenine dinucleotide phosphate oxidase (NADPH oxidase). External stimuli bind to a G protein–associated receptor, and the G protein activates phospholipase C. The phospholipase splits phosphatidylinositol 4,5-biphosphate (PIP_2) to yield sn-1,2-diacylglycerol (DAG) and myo-inositol 1,4,5-triphosphate (IP_3). DAG directly stimulates the activity of protein kinase C (PKC), while IP_3 indirectly stimulates PKC by liberating Ca^{2+} from intracellular stores. PKC then stimulates the activity of a complex of G protein, guanosine triphosphate (GTP), and NADPH oxidase. This complex converts NADPH to $NADP^+$ while donating two electrons to the membrane-bound flavocytochrome b_{558} complex. Cytochrome b_{558} then completes the process by donating the two electrons to oxygen to convert it to superoxide.

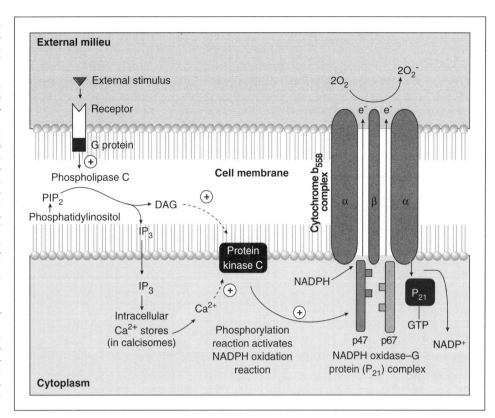

protease has been characterized as the major secretory protein of L. pneumophila and is probably an important virulence determinant. It is cytotoxic, inhibits superoxide production, inhibits PMN chemotaxis and migration, inhibits natural killer activity, inactivates α_1-antitrypsin, degrades two key inflammatory messengers (interleukin-2 and tissue necrosis factor alpha), and destroys the lymphocyte CD4 antigen. Most important, several groups have shown that if the zinc metalloprotease is introduced by inhalation into guinea pigs, it produces pulmonary lesions that are indistinguishable from those found in humans with legionellosis. The significance of the protease remains controversial, however, because some Legionella strains lack detectable amounts of the protease but can nevertheless produce disease in guinea pigs.

(e) Other Cell Products. Other Legionella products of uncertain significance are a phospholipase C; a chymotrypsinlike protease; a protein kinase that phosphorylates tubulin, histones, and phosphatidylinositol; and a hemolysin that has been named legiolysin.

(2) Pathogenic Processes. Legionellae enter the lungs via the respiratory tract without infecting the pharyngeal mucosa. The organisms are phagocytosed initially by alveolar macrophages and later by PMNs. Early studies showed that the Philadelphia 1 strain of L. pneumophila serotype 1 is phagocytosed by a process called coiling phagocytosis (Fig. 13–3). This unusual process leaves the bacterium in a whorled vacuole that is lined with ribosomes, and the

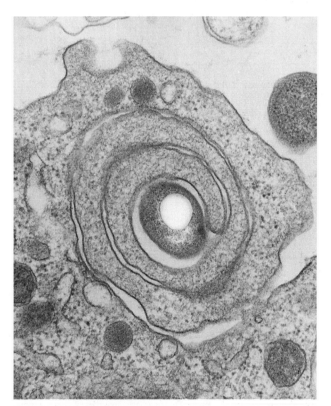

FIGURE 13–3. Phagocytosis of Legionella pneumophila (Philadelphia 1 strain) by monocytes. The process of coiling phagocytosis is shown. (Reproduced, with permission, from Horwitz, M. A. Phagocytosis of the legionnaires' disease bacterium, Legionella pneumophila, occurs by a novel mechanism: engulfment within a pseudopod coil. Cell 36:27–33, 1984. © Cell Press.)

bacterium multiplies and fills the phagocytic vacuole without eliciting degranulation. Subsequent studies have shown that coiling phagocytosis is unique to the entry of the Philadelphia 1 strain; all other legionellae (including other *L. pneumophila* serotypes) enter via **conventional phagocytosis,** and phagosomes containing these strains fuse normally with secondary granules.

Antibody and **complement components** play a critical role in the entry of legionellae into host cells (Fig. 13–4). *L. pneumophila* enters phagocytic cells efficiently only when the complement component C3 is activated by antibody to *Legionella* and binds to the MOMP and the cellular C3 receptor. In contrast, *L. micdadei* efficiently activates complement via the alternative pathway, and its entry is facilitated when it binds C3 activated in the absence of antibody. In

both cases, antibody and complement do not lyse the legionellae or augment the killing of bacteria once they are phagocytosed. Instead, recovery from legionellosis depends on the generation of a potent **cell-mediated immune response** to the organism. At least one laboratory has reported that intracellular growth of legionellae is limited by interferon-gamma and that cells activated with interferon-gamma do not kill legionellae but limit their growth by making iron unavailable to the bacteria. Others have shown that tumor necrosis factor alpha acts synergistically with interferon-gamma to stimulate nitric oxide synthesis and that nitric oxide further limits intracellular multiplication of legionellae.

Studies in vitro and in animal models have indicated that most phagocytosed legionellae do not survive, but those which do survive are capable of multi-

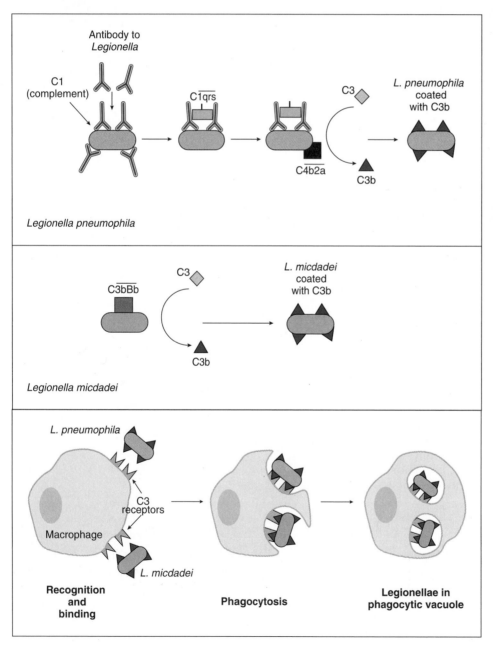

FIGURE 13–4. Entry of legionellae into host cells. *Legionella pneumophila* activates complement via the classic pathway, while *Legionella micdadei* generates C3b via the alternative pathway. In each case, C3b bound to the *Legionella* major outer membrane protein (MOMP) adheres to C3 receptors on the surface of macrophages, and the bacterium is phagocytosed. Once inside the host cell, the bacterium blocks the oxidative response and multiplies within the phagocytic vacuole.

plying rapidly and eventually destroying the host cell. Early studies demonstrated that phagocytes containing the Philadelphia 1 strain of *Legionella* could not degranulate, but it now appears that this is a unique property of this strain. Other strains apparently survive within macrophages and monocytes instead by blocking the oxidative burst so that superoxide and other cytotoxic free radicals are not formed. Within 30 minutes of ingesting legionellae, phagocytes lose their ability to kill *Staphylococcus aureus* and *Escherichia coli* and can no longer be activated by a variety of agents that usually serve as cell-activating agents. Thus, once a macrophage or monocyte has phagocytosed a *Legionella* organism, it rapidly loses its ability to participate in defensive activities.

Amebas may play a role in the course of legionnaires' disease. In vitro studies have shown that mice coinfected with *Legionella pneumophila* and the ameba *Hartmannella vermiformis* developed much higher levels of pulmonary legionellae as well as more severe lung disease than did mice infected with legionellae alone. Furthermore, mice naturally resistant to *Legionella* infection developed pulmonary legionellosis when they were coinfected with legionellae and *Hartmannella*.

Diseases Due to *Legionella*

Epidemiology. One group of investigators has estimated that between 20,000 and 50,000 cases of legionnaires' disease occur each year in the USA, while others believe that the number is even higher. *Legionella* is thought to be the cause of anywhere from 1% to 15% of cases of community-acquired pneumonia and from 1% to 40% of cases of hospital-acquired pneumonia.

Legionnaires' disease occurs mainly in people with underlying medical conditions, especially conditions that compromise immune or cardiopulmonary functions. Among the most common risk factors are advanced age, cigarette smoking, chronic obstructive pulmonary disease (COPD), tracheal intubation, use of corticosteroids or other immunosuppressive drugs (for example, by transplant patients), and the presence of hairy cell leukemia (which suppresses monocyte function). Renal transplant patients are particularly susceptible to infection with *L. micdadei*. Surprisingly, patients with acquired immunodeficiency syndrome (AIDS) or neutropenia are not unusually susceptible to legionnaires' disease.

Diagnosis

(1) History and Physical Examination. Although legionellae are occasionally the cause of soft tissue infections, endocarditis, or pericarditis, *Legionella* infection most often results in legionnaires' disease or Pontiac fever.

(a) Legionnaires' Disease. Legionnaires' disease is an acute purulent pneumonia that is clinically and radiologically indistinguishable from pneumococcal pneumonia. It occurs from 2 to 10 days after the patient is exposed to water that contains legionellae, with the shortest incubation period found in immunosuppressed patients. During the first 24–48 hours of disease, manifestations may include fever, malaise, myalgia, headache, weakness, lethargy, and loss of appetite. The patient then rapidly becomes acutely ill and complains of pleuritic or nonpleuritic chest pain, accompanied by dry cough and a high fever (often higher than 40.5 °C or 104.9 °F). Hemoptysis is rare, but patients usually develop purulent sputum over the next few days. In most cases, radiographs show an early pleural effusion that is patchy and becomes unilateral pneumonia with a lower lobe predominance. The pneumonia tends to progress for days, even after appropriate antibiotic therapy has been started.

Although legionnaires' disease is often a multisystem disease, retrospective studies have not shown that the incidence of nonpulmonary clinical manifestations is significantly higher in this disease than in pneumococcal pneumonia. Among the nonpulmonary clinical manifestations are watery diarrhea (in 25–50% of patients); nausea, vomiting, and abdominal pain (in 10–20% of patients); neurologic signs, including confusion, encephalopathy, neuropathy, cerebellar ataxia, and headache with lethargy; renal disease; sinusitis; and cardiac involvement with pericarditis and endocarditis. Many patients develop shaking chills, and about one-fifth of patients become hypotensive.

(b) Pontiac Fever. Pontiac fever usually occurs as an epidemic 24–48 hours after individuals are exposed to an environmental source of legionellae, with about 90% of those exposed developing disease. Pontiac fever is a flu-like illness that is characterized by high fever, headache, diarrhea, and malaise, but there is no pneumonia. Occasionally, patients develop a dry cough or neurologic signs. Most patients recover without treatment in 1 week.

(2) Laboratory Analysis. In cases of pneumonia, legionnaires' disease should be suspected under the following conditions: PMNs are present in the sputum, but few or no organisms can be demonstrated by Gram's stain; hyponatremia is present (serum sodium level under 130 mEq/L); the temperature is high (>39 °C or 101.8 °F); and the patient is either immunosuppressed or has COPD. Patients may also exhibit high serum levels of the liver enzymes aspartate aminotransferase (ASAT) and gamma-glutamyltransferase (GGT).

Although legionnaires' disease is bacterial in origin, legionellae do not stain well with Gram's stain, and most of the legionellae are within macrophages. This is why Gram's stains of exudative PMNs often yield negative results.

The diagnosis of legionnaires' disease is best established by culturing the organisms. Transtracheal aspirates or sputum samples are treated with acid to reduce the number of interfering bacteria and then are cultured on buffered charcoal–yeast extract agar that contains L-cysteine, antibiotics, and appropriate dyes. *L. pneumophila* will appear after 3–5 days as blue-green colonies. Transtracheal aspirates are the best samples and have a sensitivity of about 90%, while sputum samples have a sensitivity of about 70%.

Serologic tests of acute and convalescent serum samples can also be performed. To confirm the diagnosis of legionnaires' disease, there must be a four-fold or greater rise in antibody titer to at least 1:128 in convalescent sera as compared with acute sera. Unfortunately, although 25–40% of patients have antibody to *Legionella* during the first week of disease, many patients will not exhibit detectable levels of antibody until 4–8 weeks after the onset of disease. Thus, serologic tests are most useful for retrospectively confirming legionnaires' disease.

Sputum samples can be stained by the Gimenez method or can be more specifically stained for legionellae by the direct fluorescent antibody (DFA) test. *L. micdadei* often appears as a weakly acid-fast rod in sputum. The sensitivity of the DFA test is about 70%, which is lower than the sensitivity of culturing organisms in transtracheal aspirate. DNA probes can be used, but they are no more sensitive than is the DFA test. Newer tests have been developed to detect the presence of soluble *L. pneumophila* antigens in urine. These tests have a sensitivity of 75–90% and are highly specific. Unfortunately, some of the currently available urine antigen test systems recognize only serogroup 1 of *L. pneumophila*.

In summary, the diagnosis of legionnaires' disease is best established by culture of transtracheal aspirates. The diagnosis can be further substantiated by staining sputum with Gimenez stain or DFA and by testing urine for the presence of *Legionella* antigens.

A diagnosis of Pontiac fever is confirmed serologically.

Treatment and Prognosis. Patients with legionnaires' disease are usually treated with erythromycin, sometimes in combination with rifampin. Alternatively, patients have been treated successfully with trimethoprim-sulfamethoxazole, a newer macrolide, tetracycline, or doxycycline. In immunocompetent patients, antibiotics are administered for 10–14 days. In immunosuppressed patients, antibiotic therapy may be prolonged.

Patients typically show clinical improvement in 3–5 days, but reversal of abnormal radiologic findings may be fairly slow. Most immunocompetent patients respond rapidly to treatment, but the mortality rate in patients with severe underlying diseases may approach 50%. When treatment fails, it is often because a delay in diagnosis led to a delay in treatment.

Patients with Pontiac fever generally recover in about 1 week without antibiotic treatment.

Selected Readings

Abu, K. Y. The phagosome containing *Legionella pneumophila* within the protozoan *Hartmannella vermiformis* is surrounded by the rough endoplasmic reticulum. Appl Environ Microbiol 62:2022–2028, 1996.

Alary, M., and J. R. Joly. Factors contributing to the contamination of hospital water distribution systems by legionellae. J Infect Dis 165:565–569, 1992.

Brieland, J., et al. Coinoculation with *Hartmannella vermiformis* enhances replicative *Legionella pneumophila* lung infection in a murine model of legionnaires' disease. Infect Immun 64:2449–2456, 1996.

Cianciotto, N. P., et al. A *Legionella pneumophila* gene encoding a species-specific surface protein potentiates initiation of intracellular infection. Infect Immun 57:1255–1262, 1989.

Donowitz, G. R., et al. Ingestion of *Legionella micdadei* inhibits human neutrophil function. Infect Immun 58:3307–3311, 1990.

Dowling, J. N., A. K. Saha, and R. H. Glew. Virulence factors in the family Legionellaceae. Microbiol Rev 56:32–60, 1992.

Hacker, J., et al. Analysis of virulence factors of *Legionella pneumophila.* Int J Med Microbiol Virol Parasitol Infect Dis 278:348–358, 1993.

Halablab, M. A., L. Richards, and M. J. Bazin. Phagocytosis of *Legionella pneumophila.* J Med Microbiol 33:75–83, 1990.

Hart, C. A., and T. Makin. *Legionella* in hospitals: a review. J Hosp Infect 18(supplement A):481–489, 1991.

Marra, A., et al. Identification of a *Legionella pneumophila* locus required for intracellular multiplication in human macrophages. Proc Natl Acad Sci USA 89:9607–9611, 1992.

Mintz, C. S., et al. *Legionella pneumophila* protease inactivates interleukin-2 and cleaves CD4 on human cells. Infect Immun 61:3416–3421, 1993.

Rechnitzer, C., et al. Demonstration of the intracellular production of tissue-destructive protease by *Legionella pneumophila* multiplying within guinea pig and human alveolar macrophages. J Gen Microbiol 138:1671–1677, 1992.

Skerrett, S. J., and T. R. Martin. Roles for tumor necrosis factor alpha and nitric oxide in resistance of rat alveolar macrophages to *Legionella pneumophila.* Infect Immun 64:3236–3243, 1996.

Torres, A., et al. Severe community-acquired pneumonia: epidemiology and prognostic factors. Am Rev Respir Dis 144:312–318, 1991.

Wadowsky, R. M., et al. Growth-supporting activity for *Legionella pneumophila* in tap water cultures and implication of hartmannellid amoebae as growth factors. Appl Environ Microbiol 54:2677–2682, 1988.

CHAPTER FOURTEEN

TOXIGENIC BACTERIA

Aeromonas, Bacillus, Clostridium, Corynebacterium, Plesiomonas, and *Vibrio*

GENERAL PRINCIPLES OF TOXIN ACTIVITY

While earlier chapters examined bacteria that cause diseases primarily by colonizing bacterial surfaces or by invading host cells, this chapter focuses on bacteria that cause diseases primarily by producing one or more protein exotoxins. This distinction is somewhat arbitrary because toxins contribute to the pathogenesis of many infections that are traditionally considered to be extracellular invasive diseases as well as to a few infections caused by facultatively intracellular bacteria. However, microbiologists have historically considered a disease to be toxigenic if the disease manifestations can be produced by injecting a sample of the bacterial exotoxin into a susceptible host.

Exotoxins Versus Endotoxins

Exotoxins should not be confused with endotoxins. The term "endotoxin" is used to describe the toxic activities associated with bacterial envelope components. It usually refers to the activities of the lipid A moiety of the lipopolysaccharide (LPS) of gram-negative bacteria. Endotoxins are "endo" because they are part of the structure of the bacterium, while exotoxins are "exo" because they are nonstructural bacterial products released into the environment.

As Fig. 14–1 shows, endotoxins are usually released from gram-negative bacteria as blebs of outer membrane that are heavily impregnated with LPS. These blebs activate complement via the alternative pathway and elicit the formation of interleukin-1, tumor necrosis factor, platelet-activating factor, nitric oxide, and other effector molecules that are responsible for the fever, thrombosis, and hypotension that typify sepsis. In contrast, exotoxins are proteins that are manufactured by either gram-negative or gram-positive bacteria and are excreted into the environment. These toxins migrate to their cellular targets, where they bind, enter the cell, and exert toxic effects such as the killing of cells.

Actions and Types of Exotoxins

Most of the strictly toxigenic diseases follow a common pattern of infection, as shown in Fig. 14–2.

The bacterium is introduced into a site where the primary infection will develop. If a mucosal surface is involved, the bacterium must have an adherence mechanism to allow it to adhere closely to the mucosa and deliver its toxin to the target. Often the toxin is synthesized and excreted as a **toxinogen** (a relatively inactive precursor) that will subsequently be cleaved to reveal the active site and confer full activity to the toxin. Most toxins are multimeric proteins, with many composed of a single toxic moiety (termed the A subunit) and multiple copies of a subunit that binds to the host cellular receptors (termed the B subunit). The infecting bacterium is usually confined to the initial infection site and, if the toxin is not produced, will cause little local effect other than inflammation. The toxin molecules disseminate to their cellular targets, which may be local but are often well separated from the initial infection site. Once a toxin arrives at its target cell, the B subunits bind to cellular receptors, allowing the toxic A subunit to enter the host cell. When it is inside the cell, the A subunit acts as an enzyme to catalyze a cellular reaction that will kill or transform the activities of the targeted cell.

Table 14–1 lists the bacterial toxins that have catalytic (A) and binding (B) subunits and are called **type A-B bacterial exotoxins** or **catalytic unit–binding unit toxins.**

Although there are numerous toxic mechanisms, there is one mechanism that seems to recur with amazing frequency: the splitting of nicotinamide adenine dinucleotide (NAD). As shown in Table 14–2, **NADase toxins** seem to fall into four categories: (1) toxins that stimulate adenylate cyclase, (2) toxins that inactivate elongation factor 2, (3) toxins that inactivate other host enzymes, and (4) toxins that inhibit respiration by depleting adenosine diphosphate (ADP). In most cases, the toxin splits NAD into ADP-ribose (ADP-R) and nicotinamide and then alters the function of a key host protein by ADP-ribosylating it.

Bacterial exotoxins can also be categorized by their target sites. Although not all toxins fall neatly into these categories, most bacterial toxins with sys-

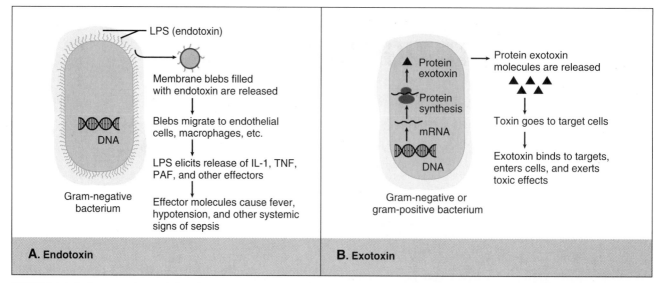

FIGURE 14–1. A comparison of the sources and activities of bacterial endotoxins (A) and bacterial exotoxins (B). Endotoxins are structural components of gram-negative bacteria, particularly the lipid A moiety of the lipopolysaccharide (LPS) of these bacteria, whose toxicity is due to their abilities to elicit the production of cytokines such as interleukin-1 (IL-1), tumor necrosis factor (TNF), and platelet-activating factor (PAF). Exotoxins are peptides that are synthesized de novo and released by gram-negative or gram-positive bacteria. The exotoxin attaches to target cells, and a portion of the toxin enters the cell, where it will exert its toxic effects.

temic effects fall into one of the following four categories, as shown in Table 14–3: (1) toxins that block protein synthesis, (2) toxins that cause hypersecretion by altering cyclic nucleotide levels, (3) toxins that stimulate vomiting neural receptors, and (4) pyrogenic exotoxins that act as superantigens.

Production and Effects of Exotoxins

The question of why bacteria produce exotoxins cannot be satisfactorily answered from the information that is now available, especially in light of the variability in the genetic sources of toxin genes. It is tempting to think of toxin genes as an intrinsic part of the genetic makeup of each toxigenic bacterium.

Indeed, as Table 14–4 shows, many toxin genes are chromosomal, but others are encoded on plasmids or are located within the genomes of bacteriophages.

Exotoxins that primarily affect the gastrointestinal system and cause vomiting or diarrhea are called **enterotoxins.** As shown in Table 14–5, examples include the toxins produced by some species of *Aeromonas, Bacillus, Campylobacter,* and *Vibrio.* In some cases, individuals ingest food that contains an enterotoxin. In other cases, the enterotoxin is released by bacteria multiplying in the intestine.

Not all exotoxins are enterotoxins. Examples of disease manifestations caused by **nonenterotoxic exotoxins** are flaccid paralysis (due to botulinum toxin) and spastic paralysis (due to tetanospasmin).

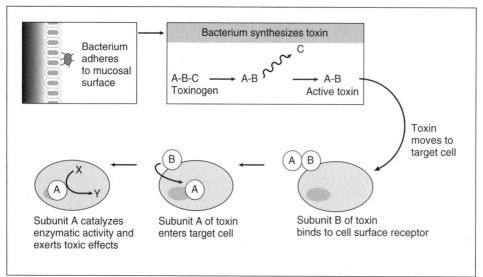

FIGURE 14–2. The general mechanism of action of type A-B bacterial exotoxins. Type A-B toxins are often synthesized as toxinogens (A-B-C). Once a portion of the toxin is cleaved in the extracellular space, the active toxin (A-B) binds to its target cell via its binding subunit (B), allowing the toxic subunit (A) to enter the cell. Once inside, subunit A catalyzes a reaction that is responsible for the toxin's effects.

TABLE 14-1.   Bacterial Toxins That Have Catalytic (A) and Binding (B) Subunits (Type A-B Bacterial Exotoxins)

Organism*	Toxin	Subunit Structure	Cellular Receptor
Bacillus anthracis	Anthrax toxin	EF/LF/PA†	Unknown
Bordetella pertussis	Adenylate cyclase	A-B	Unknown
	Pertussis toxin	A-5B	Unknown
Clostridium botulinum	Botulinum toxin	A-B	Possibly ganglioside GD_{1b}
Clostridium tetani	Tetanospasmin	A-B	Gangliosides GT_1 and GD_{1b}
Corynebacterium diphtheriae	Diphtheria toxin	A-B	Possibly glycoprotein
Escherichia coli (EHEC)	Verotoxin	A-5B	Glycoprotein or glycolipid
E. coli (ETEC)	Labile toxin	A-5B	Ganglioside GM_1
Pseudomonas aeruginosa	Pseudomonal exotoxin A	A-B	Unknown
Shigella dysenteriae	Shiga neurotoxin	A-5B	Glycoprotein or glycolipid
Vibrio cholerae	Cholera toxin	A-5B	Ganglioside GM_1

*EHEC = enterohemorrhagic strains; and ETEC = enterotoxigenic strains.
†Anthrax toxin consists of three proteins: edema factor (EF or factor I), protective antigen (PA or factor II), and lethal factor (LF or factor III). EF and LF are toxic subunits, while PA is the binding unit.

Exotoxins that cause necrosis are often detected by assessing their ability to kill monolayers of cultured cells. For example, the verotoxin of enterohemorrhagic (verotoxic) *Escherichia coli* is so named because it kills a standard fibroblastic cell line called Vero cells. Many of the enterotoxins as well as some nonenterotoxic exotoxins cause hypersecretion by altering intracellular cyclic nucleotide levels. These toxins are often identified by injecting them into ligated small intestine loops from a rabbit, guinea pig, or pig. If the material injected into the ileal loop contains such a toxin, the loop will swell as a result of hypersecretion.

Because toxins are proteins or peptides, they would generally be expected to elicit a good antibody response. Indeed, several of the standard immunizations administered to children contain **formalin-inactivated toxins,** or **toxoids,** which have no toxic activity but are fully immunogenic. These toxoids typically elicit a vigorous antibody response, and the antibody elicited will block the activity of the specific toxin against which it is directed by adhering either to the binding site or to the active site of the toxin. Some examples of toxoids used for immunizing humans include the diphtheria and tetanus toxoids contained in the standard diphtheria, tetanus, and pertussis (DTP) vaccine. The most dangerous toxins are fatal in microgram or submicrogram amounts, so a lethal dose of the native toxin for a human may be hundreds or thousands of times smaller than the dose needed to elicit an immune response. For this reason, recovery from the diseases caused by these toxins does not confer protective immunity, and immunization with toxoids is critical to prevent the disease from occurring. When nonimmune individuals are exposed to these toxins, they will need to be immunized and also given a protective dose of **antitoxin.**

Major Toxigenic Bacteria

The bacteria described in this chapter are not the only toxigenic bacteria, but they constitute the key toxigenic bacteria whose pathogenic potential lies almost entirely in the activities of the toxins they

TABLE 14-2.   Categorization of NADase Toxins by Their Mechanisms*

Category	Mechanism	Examples Organism	Toxin
Toxins that stimulate adenylate cyclase	Split NAD → attach ADP-R to regulatory protein (G_s or G_i protein) → stimulate adenylate cyclase (directly or indirectly) → increase cAMP → cause hypersecretion.	*Bacillus cereus* *Bordetella pertussis* *Clostridium perfringens* *Escherichia coli* (ETEC) *Vibrio cholerae*	Enterotoxin Pertussis toxin Enterotoxin (hypothesized) Labile toxin Cholera toxin
Toxins that inactivate elongation factor 2	Split NAD → attach ADP-R to EF-2 → halt protein synthesis.	*Corynebacterium diphtheriae* *Pseudomonas aeruginosa*	Diphtheria toxin Pseudomonal exotoxin A
Toxins that inactivate other host enzymes	Split NAD → attach ADP-R to other host proteins (precise target may be unknown) → inactivate host protein.	*Clostridium botulinum* *C. perfringens* *P. aeruginosa*	Type C_2 botulinum toxin Iota toxin Exoenzyme S
Toxins that inhibit respiration by depleting NAD	Split NAD → no ADP-ribosylation → halt respiration.	*Yersinia pestis* *Yersinia pseudotuberculosis*	Murine toxin Murine toxin

*ADP-R = adenosine diphosphate and ribose; cAMP = cyclic adenosine monophosphate; EF-2 = elongation factor 2; ETEC = enterotoxigenic strains; G_i = G protein that inhibits effector functions; G_s = G protein that stimulates effector functions; and NAD = nicotinamide adenine dinucleotide.

TABLE 14–3. Categorization of Bacterial Toxins by Their Target Sites*

Category	Examples	
	Organism	Toxin
Toxins that block protein synthesis by ADP-ribosylation of elongation factor 2	*Corynebacterium diphtheriae*	Diphtheria toxin
	Pseudomonas aeruginosa	Pseudomonal exotoxin A
Toxins that block protein synthesis by cleaving rRNA	*Escherichia coli* (EHEC)	Verotoxin
	Shigella species	Shiga neurotoxin
Toxins that cause hypersecretion by altering cyclic nucleotide levels via direct stimulation of adenylate cyclase activity	*Bacillus anthracis*	Anthrax toxin
Toxins that cause hypersecretion by altering cyclic nucleotide levels via modulation of a regulatory protein (G_s protein) to form a stable adenylate cyclase	*Bacillus cereus*	Enterotoxin
	Clostridium perfringens	Enterotoxin
	E. coli (ETEC)	Labile toxin
	Vibrio cholerae	Cholera toxin
Toxins that cause hypersecretion by losing the ability to down-regulate adenylate cyclase activity	*Bordetella pertussis*	Pertussis toxin
Toxins that cause hypersecretion by indirectly stimulating guanylate cyclase activity	*E. coli* (ETEC)	Stable toxin
Toxins that stimulate vomiting neural receptors	*B. cereus*	Heat-stable enterotoxin
	Staphylococcus aureus	Enterotoxins
Pyrogenic exotoxins that act as superantigens (cause cytokine release)	*S. aureus*	Toxic shock syndrome toxin 1
		Staphylococcal enterotoxin B
	Streptococcus pyogenes	Streptococcal pyrogenic exotoxins

*ADP = adenosine diphosphate; EHEC = enterohemorrhagic strains; ETEC = enterotoxigenic strains; G_s = G protein that stimulates effector functions; and rRNA = ribosomal RNA.

produce. They include the following: the vibrios (causing cholera and diarrhea); the clostridia (causing tetanus, botulism, pseudomembranous colitis, gas gangrene, food poisoning, and enteritis necroticans); the *Bacillus* species (causing anthrax and food poisoning); and the corynebacteria (causing diphtheria).

Other major pathogenic bacteria that are known to express an exotoxin—either as their primary pathogenic mechanism or as a major contributing factor to disease—are discussed in earlier chapters and are listed in Table 14–5.

VIBRIOS

Vibrios are gram-negative rods that are shaped like commas (see Fig. 1–1). They are actually short

helices with only a partial helical turn, and in stains of clinical samples, an aggregate of these organisms resembles a flock of sea gulls from a distance.

The most important pathogenic vibrios are *Aeromonas* (a member of the family Aeromonadaceae) and *Plesiomonas* and *Vibrio* (members of the family Vibrionaceae). Many of these vibrios live free in water, but some are there only when water is contaminated with feces. Because *Vibrio cholerae* is by far the most significant pathogen among the vibrios, it is the focus of this section of the chapter.

Vibrio cholerae

Vibrio cholerae is the cause of cholera, one of the most devastating human diseases. Cholera occurs

TABLE 14–4. Categorization of Bacterial Toxins by Genetic Encoding

Category	Examples	
	Organism*	Toxin
Toxins whose genes are encoded on bacterial chromosomes	*Bordetella pertussis*	Adenylate cyclase and pertussis toxin
	Pseudomonas aeruginosa	Pseudomonal exotoxin A
	Shigella dysenteriae	Shiga neurotoxin
	Staphylococcus aureus	Enterotoxin B (transposon), exfoliative toxin A, and toxic shock syndrome toxin 1 (transposon)
	Yersinia pestis	Murine toxin
Toxins whose genes are encoded on plasmids	*Bacillus anthracis*	Anthrax toxin
	Clostridium tetani	Tetanospasmin
	Escherichia coli (ETEC)	Labile toxin
	S. aureus	Exfoliative toxin B
Toxins whose genes are encoded within the genome of bacteriophages	*Clostridium botulinum*	Botulinum toxin and type C_2 botulinum toxin
	Corynebacterium diphtheriae	Diphtheria toxin
	E. coli (EHEC)	Verotoxin
	S. aureus	Enterotoxin A
	Vibrio cholerae	Cholera toxin

*EHEC = enterohemorrhagic strains; and ETEC = enterotoxigenic strains.

TABLE 14–5. The Major Toxigenic Bacteria and Their Associated Toxins and Pathogenic Effects

Organism*	Toxin	Pathogenic Effects and Associated Disease
Aeromonas hydrophila	Enterotoxin	Watery diarrhea
Bacillus anthracis	Anthrax toxin	Edema and necrosis (anthrax)
Bacillus cereus	Enterotoxin	Watery diarrhea (diarrheal syndrome)
	Heat-stable enterotoxin	Vomiting and diarrhea (emetic syndrome)
Bordetella pertussis	Adenylate cyclase	Edema and histamine sensitivity
	Pertussis toxin	Edema and histamine sensitivity (pertussis, or whooping cough)
Campylobacter species	Enterotoxin and cytotoxin	Diarrhea
Clostridium botulinum	Botulinum toxin	Flaccid paralysis (botulism)
	Type C_2 botulinum toxin	Cell death and necrosis
Clostridium difficile	Enterotoxin A	Watery diarrhea (pseudomembranous colitis)
	Toxin B	Necrosis (pseudomembranous colitis)
Clostridium perfringens	Alpha toxin, iota toxin, and others	Necrosis (gas gangrene)
	Beta toxin	Fatal enterocolitis (pig-bel)
	Enterotoxin	Abdominal pain and diarrhea (food poisoning)
Clostridium tetani	Tetanospasmin	Spastic paralysis (tetanus)
Corynebacterium diphtheriae	Diphtheria toxin	Death of cells, especially myocardial, renal, and nerve cells (diphtheria)
Escherichia coli (EHEC)	Verotoxin	Bloody diarrhea and hemolytic-uremic syndrome
E. coli (ETEC)	Labile toxin and stable toxin	Watery diarrhea
Pseudomonas aeruginosa	Elastase	Corneal damage during eye infections
	Exoenzyme S	Cell death in burn infections
	Pseudomonal exotoxin A	Liver damage during diverse infections
Shigella species	Shiga neurotoxin	Dysentery and hemolytic-uremic syndrome
Staphylococcus aureus	Exfoliative toxin	Scalded skin syndrome
	Heat-stable enterotoxins	Vomiting and diarrhea (food poisoning)
	Toxic shock syndrome toxin 1 and enterotoxin B	Toxic shock syndrome
Streptococcus pyogenes	Streptococcal pyrogenic exotoxins	Scarlet fever and toxic streptococcal syndrome
Vibrio cholerae	Cholera toxin, accessory cholera enterotoxin, and zonula occludens toxin	Watery diarrhea (cholera)
Vibrio mimicus	Enterotoxin	Watery diarrhea
Yersinia pestis	Murine toxin	Cell death (plague)
Yersinia pseudotuberculosis	Murine toxin	Cell death
Yersinia enterocolitica	Enterotoxin	Painful gastroenteritis with ulceration

*EHEC = enterohemorrhagic strains; and ETEC = enterotoxigenic strains.

mainly in the warmer months, when the organisms can multiply in water sources contaminated with human feces. Infection causes watery diarrhea that is isotonic with saline. During the acute phase of cholera, the patient can lose a liter of fluid per hour.

Since 1817, there have been seven cholera pandemics. The 1832–1849 pandemic was reported to have killed a total of 150,000 people, and the 1866 pandemic killed 50,000 in the USA alone. The current pandemic of cholera is the seventh one, with estimates of new cases ranging from 100,000 to 200,000 each year. During a 2-year period in the early 1980s, about 79,000 people died of cholera in 34 countries. In 1991, a new focus of cholera appeared in Peru. Since that time, tens of thousands of people have been infected, some of whom were US citizens who contracted cholera when they consumed drinks containing contaminated water or ice during international flights that originated in Peru. Most cholera during the 20th century, however, has occurred in India (particularly in West Bengal) and Bangladesh, where it is endemic.

Characteristics of V. cholerae

General Features. *V. cholerae* is a facultative anaerobe that can be grown on very simple media and at temperatures as low as 18 °C; this presages its ability to survive in water supplies. It grows optimally when the pH is between 7 and 9, and it is killed rapidly when the pH falls below 6. Thus, it is susceptible to being killed in the stomach, requiring that high numbers of the bacteria ($>10^8$) be ingested to reliably cause infection. Anything that raises the stomach pH, such as sodium bicarbonate or antacids, will cause a person to be more susceptible to cholera because raising the pH lowers the 50% infectious dose (ID_{50}) substantially. For example, routine use of bicarbonate reduces by fivefold the number of vibrios needed to initiate cholera.

V. cholerae can be isolated on special media that take advantage of the organism's preference for high pH and tolerance of bile salts. Two commonly used selective media are tellurite taurocholate gelatin agar (TTGA) and thiosulfate citrate bile salts sucrose (TCBS) agar. *V. cholerae* is an oxidase-positive vibrio and is sensitive to a dye called O/129.

Each organism has a single flagellum and is motile. Two adhesins for host cell receptors have been described. One adhesin for intestinal epithelial cells is believed to either be part of the flagellum or be expressed coordinately with it. The most important vibrio adhesin is thought to be type IV pili, also known as bundle-forming pili, which are similar to the pili of *Neisseria gonorrhoeae.* Adhesins are necessary for virulence because they bring the vibrios into close contact with the intestinal epithelium. When this close adherence does not occur, the cholera toxin is unable to exert its effects, and infection will not result in cholera.

V. cholerae has lipopolysaccharide, although it is somewhat unusual in that 2-keto-3-deoxyoctulosonic acid (KDO) has not been detected. There are six serotypes of O antigen, but most cases of cholera are caused by the O1 serotype. *V. cholerae* strains are identified by biotype and by serotype. There are four biotypes: *cholerae, eltor* (also called *El Tor*), *albensis,* and *proteus.* Both *cholerae* and *eltor* cause classic cholera and are O1 serotype; however, there are some O1 serotype vibrios that do not make cholera toxin and do not cause disease. The *albensis* and *proteus* biotypes do not agglutinate with antibody against the O1 antigen and are often called nonagglutinating (NAG) strains or noncholera vibrio (NCV) strains. Thus, there are three groups of *V. cholerae:* (1) VC O1, which causes cholera; (2) atypical or nontoxigenic O1, which does not cause cholera; and (3) NAG or NCV, which only occasionally causes cholera but more often causes bloody diarrhea.

Once a strain has been identified as O1, it can be differentiated as *cholerae* or *eltor* by its biologic activities. Biotype *cholerae* differs from biotype *eltor* in three ways: it is susceptible to Mukerjee's type IV bacteriophage; it is nonhemolytic; and it is not killed by the antibiotic polymyxin B. Finally, both *cholerae* and *eltor* can be further typed by antigens A, B, and C as follows: serotype Ogawa expresses antigens A and B; serotype Inaba expresses antigens A and C; and serotype Hikojima expresses antigens A, B, and C. An example of a complete designation for a strain is *V. cholerae* O1, biotype *eltor,* serotype Inaba. The identification of organisms in this precise manner allows epidemiologists to track the appearance of new cholera outbreaks and find out where contaminated water supplies are located so that further cases can be prevented.

For many years, almost all cholera cases were attributed to *V. cholerae* biotype *cholerae,* and when the *eltor* biotype was associated with cholera, it was as the cause of less severe disease. In 1961, however, the seventh cholera pandemic began in the Celebes (now called Sulawesi), and this pandemic was due to the *eltor* biotype. The *cholerae* biotype is still considered to be the classic biotype of cholera, but it is now apparent that both O1 biotypes can cause cholera.

Mechanisms of Pathogenicity.   Most of the key virulence genes for *V. cholerae* are clustered within a chromosomal segment known as the CTX element. This gene cluster, or "virulence cassette," is present only in virulent strains of *V. cholerae* and includes genes for three virulence factors: the **cholera toxin** (encoded by the *ctx*AB genes), the **zonula occludens toxin** (encoded by *zot*), and the **accessory cholera enterotoxin** (encoded by *ace*). The expression of the virulence cassette genes is controlled by ToxR, a

membrane protein that responds to changes in environmental pH, osmolarity, and temperature. ToxR also affects the expression of a second regulatory protein, ToxT, whose function is to up-regulate the expression of *V. cholerae* **type IV pili.** The CTX gene cluster is introduced into *V. cholerae* as a transposon that is part of the genome of a filamentous bacteriophage called ϕCTX. This phage only infects cells that express type IV pili on their surface.

Cholera toxin (also called choleragen) and type IV pili (also called toxin-coregulated pili) are key to the ability of *V. cholerae* to cause disease. Type IV pili act as adhesins and bring the vibrios into close contact with the mucosal surface so that the cholera toxin can exert its full effect. The precise roles of the zonula occludens toxin and the accessory cholera endotoxin in disease are not understood, but these two toxins are believed to play minor roles in the generation of watery diarrhea. Zonula occludens toxin affects F-actin polymerization and increases tight junction permeability, while accessory cholera endotoxin causes hypersecretion in ligated rabbit ileal loops, possibly in conjunction with ATPase activity.

Vibrios do not invade the epithelium during cholera, and there is no bacteremia. Instead, they produce cholera toxin, which is identical in mechanism to (but more potent than) *Escherichia coli* labile toxin. Cholera toxin is a typical type A-B toxin, with a single toxic A subunit per molecule and up to five B subunits that serve as receptors for GM_1 gangliosides. Subunit A has two fragments, A_1 and A_2, which are connected by a disulfide bond.

When *V. cholerae* enters the intestinal lumen, it penetrates the mucous layer over the epithelium and then adheres to the brush border enterocytes and crypt cells. Studies in animals have shown that it is not until the vibrios adhere to the crypt cells that hypersecretion begins. As Fig. 14–3 shows, the B subunits of cholera toxin released by adherent vibrios bind to GM_1 gangliosides on the surface of villous enterocytes and crypt cells, allowing the A subunit to enter the target cells. Once inside the cell, the disulfide bond connecting the A_1 and A_2 fragments is reduced and the toxic A_1 fragment is released.

The effects of cholera toxin on gastrointestinal secretion are phenomenal. An average of 9 L of fluid enters the human gastrointestinal tract daily, and healthy individuals excrete only about 100 mL of this fluid in the stools per day. In contrast, cholera patients excrete up to 1 L of fluid per hour. Unchecked, this would result in the loss of over half of the body's fluid component in 24 hours. Some of the effects of cholera toxin are due to stimulation of prostaglandin E_2 synthesis, release of 5-hydroxytryptamine, and modulation of activity of the gastrointestinal nervous system. However, hypersecretion primarily involves two processes: G protein regulation of adenylate cyclase activity and catabolite regulation of cellular ion secretion. Recent studies have suggested that stem cell factor and its receptor may also play important

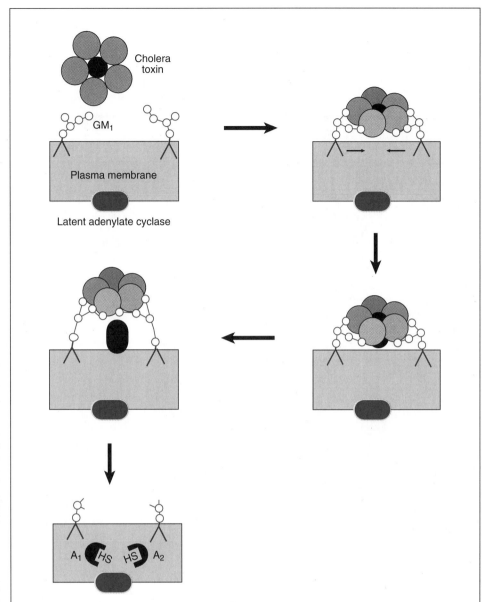

FIGURE 14–3. The mechanism of action of cholera toxin (choleragen). Each molecule of cholera toxin is composed of one A subunit and an average of five B subunits. The B subunits bind to cellular receptors (GM₁ gangliosides), allowing the single A subunit to enter the target cell. The A subunit consists of two fragments—A₁ and A₂—connected by a disulfide bond. Inside the target cell, the disulfide bond within the A subunit is reduced, releasing the catalytic A₁ fragment. HS = sulfhydryl group. (Source: Field, M., J. S. Fordtran, and G. Schultz. Secretory Diarrhea. La Jolla, Calif., Waverly, 1980. Redrawn and reproduced, with permission, from the American Physiological Society.)

roles in the intestinal response to cholera toxin. The precise nature of these roles is not known.

Many of the effects of agonists on human cells are mediated by the expression of a second messenger in response to the binding of the agonist to cell surface receptors. As Fig. 14–4 shows, the connection between the activated receptor and the enzyme that generates the second messenger is one of a series of **G proteins,** so named because their normal function is to bind guanosine triphosphate (GTP) and convert it to guanosine diphosphate (GDP) and inorganic phosphate. G proteins that stimulate effector functions are known as **Gₛ proteins,** while those that inhibit effector functions are called **Gᵢ proteins.**

Fig. 14–5 shows that intestinal cells possess a Gₛ protein whose function is to activate adenylate cyclase in response to external stimuli. Cholera toxin splits NAD to ADP-R and nicotinamide and then at-

taches the ADP-R to an arginine in the α subunit of this Gₛ protein. This causes the G protein to exchange GDP for GTP and to associate with and activate the membrane-bound adenylate cyclase. Because the G protein is permanently altered, the adenylate cyclase is also permanently turned on, and the cell accumulates huge amounts of cyclic adenosine monophosphate (cAMP). The accumulation of cAMP in crypt cells and villous enterocytes then causes massive hypersecretion.

Under normal conditions, crypt cells and villous enterocytes secrete or absorb water in response to changes in osmotic pressure, and osmotic pressure varies with changes in the rate of **ion secretion** by these cells. Fig. 14–6A depicts some of the significant ion transport mechanisms carried out by villous enterocytes and crypt cells. When cholera toxin causes these cells to accumulate excess cAMP, there are at

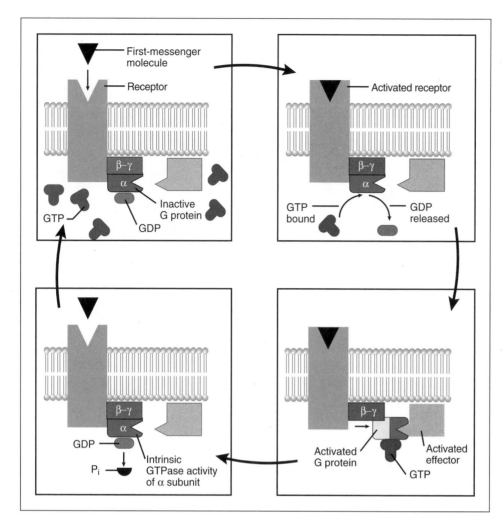

FIGURE 14–4. Summary of the general scheme of G protein–coupled signal transduction. In the absence of a first-messenger molecule, the G protein is in its inactive state. When an appropriate messenger binds to a cellular receptor, the associated G protein releases guanosine diphosphate (GDP) and binds a molecule of guanosine triphosphate (GTP). This causes the α subunit to dissociate from the receptor and to associate instead with an effector protein (such as adenylate cyclase). The activated G protein activates the effector molecule and then splits GTP to yield GDP and inorganic phosphate (P_i). When GTP is hydrolyzed, the G protein returns to its original conformation and the effector molecule is deactivated. (Redrawn and reproduced, with permission, from Spiegel, A. M. G proteins in clinical medicine. Hospital Practice 1988;23[6]:93. © 1988, The McGraw-Hill Companies, Inc. Illustration by Seward Hung.)

FIGURE 14–5. The effects of cholera toxin on G_s proteins in villous enterocytes and crypt cells. Cholera toxin hydrolyzes nicotinamide adenine dinucleotide (NAD) and attaches adenosine diphosphate and ribose (ADP-R) to the α subunit of the G_s protein. In so doing, it permanently alters the G protein, holding it perpetually in its activated state. The permanently altered G_s protein now turns on the membrane-bound adenylate cyclase, and enormous amounts of cyclic adenosine monophosphate (cAMP) are made in the absence of external stimuli. (Redrawn and reproduced, with permission, from Spiegel, A. M. G proteins in clinical medicine. Hospital Practice 1988;23[6]:93. © 1988, The McGraw-Hill Companies, Inc. Illustration by Seward Hung.)

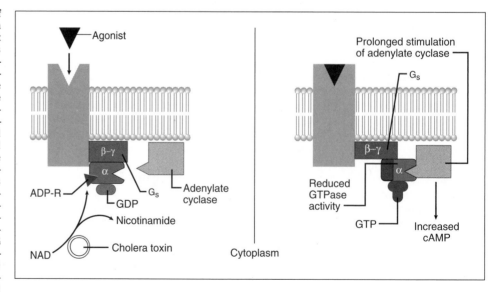

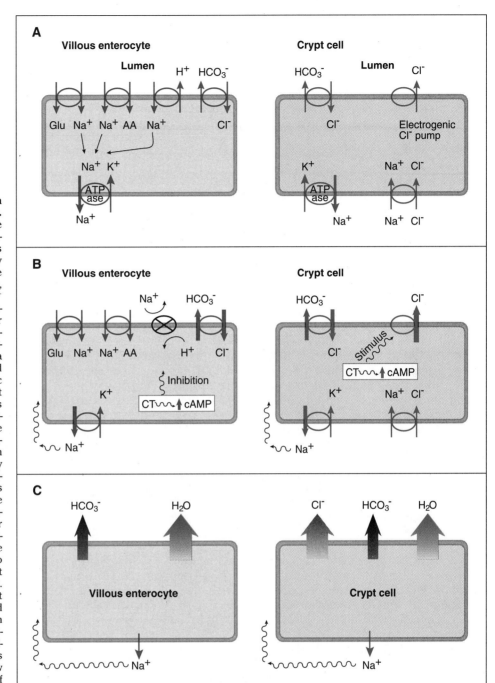

FIGURE 14–6. The mechanism of action of cholera toxin (CT). Diagram **A** shows how ions are transported in normal villous enterocytes and crypt cells. Villous enterocytes accumulate Na^+ by cotransporting it with glucose (Glu) and with amino acids (AA), while crypt cells accumulate Na^+ by cotransporting it with Cl^-. Enterocytes also exchange Na^+ for H^+ on the luminal side. Both enterocytes and crypt cells exchange HCO_3^- for Cl^- and have a basolateral Na^+/K^+ ATPase, and crypt cells have an electrogenic Cl^- pump. Diagram **B** shows that the enormous intracellular levels of cyclic adenosine monophosphate (cAMP) that result from the action of CT on the G_s protein exert their greatest direct effect on crypt cells, where they greatly stimulate the activity of the electrogenic Cl^- pump. This causes extracellular Cl^- levels to become extremely high, which in turn increases the exchange of Cl^- for HCO_3^- in both crypt cells and enterocytes. The Na^+/H^+ exchange system of the enterocytes is also inhibited, but Na^+ cotransport with Glu and AA is unaffected. Diagram **C** shows that the net massive accumulation of Cl^- and HCO_3^- in the intestinal lumen causes a great increase in osmotic pressure across the intestinal cells, and this in turn causes massive amounts of water to flow from the cells into the lumen of the intestine.

least three effects on ion migration (see Fig. 14–6B). First, the activity of the electrogenic chloride pump in crypt cells is tremendously stimulated, causing large amounts of Cl^- to leave these cells. Second, cAMP blocks the activity of the Na^+/H^+ exchange system in the villous enterocytes. Third, the accumulation of Cl^- in the lumen increases the exchange of Cl^- for HCO_3^- by both cell types, and sodium movement across the intercellular junctions into the lumen increases in response to the accumulation of anions in the lumen. How cAMP affects ion transport is not entirely clear, but it may involve phosphorylation of the permeases. The net result of these processes (see

Fig. 14–6C) is that osmotic pressure is greatly increased by the luminal accumulation of Cl^-, HCO_3^-, and Na^+, and water rushes out of the affected cells and into the lumen.

Because the sodium cotransport systems (involving glucose or amino acids) are not affected by cholera toxin, patients can be orally rehydrated using solutions that contain glucose and salts. Oral administration of these solutions does not halt Cl^- excretion but, instead, increases Na^+ absorption and, with it, water absorption. This phenomenon may be tied to putative differential effects of cholera toxin on crypt cells and villous enterocytes. As mentioned above, studies using animal models have shown that hypersecretion does not occur until vibrios adhere closely to crypt cells. Indeed, the major ion carrier effect of cholera toxin is on the electrogenic chloride pump in crypt cells. Thus, it may be that reabsorption of water occurs primarily in the villous enterocytes and that fluid loss occurs mainly through the crypt cells.

Diseases Due to *V. cholerae*

Diagnosis

(1) Cholera. Symptoms of cholera begin abruptly 8–72 hours after the patient ingests an infective dose of vibrios. In most cases, the organisms are acquired from contaminated water or ice, but there are human carriers. **Convalescent carriers** are usually individuals who are under 50 years of age and have recovered from cholera; they may spread the organisms for up to 1 year after recovery. **Chronic carriers** are usually older than 50 and shed organisms intermittently for years; the organisms apparently are carried in the gallbladder.

The major disease manifestation is watery diarrhea, which may cause the patient to lose as much as 1 L of fluid per hour during the first 24 hours. In some cases, the patient is placed on a cholera bed, which consists of a cot with an opening that drains to a bucket and allows the fluid to be captured and measured as it is eliminated from the body. Because this diarrhea is due to hypersecretion rather than to hyperactivity or inflammation of the bowel, the bowel sounds are hypoactive. The patient may also suffer from an effortless vomiting but is not nauseated.

During the acute stage of disease, the patient appears cyanotic, with sunken eyes and cheeks, scaphoid abdomen, poor skin turgor, a thready or absent peripheral pulse, and a voice that is high-pitched and barely audible. Tachycardia and tachypnea (rapid heart and breath rates) are present. The blood pressure is low (owing to loss of blood volume), and the heart sounds are distant or inaudible. In general, patients appear well oriented but extremely apathetic.

When samples of the stools (called rice water stools) of infected patients are examined by darkfield microscopy, they are found to be filled with vibrios ($>10^6$ organisms per milliliter) and are almost isotonic with saline. *V. cholerae* can be cultured rapidly in alkaline peptone water and typed by immunofluorescence. Additionally, the organisms can be isolated on TCBS agar or TTGA, but they will not grow on standard enteric media.

(2) Bloody Diarrhea. Various NAG strains of *V. cholerae* have been shown to elaborate a toxin that is similar to the *E. coli* stable toxin and to Shiga neurotoxin. Although the NAG strains rarely cause cholera, they can cause bloody diarrhea. Culture of the organism will confirm the etiologic agent.

Treatment and Prognosis

(1) Cholera. Proper rehydration is the key to treating the cholera patient effectively. This is because the primary threat posed by cholera is the loss of fluids and electrolytes, rather than sepsis, and cholera toxin does not affect the ability of the patient to be rehydrated orally.

Rehydration formulas are mixtures of electrolytes and glucose in water. While some formulas are available commercially, others have been designed and distributed by the World Health Organization (WHO). One of the most recent WHO-designed formulas uses rice and is easy to make up at home. The patient's fluid loss must be monitored, and the amount of fluid lost from the body must be replaced by drinking a rehydration formula. If the patient is too weak to drink, a rehydration formula can be administered intravenously, but care must be taken not to overrehydrate.

In addition to rehydration, patients should be treated with antibiotics to eliminate the source of cholera toxin. Tetracycline is the drug of choice to reduce the extent of infection. Alternatively, either ciprofloxacin (a fluoroquinolone) or a combination of trimethoprim and sulfamethoxazole (TMP/SMX) can be used. Although some groups have reported that prompt antibiotic therapy alone can reduce the amount of fluid loss by up to 60%, antibiotics should be used in addition to (rather than as a substitute for) rehydration.

The mortality rate in patients with untreated cholera is about 60%, but proper treatment reduces the rate to about 1%.

(2) Bloody Diarrhea. In most cases of bloody diarrhea, rehydration is not necessary. Patients can be treated on an outpatient basis with tetracycline, TMP/SMX, or a fluoroquinolone.

Prevention

Every effort should be made to prevent cholera. Water supplies should be examined for contamination. Travelers to endemic areas should avoid the following: drinking water that has not been boiled or chemically decontaminated; using ice prepared from unboiled water; eating salads or fruits washed with contaminated water; and using sodium bicarbonate and antacids, which lower the ID_{50} for *V. cholerae*. For some travelers, immunization with **cholera vaccine,** which contains killed cholera vibrios, may be indicated. Since the efficacy of the vaccine wanes rapidly, a booster injection must be given every 6 months. Because cholera patients who recover seem to be immune from further cholera for about 3 years, trials using choleragen toxoids have been attempted. Recently, a live attenuated cholera vaccine was also licensed for use in the USA.

Other Pathogenic Vibrios

Although *Vibrio cholerae* is the major pathogenic vibrio, diarrhea and other diseases are caused by a variety of other vibrios.

Vibrio fluvialis is an occasional cause of diarrhea in the USA. Patients typically have blood and polymorphonuclear leukocytes in their stools. There is no consensus recommendation for treating diarrhea caused by this organism.

Vibrio mimicus is so named because it causes

a profuse watery diarrhea that mimics cholera in its appearance. There are 6–10 cases of *V. mimicus* diarrhea reported each year in the USA. Most patients have eaten contaminated seafood that originated from the Gulf Coast. Treatment consists of rehydration and administration of tetracycline or a fluoroquinolone.

Vibrio parahaemolyticus is an enteroinvasive organism (like enteroinvasive *Escherichia coli*) and is responsible for 70% of the cases of diarrhea in Japan. Patients typically acquire the infection by eating contaminated shellfish, including crabs, oysters, and shrimp. The diarrhea is accompanied by abdominal cramping and lasts 2–3 days. Because it occurs predominantly during the warmer months, it is sometimes referred to as Japanese summer diarrhea. Patients are rehydrated as needed and treated with tetracycline or a fluoroquinolone.

Vibrio vulnificus causes wound infections that can lead to fatal sepsis in patients who have alcohol-related liver disease or altered immunity. The typical patient is a male who has cirrhosis and cuts his hand while shelling crabs or oysters from the Gulf Coast. *V. vulnificus* organisms in the wound spread to the blood, causing overwhelming sepsis. Treatment consists of a combination of tetracycline plus an antipseudomonal aminoglycoside or a combination of doxycycline plus ceftazidime. Without treatment, up to 16% of patients with sepsis die.

Aeromonas hydrophila is acquired by eating contaminated fish and causes an enterotoxin-dependent watery diarrhea in patients with preexisting hepatic or neoplastic diseases, including leukemia. Treatment consists of rehydration and administration of a fluoroquinolone.

Plesiomonas shigelloides causes bloody diarrhea in people who eat raw oysters contaminated with the organism. Patients are rehydrated as needed and treated with a fluoroquinolone or with TMP/SMX.

CLOSTRIDIA

The clostridia are gram-positive anaerobes that produce spores which allow them to persist in the soil and in other adverse environments. Some clostridia are strict anaerobes, while others are aerotolerant. Their most significant characteristic is that they produce exotoxins which are so potent that the introduction of a submicrogram amount in some cases is sufficient to kill a person.

There are four major pathogenic species of *Clostridium*: *Clostridium tetani*, which causes tetanus; *Clostridium botulinum*, which causes botulism; *Clostridium difficile*, which causes pseudomembranous colitis; and *Clostridium perfringens*, which causes gas gangrene, food poisoning, and necrotizing enteritis (pigbel). *C. perfringens* is the most important of the clostridia that are histotoxic (poisonous to tissues). Some of the other **histotoxic clostridia,** all of which cause tissue necrosis and gangrene, are *Clostridium fallax*, *Clostridium histolyticum*, *Clostridium novyi*, *Clostridium septicum*, *Clostridium sordellii*, and *Clostridium tertium*.

Clostridium tetani

Each year in the USA, there are 80–90 cases of tetanus. In over two-thirds of these cases, *Clostridium tetani* is introduced via a household wound. Although the wound may seem rather insignificant at the time, *C. tetani* spores begin to germinate in it when the tissue becomes anoxic. In about 12% of patients, tetanus results from a chronic disease (such as skin ulcers or chronic otitis media), rather than an acute wound. In 7% of patients, there is no apparent injury.

Characteristics of *C. tetani*

General Features. *C. tetani* is found in the feces of humans and animals, and the organisms grow to tremendous density in soil that is contaminated with feces. Horse manure, in particular, is an excellent source of organisms, making penetrating wounds received in a barn or a pasture where horses graze especially dangerous. In most cases, the infectious form of the organism is the endospore. There are several antigenic types of *C. tetani*, but there is only one antigenic type of tetanus neurotoxin, called **tetanospasmin.** Tetanus is entirely due to the actions of this toxin.

Mechanisms of Pathogenicity. When a person incurs a penetrating wound that contains *C. tetani* spores, the spores germinate as the site of inoculation becomes devitalized and anaerobic. As the clostridia multiply in the tissue, some of them autolyze and release tetanospasmin.

Tetanospasmin is secreted as a single peptide and is then cleaved by proteases to yield a classic type A-B dipeptide toxin. The B subunit of tetanospasmin binds to gangliosides on neuron membranes and enters the cell via receptor-mediated phagocytosis. The phagocytic vacuole becomes acidified, and this causes the B subunit to serve as a channel to allow the A subunit to enter the cytoplasm. The toxin now travels to the central nervous system via retrograde intra-axonal transport within motor, sensory, and adrenergic neurons. Toxin molecules that travel up motor neurons pass transsynaptically and bind to presynaptic membranes in the perikaryon. Here they enter and block the release of inhibitory transmitters (gamma-aminobutyric acid, or GABA, and glycine) from the presynaptic terminal, as shown in Fig. 14–7.

The means by which tetanospasmin halts the release of inhibitory substances are only now beginning to be understood. The release of neurotransmitters from synaptic vesicles requires that integral proteins in the vesicle membrane recognize and interact with docking proteins located in the cell membrane. When vesicle membrane proteins and docking proteins properly match, a structure called the SNARE complex is formed. This allows the vesicle and cell membranes to fuse, and exocytosis occurs. Tetanospasmin is a zinc-dependent endopeptidase, and investigators believe that it cleaves synaptobrevin, a vesicle membrane protein. The cleaved synaptobrevins cannot match with the membrane docking proteins, so degranulation is blocked. Some investigators

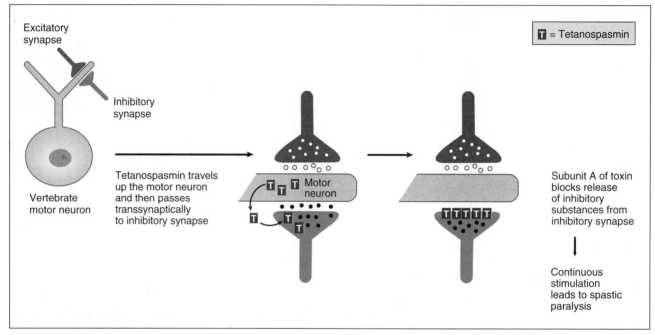

FIGURE 14–7. The mechanism of action of tetanospasmin. Tetanospasmin is secreted as a single peptide that is cleaved proteolytically to yield a dipeptide with the classic type A-B toxin structure. Subunit B binds to gangliosides on sensory nerve cells and is endocytosed. After subunit A enters the cytoplasm, the toxin is transported to the central nervous system via retrograde intra-axonal transport. It then crosses the intersynaptic space and enters inhibitory neurons, where it blocks the release of the inhibitory transmitters gamma-aminobutyric acid (GABA) and glycine.

have also reported that tetanospasmin can cleave the plasma membrane proteins SNAP 25 and syntaxin. Because these proteins are involved in vesicle docking, their cleavage interferes with exocytosis and release of neurotransmitters.

In infected patients, toxin molecules enter sensory neurons and travel to the dorsal root ganglion. Moreover, toxin in adrenergic neurons passes to the lateral gray matter in the spinal cord, where the cell bodies of the preganglionic sympathetic neurons are located. The result of these processes (Fig. 14–8) is that inhibitory pathways are blocked. This means that any stimulus that causes motor pathways to be activated will not be down-regulated by an inhibitory response but will instead result in paralyzing muscle spasms. Postsynaptic reflex pathways will not be inhibited, so stretching of agonist muscles will cause excitation of antagonist muscles and lead to reflex spasms. The sympathetic nervous system will also lose inhibitory pathways, so patients will experience greatly increased catecholamine secretion from adrenal glands. Because of this hypersympathetic activity, they will suffer from hypertension, tachycardia, profuse sweating, cardiac arrhythmia, and fever—a condition that is reminiscent of crises brought on by pheochromocytoma.

The hallmark of tetanus is the occurrence of local or generalized spastic paralysis. The sequence of onset of the muscle spasms is largely dependent on the length of the nerves affected, so spasms typically begin in the muscles controlled by the shortest nerves—namely, the cranial nerves—and proceed in

a descending pattern to affect the muscles of the trunk and then those of the limbs.

Diseases Due to *C. tetani*

Diagnosis. There are four forms of tetanus: **localized tetanus; generalized tetanus; cephalic tetanus,** which occurs after a head wound or as a consequence of chronic otitis media; and **neonatal tetanus,** which is generalized tetanus of the newborn. Of these, generalized tetanus is the most common. Cephalic tetanus is extremely rare. In some of the developing countries, neonatal tetanus occurs when a contaminated knife is used to cut the umbilical cord and the newly cut umbilicus is packed in dirt or cow manure, as dictated by folk medicine practices.

(1) History and Physical Examination. Tetanus is found most often in older persons. About two-thirds of tetanus patients in the USA are 50 years of age or older and have become susceptible to the disease because they have not been reimmunized against tetanus on a regular basis. In fact, several surveys have shown that between one-half and two-thirds of people over age 60 have no detectable antibody to tetanus. Depending on the form of tetanus, the clinical signs may begin from 3 to 21 days after clostridia are introduced into a wound.

In patients with localized tetanus, the symptoms appear late. The muscles around the wound first become rigid, and this rigidity spreads to include most of the skeletal muscles. Because the trigeminal nerve is affected, spasms of the masticatory muscles occur,

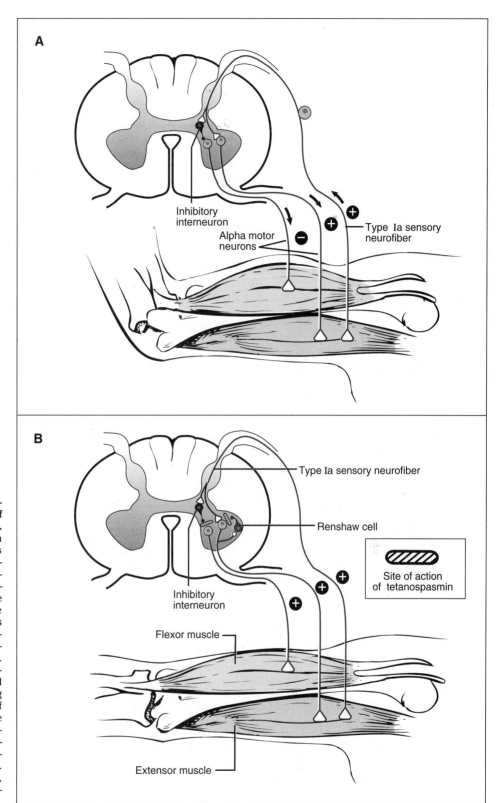

FIGURE 14–8. The effects of tetanospasmin on the flexion of biceps and triceps muscles. Diagram **A** shows that when the biceps are flexed, the triceps are stretched, stimulating the motor innervation of the triceps. Inhibitory synapses release inhibitory transmitters to prevent the stretch-induced excitation of the triceps. The extent of biceps flexion is also controlled postsynaptically by Renshaw cells releasing inhibitory transmitters. Diagram **B** shows that tetanospasmin blocks the release of all inhibitory transmitters, resulting in simultaneous hyperflexion of the biceps, reflex flexion of the triceps, and a heightened excitability of skeletal muscles. (Redrawn and reproduced, with permission, from Roos, K. L. Tetanus. Seminars in Neurology, vol. 11, pp. 206–214, 1991, Thieme Medical Publishers, Inc.)

and the patient develops **trismus (lockjaw).** Gradually, the spasms abate, and the patient recovers in 2–4 weeks.

In patients with generalized tetanus, the symptoms appear early, usually during the first 7 days after the injury. The rapidity of the onset is directly proportional to the amount of toxin that the patient has absorbed. Patients with generalized tetanus rapidly develop pronounced muscular hypertonicity that interferes with breathing. Because the toxin affects muscles controlled by shorter nerves first, muscular rigidity follows a descending pattern, beginning with the muscles of the jaw and then spreading to the trunk and limbs. Even a minor stimulus will elicit an episode of **opisthotonos,** characterized by long, violent, asphyxial, paroxysmal spasms that cause the patient's heels and head to bend back, thrust the patient's abdomen forward, and twist the patient's face into a horrible sardonic smile, called **risus sardonicus.** With each paroxysm, the heart rate and blood pressure rapidly increase. Death usually occurs from complications related to overactivity of the sympathetic nervous system, although some patients die from pneumonia or thromboembolism.

(2) Laboratory Analysis and Other Studies. In a patient with a history of a tetanus-prone wound and lack of adequate immunization, the diagnosis of tetanus is usually made on the basis of clinical signs, but assays will show that the level of circulating antibody to tetanospasmin is less than 0.01 IU/mL. Electromyography can be a valuable adjunct in establishing the diagnosis of tetanus. Cultures of the wound are not useful, since *C. tetani* cannot be isolated from most patients.

Differential Diagnosis. Tetanus must be distinguished from rabies, hypocalcemia, strychnine poisoning, dystonic reactions to dopamine-blocking agents, and peritonitis. Tetanus is unlikely in an individual who has had a complete primary series of tetanus immunizations, has received booster injections every 10 years, and has detectable serum titers of antibody to tetanus.

Treatment and Prognosis. There are three goals of tetanus therapy: to provide supportive care until the noncirculating tetanospasmin is metabolized; to neutralize the circulating toxin; and to remove the source of the toxin.

The first goal is met by isolating the patient in a darkened room where physical stimuli are kept at a minimum. Death is often due to asphyxiation, so muscle relaxants are given to reduce the severity of spasms. Benzodiazepines are the muscle relaxants of choice because they are GABA agonists. When benzodiazepines fail to control spasms, neuromuscular blocking agents can be administered, and the patient should be sedated. Hypersympathetic effects of tetanus toxin should be controlled with combination alpha-adrenergic and beta-adrenergic blockade. A respirator, oxygen therapy, and suction are used as needed.

The second goal is met by giving the patient **tetanus immune globulin** (TIG) to neutralize any toxin that is still circulating. Once the toxin binds to the central nervous system tissue, it cannot be neutralized by antibody. The patient is also immunized with **tetanus toxoid.**

The final goal is met by treating the wound that was responsible for the tetanus. The wound is debrided to remove devitalized tissue, and then penicillin G or metronidazole is given to eliminate clostridia. Note that the patient must receive TIG *before* an antibiotic is administered, because the toxin is released by autolysis. If TIG is not administered first, the patient's tetanus may be exacerbated by the lytic action of the antibiotic.

In cases of tetanus, the outcome depends on the quality of supportive care that the patient receives. The overall mortality rate is 60%, but in centers where tetanus is seen often, the fatality rate is only about 10%.

Prevention. The best approach to tetanus is, of course, to prevent its occurrence. The attack rate of tetanus among immunized persons is less than 4 per 100,000, but 5% of tetanus cases occur in people who were not properly immunized before an injury and were given TIG after the injury occurred. The series of childhood immunizations against diphtheria, tetanus, and pertussis (DTP) begins shortly after birth, usually consists of five injections of **DTP vaccine,** and is completed by 4–6 years of age. After the childhood series is completed, individuals should receive a **tetanus toxoid booster** once every 10 years. The vaccine for tetanus is a formalin-inactivated toxin (a toxoid) that has no toxic activity but is fully immunogenic. Unfortunately, recovery from tetanus does not confer immunity to the toxin, because a lethal dose of tetanospasmin is many hundreds of times smaller than the minimal amount needed to elicit antibody formation.

Clostridium botulinum

The *botulinum* species of *Clostridium* derived its name from *botulus,* the Latin word for sausage. The disease caused by this species was often called "sausage disease" because sausages were so often implicated in early accounts of botulism. In the USA, there are usually about 40–80 cases of botulism each year, but whenever the economy is poor and more people become involved in the canning of food, the incidence goes up.

There are three types of botulism. The first type, **classic botulism,** occurs when *C. botulinum* multiplies in food and the botulinum toxin is ingested. This form of botulism is actually an intoxication, rather than an infection. The second type, **wound botulism,** is an infection that occurs when *C. botulinum* is introduced into a wound. It is relatively rare. The third type, **infant botulism,** is the result of feeding honey-sweetened food or drinks to infants and is the most common form of botulism in the USA. During 1992, for example, 59 of the 81 cases of botulism reported to the Centers for Disease Control and Prevention were cases of infant botulism. Honey is often filled with botulinum spores. These spores cause no problem for children or adults, because their normal gastrointestinal flora will not be supplanted by *C. botulinum.* They do pose a risk for infants, however, if the spores germinate and produce toxin in the gastrointestinal tract. For this reason, infants should not be given honey.

Characteristics of *C. botulinum*

General Features. There are eight antigenic types of **botulinum toxin,** designated as types A, B,

C_1, C_2, D, E, F, and G. Most disease is caused by toxin types A, B, and E, with type F occurring sporadically. Types A and B are particularly associated with home canning of food, and type E is acquired most often from raw or smoked fish. In the USA, type A predominates in the western states, type B in the eastern states, and type E in the midwestern states and Alaska. Types C and D are not toxic to humans, but they are found in high concentration in the water of alkaline flats in the midwestern states, where they have killed thousands of ducks.

When food-canning processes are incomplete, vegetative *C. botulinum* organisms may be killed, but their spores survive. When containers of the incompletely processed food are sealed, the food becomes anaerobic, and the clostridial spores germinate and produce toxin. Usually, there is no outward indication that the food is spoiled, and the food may taste and smell normal. Often, the victim of botulism is the cook who tastes the food as it is being prepared. The toxin is neutralized if it is heated at 80 °C for 30 minutes or if it is boiled for 10 minutes, so the people who are served the food may be unaffected. Botulinum toxin is not neutralized by acidity. In fact, the activity of type E toxin is increased 10- to 1000-fold by partial acid hydrolysis. Only micrograms of the toxin need be ingested to produce botulism.

Mechanisms of Pathogenicity. Like tetanospasmin, botulinum toxin is synthesized as a toxinogen that is later cleaved to yield a classic type A-B toxin with a toxic subunit (A) and a binding subunit (B). Unlike tetanospasmin, which is cleaved in the tissues around a wound, botulinum toxin is cleaved in the gastrointestinal tract.

When subunit B fixes to gangliosides at the nerve terminal in the neuromuscular junction, the botulinum toxin is endocytosed and the toxic A subunit enters the nerve cell cytoplasm through a channel created by the B subunit in the phagosome membrane. Here it causes flaccid paralysis by preventing acetylcholine release (Fig. 14–9). Like tetanospasmin, botulinum toxin is a zinc-dependent endopeptidase that is capable of cleaving synaptobrevin, SNAP 25, and syntaxin. It appears that botulinum toxin has greater activity against SNAP 25 and syntaxin than does tetanospasmin. The cleavage of vesicle proteins and docking proteins blocks membrane fusion, degranulation, and release of neurotransmitters. All cholinergic synapses are affected, but the toxin does not affect nerve conduction or sensitivity of the muscle to acetylcholine. Autonomic preganglionic and parasympathetic postganglionic fibers are affected, and the cranial nerves are affected early and severely. However, the central nervous system is not affected by botulinum toxin. Deaths among botulism patients are usually due to toxin-induced paralysis of respiratory muscles, which causes respiratory failure.

Some *C. botulinum* strains produce a second toxin called the **type C_2 botulinum toxin** or **botulinum binary toxin.** This toxin is very different from standard botulinum toxin in that it is a true binary toxin (it is synthesized as two independent chains) and its effects are due to its ability to ADP-ribosylate host proteins. Thus, its general structure and its mode of action are more reminiscent of diphtheria toxin or pseudomonal exotoxin A than of botulinum toxin. Type C_2 botulinum toxin probably plays no role in human botulism.

Diseases Due to *C. botulinum*

Diagnosis

(1) History and Physical Examination. Classic (food-borne) botulism is usually due to the ingestion of improperly canned food. Clinical signs begin 6 hours to 8 days after ingestion, but the usual incubation period is 12–48 hours. The earlier the onset, the worse the disease will be.

The manifestations of classic, infant, and wound botulism are similar. The disease commonly begins with nausea and vomiting. Because the mouth, tongue, and pharynx are dry and painful, the early phase of disease may be mistaken for "strep throat" (streptococcal pharyngitis). This is quickly followed by acute symmetric impairment of cranial nerve function, with blurred vision, double vision (diplopia), difficulty in speaking (dysarthria), and difficulty in swallowing (dysphagia). Other early manifestations of disease may include drooping of the upper eyelids (ptosis), dilated and fixed pupils, and unexplained hypotension upon standing (postural hypotension). In the next phase, patients develop a descending pattern of weakness or paralysis of muscles in the extremities and trunk. If the botulism is severe, they may have difficulty in breathing because their respiratory muscles are paralyzed. There are, however, no sensory changes or paresthesias, and their mental processes remain clear. Some patients develop ileus (intestinal obstruction with abdominal pain, fever, vomiting, and dehydration), while others suffer from urinary retention. Because the onset of respiratory distress may be sudden and rapid, it is important to monitor the respiratory function of patients with botulism.

(2) Laboratory Analysis and Other Studies. Samples of food eaten by the patient and samples of the patient's serum, feces, and gastric contents can be examined for the presence of botulinum toxin. Electromyographic analysis may be helpful in some cases.

Differential Diagnosis. Botulism must be differentiated from multiple sclerosis, encephalitis, and other paralytic neurologic conditions. The diagnosis of botulism is usually made on the basis of four criteria: neurologic manifestations are symmetric and descending; mental processes are clear; there are no sensory disturbances; and there is no early fever.

Treatment and Prognosis. In patients with botulism, treatment consists of emptying the patient's stomach contents to remove the source of toxin, administering antitoxin to neutralize the circulating toxin, and giving adequate supportive care. **Trivalent antitoxin,** directed against toxin types A, B, and E, should be given immediately. Once neurologic signs

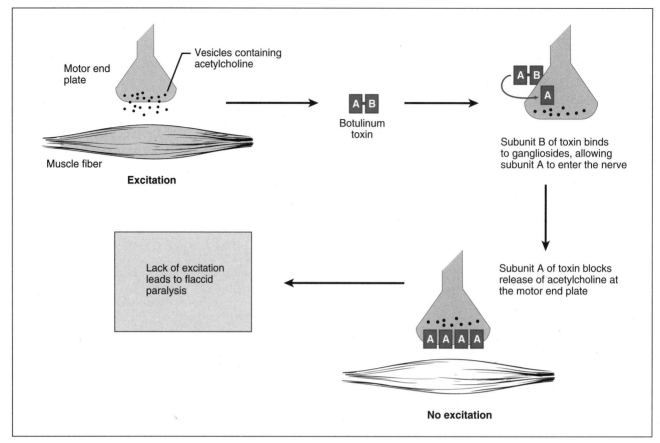

FIGURE 14–9. The mechanism of action of botulinum toxin. Like tetanospasmin, botulinum toxin is synthesized as a single protein and is then split to yield a classic type A-B toxin peptide. Subunit B of the botulinum toxin binds to gangliosides on motor neurons and is endocytosed. Subunit A is then released from the vacuole and into the cytoplasm, where it blocks the release of acetylcholine at the motor end plate and causes flaccid paralysis.

begin, anti-A toxin appears to be of minimal help, but type E toxin may be at least partially neutralized. Even if treatment is delayed, antitoxin should be given, because toxin has been detected in the serum of some patients up to 30 days after onset of the disease. For patients suffering from generalized flaccid paralysis, supportive measures may include tracheostomy, use of a respirator, and administration of guanidine hydrochloride. Reports indicate that respiratory function improved and cranial nerve palsies subsided in half of the botulism patients who were given guanidine hydrochloride, an agent believed to enhance the release of acetylcholine at the motor end plate.

The mortality rate associated with botulism was 70% before 1950 but is now about 25%.

Clostridium difficile

Clostridium difficile has been implicated as the cause of pseudomembranous colitis, a profuse diarrhea that occurs in some individuals receiving high doses of broad-spectrum antibiotics. Since *C. difficile* has been found in many asymptomatic individuals, its presence does not always result in disease.

Characteristics of *C. difficile*

General Features. *C. difficile* is a slender, gram-positive sporulating anaerobe found in small num-

bers in the gastrointestinal tract. When broad-spectrum antibiotics eliminate much of the normal gastrointestinal flora, *C. difficile* is able to proliferate in the gastrointestinal mucosa and cause disease.

Mechanisms of Pathogenicity. *C. difficile* produces two toxins: **enterotoxin A** (which causes fluid accumulation in the bowel) and **toxin B** (a cytopathic toxin). Enterotoxin A is reported to cause hypersecretion by elevating intracellular Ca^{2+} levels. As indicated earlier in this chapter (see the discussion of cholera toxin and Fig. 14–6), elevating calcium levels within intestinal cells stimulates the electrogenic chloride pump and causes hypersecretion by increasing osmotic pressure.

Diseases Due to *C. difficile*

Diagnosis. Pseudomembranous colitis may occur in patients receiving high-dose antibiotic therapy. Although it is especially associated with clindamycin or lincomycin use, it also occurs with ampicillin or cephalosporin treatment and typically has its onset about 4–8 days after antibiotic therapy begins. The patient usually presents with a profuse, watery or mucoid-green, foul-smelling diarrhea. Accompanying manifestations may include severe abdominal pain, high fever, leukocytosis, and hypoalbuminemia. If the pseudomembranous colitis goes unchecked, the patient can develop intractable colitis, intestinal perforation, and toxic megacolon.

Colonoscopy reveals that the mucosa is covered with gray, white, or yellow patches. These patches, which contain fibrin, mucus, and leukocytes, are the pseudomembranes. Stool samples are cultured on a selective agar that contains cycloserine, cefoxitin, and fructose (CCF agar) and are tested for the presence of toxin B. Toxin B production is measured by the ability of the toxin to kill cultured fibroblasts, and the toxin's identity is confirmed by determining if the toxin's cytocidal activity is blocked by specific antisera. A counterimmunoelectrophoresis test for toxin B is also available, but it is subject to frequent false-positive results. Barium studies are contraindicated because they may elicit dangerous complications, such as toxic megacolon.

Treatment and Prognosis. Treatment of pseudomembranous colitis follows a two-pronged approach. First, use of the exacerbating antibiotic must be halted; this gives other gastrointestinal flora a chance to regrow. Second, the *C. difficile* infection must be treated; this usually involves administration of vancomycin or metronidazole.

Retrospective studies indicate that death occurs in 27–44% of patients whose pseudomembranous colitis is not treated by appropriate measures. Death is most often due to hypovolemic shock, hemorrhage, secondary sepsis, or cecal perforation.

Prevention. *C. difficile* is often spread nosocomially on the hands of health care personnel and on fomites. To prevent its spread in the hospital setting, patients with pseudomembranous colitis should be placed in isolation, and disinfectants known to kill bacterial spores (such as sodium hypochlorite, chlorine dioxide, and alkaline glutaraldehyde) should be used to clean environmental surfaces as well as instruments that are inserted into the gastrointestinal tract. Because *C. difficile* spores are resistant to many disinfectants, eliminating the organism from the hospital environment may be difficult.

Clostridium perfringens

Clostridium perfringens (formerly called *Clostridium welchii*) is the most important of the histotoxic clostridia and has been implicated in three distinct diseases: gas gangrene, food poisoning, and enteritis necroticans.

In the past, gas gangrene (clostridial myonecrosis) was a major killer. During the Civil War and World War I, for example, many soldiers died of superficial wounds that became gangrenous—a fact that explains the eagerness of physicians during these wars to amputate the limbs of wounded soldiers. In recent years, about 20 of the 60 or more recognized species of clostridia have been isolated from patients with gas gangrene. However, in 80% of the cases of gas gangrene, *C. perfringens* is the causative species.

In recent surveys, *C. perfringens* has been reported to be responsible for about 15% of cases of food poisoning in Great Britain and about 7% of those in the USA. Clostridial food poisoning is often associated with outbreaks of cramping and diarrhea among people who have eaten at a banquet or a restaurant. Symptoms typically occur after ingesting poultry, fish, roasts, stews, gravies, or other meat products that have not been reheated properly.

The C type of *C. perfringens* is associated with a rapidly fatal gastrointestinal infection called enteritis necroticans. At the end of World War II, this infection was epidemic among the malnourished in Germany, where it was called darmbrand. It is now seen primarily in Papua New Guinea, where it is called pig-bel.

Characteristics of *C. perfringens*

General Features. *C. perfringens* has been isolated from the intestinal contents of every vertebrate animal tested, and its spores have been found in soils from every part of the world. The organism is fairly aerotolerant, grows as boxcar-shaped rods in media and tissue, and can multiply as often as once every 8 minutes at 43–45 °C. It forms a double zone of hemolysis on blood agar, and its growth in milk results in stormy fermentation.

C. perfringens produces 12 toxins, among which are an enterotoxin, a lecithinase, a deoxyribonuclease, a collagenase, a hyaluronidase, and several proteases. *C. perfringens* isolates are grouped into five types (A through E) according to the ability of specific antisera to neutralize toxins produced by each strain.

Mechanisms of Pathogenicity. Gas gangrene occurs when a dirty wound has a region of decreased redox potential. In this region, clostridial spores can germinate and vegetative clostridia can multiply and produce toxins. The **alpha toxin** (lecithinase C), the **iota toxin** (an NADase that ADP-ribosylates host proteins), and the **mu toxin** (a cytolytic hyaluronidase) cause the devitalized area to necrose, and they extend the anaerobic region.

The importance of predisposing local conditions to the development of gas gangrene cannot be overestimated. Studies have shown that although wounds typically contain *C. perfringens,* only a small percentage of patients with wounds will develop gangrene. Those most at risk are patients who have vascular insufficiency, patients whose wounds have become anoxic because they contain foreign bodies, and patients whose wounds have become concomitantly infected with other agents.

The "gas" in gas gangrene consists of CO_2 and H_2, which are released by the clostridia and accumulate in the tissues, along with edema fluid. This accumulation causes extensive swelling, tissue separation, and intense pain. The clostridia soon spread into the blood, where they continue to produce necrogenic toxins, spreading necrotic foci throughout the body. Although numerous toxins are produced, the key toxin is alpha toxin (Fig. 14–10). In experimental animals, alpha toxin was shown to cause extensive hemolysis, widespread capillary damage, and thrombocytopenia due to platelet destruction. Immunizing

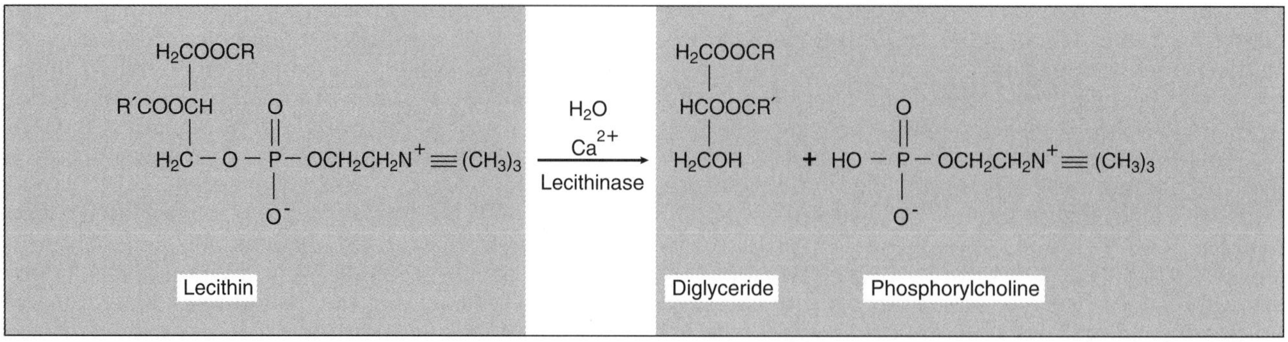

FIGURE 14–10. The mechanism of action of the alpha toxin (lecithinase C) of *Clostridium perfringens*. Lecithinase C splits the phosphate bond in lecithin to yield a diglyceride and phosphorylcholine. This disrupts the integrity of the cell membrane and kills the affected cell.

guinea pigs against alpha toxin was reported to protect them against gas gangrene.

C. perfringens is a relatively frequent cause of food poisoning. When food is heated and then cooled, the clostridial spores survive the heating process and germinate in the cooling food. The vegetative clostridial cells multiply rapidly (as fast as one division every 12 minutes) at a wide variety of temperatures. Large amounts of clostridia and **enterotoxin** can be found in food that is not properly reheated, and ingestion of this food leads to cramping and diarrhea.

The pathogenesis of enteritis necroticans is poorly understood. The strains that cause the disease all produce the necrotoxic **beta toxin,** but why only certain groups of people are susceptible to enteritis necroticans has been the subject of much speculation. Some have noted that the disease typically occurs following a large dinner of undercooked pork and have suggested roles for bacterial stasis and bowel distention. Others have pointed out that beta toxin is destroyed in most people by intestinal hydrolases. However, individuals with severe protein malnutrition lack these hydrolases, allowing the beta toxin to persist. In Papua New Guinea, adults and children typically eat a diet consisting largely of sweet potatoes, which contain trypsin inhibitors. Additionally, children typically carry unusually high burdens of *Ascaris lumbricoides,* an organism that secretes trypsin inhibitors. It may be that large amounts of these protease inhibitors block the action of the hydrolases that normally inactivate the beta toxin.

Diseases Due to *C. perfringens*

Diagnosis

(1) Gas Gangrene. There are three clinically distinguished forms of gas gangrene: **anaerobic myositis (classic gangrene),** which may occur after a traumatic injury or abdominal surgery; **anaerobic cellulitis,** which most often occurs in patients with leukemia or metastatic carcinomas; and **anaerobic puerperal sepsis,** or gangrene of the uterus, which may occur after an abortion.

Although clinical manifestations of gas gangrene may be noted as early as 4 hours after a wound, they usually have their onset 1–4 days later. The patient suddenly develops disproportionate local pain, accompanied by hypovolemia due to circulating toxin. Tachycardia, hypotension, tachypnea, and a moderate fever may be present, and the patient may begin to show signs of toxic delirium, becoming obstreperous, incoherent, and disoriented. Over the next 6 hours, the affected area of the body becomes progressively edematous and the skin covering the area undergoes several changes. The skin becomes stretched, shiny, bronze-colored, and necrotic; bullae (blisters) form; and a thin, brownish, malodorous discharge is present. Within 36 hours, the skin ruptures to reveal pallid necrotic muscle.

Gas gangrene is often difficult to distinguish from Meleney's synergistic gangrene and necrotizing fasciitis. Because the condition of patients with gas gangrene deteriorates so rapidly, the diagnosis must be made primarily on clinical grounds. X-ray or palpation may reveal that the tissues contain gas. Gram-positive rods may be found in the wound, and these can be cultured, but treatment cannot be delayed while waiting for culture results.

(2) Food Poisoning. About 50% of those who ingest food contaminated with enterotoxigenic *C. perfringens* develop food poisoning 8–24 hours later. Abdominal pain and diarrhea may be accompanied by nausea, but vomiting is rare. The symptoms and signs, which are caused by enterotoxin molecules released when *C. perfringens* germinates in the intestine, usually last 12–18 hours. However, *C. perfringens* has also been reported to be a cause of sporadic persistent diarrhea (with an average duration of 11 days), antibiotic-associated diarrhea, and diarrhea among nursing home residents.

Because clostridial food poisoning is generally a self-limited disease, its diagnosis is usually made on clinical grounds alone. If a definitive diagnosis is needed, a sample of the suspected food source can be tested for high levels of *C. perfringens* ($\geq 10^5$ organisms per gram), and a sample of the patient's stool can be checked for high levels of *C. perfringens* spores ($\geq 10^6$ spores per gram). In addition, the presence of enterotoxin in stool can be determined by enzyme-linked immunosorbent assay, latex agglutination assay, cytotoxicity assay, or similar test.

(3) Enteritis Necroticans. Abdominal pain, vomiting, and bloody diarrhea are the common manifestations of enteritis necroticans and usually have their onset 1 day after the patient eats a large dinner of contaminated pork. At this time, the clostridia are proliferating in the gastrointestinal tract and are producing beta toxin. This leads to development of patchy areas of necrosis in the upper small intestine, and the intestinal wall may become perforated. Eventually, the gastrointestinal tract becomes obstructed, and there may be dissemination of the clostridia.

The diagnosis of enteritis necroticans can be confirmed by examining the bowel wall endoscopically for necrosis. Cultures are not particularly useful, because the rate of asymptomatic carriage of *C. perfringens* in areas of endemicity is high.

Treatment and Prognosis

(1) Gas Gangrene. Treatment consists of surgical debridement of the devitalized area and administration of high-dose antibiotic therapy. In most cases, the wound is debrided extensively and penicillin G is given intravenously. There is no antitoxin, but hyperbaric oxygen may be given as adjunctive therapy.

Gas gangrene must be treated rapidly. If left untreated, the mortality rate is 100%. The relative importance of aggressive surgical intervention is evidenced by the ability of surgery alone to hold the mortality rate of gas gangrene to about 30% during the preantibiotic era. The use of antibiotics has improved the mortality rate only to 20–25%.

(2) Food Poisoning. Most patients recover without incident, but patients at risk of depletion of fluids and electrolytes should be rehydrated as needed.

(3) Enteritis Necroticans. Patients can be treated with penicillin G or chloramphenicol. About half of those with acute disease must also have 50–200 cm of their jejunum resected surgically. Most patients are children, and the mortality rate is high (15–45%).

Other Pathogenic Clostridia

About 20 other species of *Clostridium* have been sporadically implicated as causes of disease in humans. These include *Clostridium fallax, Clostridium histolyticum, Clostridium novyi, Clostridium septicum, Clostridium sordellii,* and *Clostridium tertium.*

The most significant in this group is ***Clostridium septicum,*** a sporulating gram-positive anaerobe that is part of the normal flora of the appendix in 10–60% of individuals. *C. septicum* is one of several histotoxic clostridia occasionally associated with gas gangrene. Of much greater importance, however, is that *C. septicum* can cause life-threatening bacteremia in patients with leukemia or malignant neoplasms such as carcinoma of the colon. In bacteremic patients, three toxins produced by strains of *C. septicum* have been found: alpha toxin (lecithinase C), beta toxin (DNAase), and gamma toxin (hyaluronidase).

Bacteremia caused by *C. septicum* usually has a sudden onset; is characterized by fever, abdominal pain, vomiting, and diarrhea; and initially appears similar to appendicitis. Some patients develop gangrene at metastatic sites, while others develop arthritis, meningitis, or other accompanying disorders. The cecum and adjacent gut become necrotic and edematous, and *C. septicum* can be found to have invaded the intestinal wall and to be disseminating hematogenously. The organism can be isolated from the blood and gastrointestinal tract, and the patient can be examined by laparotomy for necrosis and bacterial invasion of the intestinal wall. The treatment of choice is penicillin G, but antibiotic therapy is successful in only about one-half of the cases. When death occurs, it is usually due to hypovolemic shock.

In cancer patients, bacteremia can also be caused by several other species of *Clostridium,* of which ***Clostridium tertium*** is the most common.

BACILLUS SPECIES

Members of the genus *Bacillus* are large gram-positive rods that form spores. With the exception of *Bacillus anthracis,* the *Bacillus* species are motile. Most of the species are strict aerobes, but some are facultative anaerobes. Many of the species have been adapted for industrial use, producing antibiotics (polymyxin and bacitracin), alcohols, vitamins, solvents, and enzymes. Although various *Bacillus* species have been reported to cause sporadic cases of systemic disease in immunocompromised patients, the two most common pathogenic species affecting immunocompetent individuals are *B. anthracis,* which causes anthrax, and *Bacillus cereus,* which causes food poisoning.

Bacillus anthracis

Bacillus anthracis played a major role in the early development of microbiology. Bacteria were first discovered to be pathogens during the latter part of the 19th century. At that time, anthrax was endemic among livestock in western Europe, costing farmers and related industries millions of dollars each year. In the European textile factories, many people who handled unprocessed bales of wool died rapidly of a fulminating pneumonia that was named woolsorters' disease and is now known to be inhalational anthrax.

In 1877, Robert Koch isolated anthrax bacilli from diseased animals, and it was from his studies with *B. anthracis* that he developed the now-famous **Koch's postulates** that are used to establish the causative agent of disease: (1) the agent must always be in diseased animals but never in healthy ones; (2) the agent must be isolated in pure culture away from the animal; (3) when the agent is inoculated into susceptible animals, they must develop the original disease; and (4) the agent must be reisolated from the newly diseased animals. Although these postulates have undergone modifications in light of current knowledge concerning immunity and asymptomatic disease, the general concepts outlined by Koch are still used today.

In 1881, *B. anthracis* became the first bacterium to be used in a **vaccine.** At Pouilly-le-Fort, Louis Pasteur injected 24 sheep, 1 goat, and 6 cows with a living culture of anthrax bacilli that he had attenuated by growing the organisms at 42 °C. Two weeks later, he infected these animals and a corresponding group of controls with virulent *B. anthracis.* Within 2 days, all of the nonimmune animals were severely ill or dead from anthrax, but all of the immunized animals remained healthy. Pasteur took considerable risk in performing this experiment publicly, but because of his success, the doors were opened for further experiments such as this.

Today, anthrax in livestock is controlled by immunizing animals with a live, attenuated vaccine and also by burying animals that die of anthrax deep in the ground, so that the anthrax spores will not be consumed by grazing animals. Nevertheless, anthrax continues to be a problem in livestock in Asia, Africa, and the Middle East. In the USA, diseased livestock are seen particularly in California, Louisiana, Texas, South Dakota, and Nebraska.

Anthrax in humans also continues to be reported. In the USA, about 5 cases occur each year, mostly among veterinarians, laboratory workers, and people who handle textiles made of goat hair, wool, or animal hides. In some countries, hundreds of cases are reported annually. When public health measures break down, epidemics of anthrax may occur. For example, during the 1979–1980 civil war in Zimbabwe, more than 6000 cases of anthrax were reported.

Characteristics of *B. anthracis*

General Features. *B. anthracis* is a gram-positive rod that is about 1 μm wide and 4–10 μm long. A capsule is seen in vivo, but it is not formed in vitro unless the organism is grown in the presence of high CO_2 levels. Spores are formed, and these can be found in soil, wool, and hides, but they are not found in living tissues. *B. anthracis* is differentiated from other bacilli by its lack of motility. When grown on a standard medium, such as blood agar, and examined under a dissecting microscope, the hemolytic colonies look like tufts of curled hair and are called **Medusa's head colonies.**

Mechanisms of Pathogenicity. The capsule and the toxin of *B. anthracis* are responsible for the virulence of the organism. The capsule, composed of a polymer of D-glutamic acid, is antiphagocytic and protects the organism from the lytic action of antibody and complement. The capsule is encoded by a 60-mD plasmid that is called either pXO_2 or pBA_2 and can be passed by conjugation or transduction.

Anthrax toxin is encoded by pXO_1 or pBA_1, a plasmid that consists of three proteins: **edema factor** (EF or factor I), **protective antigen** (PA or factor II), and **lethal factor** (LF or factor III). Injecting animals with samples of these factors, alone or in combination, elicits the following response: (1) injection of any single factor (EF, PA, or LF alone) has no effect; (2) injection of EF plus LF has no effect; (3) injection of EF plus PA causes edema that is comparable to the effect of injecting choleragen into the skin; (4) injection of LF plus PA kills the animal; and (5) injection of EF plus PA plus LF causes the animal to develop subcutaneous edema and die.

In vitro studies have shown that PA is a carrier protein that binds to receptors on host cell surfaces. Once bound, a cellular protease cleaves PA, and the larger component remains attached to the surface receptor, where it will bind a molecule of either EF or LF. The EF-PA or LF-PA complex then enters the cell by endocytosis and exerts its effect. EF is an adenylate cyclase that is activated by calmodulin. Once EF is activated, massive amounts of cAMP are made, causing hypersecretion and edema. The function of LF is not known, but some investigators believe that LF may be further activated by cAMP and that EF potentiates its activity. It may, then, act as an enzyme to catalyze a reaction that is fatal to the cell. Studies in mice suggest that LF is active only against macrophages and that its effects are primarily due to its ability to induce macrophages to secrete large amounts of cytokines, particularly interleukin-1. The activities of anthrax toxin are depicted in Fig. 14–11.

To be fully virulent, both the capsule and the toxin must be produced. The capsule is apparently needed to establish an initial infection, while the toxin produces the clinical signs of the disease, including edema, hemorrhage, and capillary thrombosis. The toxin also has been reported to depress central nervous system function and to be a potent leukotoxin.

Attenuated strains that are used as vaccine in livestock have been "cured" of plasmid pXO_2 by growing the bacteria in the presence of novobiocin. These bacteria produce the toxin but cannot cause disease. Instead, they elicit protective immunity against anthrax.

Diseases Due to *B. anthracis*

Anthrax is acquired when individuals handle animal wool, fur, hides, or feces that contain anthrax spores or when they ingest meat that contains vegetative *B. anthracis.* The bacteria multiply at the site of entry, with some multiplying within leukocytes. The leukocytes are lysed when the cytoplasm fills with bacteria, and the bacteria then multiply extracellularly and produce anthrax toxin. Anthrax toxin causes marked local necrosis, tissue damage throughout the body, and shock.

Diagnosis. There are four forms of anthrax: cutaneous, pulmonary, gastrointestinal, and meningeal.

Cutaneous anthrax, which is also called **malignant pustule,** is the most common form of anthrax and is responsible for 95% of cases in the USA. The patient is infected with anthrax spores via a cut or abrasion and develops a lesion 2–5 days later. The lesion is usually painless and is located on an exposed area of the body, such as the hand, forearm, or head.

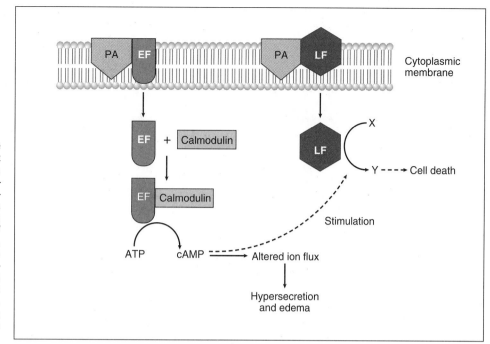

FIGURE 14–11. The putative mechanism of action of anthrax toxin. The protective antigen (PA) of the toxin binds to the surface of target cells, where it combines with a molecule of edema factor (EF) or lethal factor (LF) and facilitates the entry of the EF or LF into the cell. Once inside, EF combines with calmodulin to become a potent adenylate cyclase, while LF is believed to act as an enzyme; the exact function of LF has not been determined. ATP = adenosine triphosphate; and cAMP = cyclic adenosine monophosphate.

Although the lesion starts as an itching papule, it soon becomes an ulcer that has a raised edge, is filled with bluish-black fluid, and is surrounded by smaller vesicles. The ulcer then becomes a black eschar, and the lymph nodes that drain it become swollen and inflamed. The eschar usually heals spontaneously and leaves a scar, but some patients subsequently develop a spreading lesion, massive subcutaneous edema, bacteremia, or toxemia. Patients with systemic toxicity may also suffer from hemoconcentration and hypotension. Between 10% and 20% of untreated patients die. Cutaneous anthrax may be confused with staphylococcal pyoderma, orf, plague, or tularemia.

Pulmonary anthrax, which is also called **inhalational anthrax** or **woolsorters' disease,** occurs in individuals who handle raw wool, fur, or hides and inhale the anthrax spores. The spores go to the lower bronchi or alveoli, where they are phagocytosed by alveolar macrophages. The bacilli multiply within the macrophages and spread to the regional lymph nodes, where they cause mediastinitis. The initial symptoms are those of a typical respiratory disease and include myalgia, moderate fever, and a nonproductive cough. The patient seems to improve clinically over a period of 2–4 days but then suddenly relapses and shows signs of severe respiratory distress, cyanosis, dyspnea, stridor, subcutaneous edema of the face and neck, and pleural effusion. Death may ensue within 24 hours of the onset of these manifestations of disease.

Gastrointestinal anthrax is a disease found in developing countries. It occurs 2–5 days after ingestion of meat that contains vegetative *B. anthracis* and is initially characterized by nausea, vomiting, anorexia, fever, and abdominal pain, sometimes with bloody diarrhea. Toxemia and shock then develop and result in death.

Meningeal anthrax occurs in about 5% of cases as an extension of one of the other three forms of anthrax. As the bacteria spread hematogenously to the brain, the patient develops hemorrhagic meningitis. Death occurs in 1–6 days.

Anthrax bacilli can be isolated from the vesicular fluid of patients with malignant pustule and from the pleural fluid of patients with pulmonary disease. The organisms can also be visualized as large, boxcar-shaped bacilli in Gram-stained samples of vesicular fluid. Although serum samples can be tested for a fourfold or greater increase in titer of hemagglutinating antibodies, most anthrax cases are too fulminant to depend on antibody formation for diagnosis.

Treatment and Prognosis. Anthrax is usually treated with penicillin G, penicillin V, or ciprofloxacin. Erythromycin or doxycycline has also been used successfully. Prompt treatment of malignant pustule reduces the mortality rate from 10–20% to about 1%. Pulmonary anthrax is almost always fatal, even with treatment. The gastrointestinal and meningeal forms of anthrax do not typically respond well to antibiotic therapy. In patients with gastrointestinal anthrax, the mortality rate is 25–50%.

Prevention. There is an **anthrax vaccine,** but because of problems of legal liability, it is not widely available in the USA. Since *B. anthracis* has the potential for being used in biologic warfare against US troops, some military personnel are being immunized with anthrax vaccine.

Bacillus cereus

Bacillus cereus causes two forms of food poisoning: a diarrheal form and an emetic form. It can also cause systemic disease in immunocompetent individuals, but this is rare.

Characteristics of *B. cereus*

B. cereus is found in grains, vegetables, and dairy products. When foods prepared with these products are improperly refrigerated and are then reheated, the spores of *B. cereus* germinate and the vegetative cells produce enterotoxins. In experimental studies, the enterotoxin responsible for the diarrheal form of food poisoning has been shown to increase intracellular levels of cAMP and to cause ligated rabbit ileal loops to accumulate fluid. The toxin responsible for the emetic form is a **heat-stable enterotoxin.**

Diseases Due to *B. cereus*

The diarrheal form of *B. cereus* food poisoning is an intestinal infection, the symptoms of which result from the production of enterotoxin as the bacilli multiply in the gastrointestinal tract. Patients typically develop severe cramping and diarrhea 10–18 hours after eating fried rice, dairy products, or other food that contains *B. cereus.* Their illness is similar to the food poisoning caused by *Clostridium perfringens.*

The emetic form of *B. cereus* food poisoning is not an infection. It is characterized by nausea and vomiting that develop 1–5 hours after the ingestion of contaminated food. The vomiting lasts 1–6 hours and mimics *Staphylococcus aureus* food poisoning.

Antibiotics are not recommended for either form of the disease. Instead, fluid loss should be monitored, and fluids and electrolytes should be replenished as needed.

CORYNEBACTERIA

Members of the genus *Corynebacterium* are nonsporulating, gram-positive rods. Because they contain metachromatic granules, they tend to stain unevenly with standard bacteriologic stains. *Corynebacterium, Mycobacterium,* and *Nocardia* form the **CMN group,** consisting of gram-positive rods whose cell envelopes contain mycolic acids.

Corynebacterium diphtheriae

A number of *Corynebacterium* species are commensals in the respiratory tract; in the clinical laboratory, these are routinely identified as **"diphtheroids"** when sputum samples are examined, and their appearance is considered to be unremarkable. *Corynebacterium diphtheriae,* the agent of diphtheria, is the most significant pathogen among the corynebacteria. This organism received its name because it is club-shaped (the Greek word *korynē* means "club") and patients develop a leathery pseudomembrane in the throat (the Greek word *diphthera* means "leather").

In the USA today, people rarely think about diphtheria. This is because immunization programs have been so successful in reducing both the number of diphtheria cases and the number of disease carriers.

Only 27 cases of diphtheria were reported in the USA during the 10-year period from 1981 to 1990, in contrast to 200,000 cases reported in the year 1921. Yet diphtheria continues to plague the rest of the world, particularly developing countries in which accessibility to immunization programs is limited. Some investigators estimate that about 1 million people, most of whom are children, die each year from this disease.

Humans are the only significant reservoir for *C. diphtheriae.* On rare occasions, the organism has been isolated from the respiratory tract of horses and from diseased poultry, but these isolates are not considered to play a significant role in the epidemiology of diphtheria. In humans, *C. diphtheriae* may be carried in the upper respiratory tract or on the skin. The respiratory carriage rate varies tremendously among locales, with estimates ranging from 2% to 40% at specific sites. In the USA, respiratory carriers are extremely rare. In tropical and subtropical climates, many people carry *C. diphtheriae* on their skin. Thus, *C. diphtheriae* can be disseminated by either inhaling respiratory droplets or by contact with infected skin. *C. diphtheriae* is hardy, and dried pseudomembrane fragments from diphtheria patients have been shown to be able to harbor living diphtheroids for more than 3 months. These dried and detached fragments may be another source of infection.

Characteristics of *C. diphtheriae*

General Features. *C. diphtheriae* can be cultured on Loeffler's medium or on a medium that contains tellurite salts to inhibit the growth of streptococci and pneumococci, which are usually cultured from the same sites as corynebacteria.

When grown on an appropriate medium, *C. diphtheriae* organisms are often seen in pairs, with the organisms joined at right angles or forming shapes that look like the letter V. These forms, called Chinese letters, are distinctive for *C. diphtheriae.*

There are three colony types of *C. diphtheriae:* the *gravis, intermedius,* and *mitis* types. All three cause disease, and there seems to be no consistent association of a single colony type with a particular form of disease. Yet it appears that the percentage of strains carrying the toxin gene varies among the colony types. In one survey, about 99% of *intermedius* strains were toxigenic, compared with about 84% of *gravis* strains and 34% of *mitis* strains.

Mechanisms of Pathogenicity. To cause diphtheria, *C. diphtheriae* must colonize the upper respiratory tract, evade host defenses, and produce a toxin. There are two critical virulence factors: diphtherial cord factor and diphtheria toxin.

Diphtherial cord factor is a 6,6' diester of trehalose that contains the mycolic acids associated with corynebacteria. Like the cord factor of *Mycobacterium tuberculosis,* diphtherial cord factor is toxic to host cells and is needed for the bacteria to be virulent.

Diphtheria toxin is possibly the best studied of all the toxins. It is synthesized and excreted as a single peptide chain. It becomes activated when it is cleaved by trypsin to yield two peptides (subunits A and B) that are linked by a disulfide bond. Subunit B recognizes and binds to receptors on the host cell surface, causing the host cell to endocytose subunit A. Once inside, subunit A leaves the phagocytic vacuole and inactivates elongation factor 2 (EF-2). This factor is the eukaryotic parallel to bacterial EF-G, and its primary function is to act as the translocase enzyme. When a new amino acid is added to the growing peptide chain, EF-2 moves (translocates) the nascent peptide from the ribosomal A site to the P site and expends GTP in doing so. EF-2 contains **diphthamide,** an amino acid that is a derivative of histidine. Subunit A splits NAD to yield ADP-R and nicotinamide, and the ADP-R then becomes attached to the diphthamide residue of EF-2 molecules that are not ribosome-bound. The attachment of ADP-R to EF-2 permanently inactivates EF-2. Interestingly, mitochondrial and bacterial elongation factors do not contain diphthamide and cannot be inactivated by diphtheria toxin.

The mode of action of diphtheria toxin is depicted in Fig. 14–12. It is identical to the mode of action of *Pseudomonas aeruginosa* exotoxin A, but the latter is less potent and has different target cells. The pseudomonal toxin preferentially attacks the liver, while diphtheria toxin attacks the heart, kidneys, and nerves.

The effects of diphtheria toxin on EF-2 may not be the whole story. Some investigators have argued that diphtheria toxin has additional activities, based on experiments showing that the chromosomes of human target cells exposed to diphtheria toxin are degraded.

The control of the production of diphtheria toxin is a story unto itself. The gene for diphtheria toxin does not reside within the bacterial chromosome but is instead carried in the genome of any of a number of bacteriophages that infect *C. diphtheriae.* The best studied of these is the **beta corynephage.** The process that brings the toxin gene into a corynebacterium is called **phage conversion.** The phages are lysogenic, and the toxin gene can be expressed whether a phage is in its lytic cycle (in the prophage stage) or whether it is dormant within an "immune" corynebacterium. Yet the toxin gene is not read indiscriminately. *C. diphtheriae* produces an aporepressor that blocks the reading of the phage toxin gene unless iron concentrations are low. Iron concentrations are lowest during the late stationary or early death phase of the bacterium.

Diseases Due to *C. diphtheriae*

Diagnosis. There are two forms of diphtheria: respiratory disease and wound diphtheria.

(1) History and Physical Examination. Most cases of diphtheria in temperate climates are respiratory. The **respiratory disease** is spread via respiratory droplets and by skin carriers, and infection begins in the tonsils and oropharynx. The disease usually has its onset 2–4 days after exposure to *C. diphtheriae* and is heralded by a moderate fever and

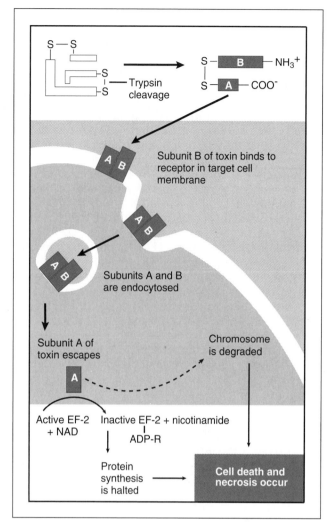

FIGURE 14–12. The mechanism of action of diphtheria toxin. Diphtheria toxin is synthesized and excreted as a toxinogen. The toxinogen is subsequently cleaved to yield a classic type A-B toxin. Subunit B of the toxin binds to target cell receptors, and both subunits of the toxin are endocytosed. Subunit A escapes the phagocytic vacuole and enters the cell cytoplasm, where it splits nicotinamide adenine dinucleotide (NAD), attaching adenosine diphosphate and ribose (ADP-R) to elongation factor 2 (EF-2). The permanently altered EF-2 is now unable to carry out its translocation functions, and protein synthesis is halted. Diphtheria toxin may also cause the chromosome to be degraded, but no mechanism for this effect has been described. As a result of the activities of diphtheria toxin, the cell dies.

sore throat. The patient may be hoarse and have a brassy cough. Over the next few days, the characteristic pseudomembrane of diphtheria forms in the throat. Early in the disease, many patients develop cervical soft tissue swelling and lymphadenopathy, a condition that is called bull neck and strongly suggests diphtheria. About 25% of patients also have headache, nausea, and vomiting.

The pseudomembrane is a fibrous mat that adheres tenaciously to the mucosa and consists of fibrin, bacteria, polymorphonuclear leukocytes, erythrocytes, and epithelial cells. If a diphtheric pseudomembrane is grasped with forceps and pulled away from the mucosa, attachment points will bleed profusely. Because the pseudomembrane may spread across the airway, the patient may be at risk for asphyxiation.

In a patient who is immune to *C. diphtheriae* or is infected with a nontoxigenic strain of the organism, there may be no pseudomembrane or only a limited pseudomembrane forms. The patient may have nosebleeds and a sore throat, but there will be no systemic toxicity. In contrast, in a nonimmune patient who is infected with a toxin-producing strain, the pseudomembrane will spread into the nose and larynx, necrotic foci will develop in the pharyngeal mucosa, the patient will be at risk of suffocation, and the toxin may cause life-threatening systemic effects. There is no spread of the bacteria into the blood. Instead, diphtheria toxin is produced in the pharynx and travels hematogenously to its target organs—the heart, the cranial and peripheral nerves, and the kidneys—where it causes myocarditis, paralysis, and nephritis.

Myocarditis occurs in 20% of diphtheria cases, but it is responsible for 50% of the deaths. Myocarditis usually appears 1 week or more after the disease begins. It is not uncommon for the disease to wane with at least partial disappearance of the pseudomembrane before cardiac symptoms begin. Patients who have toxin-induced megakaryocytic thrombocytopenia are at greatest risk of developing myocarditis.

Paralysis occurs as a result of myelin degeneration. The neurologic symptoms may appear a month or more after the infection began. The cranial nerves are most often and most severely affected, often causing dysphagia or nasal regurgitation of liquids. The palate may also become paralyzed, as can the larynx, facial muscles, and ocular muscles. Some patients develop weakness or paralysis of distal skeletal muscles. Fortunately, the neuritis is temporary, and normal functions usually return after the patient receives appropriate treatment for diphtheria.

Some patients with mild diphtheria develop a high fever and extremely sore throat—not directly from the *C. diphtheriae* infection but because the diphtheric lesion in the throat has become superinfected with group A streptococci.

In tropical and subtropical climates, **wound diphtheria** is common. Patients becomes infected when they come into contact with a person who is a skin carrier of *C. diphtheriae*. The corynebacteria grow within a minor abrasion, often in conjunction with *Staphylococcus aureus* and group A streptococci. The lesion ulcerates and is covered by a grayish pseudomembrane. Most patients do not have systemic symptoms. If systemic effects are present, they are not severe.

(2) Laboratory Analysis and Other Studies. The throat should be swabbed or a tiny piece of pseudomembrane should be obtained. The samples can be stained with methylene blue and examined directly for the presence of club-shaped bacteria. The samples should also be cultured on Loeffler's medium or tellurite medium. These media are selective for corynebacteria and will inhibit the growth of other

respiratory isolates. The laboratory should be forewarned that diphtheria is suspected so that appropriate isolation media are used.

Isolated corynebacteria can be speciated by fermentation reactions and by immunofluorescence techniques.

Once *C. diphtheriae* is isolated, it must be tested to determine if it is a toxigenic or nontoxigenic strain. The results will influence the type of treatment given. If the strain is not producing toxin, systemic symptoms will not occur. If, however, the strain is producing toxin, the patient must be treated with antitoxin. An immunoprecipitin test called the **Elek test** is used to detect toxin production.

Patients with signs of myocarditis should undergo electrocardiographic examination.

Differential Diagnosis. Mild diphtheria is most difficult to diagnose, especially when no pseudomembrane is present. Mild diphtheria must be differentiated from group A streptococcal infection, viral pharyngitis, infectious mononucleosis, and Vincent's angina.

Treatment and Prognosis. In patients with pseudomembranes that obstruct the airway, tracheostomy or cricothyrotomy is necessary. In all patients, the key to effective treatment of diphtheria is administration of **antitoxin.** Once toxin has bound to host cells, it is irreversible. Therefore, antitoxin must be administered as soon as possible. The antitoxin is an equine antiserum whose activity is primarily due to antibody against the B subunit of the toxin. Thus, it prevents binding of the toxin to its cellular receptors and prohibits entry of the toxic A subunit into the target cell. Because the antitoxin is equine, the patient should be tested for hypersensitivity to horse serum by a skin test. In some countries, a skin test called the **Schick test** is used to determine if the patient is immune to the toxin.

In addition to antitoxin, an antibiotic such as erythromycin or benzathine penicillin G is used to treat patients with diphtheria. Treatment with antibiotics is important because it prevents the formation of more diphtheria toxin, eliminates group A streptococci and other organisms that may have superinfected the diphtheric lesion, and prevents the *C. diphtheriae* organisms from persisting in the patient after recovery. When an antibiotic is not used, 1–15% of recovered patients become nasal carriers of *C. diphtheriae*.

The mortality rate in patients who are not adequately treated is about 20%. About 50% of the deaths in diphtheria patients are due to myocarditis.

Prevention. All persons should receive routine immunization against diphtheria. The **diphtheria toxoid** is usually given jointly with tetanus toxoid and pertussis vaccine as part of the DTP series given to infants and children. The series begins shortly after birth, usually consists of five injections of **DTP vaccine,** and is completed by 4–6 years of age. Unfortunately, with the carriage rate of *C. diphtheriae* now extremely low in the USA, natural boosting of immunity associated with asymptomatic infections does not regularly occur, so immunity wanes by the time an immunized person becomes an adult. Thus, medical personnel are encouraged to be reimmunized every 10 years with **Td,** a combination of tetanus toxoid and diphtheria toxoid for use in adults.

Immunization is important because it greatly diminishes the percentage of C. diphtheriae isolates that produce toxin, reduces the frequency and severity of diphtheria, and reduces the likelihood that a person will become a carrier. For example, before children were routinely immunized in Romania, surveys consistently revealed that about 86% of the isolates were toxin producers. Childhood immunization programs were begun during the late 1950s, and the percentage of isolates that were toxigenic dropped to about 11% by 1966. Between 1959 and 1970, about two-thirds of the cases of diphtheria occurred in children who had not been immunized, while 19% of the cases occurred in children who had been fully immunized. Of these, 19% of the unimmunized children died, but only 1.3% of the immunized children died. The lesson from this is clear: children must be immunized against diphtheria.

When diphtheria is diagnosed in a patient, efforts should be made to prevent infection from occurring in the patient's family members and other close contacts. Persons who have been exposed to the disease should be given a booster dose of diphtheria toxoid if they have been vaccinated in the past 5 years. Inadequately immunized or unimmunized persons should be vaccinated and should receive erythromycin or penicillin prophylactically.

Other Pathogenic Corynebacteria

Several other corynebacteria cause human diseases that are extremely rare in the USA. Three of these corynebacteria, however, deserve mention.

Corynebacterium jeikeium is a newly described bacterium that is part of the normal skin flora, especially in the axillary, inguinal, and rectal regions. The organism poses a threat to hospitalized patients who have leukemia or neutropenia, especially if the patients are receiving broad-spectrum antibiotics. The most common C. jeikeium infections are pneumonia, bacteremia, skin lesions at the sites of catheter insertions, and prosthetic valve endocarditis. Vancomycin is the antibiotic of choice, with ciprofloxacin as an alternative.

Corynebacterium minutissimum is often found as part of the normal flora in the webbing between the toes and occasionally in the groin area, but it also causes a skin infection called **erythrasma.** Erythrasma usually appears in the groin area as red or reddish-brown, glistening or greasy-looking patches that tend to scale. Erythrasma occasionally occurs between the toes, in the axillas, and under the breast folds. The lesions are usually not inflamed, and itching is minor. Although fungi cause lesions in the same areas, the fungal lesions tend to be raised and inflamed and can be differentiated from erythrasma by examining skin scrapings for the presence of organisms. A good method for visualizing the organisms is to touch a lesion with cellophane tape, place the tape on a slide, and stain the slide with methylene blue, Gram's stain, or Giemsa stain. Scrapings can also be digested with potassium hydroxide and examined under oil immersion. Erythrasma lesions will contain a mixture of cocci and filamentous rods up to 7 μm long. Erythrasma lesions also fluoresce coral red along the edges because C. minutissimum produces a porphyrin dye. Erythrasma is treated with erythromycin.

Arcanobacterium haemolyticum, a diphtheroid formerly called *Corynebacterium haemolyticum,* is often found on the skin and in the nasopharynx of healthy persons. It has been reported to cause pharyngitis. Pharyngitis due to A. haemolyticum appears similar to pharyngitis due to group A streptococci ("strep throat"), but patients who are infected with A. haemolyticum are usually older than those with strep throat and commonly have a red or pink rash that looks like scarlet fever (scarlatiniform rash). A. haemolyticum infection is treated with benzathine penicillin G or erythromycin.

Selected Readings

Ahnert-Hilger, G., and H. Bigalke. Molecular aspects of tetanus and botulinum neurotoxin poisoning. Prog Neurobiol 46:83–96, 1995.

Arduino, R. C., and H. L. DuPont. Travellers' diarrhoea. Baillieres Clin Gastroenterol 7:365–385, 1993.

Czerkinsky, C., A. M. Svennerholm, and J. Holmgren. Induction and assessment of immunity at enteromucosal surfaces in humans: implications for vaccine development. Clin Infect Dis 2(supplement 16):106S–116S, 1993.

Fayad, I. M., et al. Comparative efficacy of rice-based and glucose-based oral rehydration salts plus early reintroduction of food. Lancet 342:772–775, 1993.

Guerrant, R. L., and D. A. Bobak. Bacterial and protozoal gastroenteritis. N Engl J Med 325:327–340, 1991.

Hambleton, P. Clostridium botulinum toxins: a general review of involvement in disease, structure, mode of action, and preparation for clinical use. J Neurol 239:16–20, 1992.

Hanna, P. C., D. Acosta, and R. J. Collier. The role of macrophages in anthrax. Proc Natl Acad Sci USA 90:10198–10201, 1993.

Holmberg, S. D. Vibrios and Aeromonas. Infect Dis Clin North Am 2:655–676, 1988.

Kefer, M. P. Tetanus. Am J Emerg Med 10:445–448, 1992.

Klimpel, G. R., et al. A role for stem cell factor and c-kit in the murine intestinal tract secretory response to cholera toxin. J Exp Med 182:1931–1942, 1996.

Levine, M. M., and J. B. Kaper. Live oral vaccines against cholera: an update. Vaccine 11:207–212, 1993.

Lubran, M. M. Bacterial toxins. Ann Clin Lab Sci 18:58–71, 1988.

Peterson, J. W., et al. Molecular mediators formed in the small intestine in response to cholera toxin. J Diarrhoeal Dis Res 11:227–234, 1993.

Pfeuffer, T., and E. J. Helmreich. Structure and functional relationship of guanosine triphosphate binding proteins. Curr Top Cell Regul 29:129–216, 1988.

Poewe, W., et al. Treatment of spasmodic torticollis with local injections of botulinum toxin. J Neurol 239:21–25, 1992.

Richardson, S. H., and D. J. Wozniak. An ace up the sleeve of the cholera bacterium. Nat Med 2:853–855, 1996.

Singh, Y., et al. The carboxy-terminal end of protective antigen is required for receptor binding and anthrax toxin activity. J Biol Chem 266:15493–15497, 1991.

Spangler, B. D. Structure and function of cholera toxin and related Escherichia coli heat-labile enterotoxin. Microbiol Rev 56:622–647, 1992.

Spiegel, A. M. G proteins in clinical medicine. Hosp Pract 23:93–112, 1988.

Spiro, H. M. Small intestine disorders. *In* Spiro, H. M., ed. Clinical Gastroenterology, 4th ed. New York, McGraw-Hill, 1993.

Titball, R. W. Bacterial phospholipase C. Microbiol Rev 57:347–366, 1993.

Trucksis, M., et al. Accessory cholera enterotoxin (ACE), the third toxin of a *Vibrio cholerae* virulence cassette. Proc Natl Acad Sci USA 90:5267–5271, 1993.

Waldor, M. K., and J. J. Mekalanos. Lysogenic conversion by a filamentous phage encoding cholera toxin. Science 272:1910–1914, 1996.

Williamson, L. C., et al. Clostridial neurotoxins and substrate proteolysis in intact neurons: botulinum neurotoxin C acts on synaptosomal associated protein of 25 kDa. J Biol Chem 271:7694–7699, 1996.

Williamson, E. D., and R. W. Titball. A genetically engineered vaccine against the alpha toxin of *Clostridium perfringens* protects mice against experimental gas gangrene. Vaccine 11:1253–1258, 1993.

Wilson, B. A., and R. J. Collier. Diphtheria toxin and *Pseudomonas aeruginosa* exotoxin A: active-site structure and enzymatic mechanism. Curr Top Microbiol Immunol 175:27–41, 1992.

CHAPTER FIFTEEN

NONSPORULATING

ANAEROBIC BACTERIA

Bacteroides, Bifidobacterium, Eubacterium,
Fusobacterium, Gemella, Lactobacillus,
Mobiluncus, Peptostreptococcus, Porphyromonas,
Prevotella, Propionibacterium, and *Veillonella*

In the past, microbiologists and physicians were concerned primarily with aerobes and facultative anaerobes as causes of human infections. Strict anaerobes were largely ignored because culture techniques commonly used were not capable of isolating and identifying them. Abscesses were often mixed infections that involved both anaerobes and facultative gram-negative rods. Because these infections so often contained enteric organisms, clinicians generally assumed that these bacteria were the sole cause of the infection and prescribed treatment based on this line of reasoning. When the infections were **exogenous infections** (infections acquired from an outside source), this assumption was generally appropriate. But the importance of strict anaerobes as the cause of **endogenous infections** (infections arising from one's own microflora) was not appreciated until recently. Anaerobes are now known to constitute a major portion of the human body flora, and their presence must be suspected in any endogenous abscess.

General Characteristics and Classification

The anaerobes are bacteria that grow in the absence of atmospheric oxygen. They can be considered to fall into two broad categories: **moderate anaerobes,** which grow when the Po_2 is 3% or less; and **strict anaerobes,** which cannot grow unless the Po_2 is 0.5% or less. Anaerobes are found on any body surface that provides a low enough Po_2 for them to multiply. As Table 15–1 shows, anaerobes are found on the skin and throughout the respiratory, gastrointestinal, and genitourinary systems. In gingival crevices and the colon, the ratio of anaerobes to aerobes is 1000:1. In nasal washings and in the endocervix and vagina, the ratio is about 5:1. Anaerobes are as

prevalent as aerobes on the surfaces of teeth and in the saliva.

Some strict anaerobes are aerointolerant and are therefore rapidly killed when exposed to air. The biochemical basis of anaerobiosis is not well understood. Many strict anaerobes lack superoxide dismutase, catalase, or both. As a general rule, the lack of these enzymes makes the organisms susceptible to oxygen-derived free radicals that are formed when the cytochromes of anaerobes use oxygen as a terminal electron acceptor. Yet there are exceptions to this rule, leading many investigators to believe that anaerobiosis is a multifactorial process.

Anaerobes may be gram-positive or gram-negative, and they may be rods or cocci. In general, anaerobic rods are more pleomorphic than the commonly encountered aerobic or facultative rods, and they often have tapered ends. Most of the gram-positive anaerobic rods are members of the genus *Clostridium.* These spore-forming bacteria, which are discussed in Chapter 14, are important causes of exogenous infections and are sometimes responsible for endogenous infections. The rest of the anaerobes do not form spores, and most infections with these non–spore-forming bacteria are endogenous.

Anaerobes cause endogenous infections when a breach in the integrity of a body surface or a loss of immune function allows the anaerobic flora to enter a normally sterile body site. If the tissue involved is devitalized by trauma (for example, by penetrating injuries or surgery), anaerobes may persist and establish a nidus of infection. Abscesses are often mixed infections that involve anaerobes and facultative gram-negative rods. Anaerobic abscesses commonly occur near a mucosal surface, and the anaerobes responsible for the infection are derived from the

TABLE 15–1. Infections Commonly Caused by Anaerobic Bacteria

Site of Infection	Type of Infection	Anaerobic Genera Most Prevalent
Central nervous system	Cerebral abscess, epidural abscess, and subdural abscess.	*Fusobacterium, Peptostreptococcus,* and *Propionibacterium.*
Skin and soft tissue	Bite wounds, cellulitis, decubitus ulcer, diabetic foot ulcer, myonecrosis, necrotizing fasciitis, and perirectal abscess.	*Peptostreptococcus* and *Propionibacterium.*
Mouth, sinuses, and respiratory tract	Aspiration or nosocomial pneumonia, bronchiectasis, chronic otitis media, chronic sinusitis, dental abscesses (including root canal, periodontal, and orofacial abscesses), empyema, gingivitis, lung abscess, mastoiditis, and peritonsillar abscess.	*Actinomyces, Bacteroides, Eubacterium, Fusobacterium, Peptostreptococcus, Porphyromonas, Prevotella, Propionibacterium,* and *Veillonella.*
Gastrointestinal tract	Appendicitis, intra-abdominal abscess, liver abscess, and peritonitis.	*Lactobacillus* in stomach when fasting; *Lactobacillus, Peptostreptococcus,* and *Streptococcus* in small intestine; and anaerobic cocci, *Bacteroides, Bifidobacterium, Clostridium, Eubacterium, Fusobacterium, Porphyromonas,* and *Propionibacterium* in terminal ileum and large bowel.
Female genital tract	Bacterial vaginosis, Bartholin's gland abscess, endometritis, salpingitis, septic abortion, and tubo-ovarian abscess.	*Bacteroides, Clostridium, Eubacterium, Lactobacillus, Mobiluncus, Peptostreptococcus, Porphyromonas, Prevotella, Propionibacterium,* and *Veillonella* in vagina and cervix; and *Bacteroides, Fusobacterium, Peptostreptococcus, Prevotella,* and *Propionibacterium* in urethra.
Other sites	Postoperative abscesses at any site.	Site-specific organisms.

nearby mucosa. For example, abdominal infections usually occur when fecal matter spills into the abdominal cavity. The infection begins as peritonitis and subsequently develops into an intra-abdominal abscess.

Table 15–1 lists infections commonly caused by anaerobes. Anaerobes are involved in at least 70% of the following infections: brain abscesses; postoperative head, abdominal, and obstetric infections; peritonsillar abscesses; dental abscesses; aspiration pneumonia; lung abscesses; bronchiectasis; intra-abdominal abscesses; appendicitis and peritonitis; vulvovaginal abscesses; tubo-ovarian abscesses; septic abortions; endometritis; necrotizing fasciitis; diabetic foot ulcers; cellulitis; and perirectal abscesses.

Culture and Identification of Anaerobes

Specimens suspected of containing anaerobic bacteria must be carefully collected, placed into pre-reduced transport media, and sent to the laboratory for culture as quickly as possible. Prepackaged systems for transporting, cultivating, and identifying anaerobic bacteria are now available, and small anaerobic culture chambers are relatively easy to use. As a result, the majority of hospitals are able to culture and identify the most frequently encountered non-sporulating anaerobes.

Before clinical samples are taken from the skin and mucous membranes, the area must be decontaminated with 70% ethyl or isopropyl alcohol and tincture of iodine, and the iodine should then be removed with alcohol. Samples should be obtained with a needle and syringe, rather than with a swab.

Laboratory personnel should examine the specimen grossly for pungent odor and for evidence of purulence. Blood samples should be cultured in a standard anaerobic blood culture system, such as a BACTEC system. Other samples can be cultured on nonselective, selective, or enriched media. The enriched media allow growth of fastidious organisms and contain antibiotics to inhibit the growth of facultative anaerobes, such as enteric organisms. In most cases, an aminoglycoside (such as kanamycin) is used to inhibit gram-negative bacteria, and vancomycin is used to block the growth of gram-positive bacteria. Anaerobic media commonly used for primary isolation include CDC anaerobe blood agar (AnBAP), anaerobe phenylethyl alcohol (PEA) blood agar, anaerobe kanamycin-vancomycin (KV) blood agar, anaerobe paromomycin-vancomycin (PV) laked blood agar, cycloserine-cefoxitin fructose agar (CCFA), and enriched thioglycollate (THIO) broth. Media for culturing anaerobes should be incubated within an anaerobe jar or anaerobic glove box in an atmosphere of 85% N_2, 10% H_2, and 5% CO_2 for 4–16 hours before use.

Strict anaerobes must be grown within a chamber that provides an atmosphere containing less than 0.5% Po_2. This requirement is met by a number of commercially available systems, some of which are relatively inexpensive. Examples of popular systems are GasPak and the Oxoid Anaerobe Jar. In these systems, the jar is large and can be made airtight. Petri dishes are placed within the jar, and atmospheric oxygen is removed by use of a catalyst that combines H_2 and O_2 to form water. In most cases, the catalyst is available as palladium-coated aluminum pellets. A methylene blue indicator is also put into the jar. The indicator strip turns white when no oxygen remains in the jar, but it turns blue if oxygen leaks back in through an inadequate seal. Alternatively, a jar can be vacuum-evacuated, and the air can be replaced by a mixture of 85% N_2, 10% H_2, and 5% CO_2.

Solid media inoculated with clinical specimens should be checked after 48 hours of incubation at 35–37 °C. If there is no growth at this time, the plates should be incubated anaerobically for an additional 2–4 days and then rechecked. Colonies should be examined for aerotolerance, morphologic appearance, pitting of the culture medium, pigment production, and hemolysis. The isolates should be Gram-stained and examined for cell shape. Primary cultures can then be used to inoculate new media that will characterize the biochemical activities of the isolated bacteria. Presumpto 1, 2, and 3 agar media are commonly used to identify anaerobes. These media, which come in Petri dishes that are divided into sections and contain Lombard-Dowell medium as their base, test for 20 biochemical characteristics. Anaerobes can also be identified via rapid enzyme assays, and some anaerobes can be identified by use of gas-liquid chromatography to demonstrate the presence of the unique short-chain fatty acids that they produce.

Anaerobic Rods

The most important **gram-negative anaerobic rods** are (1) *Bacteroides fragilis* and members of the so-called DOT group, consisting of *Bacteroides distasonis, Bacteroides ovatus,* and *Bacteroides thetaiotaomicron;* and (2) *Prevotella melaninogenica* and other pigmented *Prevotella* species, including *Prevotella corporis, Prevotella denticola, Prevotella intermedia,* and *Prevotella loeschii.* Additional gram-negative rods that cause disease in humans include the pigmented *Porphyromonas* species; the nonpigmented *Prevotella bivia, Prevotella oralis,* and *Prevotella ruminicola;* and *Fusobacterium necrophorum* and *Fusobacterium nucleatum.* Of these, *B. fragilis* is the most common cause of human infection.

The **gram-positive anaerobic rods** associated with human infection include members of the following genera: *Actinomyces* (see Chapter 9), *Clostridium* (see Chapter 14), *Bifidobacterium, Eubacterium, Lactobacillus, Mobiluncus,* and *Propionibacterium.*

Table 15–1 outlines the body sites in which these organisms are commonly found.

Characteristics of Anaerobic Rods

General Features. Most of the current knowledge about the pathogenesis of infections caused by anaerobic rods is derived from studies of *B. fragilis.* This organism is a nonmotile rod that has rounded ends and is 0.5–0.8 μm wide by 1.5–9.0 μm long. *B. fragilis* has a capsule that is believed to contribute to its virulence, has many plasmids and bacteriophages, and can transmit antibiotic resistance via gene transfer. *B. fragilis* has the ability to deconjugate bile acids, and this allows it to grow in the presence of 20% bile.

P. melaninogenica derives its name from the fact that it produces a dark heme-like pigment. The organism is extremely fastidious in its growth require-

ments, and its growth is inhibited by bile acids. Several of the pigmented *Prevotella* and *Porphyromonas* species require vitamin K or hemin for growth. Unlike the *Porphyromonas* species, the *Prevotella* species are able to utilize carbohydrates as a sole source of carbon and energy. Unlike the *Bacteroides* species, the *Fusobacterium* species show susceptibility to kanamycin and are indole-positive.

Mechanisms of Pathogenicity. The capsule of *B. fragilis* inhibits phagocytosis by polymorphonuclear leukocytes, interferes with intraleukocytic killing, and causes phagocytic cells to secrete tumor necrosis factor alpha and three forms of interleukin (IL-1α, IL-8, and IL-10). *B. fragilis* has been reported to secrete an enterotoxin and to secrete succinic acid, a chemical that interferes with phagocytosis. Studies indicate that succinate produced by *B. fragilis* protects other bacteria in the vicinity from phagocytosis, and this may contribute to the propensity of *B. fragilis* to cause synergistic infections with *Escherichia coli.*

The lipopolysaccharide (LPS) of *B. fragilis* has no demonstrable endotoxic activity, but some investigators have reported that injection of *B. fragilis* LPS into tissues promotes abscess formation. In contrast, the LPS of *Fusobacterium* has endotoxic activity similar to that of the enteric bacteria. *Fusobacterium* produces a lipase and a leukocidal toxin.

The pathogenicity of *P. melaninogenica* may be potentiated by its phospholipase A activity. Phospholipase A releases arachidonic acid from cell membranes, and this substance can be converted to prostaglandins, leukotrienes, and thromboxanes.

Porphyromonas gingivalis, an agent of periodontitis, produces an extracellular protease that cleaves human complement C5. This contributes to inflammation of the periodontium by evoking neutrophil activity.

The rat model of intra-abdominal sepsis has been widely used to study the pathogenesis of *B. fragilis* infections. In this model, *B. fragilis* infections are biphasic. During the initial phase, *E. coli* establishes peritonitis, and this devitalizes tissue and reduces P_{O_2}. During the subsequent phase, *B. fragilis* multiplies in the peritoneum and establishes an anaerobic abscess. This model is believed to mirror the course of events in human infections and emphasizes the fact that antimicrobial therapy against anaerobic abscesses, especially those in the abdomen, must be effective against *E. coli* and anaerobes.

Diseases Due to Anaerobic Rods

Diagnosis. Gram-negative anaerobic rods cause abscesses and tissue destruction, particularly in patients who have undergone surgery, are being treated with aminoglycosides, are immunosuppressed, or have diabetes, leukopenia, cancer, or animal bites. The gram-negative anaerobic rods most commonly isolated from clinical specimens are *B. fragilis,* the pigmented *Prevotella* and *Porphyromonas* species, and *F. nucleatum.*

B. fragilis causes a wide variety of infections but

is especially associated with intra-abdominal abscesses and septicemias that originate in the abdomen. As described above, *B. fragilis* infections are generally biphasic synergistic infections that involve both *B. fragilis* and enteric bacilli such as *E. coli*. In women, *B. fragilis* also causes serious genital tract infections.

The pigmented *Prevotella* and *Porphyromonas* species are most commonly associated with dental infections and with other infections of the head, neck, and respiratory tract. They are also associated with pelvic and intra-abdominal infections and with a variety of soft tissue infections. Along with *Fusobacterium* species, *Prevotella* and *Porphyromonas* species are the most common causes of aspiration pneumonia, lung abscesses, necrotizing pneumonia, and empyema. *P. bivia* is often associated with obstetric infections but is also a cause of head and neck infections.

F. nucleatum is an important cause of aspiration pneumonia and lung abscesses and is also associated with oral infections, brain abscesses, chronic sinusitis, metastatic osteomyelitis, abdominal infections, and infections of the amniotic fluid. *F. necrophorum* is found primarily in the gastrointestinal tract and causes liver abscesses, abdominal infections, and periodontitis. Most *Fusobacterium* infections are mixed infections that also involve anaerobic cocci, *Bacteroides, Porphyromonas, Prevotella,* or members of the family Enterobacteriaceae.

Propionibacterium acnes is the gram-positive nonsporulating anaerobic rod most commonly isolated from clinical specimens. It is an occasional cause of endocarditis and central nervous system shunt infections, but it is best known as the principal agent of acne. *Propionibacterium propionicum* causes cervicofacial and pulmonary abscesses similar to those caused by actinomycetes. *Bifidobacterium eriksonii* causes polymicrobic lung infections. *Eubacterium* species sometimes cause periodontitis, and *Lactobacillus catenaforme* occasionally causes pleuropulmonary infections.

Mobiluncus has been implicated in the development of bacterial vaginosis, but the infection is probably mixed and also involves *Gardnerella vaginalis, Peptostreptococcus* species, and some *Bacteroides* species. Signs of bacterial vaginosis include an offensive vaginal discharge, high vaginal pH, and the presence of "clue cells" (squamous epithelial cells covered with gram-negative rods).

Treatment. For infections caused by strict anaerobes, the necrotic material should be excised, the abscesses should be drained, and antibiotics appropriate for the infecting anaerobes should be administered. In cases of abdominal abscesses, the antibiotics should be effective against both anaerobes and *E. coli*.

At one time, *B. fragilis* and *Bacteroides* in the DOT group were uniformly sensitive to penicillin G, and tetracyclines were also effective. Today, at least 50% of *B. fragilis* strains are resistant to tetracyclines, and many produce beta-lactamases. Aminoglycosides are not effective against anaerobes, because their transport is dependent on a strong proton motive force.

The drug of choice for treatment of *Bacteroides* infections is metronidazole or clindamycin. Alternatively, cefoxitin, imipenem, cefmetazole, cefotetan, or a combination of penicillin plus a beta-lactamase inhibitor can be given. For infections that involve *Bacteroides* and *E. coli,* an aminoglycoside should be added to the treatment regimen to eliminate the enteric organism.

Prevotella and *Porphyromonas* species are generally susceptible to a wide variety of antibiotics, including cefoperazone, cefotaxime, clindamycin, metronidazole, and the combination of ampicillin plus sulbactam.

Gram-positive nonsporulating anaerobic rods are sensitive to ampicillin and to penicillin G. They are generally not sensitive to metronidazole.

Anaerobic Cocci

Veillonella is the only genus of **gram-negative anaerobic cocci** isolated in cases of human disease. *Veillonella* species are found in the oral cavity and the female urogenital tract. They are reported to represent about 3% of anaerobic clinical isolates and are an occasional cause of dental and urogenital abscesses.

The most commonly isolated **gram-positive anaerobic cocci** are members of the genera *Peptostreptococcus, Streptococcus,* and *Gemella*. They are part of the indigenous flora of the mouth, genital tract, and gastrointestinal tract. Members of the genus *Peptostreptococcus* cause a wide variety of abscesses but are most often found as causes of wound infections, aspiration pneumonia, lung abscesses, brain abscesses, chronic otitis media, and obstetric and gynecologic infections.

Anaerobic cocci are sensitive to penicillin G and to clindamycin.

Selected Readings

Botta, G. A., et al. Role of structural and extracellular virulence factors in gram-negative anaerobic bacteremia. Clin Infect Dis 18(supplement 4):S260–S264, 1994.

Brook, I. Fusobacterial infections in children. J Infect 28:155–165, 1994.

Brook, I., and P. Burke. The management of acute, serous, and chronic otitis media: the role of anaerobic bacteria. J Hosp Infect 22(supplement A):75–87, 1992.

Discipio, R. G., et al. Cleavage of human complement component C5 by cysteine proteases from *Porphyromonas (Bacteroides) gingivalis:* prior oxidation of C5 augments proteinase digestion of C5. Immunology 87:660–667, 1996.

Gibson, F. C., III, et al. The capsular polysaccharide complex of *Bacteroides fragilis* induces cytokine production from human and murine phagocytic cells. Infect Immun 64:1065–1069, 1996.

Holt, S. C., and T. E. Bramanti. Factors in virulence expression and their role in periodontal disease pathogenesis. Crit Rev Oral Biol Med 2:177–281, 1991.

Makristathis, A., et al. Induction and release of prostaglandin E$_2$ from polymorphonuclear neutrophil granulocytes by *Bacteroides fragilis:* its possible role in the pathogenesis of mixed infections. Int J Med Microbiol Virol Parasitol Infect Dis 279:505–511, 1993.

Peterson, L. J. Contemporary management of deep infections of the neck. J Oral Maxillofac Surg 51:226–231, 1993.

Salyers, A. A., and N. B. Shoemaker. Chromosomal gene transfer elements of the *Bacteroides* group. Eur J Clin Microbiol Infect Dis 11:1032–1038, 1992.

Sobel, J. D. Bacterial vaginosis. Br J Clin Pract Symp Suppl 71:65–69, 1990.

SECTION II

FUNGI AND

FUNGAL DISEASES

OVERVIEW OF MYCOLOGY

AND ANTIFUNGAL AGENTS

Fungal diseases in humans can be divided into four groups: superficial mycoses, cutaneous mycoses, subcutaneous mycoses, and deep (systemic) mycoses. Chapter 17 discusses the first three groups, while Chapter 18 discusses the fourth group of diseases. This chapter provides introductory information on the classification, structure, reproduction, metabolism, and laboratory identification of fungal organisms and reviews the types of antifungal agents available for the treatment of mycoses.

CLASSIFICATION AND STRUCTURE OF FUNGI
Classification as Eukaryotes

Unlike bacteria, which are prokaryotes, fungi and human cells are eukaryotes. Bacteria are single-celled organisms that do not have membrane-bound organelles and have cellular structures quite different from those of human cells. Thus, it is possible to design antibacterial strategies that target the key differences between bacteria and human cells. In contrast, fungi hold much in common with human cells. Each fungus has a Golgi apparatus, mitochondria, ribosomes, endoplasmic reticula, and a cell membrane, making it difficult to develop antibiotics that are selectively toxic for fungi. Fungi do differ, however, in several respects from human cells. Two important differences involve the constituents of the cell membrane and the cell wall of fungi.

The fungal **cell membrane** contains unusual steroids. Human cell membranes contain cholesterol, but the cell membranes of fungi contain **ergosterol** and **zymosterol.**

The fungal **cell wall** is composed of cross-linked polysaccharides, proteins, and glycoproteins, and it provides the fungus with osmotic stability and rigidity. Some fungal walls have also been reported to mediate attachment to host cells by containing **adhesins** that bind to host cell receptors. The **polysaccharides,** which make up about 80% of the cell wall, are polymers of simple sugars and include **chitin,** consisting of N-acetylglucosamines linked by $\beta1,4$ bonds; **glucan,** consisting of glucoses linked by $\beta1,6$ bonds, with occasional $\beta1,3$ branches; and **mannan,** consisting of mannoses linked by $\alpha1,6$ bonds, with occasional $\alpha1,2$ and $\alpha1,3$ branches. **Cellulose** and **chitosan,** two other polysaccharides, make the fungal

wall resistant to the degradative effects of acids and alkalies. Thus, when technicians look for fungi in tissue or sputum samples, they routinely "clear" the samples with potassium hydroxide (KOH). This process digests tissues and bacteria, but it does not damage the fungi.

Classification by Morphologic Characteristics

Some fungi arrange themselves into multiple-cell structures called molds and mushrooms; other fungi grow as single cells called yeasts; and still other fungi are thermally dimorphic, growing as a mold at 25 °C (room temperature) and as a yeast at 37 °C.

Molds

A mold is a mat of filamentous fungal cells. An individual fungal filament is called a **hypha,** and the mass of intertwined hyphae (the Greek word *hyphe* means "web") is called a **mycelium.** The hyphal mass gives the mold its fuzzy appearance. Each hypha is a rectangular or tube-shaped cell.

The hyphae of some fungi have numerous cross-walls, or **septa,** which separate the individual cells. The cross-walls of these **septate hyphae** are not absolute barriers; rather, each septum has holes that allow protoplasm and cellular organelles to stream between adjacent hyphae. Thus, septate hyphae are said to be coenocytic. In fungi with **aseptate hyphae,** each hypha is a long tube that contains many nuclei. Septate and aseptate hyphae are compared in Fig. 16–1.

Hyphae grow apically (at their tips) and can be classified as either vegetative or aerial. **Vegetative hyphae** (Fig. 16–2) make up the bulk of the mycelium and are merely long tubes whose individual cells are absorbing nutrients and reproducing asexually. **Aerial hyphae** are specialized hyphae that are pedestals for fungal spores. They are called aerial hyphae because they so often extend upward from the mycelium.

Yeasts

Yeasts are oval or spherical cells that are usually about 5 μm in diameter and look somewhat like bacte-

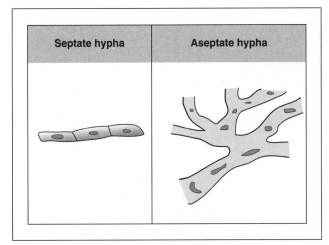

FIGURE 16–1. A comparison of the typical appearance of a septate hypha and an aseptate hypha.

rial cocci. Most medically important bacteria multiply by transverse binary fission. Although a few yeasts also multiply this way, most reproduce by **budding.** As shown in Fig. 16–3, this process leaves the daughter cell with a convex **birth scar** and leaves the mother cell with a concave **budding scar.** Although each yeast cell has a single birth scar, it may have many budding scars.

Some yeasts form an elongated bud called a **germ tube.** When a series of germ tubes are lined up end to end, they look like a hypha. However, these structures are not true hyphae, because there are no interconnecting cytoplasmic bridges between individual cells. For this reason, the structures are referred to as **pseudohyphae** (see Fig. 16–2).

Classification by Types of Reproduction and Spores

Fungi can reproduce asexually, sexually, parasexually, or by more than one of these methods. Dur-

ing reproduction, all fungi generate specialized reproductive structures called **spores** or **conidia** (from the Greek *konis,* meaning "dust"). Mycologists depend heavily upon recognition of characteristic **sexual and asexual spores** both to classify fungi and to identify fungi isolated from clinical samples. Based on the types and characteristics of spores produced by fungi (Table 16–1), the organisms can be divided into four classes: Ascomycetes, Basidiomycetes, Deuteromycetes, and Zygomycetes.

The **sexual form** of a fungus is often called its **perfect state,** and the **asexual form** is the **imperfect state.** Since they have no sexual state, fungi in the Deuteromycetes class are often referred to as the **imperfect fungi (Fungi Imperfecti).** Most of the fungi that cause human diseases are imperfect fungi. For example, members of the three genera *Epidermophyton, Microsporum,* and *Trichophyton*—a group of organisms that cause skin disease and are called **dermatophytes**—are imperfect fungi.

The nomenclature of mycology is difficult to fathom for most people outside the field. Because the asexual and sexual forms of many fungi were discovered independently, these forms received separate names. For example, the organism that is called *Malassezia furfur* in its asexual form is called *Pityrosporum orbiculare* in its sexual form. The fact that two names are assigned may seem odd, but mycologists are quick to point out that some sexual forms are produced by more than one fungal species, and these cannot be distinguished on the basis of morphology. Thus, fungi other than those in the Deuteromycetes class have two names, and it is necessary to know both names.

REPRODUCTION OF FUNGI
Asexual Reproduction

While some fungi reproduce by more than one means, all fungi reproduce asexually via processes that involve mitosis and cytokinesis, and all fungi

FIGURE 16–2. A comparison of true hyphae and pseudohyphae. True hyphae, which are formed by molds, are coenocytic tubes that may occur as vegetative or aerial hyphae. Pseudohyphae, which are formed by some yeasts, are elongated yeasts and contain no intercellular cytoplasmic bridges.

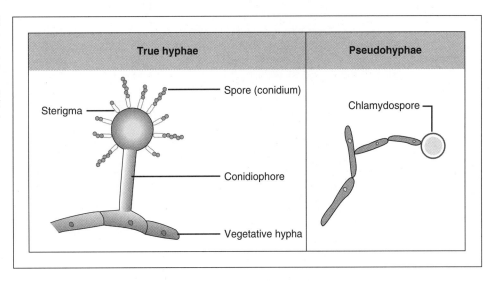

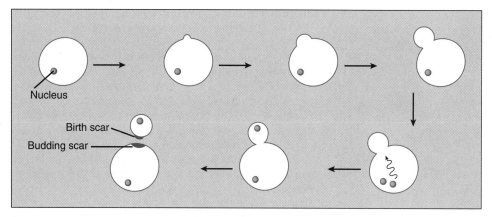

FIGURE 16–3. Formation of a bud by a typical yeast. Budding begins when a restricted autolytic process damages a section of the yeast wall. A portion of cell membrane bulges out through the damaged wall to form a small bud; the nucleus of the mother cell divides; and one copy of the nucleus is segregated into the bud. The bud wall is synthesized, and the bud breaks away from the mother cell. The daughter cell has a convex birth scar, and the mother cell is left with a concave budding scar. Thus, each yeast has a single birth scar but may have many budding scars.

form conidia, or spores. These spores should not be confused with the dormant, environmentally resistant endospores of bacteria.

In fungi, **asexual spores** can arise by two methods. Some spores are formed by altering the structure of a hyphal segment. Because they arise from the body of the fungus, they are said to be **thallic conidia** (from the Greek *thallos,* meaning "a green twig or shoot"). Other spores arise from only a portion of the hypha and are referred to as **blastic conidia** (from the Greek *blastos,* meaning "a bud"). Aleuriospores, arthrospores, and chlamydospores are examples of thallic conidia (Fig. 16–4A), while blastospores, conidiospores, and sporangiospores are examples of blastic conidia (Fig. 16–4B). These represent the asexual spores most often used to identify medically important fungi.

Aleuriospores are also called microconidia and macroconidia. Some occur singly or in groups on short lateral branches from the hyphae, and others occur directly on the hyphae. They may be large (macroaleuriospores) or the size of a yeast cell (microaleuriospores). The dermatophytes are identified largely by the aleuriospores they form when cultured on agar.

Arthrospores arise when hyphae form double septa. The spores are released when the fungal hypha breaks apart, and they can be highly infectious. An important arthrospore-forming fungus is *Coccidioides immitis,* the agent of San Joaquin Valley fever.

Chlamydospores are thick-walled spores that form at the end of hyphae or between hyphal segments. They are uniquely resistant to heat and to drying. *Candida albicans,* which causes candidiasis (thrush), forms chlamydospores.

Blastospores are formed by yeasts during budding, a process discussed above and depicted in Fig. 16–3. Blastospores can be formed by spherical yeasts and by elongated pseudohyphae. Two important fungi that form blastospores are *Candida* and *Blastomyces.*

Conidiospores occur singly or in groups at the ends of specialized structures called **conidiophores** (see Fig. 16–2). The fact that conidiospores are often referred to only as conidia sometimes causes confusion, because the term "conidia" is used by many to refer to all fungal spores. *Aspergillus* and *Penicillium* are two medically important fungi that reproduce via conidiospores.

Sporangiospores form within saclike structures known as **sporangia** and are found at the end of specialized hyphae called **sporangiophores.** Fungi of the Zygomycetes class form sporangiospores.

Sexual Reproduction

Most medically important fungi are in the Deuteromycetes class and have no sexual reproductive cycle. However, several of the pathogenic yeasts are in the Ascomycetes class, and the molds that cause

---

TABLE 16–1. Characteristics of the Four Classes of Fungi

Class	Sexual Spores	Asexual Spores*	Hyphae	Examples
Ascomycetes	Ascospores in sacs (asci).	Exogenous.	Septate.	*Aspergillus, Penicillium,* morels, puffballs, true yeasts, and truffles.
Basidiomycetes	Basidiospores on the surface of the basidium.	Exogenous.	Septate.	Mushrooms, rusts, and smuts.
Deuteromycetes (Fungi Imperfecti)	None.	Exogenous.	Septate.	Most human pathogens.
Zygomycetes	Variable.	Endogenous.	Aseptate.	*Mucor* and *Rhizopus.*

*Exogenous spores form at ends or sides of hyphae. Endogenous spores form in sacs.

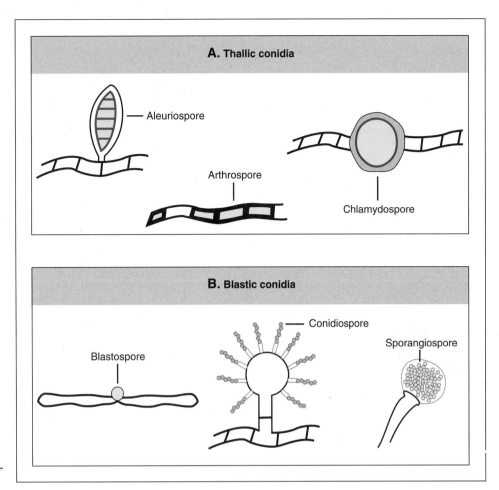

FIGURE 16–4. Examples of asexual spores formed by fungi.

opportunistic infections in diabetics are in the Zygomycetes class.

Fungal sexual reproduction has been most completely studied in *Neurospora,* a genus in the Ascomycetes class. *Neurospora* forms **ascospores,** which are packaged within a small sac known as an **ascus** (Fig. 16–5). Hundreds of asci are located within a larger sac called a **cleistothecium.** Sexual reproduction is initiated when the haploid nucleus of a donor cell enters the cytoplasm of a recipient cell. The nuclei of the donor and recipient cells then fuse to form a diploid zygotic nucleus. The cell undergoes meiosis to yield four haploid ascospores, which subsequently undergo mitosis to yield the eight ascospores packaged within each ascus.

Some of the other fungi have distinct sex organs and gametes, and these forms are used to classify them.

Parasexual Reproduction

A few fungi produce progeny of mixed inheritance, using an unusual reproductive cycle called parasexual reproduction. This process, which is also called **mitotic recombination** and is somewhat reminiscent of bacterial recombination processes, is depicted in Fig. 16–6. The process involves no discrete mating types. Instead, two adjacent hyphae fuse to

form a single hyphal segment with two nuclei. In most cases, the two nuclei coexist stably as a **heterokaryon.** On rare occasions, the nuclei fuse to form a single diploid nucleus. The chromosomes in most diploid nuclei remain segregated, but rarely (once in every 10,000 mitoses) a single crossover event occurs

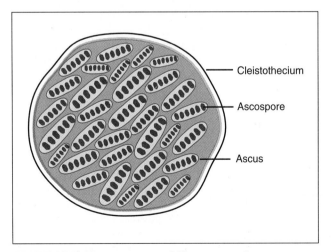

FIGURE 16–5. The ascospores of *Neurospora.* Ascospores are enclosed within a small sac called an ascus, and many asci are contained within a larger sac called a cleistothecium.

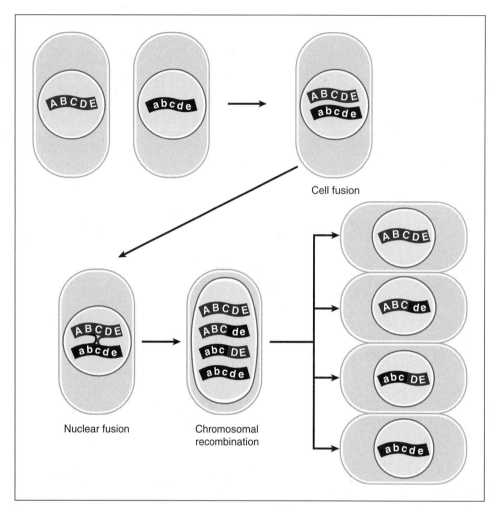

Cell fusion

Nuclear fusion

Chromosomal
recombination

FIGURE 16–6. Parasexual reproduction (mitotic recombination). The process shown involves the following steps: (1) cell fusion to form a heterokaryon, (2) nuclear fusion, (3) and chromosomal recombination. The mitotic progeny have recombined nuclei.

between chromosomes during mitosis, and chromosomes with partially mixed inheritance are generated. Later, when the nuclei yield haploid progeny, half will contain recombined chromosomes.

METABOLISM, CULTURE, AND IDENTIFICATION OF FUNGI

Fungi are aerobes and facultative anaerobes, but there are no strictly anaerobic fungi. Some fungi have simple nutritional requirements and are capable of multiplying in cold temperatures (for example, in a kitchen refrigerator). Most of the medically important fungi are fastidious, however, and require special media for their isolation.

Culture Media

Dermatophytes and environmental fungi are the least fastidious of the medically important fungi and can be cultivated on Sabouraud's dextrose agar. For many years, this was the medium of choice for all medically important fungi. Now, however, media that allow better selective culture of the more fastidious fungi are available. These media may contain serum and other growth factors, and antibiotics are added

to ensure that the slow-growing fungi are not overgrown by bacteria. Bacterial overgrowth can be a problem, because weeks are needed to obtain a culture of some of the fungi. Three important selective fungal media are inhibitory mold agar, Sabhi agar, and brain-heart infusion agar containing antibiotics.

Yeasts and molds can be cultivated on media that contain a series of carbohydrate-impregnated disks. This carbohydrate assimilation test determines carbohydrate requirements of fungi by identifying fungal growth around the individual disks.

True yeasts are identified using special media to produce chlamydospores and germ tubes.

Culture, Staining, and Other Laboratory Techniques

If cultures are performed, the sample should be cultured at both 25 °C and 37 °C to determine if the fungus is thermally dimorphic, and the rate at which the fungus grows should be noted. The undersides of plates that grow molds should be examined for characteristic coloration and for growth patterns. A portion of the mold should be teased out of the mycelium with a needle, placed on a slide, stained, and examined for the presence of septate or aseptate hyphae and reproductive structures. Teased samples of mycelia are generally stained with lactophenol aniline blue ("cotton" blue) stain or with calcofluor white reagent.

Mold samples can also be cultivated directly on slides, a technique that produces beautifully preserved mycelia.

After yeasts are cultured, they should be examined microscopically for their morphology, including the types and numbers of buds formed.

Clinical samples can be examined directly for the presence of some fungi. Except in the case of thrush, which is caused by *Candida albicans,* Gram's stain preparations are not helpful in identifying fungi in these samples. Instead, clinical samples are digested with potassium hydroxide (KOH) or *N*-acetyl-L-cystine to remove extraneous material, and the samples are stained. Biopsy samples are generally stained with Grocott-Gomori methenamine–silver nitrate stain or periodic acid–Schiff stain. Cerebrospinal fluid samples suspected of containing the encapsulated yeast *Cryptococcus neoformans* can be stained with India ink or nigrosin.

ANTIFUNGAL AGENTS

Various types of agents used in the treatment of fungal infections are discussed below. The problems of developing selectively toxic antifungal antibiotics have been partially solved by looking for agents that bind to or inhibit the synthesis of unique components of the cell membranes and walls of fungi. Thus, most effective antifungal agents bind to or inhibit the synthesis of ergosterol. A few antifungal agents inhibit mitosis, synthesis of glucan and mannan, or fungal protein synthesis. Yet many antibiotics that kill fungi are toxic for human cells when used systemically at high concentrations, a factor that makes treating systemic fungal diseases a difficult task.

Polyene Antibiotics

Amphotericin B and nystatin (Fig. 16–7) are polyene antibiotics. These fungistatic agents are selectively toxic for fungi because they preferentially bind to ergosterol, a steroid found only in fungal membranes. The binding of these antibiotics to the fungal membrane disorganizes the bilayer, and metabolites leak into the environment from the fungal cytoplasm. Although their greatest affinity is for ergosterol, polyenes will also bind to cholesterol in human cell membranes. For this reason, amphotericin B is toxic when used intravenously, and high-dose therapy may permanently damage the renal basement membrane. This is not a problem with nystatin, because it is not administered intravenously.

Because of its propensity to cause renal damage, amphotericin B is often called "amphiterrible." Until the azole antibiotics were developed, amphotericin B was the only antibiotic effective in the treatment of systemic fungal infections, and it remains the drug of choice in treating systemic forms of aspergillosis, blastomycosis, candidiasis, coccidioidomycosis, cryptococcosis, histoplasmosis, mucormycosis, and sporotrichosis. In some cases, amphotericin B is administered with flucytosine, a nucleic acid analogue.

Nystatin is used topically to treat cutaneous and mucocutaneous *Candida* infections. It is sometimes given orally to treat gastrointestinal candidiasis. The drug is not absorbed in the gut.

Azole Antibiotics

Two groups of azole antibiotics have been developed: the imidazoles and the bistriazoles. Both groups are fungistatic. Azoles inhibit the synthesis of ergosterol, the essential fungal membrane steroid, by inhibiting the activity of a cytochrome P-450 enzyme called lanosterol-14-demethylase. With less ergosterol available, the permeability properties of the fungal cell membrane are altered, and growth of the susceptible fungus is inhibited.

The imidazole antibiotics include ketoconazole (Fig. 16–8), butoconazole, clotrimazole, econazole, miconazole, oxiconazole, sulconazole, and tioconazole. Imidazoles are used topically to treat dermatophyte infections, and some are used systemically to treat deep fungal infections. Ketoconazole is recommended in the treatment of chronic mucocutaneous candidiasis and is a second choice in the treatment of a wide variety of deep fungal infections.

The bistriazole antibiotics include fluconazole (see Fig. 16–8), itraconazole, and terconazole. Because fluconazole and itraconazole have a high affinity for lanosterol-14-demethylase, they have proved to be less toxic than other azoles when administered intravenously. They are used to treat candidiasis in immunocompromised patients, chromoblastomycosis, paracoccidioidomycosis, and cutaneous and lymphatic sporotrichosis.

Nucleoside Analogues

Flucytosine (Fig. 16–9) is the only nucleoside analogue currently used in treating fungal diseases. It is converted by susceptible fungi to fluorouracil and fluorodeoxyuridine monophosphate, and these agents inhibit protein synthesis when incorporated into fungal RNA. Flucytosine is used alone to treat *Candida* infections of the urinary tract, and it is administered in combination with amphotericin B to treat systemic candidiasis or cryptococcosis. Unfortunately, up to 15% of isolates of fungi rapidly become resistant to flucytosine when it is administered alone. Flucytosine is toxic, and some patients become dangerously leukopenic or thrombocytopenic.

Allylamine Antibiotics

The allylamines are relatively new antibiotics and include naftifine and terbinafine. They are used topically to treat dermatophyte infections, such as ringworm and athlete's foot. The allylamines are fungicidal, and their activity is due to allosteric inhibition of squalene epoxidase, which leads to accumulation

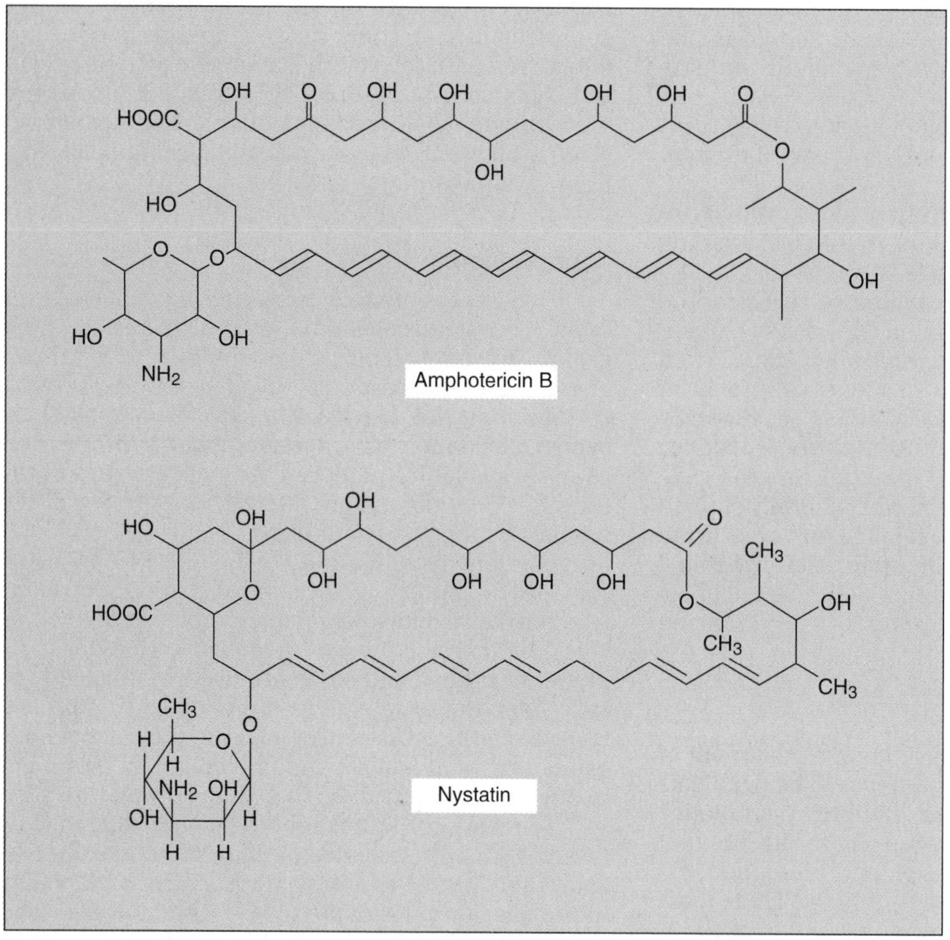

FIGURE 16–7. Structures of amphotericin B and nystatin, two polyene antibiotics.

FIGURE 16–8. Structures of ketoconazole, an imidazole antibiotic, and fluconazole, a bistriazole antibiotic.

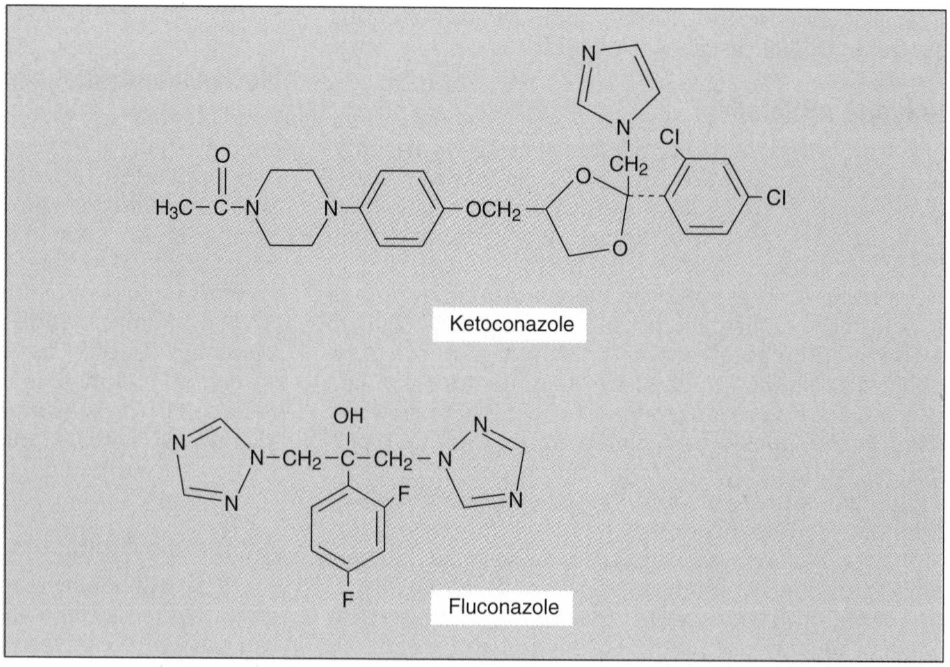

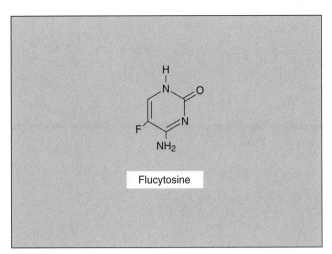

FIGURE 16–9. Structure of flucytosine, an antifungal antibiotic.

of toxic quantities of squalene and inhibition of the synthesis of ergosterol.

Griseofulvin

Griseofulvin is a fungistatic antibiotic that is produced by *Penicillium* species and is used in the treatment of dermatophyte infections that do not respond to topical antibiotics. It is unusual in that it is administered orally to eradicate infections that are in the stratum corneum. This is possible because griseofulvin accumulates in sweat, and when the sweat evaporates, it leaves griseofulvin in the keratinized layer of the epidermis.

Griseofulvin acts as a colchicine-like agent, inhibiting fungal mitosis and causing the affected fungi to assume odd shapes. Both of these effects are believed to result from the ability of griseofulvin to interfere with microtubule assembly. In some fungi, griseoful-

vin has also been shown to interfere with the synthesis of glucan and chitin, which are polysaccharides in the walls of the organisms.

Although effective against dermatophytes, griseofulvin is not effective for the treatment of tinea versicolor or tinea nigra. Griseofulvin is well tolerated, and headache is the most commonly reported adverse reaction.

Other Antifungal Agents

Among the other agents available for topical use are the following: ciclopirox olamine, which inhibits fungal transport; tolnaftate, which inhibits squalene epoxidation and lipid biosynthesis; and haloprogin, undecylenic acid, selenium sulfide, and clioquinol, which have mechanisms of action that are not well understood. These antifungal agents are used primarily to treat dermatophyte infections, although some are also used in the treatment of tinea versicolor.

Selected Readings

Fromtling, R. A. Fungi. *In* Balows, A., et al., eds. Manual of Clinical Microbiology, 5th ed. Washington, D. C., American Society for Microbiology, 1991.

Haria, M., et al. Itraconazole: a reappraisal of its pharmacological properties and therapeutic use in the management of superficial fungal infections. Drugs 51:585–620, 1996.

Haynes, M. P., et al. Fluorescence studies on the molecular action of amphotericin B on susceptible and resistant fungal cells. Biochemistry 35:7983–7992, 1996.

Koneman, E. W., et al. Mycology. *In* Koneman, E. W., et al., eds. Diagnostic Microbiology, 4th ed. Philadelphia, J. B. Lippincott Company, 1992.

Larone, D. H. Medically Important Fungi: A Guide to Identification, 2nd ed. Washington, D. C., American Society for Microbiology, 1993.

Rashid, A. New mechanisms of action with fungicidal antifungals. Br J Dermatol 134(supplement 46):1–6, 1996.

Rippon, J. W. Medical Mycology: The Pathogenic Fungi and the Pathogenic Actinomycetes, 3rd ed. Philadelphia, W. B. Saunders Company, 1988.

CHAPTER SEVENTEEN

FUNGI THAT CAUSE SUPERFICIAL, CUTANEOUS, AND SUBCUTANEOUS MYCOSES

Basidiobolus, Cladosporium, Conidiobolus, Epidermophyton, Fonsecaea, Loboa, Malassezia, Microsporum, Phaeoannellomyces, Phialophora, Piedraia, Rhinocladiella, Rhinosporidium, Sporothrix, Trichophyton, and *Trichosporon*

THE SUPERFICIAL AND CUTANEOUS MYCOSES

Tinea versicolor, tinea nigra, black piedra, and white piedra are examples of superficial mycoses, while the various dermatophytoses discussed below are examples of cutaneous mycoses.

Tinea Versicolor and *Malassezia furfur*

Tinea versicolor is a fairly common fungal infection of the skin and is caused by *Malassezia furfur*. The infection, which is also called **pityriasis versicolor,** is marked by the appearance of brownish-yellow scaling lesions. The term "versicolor" refers to the tendency of the lesions to vary somewhat in their color. The term "tinea," used to describe many of the fungal skin infections, comes from the Romans, who believed that the red ring of "ringworm" infections was, in fact, a worm lying under the skin (the Latin word *tinea* means "worm"). Today, clinicians know that this ring is merely an advancing area of inflammation and that all "ringworms" are fungal infections.

Characteristics of *M. furfur*

M. furfur is the asexual form of a lipid-loving fungus whose sexual form is known as *Pityrosporum orbiculare.* The organism is a commensal of the skin, and it spreads and initiates the lesions of tinea versicolor when the skin is not washed for a prolonged time. The characteristic changes in skin pigmentation may be due to oxidation of fatty acids to dicarboxylic acids. The latter acids act as competitive inhibitors of tyrosinase. On rare occasions, *M. furfur* has been the cause of systemic infections in patients who have deep-line vascular catheters and are receiving intravenous therapy with oil-rich emulsions. The organisms multiply at the site of entry and then deposit in the lungs, where they cause bronchopneumonia.

M. furfur can be cultivated on Sabouraud's dextrose agar that has been overlaid with olive oil. The cultures must be incubated at 30 °C because the organism will not grow at 25 °C. *M. furfur* grows as bottle-shaped yeasts with broad-based buds.

Management of Tinea Versicolor

Diagnosis. Tinea versicolor is characterized by oval or round patches of scaling skin that can be either hypopigmented or hyperpigmented. The patches are often brownish-yellow, but the color varies with the patient's skin color. The lesions are most often on the trunk, and they sometimes burn and itch. There is little if any inflammation, and many patients are unaware of the infection until they tan unevenly. If the lesions are due to *M. furfur*, they will have a characteristic yellowish fluorescence when they are examined under a Wood's lamp. Rarely, patients develop a more severe dermatosis, forming pustules that contain *M. furfur*. A second organism, *Malassezia ovalis,* may also be found in these lesions, but it is uncertain if *M. ovalis* is a pathogen.

Laboratory confirmation of tinea versicolor is based on culturing *M. furfur* on Sabouraud's dextrose agar and directly observing the organism in skin scrapings that are digested with 10% potassium hydroxide (KOH). A collection of blastospores and hyphae will be seen in the scrapings and will look like spaghetti and meatballs (Fig. 17–1). In some cases, the skin can be lifted off the lesion as a single sheet, and the organisms will be seen in the most superficial layer of the skin.

Treatment. Treatment with ketoconazole has been reported to be effective in about 95% of cases. Alternative treatments include creams or lotions containing selenium sulfide, ciclopirox olamine, miconazole, tolnaftate, econazole, or sulconazole. Griseofulvin is ineffective.

Tinea Nigra and *Phaeoannellomyces werneckii*

Tinea nigra is a fungal infection of the skin and is caused by *Phaeoannellomyces werneckii,* an organism that has also been called *Cladosporium werneckii* and *Exophiala werneckii.* Tinea nigra was first described in Bahia, a Brazilian port city, and is now known to occur in other parts of South America and in the Caribbean islands. Vacationers from the USA sometimes return from their island paradise only to discover that they brought this infection home as an unexpected memento.

Tinea nigra begins as a single flat brown macule. The lesion slowly spreads centrifugally (outward) and darkens. Most lesions are on the palms or fingers, but they occasionally occur on the neck, plantar surface, or thorax. The lesions are not painful and do not itch. Their greatest significance lies in the fact that they are often misdiagnosed as melanomas.

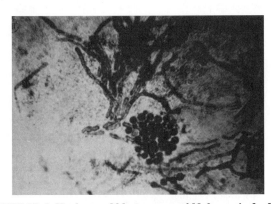

FIGURE 17–1. Hyphae and blastospores of *Malassezia furfur* in skin scrapings from a patient with tinea versicolor. (Reproduced, with permission, from Rippon, J. W. Medical Mycology: The Pathogenic Fungi and the Pathogenic Actinomycetes, 3rd ed. Philadelphia, W. B. Saunders Company, 1988.)

Laboratory diagnosis of tinea nigra is made by examining a KOH-hydrolyzed skin scraping. The stratum corneum will contain a mixture of hyphae and yeastlike cells, similar to that seen in tinea versicolor. The hyphae of *P. werneckii,* however, have a distinct twisted and pigmented appearance.

Tinea nigra is treated effectively with tincture of iodine or with a cream that contains 2% salicylic acid or 3% sulfur. Griseofulvin is ineffective.

Black Piedra and *Piedraia hortae*

The piedras are fungal infections of the hair shaft. Black piedra occurs commonly in tropical South America, Asia, and the Pacific islands and is caused by *Piedraia hortae.* This fungus is found in the soil and on plants and often grows as hard masses on trees.

Black piedra is characterized by the formation of hard black nodules on the outside of the hair shaft. In some geographic regions, the nodules of black piedra are considered to be attractive, so individuals who wish to become infected will forgo oiling their hair (which they normally do to control head lice) and will sleep with their head in a depression in the dirt. This exposes their scalp hair and beards to infection with the fungi that grow in the soil.

The nodules of black piedra must be distinguished from the eggs (nits) of head lice. When KOH-digested hair samples are examined, black piedra can be diagnosed by finding branching hyphae and asci outside the hair shaft.

Black piedra is treated by cutting or shaving the hair or beard.

White Piedra and *Trichosporon beigelii*

White piedra is a fungal infection of the hair and is caused by *Trichosporon beigelii.* It is most commonly found in temperate and subtropical regions in Asia and South America, but it also occurs in the USA and Europe. It is not known how the infection is acquired by humans, but some cases have been associated with swimming in stagnant water.

White piedra occurs most often on the beard and in the hair of the axillas and groin. Patients develop white to light brown soft fungal masses on the hair, and the fungi often grow into the hair shaft. Unlike the nodules of black piedra, the nodules of white piedra can be easily stripped from the hair.

Laboratory confirmation of white piedra involves examination of KOH-digested samples of the affected hair.

White piedra is treated by cutting or shaving the hair.

Dermatophytoses and the Dermatophytes

The fungi that cause superficial mycoses, or dermatophytoses, are called dermatophytes. The dermatophytes are a group of 40 fungal species that fall into three genera: *Trichophyton, Microsporum,* and *Epidermophyton.* These fungi were discovered and described as the causes of "ringworm" infections 40 years before Koch used anthrax to develop his postulates.

The ancient Greeks noticed that common skin lesions tended to spread slowly, so they called the infections *herpes* (from *herpō*, meaning "to creep") and attached the name of the site to each infection. For example, they used the name herpes tonsurans to designate lesions of the scalp. The Romans believed the infections were due to insect larvae or worms, so they called the infections *tineas* (meaning "worms"). In the 20th century, ringworm infections began to be called dermatophytoses and were commonly designated by names that combined the Roman and Greek systems. For example, herpes tonsurans became tinea tonsurans. Today, tinea tonsurans is more commonly referred to as tinea capitis. Some of the designations for various forms of dermatophyte infections are listed in Table 17–1.

Characteristics of the Dermatophytes

Although there are about 40 species of dermatophytes, 7 species cause about 90% of the cases of dermatophyte infection seen in the USA. Some urban health clinics have reported that as much as 5% of their caseload involves dermatophyte infections.

General Features.   *Trichophyton, Microsporum,* and *Epidermophyton* are not thermally dimorphic. They always grow as molds. They are identified primarily by the types of macro- and microconidia (also called macro- and microaleuriospores) that they form when cultured on Sabouraud's dextrose agar or mycosel agar.

(1) *Trichophyton.*   When grown on Sabouraud's dextrose agar, cultures of *Trichophyton* exhibit septate hyphae, many microconidia, and a few long,

TABLE 17–1. Usual Site of Infection and Causative Organisms in Various Common Dermatophytoses

Dermatophytosis	Usual Site of Infection	Organisms Most Frequently Isolated in the USA
Favus	Scalp.	*Trichophyton schoenleinii* and *Trichophyton violaceum.*
Tinea barbae	Beard.	*Trichophyton mentagrophytes* and *Trichophyton verrucosum.*
Tinea capitis	Scalp.	*Microsporum audouinii, Microsporum canis,* and *Trichophyton tonsurans.*
Tinea corporis	Trunk.	*T. mentagrophytes* and *Trichophyton rubrum.*
Tinea cruris	Groin.	*Epidermophyton floccosum, T. rubrum,* and *T. mentagrophytes.*
Tinea manus	Hands and fingers.	*T. mentagrophytes, T. rubrum,* and *E. floccosum.*
Tinea pedis	Feet.	*E. floccosum, T. mentagrophytes,* and *T. rubrum.*
Tinea unguium	Nails.	*T. mentagrophytes, T. rubrum,* and *E. floccosum.*

thin macroconidia (Fig. 17–2A). The appearance of the underside of the fungal mass on agar is helpful in identifying some species. For example, *Trichophyton rubrum* is named for the fact that it forms reddish colonies (hence, "rubrum") on cornmeal agar. *Trichophyton schoenleinii,* which causes a scalp infection called favus, can be identified by its unusual pectinate (comb-shaped) hyphae, which look much like the antlers of a reindeer.

Of the more common *Trichophyton* species, *T. rubrum, Trichophyton mentagrophytes,* and *Trichophyton tonsurans* cause infection of nails (onychomycosis), but *Trichophyton verrucosum* does not. *T.*

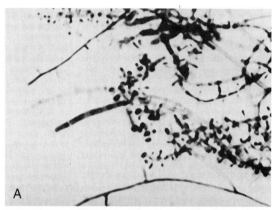
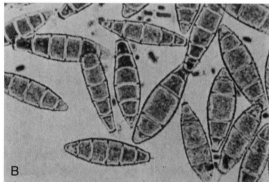
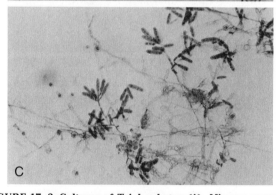

FIGURE 17–2. Cultures of *Trichophyton* (A), *Microsporum* (B), and *Epidermophyton* (C), showing the typical conidia (aleuriospores) of each genus. *Trichophyton* produces many microconidia and few macroconidia; *Microsporum* produces many macroconidia and few microconidia; and *Epidermophyton* produces only macroconidia. (Reproduced, with permission, from Rippon, J. W. Medical Mycology: The Pathogenic Fungi and the Pathogenic Actinomycetes, 3rd ed. Philadelphia, W. B. Saunders Company, 1988.)

rubrum is unusual in that it does not infect hairs. The other *Trichophyton* species do infect hairs, but they vary in their abilities to invade the hair shaft. Some exhibit **endothrix growth,** or growth inside hair shafts, while others exhibit only **ectothrix growth,** remaining on the outside of hair shafts.

(2) *Microsporum.* The *Microsporum* species grow as septate hyphae with many large, rough macroconidia and a few microconidia (Fig. 17–2B). Although they do not infect nails, they do infect the outside of the hair. Species include *Microsporum audouinii, Microsporum canis,* and *Microsporum gypseum.*

(3) *Epidermophyton.* There is only one clinically significant species of *Epidermophyton*—namely, *Epidermophyton floccosum.* This septate mold infects the nails but does not infect the hair. It has no microconidia and forms banana-shaped clusters of large, smooth macroconidia (Fig. 17–2C).

Mechanisms of Pathogenicity. Dermatophyte infections follow a two-phase process that has two possible outcomes. During the **invasion phase,** the patient is inoculated with spores, and the fungi grow without impediment because there is not yet an effective immune response. During the **immune phase,** when the patient develops a cell-mediated immune response to the fungus, the lesion becomes inflamed. After these phases, some patients recover and their lesions heal, while other patients suffer from chronic infection.

Inoculation with spores can be via contact with soil, animals, people, or fomites. *M. gypseum* is a geophilic fungus that is acquired from the soil. *M. canis, T. verrucosum,* and *T. mentagrophytes* are zoophilic dermatophytes that can be acquired through contact with animals. For example, *M. canis* infections are usually acquired via contact with an infected kitten, and *T. verrucosum* infections are acquired from cattle. The other fungi are acquired through contact with infected people or with the objects or surfaces that infected people have recently touched (clothing, the floors of shower stalls, and so forth). People who are often exposed to moisture, who have large skin folds (due to obesity), or who are constantly exposed to heavily infected environments may become repeatedly infected with dermatophytes. Individuals who use topical corticosteroids for prolonged periods of time are also at high risk of developing dermatophytoses.

Because the dermatophytes metabolize keratin, they grow within keratin-containing structures such as the nails, hair, and the stratum corneum of the skin. When fungal spores are introduced onto the skin, they germinate to yield hyphae that spread laterally within the stratum corneum for 10–35 days. Iron is freely available to the dermatophytes in the stratum corneum, but the extension of organisms into the tissues is limited by their inability to compete with transferrin for iron in the deeper tissues.

Dermatophytes produce no toxins, and the skin looks normal or only slightly inflamed during the early colonization period. However, about 2–3 weeks into the infection, the fungi elicit a cellular immune response, and the advancing border of the area of fungal colonization becomes inflamed. Two defensive factors are brought to bear during the immune phase: macrophages invade the infected area, and transferrin is leaked into the stratum corneum. If the response is vigorous, the combined actions of cell-mediated immunity and transferrin will eliminate the infection in 1–2 weeks. If, however, the response is suboptimal, the inflammation will persist, resulting in a dry red lesion that scales, itches, cracks, and may develop deep fissures.

Chronic infections are particularly common in patients with tinea pedis (athlete's foot) and in patients infected with *T. rubrum.* Some children suffer from repeated ringworm infections, but this condition spontaneously improves when they reach puberty, probably because of changes that occur in the fatty acid composition of the skin oils.

Management of Dermatophytoses

Diagnosis. Diagnosis is based on the gross appearance of the lesion, microscopic examination of a KOH-digested skin scraping, and culture of the organism.

(1) History and Physical Examination. The patient's lesions are examined carefully for their gross appearance. Figs. 17–3 and 17–4 show the gross appearance of four types of dermatophyte infections: **tinea corporis, tinea capitis, tinea barbae,** and **favus.**

In patients with tinea capitis, a Wood's lamp may be used to determine if the hair fluoresces. *M. canis* and *M. audouinii* are common causative organisms of tinea capitis, and these organisms synthesize pteridine, which penetrates the hair and causes it to fluoresce under ultraviolet illumination.

Dermatophytoses caused by zoophilic fungi such as *M. canis* and *T. mentagrophytes* are usually more inflammatory than those caused by other dermatophytes. In patients with zoophilic dermatophytoses, the lesions may develop into boggy, red, tender, draining nodules known as **kerions,** and the cutaneous manifestations are sometimes accompanied by systemic symptoms, such as fever, lymphadenopathy, and malaise.

With some types of dermatophytoses, the patient may develop small, itching blisters or bumps that contain serous fluid, usually on the fingers but sometimes on the trunk. This is an allergic reaction to fungal antigens and is called a **dermatophytid** or **id reaction.**

Favus is an unusual dermatophytosis, usually caused by *T. schoenleinii.* Patients develop **scutula,** which are yellowish, cup-shaped crusts on the scalp (see Fig. 17–4). Each scutulum forms at a hair follicle, and removal of the crust reveals a red and oozing hair follicle. Eventually, the affected skin atrophies and scars, resulting in hair loss (alopecia).

(2) Laboratory Analysis. Scrapings from the lesions are digested with 10% KOH, stained, and examined for the presence of septate hyphae and ar-

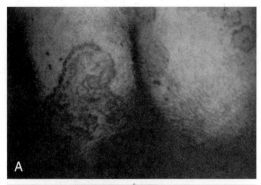

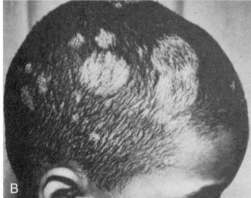

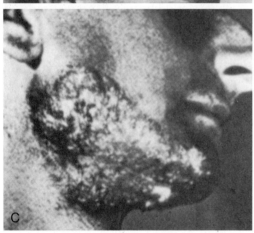

FIGURE 17–3. The lesions of tinea corporis (A), tinea capitis (B), and tinea barbae (C). (Reproduced, with permission, from Rippon, J. W. Medical Mycology: The Pathogenic Fungi and the Pathogenic Actinomycetes, 3rd ed. Philadelphia, W. B. Saunders Company, 1988.)

throspores. When hair is examined, only *Microsporum* and *Trichophyton* species will be found, since *Epidermophyton* does not infect the hair. Dermatophytes can also be cultivated on appropriate agar, usually Sabouraud's dextrose agar. The species most often associated with the major dermatophytoses are listed in Table 17–1.

Treatment. Many antifungal creams and powders are available over the counter, and some are moderately effective. The best of these contain miconazole or clotrimazole. Tolnaftate is sometimes effective, but clinical tests suggest that its efficacy in vivo is less than predicted by in vitro tests. Haloprogin is

also effective in treating some infections. Tinea pedis (athlete's foot) often responds to treatment with undecylenic acid, a fatty acid found in several powders.

When dermatophytoses do not respond well to topical treatments, oral griseofulvin can be used. This antibiotic accumulates in sweat, so it is deposited in the stratum corneum when the sweat evaporates. In some cases, griseofulvin is used in combination with miconazole. Nystatin has occasionally been used to treat difficult dermatophytoses.

Dermatophytoses caused by *T. rubrum* tend to be more severe than those caused by other organisms and do not respond as well to antibiotic therapy.

THE SUBCUTANEOUS MYCOSES

The fungi that cause subcutaneous mycotic infections usually infect only the submucosa and rarely disseminate to ectopic sites unless the patient has a T cell immunodeficiency. Immunosuppressed individuals are not, however, unusually susceptible to developing subcutaneous mycoses.

The five major subcutaneous mycoses are chromomycosis, entomophthoromycosis, lobomycosis, rhinosporidiosis, and sporotrichosis. Because sporotrichosis is the only one of these that is not rare in the USA, it is the focus of this section.

Sporotrichosis and *Sporothrix schenckii*

Sporotrichosis is caused by *Sporothrix schenckii,* a saprophytic fungus. Because the fungus grows in decaying vegetation, soil, peat moss, thorns, and mining timbers, sporotrichosis is an occupational hazard for agricultural workers, florists, and miners. In fact, sporotrichosis is often called **rose thorn disease** because so many patients become infected after being pricked by a rose thorn. Infection usually occurs following a puncture with a splinter or thorn but sometimes occurs through abrasions or via person-to-person contact.

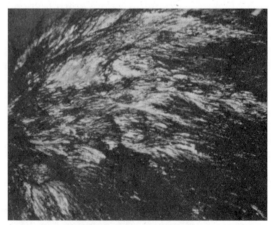

FIGURE 17–4. The lesions of favus. (Reproduced, with permission, from Rippon, J. W. Medical Mycology: The Pathogenic Fungi and the Pathogenic Actinomycetes, 3rd ed. Philadelphia, W. B. Saunders Company, 1988.)

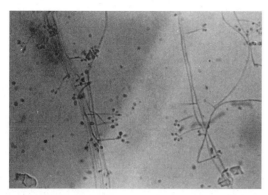

FIGURE 17–5. Culture of *Sporothrix schenckii*. (Reproduced, with permission, from Rippon, J. W. Medical Mycology: The Pathogenic Fungi and the Pathogenic Actinomycetes, 3rd ed. Philadelphia, W. B. Saunders Company, 1988.)

Although sporotrichosis is found throughout the world, there are pockets where the disease is more prevalent. It is endemic in France and Mexico, and it affects many thousands of individuals working in gold mines in South Africa. In the USA, it is most common along the valleys of the Missouri and Mississippi Rivers. In general, sporotrichosis is most frequently found in temperate plateaus where rainfall is not heavy.

Characteristics of *S. schenckii*

General Features. *S. schenckii* is a thermally dimorphic fungus. When cultivated at 25 °C on blood agar or mycosel agar, *S. schenckii* grows as a white to yellow mold that develops a folded or wrinkled appearance as the fungal colony matures. The hyphae are twisted and thin (1–2 μm in diameter), and they bear many delicate conidia arranged in "flowerettes" at right angles to the hyphae (Fig. 17–5). When cultivated at 37 °C, the fungi grow as yeasts that are 2–4 μm in diameter and may bear a single broad-based bud. Some yeasts assume a characteristic cigar shape.

Mechanisms of Pathogenicity. Sporotrichosis is an infection of the subcutaneous tissues and the draining lymph vessels. The organisms enter the skin through an abrasion or puncture wound, multiply locally, and produce a primary lesion that contains masses of epithelioid histiocytes with an admixture of neutrophils, plasma cells, and lymphocytes. Few fungi can be seen within the lesion. The fungi spread to the draining lymph vessels and produce a series of suppurative or granulomatous lesions. The cell-mediated immune reaction restricts the fungi to these tissues unless the patient has a T cell immunodeficiency.

Management of Sporotrichosis

Diagnosis. Diagnosis is based on the gross appearance of the lesions, microscopic examination of material biopsied from lesions, and culture of the organism.

(1) History and Physical Examination. Sporotrichosis may be either cutaneous or systemic. Cutaneous sporotrichosis occurs in patients with normal cellular immune responses and may be lymphocutaneous, fixed cutaneous, or mucocutaneous. The organisms disseminate in patients with depressed T cell function and may infect the lungs, bone, meninges, or multiple organs.

More than 75% of patients develop lymphocutaneous sporotrichosis (Fig. 17–6). A granulomatous lesion develops at the initial cutaneous inoculation site (for example, at the site of a thorn prick) 3 weeks to 6 months after the patient is infected. The primary lesion is most often on the hand or finger. The lesion begins as an ulcer or lump (bubo) and gradually develops into a necrotic lesion known as the sporotrichotic chancre. Within a few days or weeks after the appearance of the initial lesion, multiple subcutaneous nodules appear along the course of the draining lymph vessels. These lesions are moveable at first, but they soon become firmly attached to the skin that covers them. They may ulcerate and look somewhat like the gumma of tertiary syphilis or yaws. Typically, there is a series of draining or gummatous lumps radiating up the arm from an ulcer on the hand.

The primary lesion may be misdiagnosed as malignant pustule (cutaneous anthrax) or tularemia. Differentiation of sporotrichosis from these diseases is not difficult; patients with anthrax or tularemia are

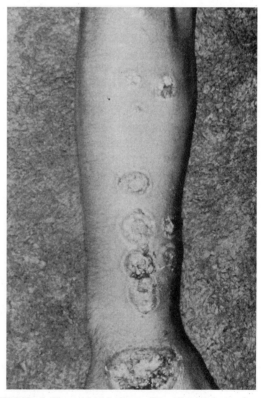

FIGURE 17–6. The typical lesions of lymphocutaneous sporotrichosis. (Reproduced, with permission, from Rippon, J. W. Medical Mycology: The Pathogenic Fungi and the Pathogenic Actinomycetes, 3rd ed. Philadelphia, W. B. Saunders Company, 1988.)

TABLE 17–2. Uncommon Subcutaneous Mycoses

Disease	Causative Agent	Source	Clinical Manifestations	Laboratory Analysis	Treatment
Chromomycosis	Various soil fungi, including *Cladosporium, Fonsecaea, Phialophora,* and *Rhinocladiella.*	Soil; enters through cut or abrasion.	Granulomas on limbs.	Biopsy.	Surgery plus itraconazole.
Entomophthoromycosis basidiobolae	*Basidiobolus ranarum.*	Leaf detritus, amphibians, and reptiles.	Massive subcutaneous growths.	Culture.	Saturated potassium iodide.
Entomophthoromycosis conidiobolae	*Conidiobolus coronatus.*	Spiders and termites.	Massive nasal polyps.	Culture.	Saturated potassium iodide.
Lobomycosis	*Loboa loboi.*	Unknown; enters through cut or abrasion.	Keloidal or verrucous lesions. Some crust.	Biopsy.	Surgery plus sulfonamide and clofazimine.
Rhinosporidiosis	*Rhinosporidium seeberi.*	Unknown; perhaps water.	Disfiguring mucocutaneous growths.	Biopsy.	Surgery.

acutely ill, but patients with lesions caused by *S. schenckii* are otherwise healthy. The primary lesion persists for weeks or months and heals without scarring. Buboes may reappear at the site intermittently for years.

In patients with depressed T cell function, the most common ectopic focus is the lung, but some patients develop disseminated lesions similar to those seen in miliary tuberculosis. These destructive lesions most frequently occur in the bones or joints but sometimes affect the sinuses, visceral organs, or meninges.

(2) Laboratory Analysis. Suspected sporotrichotic lesions should be biopsied, and the biopsy samples should be examined microscopically and cultured. *S. schenckii* is usually difficult to locate within lesions, but characteristic asteroid bodies, consisting of yeasts surrounded by a mass of amorphous eosinophilic material, may be seen (Fig. 17–7). Asteroid bodies are also associated with some other granulomatous fungal diseases as well as a few bacterial granulomas, so their presence is not diagnostic in the absence of other evidence of sporotrichosis.

Treatment. Cutaneous sporotrichosis can be treated with oral potassium iodide. Disseminated sporotrichosis is usually treated with amphotericin B. Itraconazole has been used successfully to treat both cutaneous and disseminated sporotrichosis. Because patients with disseminated disease are immunosuppressed, treatment is often unsuccessful.

Uncommon Subcutaneous Mycoses and Their Agents

Information concerning the acquisition and management of chromomycosis, entomophthoromycosis, lobomycosis, and rhinosporidiosis is presented in Table 17–2.

Selected Readings

Blitzer, A., and W. Lawson. Fungal infections of the nose and paranasal sinuses. Otolaryngol Clin North Am 26:1007–1035, 1993.

DeLuca, C., et al. Lipoperoxidase activity of *Pityrosporum:* characterization of by-products and possible role in pityriasis versicolor. Exp Dermatol 5:49–56, 1996.

Elewski, B. E. Cutaneous mycoses in children. Br J Dermatol 134(supplement 46):7–11, 1996.

Esterre, P., et al. Treatment of chromomycosis with terbinafine: preliminary results of an open pilot study. Br J Dermatol 134(supplement 46):33–36, 1996.

Fothergill, A. W. Identification of dematiaceous fungi and their role in human disease. Clin Infect Dis 22(supplement 2):S179–S184, 1996.

Gaines, J. J., Jr., et al. Rhinosporidiosis: three domestic cases. South Med J 89:65–67, 1996.

Ibrahim-Granet, O., et al. Expression of PZ-peptidases by cultures of several pathogenic fungi: purification and characterization of a collagenase from *Trichophyton schoenleinii.* J Med Vet Mycol 34:83–90, 1996.

Koneman, E. W., et al. Mycology. *In* Koneman, E. W., et al., eds. Diagnostic Microbiology, 4th ed. Philadelphia, J. B. Lippincott Company, 1992.

McGinnis, M. R. Chromoblastomycosis and phaeohyphomycosis: new concepts, diagnosis, and mycology. J Am Acad Dermatol 8:1–15, 1983.

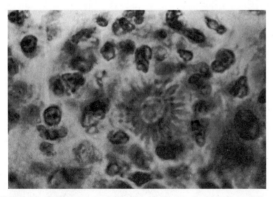

FIGURE 17–7. The asteroid body of *Sporothrix schenckii*, seen in a biopsy specimen from a sporotrichotic lesion. (Reproduced, with permission, from Rippon, J. W. Medical Mycology: The Pathogenic Fungi and the Pathogenic Actinomycetes, 3rd ed. Philadelphia, W. B. Saunders Company, 1988.)

Morgan, M. A., et al. Disseminated sporotrichosis with *Sporothrix schenckii* fungemia. Diagn Microbiol Infect Dis 2:151–155, 1984.

Odom, R. B. New therapies for onychomycosis. J Am Acad Dermatol 35:S26–S30, 1996.

Radentz, W. H. Fungal skin infections associated with animal contact. Am Fam Physician 43:1253–1256, 1991.

Richet, H. M., et al. Cluster of *Malassezia furfur* pulmonary infection in infants in a neonatal intensive care unit. J Clin Microbiol 27:1197–1200, 1989.

Rippon, J. W. Medical Mycology: The Pathogenic Fungi and the Pathogenic Actinomycetes, 3rd ed. Philadelphia, W. B. Saunders Company, 1988.

Savin, R. Diagnosis and treatment of tinea versicolor. J Fam Pract 43:127–132, 1996.

CHAPTER EIGHTEEN

FUNGI THAT CAUSE DEEP

(SYSTEMIC) MYCOSES

Aspergillus, Blastomyces, Candida, Coccidioides, Cryptococcus, Histoplasma, Mucor, Paracoccidioides, Rhizopus, and Other Fungi

PATHOGENIC AND OPPORTUNISTIC FUNGI

The deep mycoses are systemic infections caused by two groups of fungi found in the environment: fungi that are true human pathogens and fungi that are opportunistic.

The **pathogenic fungi** cause disease both in immunocompetent hosts (persons with normal immune responses) and in immunocompromised hosts (persons whose immunity is altered because of the presence of a debilitating disease or because of the use of immunosuppressive drugs). These fungi include *Blastomyces dermatitidis, Coccidioides immitis, Histoplasma capsulatum,* and *Paracoccidioides brasiliensis.* The organisms show no predilection for immunocompromised hosts, but they cause more severe disease in these individuals than in immunocompetent hosts. Most of the pathogenic fungi are geographically restricted and are thermally dimorphic. The organisms are acquired by breathing spores, so patients must be present when the fungi are fruiting. The initial site of infection is usually the lungs. About 99% of the infections resolve spontaneously, and 90% are either asymptomatic or cause mild symptoms. The lesions formed when the infection disseminates are granulomas and are similar to those formed in disseminated tuberculosis. Patients who recover have protective cell-mediated immune responses and are not likely to develop disease again.

The **opportunistic fungi** are only rarely pathogenic in immunocompetent hosts but cause life-threatening disease in immunocompromised hosts, including those being treated with immunosuppressive drugs (such as cancer and organ transplant patients) and those with serious diseases (such as acquired immunodeficiency syndrome [AIDS], diabetes, and lymphoma). Among the opportunistic fungi are some species of *Aspergillus, Candida, Cryptococcus,*

Mucor, and *Rhizopus.* These fungi are not geographically restricted (they are ubiquitous) and are not thermally dimorphic. The site of entry may be respiratory, but it is often through some other breach in the body's defenses. The lesions are pyogenic and necrotic, and a poorly organized granuloma may form. Because opportunistic infections are difficult to control, they are often fatal if untreated. Patients who recover are usually not immune and may develop disease again.

DEEP MYCOSES CAUSED BY PATHOGENIC FUNGI

Histoplasmosis and
Histoplasma capsulatum

Histoplasmosis is caused worldwide by *Histoplasma capsulatum* but is most prevalent in locales with warm, humid summers. In most of the world, disease is due to *H. capsulatum* var. *capsulatum.* In Africa, however, infections due to *H. capsulatum* var. *duboisii* are often seen.

In the USA, histoplasmosis is endemic in the Midwest. The mold form of *Histoplasma* is found in the soil throughout the region, but it grows to tremendous density in the droppings of starlings, chickens, and bats, possibly because of their high nitrogen content. *H. capsulatum* will also grow on the feathers of birds, but the birds do not become internally infected with the organism. At one time, histoplasmosis was considered to be a rare disease in the Midwest, and researchers claimed that it was always fatal. But skin testing of large numbers of people with **histoplasmin,** an antigen of *H. capsulatum,* has shown that 85–90% of those living in the Midwest have been infected by 20 years of age and that the infection is mild or asymptomatic in almost all cases.

This high level of endemicity in the Midwest can be largely placed at the feet of one man: Eugene Schieffelin. A member of a society of Swiss immigrants living in New York City, Schieffelin was devoted to birds and the arts. He noted that there were no starlings in the USA, despite the fact that they were mentioned by Shakespeare in *Henry IV, Part One:* "Nay, I'll have a starling shall be taught to speak / Nothing but 'Mortimer' and give it to [Mortimer], / To keep his anger still in motion." What Schieffelin failed to notice was that the starling mentioned here was meant to *torment* Mortimer. In any case, Schieffelin imported 80 pairs of starlings and released them in 1890 and 1891 in the USA. The timing was perfect because the disappearance of the passenger pigeons soon thereafter left an ecologic niche for the starlings. Within a handful of years, there were so many starlings that homeowners in Cincinnati and Indianapolis were using shovels to clear the starling droppings from their yards. There had previously been histoplasmosis in the Midwest, but epidemics of the disease began to occur because of the rapid multiplication and congregation of starlings into "roosts."

More than 100 outbreaks of histoplasmosis have been documented in the last 50 years in the Midwest. In 1970, a major outbreak occurred in Ohio when 294 children and teachers decided to rake and sweep a schoolyard on Earth Day. Two large trees in the schoolyard served as blackbird roosts, and the soil was filled with blackbird droppings. Everyone involved in the project developed histoplasmosis. In 1978, an outbreak affecting almost 400 people occurred in Indianapolis when Riverside Amusement Park was disassembled.

Characteristics of *H. capsulatum*

General Features. *H. capsulatum* var. *capsulatum* is a thermally dimorphic fungus that lives in the topmost layer of soil. When cultivated at 25 °C on Sabouraud's dextrose agar, *H. capsulatum* grows as a mold with smooth microconidia that are 1–3 μm in diameter and tuberculate macroconidia that are 5–15 μm long (Fig. 18–1A). At 37 °C, *H. capsulatum* becomes an unencapsulated yeast that is 2–4 μm in diameter (Fig. 18–1B). The yeasts are characteristic in having a single bud that is attached via a slender neck.

In vivo, *H. capsulatum* organisms are generally seen as small yeasts, but in deep tissues, larger yeast variants (as large as 25 μm in diameter) are occasionally seen. These may be cigar-shaped, and both germ tubes and hyphae may be identified.

The sexual form of *H. capsulatum* is called *Ajellomyces capsulatus.*

Mechanisms of Pathogenicity. The key pathogenic characteristic of *H. capsulatum* is its ability to invade and survive within host cells, particularly within fixed and migrating macrophages and monocytes. Recovery and immunity to infection require development of an effective cell-mediated immune

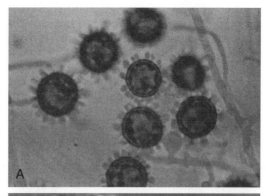
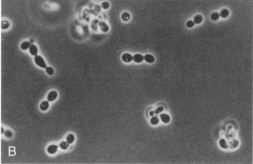

FIGURE 18–1. The tuberculate macroconidia (A) and yeasts (B) of *Histoplasma capsulatum*. (Reproduced, with permission, from Rippon, J. W. Medical Mycology: The Pathogenic Fungi and the Pathogenic Actinomycetes, 3rd ed. Philadelphia, W. B. Saunders Company, 1988.)

response, and the pathologic hallmark of histoplasmosis is the formation of granulomas.

The arthrospores and microconidia of *H. capsulatum* are infective. The macroconidia are not infective, because they are unable to reach the lower lung fields, where productive infection begins. *Histoplasma* spores are phagocytosed by polymorphonuclear leukocytes and macrophages within 4–6 hours, and the spores become yeasts within 24–72 hours. The transition from mold to yeast requires the relatively high temperatures of the body and the presence of cysteine. The yeasts multiply within macrophages and are transported throughout the body as the macrophages wander. The yeasts infect new macrophages and monocytes by adhering to specific receptors of the CD18 family on host cell surfaces. Adherence may be biphasic, involving coadherence to the receptor for the inactivated C3b complement component (the CR3 receptor) and to a membrane glycosphingolipid. Adherent yeasts are phagocytosed and then multiply within the phagocytic vacuole. *Histoplasma* organisms have also been shown to invade and multiply within epithelial cells and endothelial cells.

In vitro studies have demonstrated that isolated *Histoplasma* yeasts and hyphae are killed by the oxidative products and lysosomal contents of granulocytes. Yet the unstimulated macrophage or monocyte is the normal home for *Histoplasma*. It is believed that *H. capsulatum* survives within macrophages by failing to trigger the oxidative burst and by either resisting or inactivating the fungicidal activities of macrophage lysosomes. Activated macrophages do not kill *Histoplasma* organisms but restrict their ability to multiply.

H. capsulatum is disseminated from the lungs within monocytes. The organisms deposit primarily (but not exclusively) in lymphoid tissue and multiply within fixed macrophages and endothelial cells. Within 3 weeks, a cell-mediated immune response develops and causes a granuloma to form around the infection focus. The lesion necroses and calcifies, and the infection is limited. Although disease is quiescent in most cases, about 70% of patients exhibit multiple healed calcifications in their spleen and liver. If an adequate cell-mediated immune response does not occur, patients develop progressive disseminated disease. Patients highly likely to develop this form of histoplasmosis include those with Hodgkin's disease, AIDS, an organ transplant, or other condition requiring immunosuppressive therapy. Thus, all patients with histoplasmosis develop disseminated disease, but those with depressed T cell immunity develop *progressive* disseminated disease.

Management of Histoplasmosis

Diagnosis
(1) History and Physical Examination. Most patients with histoplasmosis are asymptomatic or suffer from a mild acute disease that is often called summer flu, summer fever, or fungus flu. Histoplasmosis occurs more frequently in children than in adults and is generally more severe in children. In most cases, histoplasmosis resolves spontaneously with no sequelae, but about 1% of untreated patients develop chronic histoplasmosis in the form of progressive disseminated histoplasmosis, chronic cavitary histoplasmosis, or chronic ocular histoplasmosis.

(a) Primary Acute Histoplasmosis. Primary infection is most often seen when large numbers of individuals are simultaneously infected with moderately large doses of *Histoplasma* conidia, usually as a consequence of disturbing bird droppings. Patients develop a fever, nonproductive cough, headache, chest pain, and sore muscles and joints. In white women, erythema multiforme or erythema nodosum has also been reported. Some patients with arthralgia and myalgia develop acute pericarditis. Most patients do not develop lung consolidation or pleural effusion, but radiographic examination may reveal a patchy nonsegmented infiltrate and ipsilateral mediastinal or hilar lymphadenitis. More than 95% of the patients with primary acute infection recover spontaneously, but most will have calcified lesions in the lung, liver, or spleen.

(b) Primary Cutaneous Histoplasmosis. Cutaneous histoplasmosis is rare. It occurs mainly in laboratory workers, pathologists, or others who have accidentally inoculated themselves with *Histoplasma* via injection or a cut. The lesions ulcerate and may become quite large, but most heal spontaneously without antibiotic therapy.

(c) Progressive Disseminated Histoplasmosis. Disseminated disease occurs primarily in infants, young children, and older men and is characterized by hepatomegaly, splenomegaly, generalized lymphadenopathy, fever, and weight loss. It is not uncommon for one organ or system to be predominantly affected. The initial infection site is the lung, but the fungi travel within macrophages to establish new infection foci. Many patients develop ulceration of the tongue, palate, or larynx. The fatality rate of untreated progressive disseminated histoplasmosis is about 90%.

(d) Chronic Cavitary Histoplasmosis. Chronic cavitary histoplasmosis is very similar to chronic cavitary tuberculosis. Most of the cavitary lesions develop in the upper lung. As with tuberculosis, the cavitary lesions cause lung damage and necrosis, and they may promote the dissemination of organisms to ectopic foci if the cavity involves a blood vessel. Without antibiotic therapy, about 20% of patients die in 1 year and 50% die in 5 years.

(e) Chronic Ocular Histoplasmosis. In rare cases, patients develop chronic uveitis that may interfere with sight and require treatment. The uveitis is due to a repair response to the presence of organisms rather than to granuloma formation.

(2) Laboratory Analysis. Laboratory diagnosis of histoplasmosis depends on demonstrating *Histoplasma* yeasts in tissues, culturing *H. capsulatum* on an appropriate medium, and demonstrating a rising titer of antibody to *Histoplasma* in serum samples. In patients with disseminated disease, *Histoplasma* polysaccharide antigens may be found in urine and blood samples.

A variety of histologic stains can be used to visualize *Histoplasma* yeasts, including Giemsa stain and hematoxylin-eosin stain. Immunofluorescence can be used to identify the yeasts in situ. In stained samples of blood or tissue, *H. capsulatum* yeasts are 2–4 μm in diameter and have a single bud attached by a narrow neck. Samples from deep tissues may contain larger yeast forms, some of which are oblong or exhibit germ tubes.

H. capsulatum is often difficult to culture, and definitive identification may take 4 weeks or longer. Clinical samples are cultured on Sabouraud's dextrose agar at 25 °C and yield downy white or brown mycelia with tuberculate macroconidia. Because they so closely resemble several saprophytic fungi, the organisms must be converted to yeast form, a process that may take as long as 4–6 weeks. Alternatively, the hyphal or yeast forms can be identified by an exoantigen test or by use of a commercially available DNA probe assay. The exoantigen test takes 48–72 hours, and the DNA probe can identify the organisms in about 2 hours.

Antibody to *H. capsulatum* can be detected in serum samples by complement fixation (CF), immunodiffusion, latex agglutination, or radioimmunoassay. In the CF test, which is widely used, a fourfold or greater rise in antibody titer indicates an active *Histoplasma* infection. Because the CF test does not detect antibody during the first 4–6 weeks of infection, the test often yields false-negative results. Thus, although a positive CF test result confirms the diagnosis, a negative CF test result does not rule out histoplasmosis. The immunodiffusion test is highly specific but lacks sensitivity. It has been useful, however, in diagnosing meningeal histoplasmosis on the basis of antibody detected in cerebrospinal fluid samples. The latex agglutination test is useful in diagnosing early acute histoplasmosis, but many patients with chronic disease show negative results in this test.

H. capsulatum polysaccharide antigens appear in the urine of about 90% of patients with disseminated histoplasmosis and in the blood of about 50% of these patients. The antigens are present very early in infection and can be found in some patients without disseminated disease. Antigen detection has been useful in the diagnosis of histoplasmosis in patients with underlying T cell deficiencies, such as AIDS patients.

Treatment. Because histoplasmosis is self-limited in more than 95% of cases, most patients do not require treatment. Amphotericin B is generally used to treat patients with progressive disease and is always indicated in cases of aggressive disease. Ketoconazole has been used to treat some patients with moderately progressive histoplasmosis.

Blastomycosis and *Blastomyces dermatitidis*

Blastomycosis was once called Chicago disease because so many of the early cases, which were described around 1900, occurred in people living or working in Chicago. Although cases have been reported all over the world, most are found in the USA, particularly along the valleys of the Mississippi, Ohio, and Tennessee Rivers, along the shores of the Great Lakes, and near the Blue Ridge and Smoky Mountains. A large number of cases have recently been described in Wisconsin. The disease is sometimes called **North American blastomycosis** to distinguish it from paracoccidioidomycosis, which is also called South American blastomycosis.

The agent of North American blastomycosis is *Blastomyces dermatitidis*. Although the organism has rarely been isolated from environmental samples, the conidia of *B. dermatitidis* are believed to be in the soil, and human exposure is thought to occur when the top layers of soil are disturbed. Recent surveys in Wisconsin have suggested that *Blastomyces* grows in the topmost layers of soil that is rich in bird droppings or animal droppings. Bird droppings are high in nitrogen content and therefore promote the growth of *Blastomyces*. The peak time of exposure to organisms is autumn and early winter, and clinical signs of disease begin most often during the period from December through April. In endemic areas, individuals at greatest risk are those who live along a waterway and pursue outdoor activities. In 90% of cases, the patient is a male, usually between the ages of 30 and 50 years. Unlike histoplasmosis, blastomycosis is rare in children.

Characteristics of *B. dermatitidis*

General Features. Blastomycosis is caused by an ascomycete whose imperfect state is known as *B. dermatitidis* and whose perfect state is called *Ajellomyces dermatitidis*. The organism is thermally dimorphic, growing as a mold at 25 °C and as a yeast at 37 °C. On Sabouraud's dextrose agar, the hyphal colonies of *B. dermatitidis* usually appear fluffy and white (although colonies with many conidia may look brown) and contain septate hyphae bearing oval or dumbbell-shaped microconidia that are 2–10 μm in diameter. The yeasts (Fig. 18–2) are thick-walled and unencapsulated, and each yeast has a single broad-based bud. The yeasts range in size from 2 to 20 μm, but most are between 5 and 15 μm in diameter. *Blastomyces* will form ascospores when it is grown on a medium containing oatmeal.

Mechanisms of Pathogenicity. *B. dermatitidis* is difficult to locate in the environment, but it is found sporadically in rotting wood, dust, pigeon droppings, and soil that is moist and enriched with animal and bird droppings. Humans become infected with *B. dermatitidis* when they breathe conidia that enter the lower lung fields. The conidia become yeasts in the alveolar spaces and elicit an inflammatory response. The early cellular response consists primarily of polymorphonuclear leukocytes; however, with the development of cell-mediated immunity, macrophages congregate in the infection focus. Unlike in histoplasmosis, in blastomycosis the polymorphonuclear leukocytes persist in the lesion and the cellular response is pyogranulomatous. That is, the granuloma formed in blastomycosis is noncaseating and contains both macrophages and polymorphonuclear leukocytes.

Blastomyces is found both within macrophages and in alveolar fluid. If the cell-mediated immune response is sufficiently vigorous, the infection is restricted to the lungs and is manifested as localized pneumonitis with hilar lymph node involvement. If the immune response is not sufficient to control the infection, the organisms disseminate to establish ectopic foci, most often in the skin, bones, genitourinary

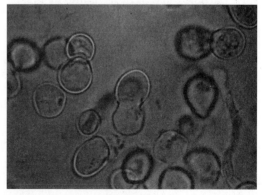

FIGURE 18–2. The yeasts of *Blastomyces dermatitidis* with their typical broad-based buds. (Reproduced, with permission, from Rippon, J. W. Medical Mycology: The Pathogenic Fungi and the Pathogenic Actinomycetes, 3rd ed. Philadelphia, W. B. Saunders Company, 1988.)

tract, and central nervous system. Growth of *Blastomyces* in these sites results in the formation of suppurative granulomas.

Whereas almost all cases of histoplasmosis in immunocompetent patients resolve spontaneously, the picture is not so clear-cut with blastomycosis. Early studies suggested that almost all patients with blastomycosis develop life-threatening disease and that more than 90% of them die without treatment. Recent serologic surveys and clinical studies in Wisconsin have turned this view of blastomycosis upside down. According to these studies, many individuals who have never had overt symptoms of blastomycosis have been infected. Furthermore, one study of 44 patients showed that only 9 (20%) required treatment and that infection in the other 35 (80%) resolved spontaneously without relapse or progressive infection. Thus, although the jury is still out on the percentage of patients who are asymptomatic, it appears that most patients experience mild acute disease or none at all and that relatively few patients develop life-threatening disease.

Management of Blastomycosis

Diagnosis

(1) History and Physical Examination. Blastomycosis may be subclinical, acute, or chronic, and patients may develop chronic blastomycosis with or without suffering from an initial acute episode. Chronic blastomycosis is rare in patients younger than 15 years of age.

(a) Acute Blastomycosis. Acute blastomycosis begins about 6 weeks (range is from 21 to 106 days) after exposure to the conidia of *B. dermatitidis*. Patients suffer from a flu-like syndrome, with fever, arthralgia, myalgia, headache, a cough productive of mucopurulent sputum, and pleuritic chest pain. In some cases, the sputum is tinged with blood. Erythema nodosum may be present, and weight loss may be noted. Acute blastomycosis usually resolves spontaneously.

(b) Inoculation Blastomycosis. Laboratory workers, pathologists, or other individuals who accidentally inject themselves with *Blastomyces* may develop inoculation blastomycosis. The disease is localized and self-limited.

(c) Chronic Blastomycosis. Most patients first seek medical intervention when blastomycosis has already become chronic and organisms have invaded the lungs, skin, bones, genitourinary tract, or central nervous system.

Chronic pulmonary disease is the most common form of chronic blastomycosis and is characterized by pneumonia with night sweats, weight loss, fatigue, chest pain, fever, and a cough productive of mucopurulent sputum. The disease is similar in appearance to acute pulmonary blastomycosis but is of longer duration and may be more severe. Its manifestations are also similar to those of pulmonary tuberculosis or lung cancer.

Cutaneous blastomycosis (Fig. 18–3) is the second most common form of chronic blastomycosis. It often begins as a pustular nodule on the face or extremities. In weeks or months, it develops into an ulcerative or verrucous (wartlike) granuloma with serpiginous advancing borders. The lesion may become quite large and elevated, and the center will become covered with a crust that is speckled with black dots. A subcutaneous abscess lies below the lesion. Over several years, the lesion becomes deforming and will leave a thin, depigmented, atrophic scar. The fungi may spread to underlying bony structures and may disseminate.

About 25% of patients with extrapulmonary blastomycosis develop osteomyelitis. The bones most often affected are the vertebrae, ribs, pelvis, sacrum, cranium, and long bones. The bones contain granulomas that may be purulent or necrotic. Osteomyelitis is often a sign of widespread dissemination of fungi and carries a poor prognosis.

Between 5% and 22% of patients with extrapulmonary blastomycosis develop urogenital disease. Patients most often develop epididymitis, and there may be testicular and prostate involvement. Urogenital blastomycosis is rare in women.

Between 5% and 10% of patients with extrapulmonary blastomycosis develop central nervous system disease, often accompanied by granulomas in the liver or spleen. Manifestations may include headache, confusion, convulsions, slight paralysis of the extremities on one or both sides, loss of speech or the ability to speak coherently, and personality changes.

(2) Laboratory Analysis. Laboratory confirmation of blastomycosis has traditionally been based on the direct identification of *Blastomyces* in sputum or tissue samples and the culture of *Blastomyces* on a standard fungal medium.

Sputum samples can be digested with 10% potassium hydroxide, stained, and examined for the presence of thick-walled yeasts with broad-based buds. Sputum samples should be stained with periodic acid–Schiff stain, rather than hematoxylin-eosin stain. *Blastomyces* is best visualized in tissue or exudate samples stained with Grocott-Gomori methenamine–silver nitrate stain. The organism is easy to find in sputum and tissue samples, but samples stained

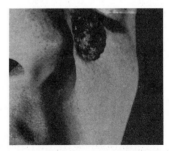

FIGURE 18–3. A cutaneous lesion caused by *Blastomyces dermatitidis*. (Reproduced, with permission, from Rippon, J. W. Medical Mycology: The Pathogenic Fungi and the Pathogenic Actinomycetes, 3rd ed. Philadelphia, W. B. Saunders Company, 1988.)

with Papanicolaou's stain may be misidentified as indicative of lung carcinoma. Samples taken from skin lesions should be obtained from the advancing edge of the lesion, where the fungi are in greater concentration.

Blastomyces can be cultivated initially in about 5 days on Sabouraud's dextrose agar, but complete identification may take about 30 days. Recent advances have shortened the identification process considerably. Cultivated fungi can be tested by an exoantigen test or a single-stranded DNA probe test to confirm the identity of *B. dermatitidis*. The exoantigen test can be performed in 24 hours, and the DNA probe takes 2 hours. Both are highly specific for *Blastomyces*.

There is no reliable test available to detect circulating antibody to *Blastomyces*. The complement fixation test, immunodiffusion test, and enzyme immunoassay are available. However, the complement fixation and immunodiffusion tests are not sensitive or specific, and the enzyme immunoassay yields many false-positive results when antibody titers are low.

Treatment.   Most patients with primary disease recover spontaneously without treatment. Patients with mild chronic disease can be treated with ketoconazole. Severely ill patients with progressive chronic disease, especially those with noncutaneous lesions, should receive amphotericin B. Nonprogressive skin lesions have been treated successfully with hydroxystilbamidine isethionate. Pulmonary blastomycosis is often treated effectively with surgery alone.

Coccidioidomycosis and *Coccidioides immitis*

Coccidioidomycosis is prevalent in the southwestern USA, northern Mexico, and Argentina. Each year, an estimated 100,000 cases occur in the USA, and 70 result in death. The disease most often affects people living in hot and semiarid environments, such as the San Joaquin Valley, San Diego, Phoenix, and Tucson. For this reason, coccidioidomycosis is often known as **San Joaquin Valley fever, valley fever, and desert rheumatism.**

Coccidioidomycosis is caused by *Coccidioides immitis,* a fungus that grows in the soil of semiarid desert regions that experience short but intense rains, followed by rapidly rising temperatures. The fungi grow most prolifically in rodent burrows, possibly because of the presence of nitrogen-rich rodent droppings. Humans are infected when they breathe *C. immitis* arthrospores. Because arthrospores are not formed in the lungs, there is no person-to-person spread of coccidioidomycosis. Outbreaks often occur when the soil is disturbed by farming, archaeologic digging, excavating, or house construction.

Characteristics of *C. immitis*

General Features.   *C. immitis* is unusual among the pathogenic deep fungi in that it is nutritionally

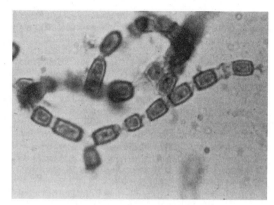

FIGURE 18–4. The highly infectious arthrospores of *Coccidioides immitis*. (Reproduced, with permission, from Rippon, J. W. Medical Mycology: The Pathogenic Fungi and the Pathogenic Actinomycetes, 3rd ed. Philadelphia, W. B. Saunders Company, 1988.)

dimorphic but not thermally dimorphic. When growing in the soil or on a standard medium at 25–30 °C, *C. immitis* appears as a grayish-white mold with branched septate hyphae that are 2–4 μm in diameter. The hyphal mass contains many rectangular and barrel-shaped arthrospores (Fig. 18–4). The arthrospores are typically interdigitated between empty hyphal segments and are highly infectious, making culture of the organisms dangerous. When *C. immitis* is growing in its mammalian hosts, some hyphae may be seen, but *C. immitis* grows primarily as spherules (Fig. 18–5). The spherules are 20–200 μm in diameter and contain many endospores, each of which is 2–5 μm in diameter. Because the spherules are also infectious, clinical samples should be handled carefully during testing.

Mechanisms of Pathogenicity.   Infection occurs when humans breathe the arthrospores of *C. immitis*. The arthrospores, which are converted to spherules in the lung, elicit an inflammatory response

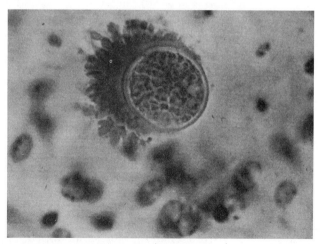

FIGURE 18–5. A tissue spherule of *Coccidioides immitis* surrounded by amorphous eosinophilic material. (Reproduced, with permission, from Rippon, J. W. Medical Mycology: The Pathogenic Fungi and the Pathogenic Actinomycetes, 3rd ed. Philadelphia, W. B. Saunders Company, 1988.)

that produces the pneumonia or pneumonitis of coccidioidomycosis. The early response consists mainly of polymorphonuclear leukocytes, but macrophages and monocytes are soon attracted to the infection focus. As in blastomycosis, in coccidioidomycosis the polymorphonuclear leukocytes persist in the infection focus, and a pyogranuloma is formed. Pleural effusion develops, and the inflammatory exudate contains many eosinophils. Primary coccidioidomycosis is usually self-limited in immunocompetent patients, but individuals who are exposed to extremely large inocula of arthrospores may develop secondary (disseminated) coccidioidomycosis.

In patients with T cell immunodeficiencies, including those with AIDS, Hodgkin's disease, and renal transplants, the spherules of *C. immitis* may disseminate, and the presence of spherules in various organ systems is heralded by symptoms consistent with the formation of pyogranulomas in the affected organ. In these patients, secondary coccidioidomycosis is often life-threatening.

Management of Coccidioidomycosis

Diagnosis

(1) History and Physical Examination. About 60% of individuals infected with *C. immitis* have subclinical infections. Fewer than 40% develop acute pulmonary disease, which generally resolves spontaneously. Only 1–2% of patients develop disseminated disease. Males and females are infected equally with *C. immitis,* but men are about four times as likely as women to have disseminated disease. There appears to be a genetic predilection for disease dissemination, with unusually high rates reported in blacks and Filipinos.

(a) Primary Coccidioidomycosis. Acute pulmonary coccidioidomycosis begins 1–4 weeks (mean onset is 10–16 days) following exposure. Patients have a dry cough, fever, malaise, pleuritic chest pain, night sweats, anorexia, arthralgia, myalgia, and headache. The pleuritic pain is severe in many patients, and a weight loss of 9–13 kg (about 20–30 lb) is not unusual. Radiographic examination reveals the presence of pleural effusion that is often accompanied by hilar lymphadenopathy. Thin-walled cavitary lesions are often seen.

About 1–2 days after the onset of symptoms, children often develop a fine rash that looks like scarlet fever. From 3 days to 3 weeks after the onset of symptoms, about 25% of women and 5% of men develop erythema nodosum, erythema multiforme, or toxic erythema. These cutaneous manifestations are probably allergic reactions to coccidioidin antigens, and their appearance seems to correlate with the development of a measurable cell-mediated immune response to *C. immitis.* Erythema nodosum is characterized by red, tender nodules that appear on the lower extremities (usually on the shins but sometimes around the knees or on the thighs), are filled with serous fluid, have a bluish cast to them, and will regress in a few days. Erythema multiforme is

characterized by red to purple nodules, papules, or vesicles that appear on the upper part of the body. Toxic erythema is a fine rash. The appearance of these allergic manifestations is usually a signal that the patient is recovering and will not suffer from disseminated disease.

(b) Secondary (Disseminated) Coccidioidomycosis. Secondary pulmonary coccidioidomycosis is rare in immunocompetent patients but relatively common in immunocompromised patients. One study, for example, found that about 50% of patients with AIDS and 16% of other immunocompromised patients developed secondary pulmonary disease as a consequence of coccidioidomycosis, and more than half of these immunocompromised patients died within 1 month.

Secondary pulmonary coccidioidomycosis occurs when patients hematogenously reseed their lungs with the spherules of *C. immitis.* This may produce a single granulomatous mass or diffuse reticulonodular infiltrates. Patients may suffer from progressive pneumonia or from an acute miliary type of pneumonia. Progressive pneumonia gradually develops over several years; is characterized by persistent cough, chest pain, hemoptysis, and anorexia; and is clinically and pathologically similar to chronic cavitary tuberculosis and chronic cavitary histoplasmosis. In contrast, the miliary type of pneumonia is rapidly progressive and has a high fatality rate.

Other disseminated forms of coccidioidomycosis include chronic granulomatous meningitis, which is similar to meningitis caused by *Mycobacterium tuberculosis* or *Cryptococcus neoformans;* chronic cutaneous coccidioidomycosis; and generalized disseminated coccidioidomycosis.

(2) Laboratory Analysis. Laboratory confirmation of coccidioidomycosis rests on directly demonstrating the presence of spherules in tissue and sputum samples and showing that the patient has specific antibodies to *C. immitis.* Cultures and skin tests with *Coccidioides* antigens may be helpful.

A variety of clinical samples, including sputum, biopsies, and exudates, can be examined microscopically for the presence of spherules. The samples are treated with 10% potassium hydroxide and are examined using subdued lighting. The spherules are typically 30–60 μm in diameter, although spherules as large as 200 μm are occasionally seen. Spherules can be further positively identified by immunofluorescence.

Antibody to *Coccidioides* can be detected by a variety of tests. The complement fixation test and the enzyme immunoassay detect IgG antibodies to *Coccidioides.* In contrast, the immunodiffusion tube precipitin test and the latex agglutination test detect IgM antibodies, which appear during the second or third week of illness, peak at about 1 month, and disappear within 6 months. The primary disadvantage of the immunodiffusion and latex agglutination tests is that false-positive results occur in about 6% of individuals who are tested.

Skin tests using coccidioidin or spherulin are

available, but their use in adults in endemic areas is not useful unless it can be established that results in the adult being tested have recently converted from negative to positive. About 70–90% of adults living in the San Joaquin Valley show positive results in skin tests.

Culturing *C. immitis* is dangerous and should only be done in facilities whose technicians follow special precautions. Laboratory workers should be warned that the sample is suspected of containing *C. immitis*. The mycelial form of *C. immitis* can be grown in 3–14 days on Sabouraud's dextrose agar, and the identity of the fungus can be confirmed by one of the following methods: inoculating animals or utilizing special media to develop the characteristic spherules, using a DNA probe assay, or using an exoantigen test. Media containing cycloheximide will inhibit the growth of most saprophytic fungi that might be confused with *C. immitis*.

Treatment. Most patients who have primary coccidioidomycosis recover spontaneously without treatment. Antibiotic therapy is indicated for secondary (disseminated) infection. Amphotericin B is the antibiotic of choice for nonmeningeal coccidioidomycosis in all patients and for meningeal coccidioidomycosis in adults. A combination of ketoconazole and miconazole is used for meningeal coccidioidomycosis in children. Other drugs that have been used are fluconazole and itraconazole. In patients with nonmeningeal coccidioidomycosis, the cure rate is 50–70% for amphotericin B, 61% for fluconazole, and 57% for itraconazole. Relapses are seen in 25% of children and 40–50% of adults with meningeal coccidioidomycosis.

Paracoccidioidomycosis and *Paracoccidioides brasiliensis*

Paracoccidioidomycosis is an uncommon disease that occurs from Mexico to Argentina and Paraguay. Often called **South American blastomycosis,** it begins as a pulmonary infection and then disseminates, resulting in the formation of cutaneous and visceral granulomas. Patients generally seek treatment when the characteristic skin lesions appear. The agent of paracoccidioidomycosis is *Paracoccidioides brasiliensis*. Diagnosis is by culture, biopsy, and antibody tests, and patients are treated with itraconazole or ketoconazole.

DEEP MYCOSES CAUSED BY OPPORTUNISTIC FUNGI

As mentioned at the beginning of the chapter, the opportunistic fungi rarely affect immunocompetent individuals but cause life-threatening disease in immunocompromised patients.

Cryptococcosis and *Cryptococcus neoformans*

Cryptococcosis occurs primarily in patients with T cell immunodeficiencies and is caused by *Cryptococcus neoformans,* a fungus found in all parts of the world. Because the presence of cryptococcosis may herald an underlying immunosuppressive disease, such as cancer or AIDS, cryptococcosis is sometimes known as **signal disease.**

Characteristics of *C. neoformans*

General Features. *C. neoformans* is an encapsulated yeast (Fig. 18–6) that is not thermally dimorphic. There are several *Cryptococcus* species, but only *C. neoformans* causes systemic disease in humans. In vitro studies have shown that *C. neoformans* is the asexual form of the basidiomycete *Filobasidiella neoformans*.

Cryptococci grow to tremendous densities (about 5×10^7 yeasts per gram) in the feces of pigeons, starlings, blackbirds, and turkeys that pick up food in contaminated soil. These feces serve as excellent habitats not only for *Cryptococcus* but also for *Candida, Geotrichum,* and *Rhodotorula* because of their alkalinity and high content of nitrogen and salt.

When *C. neoformans* is growing in soil, little capsule is made unless nitrogen and moisture become limiting factors. Under these conditions, more capsule is synthesized, but it dehydrates and forms a thin protective layer around the yeast. This protects the yeast from becoming too dry and reduces the effective size of the yeast to about 5 μm—an ideal size to allow the yeast to enter the lower lung fields when an individual comes into contact with infected soil or feces. Once the yeast is inside the body, its capsule rehydrates and its effective size is increased to about 20 μm.

C. neoformans grows as a mucoid yeast on standard media such as Sabouraud's dextrose agar. The capsule can be easily demonstrated by India ink or nigrosin capsule stain. No pseudohyphae are formed, and serial subcultures can result in loss of the capsule. *C. neoformans* has urease activity that can be demonstrated using a rapid urease test. *C. neoformans* does not reduce nitrate to nitrite, and it produces a red-brown or maroon pigment when cultivated on niger seed agar. *C. neoformans* is distin-

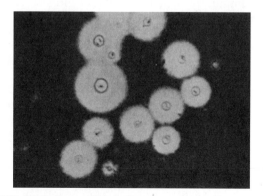

FIGURE 18–6. Encapsulated *Cryptococcus neoformans* organisms. (Reproduced, with permission, from Rippon, J. W. *In* Freeman, B. A. Burrows Textbook of Microbiology, 22nd ed. Philadelphia, W. B. Saunders Company, 1985.)

guished from other *Cryptococcus* species by its carbohydrate assimilation and fermentation reactions.

Mechanisms of Pathogenicity. The key virulence structure of *C. neoformans* is its capsule. The capsule inhibits phagocytosis and inhibits the ability of macrophages to process and present antigens. This protects the fungus from being internalized and destroyed by macrophages, monocytes, and polymorphonuclear leukocytes, and it diminishes the cellular immune response to cryptococci.

The capsule is composed primarily of a polysaccharide that is known as **glucuronoxylomannan** and is a complex of glucuronic acid, xylose, and mannan. Four serotypes of *C. neoformans* have been described. Serotypes A and D are designated as *C. neoformans* var. *neoformans,* while serotypes B and C are called *C. neoformans* var. *gattii* by some investigators. Serotype A has been implicated in 99% of AIDS-related cases of cryptococcosis in the USA, but serotypes B and C predominate in Europe. Glucuronoxylomannan has been reported to do the following: inhibit the alternative pathway of complement activation; cause neutrophils to shed L-selectin and reduce their expression of receptors for tumor necrosis factor; and cause monocytes to secrete interleukin-10, which down-regulates the production of proinflammatory cytokines.

Two other polysaccharide antigens have been described: **mannoprotein** and **galactoxylomannan.** Mannoprotein appears to be the key antigen in eliciting a cell-mediated immune response, but the function of galactoxylomannan is not understood.

C. neoformans releases mannitol into its environment. Investigators believe that the mannitol scavenges reactive oxygen intermediates and thereby protects intracellular cryptococci from being killed within phagosomes.

Cryptococcosis begins as an asymptomatic pulmonary infection. In immunocompetent hosts, the infection usually resolves when opsonizing antibody appears and a cell-mediated immune response occurs, causing the cryptococci to be phagocytosed and destroyed. Antibody-dependent cellular cytotoxicity, phagocytosis, and natural killer cell activities participate in clearing cryptococci. In patients whose T cell immunity is deficient, the cryptococci spread hematogenously and disseminate to a variety of organs, including the lungs, bones, kidneys, liver, and skin, but the central nervous system is most profoundly involved. In some cases, the cryptococci grow diffusely throughout the meninges and brain, producing cystic lesions called **pseudocysts.** Less commonly, a granulomatous lesion called a **cryptococcoma** develops. Some investigators have suggested that cryptococci grow well in the central nervous system because the granulocytic response there is poor and because the high concentrations of creatinine and asparagine in the brain are good sources of nitrogen for cryptococci.

Studies using a mouse model suggest that interleukin-12 plays a key role in protection against *C. neoformans* infections.

Management of Cryptococcosis

Diagnosis

(1) History and Physical Examination. Cryptococcosis occurs in four forms, as described below. The central nervous system disease is particularly associated with AIDS, and cryptococcal meningitis is estimated to occur in about 10% of AIDS patients. Males with meningoencephalitis outnumber females by 3 to 1.

(a) Pulmonary Cryptococcosis. Cryptococci grow initially in the lower lung fields, and the encapsulated yeasts resist phagocytosis until antibody appears. Most patients have no pulmonary symptoms. However, some patients develop a nonproductive cough, pleuritic pain, and weight loss, and a few exhibit an infiltrate and signs of pneumonia. Gelatinous nodules of encapsulated fungi can be found in the lung, but little inflammation occurs. A granuloma may be formed, but pulmonary cryptococcosis usually resolves spontaneously in patients with normal immune responses. Cryptococci disseminate in patients with T cell deficiencies.

(b) Cryptococcosis of the Central Nervous System. Cryptococcal meningoencephalitis occurs more frequently than cryptococcoma. Symptoms and signs of cryptococcal meningoencephalitis generally develop gradually over weeks or months. Severe headache is the first significant symptom and is followed by manifestations such as fever, nausea, vomiting, papilledema, nuchal rigidity, personality changes, slurred speech, clumsiness, and paralysis. Hydrocephalus is a common sequela. Patients with cryptococcoma suffer from focal neurologic changes including seizures.

(c) Cutaneous and Mucocutaneous Cryptococcosis. About 10–15% of European patients with cryptococcosis develop cutaneous and mucocutaneous lesions that begin as papules, pustules, or abscesses. These infections are caused by serotypes B and C of *C. neoformans.*

(d) Generalized Disseminated Cryptococcosis. Rarely, patients develop generalized disseminated disease, with cryptococcal granulomas in the bones, vertebrae, and viscera.

(2) Laboratory Analysis. Laboratory confirmation of cryptococcosis is based on direct examination of cerebrospinal fluid for the presence of cryptococci, on culture of the organisms, and on demonstration of the presence of cryptococcal antigens in body fluids.

The cerebrospinal fluid sample usually contains lymphocytes and shows elevated protein levels and depressed glucose levels. When cerebrospinal fluid is examined by India ink staining for the presence of encapsulated yeasts, positive results are found in about 50% of patients who have cryptococcosis but not AIDS and in 75% of patients who have both cryptococcosis and AIDS.

Cryptococci can be cultured from the cerebrospinal fluid of about 95% of patients with cryptococcosis of the central nervous system. A latex agglutination test that detects the presence of cryptococcal capsule antigens in cerebrospinal fluid is highly sensitive and specific, yielding positive results in about 90% of these patients.

Although antibody tests are not useful for diagnosis of cryptococcosis, such tests can be used along with the latex agglutination test to monitor a patient's response to treatment. If antigen levels increase but antibody levels drop, the prognosis is poor.

Treatment. Mild pulmonary cryptococcosis is not treated with antibiotics unless there is evidence that dissemination is occurring. Cryptococcal meningitis is usually treated with amphotericin B plus flucytosine, and fluconazole may also be used. This treatment causes improvement in 75% and cure in about 60% of patients. Cryptococcal infections of the central nervous system are uniformly fatal if untreated. Nonmeningeal cryptococcosis is usually treated with fluconazole; if this is ineffective, amphotericin B plus flucytosine may be administered.

Candidiasis and *Candida* Species

A variety of yeasts grow as normal flora on mucosal surfaces. These yeasts are controlled by the immune response, pH, and carbohydrate availability, as well as by bacteria that compete with yeasts for mucosal surfaces. When normal conditions change, yeasts may spread across the mucosal surface, and they may disseminate in immunocompromised patients. Opportunistic yeast infections are caused by a number of fungi that are not thermally dimorphic, including *Candida*, *Geotrichum*, *Rhodotorula*, *Trichosporon*, and *Cryptococcus* species other than *Cryptococcus neoformans*. Because the vast majority of opportunistic yeast infections are caused by *Candida albicans*, the discussion that follows will focus on this organism.

At least five conditions favor the development of candidiasis: (1) extreme youth; (2) physiologic changes, such as diabetes and pregnancy; (3) prolonged antibiotic usage; (4) general debility or constitutional inadequacy; and (5) penetration of the skin. Hippocrates was one of the first to describe yeast infections in debilitated patients, and Galen told how a yeast infection known as thrush was common among "sickly" children. Samuel Pepys described candidiasis in his now-famous diary, which was written in the 1660s.

Characteristics of *Candida* Species

General Features. Although *C. albicans* is the most common and pathogenic of the *Candida* species, other species have been identified in clinical specimens and include *Candida glabrata* (*Torulopsis glabrata*), *Candida guilliermondii*, *Candida krusei*, *Candida lusitaniae*, *Candida parapsilosis*, *Candida pseudotropicalis*, *Candida tropicalis*, and *Candida utilis*.

When cultivated on Sabouraud's dextrose agar at 37 °C, *C. albicans* grows within 24–48 hours as opaque white or cream-colored yeast colonies. The colonies of *C. albicans* are not distinctive, so identification of *C. albicans* rests on biochemical and other cultural characteristics. Carbohydrate assimilation and fermentation tests are also used to differentiate among the *Candida* species.

When grown on standard media, *C. albicans* grows as a yeast. In tissues, however, a mixture of yeasts, hyphae, pseudohyphae, and germ tubes is seen. These nutritionally based morphologic variations can be used to identify *C. albicans*. When placed in rabbit or human serum, *C. albicans* will form germ tubes (Fig. 18–7) within 2 hours. *Candida* species in general will form blastospores and hyphae when grown on cornmeal agar that contains polysorbate 80 (Tween 80), but only *C. albicans* will form chlamydospores.

Mechanisms of Pathogenicity. *C. albicans* is an opportunistic pathogen. It is normally found in small numbers on mucosal surfaces and spreads when conditions become favorable for it to do so. Several *C. albicans* adhesins have been identified, and these are believed to promote colonization by allowing *Candida* to persist on body surfaces. For example, a receptor analogous to complement receptor 3 (CR3) has been identified, and this receptor binds inactivated C3b (iC3b). Mannan and glycoprotein adhesins for host cells have also been identified. Some isolates of *C. albicans* are unusually hydrophobic and adhere tenaciously to catheters and other plastic surfaces.

Several *C. albicans* enzymes are believed to be

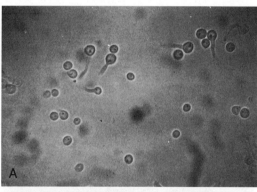
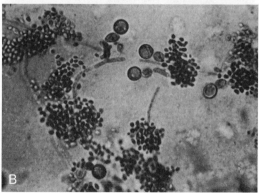

FIGURE 18–7. The germ tubes (A) and the chlamydospores and blastospores (B) of *Candida albicans*. (Reproduced, with permission, from Rippon, J. W. Medical Mycology: The Pathogenic Fungi and the Pathogenic Actinomycetes, 3rd ed. Philadelphia, W. B. Saunders Company, 1988.)

involved in the pathogenesis of candidiasis. Among these are various proteases, phospholipases, and lysophospholipases. In addition, the ability of *C. albicans* organisms to persist in tissue or to infect certain hosts may be related to their production of receptor proteins for steroids and their production of iron receptors known as siderophores.

Growth of *C. albicans* results in a profound immune response that is responsible for many of the clinical manifestations of candidiasis. This response, which is primarily cell-mediated, is depressed in patients who develop chronic mucocutaneous candidiasis. It is thought that circulating mannan fragments released by *Candida* suppress cellular immunity.

Management of Candidiasis

Diagnosis

(1) History and Physical Examination. *C. albicans* can cause a variety of mucocutaneous, cutaneous, systemic, and allergic manifestations of disease.

(a) Mucocutaneous Candidiasis. Oral candidiasis, or thrush, is the most common type of *Candida* infection. It occurs often in newborn infants born to mothers with vaginal candidiasis. It also occurs as a chronic infection in children with polyendocrine problems or immune response defects; in adults with AIDS, riboflavin deficiency, diabetes, or cancer; and in adults using corticosteroids or undergoing long-term antibiotic therapy. White pseudomembranes appear on the tongue, soft palate, and buccal mucosa (Fig. 18–8). These may crumble and look much like milk curds. If ulceration occurs, the lesions may be quite painful.

Esophageal candidiasis is usually an extension of oral thrush, especially in newborn infants, but is also occasionally seen in patients who have diabetes or are being treated with broad-spectrum antibiotics.

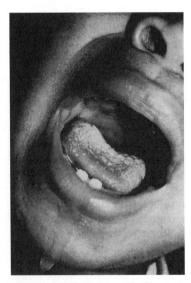

FIGURE 18–8. Oral candidiasis (thrush). (Reproduced, with permission, from Rippon, J. W. Medical Mycology: The Pathogenic Fungi and the Pathogenic Actinomycetes, 3rd ed. Philadelphia, W. B. Saunders Company, 1988.)

More than half of patients with AIDS develop oral and esophageal candidiasis. Manifestations of esophageal candidiasis include dysphagia, retrosternal pain, nausea, and vomiting.

Vaginal candidiasis may occur with conditions that change the vaginal pH, such as antibiotic use, oral contraceptive use, diabetes, and pregnancy (especially during the third trimester). Patients develop a thick yellow or milky discharge and have patches of gray-white pseudomembranes on the vaginal mucosa. Vaginal candidiasis is accompanied by itching and may be particularly severe just before menstruation. The source of infection is usually the gastrointestinal tract.

Intra-abdominal candidiasis is an infection of the stomach and may be seen in patients with disseminated candidiasis. Candidal peritonitis sometimes occurs in patients who have perforated ulcers, are receiving peritoneal dialysis, have undergone abdominal surgery, or have an abdominal neoplasm. Enteric candidiasis occasionally occurs as an overwhelming infection of the intestines during high-dose and prolonged use of broad-spectrum antibiotics.

Many deep fungal infections originate in the lungs. This is not so with *Candida* infections, because *C. albicans* is not a saprobe that releases spores into the environment and is inhaled. Thus, respiratory infections caused by *Candida* are rare. When they occur, they usually take the form of chronic bronchitis or pneumonia. Patients with chronic bronchitis have rales and curdlike patches in the bronchi. Candidal pneumonia occurs only in immunocompromised patients.

Chronic mucocutaneous candidiasis is an overwhelming mucocutaneous infection that occurs in children with familial defects of cell-mediated immunity or polymorphonuclear leukocytes, children with hypoadrenocorticism, and adults with thymomas.

(b) Cutaneous Candidiasis. Intertriginous candidiasis may occur in the groin, axillas, or intergluteal folds; beneath the breasts; or between the fingers and toes. The skin looks as if it has been scalded and has a red base and scalloped edges. The primary lesion is usually surrounded by smaller satellite lesions. Intertriginous candidiasis occurs most often in individuals who are obese, are chronic alcoholics, are often wet or sweat profusely, have skin areas that are continually macerated, or have burns. Candidiasis in burn victims may lead to fatal candidemia.

Candidal paronychia (infection of the cuticle) often appears as a painful red swelling of the nail cuticle. The infection may persist and spread to the nail itself, causing onychomycosis.

Cutaneous candidiasis is often seen in infants with diaper rash. The rash begins as irritation dermatitis, becomes infected with *Candida,* and is characterized by lesions that are red and painful. The infection may spread to other sites.

(c) Systemic Candidiasis. Patients with terminal debilitating conditions can develop several types of disseminated candidiasis, including urinary tract infections, endocarditis, meningitis, and septicemia.

Examples of predisposing conditions include AIDS, leukemia, corticosteroid use, organ transplant, and major surgery.

(d) Allergic Candidiasis. Patients with *C. albicans* infection can develop a number of types of allergic reactions to the yeast, including id reactions, asthma, allergic eczema, and gastritis. Allergic balanitis (inflammation of the glans penis) sometimes occurs following intercourse with a woman who has vaginal candidiasis.

(2) Laboratory Analysis. Laboratory diagnosis of candidiasis involves direct demonstration of *Candida* in clinical specimens and cultivation of *C. albicans.*

A wide variety of specimens, ranging from crusts to exudates to tissue sections can be examined directly for the presence of *C. albicans.* Samples are generally cleared by pretreatment with 10% potassium hydroxide and are then stained with standard biologic stains. When crusts of fungal growth are examined, the sample can be stained with Gram's stain. *C. albicans* will appear as a mixture of yeasts, hyphae, and pseudohyphae.

C. albicans can be cultivated on Sabouraud's dextrose agar. Demonstration that the yeasts produce germ tubes in serum will presumptively identify the yeast as *C. albicans.* The isolate should then be tested for blastospore and chlamydospore formation to place it within the genus *Candida,* and carbohydrate assimilation and fermentation tests can be used to speciate the organism. If the yeast forms arthrospores and no blastospores, it is likely to be a *Trichosporon* or *Geotrichum* species. These organisms can be differentiated by performing a urease test (*Trichosporon* is urease-positive).

Treatment. See Table 18–1. In general, systemic candidiasis is treated with amphotericin B, and localized *Candida* infections are treated with nystatin or azole antibiotics.

TABLE 18–1. Recommended Antifungal Agents for the Treatment of Mucocutaneous, Cutaneous, and Systemic Candidiasis

Disease	Recommended Treatment
Mucocutaneous candidiasis	
Oral candidiasis (thrush)	Nystatin or clotrimazole.
Esophageal candidiasis	Fluconazole, nystatin, or clotrimazole.
Vaginal candidiasis	Topical miconazole, clotrimazole, butoconazole, tioconazole, or terconazole; or oral fluconazole.
Intra-abdominal candidiasis	Amphotericin B plus flucytosine.
Chronic mucocutaneous candidiasis	Ketoconazole or amphotericin B.
Cutaneous candidiasis	Topical amphotericin B, clotrimazole, econazole, ketoconazole, miconazole, or nystatin.
Systemic candidiasis	Amphotericin B or fluconazole.

Aspergillosis and *Aspergillus* Species

About 700 species of *Aspergillus* are distributed throughout almost every known environment. They are in the soil, on decaying vegetation, on hay and straw, in the dust found in air-conditioning vents, and in rotting bird feces. They are the bottle imps floating in "old" bottles of reagents or media. Not only have the organisms been found by scientists in the Sahara and the Antarctic, but their spores have been encountered by balloonists in the upper atmosphere. Their ubiquity prompted W. B. Cook to refer to the planet as "this moldy earth."

With so many aspergilli around, it would not be surprising if *Aspergillus* either infected every human being or infected no human beings at all. In fact, however, the organism rarely causes infection in healthy people. Aspergillosis usually occurs in immunocompromised patients, particularly those with depressed cell-mediated immunity or chronic cavitary disease.

Characteristics of *Aspergillus* Species

General Features. The four *Aspergillus* species most often responsible for human disease are *Aspergillus flavus, Aspergillus fumigatus, Aspergillus niger,* and *Aspergillus terreus.* When cultivated on standard mycologic media, *Aspergillus* species grow as molds that exhibit septate hyphae and specialized fruiting bodies known as conidiophores. The fungus was named *Aspergillus* because each fruiting body (Fig. 18–9) resembles an aspergillum, which is a perforated globe used to sprinkle holy water during Catholic religious ceremonies. The term comes from the Latin word *aspergo,* which means "to sprinkle."

The individual *Aspergillus* species are identified by the color and gross appearance of the mycelial mass and by the microscopic appearance of the characteristic fruiting bodies. Two *Aspergillus* species that are occasionally isolated from humans—*Aspergillus glaucus* and *Aspergillus nidulans*—form ascospores.

Mechanisms of Pathogenicity. The pathogenesis of invasive diseases due to *Aspergillus* species is not well described. Cell wall glycoproteins of *A. fumigatus* and *A. flavus* have been shown to have endotoxinlike activity and are able to elicit hemorrhage and necrosis. The ability of *A. fumigatus* to cause invasive disease in mice has been linked with production of elastase. The ability of the various *Aspergillus* species to invade tissue is also likely assisted by their production of siderophores that allow them to compete for iron.

Allergic aspergillosis (farmer's lung) occurs in individuals who have inhaled a large number of *Aspergillus* spores. The allergic response is believed to involve three types of immunologic reactions to *Aspergillus* antigens: a type I (IgE or immediate-type hypersensitivity) reaction, a type III (IgG or Arthustype) reaction, and a type IV (delayed-type hypersensitivity) reaction.

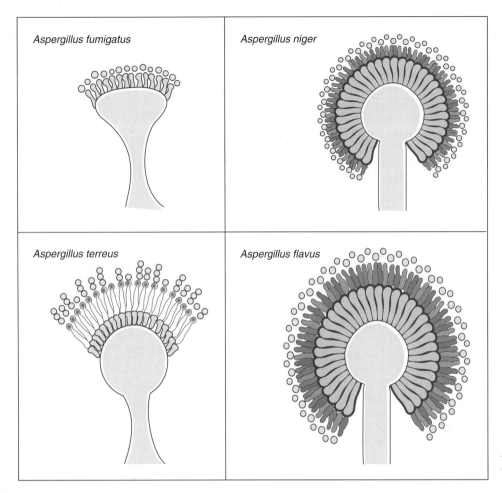

Aspergillus fumigatus

Aspergillus niger

Aspergillus terreus

Aspergillus flavus

FIGURE 18–9. Fruiting bodies of *Aspergillus fumigatus, Aspergillus niger, Aspergillus terreus,* and *Aspergillus flavus.*

Management of Aspergillosis

Diagnosis

(1) History and Physical Examination. There are numerous localized and disseminated forms of *Aspergillus* infection. Seven major forms of infection are discussed here.

(a) Mycetoma. When a large number of *Aspergillus* (usually *A. fumigatus*) conidia are inhaled, the fungi may grow in the lung, eventually forming a ball of fungal mycelia and conidia in a cavity in the tissues. Mycetoma (fungus ball) is rarely seen in healthy individuals and most often occurs in patients who have an immunosuppressive disease or have pulmonary cavities left by tuberculosis or histoplasmosis. The range of clinical manifestations is large. In some cases, the mycetoma causes no symptoms and is discovered incidentally on x-ray. In other cases, mycetoma causes hemoptysis, bronchiectasis, eosinophilia, thrombogenesis, and allergic symptoms and may have a fatal outcome.

(b) Invasive Aspergillosis. Invasive aspergillosis may occur as a sequela of mycetoma or arise independently of mycetoma. Patients with invasive aspergillosis typically suffer from pneumonia, respiratory distress, fever, cough, and leukocytosis. There are fungi in the sputum, and the disease can progress rapidly. The typical x-ray picture is that of broncho-

pneumonia with multiple peripheral patchy focal infiltrates. The fungi invade the tissues and the vasculature, causing thrombosis and ischemia. Emboli can break off and be spread throughout the body, carrying aspergilli with them. Patients with severe disease develop fulminating necrotizing pneumonia.

(c) Disseminated Aspergillosis. Disseminated aspergillosis occurs sometimes as an extension of a pulmonary infection with *Aspergillus*. Almost all patients have an underlying condition such as hepatitis, leukemia, diarrhea, eclampsia, or pneumonia, and some have been receiving high-dose treatment with antibiotics or corticosteroids. The signs and symptoms of disseminated aspergillosis are consistent with the occurrence of *Aspergillus* infection in specific organs.

(d) Otitis Externa. Infection of the outer ear canal (otitis externa) is often accompanied by itching, scaling, and a foul odor. Otitis externa is sometimes caused by bacteria and may be caused by many saprophytic fungi, but *A. niger* is one of the agents found in about 90% of the cases.

(e) Endophthalmitis. Endophthalmitis may appear 2–3 weeks after an eye injury and be caused by *Aspergillus*. The patient's vision becomes clouded, and the conjunctiva appears red. Pain is caused by the accumulation of pus in the anterior chamber (hypopyon).

(f) Allergic Aspergillosis.   Individuals exposed to large doses of spores may develop an allergic reaction that can be life-threatening. This condition, known as farmer's lung, is frequently caused by the spores of *Aspergillus* (particularly *A. flavus, A. fumigatus, and A. niger*), *Penicillium,* or other fungi. However, it may be caused by the spores of actinomycetes such as *Micromonospora faeni, Micromonospora vulgaris,* and *Thermopolyspora polyspora.* These agents are bacteria, rather than fungi.

Farmer's lung can be acute, subacute, or chronic. Typical manifestations include shallow breathing, dyspnea following exertion, discolored lips, cough, and weakness. Acute attacks are sometimes fatal, and chronic disease can also lead to death. The lungs undergo fibrotic changes, and there may be interstitial edema, lymphocyte infiltration, vasculitis, and bronchiolitis. Granulomas resembling sarcoid may develop and sometimes become quite large and calcified.

Similar allergic syndromes are elicited by other fungi: bird fancier's lung, caused by *Aspergillus* or *Penicillium;* maple bark stripper's disease, caused by *Cryptostroma,* a fungus that grows under maple bark; allergic scopulariopsosis, caused by a fungus that grows on opium; bagassosis, caused by breathing the conidia of fungi that grow on sugar cane; byssinosis, caused by breathing fungi that grow on cotton plants; and lycoperdonosis, caused by breathing conidia of puffball mushrooms.

(g) Aflatoxin-Related Diseases.   When *A. flavus* grows on peanuts, wheat, or rice, it produces a toxin known as aflatoxin (Fig. 18–10). There are six different aflatoxin types, all of which are structurally similar and structurally related to the coumarins. The ingestion of foods containing aflatoxin is a major risk factor for the development of primary hepatocellular carcinoma and is also a risk factor for Reye's syndrome, which is an acute encephalopathy accompanied by fatty degeneration of the liver and renal tubules. In the USA, Reye's syndrome is normally associated with viral infections. In Thailand, however, aflatoxin

was implicated as the agent responsible for a major outbreak of Reye's syndrome, and it was found that children who snacked on bowls of moist rice infected with *Aspergillus* often developed fatal Reye's syndrome.

(2) Laboratory Analysis.   Laboratory confirmation of localized and invasive *Aspergillus* infections is based on visualizing the characteristic hyphae in tissues or exudate samples and on culturing the organisms on standard mycologic media. The presence of antibody may assist in the diagnosis of some types of aspergillosis.

Aspergillus can be visualized in clinical specimens stained with periodic acid–Schiff stain or with Grocott-Gomori methenamine–silver nitrate stain. The septate hyphae can often be seen growing within infarcted blood vessels, and calcium oxalate crystals may be seen in the surrounding tissues. Samples taken from pulmonary mycetomas contain poorly staining and lifeless-looking hyphae with abundant conidia.

Aspergillus should be cultivated on a medium that does not contain cycloheximide. The fungi are identified by their colony color and morphology and by their characteristic fruiting bodies.

Patients with allergic aspergillosis are eosinophilic and have IgE antibodies to *Aspergillus.* These antibodies can be demonstrated by a radioallergosorbent test. A skin test can also be used to diagnose allergic aspergillosis. Intradermal injection of antigen elicits a type I hypersensitivity reaction (IgE-mediated wheal and flare) followed several hours later by a type III reaction. *Aspergillus* may also be cultured from patients with allergic aspergillosis.

Treatment.   Treatment of mycetoma with antibiotics has not proved to be highly successful. Mycetomas can be surgically removed, and oral itraconazole has been used with some success. Invasive and disseminated *Aspergillus* infections are treated with amphotericin B, sometimes with rifampin given as an adjunct. Otitis externa can be treated with aluminum subacetate irrigation or with creams that contain nystatin or clotrimazole. Endophthalmitis is treated by removing the infected eye. Allergic aspergillosis is treated with corticosteroids and itraconazole.

Mucormycosis and the Zygomycetes

Mucormycosis is an invasive infection caused by saprophytic organisms of the order Mucorales. The most common mucormycoses are opportunistic infections of the blood vessels of the paranasal sinuses and the brain. These infections were once called **phycomycoses** and are referred to by some investigators as **zygomycoses.** The infections can be caused by a wide variety of fungi, including *Absidia, Aphophysomyces, Cunninghamella, Mortierella, Mucor, Rhizomucor, Rhizopus,* and *Saksenaea.*

Characteristics of the Zygomycetes

General Features.   The Mucorales are zygomycetes and are ubiquitous in the environment. They

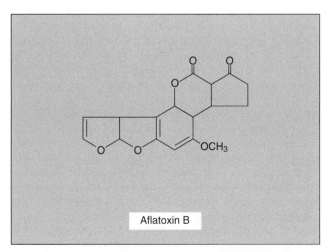

Aflatoxin B

FIGURE 18–10. Molecular structure of aflatoxin B.

are not thermally dimorphic. Although they grow as molds at a wide range of temperatures (25–55 °C), the optimum temperature for most of them is 25–30 °C. Zygomycetes grow rapidly and prolifically on standard mycologic media, forming fluffy colonies that have no definite edge. They are sometimes referred to as "lid lifters" because their prolific growth pushes up the lid of the Petri dish.

Rhizopus (Fig. 18–11) and other zygomycetes are

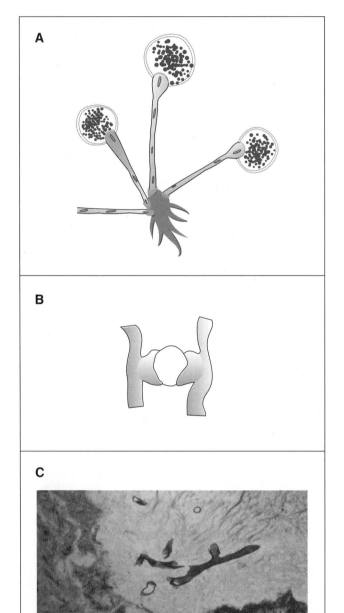

FIGURE 18–11. Sporangiophore (A), sexual ascospore (B), and broad aseptate hyphae (C) of *Rhizopus*. (Photomicrograph reproduced, with permission, from Rippon, J. W. Medical Mycology: The Pathogenic Fungi and the Pathogenic Actinomycetes, 3rd ed. Philadelphia, W. B. Saunders Company, 1988.)

identified by their gross and microscopic morphologies. Zygomycetes have broad aseptate hyphae and both zygospores and sporangiospores. *Rhizopus* and *Absidia* exhibit specialized rootlike structures called rhizoids at the base of each sporangiophore.

Mechanisms of Pathogenicity. Infections are acquired by breathing the spores of zygomycetes. Most individuals are not colonized by zygomycetes, but individuals with risk factors that affect immune responsiveness develop diseases specific to their immune defect. Thus, diabetic patients with ketoacidosis develop rhinocerebral mucormycosis; leukemic patients with neutropenia develop rhinocerebral, pulmonary, or disseminated mucormycosis; children with protein-calorie malnutrition (kwashiorkor) develop gastrointestinal or abdominal-pelvic mucormycosis; and patients receiving deferoxamine in conjunction with hemodialysis develop disseminated mucormycosis.

It is not well understood why zygomycetes tend to invade blood vessels or how they cause necrosis and hemorrhage. Studies have shown that alveolar macrophages from healthy mice block the germination of *Rhizopus* spores but that macrophages from diabetic mice allow the spores to germinate normally. Diabetic mice rapidly develop rhinocerebral mucormycosis when they breathe *Rhizopus* spores. Some investigators believe that *Rhizopus* preferentially infects the rhinocerebral blood vessels of diabetics because the organism thrives at 39 °C, grows well in the presence of an acid pH, and has an active ketoreductase.

Management of Mucormycosis

Diagnosis

(1) History and Physical Examination. The three most prevalent forms of mucormycosis are discussed below. Mucormycosis also occurs as disseminated or central nervous system disease.

(a) Rhinocerebral Mucormycosis. Rhinocerebral mucormycosis is the most fulminating of fungal diseases, with death sometimes occurring as early as 2 days after infection. Almost all cases are caused by *Rhizopus arrhizus (Rhizopus oryzae)*. The infection begins with the germination of *Rhizopus* spores in the nose or nasal sinuses. The hyphae invade vascular channels, particularly those of the arterial series, and pass through them to the cerebral circulation and the brain. Their progression is marked by thrombosis, infarction, and necrosis. The brain itself becomes necrotic, and the frontal lobes are softened.

Clinical manifestations include facial pain, headaches, fever, and a dark bloody nasal discharge. Invasion down to the mouth is evidenced by the formation of a black, necrotic eschar on the palate. The eyes may bulge outward (exophthalmos), and the conjunctivas may swell around the cornea (chemosis). The patient rapidly develops seizures, and death generally occurs between days 7 and 10. Computed tomography scans and x-rays reveal soft tissue swelling and bone destruction.

(b) Pulmonary Mucormycosis. Those most likely to develop pulmonary mucormycosis are neutropenic patients who have leukemia or lymphoma and patients who have received bone marrow transplants. Pulmonary mucormycosis often begins suddenly with chest pain due to progressive pneumonia. Fever and dyspnea are also noted. There may be extensive pulmonary infarction, and some patients develop massive cavitary lesions. Chest x-rays do not adequately demonstrate the severity of the disease, because patients develop little inflammatory infiltrate.

(c) Gastrointestinal Mucormycosis. Children with severe protein-calorie malnutrition (kwashiorkor) are those most likely to develop gastrointestinal mucormycosis. The extent of infection and sites of infection within the gastrointestinal tract vary greatly among patients. The stomach, ileum, and colon are most often affected. Patients have signs of intraabdominal abscess and often pass bloody (rather than tarry) stools (hematochezia). Gastrointestinal mucormycosis generally spreads to the peritoneum, and death occurs after an average of 70 days. The diagnosis is usually made postmortem.

(2) Laboratory Analysis. Zygomycetes can be cultured from tissue samples, but diagnosis of the fulminating diseases rests on observing the aseptate hyphae of the zygomycetes in tissue samples (see Fig. 18–11C).

Treatment. Mucormycoses are treated by surgically debriding devitalized and infected tissues, instituting aggressive antibiotic therapy, and correcting the patient's predisposing condition. Debridement may have to be performed on several consecutive days. Intravenous amphotericin B is the antibiotic of choice. The mortality rate for untreated rhinocerebral mucormycosis is about 90%, but aggressive surgical and antibiotic treatment coupled with appropriate management of diabetes can reduce this rate to about 20%.

Selected Readings

Bradsher, R. W. Blastomycosis. Clin Infect Dis 14(supplement 1):S82–S90, 1992.

Bradsher, R. W. Histoplasmosis and blastomycosis. Clin Infect Dis 22(supplement 2):S102–S111, 1996.

Butugan, O., et al. Rhinocerebral mucormycosis: predisposing factors, diagnosis, therapy, complications, and survival. Rev Laryngol Otol Rhinol (Bord) 117:53–55, 1996.

Chaturvedi, V., et al. Oxidative killing of *Cryptococcus neoformans* by human neutrophils: evidence that fungal mannitol protects by scavenging reactive oxygen intermediates. J Immunol 156:3836–3840, 1996.

Cherniak, R., and J. B. Sundstrom. Polysaccharide antigens of the capsule of *Cryptococcus neoformans.* Infect Immun 62:1507–1512, 1994.

DeRepentigny, L. Serodiagnosis of candidiasis, aspergillosis, and cryptococcosis. Clin Infect Dis 14(supplement 1):S11–S22, 1992.

Dong, Z. M., and J. W. Murphy. Cryptococcal polysaccharides induce L-selectin shedding and tumor necrosis factor receptor loss from the surface of human neutrophils. J Clin Invest 97:689–698, 1996.

Eissenberg, L. G., and W. E. Goldman. *Histoplasma* variation and adaptive strategies for parasitism: new perspectives on histoplasmosis. Clin Microbiol Rev 4:411–421, 1991.

Goldman, D., S. C. Lee, and A. Casadevall. Pathogenesis of pulmonary *Cryptococcus neoformans* infection in the rat. Infect Immun 62:4755–4761, 1994.

Gurney, J. W., and D. J. Conces. Pulmonary histoplasmosis. Radiology 199:297–306, 1996.

Kaufman, L. Laboratory methods for the diagnosis and confirmation of systemic mycoses. Clin Infect Dis 14(supplement 1):S23–S29, 1992.

Kawakami, K., et al. Interleukin-12 protects mice against pulmonary and disseminated infection caused by *Cryptococcus neoformans.* Clin Exp Immunol 104:208–214, 1996.

Levitz, S. M., and E. A. North. Gamma interferon gene expression and release in human lymphocytes directly activated by *Cryptococcus neoformans* and *Candida albicans.* Infect Immun 64:1595–1599, 1996.

Magee, D. M., and R. A. Cox. Interleukin-12 regulation of host defenses against *Coccidioides immitis.* Infect Immun 64:3609–3613, 1996.

Retini, C., et al. Capsular polysaccharide of *Cryptococcus neoformans* induces proinflammatory cytokine release by human neutrophils. Infect Immun 64:2897–2903, 1996.

Rippon, J. W. Medical Mycology: The Pathogenic Fungi and the Pathogenic Actinomycetes, 3rd ed. Philadelphia, W. B. Saunders Company, 1988.

Sposto, M. R., et al. Oral paracoccidioidomycosis: a study of 36 patients. Oral Surg Oral Med Oral Pathol 75:461–465, 1993.

Stansell, J. D. Pulmonary fungal infections in HIV-infected persons. Semin Respir Infect 8:116–123, 1993.

Sugar, A. M. Mucormycosis. Clin Infect Dis 14(supplement 1):S126–S129, 1992.

Sugar, A. M., and M. Picard. Macrophage- and oxidant-mediated inhibition of the ability of live *Blastomyces dermatitidis* conidia to transform to the pathogenic yeast phase: implications for the pathogenesis of dimorphic fungal infections. J Infect Dis 163:371–375, 1991.

Treseler, C. B., and A. M. Sugar. Fungal meningitis. Infect Dis Clin North Am 4:789–808, 1990.

Vartivarian, S. E. Virulence properties and nonimmune pathogenetic mechanisms of fungi. Clin Infect Dis 14(supplement 1):S30–S36, 1992.

Vecchiarelli, A., et al. Purified capsular polysaccharide of *Cryptococcus neoformans* induces interleukin-10 secretion by human monocytes. Infect Immun 64:2846–2849, 1996.

Wheat, L. J. Histoplasmosis in Indianapolis. Clin Infect Dis 14(supplement 1):S91–S99, 1992.

Zhong, Z., and L. A. Pirofski. Opsonization of *Cryptococcus neoformans* by human anticryptococcal glucuronoxylomannan antibodies. Infect Immun 64:3446–3450, 1996.

VIRUSES AND

VIRAL DISEASES

OVERVIEW OF VIROLOGY

AND ANTIVIRAL AGENTS

The science of virology was founded in 1892, when Dmitri Ivanovski discovered that mosaic disease of tobacco plants could be transmitted and that the agent of the disease was not a bacterium, since it could be passed through a filter capable of trapping bacteria. Shortly thereafter, Martinus Beijerinck showed that the filterable agent of tobacco mosaic disease could diffuse through an agar gel or could be precipitated in alcohol and that the precipitated agent was still infectious. Because these properties were unknown in any living microbe, Beijerinck concluded that mosaic disease was caused not by a live agent but by a "fluid infectious principle." It was not until 1935 that W. M. Stanley showed that the disease was caused by tobacco mosaic virus, an organism composed mostly of a crystallizable protein.

The first viruses to be thoroughly studied were not agents of human or animal disease but instead were viruses that infect bacteria. In 1915, Frederick Twort and Félix d'Herelle independently reported the existence of bacterial viruses, or **bacteriophages** (often shortened to "phages"). At this time, studies using animal viruses were extremely difficult because cell cultures had not yet been developed. Nevertheless, the early studies of Twort, d'Herelle, and others concerning bacteriophage structure and replication laid the groundwork for subsequent work on human and animal viruses.

HUMAN VIRUSES
Classification of Viruses

Viruses are nucleic acid fragments that are enclosed within a protein shell. They are obligately intracellular parasites because they are absolutely dependent on host cells to complete their replication. When they enter a host cell, they disassemble and construct new viruses by using a combination of host- and virus-encoded enzymes. Viruses cannot produce their own energy and have no endogenous metabolic activity. Thus, they are fundamentally different from all bacteria, including obligately intracellular bacteria.

Classification as Infectious Entities

The structure and composition of viruses were not known until scientists understood the nature of nucleic acids and developed the techniques of electron microscopy, which allowed viral particles to be seen. Thus, early attempts to name and classify viruses were based on the diseases they caused. For example, viruses that caused measles and influenza were simply named measles virus and influenza virus. Then epidemiologic information, such as mode of transmission and site of infection, was used to classify the various viruses as arboviruses (in which *arbo* stands for *ar*thropod-*bo*rne), enteric viruses, hepatitis viruses, respiratory viruses, and sexually transmitted viruses, as shown in Table 19–1.

Classification by Structure

During the 1950s, electron microscopy was used extensively to examine viral particles, and molecular biology was born, allowing the structure and significance of viral nucleic acid to be appreciated. Electron microscopic studies not only expanded the body of knowledge concerning the nature of viruses but also led to new ways of classifying viruses, based on their shapes, structures, and content.

Fig. 19–1 shows the general structures of several representative viruses. Viruses are pieces of DNA or RNA that are packaged within a protein shell known as a **capsid.** This shell may also enclose enzymes that are needed to replicate the virus, and some viral capsids contain histones or histone-like proteins. Capsids that contain nucleic acid are known as **nucleocapsids.** Each nucleocapsid contains DNA or RNA, but never both. The nucleic acid may have a single or double strand, and all viruses except retroviruses are haploid. Some RNA viruses contain multiple RNA fragments and are said to have a **segmented genome.**

Viruses are extremely small, with the genomes of some viruses encoding fewer than five genes. Thus, the relatively large viral capsid must be constructed from many copies of a few types of subunits, or **protomers.** To accomplish this, most animal viruses construct **helical capsids** or **icosahedral capsids.** A few large animal viruses and some bacteriophages are enclosed within **complex capsids.**

Viruses may be nonenveloped ("naked"), or they may acquire an **envelope** by budding through a host

TABLE 19–1. Classification of Viruses on the Basis of Mode of Transmission or Site of Infection

Virus Group	Characteristics	Examples
Arboviruses	Spread by the bites of mosquitoes, ticks, or sandflies.	Bunyaviruses; flaviviruses; some reoviruses (orbiviruses); some rhabdoviruses; and togaviruses.
Enteric viruses	Infect the gastrointestinal tract; may cause local or systemic infection, with or without gastrointestinal symptoms.	Some adenoviruses; astroviruses; caliciviruses; some coronaviruses; picornaviruses; and rotaviruses.
Hepatitis viruses	Infect the liver.	Hepatitis viruses A, B, C, D, and E.
Respiratory viruses	Generally cause upper respiratory tract disease, but some infect the lungs.	Some adenoviruses; some coronaviruses; orthomyxoviruses; some paramyxoviruses; and rhinoviruses.
Sexually transmitted viruses	Spread by sexual contact; may cause local or systemic infection.	Some hepatitis viruses; some herpesviruses; some papillomaviruses; and some retroviruses.

membrane. Although most enveloped viruses bud through the cell membrane, the flaviviruses, coronaviruses, and bunyaviruses bud through the Golgi complex or rough endoplasmic reticulum, and the herpesviruses bud through the nuclear membrane. The viral envelope contains **lipids** from the host and **proteins** that are encoded by viral genes. Depending on the virus, two types of proteins may be found within the envelope: matrix proteins and glycoproteins.

Some of the enveloped RNA viruses contain **matrix proteins** that are inserted into the cytoplasmic side of the cell membrane. Matrix proteins act as a link between the viral capsid and its envelope. Enveloped viruses that have a matrix protein are rigid, while those that lack matrix proteins are pleomorphic.

Glycoproteins are the major external antigen of enveloped viruses and are inserted at membrane sites where budding will take place. The glycoproteins, which are also known as **peplomers,** often appear as spikes on the surface of the virus. As Fig. 19–2 shows, their hydrophobic end is inserted into the membrane, and a glycosylated hydrophilic portion of the protein extends into the external environment. Viral glycoproteins may serve as hemagglutinins, cell fusion promoters, or adhesins, or they may have neuraminidase activity.

Virologists have used these characteristics to classify viruses by shape and by nucleic acid content.

Classification by Shape and Envelope. As outlined in Table 19–2, viruses have been separated into three major groups on the basis of whether they have icosahedral, helical, or complex capsids. These groups are further subdivided on the basis of whether the viruses are nonenveloped or enveloped. The purposes of the capsid are to protect the viral DNA from digestion by nucleases and to provide adhesins that will allow nonenveloped viruses to attach to and invade host cells. The envelope influences the stability of the virus under various environmental conditions. For example, all enteroviruses are nonenveloped; viruses with envelopes are inactivated when they pass through the gastrointestinal tract.

(1) Helical, Enveloped Viruses. The tobacco mosaic virus was the first helical virus that was described. The RNA of this virus is wound as a helix, and the protomers of the capsid are attached to the RNA (Fig. 19–3). All helical animal viruses are RNA viruses, and all are enclosed within a lipid envelope derived from the host cell membrane. In each case, the diameter of the capsid is determined by the physi-

FIGURE 19–1. Structures of some representative viruses. Picornaviruses and adenoviruses show the typical shape of icosahedral, nonenveloped viruses. The herpes simplex virus has the typical shape of icosahedral, enveloped viruses. Parainfluenza virus is a helical, enveloped virus. Bacteriophage T4 shows the complex structure seen among the T-even bacteriophages. Viruses are not drawn to scale.

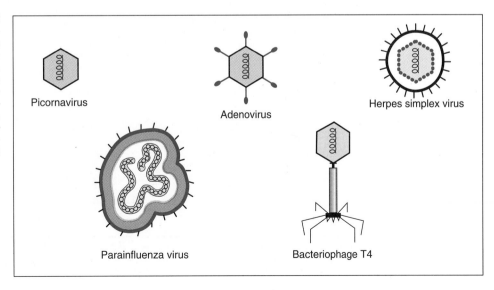

Picornavirus

Adenovirus

Herpes simplex virus

Parainfluenza virus

Bacteriophage T4

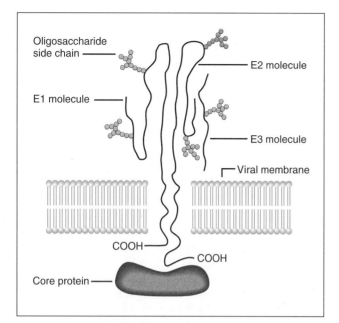

FIGURE 19–2. The structure of the peplomer (glycoprotein spike) of a togavirus. The spike is constructed from three virus-encoded glycoprotein molecules (E1, E2, and E3), two of which extend from the host membrane into the environment, with their carboxyl ends passing through the cell membrane into the interior of the cell.

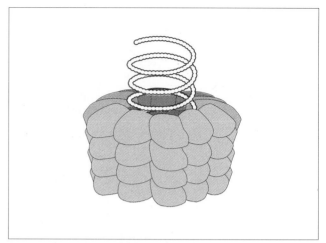

FIGURE 19–3. The structure of tobacco mosaic virus. The viral proteins are arranged around the helically coiled RNA.

cal characteristics of the protomers, and the length of the virus is determined by the length of the RNA helix. When viewed by electron microscopy, helical viruses may appear spherical, filamentous, or bullet-shaped; the general shape of the virus is determined by the shape of the envelope that encloses the nucleocapsid. Helical viruses that possess a matrix protein have a distinct shape, while those that lack matrix proteins tend to be pleomorphic.

(2) Icosahedral, Enveloped and Nonenveloped Viruses. An icosahedron is a regular polyhedron with 20 triangular faces and 12 corners. Icosahedrons are roughly spherical and are the geometric basis for the architectural structure known as a geodesic dome. Most DNA and some RNA viruses have icosahedral capsids. The icosahedral shape of the capsid is constructed from many subunits that are known as **capsomers** and are actually short ribbons of identical protomers arranged in a circular fashion with a central pore (Fig. 19–4). Two types of capsomers exist: **pentons,** which contain 5 protomers, and **hexons,** which contain 3 or 6 protomers. Most icosahedral

TABLE 19–2.   **Classification of DNA and RNA Viruses on the Basis of Shape, Envelope, and Diameter**

Virus Group	Shape and Envelope	Example	Diameter (nm)
DNA viruses	Icosahedral, nonenveloped	*Adenoviridae*	80–90
		Hepadnaviridae	42
		Papovaviridae	45–55
		Parvoviridae	18–26
	Icosahedral, enveloped	*Herpesviridae*	120–200
	Complex, enveloped	*Poxviridae*	200–300*
RNA viruses	Icosahedral, nonenveloped	*Astroviridae*	28–30
		Caliciviridae	27–40
		Deltavirus	32
		Picornaviridae	25–30
		Reoviridae	70–80
	Icosahedral, enveloped	*Flaviviridae*	40–50
		Retroviridae	80–100
		Togaviridae	60–70
	Helical, enveloped	*Arenaviridae*	110–130
		Bunyaviridae	90–100
		Coronaviridae	60–220
		Filoviridae	800–1400†
		Orthomyxoviridae	80–120
		Paramyxoviridae	150–300
		Rhabdoviridae	170–200

* Members of the *Poxviridae* family are brick-shaped and generally measure about 250 nm by 200 nm.
† Members of the *Filoviridae* family are oblong and generally measure about 800–1400 nm by 80 nm. Some individual virions may reach up to 14,000 nm in length.

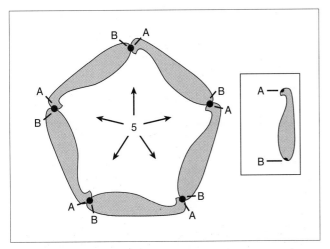

FIGURE 19–4. Arrangement of five asymmetric protomers into a closed ring. The capsomer formed by these protomers has fivefold rotational symmetry. A and B are recognition sites that allow the protomer to form a closed ring.

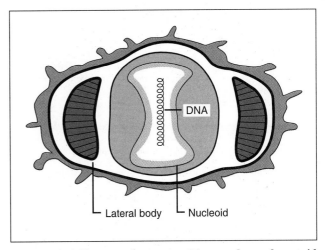

FIGURE 19–6. The general structure of the complex nucleocapsid of poxviruses. The poxvirus depicted here is vaccinia virus. Poxvirus DNA lies coiled within the nucleoid, which is surrounded by a virus-encoded membrane that also encloses two large lateral bodies.

viruses contain both pentons and hexons, but the smallest icosahedrons are constructed from 12 pentons alone. When an icosahedron is rotated in various directions, it is possible to see that each icosahedron has fivefold, threefold, and twofold symmetry (Fig. 19–5). As shown in Table 19–2, icosahedral viruses may be enveloped or nonenveloped.

(3) Complex, Enveloped Viruses. Among the animal viruses, only poxviruses are packaged within complex nucleocapsids (Fig. 19–6). Poxvirus capsids are roughly brick-shaped, have a host-derived envelope, and appear to contain many rodlets. The capsid core is dumbbell-shaped, and two lateral bodies can be seen within the nucleocapsid.

Classification by Nucleic Acid Characteristics. Table 19–3 classifies the viruses by their nucleic acid characteristics and nucleocapsid contents. As noted earlier, viruses can contain DNA or RNA, but not both. The nucleic acid may be double-stranded (ds) or single-stranded (ss), and some RNA viruses contain multiple unique RNA segments. Although the retroviruses are diploid, the other viruses are haploid.

Taxonomic Classification

Since 1966, the animal viruses have been systematically classified on the basis of a variety of characteristics, including nucleic acid composition, capsid shape, presence of envelope, and genetic homology. Under this scheme, viruses are organized into orders (designated by the suffix -*virales*), families (-*viridae*), subfamilies (-*virinae*), and genera (-*virus*). The viral species are designated by their common names. Table 19–4 organizes the various viruses by their taxonomic classifications and lists specific diseases associated with the viruses.

Replication of Viruses

To be replicated, a virus must undergo the following processes: (1) attachment to a host cell, (2) entry into the host cell, (3) uncoating, (4) replication of parts, (5) assembly into new viruses, and (6) escape from the host cell.

Fig. 19–7 depicts a one-step replication curve for a typical virus. To produce this growth curve, a monolayer of cultured cells is overlaid with a viral suspension that contains hundreds or thousands of

FIGURE 19–5. The fivefold (A), threefold (B), and twofold (C) rotational symmetry of an icosahedron.

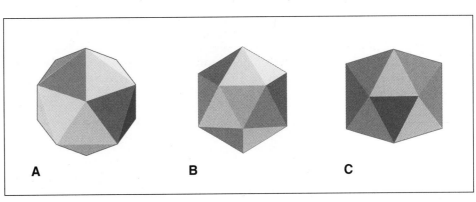

A   B   C

TABLE 19–3. Classification of DNA and RNA Viruses on the Basis of Nucleic Acid Characteristics and Nucleocapsid Contents

Virus Group and Class	Nucleic Acid Characteristics	Examples	Number of Segments	Nucleocapsid Encloses Transcriptase
DNA viruses				
Class I	Double-stranded, linear	*Adenoviridae*	—	No
		Herpesviridae	—	No
		Poxviridae	—	Yes
Class II	Double-stranded, circular	*Papovaviridae*	—	No
Class III	Single-stranded, negative-sense, linear	*Parvoviridae*	—	No
Class IV	Partially double-stranded, circular	*Hepadnaviridae*	—	Yes
RNA viruses				
Class I	Single-stranded, positive-sense, nonsegmented	*Astroviridae*	—	No
		Caliciviridae	—	No
		Coronaviridae	—	No
		Flaviviridae	—	No
		Picornaviridae	—	No
		Togaviridae	—	No
Class II	Single-stranded, negative-sense, nonsegmented	*Deltavirus*	—	Yes
		Filoviridae	—	Yes
		Paramyxoviridae	—	Yes
		Rhabdoviridae	—	Yes
Class III	Single-stranded, negative-sense, segmented	*Arenaviridae*	2	Yes
		Bunyaviridae	3	Yes
		Orthomyxoviridae	6–8	Yes
Class IV	Double-stranded, segmented	*Reoviridae*	10–12	Yes
Class V	Single-stranded, positive-sense, nonsegmented, diploid	*Retroviridae*	—	Yes*

* The nucleocapsid of *Retroviridae* contains reverse transcriptase.

viruses per cultured cell and therefore is considered to have a high **multiplicity of infection** (MOI). A high MOI ensures that essentially all cells in the culture will be infected with viruses. The viruses attach to and enter the host cells, and then they become undetectable for 10–20% of the infection cycle. During this part of the cycle, called the **eclipse period,** the virus is uncoated (disassembled), the viral nucleic acid is used to produce viral proteins and nucleic acid, and the viral parts are reassembled to form new viruses. Once new viruses are assembled, intracellular viruses can be detected and the eclipse period is completed. Depending on the type of virus, the viral particles may egress individually by budding through a membrane, or the cell may fill with viral particles until cell lysis releases a "burst" of viruses. The portion of the viral growth curve between the infection of a host cell and the appearance of infectious extracellular viruses is known as the **latent period.**

Attachment to Host Cells

Each virus can invade a restricted number of cell types. The specificity of infection is controlled largely by the availability of **receptors,** which are located on host cell surfaces and can be recognized by viral surface proteins. As Fig. 19–8 shows, the viral **adhesin** recognizes a glycoprotein on the host cell surface, binds to the receptor, and initiates the internalization process. Viruses cannot recognize cells that lack appropriate receptors, so these cells will not be infected.

Cellular receptors for viruses include molecules as diverse as growth factor receptors, intercellular adhesion molecules, and gangliosides. There is evidence that some viruses recognize multiple receptors, binding loosely to an initial receptor and then binding tightly to a second receptor that triggers the process of entry into the target cell.

Adhesins, which are also called **attachment proteins** or **antireceptors,** may be capsid proteins or envelope proteins. The best-studied viral adhesins are the hemagglutinins of the orthomyxoviruses and paramyxoviruses. When these adhesins bind to cellular receptors but the virus is not internalized, a viral neuraminidase will cleave neuraminic acid and allow the virus to move to another target cell that internalizes viruses.

Entry Into Host Cells

Once the virus has bound to its receptor, the virus penetrates into the host cell cytoplasm. The term "penetration," which is widely used, carries with it the unfortunate connotation that the virus actively (using its own energy) forces its way into the target cell. This is not the case. Instead, binding of the adhesin and receptor triggers one of two processes (see Fig. 19–8) that move the adherent virus into the target cell.

Nonenveloped (naked) viruses generally adhere to receptors that cluster within clathrin-coated pits, and then they are phagocytosed in a process known as **viropexis.** When the phagocytic vacuole fuses with lysosomes, the resulting acidification of the phagosome may cause the viral particle to be partially disassembled, and parts of the virus needed for viral replication escape into the cell cytoplasm.

Some enveloped viruses undergo viropexis. Others enter the host cell via a process of **fusion.** In

TABLE 19–4.   Taxonomic Classification of the Human Viruses

DNA VIRUSES
Family: *Adenoviridae* (adenoviruses)
  Subfamily: None
    Genus: *Mastadenovirus*
      Example: Human adenovirus serotypes 1–47.
      Diseases: Acute respiratory disease; cervicitis;
          encephalitis; epidemic keratoconjunctivitis;
          gastroenteritis; hemorrhagic cystitis;
          pharyngitis; pharyngoconjunctival fever;
          pneumonia.

Family: *Hepadnaviridae* (hepatitis B–like viruses)
  Subfamily: None
    Genus: *Orthohepadnavirus*
      Example: Hepatitis B virus.
      Diseases: Cirrhosis; hepatitis B; primary hepatocellular
          carcinoma.

Family: *Herpesviridae* (herpesviruses)
  Subfamily: *Alphaherpesvirinae*
    Genus: *Simplexvirus*
      Example: Herpes simplex virus.
      Diseases: Blepharitis; congenital herpes infection;
          conjunctivitis; disseminated herpes infection;
          encephalitis; genital herpes infection;
          gingivostomatitis; herpes gladiatorum; herpes
          labialis; herpetic whitlow; keratitis;
          keratoconjunctivitis; pharyngitis.
    Genus: *Varicellovirus*
      Example: Varicella-zoster virus.
      Diseases: Herpes zoster (shingles); varicella
          (chickenpox).
  Subfamily: *Betaherpesvirinae*
    Genus: *Cytomegalovirus*
      Example: Human cytomegalovirus.
      Diseases: Cytomegalic inclusion disease (prenatal);
          encephalitis (in patients with acquired
          immunodeficiency syndrome, or AIDS);
          gastroenteritis (in patients with AIDS); mild
          hepatitis; mild mononucleosis; pneumonitis;
          retinitis.
    Genus: *Roseolovirus*
      Example: Human herpesvirus 6.
      Diseases: Roseola infantum (sixth disease).
  Subfamily: *Gammaherpesvirinae*
    Genus: *Lymphocryptovirus*
      Example: Epstein-Barr virus.
      Diseases: Burkitt's lymphoma; infectious
          mononucleosis; nasopharyngeal carcinoma;
          progressive lymphoproliferative disease (in
          patients with AIDS or transplants); some non-
          Burkitt's B cell lymphomas.
    Genus: Unnamed
      Example: Human herpesvirus 8 (Kaposi's
          sarcoma–associated herpesvirus).
      Diseases: Kaposi's sarcoma; non-Hodgkin's lymphoma
          (in patients with AIDS).

Family: *Papovaviridae* (papovaviruses)
  Subfamily: None
    Genus: *Papillomavirus*
      Example: Papillomaviruses.
      Diseases: Cervical and anogenital carcinoma; squamous
          cell carcinoma; a wide variety of warts,
          including anogenital warts, plantar warts,
          other skin warts, and respiratory warts. Type
          of wart is strain-specific.
    Genus: *Polyomavirus*
      Example: BK virus.
      Diseases: Kidney infections.
      Example: JC virus.
      Diseases: Kidney infections; progressive multifocal
          leukoencephalopathy.

Family: *Parvoviridae* (parvoviruses)
  Subfamily: *Parvovirinae*
    Genus: *Dependovirus*
      Example: Adeno-associated viruses.
      Diseases: None.
    Genus: *Erythrovirus*
      Example: Parvovirus B19.
      Diseases: Erythema infectiosum (fifth disease);
          transient aplastic crisis (in patients with
          anemia).

Family: *Poxviridae* (poxviruses)
  Subfamily: *Chordopoxvirinae*
    Genus: *Molluscipoxvirus*
      Example: Molluscum contagiosum virus.
      Diseases: Molluscum contagiosum.
    Genus: *Orthopoxvirus*
      Example: Cowpox virus.
      Diseases: Cowpox.
      Example: Monkeypox virus.
      Diseases: Monkeypox.
      Example: Vaccinia; vaccinia-like viruses.
      Diseases: Buffalopox; smallpox (variola major and
          variola minor); vaccinia.
    Genus: *Parapoxvirus*
      Example: Milker's nodule virus.
      Diseases: Milker's nodule.
      Example: Orf virus.
      Diseases: Orf (contagious pustular dermatitis).
    Genus: *Yatapoxvirus*
      Example: Tanapox virus.
      Diseases: Tanapox.
      Example: Yabapox virus.
      Diseases: Yabapox.

RNA VIRUSES
Family: *Arenaviridae* (arenaviruses)
  Subfamily: None
    Genus: *Arenavirus*
      Example: Guanarito virus.
      Diseases: Venezuelan hemorrhagic fever.
      Example: Junin virus.
      Diseases: Argentinean hemorrhagic fever.
      Example: Lassa virus.
      Diseases: Lassa fever (hemorrhagic fever).
      Example: Lymphocytic choriomeningitis virus (LCM
          virus).
      Diseases: Aseptic meningitis; encephalitis; flu-like
          illness; lymphocytic choriomeningitis.
      Example: Machupo virus.
      Diseases: Bolivian hemorrhagic fever.

Family: *Astroviridae* (astroviruses)
  Subfamily: None
    Genus: *Astrovirus*
      Example: Astroviruses.
      Diseases: Mild childhood gastroenteritis.

Family: *Bunyaviridae* (bunyaviruses)
  Subfamily: None
    Genus: *Bunyavirus*
      Example: Bunyamwera supergroup of viruses, which
          includes Bunyamwera virus, California
          encephalitis virus, La Crosse encephalitis virus,
          Oropouche virus, and over 150 additional
          viruses.
      Diseases: Encephalitis; febrile viremia; Oropouche
          fever.
    Genus: *Hantavirus*
      Example: Belgrade hantavirus.
      Diseases: Hantavirus respiratory disease.
      Example: Hantaan virus.
      Diseases: Hantaan.

Continued

TABLE 19-4. **Taxonomic Classification of the Human Viruses** (*Continued*)

Family: *Bunyaviridae* (bunyaviruses) (*continued*)
   Example: Korean hemorrhagic fever virus.
      Diseases: Korean hemorrhagic fever.
   Example: Puumala virus.
      Diseases: Puumala.
   Example: Sinnombre virus.
      Diseases: Sinnombre fever (Muerto Canyon fever).
   Genus: *Nairovirus*
      Example: Crimean-Congo hemorrhagic fever virus.
         Diseases: Crimean-Congo hemorrhagic fever.
   Genus: *Phlebovirus*
      Example: Rift Valley fever virus.
         Diseases: Rift Valley fever.
      Example: Sandfly fever virus.
         Diseases: Sandfly fever.

Family: *Caliciviridae* (caliciviruses)
   Subfamily: None
   Genus: *Calicivirus*
      Example: Norwalk virus.
         Diseases: Acute gastroenteritis.
      Example: Hepatitis E virus.
         Diseases: Acute hepatitis E with cholestasis.

Family: *Coronaviridae* (coronaviruses)
   Subfamily: None
   Genus: *Coronavirus*
      Example: Human coronaviruses.
         Diseases: Upper respiratory tract infection (common cold); gastroenteritis(?).
   Genus: *Torovirus*
      Example: Toroviruses.
         Diseases: Gastroenteritis(?).

Family: *Filoviridae* (filoviruses)
   Subfamily: None
   Genus: *Filovirus*
      Example: Ebola virus.
         Diseases: Ebola disease.
      Example: Marburg virus.
         Diseases: Marburg disease.

Family: *Flaviviridae* (flaviviruses)
   Subfamily: None
   Genus: *Flavivirus*
      Example: Group B arboviruses, which include dengue virus; encephalitis viruses (Japanese encephalitis virus, Kunjin virus, louping ill virus, Murray Valley encephalitis virus, Powassan virus, Rocio virus, and St. Louis encephalitis virus); tick-borne hemorrhagic viruses (Kyasanur Forest disease virus and Omsk hemorrhagic fever virus); West Nile fever virus; and yellow fever virus.
         Diseases: Dengue; encephalitis; fever with arthritis, mylagia, and rash; hemorrhagic fever; yellow fever.
   Genus: *Hepatitis C virus*
      Example: Hepatitis C virus.
         Diseases: Acute and chronic hepatitis C; primary hepatocellular carcinoma.

Family: *Orthomyxoviridae* (orthomyxoviruses)
   Subfamily: None
   Genus: *Influenzavirus A,B*
      Example: Influenza A and B viruses.
         Diseases: Influenza.
   Genus: *Influenzavirus C*
      Example: Influenza C virus.
         Diseases: Mild influenza.
   Genus: Unnamed (tick-borne Thogoto-like viruses)
      Example: Dhori virus and Thogoto virus.
         Diseases: Asymptomatic viremia.

Family: *Paramyxoviridae* (paramyxoviruses)
   Subfamily: *Paramyxovirinae*
   Genus: *Morbillivirus*
      Example: Measles virus.
         Diseases: Acute postinfectious measles encephalitis; giant cell pneumonia; measles; subacute measles encephalitis; subacute sclerosing panencephalitis (SSPE).
   Genus: *Paramyxovirus*
      Example: Parainfluenza virus types 1 and 3.
         Diseases: Bronchiolitis; croup; pneumonia; upper respiratory tract infection (coldlike symptoms).
   Genus: *Rubulavirus*
      Example: Mumps virus.
         Diseases: Epididymo-orchitis; mumps; mumps encephalitis.
      Example: Parainfluenza virus types 2, 4a, and 4b.
         Diseases: Croup; upper respiratory tract infection.
   Subfamily: *Pneumovirinae*
   Genus: *Pneumovirus*
      Example: Respiratory syncytial virus.
         Diseases: Pharyngitis; respiratory syncytial bronchiolitis (in newborn infants); rhinitis.

Family: *Picornaviridae* (picornaviruses)
   Subfamily: None
   Genus: *Enterovirus*
      Example: Coxsackieviruses.
         Diseases: Acute hemorrhagic conjunctivitis; colds; hand-foot-and-mouth disease; herpangina; myocarditis; paralysis; pleurodynia; systemic neonatal disease.
      Example: Echoviruses.
         Diseases: Chronic meningoencephalitis; colds; maculopapular exanthems; myocarditis; neonatal carditis; neonatal encephalitis; neonatal hepatitis.
      Example: Enteroviruses.
         Diseases: Acute hemorrhagic conjunctivitis; hand-foot-and-mouth disease; paralysis.
      Example: Poliovirus types 1, 2, and 3.
         Diseases: Poliomyelitis.
   Genus: *Hepatovirus*
      Example: Hepatitis A virus.
         Diseases: Acute hepatitis A.
   Genus: *Rhinovirus*
      Example: Rhinoviruses (over 100 serotypes).
         Diseases: Common cold.

Family: *Reoviridae* (reoviruses)
   Subfamily: None
   Genus: *Coltivirus*
      Example: Colorado tick fever virus.
         Diseases: Colorado tick fever.
      Example: Eyach virus.
         Diseases: Eyach meningoencephalitis(?); hemorrhagic fever.
   Genus: *Orbivirus*
      Example: Kemerovo virus.
         Diseases: Meningoencephalitis.
   Genus: *Orthoreovirus*
      Example: Reoviruses.
         Diseases: Unknown; mild respiratory tract infection(?).
   Genus: *Rotavirus*
      Example: Rotaviruses.
         Diseases: Diarrhea (in children).

Continued

TABLE 19–4. Taxonomic Classification of the Human Viruses (*Continued*)

Family: *Retroviridae* (retroviruses)
Subfamily: *Lentivirinae*
  Genus: *Lentivirus*
    Example: Human immunodeficiency virus (HIV) types 1 and 2.
    Diseases: Acquired immunodeficiency syndrome (AIDS).
Subfamily: *Spumavirinae*
  Genus: *Spumavirus*
    Example: Human "foamy" viruses.
    Diseases: Unknown.
Subfamily: *Oncovirinae*
  Genus: *Oncovirus*
    Example: Human T cell lymphotropic virus (HTLV) types I and II.
    Diseases: Adult T cell leukemia or lymphoma; tropical spastic paraparesis.

Family: *Rhabdoviridae* (rhabdoviruses)
Subfamily: None
  Genus: *Lyssavirus*
    Example: Duvanhage virus, Lagos bat virus, Mokola virus, and rabies virus.
    Diseases: Rabies, rabieslike neurologic diseases.
  Genus: *Vesiculovirus*
    Example: Vesicular stomatitis virus.
    Diseases: Vesicular stomatitis.

Family: *Togaviridae* (togaviruses)
Subfamily: None
  Genus: *Alphavirus*
    Example: Group A arboviruses, which include encephalitis viruses (eastern equine encephalitis virus, Venezuelan equine encephalitis virus, and western equine encephalitis virus); and viruses that cause fever with arthritis, myalgia, and rash (chikungunya virus, Mayaro virus, o'nyong-nyong virus, Ross River virus, and Sindbis virus).
    Diseases: Encephalitis; fever with arthritis, myalgia, and rash.
  Genus: *Rubivirus*
    Example: Rubella virus.
    Diseases: Acquired rubella; congenital rubella syndrome.

OTHER VIRUSES OR VIRUSLIKE AGENTS
  Genus: *Deltavirus* (RNA hepatitis virus)
    Example: Hepatitis D virus.
    Diseases: Cofactor in hepatitis B.

  Prions (proteinaceous infectious particles)
    Example: Agents for spongiform encephalopathies.
    Diseases: Creutzfeldt-Jakob disease; fatal familial insomnia; Gerstmann-Sträussler-Scheinker disease; kuru.

---

this process, the viral envelope fuses with the host membrane, allowing the nucleocapsid to be shuttled into the cell cytoplasm. A similar fusion process can allow enveloped viruses to escape host cell phagosomes.

Uncoating

In order for new viruses to be produced, the viral nucleic acid must be released from the nucleocapsid or else the nucleocapsid must be partially degraded to allow cellular enzymes to reach the viral nucleic acid. This process, which is known as uncoating, is responsible for the apparent disappearance of identifiable viral particles during the eclipse period of the viral replication cycle (see Fig. 19–7).

Several patterns of uncoating are seen. Enveloped RNA viruses undergo the least extensive uncoating, with their RNA being transcribed while associated with the nucleocapsid. Reoviruses are also partially uncoated, and poxviruses undergo a complex two-stage uncoating that requires the assistance of virus-encoded enzymes to release the viral DNA from the nucleocapsid. Most other viruses are disas-

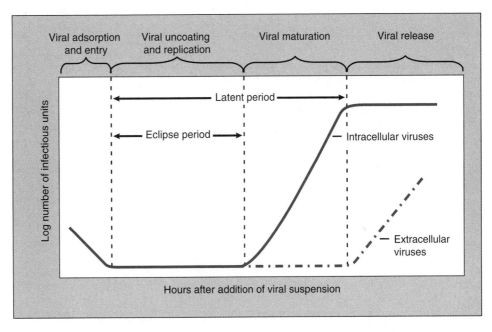

FIGURE 19–7. A one-step viral replication curve for a typical virus replicating within cultured mammalian cells. To ensure that essentially all cells are infected, a viral suspension with a high multiplicity of infection (MOI) is added to the host cell monolayer. The viruses adsorb to the host cells, are internalized, and are then uncoated. The eclipse phase begins with uncoating and ends when the infectious viral nucleocapsids are assembled spontaneously within the cell.

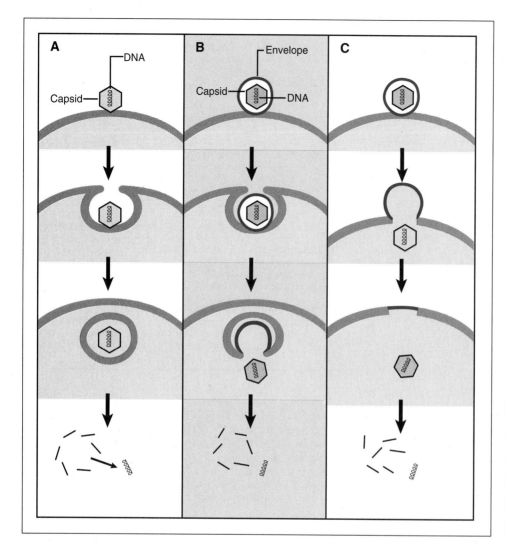

FIGURE 19–8. **Examples of means by which viruses invade host cells.** As shown in diagram **A,** nonenveloped viruses typically adsorb to the cell surface via adhesins and induce their own phagocytosis. When the phagocytic vacuole is acidified, the virus is uncoated and the viral nucleic acid enters the cell cytoplasm. This process is known as viropexis. As shown in diagram **B,** some enveloped viruses also enter host cells via viropexis, but the nucleocapsid escapes the phagosome when the viral envelope fuses with the phagosomal membrane. As shown in diagram **C,** other enveloped viruses enter the cell when the viral envelope fuses with the cell membrane.

sembled in either the cytoplasm or the nucleus by host enzymes, and their nucleic acid is fully liberated from the nucleocapsid.

Replication

Viruses are replicated within the cytoplasm or nucleus of **permissive host cells.** A host cell is characterized as permissive if it fulfills two requirements: the cell expresses receptors that allow the virus to enter it, and the cell contains enzymes or other factors that support the replicative needs of the virus. Some cells that have appropriate viral receptors will not support viral replication and are therefore called **nonpermissive host cells.**

Four processes must occur before new viral particles can be assembled. First, messenger RNA (mRNA) must be produced from viral genes. The genomes of viruses that contain a positive-sense strand of RNA can be used directly as mRNA, but a variety of schemes must be used to produce mRNA from other types of genomes. One scheme involves standard transcription of mRNA from DNA, using cellular enzymes; another involves conversion of RNA to DNA by viral reverse transcriptase, followed by standard

transcription; and yet another entails the use of viral enzymes to copy a negative-sense strand of viral RNA into mRNA. Details of these schemes are presented in Chapters 20 and 21. Second, any proteins needed for replication of the viral genome must be encoded by the virus. These proteins, which are usually DNA or RNA polymerases, are synthesized early during the eclipse phase. Third, the viral nucleic acid must be replicated. In many cases, host polymerases are used for this task, but other viruses carry special polymerases within their nucleocapsid or encode genes for special polymerases that will be produced early during the replication cycle. Fourth, viral structural proteins must be synthesized, along with any other proteins (such as histone-like proteins) that will be packaged within the nucleocapsid.

Viruses that contain double-stranded DNA typically replicate under strict **temporal control** (time control), with distinct sets of genes read at specific times. These genes are divided into **early genes** and **late genes,** with the early genes being subdivided into immediate early and delayed early genes. Although the replication of other viruses is not under such rigid temporal control, there still exists a general pattern of early and late replicative events for most viruses.

Early events are those needed to replicate the viral nucleic acid. These events may include shutdown of host nucleic acid and protein production, synthesis of viral nucleic acid polymerases, and synthesis of other proteins needed to complete replication of the viral genome. Once the viral genome is replicated, the expanded genomic pool can be used to synthesize mRNA encoding the proteins that form the capsid.

Assembly

Once capsid proteins are synthesized, the capsids are assembled via spontaneous self-assembly in a process known as **morphogenesis.** In some cases, morphogenesis is initiated by limited proteolytic cleavage of capsid proteins. The partially cleaved proteins assemble first into capsomers and then into capsids. The viral nucleic acid is not needed for this spontaneous process to occur. In fact, fully assembled icosahedral capsids often contain no nucleic acid, and these empty capsids (known as defective interfering particles) interfere with the viral replication.

The means by which viral nucleic acid is packaged into the capsid have been determined for only a few types of viruses. In adenoviruses, for example, packaging takes place in a specific nucleic acid sequence at one end of the DNA. A protein binds to this so-called **packaging sequence,** and the nucleic acid–protein complex then binds to basic core proteins within the procapsid. The final version of the nucleocapsid is constructed by further proteolytic cleavage of the capsid proteins.

The construction of viral particles and the association of nucleic acid with the assembled capsid are two events that are separated by hours during the replication of most DNA viruses. However, the two events occur within minutes of each other when nonenveloped, icosahedral RNA viruses replicate.

Escape From Host Cells

The means by which viruses escape from host cells are depicted in Fig. 19–9. Nonenveloped viruses generally accumulate within the cytoplasm or nucleus of the host cell, and then they are released as a **burst** when the host cell autolyzes. In contrast, enveloped viruses generally escape the cell one at a time by **budding** through a host membrane. Depending on the virus, the nucleocapsids may bud through the rough endoplasmic reticulum, Golgi apparatus, nuclear membrane, or cytoplasmic membrane. In each case, the viral particles bud through sites containing virus-encoded glycoproteins that will serve as adhesins for the next infection cycle. For viruses that are not pleomorphic, deposits of matrix protein on the inner aspect of the cytoplasmic membrane allow the virus to recognize sites where budding should occur.

Viral Effects on Host Cells

When viruses infect a target cell, viral replication may result in cytopathic effects, hyperplastic effects, or viral latency within host cells.

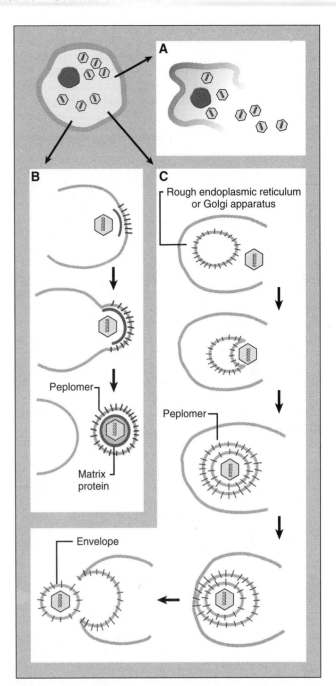

FIGURE 19–9. Means by which viruses escape from host cells. When viral maturation is completed, virulent viruses often exit host cells by causing the cell to autolyse, releasing virions in a single burst (diagram **A**). Enveloped viruses may bud through the cell membrane at a site where matrix protein and peplomers have been concentrated (diagram **B**). Enveloped viruses that do not contain matrix protein may bud through the rough endoplasmic reticulum or Golgi apparatus (diagram **C**). The viruses here are depicted as icosahedrons, but many viruses are helical.

Cytopathic Effects

Cytopathogenic viruses cause readily apparent changes in the shape, functions, or viability of the host cell. These changes are known as cytopathic effects and are distinctive for each combination of virus and target cell.

Some cytopathic effects can be seen easily in

unstained cells at low-power magnification, while others are seen only when cells are stained with special dyes that react with acidic or basic molecules. The most commonly seen cytopathic effects are cell rounding, syncytium formation (giant cell formation), cell destruction, hemadsorption, cytoplasmic vacuolation, and generation of cytoplasmic or nuclear inclusion bodies.

At least six types of molecular events are responsible for cytopathic effects: (1) altered synthesis of cellular macromolecules, (2) alterations in lysosomal integrity, (3) changes in cell membrane glycoproteins, (4) cell damage from without, (5) deposition of viral proteins as cellular inclusions, and (6) virus-induced chromosomal damage.

The DNA viruses typically inhibit cellular DNA synthesis so that viral DNA will be replicated preferentially. With most DNA viruses, the effects are due to viral proteins that are synthesized early during the infection cycle and specifically affect DNA synthesis rather than RNA or protein synthesis. With adenoviruses, however, the penton fiber poisons almost all cellular macromolecular synthetic processes.

The RNA viruses generally shut off protein and RNA synthesis early in the infection cycle. For example, poliovirus shuts off host protein synthesis by inhibiting the capping of host mRNA. Because uncapped poliovirus RNA can be translated, the host cell ignores its own mRNA and shows preference for poliovirus mRNA. In contrast, the S4 protein of reovirus disrupts the vimentin–intermediate filament cytoskeletal system, resulting in a complete shutdown of host cell DNA, RNA, and protein synthesis.

Various viruses change the permeability of host lysosomes by unknown mechanisms. When changes in lysosomal permeability do not result in lysosomal enzyme leakage, the altered lysosomes stain red with neutral red, producing what are known as **red plaques.** When changes are extensive enough to result in leakage of the lysosomal contents, the lysosomes can no longer be stained with neutral red and the cell cytoplasm is said to contain **white plaques.**

The insertion of peplomers into the host cell membrane can significantly alter the way in which the infected cell interacts with its environment. For example, herpesviruses are particularly known for their ability to cause infected cells to fuse with adjacent cells and form polynucleated giant cells. In the case of influenza virus, the insertion of hemagglutinin molecules into the host cell membrane allows erythrocytes to adhere to monolayers of virus-infected cultured cells.

Some viruses can cause cell damage from without—that is, while they are adhering to the surface of the cell and before viral replication occurs. For example, when a concentrated suspension of a paramyxovirus (such as parainfluenza virus) is added to a monolayer of cultured cells, the fusion protein on virions adhering to the surfaces of cultured cells causes the cell membranes to rapidly fuse and form syncytia. Adenoviruses kill a variety of cells from without, and vaccinia virus quickly kills macrophages.

Inclusion bodies can be cytoplasmic or nuclear. Cytoplasmic inclusion bodies are seen most often in cells infected with rabies virus, paramyxoviruses, poxviruses, or reoviruses. Nuclear inclusion bodies are associated most often with adenoviruses, herpesviruses, or parvoviruses. Inclusion bodies may take the form of accumulations of nucleocapsids (as occurs with measles virus), viral "factories" that contain viral proteins and nucleic acids (as occurs with poxviruses), or masses of degraded chromatin (as occurs with herpesviruses). Based on their staining characteristics, inclusion bodies are classified as either acidophilic (stainable with eosin) or basophilic (stainable with hematoxylin).

Some DNA and RNA viruses cause site-specific breaks in host cell chromosomes. Measles virus, for example, causes anergy by causing specific DNA breaks in infected immunocompetent cells. Other viruses that cause chromosomal damage include adenoviruses, herpesviruses, polyomaviruses, mumps virus, parainfluenza virus, and rubella virus.

Hyperplastic Effects

Some viruses cause host cell hyperplasia. When hyperplasia leads to focal cell death, pocks are formed. **Pock formation** is especially associated with poxvirus infections.

Other viruses cause infected cells to markedly transform their growth patterns so that they are no longer subject to contact inhibition (topoinhibition). Cells that have undergone **cell transformation** will multiply without constraint and are similar to malignant cells in their characteristics. In contrast to nontransformed cells, transformed cells are less dependent on serum transport and tend to adhere poorly to surfaces. These properties make them capable of growing into large masses and allow them to move freely wherever fluid flow might take them.

Transforming viruses, which are also referred to as **oncogenic viruses** or **tumor-producing viruses,** have been found to (1) stimulate host cell DNA synthesis; (2) cause transformed cells to express new, virus-encoded surface antigens; (3) disrupt the cell cytoskeletal system; (4) change host cell gene expression; and (5) eliminate the cellular topoinhibition response.

DNA viruses transform only nonpermissive cells, so a transforming infection yields no progeny virions. In contrast, RNA viruses transform permissive cells, so the infected cell is transformed and produces virions. The DNA viruses known to be oncogenic include adenoviruses, hepadnaviruses, herpesviruses, papillomaviruses, and polyomaviruses. The only RNA viruses known to be oncogenic are the retroviruses. The processes of transformation and oncogenesis are discussed more completely in Chapter 22.

Viral Latency Within Host Cells

People usually associate viruses with the rapid onset of symptoms and signs of infection. However, some viruses cause manifestations of infection after remaining dormant for years (latent viral infections), and others cause slowly progressive disease (slow viral infections).

Latent Viral Infections. At least two groups of human viruses—namely, herpesviruses and adenoviruses—are known to cause latent viral infections.

Herpesviruses are notorious for their ability to cause recurrent disease after long periods of latency. Herpes simplex and varicella-zoster viruses lay dormant for years within sensory ganglia. The latent viruses persist there as episomes or, possibly, as intact virions. When the viruses are reactivated, they multiply within cells of ectodermal origin. Reactivation disease likely occurs when an agent or factor alters the host's immune response to the virus, allowing the organisms to spread to adjacent cells. While patients with type 2 herpes simplex infection develop genital lesions, patients with type 1 infection typically develop fever blisters, sometimes accompanied by keratitis and other herpetic skin lesions. Patients with reactivated varicella infection develop herpes zoster (shingles). Other herpesviruses, including cytomegalovirus and Epstein-Barr virus, also cause latent infections in humans.

Adenoviruses can cause conjunctivitis or respiratory disease in children and young adults, but many of those infected develop no noticeable manifestations. Instead, the viruses persist in the tonsils and adenoids, where they remain undetected for years. Investigators believe that the adenovirus DNA persists as a linear episome within infected cells during the years of latency. When the viruses reactivate, they become detectable. Reactivation does not cause disease in an immunocompetent individual but can have serious consequences in an immunocompromised individual, such as a patient with acquired immunodeficiency syndrome (AIDS).

Slow Viral Infections. A small number of conventional and unconventional viruses cause infections that progress extremely slowly. In some cases, the infection is clinically inapparent for many years, although the virus can be demonstrated in the infected tissues.

(1) Conventional Slow Viruses. Among the conventional viruses, the usual causes of slow infection are enveloped viruses such as arenaviruses, coronaviruses, paramyxoviruses, retroviruses, and togaviruses.

One of the best-studied slow viral infections in humans is subacute sclerosing panencephalitis (SSPE), a progressive degenerative neurologic disease that occurs in patients who previously have suffered from measles. SSPE is characterized by high titers of antibody to measles virus and the presence of infected brain cells that contain inclusion bodies identical to those seen during measles.

Studies have shown that antibody directed specifically against measles virus antigens reacts with antigens found in the brain lesions of patients with SSPE. The RNA of the virions found in SSPE tissues is identical to the RNA of measles virus except that it contains additional sequences that increase the RNA length by about 10%. Some have suggested that the additional sequences have been acquired by recombination of the RNA of measles virus with the RNA of another virus. The precise nature of this slow viral infection is not well understood, but it has been noted that little or no matrix protein is made in SSPE-derived virus-infected cells. Without matrix protein, the virions cannot bud from the infected cells. Additionally, there is some evidence that antibody to measles virus glycoproteins may cause the glycoproteins to aggregate on the cell surface and then be shed. Thus, measles virus may persist in neural tissue because the immune response is unable to adequately recognize and eliminate infected cells.

Other examples of diseases that are due to conventional slow viruses are progressive rubella panencephalitis, which is caused by rubella virus, and progressive multifocal leukoencephalopathy, which is caused by a polyomavirus called JC virus.

(2) Unconventional Slow Viruses. During the late 1950s, Carleton Gajdusek and his colleagues investigated a bizarre disease that was decimating the Fore people in the highlands of Papua New Guinea. This disease, known as kuru (which is Fore for "trembling"), most often afflicted women and children and resulted in death 6–12 months after onset. Patients initially developed tremors of the head and extremities and became uncoordinated in their movements. Over the next few months, they developed speech impairments, muscle spasms, paralysis of the eye muscles, emotional outbursts, and dementia. The faces of many patients became distorted, giving rise to the names "laughing disease" and "laughing death."

Subsequent studies showed that kuru was one of several diseases classified as spongiform encephalopathies. In humans, these include Creutzfeldt-Jakob disease, Gerstmann-Sträussler-Scheinker disease, and fatal familial insomnia. In animals, they include scrapie and maedi in sheep, mad cow disease in cows, and transmissible encephalopathy in minks, mules, deer, and elk. In each spongiform encephalopathy, autopsy reveals cerebral atrophy; patchy, diffuse loss of neurons; diffuse vacuolation of neuropils; astroglial hypertrophy; and bilateral degeneration of the corticospinal tracts. Most important, affected humans and animals develop visible holes in the brain—a condition known as status spongiosus—and accumulate amyloid proteins.

In humans, kuru is transmitted via cannibalism, and Creutzfeldt-Jakob disease is transmitted via use of pituitary-derived human growth hormone, use of human pituitary gonadotropin, neurosurgical procedures, dura mater grafts, implantation of contaminated electroencephalographic electrodes, and corneal transplants. In about 10% of the cases of Creutzfeldt-Jakob disease and most or all of the cases of Gerstmann-Sträussler-Scheinker disease and fatal familial insomnia, the disease is inherited. Laboratory studies have shown that the agent of scrapie can be passed to a variety of experimental animals and that kuru can be passed to primates.

Early studies focused on the possibility that the agent of these diseases was a conventional virus. It was soon evident that it was not. Electron microscopy showed no viral particles in the affected tissues. The agent was not inactivated by heat (80 °C), β-propiolactone, formaldehyde, nucleases, some proteases, or ultraviolet radiation at 254 nm. The agent was inactivated, however, by autoclaving, phenol treatment, and prolonged exposure to 1 N sodium hydroxide.

Extensive investigations failed to locate any RNA or DNA in infectious preparations. Instead, transmissibility seemed to be associated with amyloid protein fibrils known as scrapie-associated fibrils. This led Stanley Prusiner and his associates to consider the possibility that the agents of kuru and scrapie were proteins. Prusiner discovered a 27- to 30-kD protein that copurified with infectivity. This protein, which he called **prion protein** or **PrP,** was derived from a larger (33- to 35-kD) protein that was named PrP^{Sc} (for prion protein of scrapie). Further studies showed that PrP^{Sc} was the actual infectious agent or was so closely associated with it that the two could not be differentiated.

The greatest surprise, however, was yet to come. It was found that one form of PrP, known as PrP^C, is a normal component of the central nervous system and is concentrated in neuronal membranes. The primary sequences of PrP^{Sc} and PrP^C are identical, and PrP is encoded on the short arm of human chromosome 20. The two types of PrP molecules differ only in the way that they are folded. While most of the PrP^C molecule is folded into alpha helices, more than 40% of the PrP^{Sc} molecule is folded as beta sheets. When PrP^{Sc} comes into contact with a molecule of PrP^C from the same species, the PrP^{Sc} acts as a template that causes the PrP^C molecules to refold themselves and become PrP^{Sc} molecules. This process is autocatalytic. One molecule of PrP^{Sc} yields two, which yields four, which yields eight, and so on. Transgenic mice that lack PrP^C are unable to develop scrapie when administered PrP^{Sc}.

Investigators have long believed that there is a "species barrier" preventing transmission of scrapie to humans. But scrapie has been passed from sheep to mice and cattle, so there must be a factor that controls the host range of prion diseases. The limiting factor is the amino acid sequence of the PrP molecules. The primary sequences of sheep and bovine PrP differ by only 7 amino acids, but human PrP differs from sheep PrP by more than 30 amino acids. Thus, scrapie is passed from sheep to cattle as mad cow disease, but humans are unaffected. This is because the sheep PrP^{Sc} matches human PrP^C too poorly to serve as a template for conformational change. During 1996, however, investigators presented evidence suggesting an epidemiologic link between mad cow disease and human Creutzfeldt-Jakob disease. Although this link has not been proved, the European Union banned the importation of beef from Great Britain because of fears that the beef contained the agent of this disease.

This leaves the problem of the etiology of inherited prion diseases. Humans with familial spongiform encephalopathies have prions with specific point mutations in their PrP. Eighteen different PrP point mutations have been identified within the four PrP alpha helices or at their borders. Investigators believe that these mutations destabilize the helices, making them more likely to spontaneously refold into a beta structure. Once such refolding occurs, the process is autocatalytic. Introduction of such genes into transgenic mice results in spontaneous development of spongiform encephalopathies.

The possibility still remains that prions are not the agents of spongiform encephalopathies but are, instead, cofactors of infection. Virologists continue to search for viroids and other subviral agents, including nonenveloped branched-chain nucleic acid fragments. To date, there is no direct evidence that these other agents exist.

The means by which prions cause disease are not well understood. PrP molecules accumulate within neuronal lysosomes and are found in greatest concentration in the neuropil. They are also found in and around astrocytes and within microglia. Investigators believe that intracellular accumulation of the nondegradable PrP^{Sc} kills neurons and leads to the status spongiosis that characterizes prion-associated diseases. No inflammatory processes are associated with these diseases, and the agents elicit no immune response in patients.

Antiviral Strategies
Dynamics of Viral Infection and Immunity

The nature and effectiveness of the immune response to viruses are largely related to the dynamics of each viral infection. For example, the site of entry of the virus greatly influences the ability of the immune response to contain the virus. Viruses that enter through the respiratory or intestinal mucosa are more likely to be influenced by available secretory IgA (sIgA) than are viruses that enter the body via an arthropod or animal bite. Other factors that influence the impact of the immune response on the outcome of infection are (1) whether primary viremia occurs; (2) whether the infection is cytolytic or noncytolytic; (3) whether the infection is active, slow, or latent; (4) whether the virus spreads via secondary viremia or directly from cell to cell; (5) whether infected cells express viral antigens on their surfaces; and (6) whether the virus is enveloped or nonenveloped.

In general, after viruses enter the body, they are replicated locally and then disseminate to new sites, where they will be further replicated. In some cases, the primary effects of viruses are greatest at the site of entry. In other cases, an infection is not clinically evident until the viruses disseminate. At each point, the outcome of infection can be altered by various components of the immune response.

The Antibody Response

Viruses are susceptible to the actions of antibodies when the organisms lie within mucosal secretions, are free in the blood, or are within cells that express viral glycoproteins on their surfaces. Fig. 19–10 summarizes some of the ways in which antibodies protect against viral infections.

Viruses that are invading mucosae may be recognized by IgG or sIgA antibodies present within mucinous secretions. IgA is believed to act primarily as a blocking agent that binds to viral adhesins, making them unable to bind to cellular receptors (see Fig. 19–10A). IgG, in contrast, may opsonize viruses (see Fig. 19–10B) or may activate complement to lyse enveloped viruses.

Once in the blood, viruses are susceptible to neutralization by IgG and IgM antibodies. The binding of these antibodies to viral surface proteins may prevent adherence to target cells, may prevent entry into target cells after adherence, or may prevent uncoating after entry into the host cell cytoplasm (see Fig. 19–10D). The way in which antibodies carry out these steps is not fully understood but may involve conformational changes in the targeted viral proteins. Antibody-mediated complement activation (see Fig. 19–10C) probably also plays a key role in controlling infections caused by enveloped viruses. Complement

FIGURE 19–10. The role of IgG, IgA, and IgM antibodies in antiviral immunity. IgA and probably IgG block adherence of viruses to mucosal surfaces (diagram **A**). IgG may be directly opsonic (diagram **B**); may block viral adsorption, entry, or uncoating (diagram **D**); or may act as a bridge for expression of ADCC (diagram **E**). IgM is an efficient activator of complement, which may opsonize viruses (diagram **C**), lyse viral envelopes (diagram **C**), or lyse virus-infected cells that express viral antigens on their surfaces (diagram **E**). IgG can also activate complement (not shown). ADCC = antibody-dependent cellular cytotoxicity.

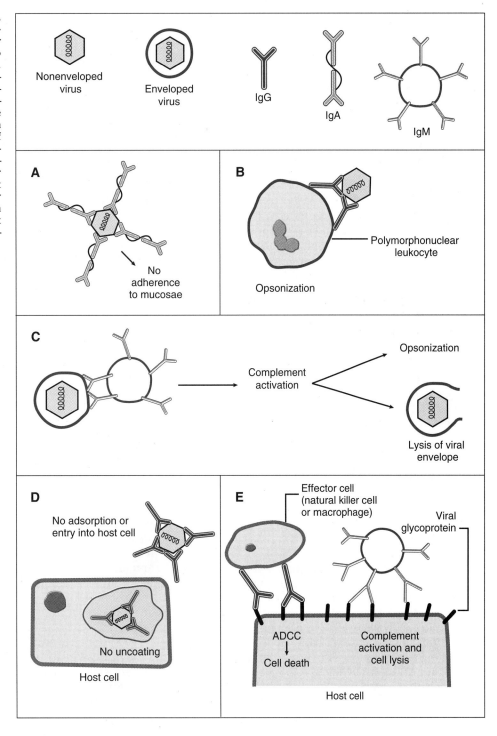

components activated by antibodies can form a terminal attack complex on the surface of the viral envelope. Subsequent lysis of the envelope renders the virus noninfectious because viral glycoproteins needed for cell recognition are lost in the lytic process.

Influenza, poliomyelitis, and other viral infections that depend on a primary or secondary viremic phase are particularly susceptible to antibody-mediated neutralization. Thus, recovery from or immunity to these diseases depends largely on the ability to form antibodies to the responsible viruses. Nonimmune individuals usually form antibodies during days 3–10 of a systemic viral infection, but previously immune patients may exhibit antibodies during the first day of infection. This is the rationale for immunizing individuals against systemic viral illnesses such as influenza, mumps, measles, and chickenpox.

Antibodies can also kill cells infected with viruses if the infected cells express viral antigens on their surfaces. In some cases, cell lysis is complement-dependent, but virus-infected cells may also be destroyed by antibody-dependent cellular cytotoxicity, or ADCC (see Fig. 19–10E).

Cellular Immune Responses

T lymphocytes play a critical role in recovery from viral infections. All antibodies formed against viruses are T-dependent antibodies, and various subclasses of T cells can act directly against virus-infected cells. Which subclass of T cell will respond to a particular virus depends largely upon whether the viral antigens are expressed in conjunction with class I or class II major histocompatibility complex (MHC) antigens.

"Exogenous" viral antigens are those antigens which come from viruses that have been phagocytosed by antigen-presenting cells (APCs) such as macrophages, have been processed, and are now expressed on the surfaces of APCs. Because exogenous antigens are presented to T cells in association with class II MHC antigens, they activate CD4$^+$ T cells. The CD4$^+$ T cells can serve as helper T cells (T$_H$) that elicit the formation of antibody, or they can act as delayed-type hypersensitivity T cells (T$_{DTH}$) that secrete cytokines and activate macrophages. Thus, viral activation of CD4$^+$ T cells turns on the classic antibody and cell-mediated immune systems to eliminate viruses. This process is summarized in Fig. 19–11A.

"Endogenous" viral antigens are those antigens which are expressed on the surfaces of virus-invaded target cells such as fibroblasts or endothelial cells. Because endogenous viral antigens are expressed in conjunction with class I MHC antigens, they activate CD8$^+$ T cells (see Fig. 19–11B). The CD8$^+$ T cells include cytotoxic T cells (CTLs or T$_C$) and suppressor T cells (T$_S$). CTLs are believed to play a major protective role in many viral infections, owing to their ability to directly kill virus-infected cells.

Interferons

Discovery, Classification, and Terminology. In 1957, A. Isaacs and J. Lindenmann reported that supernatant from chick allantoic membrane fragments which had been exposed to ultraviolet light–inactivated influenza virus blocked the replication of influenza viruses within other cells. They dubbed the new antiviral substance "interferon."

Since that time, close to 20 interferons have been identified and have been placed into three groups, known as **interferon-alpha** (IFN-α), **interferon-beta** (IFN-β), and **interferon-gamma** (IFN-γ). Most of the interferons have been identified as IFN-α. IFN-γ is also sometimes called **immune interferon.**

While IFN-α and IFN-β are often referred to as **type I interferons,** IFN-γ is referred to as **type II interferon.** These molecules are so grouped because all type I interferons bind to the same host cellular receptors and are primarily antiviral in their activity, while the most important activities of type II interferon are related to its function as a cytokine and lymphokine.

Although interferons were discovered as antiviral agents, their synthesis can be induced by a wide variety of agents, including viruses, intracellular bacteria, lipopolysaccharides, cytokines, and tumor cells. IFN-γ production can also be induced by T cell mitogens and various antigens. Unless otherwise specified, when virologists speak of interferon, they are referring to the **antiviral type I interferons.** The synthesis of these interferons is most efficiently induced by double-stranded RNA (dsRNA). Thus, RNA viruses that produce dsRNA replicative intermediates are excellent inducers of interferon expression. Some DNA viruses that produce opposite-sense RNA transcripts from adjacent genes are also good interferon inducers, but many DNA viruses fail to induce the synthesis of interferons.

General Characteristics. Several general statements can be made about the characteristics and activities of the interferons. First, interferons are not virus-specific. That is, interferons induced by one virus are fully potent against any virus normally susceptible to the activity of interferons. Second, interferons are cell-specific in their production and effects. That is, different cells produce different interferons or amounts of interferons, and the availability of receptors for the interferons determines if a cell will respond to the presence of an interferon. Third, interferons are relatively species-specific. That is, although interferons from one animal may affect cells from another animal, their effects are greatest in the animal of origin; many animals may be unresponsive to interferons from other species because they lack receptors for those interferons. Finally, interferons are extremely potent. Viral resistance can be conferred by as few as 10–20 molecules of an interferon.

Production and Activities. Human interferons are synthesized as proteins with 166 amino acids and are subsequently cleaved to yield proteins of about 145 amino acids. IFN-α is synthesized by leukocytes and is most active as a monomer. IFN-β is synthesized

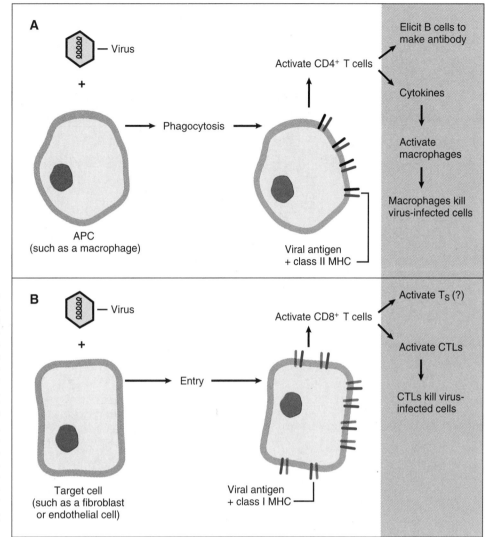

FIGURE 19–11. Cellular immunity to viruses. Exogenous viral antigens (diagram **A**) are antigens expressed on the surfaces of antigen-presenting cells (APCs) in conjunction with class II major histocompatibility complex (MHC) antigens. This process activates CD4+ T cells, which may act as helper T cells (T$_H$) or as delayed-type hypersensitivity T cells (T$_{DTH}$). Endogenous viral antigens (diagram **B**) are antigens expressed on the surfaces of virus-infected target cells in conjunction with class I MHC antigens. This process activates CD8+ T cells, which in turn activate cytotoxic T cells (CTLs) and may also activate suppressor T cells (T$_S$).

by a wide variety of cells, including fibroblasts and epithelial cells, and is most active as a dimer. IFN-γ, which is most active as a tetramer, is synthesized primarily by T lymphocytes, but null cells, natural killer cells, and endothelial cells have also been reported to secrete IFN-γ. IFN-β and IFN-γ are glycoproteins.

Interferon synthesis is induced when an appropriate virus replicates within a nucleated host cell. Interferon is synthesized and exported from the cell for 20–50 hours, and then interferon synthesis is halted. The cell is unable to produce additional interferon until it passes through two or more cell doublings. The interferon itself has no antiviral activity. Instead, it binds to specific cell surface receptors, is internalized, and induces the expression of several antiviral proteins. The details of these processes are described below and are summarized in Fig. 19–12.

(1) Induction of Interferon Synthesis. The genes for IFN-α and IFN-β are located on chromosome 9, while the gene for IFN-γ is on chromosome 12. Synthesis of IFN-β is controlled by a DNA segment known as the interferon regulatory element (IRE).

The precise nature of the inducing event is not well characterized, but investigators believe that both dsRNA and viral inhibition of cellular protein synthesis are involved. The best interferon inducers are slowly multiplying viruses that produce dsRNA replicative intermediates and do not completely inhibit cellular protein synthesis during the early phase of viral replication.

(2) Expression of Antiviral Proteins. Interferon molecules are exported from the cell and bind to specific receptors. The receptors for type I interferons contain gangliosides (glycosylated phospholipids). The receptor-bound interferon is rapidly internalized and mobilized to the nucleus, where it induces the expression of several antiviral proteins. As mentioned above, interferon does not, itself, have antiviral activity.

Type I interferons induce the expression of numerous antiviral proteins, the most important of which are thought to be 2′,5′-oligo(A) synthetase and P1/eIF-2α protein kinase. Type II interferon also induces the expression of class I and II MHC molecules, β$_2$ microglobulin, Fc receptors, and a variety of cyto-

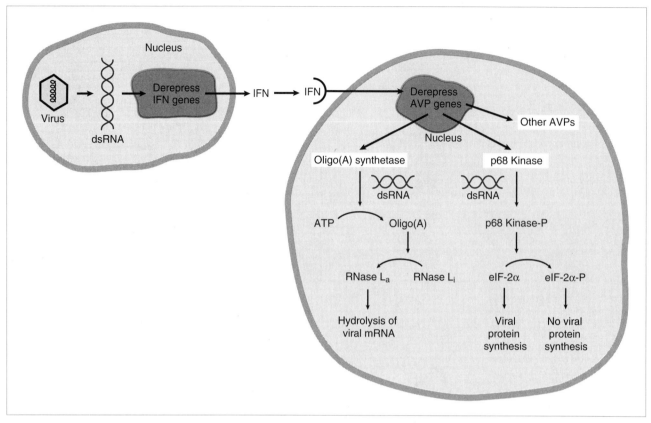

FIGURE 19–12. The induction and activities of type I interferons. Interferon (IFN) synthesis is induced when double-stranded RNA (dsRNA) or another inducing agent is present. The interferon molecules are exported and bind to specific interferon receptors on host cell surfaces. Receptor-bound interferon is rapidly internalized and taken to the nucleus, where it induces the expression of a variety of antiviral proteins (AVPs), the two most important of which are 2′,5′-oligo(A) synthetase and P1/eIF-2α protein kinase—also called oligo(A) synthetase and p68 kinase, respectively. In the presence of dsRNA, oligo(A) synthetase and p68 kinase are activated, causing hydrolysis of viral mRNA and inhibition of viral protein synthesis. ATP = adenosine triphosphate; RNase L_a = activated RNase L; RNase L_i = inactivated RNase L; and P = phosphate.

kines. The net effect of interferon activity is the selective inhibition of viral protein synthesis. It is not known why viral protein synthesis is selectively inhibited.

(a) 2′,5′-Oligo(A) Synthetase. In the presence of dsRNA, oligo(A) synthetase converts adenosine triphosphate (ATP) to 2′,5′-linked oligo(A) molecules up to 15 residues long, although the most abundant products are trimers. These molecules activate an endoribonuclease (RNase L) that hydrolyzes viral but not host mRNA. Type I interferons may cause up to a 20-fold increase in RNase L activity within virus-infected cells.

(b) P1/eIF-2α Protein Kinase. This enzyme induced by interferons is also known as p68 kinase. When dsRNA is present, p68 kinase phosphorylates itself, and then it passes the phosphate group to the small (α) subunit of initiation factor eIF-2. Once phosphorylated, eIF-2 can no longer initiate viral protein synthesis. Some viruses are resistant to the action of p68 kinase. For example, adenoviruses and influenza virus produce an inhibitor of p68 kinase, and vaccinia virus produces molecules that inhibit the activities of both p68 kinase and oligo(A) synthetase.

(3) Other Biologic Effects. IFN-γ differs from the other interferons in that it functions primarily as a cytokine rather than as an inducer of antiviral proteins. Although the monomer of IFN-γ is similar in size to that of the other interferons, it shares little sequence homology with them.

IFN-γ expression is induced in T lymphocytes by a variety of antigens, alloantigens, and mitogenic lectins. Moreover, CD4+ and CD8+ cells have been shown to synthesize IFN-γ after being stimulated with recombinant interleukin-2 or with anti-CD3 antibodies. IFN-γ is produced at least occasionally by null cells, natural killer cells, and endothelial cells.

IFN-γ exerts its activities by binding to specific type II interferon receptors on the surfaces of endothelial cells, fibroblasts, lymphocytes, mast cells, melanocytes, myelomonocytic cells, and neuronal cells. Like the other interferons, IFN-γ may elicit antiviral activity, but its greatest significance is related to its activities as a cytokine. Among the activities associated with IFN-γ are induction of B cell differentiation, induction of interleukin-6 production, induction of expression of class I and II MHC antigens, priming of macrophages to kill tumor cells, enhancement of the cytotoxic activity of natural killer cells, induction of intercellular adhesion molecule expression, up-regulation of interleukin-2 receptor activity, up-regulation of production of secretory component, and induction of expression of Fc receptors by polymorphonuclear leukocytes. Because of its potent activities as an immunomodulator, IFN-γ has been used experimentally to treat various tumors and viral infections.

Antiviral Therapy

Although antibacterial antibiotics have been used since the introduction of salvarsan at the turn of the century and Prontosil during the 1930s, few effective antiviral drugs are available even today, and most of those in use are at least somewhat toxic to humans. Viruses are parasitic genes that use much of the host cell's nucleic acid replicative machinery and are replicated freely within the cell cytosol or nucleus. Thus, drugs that interfere with viral replication are likely to have at least some effect on the health of the host. Virologists have, however, capitalized on differences between host and viral replicative needs and on unique properties of virus-infected cells to identify drugs that target viruses, to explore methods of treatment based on immunotherapy, and to develop vaccines against common systemic viral diseases.

Antiviral Drugs

Based on their primary modes of action, the antiviral antibiotics can be divided into several groups: viral DNA polymerase inhibitors, viral reverse transcriptase inhibitors, ion channel blockers, and protease inhibitors.

Viral DNA Polymerase Inhibitors. Foscarnet, acyclovir, ganciclovir, and ribavirin are drugs that inhibit the activities of viral DNA polymerases. Their structures are shown in Fig. 19–13.

The first of these antibiotics to be developed was **foscarnet,** which is also known as **trisodium phosphonoformate.** Initially, foscarnet was found to inhibit the DNA polymerases of herpesviruses and hepatitis B virus by blocking the pyrophosphate binding site on these enzymes. More recently, it was also found to inhibit the replication of hepatitis B virus and the human immunodeficiency virus (HIV) through its effects on reverse transcriptase activity. Foscarnet has been used topically to treat herpesvirus skin lesions and intravenously to treat cytomegalovirus infections in immunocompromised patients. It is used intravenously only against life-threatening infections, because it accumulates within the bone marrow and kidneys, where it inhibits cellular DNA replication.

Acyclovir was developed in 1977 and is also known as **acycloguanosine** or 9-(2-hydroxyethoxymethyl)guanine. It is a prodrug that is converted to its active form in herpesvirus-infected cells. The thymidine kinase of herpesvirus (but not that of host cells) phosphorylates acyclovir intracellularly to acycloguanosine monophosphate, and cellular guanosine monophosphate kinase then converts the

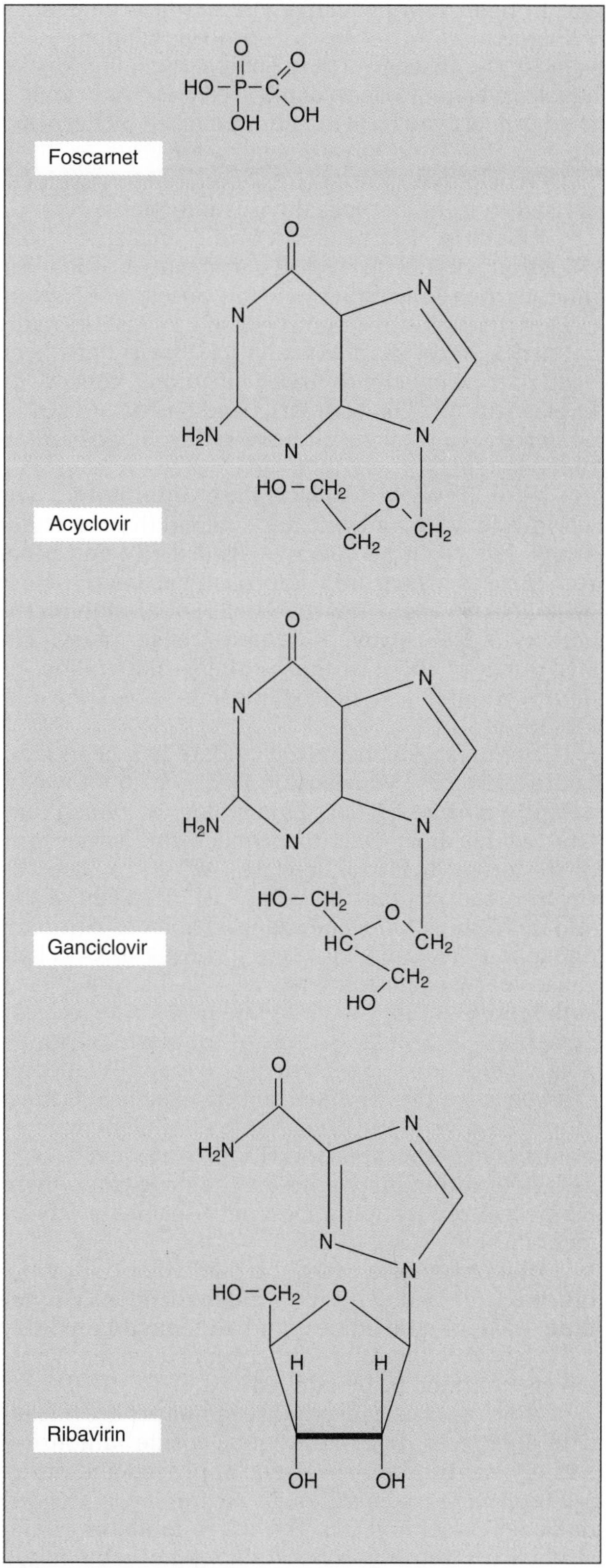

FIGURE 19–13. Structures of foscarnet, acyclovir, ganciclovir, and ribavirin. These antiviral agents are inhibitors of viral DNA polymerases.

drug to its active form (acycloguanosine triphosphate), which inhibits the herpesvirus DNA polymerase 10 times more effectively than does the cellular DNA polymerase. Because the prodrug cannot be activated in the absence of herpesvirus thymidine kinase, acyclovir is nontoxic to uninfected cells. Acyclovir is used primarily to treat infections caused by herpesviruses 1 and 2 and by varicella-zoster virus.

Ganciclovir, a drug closely related to acyclovir, is used to treat cytomegalovirus infections.

Ribavirin is the nucleoside analogue 1-β-D-ribofuranosyl-1,2-4-triazole-3-carboxamide. Ribavirin inhibits the replication of a wide variety of RNA and DNA viruses, but it is not licensed for use in many countries, because of its toxicity. Ribavirin has been used intravenously to treat infections caused by Lassa virus and Hantaan virus and has been used as an aerosol to treat respiratory syncytial virus infections in infants.

Viral Reverse Transcriptase Inhibitors. The worldwide AIDS epidemic has spurred the search for drugs that might be effective against HIV and other retroviruses. One fruitful approach has been the use of nucleoside analogues that preferentially inhibit the activity of the retroviral reverse transcriptase. The structures of three of these drugs—zidovudine, dideoxycytidine, and dideoxyinosine—are shown in Fig. 19–14.

The most effective drug to date has been **zidovudine,** a dideoxynucleoside that is also known as **azidothymidine** (AZT). Zidovudine is phosphorylated within host cells to produce the active form of the drug, AZT triphosphate (AZT-PPP). The HIV reverse transcriptase utilizes AZT-PPP in lieu of thymidine triphosphate, and the insertion of AZT monophosphate (AZT-P) into the growing DNA chain causes early chain termination. AZT-P also acts as a competitive inhibitor of thymidine kinase, causing depletion of cellular stores of adenosine triphosphate. Zidovudine is selectively toxic to HIV-infected cells because the reverse transcriptase is 100 times more sensitive to the drug than are cellular enzymes. Unfortunately, because the HIV provirus persists indefinitely within infected cells, the drug can only inhibit viral replication and cannot eliminate HIV infection.

Dideoxycytidine (ddC or zalcitabine), **dideoxyinosine** (ddI or didanosine), **didehydrodeoxythymidine** (d4T or stavudine), and **dideoxythiacytidine** (3TC or lamivudine) are dideoxynucleosides whose effects continue to be studied.

Most reverse transcriptase inhibitors are nucleoside analogues, but one nonnucleoside inhibitor—namely, **nevirapine**—has been approved and others are in clinical trials. Although nevirapine is a dipyridodiazepinone, some of the other inhibitors being studied are tetrahydrobenzodiazepine compounds. Nevirapine binds to a site that is away from the active site of the reverse transcriptase but communicates with it. When nevirapine is bound to reverse transcriptase, the correct nucleoside triphosphate is able to bind to the active site, but catalysis is inhibited.

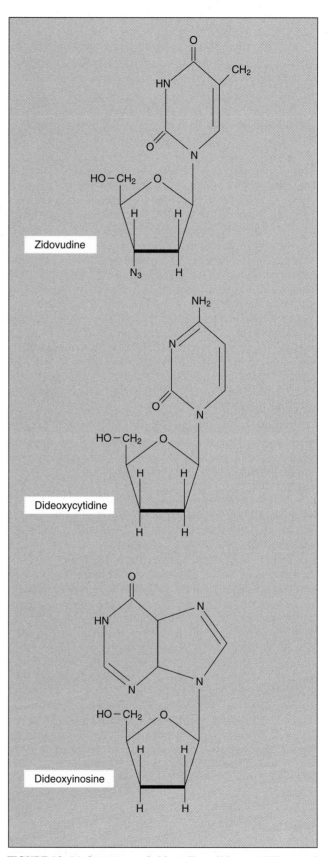

FIGURE 19–14. Structures of zidovudine, dideoxycytidine, and dideoxyinosine. These antiviral agents are inhibitors of viral reverse transcriptases.

Nevirapine also alters the cleavage specificity of the RNase H activity of reverse transcriptase. Nevirapine has been used in combination with other drugs for the treatment of AIDS, but HIV resistance to nevirapine appears rapidly.

Ion Channel Blockers. Amantadine and rimantadine are ion channel blockers whose structures are shown in Fig. 19–15.

The first antiviral ion channel blocker, called **amantadine** or **1-adamantanamine hydrochloride,** was developed during the 1960s as a possible treatment for influenza, but it turned out to be less effective in the cure of influenza than in the prevention of it. Amantadine is currently used in the prevention of influenza A during epidemics and in ameliorating early symptoms of influenza A. It is not effective against influenza B. Amantadine inhibits the replication of influenza virus at two points by preventing the M-2 capsid protein from acting as an ion channel. The drug raises the pH of the parasitized endosome, and this blocks conformational changes in the viral hemagglutinin needed for the viral envelope to fuse with host membranes. It also prevents the hemagglutinin from assuming the conformation needed to be incorporated into budding virions.

Rimantadine is similar to amantadine in its efficacy against influenza A and may be somewhat effective against influenza B. Because it is less toxic than amantadine, it is the preferred ion channel blocker.

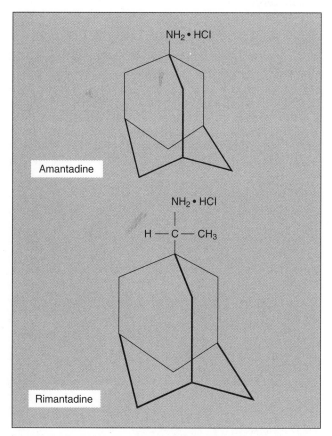

FIGURE 19–15. Structures of amantadine and rimantadine. These antiviral agents are ion channel blockers.

Protease Inhibitors. For mature HIV virions to be produced, the HIV protease must cleave the *gag* and *pol* gene products, which are polyproteins. A newly developed group of antiviral drugs is capable of inhibiting the activity of the HIV protease. Because the Gag and Pol polyproteins are not cleaved efficiently in the presence of these drugs, few infective virions are produced. Even though the net number of virions produced per infection cycle is not altered, a high percentage of the virions produced are noninfective. In the long term, this reduces the number of rounds of infection. Among the protease inhibitors approved for use in the USA are **indinavir, ritonavir,** and **saquinavir.** Protease inhibitors are effective against HIV when used in combination with a reverse transcriptase inhibitor, but resistance develops rapidly.

Antiviral Immunotherapy

Immune globulin, prepared from pooled human gamma globulin fractions, contains antibodies to hepatitis B and other viruses and has long been used to prevent or treat hepatitis B infections. With the development of a recombinant hepatitis B vaccine (see below), the importance of immune globulin in preventing hepatitis has diminished. However, the worldwide AIDS epidemic has encouraged many investigators to look again at immunotherapy as a possible therapeutic approach to the treatment of viral diseases.

Among the many immunotherapeutic approaches now being investigated are those based on using the following: (1) RNA fragments to induce the production of interferons, (2) interferons and interleukins to turn on the immune response, (3) lymphokine-activated cells to kill virus-infected cells or tumors, (4) drugs that alter the extent of the immune response, and (5) cellular receptors recognized by viral adhesins to prevent viral entry into host cells. Of these, only one has received approval for nonexperimental use. **Interferon alfa-2b,** a synthetic form of IFN-α, has been approved for the treatment of anogenital warts caused by human papillomaviruses.

Immunization Against Viral Diseases

Because few safe and effective antiviral drugs have been developed, the most important weapon against viral diseases has been that of prevention. Public health measures have been somewhat effective in reducing the spread of numerous viral diseases, particularly vector-borne and water-borne types. Many countries have made a great effort to reduce mosquito populations, and water sanitation has reduced the spread of enteric viruses quite substantially. But the most effective weapon against viruses that have a viremic phase has been immunization.

Table 19–5 lists the viral vaccines currently available in the USA. Some are composed of **live, attenuated viruses,** while others are composed of **killed**

TABLE 19–5. **Viral Vaccines Available in the USA**

Live, Attenuated Vaccines	Killed or Subunit Vaccines
Chickenpox	Hepatitis A
Measles	Hepatitis B
Mumps	Influenza
Poliomyelitis	Rabies
Rubella	
Yellow fever	

(inactivated) viruses or viral subunits. The smallpox vaccine, consisting of live vaccinia, is no longer administered.

The most effective viral vaccines are the ones that contain live, attenuated viruses. Those available in the USA are the chickenpox, measles, mumps, poliomyelitis, rubella, and yellow fever vaccines. Why live, attenuated vaccines are more effective than killed vaccines is still a matter of speculation, but their efficacy is probably related to at least two factors. First, after a live, attenuated vaccine is administered, the attenuated viruses continue to replicate. This expands the amount of immunogen that can be recognized by the immune system. Second, replicating viruses can be presented to the immune system in a variety of means that involve both class I and class II MHC restriction, with the activation of both CD4+ and CD8+ T cells. In contrast, killed vaccines do not replicate and are probably presented to T cells only via class II MHC restricted processes.

Live, attenuated vaccines present two major problems. First, there is some risk that "living" viruses can revert to virulence. Thus, great care must be taken to develop a vaccine that will not revert. Second, attenuated vaccines must be kept viable to be useful. This is a problem when the population to be vaccinated lives in a remote village in a developing country and no refrigeration is available to ensure the viability of the vaccine. Nevertheless, live vaccines have had a great impact on many viral diseases. The smallpox vaccine was so successful that smallpox was eradicated throughout the world, and the measles vaccine has resulted in a dramatic reduction in the number of cases of measles in industrialized countries.

The vaccines directed against hepatitis A, hepatitis B, influenza, and rabies are killed or subunit vaccines. That is, the viruses have been inactivated with formalin or β-propiolactone, or the vaccine has been constructed from specific parts of the virus. Some subunit vaccines contain viral glycoproteins harvested from intact virions, while others are composed of recombinant viral subunits produced within yeast cells. The hepatitis B vaccine was the first recombinant viral vaccine. Its development allowed patients to avoid using a vaccine derived from human blood. Inactivated vaccines carry no risk of reversion, but the immune response to them is lower than the response to attenuated viruses. In the case of influ-

enza vaccine, the vaccine must be administered annually just before the onset of "flu season."

New approaches to vaccine development have capitalized on using recombinant DNA technology to construct chimeric attenuated virus vaccines. Vaccinia virus has been envisioned by many as an ideal vector for such vaccines. If genes for a variety of virus subunits were placed successfully within the genome of vaccinia virus, in the future it might be possible to immunize a child against measles, mumps, rubella, chickenpox, and additional viruses with a single injection of the new vaccine.

NONHUMAN VIRUSES

Although people tend to think of viruses primarily as causes of human and animal diseases, viruses infect almost every known type of creature. Additionally, not all viruses have the familiar icosahedral or helical shape associated with animal viruses. This section of the chapter discusses two important groups of nonhuman viruses: bacterial viruses (bacteriophages) and viroids.

Bacteriophages

Bacteriophages were among the first viruses discovered. Because mammalian cell culture is such a recent development, most early studies that examined interactions between host cells and viruses involved *Escherichia coli* and the so-called T-even bacteriophages.

Phage Structure

Fig. 19–16 depicts a typical **T-even bacteriophage.** This type of bacteriophage has a complex structure, with a head that is composed of two half-icosahedrons connected by a short hexagonal prism. The head is attached to a tail that contains a tube which passes through a protein sheath. At the base of the tail are pins that serve as adhesins for the host bacterium, as well as a set of tail fibers that act as

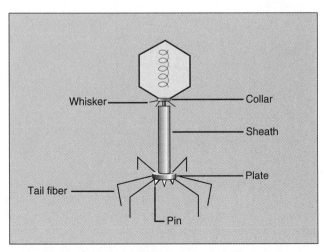

FIGURE 19–16. The complex structure of bacteriophage T4.

adhesins. Most bacteriophages exhibit this general structure, although a few phages do not have a tail. Most phages are icosahedral and are DNA viruses, but helical phages exist and some small phages contain RNA.

Phage Replication

When a bacteriophage interacts with a susceptible bacterium, it begins by attaching temporarily to lipopolysaccharides or host proteins via its tail fibers. The adhesion is then made permanent when the pins bind to receptors. The sheath contracts, and the phage nucleic acid is injected from the nucleocapsid through the tube into the recipient bacterium.

In 1952, A. D. Hershey and M. Chase used the phage infection cycle to determine that the information to replicate bacteriophages was associated with DNA. They labeled bacteriophage proteins with ^{35}S and labeled DNA with ^{32}P, allowed T2 bacteriophages to adsorb to *E. coli*, and then blended the suspension to separate the phages and bacteria. They found that the protein phage heads remained on the bacterial surface, the DNA entered the target bacterium, and the phages replicated when phage DNA alone was inside the host bacterium.

Once the phage nucleic acid enters the host bacterium, it begins a replication cycle similar to that seen with the animal viruses. Replication of the phage is under temporal control, and some phages have relatively elaborate DNA replication schemes.

Phage Infection Cycles

Based on the type of infection cycle they produce, phages may be characterized as lytic or lysogenic. With **lytic phages,** or **virulent phages,** infection results immediately in the production of new virions that are released by cell lysis. With **lysogenic phages,** or **temperate phages,** the phages infect bacteria and enter a state of dormancy in which their nucleic acid persists in the bacteria without producing progeny for long periods of time. This phenomenon is known as **lysogeny.** Occasionally, lysogenic phages revert to a lytic cycle and progeny phages are produced.

The best-studied lytic phages are the **T-even phages of *E. coli*,** while the best-studied lysogenic phage is the **lambda phage.** The nucleic acid of lytic phages remains separate from the bacterial chromosome and is replicated soon after entry. In contrast, the nucleic acid of lysogenic phages either remains separate from the chromosome (and enters a lytic cycle) or is inserted into the chromosome, where it becomes a **prophage** and remains until an inducing factor (such as ultraviolet light) causes it to exit the chromosome. Once the phage DNA is episomal, it is replicated and the lytic cycle begins.

When lytic phages are mixed with a suspension of susceptible bacteria and a sample is spread across an agar surface, the bacteria will grow as a lawn, but **clear plaques** will appear wherever there is a focus of phage infection. In contrast, lysogenic phages produce **cloudy plaques** because only occasional bacteria in the focus of infection undergo phage-induced lysis.

Significance and Application of Phages in Medicine

During the early part of the 20th century, scientists hoped that bacteriophages would prove to be effective antimicrobial agents. Volunteers with bacterial infections were injected with bacteriophages, but the results were disappointing. With the advent of antibiotics during the 1930s and 1940s, the impetus for experiments with phage treatment disappeared, but other uses of phages continued to be explored.

Bacteriophages have been shown to be significant to medicine in at least four ways. First, via the process of **transduction,** many bacteria transmit genes that are associated with disease virulence and antibiotic resistance. These genes are located on nonconjugative plasmids and are packaged into phage heads during spontaneous self-assembly (maturation) of the progeny phage. Second, some toxin genes are permanent residents of lysogenic phage chromosomes and are introduced into bacteria via the process of **phage conversion.** (See Chapter 3 for a discussion of transduction and phage conversion.) Third, bacteriophages have proved to be suitable agents for introducing pieces of DNA into susceptible bacteria as part of the process of **genetic engineering.** DNA segments that contain the *cos* site needed for efficient packaging into phage heads are created and then introduced into recipient bacteria via transduction. Fourth, bacteriophages have been helpful in the process of **bacterial typing.** Some bacteria, such as staphylococci, are typed by their susceptibility to specific sets of lysogenic bacteriophages. This is possible because phage susceptibility is related to the appearance of specific receptors that are located on the bacterial surface and match with the phage adhesin.

Viroids and Virusoids

Viroids are segments of single-stranded RNA that infect plant cells. Viroids have no capsids and are protected from degradation by being tightly wrapped like rods. They behave like segments of double-stranded RNA that have many short noncomplementary bubbles. Viroids lack initiation codons for protein synthesis and are probably not translated. They are replicated in the nucleus of host cells, but they are not copied into DNA like the retroviruses are. Some investigators believe that viroids originated from introns and that they cause diseases in plants by interfering with the splicing of host cell introns.

There are no known animal viroids. There are, however, defective viruses that are known as virusoids, have capsids, and act as satellites of other viruses. The human hepatitis D virus (see Chapter 20) is considered by some to be a virusoid.

Selected Readings

Adair, J. C., M. Gold, and R. E. Bond. Acyclovir neurotoxicity: clinical experience and review of the literature. South Med J 87:1227–1231, 1994.

Arnold, A., and G. F. Arnold. Human immunodeficiency virus structure: implications for antiviral design. Adv Virus Res 39:1–87, 1991.

Brown, P. The "brave new world" of transmissible spongiform encephalopathy (infectious cerebral amyloidosis). Mol Neurobiol 8:79–87, 1994.

Bruce, M. E., et al. PrP in pathology in scrapie-infected mice. Mol Neurobiol 8:105–112, 1994.

Coen, D. M. Acyclovir-resistant, pathogenic herpesviruses. Trends Microbiol 2:481–485, 1994.

Dudley, M. N. Clinical pharmacokinetics of nucleoside antiretroviral agents. J Infect Dis 171(supplement 2):S99–S112, 1995.

Easterbrook, P., and M. J. Wood. Successors to acyclovir. J Antimicrob Chemother 34:307–311, 1994.

Fields, B. N. Virology. New York, Raven Press, 1985.

Hammer, S. M., H. A. Kessler, and M. S. Saag. Issues in combination antiretroviral therapy: a review. J Acquir Immune Defic Syndr Hum Retrovirol 7(supplement 2):S24–S35, 1994.

Hayden, F. G., and A. J. Hay. Emergence and transmission of influenza A viruses resistant to amantadine and rimantadine. Curr Top Microbiol Immunol 176:119–130, 1995.

Hoover, D. R. The effects of long-term zidovudine therapy and *Pneumocystis carinii* prophylaxis on HIV disease: a review of the literature. Drugs 49:20–36, 1995.

Jacobson, M. A. Current management of cytomegalovirus disease in patients with AIDS. AIDS Res Hum Retroviruses 10:917–923, 1994.

Larson, S. B., et al. Three-dimensional structure of satellite tobacco mosaic virus at 2.9-A resolution. J Mol Biol 231:375–391, 1993.

Lee, S. Y., and D. Pavan-Langston. Role of acyclovir in the treatment of herpes simplex virus keratitis. Int Ophthalmol Clin 34:9–18, 1994.

Leonard, J. M. Perspectives in HIV protease inhibitors. Adv Exp Med Biol 394:319–325, 1996.

Lipsky, J. J. Zalcitabine and didanosine. Lancet 341:30–32, 1993.

Markham, A., and D. Faulds. Ganciclovir: an update of its therapeutic use in cytomegalovirus infection. Drugs 48:455–484, 1994.

Marsh, M., and A. Helenius. Virus entry into animal cells. Adv Virus Res 36:107–151, 1989.

Metcalf, P., M. Cyrklaff, and M. Adrian. The three-dimensional structure of reovirus obtained by cryo-electron microscopy. EMBO J 10:3129–3136, 1991.

Murphy, F. A., et al. Virus Taxonomy: The Classification and Nomenclature of Viruses. Sixth Report of the International Committee on Taxonomy of Viruses. New York, Springer-Verlag, 1994.

Palaniappen, C., et al. The cleavage specificity of ribonuclease H of human immunodeficiency virus 1 reverse transcriptase. J Biol Chem 270:4861–4869, 1995.

Prusiner, S. B. Biology and genetics of prion diseases. Annu Rev Microbiol 48:655–686, 1994.

Reichard, O., et al. Two-year biochemical, virological, and histological follow-up in patients with chronic hepatitis C responding in a sustained fashion to interferon alfa-2b treatment. Hepatology 21:918–922, 1995.

Richman, D. D. Antiretroviral drug resistance: mechanisms, pathogenesis, and clinical significance. Adv Exp Med Biol 394:383–395, 1996.

Spence, R. A., et al. Mechanism of inhibition of HIV-1 reverse transcriptase by nonnucleoside inhibitors. Science 267:988–993, 1995.

Stephens, E. B., and R. W. Compans. Assembly of animal viruses at cellular membranes. Annu Rev Microbiol 52:489–516, 1988.

Whitley, R. J. Neonatal herpes simplex virus infections: is there a role for immunoglobulin in disease prevention and therapy? Pediatr Infect Dis J 13:432–439, 1994.

Zaretsky, M. D. AZT toxicity and AIDS prophylaxis: is AZT beneficial for HIV-positive asymptomatic persons with 500 or more T4 cells per cubic millimeter? Genetica 95:91–101, 1995.

CHAPTER TWENTY

DNA VIRUSES

Adenoviruses, Hepadnaviruses, Herpesviruses, Papovaviruses, Parvoviruses, and Poxviruses

Chapter 19 presented an overview of viral replication. In addition to discussing diseases caused by DNA and RNA viruses, Chapters 20 and 21 will focus on two events that occur during the **eclipse phase:** the production of viral proteins and the replication of the viral genome. Three key processes must occur during the eclipse phase of DNA or RNA viruses.

First, messenger RNA (mRNA) must be generated to allow viral proteins to be synthesized. RNA viruses that are of positive polarity can be used directly as mRNA, but negative-sense RNA viruses must carry replicases within the nucleocapsid to synthesize mRNA. DNA viruses can, in general, use the host cell machinery to generate mRNA from their genomes.

Second, replicative enzymes and structural proteins must be synthesized. In some cases, the production of viral proteins is under temporal control, with replicative enzymes being the earliest proteins synthesized and structural genes being read late during the replication cycle. For some viruses, however, synthesis of replicases and structural proteins is the first molecular event after uncoating occurs.

Third, the viral nucleic acid must be replicated. The nucleic acid must be of the proper size, number of fragments, configuration, and polarity. Because of the variety of types of nucleic acid carried by viruses, numerous replication schemes exist, many of which require the participation of virus-encoded replicases.

Once viral proteins are made and the nucleic acid is replicated, the parts are used to construct nucleocapsids. This process, known as **maturation** or **morphogenesis,** occurs via spontaneous self-assembly.

CLASSIFICATION AND REPLICATION OF DNA VIRUSES

DNA viruses can be divided into four major classes, based on the structure of their DNA (see Table 19–3). Class I viruses have linear double-stranded DNA (dsDNA) genomes; class II viruses have circular dsDNA; class III viruses have linear single-stranded DNA (ssDNA); and class IV viruses have circular dsDNA with an incomplete strand.

General Concepts of Replication

Several general statements can be made about the various DNA classes.

First, in most DNA viruses, the DNA is infectious. That is, the viral genome can be used to directly infect cells when not enclosed within a capsid. This is possible because replication of DNA viruses does not generally depend on replicases packaged within the nucleocapsid, as it does with some RNA viruses. Instead, the host cell replication machinery can be used, and any additional enzymes needed for replication can be synthesized after the virus enters the host cell.

Second, the transcription and translation of DNA viruses are not linked, and viral messages are monocistronic. Thus, the molecular events of viral protein synthesis are much like those of eukaryotic cells, rather than those of prokaryotes. In some cases, the initial messages are much larger than the final messages translated at the ribosome, and the messages undergo posttranscriptional modification to remove introns.

Third, inverted repetitions are found in all DNA viruses that have linear DNA. These are found at the terminus of the genome in some viruses (for example, adenoviruses) but are found within the DNA substructure in others (for example, herpesviruses).

Fourth, except for the herpesviruses, parvoviruses, and hepadnaviruses, the replication of DNA viruses is under temporal control. Thus, only a portion of the DNA is transcribed before the genome is replicated. Early genes are generally those needed to assist in the DNA replication process. Once the viral genome is replicated, late genes are transcribed to produce capsid structural proteins.

Fifth, DNA viruses other than poxviruses replicate within the cell nucleus. It is here that the machinery needed to replicate the viral genome is available.

Poxviruses circumvent this process by carrying a DNA replicase within their nucleocapsid.

Sixth, most DNA viruses replicate semiconservatively. Because each viral genome has a unique structure, each virus generates a unique set of replicative intermediates during the replication process.

Specific Replication Schemes
Class I DNA Viruses

Adenoviruses, herpesviruses, and poxviruses are class I DNA viruses.

Adenoviruses. The adenovirus genome is about 3600 base pairs (bp) in length, and its replication occurs in two periods. During the early period, genes needed for viral replication are read and the viral genome is copied. This process takes about 8 hours. During the late period, proteins turn off host macromolecular synthesis and serve as structural proteins needed to build new capsids. This takes from 28 to 40 hours.

The adenovirus genome (Fig. 20–1A) is a linear dsDNA that has a **terminal protein** attached to a deoxycytosine at each 5′ end. This protein serves as a primer during DNA replication. Inverted repetitive nucleotide sequences occur at each end of both DNA strands. Because of these terminal repeats, when the DNA strands are separated they tend to form panhandle structures similar in appearance to those formed by insertion sequences.

During replication (see Fig. 20–1B), the adenovirus partially uncoats after entering the cell, and the nuclear core of the virus then releases the viral genome into the cell nucleus. During the first 8 hours, four sets of early genes (E1 through E4) are transcribed. Each transcript is capped at the 5′ end with guanine and a methyl group and is polyadenylated. Then introns are removed to complete the conversion of the transcript to usable mRNA. Capping the RNA transcript increases its affinity for the ribosome and makes its translation more efficient. E1 gene products are transcription and translation cofactors that activate the reading of various sets of adenovirus genes. E2 genes include those for a DNA polymerase, a terminal protein, and a DNA-binding protein. E3 gene products generally are glycoproteins that protect adenoviruses from various aspects of the immune response, and E4 genes encode proteins used during the late period of adenovirus replication.

Once E1 and E2 proteins are made, the adenovirus genome is replicated. Late genes are then read from the progeny DNA. Most late genes are capsid structural proteins, but some serve as **scaffolding proteins.** Scaffolding proteins assist in construction of the capsid but do not appear in the completed nucleocapsid.

Two additional RNA segments known as VA RNA$_I$ and VA RNA$_{II}$ are made from the adenovirus chromosome. These small RNA segments prevent the activation of a cellular protein kinase that would otherwise interfere with adenovirus replication.

Replication of the adenovirus genome (see Fig. 20–1C) requires the participation of terminal protein, DNA-binding protein, the adenovirus DNA polymerase, and a cellular nuclear factor. Replication begins with formation of a complex of terminal protein and deoxycytosine monophosphate (the TP-dCMP complex) at the 3′ end of the negative-sense DNA strand. This displaces the positive-sense strand, and continuous replication of the negative strand begins. Meanwhile, the positive strand cyclizes because of the terminal repeats, and a new replication cycle begins and uses the cyclized positive strand. Thus, replication is both asymmetric and semiconservative, and no Okazaki fragments are generated during replication.

Replication of the adenovirus genome takes place in the nucleus, but protein synthesis occurs in the cell cytoplasm. Viral proteins migrate back to the nucleus and are assembled there into capsids. Viral proteins inhibit the synthesis of host cell macromolecules. The replication of host DNA halts 8–10 hours after infection is initiated, and the synthesis of host RNA and protein stops 6–19 hours later. Only 10–15% of viral capsid proteins and DNA copies are assembled into complete virions, so the nuclei of infected cells typically contain paracrystalline arrays of viral macromolecules and other inclusion bodies. About 1% of the viral particles escape the cell, and no virus-induced cell lysis occurs.

Herpesviruses. Herpesviruses have a dsDNA genome that contains both terminal and internal repeat sequences (Fig. 20–2). Herpesviruses are uncoated at the nuclear pores, and the viral genome enters the nucleoplasm. Replication of herpesviruses begins about 4 hours after infection is initiated, peaks in about 6–8 hours, and halts after about 36 hours.

Herpesviruses differ from many DNA viruses in that their transcription is not controlled by replication of the viral genome. Thus, rather than being under true temporal regulation, the sequence of herpesvirus gene expression is controlled by posttranscriptional processing of mRNA. Genes needed for genome and capsid replication of herpesviruses are all read during the early phase, but only about 10% are translated at this time. Posttranscriptional processing mechanisms cause various genes to be translated at later times as they are needed. The translation of herpesvirus genes occurs in three stages and involves three types of genes: alpha genes in the immediate early stage, beta genes in the delayed early stage, and gamma genes in the late stage.

Alpha mRNAs are the first transcripts that are translated. Their expression is regulated by a component that is carried within the viral capsid and is called the alpha transduction factor. Each herpesvirus capsid carries between 500 and 1000 copies of this factor. Alpha proteins are phosphorylases, and several are *trans*-acting transcriptional activators of beta genes. Once the beta proteins are made, they inactivate the alpha genes and promote expression of the gamma genes. Among the beta genes are those that encode thymidine kinase, a DNA polymerase, and a DNA-binding protein. The gamma genes include

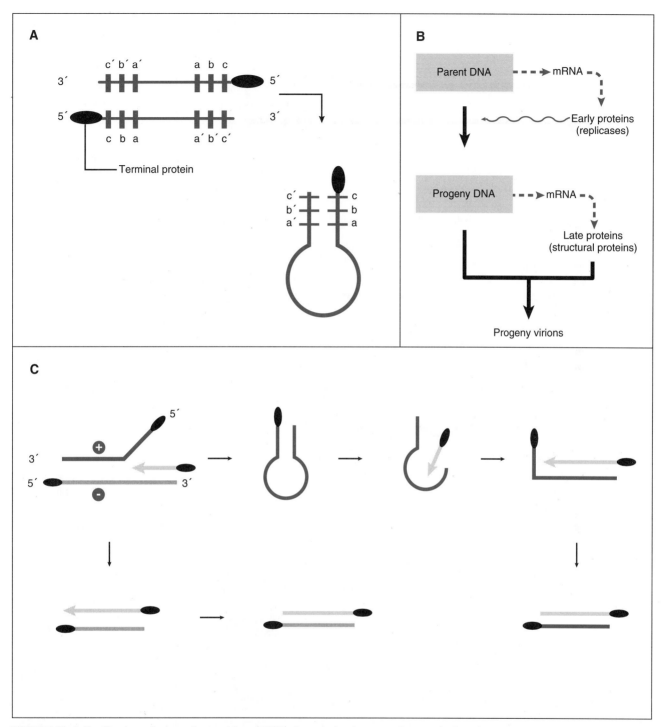

FIGURE 20–1. Replication of adenoviruses (class I DNA viruses). As shown in diagram **A,** the adenovirus genome is a linear double-stranded DNA with inverted repeat sequences at the end of each strand and with a terminal protein (TP) attached to each 5′ end. Diagram **B** shows that early proteins are synthesized from parent DNA and that late proteins are synthesized from progeny DNA. The hypothetical adenovirus DNA replication scheme is presented in diagram **C.** A complex of TP and deoxycytosine monophosphate (TP-dCMP complex) displaces the positive-sense DNA strand, and the negative-sense strand is copied continuously. The positive-sense strand probably forms a panhandle structure and is then copied continuously by another molecule of DNA polymerase.

envelope glycoproteins, the virus core protein, and capsid structural proteins.

As shown in Fig. 20–2, each set of proteins affects the expression of the next set of genes. The herpesvirus genome is replicated through the action of beta proteins. It is believed that the herpesvirus DNA is copied via a rolling circle mechanism that generates concatamers. The concatamers are later cleaved to yield genome-length DNA segments. Eventually, the nucleocapsids are assembled in the cell nucleus, and the viruses bud through the nuclear membrane and Golgi apparatus. When the viruses are replicating,

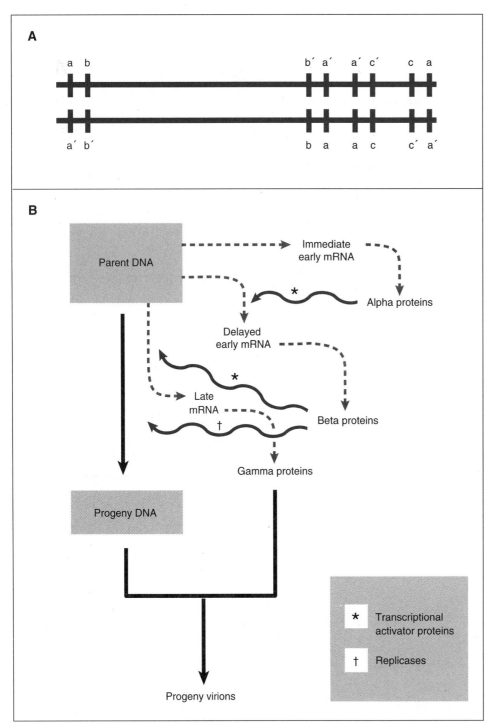

FIGURE 20–2. **Replication of herpesviruses (class I DNA viruses).** As shown in diagram **A,** the herpesvirus genome is a linear double-stranded DNA that contains several repeat sequences. Diagram **B** shows that the viral genome is transcribed to produce separate mRNA transcripts for immediate early, delayed early, and late genes. The alpha proteins allow expression of the beta proteins and shut off transcription of mRNA for their own synthesis (not shown). Beta proteins promote expression of gamma proteins and replicate the viral genome. Finally, gamma proteins are structural proteins used to construct progeny virions.

the nuclei of infected cells develop Feulgen-positive granular inclusion bodies. As the viral particles leak into the cytoplasm, the nuclear inclusion bodies become eosinophilic and Feulgen-negative. Thus, the eosinophilic nuclear inclusion bodies typically seen in herpesvirus-infected cells are burned-out remnants of viral factories.

Poxviruses. Poxviruses are extremely large brick-shaped viruses that are unusual among the DNA viruses in several respects. First, the DNA strands of poxviruses are linked covalently at or near the terminus. Second, the virus is uncoated in a two-stage process, with immediate early genes being read within the nucleocapsid core. Third, poxviruses are the only DNA viruses that replicate within the cytoplasm of host cells rather than within the nucleus.

The replication sequence of poxviruses is presented in Fig. 20–3. Poxviruses enter the cell via membrane fusion, and a host cytoplasmic enzyme then carries out the first stage of uncoating. This process leaves the viral genome within the nucleocapsid core, but it allows precursors and mRNA to go in and out

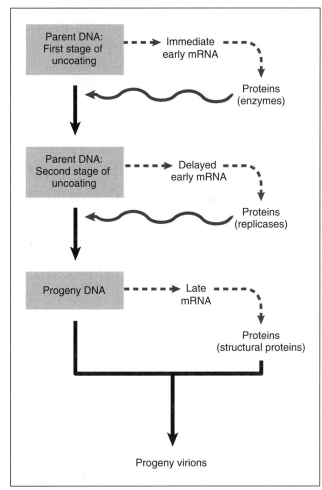

FIGURE 20–3. Replication of poxviruses (class I DNA viruses).
Poxviruses undergo a two-stage uncoating process during replication. The first stage of uncoating leaves the viral genome within the nucleocapsid core but allows precursors and mRNA to go in and out of the virus. During the second stage, immediate early mRNA is transcribed, and this produces proteins needed to complete the uncoating process. The viral DNA is released, and delayed early mRNA and proteins are produced. Among the delayed early proteins are replicases needed to produce progeny DNA. The progeny genomes are read to produce structural proteins, and progeny virions are constructed. The entire process takes place within the cell cytoplasm.

of the virus. After about 1 hour, the second stage of uncoating begins. This stage involves the transcribing and translation of about 100 immediate early genes, some of which are required to complete the uncoating process. Transcription of the early genes is initiated by a virus early transcription factor (VETF). Once the DNA is released into the cytoplasm, delayed early genes are read to provide factors necessary for replication of the viral genome.

The poxvirus genome is replicated semiconservatively and bidirectionally, resulting in the formation of lariat-shaped structures that must be cleaved by an endonuclease. The progeny DNA can then be used to produce intermediate and late proteins (sometimes called, instead, immediate late and delayed late proteins), many of which are structural

capsid and envelope proteins. About 60% of the very large poxvirus genome is read as late genes. The poxviruses are assembled within the cytoplasm and are subsequently released individually via cellular villi. Fewer than 10% of the assembled viruses are released from the cell.

Poxviruses process many of their proteins post-translationally. Some of the proteins are glycosylated or phosphorylated, but others are cleaved by proteases. This cleavage process is inhibited by the antibiotic rifampin, making poxviruses unique among the viruses in being sensitive to an antibacterial antibiotic.

Class II DNA Viruses

Papovaviruses constitute the class II DNA viruses. These viruses, which have circular dsDNA, are known for their ability either to enter a productive cycle or to transform cells. When papovaviruses encounter permissive host cells, they enter a cycle that results in the production of progeny virions and the lysis of the host cell. In contrast, in the presence of nonpermissive host cells, papovaviruses integrate their genome into that of the host cell, and the host cell is transformed without producing new virions.

Most of what is known about papovavirus replication comes from studies using simian virus 40 (SV40), but similar replication patterns are seen in two closely related polyomaviruses: JC virus and BK virus.

Papovaviruses have a circular genome that contains two DNA strands. Early genes are transcribed from one strand, while late genes are transcribed entirely from the other (Fig. 20–4A). The early phase begins shortly after the viral DNA enters the host cell nucleus and lasts from 14 to 18 hours. During this time, two or three early genes are generated from the "early" DNA strand. The first and most important of these is called **large T antigen.** This antigen is a multifunctional protein that uses adenosine triphosphate and can unwind DNA (helicase activity). Accumulation of large T antigen is needed to initiate both DNA replication and late gene transcription. Moreover, large T antigen serves as a surface glycoprotein on infected cells (known as tumor-specific transplantation antigen, or TSTA), stimulates cells in the G0 phase to enter S phase, inactivates host proteins that suppress cell growth, and is the SV40 oncogene. The second gene product generated during the early phase is called **small t antigen** and is involved in cell transformation. In the case of polyomaviruses, a third gene product, called **middle t antigen,** is also produced during the early phase and is oncogenic.

Once enough large T antigen accumulates, it binds to a 72-bp sequence that is repeated twice in tandem. This region is a **superpromoter,** and binding of T antigen both shuts down early gene transcription and activates the transcription of late genes from the "late" strand of the genome. Binding of the large T antigen to another site near this region also initiates the DNA replication process. Late genes encode three

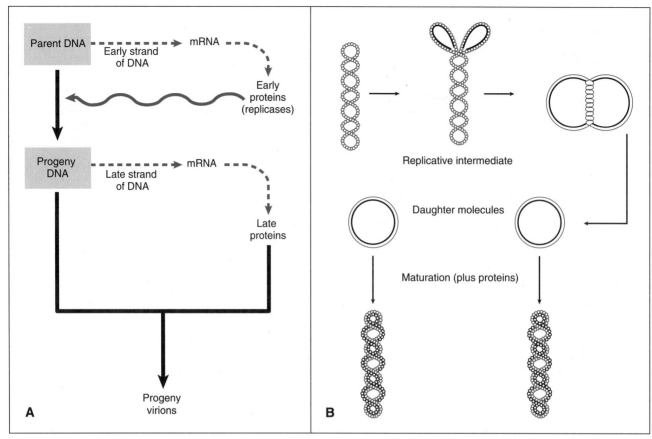

FIGURE 20–4. Replication of papovaviruses (class II DNA viruses). Papovaviruses contain circular double-stranded DNA. As shown in diagram **A,** early genes are transcribed from one strand, while late genes are transcribed from the other. The early genes are transcribed shortly after viral entry to produce large T and small t antigens. These proteins initiate DNA replication and late gene transcription, and they also serve as surface glycoproteins. Late proteins are capsid structural proteins. As shown in diagram **B,** replication of papovavirus DNA involves the formation of supercoiled replicative intermediates, and replication is bidirectional and semiconservative. (Source of diagram B: Davis, B. D., et al. Microbiology, 4th ed. Philadelphia, J. B. Lippincott Co., 1990. Redrawn and reproduced, with permission, from Lippincott-Raven Publishers.)

capsid proteins called VP1 (the major capsid protein), VP2, and VP3. These proteins overlap extensively on the viral genome.

Fig. 20–4B shows the mechanisms by which papovaviruses are believed to replicate. Replication is initiated by the binding of large T antigen to a 17-bp region composed entirely of pairs of adenine and thymine. Supercoiled replicative intermediates are formed, and the DNA is copied bidirectionally and semiconservatively. One strand is copied continuously while the other generates Okazaki fragments. Once the DNA has been copied, it quickly associates with histones to form chromatinlike structures. The progeny virions are assembled in the nucleus, and the virions escape the host cell via cell lysis.

Class III DNA Viruses

Parvoviruses are the class III DNA viruses. Parvoviruses fall into two general groups: (1) independent parvoviruses, which can replicate autonomously within permissive cells, and (2) dependoviruses, which cannot replicate unless certain key missing replicative factors are supplied by coinfecting the host cells with an adenovirus or herpesvirus. Only one parvovirus, B19, has been shown to cause disease in humans.

Parvoviruses have a single DNA strand with extensive palindromic sequences at each end that allow the DNA to form terminal hairpin loops (Fig. 20–5A). Individual parvoviruses may contain negative-sense DNA or positive-sense DNA but not both. Five genes are located on the parvovirus genome: VP1, VP2, and VP3 are capsid proteins, and NS1 and NS2 are noncapsid proteins that may be involved in regulation of DNA replication. Viral replication follows a simple pattern (see Fig. 20–5B), and transcription of parvovirus genes does not appear to be under temporal control.

Replication of parvovirus DNA requires helper functions that must come from the host cell or other viruses that have coinfected the target cell. Parvoviruses that are not dependoviruses obtain needed help by being replicated only within multiplying cells. The terminal hairpin turns of the parvovirus genome act as primers for DNA synthesis, and DNA replication follows a rolling hairpin mechanism (see Fig. 20–5C) that generates multiple genome-length replicative in-

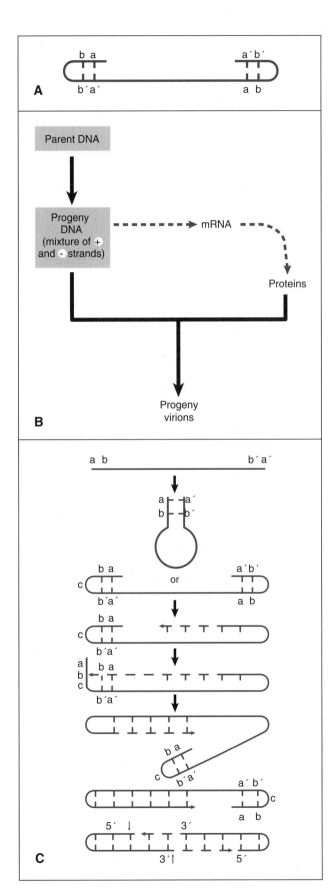

termediates. These are nicked to produce positive-sense and negative-sense DNA pieces that will subsequently be packaged into capsids within the nucleus.

Class IV DNA Viruses

Hepadnaviruses are the class IV DNA viruses. Hepatitis B virus (HBV) is an example. Hepadnaviruses contain circular DNA consisting of one complete strand that is 3200 bp and one incomplete strand that is 1700–2600 bp. The hepadnavirus genome encodes four genes, known as S, C, X, and P. The S gene encodes surface antigen (HBsAg); C encodes core antigen (HBcAg); X codes for a *trans*-active transcriptional activator protein; and P encodes HBV polymerase. HBV polymerase is unusual in that it can transcribe both RNA and DNA.

The replication cycle of HBV is shown in Fig. 20–6. The HBV core migrates to the nucleus, where the incomplete positive-sense strand of the HBV genome is completed by a cellular polymerase. The now-complete dsDNA is used to produce four species of mRNA as well as an RNA copy of the genome. The positive-sense RNA genome copy is then encapsulated by the addition of HBcAg. Within the nucleocapsid, the HBV polymerase copies the RNA strand to produce negative-sense DNA. HBsAg is then added to complete the nucleocapsid, and HBV polymerase copies the negative-sense DNA to complete the dsDNA genome of the virus. Thus, HBV gene expression is not under temporal control, and HBV is unique among the DNA viruses in that it utilizes a reverse transcriptase activity during viral replication.

CHARACTERISTICS AND EFFECTS OF DNA VIRUSES
Adenoviruses

Adenoviruses were first reported in the literature in 1953 and derived their name from the fact that they were initially found to cause cytopathic effects in adenoid tissues. The adenoviruses are now known to be a large group of icosahedral DNA viruses and have been found to cause infections of the respiratory tract, eye, urinary bladder, and intestines.

Characteristics of Adenoviruses

General Features.   Members of the family ***Adenoviridae*** are divided into two genera: ***Mastadenovirus*** (animal adenoviruses, including human adenovi-

FIGURE 20–5. Replication of parvoviruses (class III DNA viruses). The parvovirus genome (diagram **A**) is a single strand of DNA that can be of negative or positive polarity. Each strand has palindromic terminal sequences that allow the formation of hairpin loops. Viral replication follows a simple pattern (diagram **B**) with progeny DNA being transcribed to produce viral proteins. DNA replication (diagram **C**) follows a rolling hairpin pattern. (Source of diagram C: Davis, B. D., et al. Microbiology, 3rd ed. Hagerstown, Md., Harper and Row, 1980. Redrawn and reproduced, with permission, from Lippincott-Raven Publishers.)

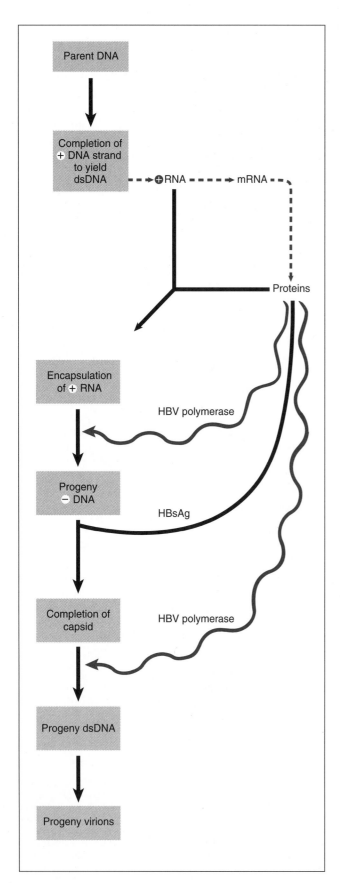

ruses) and ***Aviadenovirus*** (avian adenoviruses). The genus *Mastadenovirus* is further divided into six subgenera and various serotypes, based on biochemical and serologic criteria (Table 20–1). Human adenovirus types 40 and 41, which cause gastroenteritis, are considered to be fastidious because they were not cultivated successfully in cell cultures until recently. They can now be propagated in a transformed human embryonic kidney cell line known as cell line 293. The presence of adenovirus type 5 in cell line 293 makes the cells permissive for defective adenovirus types 40 and 41.

The capsids of adenoviruses are constructed from 240 hexamers and 12 pentons. Hexamers make up the triangular faces of the icosahedron, and pentons form the vertices. Emanating from each penton is a fiber, which makes the icosahedral virus look much like a satellite. The nucleocapsid, which is about 80–90 nm in diameter, contains a single piece of double-stranded DNA. The adenoviruses use their penton fibers to attach to host cells. After attachment, the entire virus is endocytosed, the outer capsid is removed, and the core enters the cell nucleus, where the virus is replicated by mechanisms described earlier in this chapter (see Specific Replication Schemes and Fig. 20–1).

Mechanisms of Pathogenicity. In immunocompetent patients, adenoviruses multiply at the point of entry (usually the pharynx, conjunctiva, or intestine) and remain localized within lymphoid tissue. Thus, adenovirus infections occur primarily within the lymph nodes that drain the initial infection sites. In immunocompromised patients, however, adenoviruses may spread throughout the body, and characteristic inclusions may be seen within samples taken from the brain, kidney, liver, and other major organs.

Adenoviruses responsible for acute disease in humans cause productive infections within parasitized host cells. The penton fibers of the virus are toxic to some host cells, shutting down almost all macromolecular synthesis in these cells. Thus, the presence of adenoviruses in a tissue is generally heralded by the appearance of focal necrosis, likely due to toxic effects of the adenoviruses and to immune-mediated damage of virus-infected host cells.

Some adenoviruses can enter a latent cycle in which the virus persists for years within a tissue but produces few progeny virions. This cycle occurs most often within lymphoid tissue and results in an inapparent infection.

FIGURE 20–6. Replication of hepadnaviruses (class IV DNA viruses). Hepadnaviruses such as hepatitis B virus (HBV) contain circular double-stranded DNA (dsDNA) with an incomplete strand. Replication of the virus begins with completion of the positive-sense DNA strand. This is followed by production of mRNA. The hepatitis B core antigen (HBcAg) partially encapsulates the positive-sense RNA, and HBV polymerase produces a DNA copy from the RNA. Hepatitis B surface antigen (HBsAg) is added to complete the nucleocapsid, and the HBV polymerase then copies the negative-sense DNA strand to produce dsDNA.

TABLE 20-1. The Adenoviruses and Their Associated Diseases

Subgenus	Serotypes	Oncogenic in Rodents	Latent in Humans	Human Diseases*
A	12, 18, and 31	Yes	No	None described.
B	3, 7, 11, 14, 16, 21, 34, and 35	Yes	No	Acute respiratory disease in military recruits (3, 7, 14, and 21); pneumonia (3 and 7); pharyngitis (3 and 7); pharyngo-conjunctival fever (3, 7, and 14); epidemic keratoconjunctivitis (11); and hemorrhagic cystitis (11 and 21).
C	1, 2, 5, and 6	No	Yes	Pharyngitis (1, 5, and 6); and pneumonia in children (1 and 2).
D	8–10, 13, 15, 17, 19, 20, 22–30, 32, 33, 36–39, and 42–47	No	No	Epidemic keratoconjunctivitis (8, 19, and 37).
E	4	No	No	Acute respiratory disease and pneumonia in military recruits (4); and epidemic keratoconjunctivitis (4).
F	40 and 41	No	No	Gastroenteritis (40 and 41).

*Serotypes responsible for each disease are in parentheses.

Although some adenoviruses are oncogenic in rodents, none has been shown to be oncogenic in humans.

Diseases Due to Adenoviruses

Epidemiology. Most individuals are infected with adenoviruses early in life, and many develop latent infections of the tonsils and adenoids that persist for years. Epidemics of adenovirus disease have been reported in military recruits, among whom spread is probably via respiratory secretions and is augmented by crowded conditions within barracks. Pharyngoconjunctival fever is an eye infection acquired by swimming in pools or ponds contaminated with adenovirus, and other eye infections are spread on hands or during tonometry. Eye infections are extremely contagious because the adenovirus can persist on fomites (such as instruments, toys, or doorknobs) for up to 2 months. The means by which adenovirus infections of the urinary and gastrointestinal tract are spread are not known.

Diagnosis. Adenoviruses most commonly cause diseases that affect the respiratory tract (acute respiratory disease, pneumonia, and pharyngitis); eyes (pharyngoconjunctival fever and epidemic keratoconjunctivitis); urinary bladder (hemorrhagic cystitis); and gastrointestinal tract (gastroenteritis).

(1) History and Physical Examination

(a) Respiratory Tract Disease. Adenoviruses are a common cause of acute febrile **pharyngitis** in children, causing up to 10% of childhood respiratory infections. In military recruits, adenoviruses are an important cause of **acute respiratory disease** (ARD), which usually occurs during the early weeks of basic training and is heralded by the rapid onset of fever (temperature up to 40 °C or 104 °F), cough, sore throat, malaise, and rhinorrhea. Physical examination may reveal rales, rhonchi, and pharyngitis; and x-rays may reveal patchy infiltrates. The disease usually runs its course in less than a week, but it may progress to **pneumonia.** Patients with pneumonia de-

velop a nonproductive cough that leads to dyspnea and tachypnea. Radiographic examination may reveal infiltrates and pleural effusions. Adenovirus pneumonia may also occur in children.

(b) Eye Infections. At summer camps for children, adenoviruses have been reported to cause outbreaks of **pharyngoconjunctival fever,** also called swimming pool conjunctivitis. Affected children develop a low-grade fever (temperature up to 38 °C or 100.4 °F), conjunctivitis, pharyngitis, rhinitis, and cervical adenitis. They may also suffer from malaise, vomiting, headache, and diarrhea. The blood vessels of the eye are hyperemic, and small hemorrhages may develop. In some cases, the eyes become quite crusted. Although the disease begins rapidly and generally runs its course without sequelae in 3–5 days, it may persist for up to 10 days.

Adenoviruses sometimes cause **epidemic keratoconjunctivitis.** This disease is also called shipyard eye because it was first described among shipyard workers who developed severe conjunctivitis in eyes traumatized by paint and rust chips. In individuals infected by adenovirus, conjunctivitis begins 4–24 days after exposure to the virus and initially causes one eye to become painful, red, and watery. Itching and preauricular adenopathy may also be noted. If the second eye becomes involved, it is usually less severely affected. Eye examination reveals hyperemia, lid edema, ptosis, follicles, and the presence of a pseudomembrane or membrane. The conjunctivitis wanes after 1–4 weeks and is replaced by keratitis that may disturb vision for several months. This contrasts with bacterial conjunctivitis, which is of much shorter duration and is not generally followed by keratitis. About 10% of patients spread the disease to household contacts, and nosocomial outbreaks sometimes occur in eye clinics.

(c) Bladder Infections. Adenovirus types 11 and 21 cause **hemorrhagic cystitis** in children, with infected boys outnumbering infected girls by almost 3:1. Symptoms and signs include urinary frequency, dysuria, and hematuria, and these clinical manifestations usually resolve spontaneously in less than a week. However, the kidneys of some patients become persistently infected with adenovirus. Although these patients suffer from no ill effects from their latent infection, they may shed the virus in their urine for months or years.

(d) Gastrointestinal Infections. Adenovirus types 40 and 41 cause **gastroenteritis,** accompanied by diarrhea and fever. While rotavirus is the most common cause of gastroenteritis in infants and young children, adenovirus is the second most common cause. Rotavirus and adenovirus cause similar manifestations, but gastroenteritis due to adenovirus is accompanied by less vomiting and dehydration than that due to rotavirus. The adenovirus disease generally resolves spontaneously in 8–12 days.

(e) Other Adenovirus Infections. Adenoviruses have caused sporadic cases of disseminated infection in severely immunocompromised patients. They have also been reported to cause meningitis, encephalitis, pericarditis, chronic interstitial fibrosis, and congenital abnormalities. Adenovirus types 1, 2, 3, and 5 have been circumstantially implicated as possible causes of intussusception.

(2) Laboratory Analysis. The diagnosis of adenovirus diseases is generally made on clinical grounds. When a specific diagnosis is needed, cell cultures can be inoculated with an appropriate clinical sample, such as sputum, stool, fresh urine, conjunctival scrapings, or mucosal scrapings. Adenoviruses can be cultivated within primary monkey kidney cells, human diploid fibroblasts, HEp-2 cells, and cell line 293. HEp-2 cells are preferred for most adenoviruses, but cell line 293 should be used to propagate gastrointestinal adenoviruses. Cytopathic effects due to viral replication within the cells are seen in 2–7 days. Isolated viruses can be identified by electron microscopy, grouped by hemagglutination, and specifically serotyped with antibody.

Diagnosis can also be made by demonstrating that the patient has a fourfold or greater rise in the level of serum antibody to a specific adenovirus. Immunologic tests used to detect antibody include complement fixation, virus neutralization, hemagglutination inhibition, enzyme-linked immunosorbent assay (ELISA), and radioimmunoassay. Antibodies appear about 1 week after the adenovirus infection begins. Antibodies detected by complement fixation wane in about a year, but those detected by virus neutralization may persist for years. Eye infections can be diagnosed by examining material from conjunctival scrapings using an enzyme immunoassay that detects the presence of adenovirus antigens.

Treatment. There are no antibiotics available to eradicate adenoviruses, so treatment is designed to alleviate the symptoms of disease.

Prevention. There is no vaccine to prevent adenovirus diseases. The spread of some adenovirus infections can be slowed by using proper hygiene, such as washing hands. Equipment used in eye examinations (especially tonometers) should be properly cleaned. Children with epidemic keratoconjunctivitis should be excused from school. Ocular secretions are infectious for up to 2 weeks after the onset of symptoms of conjunctivitis.

Herpesviruses
Classification, Structure, and Viral Replication

The herpesviruses are members of a large group of enveloped icosahedral viruses that contain dsDNA as their genome. Although there are about 80 members of the family *Herpesviridae,* only 9 have been identified as causing disease in humans. Based on their biologic characteristics, the 9 herpesviruses have been placed into three subfamilies (Table 20–2). The *Alphaherpesvirinae* include herpes simplex viruses 1 and 2, varicella-zoster virus, and simian herpesvirus B. These organisms are cytolytic viruses that grow rapidly and form latent infections in neurons. The *Betaherpesvirinae* include cytomegalovirus and human herpesviruses 6 and 7. These organisms grow slowly as noncytolytic viruses and cause latent infections in a variety of cells. The *Gammaherpesvirinae* include Epstein-Barr virus and human herpesvirus 8. Epstein-Barr virus not only causes active infections in squamous pharyngeal epithelial cells but also causes persistent lymphoproliferative infections in B cells. Human herpesvirus 8 infects endothelial cells and is associated with Kaposi's sarcoma and non-Hodgkin's lymphoma in patients with acquired immunodeficiency syndrome (AIDS).

Fig. 20–7 shows the structure of a typical herpesvirus. The herpesvirus genome is closely associated with a toroidal (doughnut-shaped) core protein and is enclosed within an icosahedral capsid constructed from 162 hollow capsomers. The capsid is surrounded by an amorphous protein structure known as the tegument, and the nucleocapsid is enclosed within a typical lipoprotein envelope that contains numerous glycoprotein peplomers or spikes. The entire virion is large, with a diameter of 120–200 nm. The genome, which contains reiterated sequences, encodes 70–200 proteins in its 125–229 bp. Thus, herpesviruses are, after the poxviruses, the largest viruses known.

Herpesviruses adsorb to host cells via envelope glycoproteins and enter the cells via viropexis. The virus is uncoated, and the DNA moves to the nucleus, where it is replicated by mechanisms described earlier in this chapter (see Specific Replication Schemes and Fig. 20–2). Once the nucleocapsids are constructed in the nucleus, they must first gain a coating of tegument and then be surrounded by a lipid envelope that contains viral glycolipids. Some herpesviruses seem to gain their envelope by budding through the nuclear membrane, with peplomers being added to the envelope later as the virus-containing vacuole travels through the cytoplasm (Fig. 20–8A). Studies suggest that the varicella-zoster virus buds through the inner nuclear membrane to gain a primary envelope but then loses this coating when it buds through the rough endoplasmic reticulum and into the cyto-

TABLE 20–2.   The Herpesviruses and Their Associated Diseases

Subfamily and Genus	Common Name	Primary Infections	Latent or Persistent Infections
Alphaherpesvirinae *Simplexvirus*	Herpes simplex viruses 1 and 2 (human herpesviruses 1 and 2).	Gingivostomatitis (1); pharyngitis (1 > 2); eye infections (1 > 2); skin infections (1 or 2); genital herpes infection (2 > 1); congenital herpes infection (2 > 1); encephalitis (1 > 2); and disseminated herpes infection (1 > 2).	Herpes labialis (1 > 2); eye infections (1 > 2); skin infections (1 or 2); genital herpes infection (2 > 1); encephalitis (1 > 2); and disseminated herpes infection (1 > 2).
	Simian herpesvirus B (cercopithecine herpesvirus 1).	Myelitis and hemorrhagic encephalitis with multiorgan involvement.	Unknown; possible zosteriform skin infections.
Varicellovirus	Varicella-zoster virus (human herpesvirus 3).	Varicella (chickenpox).	Herpes zoster (shingles).
Betaherpesvirinae *Cytomegalovirus*	Cytomegalovirus (human herpesvirus 5).	Cytomegalic inclusion disease in newborns; mononucleosis; pneumonitis; hepatitis; and disseminated disease in immunocompromised patients.	Similar to primary infections but generally milder.
Roseolovirus	Human herpesvirus 6.	Roseola infantum, mononucleosis, pneumonitis, and hepatitis.	Unknown.
	Human herpesvirus 7.	May be similar to infections due to human herpesvirus 6.	Unknown.
Gammaherpesvirinae *Lymphocryptovirus*	Epstein-Barr virus (human herpesvirus 4).	Infectious mononucleosis.	Burkitt's lymphoma and nasopharyngeal carcinoma.
Unknown	Human herpesvirus 8 (Kaposi's sarcoma–associated herpesvirus).	Unknown.	Kaposi's sarcoma and non-Hodgkin's lymphoma in patients with acquired immunodeficiency syndrome (AIDS).

plasm (see Fig. 20–8B). The now-naked virion enters the *trans*-Golgi network, where it becomes wrapped within a membrane that contains both tegument proteins and peplomers. These prelysosomes eventually carry the newly enveloped virions to the cell membrane, where they are released when the prelysosomal membrane fuses with the cell membrane.

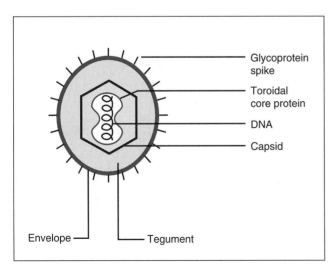

FIGURE 20–7. Typical structure of the herpesviruses.

Glycoprotein spike
Toroidal core protein
DNA
Capsid
Envelope
Tegument

Characteristics of Herpes Simplex Viruses 1 and 2

Infections with herpes simplex viruses (HSV) are some of the most common infections known. The name "herpes" comes from the Greek word meaning "to creep," and the earliest descriptions of herpetic lesions come from the Greek physician Hippocrates. HSV-1 and HSV-2 cause similar infections, but HSV-1 most commonly causes infections above the waist, and HSV-2 is most often associated with infections below the waist.

General Features.   HSV-1 and HSV-2 are 150–200 nm in diameter. Although the two viruses are very similar, they can be differentiated by their biologic properties. HSV-1 differs from HSV-2 in that it forms small (rather than large) pocks on chick chorioallantoic membranes, does not form plaques on chick embryo cell monolayers, is not sensitive to high temperature (40 °C), is sensitive to the presence of heparin, and does not form syncytia on human embryonic kidney cell monolayers. HSV-1 is less neurotropic in mice than is HSV-2, and the base composition of its DNA differs from that of HSV-2. The two viruses can also be differentiated by their reactivities with monoclonal antibodies directed against HSV glycoprotein G.

Mechanisms of Pathogenicity.   HSV organisms multiply in parabasal and intermediate epithelial cells

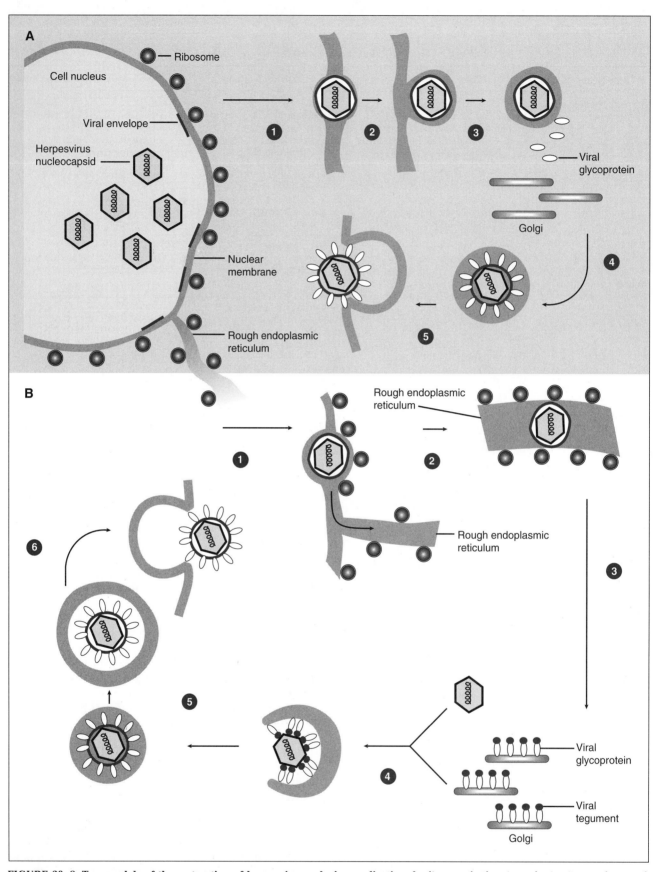

FIGURE 20–8. Two models of the maturation of herpesviruses during replication. In diagram **A,** the virus obtains its envelope and tegument by budding into the nuclear membrane (step 1). The nuclear membrane breaks away to form a vacuole (steps 2 and 3), and viral glycoproteins are added by the Golgi apparatus (step 4). Following fusion of the vacuole with the cell membrane, the virus escapes (step 5). In diagram **B,** the virus receives a primary envelope from the inner aspect of the nuclear membrane (step 1), migrates into the rough endoplasmic reticulum (step 2), and then loses the primary envelope when it buds into the cytoplasm (step 3). When it reaches the *trans*-Golgi network, the virus is enveloped and coated with tegument and glycoproteins (steps 4 and 5). The prelysosome eventually migrates to the cell membrane, where it fuses and releases viruses into the extracellular space (step 6).

at the site of their entry into the body, which is usually a mucosal surface or a break in the skin surface. As the viruses are replicated, infected cells may fuse with adjacent cells to form syncytia, but viral replication invariably results in cell lysis. These processes lead to the formation of a thin-walled vesicle with an inflammatory base. The lesion contains multinucleated giant cells that exhibit ballooning degeneration and intranuclear inclusions. Individuals with a normal immune response control viral dissemination and recover from primary infection because they elicit a vigorous CD8$^+$ T cell (cytotoxic T lymphocyte, or CTL) response. Immunocompromised patients who fail to generate an adequate CTL response can suffer from disseminated HSV disease at this time.

Unfortunately, recovery from primary HSV infection does not eradicate the virus. Instead, the virus enters the sensory nerve that innervates the site of infection. It then travels via retrograde intra-axonal transport to the dorsal root ganglion, where it enters a latent state. This latent state seems to be promoted by the production of antiviral cytokines by CTLs. Because the infected neurons do not express significant amounts of major histocompatibility complex (MHC) class I or II glycoproteins, the infected nerve is not killed. Instead, cytokines reduce the expression of so-called immediate early (alpha) genes, whose expression is required for other HSV genes to be expressed. Thus, no viral progeny are made, but the cell body retains 10–100 nonintegrated copies of the viral genome. Meanwhile, the latently infected neuron produces thousands of copies of nonpolyadenylated antisense transcripts known as **latency-associated transcripts** (LATs). Some of the LAT species may be involved in the activation of HSV genes when the HSV infection is reactivated.

HSV reactivation is poorly understood, but infection often recurs when the patient is stressed or immunodepressed. The virus travels back down the axon to the periphery, where it multiplies within epithelial cells and produces a lesion similar to that formed during primary HSV infection. The recurrent infection is generally less severe and of shorter duration than the primary infection.

Diseases Due to Herpes Simplex Viruses 1 and 2

Epidemiology.   HSV-1 and HSV-2 infect only humans, and patients are infected via direct contact with infected secretions. Because HSV-1 is most often the cause of gingivostomatitis, it is passed most frequently in oral secretions. HSV-1 is usually acquired during childhood, and most children in poorer populations have been infected by the time they reach adolescence. HSV-1 can also be passed through breaks in the skin and represents an occupational hazard for dental and medical personnel and for athletes competing in contact sports. In contrast, HSV-2 is usually transmitted during sexual contact, and most primary infections occur after puberty.

A pregnant woman with a genital HSV infection can transmit the virus to her offspring. During late pregnancy or at parturition, an estimated 1 in every 2000–10,000 infants is infected with HSV—usually HSV-2. The infant's chance of becoming infected is 3–4% if the mother's disease is recurrent, but it is 30–40% if the mother's infection is a primary genital infection. Premature infants are at greatest risk, and use of scalp electrodes during fetal monitoring increases the risk of congenital infection.

HSV can be found in the oral or genital secretions of many individuals who have no apparent herpetic lesions. Dissemination of the virus by asymptomatic patients is an important epidemiologic problem because infected individuals generally assume that they are not infectious when asymptomatic. This incorrect assumption leads them to take fewer precautions.

Diagnosis
(1) History and Physical Examination
(a) Primary Herpes Infections.   HSV-1 primary infections can be asymptomatic, but many patients develop mucosal or cutaneous lesions, especially on the mouth or other parts of the face and head. The most common clinical manifestations associated with HSV-1 primary infections are gingivostomatitis, pharyngitis, follicular conjunctivitis, blepharitis, and herpetic whitlow. Although genital infections due to HSV-1 occur, the vast majority of genital herpes infections are caused by HSV-2.

In many cases, primary infection with HSV-1 occurs when the patient is under 5 years of age and presents as **gingivostomatitis** accompanied by **pharyngitis.** Between 2 and 12 days after contact with a person shedding HSV-1, the patient develops a fever and sore throat, followed by the appearance of crops of vesicular lesions throughout the mouth. The lesions may spread to the skin around the mouth, and the patient's oral mucous membranes become extremely tender. The breath at this time is malodorous, the gums may bleed, and the draining lymph nodes are swollen. The disease will run its course within 2 weeks. Older children and adults often develop pharyngitis without gingivostomatitis. After the primary infection resolves, the virus becomes latent within the trigeminal ganglion. In at least 50% of these cases, the patient later develops recurrent attacks of herpes labialis.

HSV-1 (and, rarely, HSV-2) can infect the eye, causing either unilateral follicular **conjunctivitis** or **blepharitis.** Manifestations of conjunctivitis include photophobia, edema of the eyelid, and regional lymphadenopathy. Blepharitis is characterized by vesicular lesions on the lid margin of the eye. Most patients recover completely within 2–3 weeks, but if the disease spreads to the stroma, recovery may be a slow process.

Herpetic whitlow is a skin infection that is usually seen in medical and dental health care workers who come in contact with HSV-infected mucosae. In most cases, a single finger is involved, and itching and pain precede the development of one or more vesicular lesions (Fig. 20–9). The draining lymph nodes swell, and there may be systemic symptoms of infection. Wrestlers and football players may have

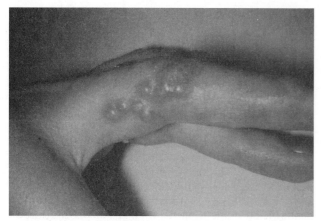

FIGURE 20–9. The lesions of herpetic whitlow. (Reproduced, with permission, from Callen, J. P., et al. Color Atlas of Dermatology. Philadelphia, W. B. Saunders Company, 1993.)

similar lesions that occur on other areas of the skin and are known as **herpes gladiatorum.** Nosocomial herpetic whitlow is almost always due to HSV-1, but community-acquired whitlow is commonly due to HSV-2.

HSV-2 is the cause of 70–95% of **primary genital herpes infections.** Patients develop vesicular lesions on the penis, vulva, perineum, buttocks, cervix, or vagina 2–7 days after sexual contact with a person shedding the virus. At this time, the patient may experience fever, malaise, localized pain, anorexia, inguinal lymphadenopathy, dysuria, and discharge. The infection is often more severe in women than in men and may lead to myeloradiculitis, urinary retention, and obstipation. About 5–10% of patients develop mild meningitis. Primary attacks of genital herpes generally resolve within 3 weeks.

(b) Recurrent Herpes Infections. Because HSV-1 and HSV-2 become dormant within sensory root ganglia, most patients who recover from the primary herpes infection later develop recurrent herpes disease. The most commonly seen recurrent infections are herpes labialis, herpes keratitis, and genital herpes infection.

Herpes labialis occurs when stressors activate the replication of HSV within the trigeminal ganglion. The viruses infect the epithelial cells over the nerve and most often cause vesicles to appear along the vermilion border of the outer lip. The lesions are painful and progress from vesicles to crusted ulcers within 48 hours. Many patients complain of prodromal symptoms such as localized pain, burning, or itching 6–48 hours before the lesions appear. Although there may be a localized lymphadenopathy, most patients do not experience systemic symptoms. Recurrent herpes labialis is much milder than is primary oral herpes infection.

Although **keratitis** is the most common recurrent ocular herpes infection, some patients develop **blepharitis** or **keratoconjunctivitis.** Most patients develop branching dendritic ulcers that stain with fluorescein. If the stroma becomes involved and uveitis

develops, recurrent attacks may lead to loss of visual acuity. Some patients may completely lose sight in the affected eye if there are several attacks with deep stromal involvement.

Episodes of **recurrent genital herpes infection** are less severe than the primary infection, but their psychologic effects can be devastating. The episodes may be preceded by a prodrome of tingling or burning sensations, and the lesions generally heal within 6–10 days. Patients may continue to shed the viruses, however, even after the lesions have healed.

(c) Complications of Herpes Infections. The most frequent complications of herpes infections in adults are the congenital spread of HSV to infants, herpes encephalitis, and dissemination of HSV in immunocompromised patients.

Many infants with **congenital herpes infection** have mild manifestations. Others suffer from jaundice, microcephaly, seizures, chorioretinitis, temperature instability, and herpetic skin vesicles. Disseminated and encephalitic herpetic infections in newborns have a high mortality rate, but infants with only localized skin or mucous membrane lesions rarely die.

Encephalitis due to HSV rarely occurs, but it is the most common sporadic cause of encephalitis in the USA. The virus is believed to travel via neural routes to the brain during either primary or recurrent infection, resulting in a necrotizing hemorrhagic encephalitis. Patients develop headache, fever, olfactory hallucinations, focal seizures, behavior disorders, and speech difficulties. Death occurs in 60–80% of untreated patients. Neurologic sequelae are found in more than 90% of those who recover.

In immunocompromised patients, HSV may cause colitis, pneumonia, perianal ulcers, esophagitis, tracheobronchitis, or hepatitis. Patients with AIDS are extremely susceptible to these infections.

(2) Laboratory Analysis. Scrapings from a lesion can be fixed and stained with Wright's or Giemsa stain. Lesions caused by HSV should contain multinucleated giant cells. Because lesions caused by varicella-zoster virus are histologically indistinguishable, a precise diagnosis requires cultivation of the virus in tissue culture. Cytopathic effects can generally be seen 24–48 hours after inoculation of the monolayer. The virus can then be further typed using immunohistochemical or microneutralization techniques. In the future, diagnosis will likely involve using polymerase chain reaction (PCR) or DNA hybridization technology to identify viral DNA in samples from infected patients. PCR is already the method of choice for demonstrating the presence of HSV in the cerebrospinal fluid of patients with HSV encephalitis.

Treatment. Latent viruses are not affected by antiviral antibiotics, but active HSV infections can be treated with acyclovir. This drug has been shown to offer only modest help for those suffering from recurrent attacks of genital herpes or herpes labialis. Patients infected with HSV that is resistant to acyclovir can be treated with foscarnet. Vidarabine has been used with some success in the treatment of herpes simplex encephalitis and neonatal herpes infection.

Prevention.   No vaccines are available for the prevention of HSV infections.

Sexually active individuals can prevent the acquisition of genital herpes by using a condom during sexual intercourse with a partner who has a history of HSV infection, even if that partner has no current symptoms of infection.

Any pregnant woman suspected of having genital herpes infection should be examined for viral shedding or the presence of lesions when labor begins. If an infant is at risk, delivery should be by cesarean section and should occur not more than 4 hours after the membranes rupture. If the infant is born vaginally and vaginal swabs from the mother are later shown to be HSV-positive, the infant's eyes, nose, throat, umbilicus, and anus should be swabbed and cultured for the presence of HSV.

Medical and dental health care workers can prevent occupational HSV infection by wearing gloves when they examine the mucous membranes of patients.

Characteristics of Simian Herpesvirus B

Simian herpesvirus B is a natural pathogen of rhesus and cynomolgus monkeys. These monkeys often experience asymptomatic infections, and recurrent infections similar to recurrent human herpes infections occur when the monkeys are under stress. Humans are infected when they come into contact with the oral or genital secretions of infected monkeys.

Diseases Due to Simian Herpesvirus B

The initial case of human simian herpesvirus B disease occurred in 1932, when an investigator involved in poliovirus experiments was bitten by a rhesus monkey. Three days later, vesicles appeared in the area of the bite. The investigator had severe abdominal cramps on the 10th day and died soon after from progressive ascending myelitis. Since that time, there have been reports of about 40 cases of simian herpesvirus B disease in humans. Lesions developed 2–14 days after contact with secretions of infected monkeys and usually resulted in death.

Serologic studies of monkey handlers suggest that asymptomatic human infections do not occur. Abdominal pain is a common complaint early in the disease. Other manifestations include severe headache, fever, malaise, regional lymphadenopathy, myelitis, and hemorrhagic encephalitis with multiorgan involvement. Diagnosis requires culture of the virus. Because the virus is a biosafety level 4 agent, samples must be sent to an appropriate facility with level 4 protection capabilities.

To prevent infection, individuals who have been scratched or bitten by a monkey should immediately clean the area vigorously with soap, iodine, or bleach solutions. Patients with suspected primary herpesvirus B lesions should be treated with acyclovir or ganciclovir. Infections have remained localized with early treatment, but patients with encephalitis have not responded well to acyclovir treatment.

Characteristics of Varicella-Zoster Virus

The varicella-zoster virus (VZV) causes two clinically distinct diseases. Chickenpox, also called varicella, is a primary VZV infection and occurs mainly in children. Herpes zoster, also called shingles, is a recurrent VZV infection that occurs in some individuals who have recovered from chickenpox.

General Features.   VZV is very similar to HSV-1 and HSV-2. Each enveloped VZV is 150–200 nm in diameter, and the icosahedral capsid encloses a genome that encodes about 75 proteins. Only enveloped virions are infectious, and the envelope is highly sensitive to air drying and to detergents.

Mechanisms of Pathogenicity.   VZV organisms multiply rapidly at the site of entry into the body (probably the respiratory mucosa) and then are disseminated throughout the body via the blood and lymphatic vessels. The virions multiply within monocytes, capillary endothelial cells, and epithelial cells. Their multiplication within the epithelium results in the development of the characteristic vesicular rash of chickenpox. The lesions contain VZV and involve the corium and dermis. Some epithelial cells within the lesion fuse to form polynucleated giant cells. Others merely show balloon degeneration and eosinophilic intranuclear inclusions.

After the primary infection is controlled by virus-specific T lymphocytes, the organisms can enter sensory nerves in the affected skin and travel to the dorsal root ganglia, where they become dormant. Years later and by mechanisms not understood, the organisms can reactivate, travel up the sensory nerve to the dermatome, and cause a vesicular eruption along the skin that overlies the nerve. Reactivation of VZV infection is much less common than reactivation of HSV infection.

Diseases Due to Varicella-Zoster Virus

Epidemiology.   In the past, the incidence of chickenpox in the USA has been similar to the birth rate (3–4 million cases per year), but with the recent introduction of the varicella vaccine, this is likely to plummet. Currently, about 20% of people in the USA can expect to develop herpes zoster during their lifetime.

Chickenpox is primarily a disease of childhood, with about 90% of the cases occurring among children under 13 years of age. Investigators believe that the disease is spread via respiratory secretions or via contact with infected vesicular material. Patients with chickenpox become infectious about 48 hours before the vesicular rash begins, and they remain infectious until the vesicles have crusted (usually after 4–5 days). Although unusual, some children develop chickenpox more than once, with the second infection much milder than the first. Chickenpox can also be acquired via contact with patients who have herpes zoster. More than 90% of nonimmune individuals exposed to patients with chickenpox or active herpes zoster will develop chickenpox.

Herpes zoster is due to reactivation of latent virions and is not acquired from other individuals.

Diagnosis

(1) History and Physical Examination

(a) Varicella (Chickenpox). In most cases, chickenpox begins suddenly (without prodrome) 14–15 days after exposure to a person shedding VZV. The disease begins with the appearance of a handful of maculopapules on the trunk, neck, or face. Occasional patients suffer from a brief prodrome of fever and malaise during the day preceding the appearance of the rash. Over the next few hours, the number of lesions increases dramatically, and the eruption spreads centrifugally. Pruritus and lethargy are usually accompanied by a temperature of 37.8–39.5 °C (100–103 °F). The lesions rapidly progress from maculopapules to vesicles that look like dewdrops on a rose petal. The vesicles may rupture, or they may become purulent as polymorphonuclear leukocytes are attracted to the center of the lesion.

All stages of lesion development can be seen at any time because successive crops of new lesions appear over the course of 2–4 days. The eruption of chickenpox sometimes seems to cover every body surface, and the oral and genital mucous membranes are often covered with vesicles. If vesicles are scratched, bacterial superinfection may develop. Otherwise, the fluid within a lesion soon dries up, and a crust forms over the lesion.

In most children, chickenpox is a fairly benign disease. The fever lasts only 3–5 days, and crusted lesions are generally gone within 1–2 weeks. Yet a small but significant number of patients with chickenpox develop life-threatening disease, resulting in 50–100 deaths each year in the USA. The risk of death in immunocompetent children is low (1 death per 100,000 cases) compared with that in immunocompetent adults (30 deaths per 100,000 cases) and in immunocompromised patients.

(b) Complications of Varicella. The most dangerous complications of chickenpox are acute cerebellar ataxia, encephalitis, pneumonitis, visceral or disseminated infection, and neonatal chickenpox.

About 1 in 4000 patients who have chickenpox and are 15 years or under develop **cerebellar ataxia,** and 1 in 1000 develop **encephalitis.** After age 15, the risk of encephalitis increases dramatically. Cerebellar ataxia occurs 7–21 days after the appearance of the chickenpox exanthem; is characterized by impaired muscle coordination, speech defects, tremor, vertigo, fever, and vomiting; and generally resolves spontaneously in 2–4 weeks. More dangerous is encephalitis, which is accompanied by seizures, hallucinations, headaches, fever, and vomiting. In some patients, encephalitis resolves in about 2 weeks. The mortality rate is 5–20%, with about 15% of the survivors suffering from permanent neurologic sequelae. Rarer neurologic complications of chickenpox include **Guillain-Barré syndrome** and **Reye's syndrome.** Because the

use of aspirin during chickenpox has been associated with the development of Reye's syndrome in children, aspirin should not be given to children.

Varicella **pneumonitis** is the most common complication of chickenpox in adults, occurring in about 1 in 400 cases. Women in their second or third trimester of pregnancy are at greatest risk. Manifestations of nodular or interstitial pneumonitis usually occur 3–5 days after the eruption of chickenpox and include cough, dyspnea, and tachypnea.

Immunocompromised patients and neonates are at risk of developing **disseminated or visceral chickenpox.** The eruption may become hemorrhagic and necrotic, and the virus may spread throughout the viscera, including the brain, liver, and lungs. Congenital infection may occur if a pregnant woman develops chickenpox 5 or fewer days before delivery. Severe neonatal infections also occur in infants infected during the first 48 hours postpartum. The unusual susceptibility of newborns to chickenpox appears to be related to their failure to receive maternal antibodies to VZV.

(c) Herpes Zoster (Shingles). Herpes zoster is due to reactivation of VZV organisms that have remained latent for years within a sensory root ganglion. The thoracic and lumbar dermatomes are most frequently involved, but the ophthalmic branch of the trigeminal nerve is also a common source of shingles. The disease is most often seen in the elderly but can occur at any age. Herpes zoster is generally associated with little pain in children, but older adults may experience intense neuritis and postherpetic neuralgia.

Most patients report feeling pain within the affected dermatome for 48–72 hours before the appearance of crops of red maculopapular lesions that rapidly vesiculate. The lesions follow the pattern of the nerve under the skin and often extend around one side of the patient's chest, face, or abdomen. Some lesions may coalesce to form a bullous eruption. The lesions generally continue to form for 3–5 days, remain vesicular for up to 2 weeks, and heal completely within 2–4 weeks. If the anterior horn cells are involved, the patient may feel intense pain during the eruption, and some patients experience a degree of motor paralysis.

(d) Complications of Herpes Zoster. After the eruption has disappeared, about 25–50% of patients over age 50 experience **postherpetic neuralgia.** This condition is marked by intense pain that can be debilitating and sometimes lasts for over a month. Some patients with shingles of the trigeminal nerve develop **ophthalmia,** which can result in the loss of sight in the affected eye. Other dangerous complications of herpes zoster include **encephalitis, meningoencephalitis,** and **granulomatous cerebral angiitis.** Immunocompromised patients, including those with AIDS, may develop **chronic herpes zoster.**

(2) Laboratory Analysis. Chickenpox and herpes zoster can usually be identified on the basis of clinical manifestations alone, but definitive diagnosis is necessary in some patients. A scraping can be made of the vesicular lesions and stained to identify the presence of multinucleated giant cells. Tissue culture can be used to cultivate viruses from vesicular fluid, and direct fluorescent antibody tests can be used to show that VZV organisms are present in the lesions. Infected cell cultures take about 2 weeks to show characteristic VZV cytopathic effects, but lesion scrapings can be shown to be positive for VZV during the first week of the eruption. An enzyme immunoassay can be used to show a rising titer of IgM antibody to VZV, indicating recent infection with the virus.

Treatment. Most children with chickenpox are treated symptomatically to make the course of the disease more comfortable and to reduce the risk of complications. Fingernails are closely clipped, and antipruritic agents are used to prevent scratching and the development of secondary infections. Patients with pneumonitis or other potentially life-threatening complications are administered intravenous acyclovir. Oral acyclovir is used to treat herpes zoster. Acyclovir speeds healing and reduces the pain of herpes zoster, but it has been relatively ineffective in reducing postherpetic neuralgia.

Prevention. A **varicella vaccine** is now available in the USA and is recommended for nonimmune children at 12 and 18 months of age and for high-risk nonimmune adults. The vaccine consists of an active varicella virus that has been attenuated by passing it through tissue culture. Nonimmune adults who are exposed to VZV can also be protected from infection by the use of **varicella-zoster immune globulin** (VZIG) or **zoster immune globulin** (ZIG).

Characteristics of Cytomegalovirus

Disease caused by cytomegalovirus (CMV) was first described in 1881, when H. Ribbert reported the presence of "protozoanlike" cells in the kidney of a stillborn infant. By the 1930s, cytomegalic inclusion disease was found to be a relatively common cause of infant mortality. In the mid-1950s, three groups independently isolated the virus in cultured cells. The virus was named cytomegalovirus because of the cytomegalic inclusions formed within infected cells.

General Features. Like the other herpesviruses, CMV is a large, enveloped virus and is constructed from 30–35 structural proteins. Strains vary somewhat in their antigenic characteristics, but the differences seen are too small to divide CMV into immunologic types. CMV strains are species-specific, and human CMV infects only humans. In vitro, productive infections can be formed in human fibroblasts, and abortive infections can be initiated within cultured monocytes and lymphocytes.

Mechanisms of Pathogenicity. CMV causes clinically apparent disease primarily in neonates and immunosuppressed patients. Most other infected people remain asymptomatic. The virus can lie dormant for years within several cell types, possibly including peripheral blood monocytes, endothelial cells, vascular smooth muscle cells, ductal epithelial cells, and CD8$^+$ T cells. Infection is usually lifelong.

The virus periodically reactivates in immunocompetent individuals but produces no outward signs of infection. Reactivation in the immunosuppressed, however, can result in life-threatening disease.

Cytotoxic T cells are likely the key factor in controlling CMV disease, although natural killer cells are probably important during the early days of infection. CMV avoids being destroyed by the immune response by moving directly from cell to cell and by reducing the expression of MHC class I antigens on infected cells. The CMV protein UL18 protects the virus from T cell recognition and antibody in two ways: it mimics the heavy chain of the MHC class I molecule, and it accumulates a protective coat of β_2 microglobulin around the free virus. The virus also expresses an envelope protein that acts as an Fc receptor for antibody.

Diseases Due to Cytomegalovirus

Epidemiology. Most CMV infections are acquired during two periods of life: infancy and the reproductive years. Infants may acquire CMV infection congenitally or perinatally, and adults may be infected through sexual or other intimate contact, blood transfusion, or organ transplantation.

Serologic surveys in various parts of the world have shown that between 40% and 100% of adults have been infected with CMV at some time in their life. Adults in industrialized countries have a lower rate of seropositivity and are more likely to acquire the infection after childhood, while most adults in developing countries in Asia and Africa have been infected since infancy or childhood.

In developing countries, CMV infections are most often acquired during the perinatal period. Some infants become infected during passage through the birth canal or via contact with other infected infants, but breast milk is thought to be the most significant source of infection. About 10–20% of nursing mothers shed CMV in their milk, and infants who ingest CMV-contaminated milk have a 50% chance of being infected themselves. Perinatal CMV infections are almost always asymptomatic, probably because the infected infants have acquired maternal antibodies to CMV.

In industrialized countries, congenital transmission of CMV often occurs. Pregnant women who have recurrent CMV infection transmit the virus to 0.5–1.0% of their offspring, but infected infants do not suffer severe consequences from their infection. In contrast, pregnant women who acquire primary CMV infection during the first two trimesters of pregnancy transmit the virus to 30–40% of their offspring, and 10–15% of these infected infants have significant birth defects. Congenital infections are probably more severe in children born to mothers with primary infection because the amount of virus transmitted from mother to fetus is much higher during the primary infection. Congenital CMV infection is the most common viral cause of birth defects and is a major cause of congenitally acquired hearing loss and mental retardation. About 1 in 2000 infants born in the USA has signs of cytomegalic inclusion disease.

Some adults acquire CMV infection through blood transfusions or organ transplants, but most acquire it through contact with cervical secretions, semen, or saliva containing CMV. In the USA, surveys indicate that CMV is found in the cervix of only 1–2% of women in the general population but in more than 30% of women treated at sexually transmitted disease clinics. More than 40% of homosexual males shed CMV in their semen, and almost all adult homosexual males have been infected with CMV. Individuals most likely to be infected with CMV have multiple sexual partners, began sexual activity young, or practice anal sex. This has profound implications because CMV infection is a major cause of illness and death in patients who have AIDS.

The risk of acquiring CMV infection during blood transfusion has been estimated to be between 2.4% and 12% for each unit of blood transfused, although several recent studies favor the lower risk figure. Most transfusion-acquired infections are asymptomatic, but some patients develop mononucleosis. The risk of transmitting CMV via granulocyte transfusions can be decreased by transfusing cryopreserved blood, blood from CMV-seronegative donors, or granulocyte-poor blood. Almost all recipients of organ transplants become infected with CMV. This can have severe consequences because the recipients are immunosuppressed. The most severe infection is among bone marrow transplant recipients who develop interstitial pneumonia, a disease that has a mortality rate of 70–90% in those who are not treated.

Diagnosis

(1) History and Physical Examination

(a) Perinatal and Congenital Cytomegalovirus Infections. Most infants who are infected perinatally with CMV have no recognizable symptoms of disease. In contrast, 10–15% of infants who are infected in utero develop **cytomegalic inclusion disease.** Some congenitally infected infants are stillborn, while others die days or weeks after birth. Infants with cytomegalic inclusion disease generally are small and lethargic and develop respiratory distress and seizures soon after birth. Jaundice, petechial rash, and enlargement of the spleen and liver are present. Because the central nervous system, the inner ear, and the eye are unusually susceptible to infection, common manifestations include microcephaly, cerebral calcification, deafness or hearing impairment, and chorioretinitis or visual impairment. Mental impairment and motor disabilities may be noted. Some children show no outward effects of the infection initially but develop epilepsy, hearing loss, behavioral problems, and mental retardation between the ages of 2 and 4 years.

(b) Mononucleosis. Blood transfusion recipients and young adults may develop CMV-induced mononucleosis. Unlike patients with infectious mononucleosis caused by Epstein-Barr virus, patients with CMV mononucleosis feel rather well and usually do not have pharyngitis, tonsillitis, or lymphadenopa-

thy. Moreover, they tend to be older than those with infectious mononucleosis (mean age of 28 years versus 19 years) and are febrile for a longer time (19 days versus 10 days, on average). Findings in CMV mononucleosis include lymphocytosis with many atypical lymphocytes, hepatosplenomegaly, abnormal results in liver function tests, and negative results in heterophile antibody tests. Although CMV mononucleosis is usually a self-limiting disease, some patients develop hepatitis, Guillain-Barré syndrome, myocarditis, or thrombocytopenia and hemolytic anemia.

(c) Other Cytomegalovirus Infections. Recipients of bone marrow transplants may develop life-threatening interstitial pneumonitis, and recipients of liver transplants may develop CMV hepatitis. Patients with AIDS are at risk of developing a variety of diseases, including CMV colitis, chorioretinitis, adrenalitis, epididymitis, and infections of the central nervous system.

(2) Laboratory Analysis. A diagnosis of CMV disease must differentiate between primary and recurrent CMV infection. In infants with suspected cytomegalic inclusion disease, urine or saliva samples can be examined for evidence of the virus, or serum samples can be tested for IgM antibody to CMV. In older patients, primary infection is confirmed by looking for the virus in peripheral blood leukocytes, since recurrent infection may result in viral shedding in urine, saliva, cervical secretions, and semen. Samples from patients can be inoculated in human fibroblast monolayers, and a cytospin test that utilizes immunofluorescent monoclonal antibody to CMV can detect the presence of CMV after about 48 hours. Alternatively, the cultures can be observed for up to 1 month for the appearance of cells with large amphophilic nuclear inclusions (cytomegalic inclusions) and smooth, round acidophilic cytoplasmic masses. Polymerase chain reaction assays are being developed and may be used commonly in the future.

Treatment. Ganciclovir has been shown to be effective in treating CMV retinitis in AIDS patients and in preventing CMV disease in transplant recipients. Other severe CMV infections have not responded well to treatment. Foscarnet is a more toxic drug but is a suitable alternative when ganciclovir is contraindicated.

Characteristics of Human Herpesviruses 6 and 7

In 1986, S. Z. Salahuddin and his colleagues reported that they had isolated a new lymphotropic virus, which they named human B-lymphotropic virus. When the virus was subsequently discovered to be a herpesvirus, it was designated as human herpesvirus 6 (HHV-6). Two years later, K. Yamanishi and coworkers isolated HHV-6 from four children with roseola infantum. Today, HHV-6 is known to be a common cause of febrile illness in young children, about 10% of whom develop the rash associated with roseola.

Although HHV-6 infects a variety of cells, it primarily infects dividing CD4$^+$ T cells. Persistently infected macrophages may serve as an important reservoir. Two variants of HHV-6 have been identified by serologic typing and restriction endonuclease mapping. HHV-6A has been isolated primarily from adults, while HHV-6B has been isolated mainly from febrile children.

In 1991 and 1992, investigators from two laboratories announced that they had isolated a second lymphotropic herpesvirus, which they named human herpesvirus 7 (HHV-7). This virus seems to be very similar to HHV-6 and has also been isolated from children with roseola infantum.

Diseases Due to Human Herpesviruses 6 and 7

HHV-6 has been shown to persist within salivary glands and is probably spread via the saliva of infected individuals. More than 80% of adults have serologic evidence of past HHV-6 infection. Maternal antibody is believed to protect infants from infection during the first 6 months of life. About 70% of the new cases of HHV-6 infection occur in infants between 6 and 12 months of age.

In adults, HHV-6 infection usually does not cause symptoms, but in rare cases it has been associated with the occurrence of mononucleosis, severe pneumonitis, or fulminant hepatitis.

In children, febrile illness develops 6–15 days after exposure to a person shedding HHV-6. The fever starts suddenly, peaks at 39–41 °C (about 103–106 °F), continues for 3–5 days, and may be accompanied by malaise, irritability, signs of a mild upper respiratory tract infection, and a nonspecific enanthema that is seen on the uvula and soft palate and is due to lymphoid hyperplasia. Most children are not severely ill, but a few develop convulsions owing to high fever. After the fever abates, about 10% of infected children develop **roseola infantum,** a pale red macular rash that is also called exanthema subitum, sixth disease, and Zahorsky's disease. Roseola infantum may resemble the rash of rubella and may last only minutes or persist for 1–2 days.

Roseola infantum is usually diagnosed on clinical grounds alone. HHV-6 infection can be confirmed, however, by serum antibody tests that show the presence of IgM antibody to HHV-6 during the acute phase of disease and demonstrate a fourfold or greater rise in the titer of IgG antibody to HHV-6 during convalescence. The presence of HHV-6 can also be demonstrated by polymerase chain reaction assay. Isolation of HHV-6 from blood and saliva samples is probably not useful, because many asymptomatic individuals carry the virus in their blood and saliva.

Children with roseola infantum are treated symptomatically. Patients with life-threatening disease can be treated with ganciclovir or foscarnet.

Characteristics of Epstein-Barr Virus

Epstein-Barr virus (EBV) is one of the most prevalent human viruses and is responsible for infectious mononucleosis, a disease formerly known as glandular fever. The first reports of glandular fever came during the late 1800s, but they were not well accepted by the medical community until after the turn of the century. In 1920, T. P. Sprunt and F. A. Evans documented fever, lymphadenopathy, and prostration in six young adults who were previously healthy. In 1932, J. R. Paul and W. Bunnell reported that patients with glandular fever typically formed antibodies against erythrocytes from a variety of animals. These heterophile antibodies could be distinguished from the Forssman antibodies formed during serum sickness by adsorbing sera with guinea pig kidney tissue. Today, glandular fever is called infectious mononucleosis and is known to be caused by EBV. The virus has also been strongly associated with the development of two cancers: Burkitt's lymphoma and nasopharyngeal carcinoma.

General Features. The enveloped virion of EBV is 180–200 nm in diameter and carries within it a genome that encodes about 80 proteins. Two classes of EBV have been identified. EBV-A is found primarily within the B cells of immunocompetent individuals, while EBV-B is isolated mainly from immunocompromised patients suffering from a wide variety of EBV-related diseases.

Mechanisms of Pathogenicity. During infectious mononucleosis, **heterophile antibodies** are produced, and the patient develops a form of lymphocytosis characterized by the appearance of many **atypical lymphocytes** in the blood. Heterophile antibodies are a result of the effects of EBV on B lymphocytes, while the atypical lymphocytosis is associated with the cellular immune response to the presence of virus-infected B lymphocytes.

EBV initially infects the oropharyngeal epithelium but soon spreads to B cells in the lymphoid tissue of the oropharynx. Then the virus replicates and disseminates throughout the reticuloendothelial system during the 30- to 50-day incubation period of the disease.

EBV will replicate only within B lymphocytes and nasopharyngeal epithelial cells. No overt cytopathic effects are seen, but EBV transforms (immortalizes) B cells. The infection cycle begins when the EBV envelope glycoprotein gp350/220 recognizes and binds to the receptor for C3d (variously known as CR2 or CD21) on the surface of its target cells. Like other herpesviruses, the EBV enters and is replicated in the nucleus, as described earlier in the chapter (see Specific Replication Schemes and Fig. 20–2).

In B lymphocytes, EBV often enters a latent state that transforms the B cell. This process does not require that the EBV genome be integrated into the host chromosome. Limited integration may occur, but cells in which the EBV genome is entirely episomal are transformed fully. The latent cycle begins when a viral protein known as Epstein-Barr nuclear antigen 1 (EBNA-1) binds to the viral promoter *ori*P. This activates EBNA-2, which starts a process that immortalizes the B cell. B cell growth factor is produced, and the transformed B cell produces monoclonal antibodies. These antibodies, which are usually but not always IgM, are the heterophile antibodies of infectious mononucleosis. Two types are seen: (1) **Paul-Bunnell antibodies,** which specifically react with erythrocytes, and (2) **Forssman antibodies,** which react with many types of cells, are not specific for mononucleosis, and can be removed by adsorbing serum samples with guinea pig kidney cells.

The immune response to EBV infection involves the production of antibody and the elicitation of a cellular response. Antibodies to EBNA persist for life, and antibodies to viral capsid antigens (VCA) appear during active disease. $CD8^+$ T cells (mostly cytotoxic T lymphocytes, or CTLs) directed against latent membrane protein 1 (LMP-1) and five types of EBNA (EBNA-2 through EBNA-6) are activated. These CTLs destroy infected B cells, control viral replication, and are the atypical lymphocytes of infectious mononucleosis. Their significance is apparent from observations that unrestrained replication and dissemination of EBV often occur in patients with T cell immunodeficiencies and result in the development of an overwhelming B cell lymphoma.

Diseases Due to Epstein-Barr Virus

Epidemiology. Serologic surveys show that 90–95% of adults in industrialized countries have been infected with EBV. Most EBV infections during childhood are asymptomatic, but adolescents and adults infected with EBV develop infectious mononucleosis.

In the USA, there are about 45 cases of infectious mononucleosis per 100,000 population per year. The highest incidence of the disease is between the ages of 15 and 24 years, and the risk of infectious mononucleosis is 30 times higher among whites than among blacks. This is believed to reflect socioeconomic differences that result in whites being infected most often during adolescence or later, while blacks are more often infected during early childhood, when infections tend to be asymptomatic.

EBV is not easy to transmit. The virus is rather fragile, and there is no evidence that it is spread on fomites. Instead, the virus is thought to be spread mainly in saliva during intimate contact. Thus, the characterization of infectious mononucleosis as "kissing disease" is usually correct. EBV can be found within throat washings of patients with active mononucleosis, although the titers of EBV are not high. Up to 18 months after recovery from infectious mononucleosis, individuals may shed EBV in their saliva. EBV can also be spread via blood transfusion, although posttransfusion mononucleosis is usually due to cytomegalovirus.

Diagnosis

(1) History and Physical Examination. The symptoms of **infectious mononucleosis** begin 30–50 days after a nonimmune individual is exposed to the saliva of a person shedding EBV. Many patients experience a prodrome that lasts for several days and

consists of low-grade fever, chills, anorexia, fatigue, malaise, myalgia, retro-orbital headache, and a feeling of abdominal fullness. Most patients with infectious mononucleosis have a sore throat and lymphadenopathy. Fever ranges from temperatures of 38 to 40 °C (100.4 to 104 °F), usually peaks during the late afternoon or evening, and continues for 7–14 days. About 50% of patients develop tonsillitis with a grayish-white exudate that persists for 6–10 days; 25–60% develop palatal petechiae; 10–15% develop hepatomegaly; and 5–10% develop a rash that may be petechial, scarlatiniform, macular, urticarial, or similar to erythema multiforme. Curiously, almost all patients will develop a rash if administered ampicillin.

In immunocompetent patients, infectious mononucleosis generally resolves in 2–3 weeks without incident, but rare patients develop severe complications, including autoimmune hemolytic anemia (with cold agglutinins), splenic rupture, Guillain-Barré syndrome, and encephalitis. Although EBV encephalitis is acute and severe, most patients recover completely from it. In patients with T cell immunodeficiencies, the course of disease is quite different. These patients may develop progressive lymphoproliferative disease and may suffer from pneumonitis or hepatitis.

As discussed in Chapter 22, EBV infection is closely associated with the development of Burkitt's lymphoma and nasopharyngeal carcinoma.

(2) Laboratory Analysis. Laboratory confirmation of infectious mononucleosis rests on the findings of lymphocytosis, heterophile antibodies, and EBV-specific antibodies.

The circulating lymphocytosis of infectious mononucleosis peaks during the second or third week of illness. White blood cell counts usually peak at 12,000–18,000/μL with 60–70% lymphocytes, but some patients have counts as high as 50,000/μL. About 30% of the lymphocytes are atypical in most patients, but as many as 90% of the circulating lymphocytes are atypical in a few. In addition to being larger than normal lymphocytes, atypical lymphocytes have a curled edge, a vacuolated cytoplasm that stains basophilic, and a lobulated and eccentrically placed nucleus. Between 60% and 90% of patients are also neutropenic, and about half are thrombocytopenic.

At some point during their disease, 90% of patients with infectious mononucleosis develop heterophile antibodies, although preadolescent children often have negative results in heterophile antibody tests. Patients with symptoms and a heterophile antibody titer of 40 or greater are considered to have infectious mononucleosis. Antibodies that agglutinate sheep red blood cells drop below a titer of 40 within 1 year in about 70% of patients, but antibodies that agglutinate horse red blood cells persist for years.

The best and most specific test for EBV infection is the detection of IgM antibodies to VCA. These antibodies, which are not found in the general population, are present early during infection and persist only during the acute phase. In contrast, antibodies to EBNA appear late during the acute phase or during early convalescence and persist for life.

Because of the ubiquity of EBV infection, culture of EBV from oropharyngeal washings or blood is not considered clinically useful.

Treatment. Most EBV infections are mild and require no therapeutic intervention other than supportive measures. EBV does not respond well to treatment with ganciclovir, acyclovir, or foscarnet.

Poxviruses

Classification, Structure, and Viral Replication

The poxviruses are the largest and most complex viruses known. The family *Poxviridae* has been divided into eight genera, four of which contain viruses associated with human disease. Table 20–3 lists the human poxviruses and their associated diseases. Most of these poxviruses cause localized infections in animals and are only occasionally spread to humans.

The best-known poxvirus is variola virus, the cause of the now-extinct disease smallpox.

Poxviruses do not exhibit the icosahedral or helical symmetry seen with other viruses. Instead, they are brick-shaped and have a complex structure. Fig. 20–10 shows two different models of the poxvirus structure. The revised model (see Fig. 20–10B) is based on recent work, which indicates that many of the features shown in the earlier model (see Fig. 20–10A) may be artifacts of the dehydration process used in preparation of the viruses for electron microscopy.

Poxvirus virions may be as large as 300 nm in length and contain a linear dsDNA genome and close to 100 core proteins, some of which are needed for replication. The genome of parapoxviruses is about 130 kilobase pairs (kbp), while that of orthopoxviruses is about 170–250 kbp.

The general replication scheme of poxviruses is described earlier in this chapter (see Specific Replication Schemes and Fig. 20–3). Poxviruses are unique among the DNA viruses in that they replicate entirely within the host cell cytoplasm. Poxviruses are repli-

TABLE 20–3. The Poxviruses and Their Associated Diseases

Genus	Virus	Reservoir	Disease	Clinical Description
Molluscipoxvirus	Molluscum contagiosum virus.	Humans.	Molluscum contagiosum.	Dome-shaped, waxy papules with a white core; usually found on the exposed skin of children or the genitals of adults; not found on the soles or palms.
Orthopoxvirus	Buffalopox virus (may be a variant of vaccinia virus).	Water buffaloes.	Buffalopox.	Pustular lesions on the hand.
	Cowpox virus.	Rodents, cattle, and other large animals, including elephants and large cats.	Cowpox.	Localized ulcerating lesion; usually found on the hand but may also affect the eye through autoinoculation.
	Monkeypox virus.	Monkeys.	Monkeypox.	Generalized eruption of pustules similar to the lesions of smallpox.
	Vaccinia virus.	Cows, pigs, and rabbits.	Vaccinia gangrenosa, generalized vaccinia, and eczema vaccinatum.	Complications of vaccinia immunization in immunodeficient individuals.
	Variola virus.	Humans.	Smallpox.	Disease has been eradicated throughout the world; was characterized by generalized eruption of pustules and life-threatening illness.
Parapoxvirus	Milker's nodule virus.	Cattle.	Milker's nodule.	Small, nonulcerating lesion on the hand.
	Orf virus.	Sheep and goats.	Orf (contagious pustular dermatitis or ecthyma contagiosum).	Vesicular lesion on the hand or forearm; lesion has a red center surrounded by a white ring within an area of inflammation.
Yatapoxvirus	Tanapox virus.	Unknown; may be acquired from arthropod bites.	Tanapox.	Umbilicated papule at the site of an arthropod bite.
	Yabapox virus.	Monkeys.	Yabapox.	Formation of a benign tumor (histiocytoma) at the site of viral entry.

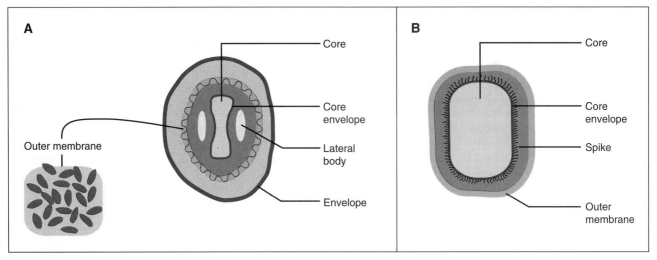

FIGURE 20–10. The structure of poxviruses. Diagram **A** shows the widely accepted model of poxvirus structure. The virus contains a core surrounded by a core envelope, two lateral bodies, an outer membrane constructed from tubules, and an outer envelope. Diagram **B** shows a revised model based on electron microscopic techniques that seek to reduce dehydration artifacts. In this model, the viral core is surrounded by a core envelope filled with hollow spikes, and there are no lateral bodies.

cated within cytoplasmic "factories" that appear as acidophilic inclusions known as **Guarnieri's bodies.** Some mature poxviruses also form intracytoplasmic aggregates that are visualized as eosinophilic cytoplasmic inclusions.

Characteristics of Orthopoxviruses

As shown in Table 20–3, the orthopoxviruses include variola, vaccinia, cowpox, buffalopox, and monkeypox viruses and are found in a variety of animal reservoirs.

There are two strains of variola virus: (1) variola major, which was usually the cause of severe smallpox, a disease with a mortality rate of 25–50%; and (2) variola minor, which was the cause of alastrim, a less severe disease with a mortality rate of about 1%. Now that smallpox has been eliminated through universal immunization efforts, variola virus exists only within the ultralow-temperature freezers of two research facilities, one in the USA and one in Russia.

Vaccinia virus is the agent that was used for smallpox immunization. It is probably an attenuated strain of the cowpox virus. However, the vaccinia virus has been maintained as a laboratory virus for so long that it may be quite different from the virus that was originally developed for vaccine use. Many strains of vaccinia exist around the world, and these differ appreciably from one another. For example, while the strain used in the USA to immunize against smallpox produced postimmunization encephalitis in only 2.3–2.9 per million vaccinated persons, the strain used in the Netherlands caused encephalitis in 1 per 4000 vaccinated persons. These observations have become important once again because vaccinia is being studied as a possible live recombinant vector for immunizing children simultaneously against multiple agents.

Diseases Due to Orthopoxviruses

Variola Virus and Smallpox. The earliest recorded victim of smallpox was Pharaoh Ramses V, who died of the disease around 1157 B.C. After smallpox was brought to Europe during the 6th century A.D., it soon became one of the greatest scourges known, along with typhus and the plague. The horror of smallpox is memorialized in T. B. Macaulay's description of England at the time of the accession of James II: "The smallpox was always present, filling the churchyards with corpses, tormenting with constant fears all whom it had stricken, leaving on those whose lives it spared the hideous traces of its power, turning the babe into a changeling at which the mother shuddered, and making the eyes and cheeks of the betrothed maiden objects of horror to the lover."

Variola virus was transmitted via respiratory tract secretions and the scabs of pustules, in which the virions could persist for months. The disease began 12–14 days after exposure and was heralded by a high fever, prostration, headache, chills, and back pain. In the typical case, a maculopapular rash then appeared on the face, hands, or forearms and spread quickly to the trunk and legs. By days 7–9, the lesions became pustules, and scabs formed over the pustules during the next week. Eventually, the crusts fell off the lesions, commonly leaving dozens or hundreds of pockmarks. There was no specific treatment for smallpox, and the mortality rate was high. For example, smallpox killed 18,000 of Iceland's 50,000 inhabitants in 1707.

The seeds for the demise of smallpox were first sown in 1786, when Edward Jenner immunized 8-year-old James Phipps with cowpox taken from the hand of a milkmaid. Seven weeks later, Jenner inoculated Phipps with smallpox, and the boy remained well. Although "variolation" had been practiced before and practitioners of folk medicine had recognized the protective effect of cowpox infections against smallpox, Jenner moved smallpox immunization into the mainstream of the medical community. Jenner's goals of eradicating the disease were finally realized in 1977 and 1978 with the resolution of the final three cases of smallpox.

Smallpox was eliminated through universal immunization efforts, but this was made possible by the fact that smallpox was a uniquely human disease, had no asymptomatic carriers, and had a secondary attack rate of only 26–44%. The presence of symptoms made it easy to identify infected individuals, and everyone else could be protected from infection by immunization with smallpox vaccine, a live vaccinia virus vaccine.

Vaccinia Virus and Associated Effects. Vaccinia virus can be administered as an immunogen via scarification, injection, or air jet. After 3–4 days, a papule usually develops at the site of inoculation. After the papule becomes a pustule, it develops a crust. The crust then drops off, leaving a pockmark. The entire process typically lasts about 3 weeks. However, an accelerated response, or vaccinoid response, occurs in patients with preexisting immunity.

Complications of immunization with vaccinia include encephalitis, vaccinia gangrenosa, generalized vaccinia, and eczema vaccinatum. Generalized **encephalitis** may occur 1–2 weeks after immunization and is associated with a mortality rate of 10–30%. **Vaccinia gangrenosa** occurs in patients with defective immune systems. The dermal lesion at the site of inoculation spreads inexorably and necroses, and the patient develops metastatic necrotic lesions throughout the body. Vaccinia gangrenosa is fatal. **Generalized vaccinia** is seen most often in children who are under 1 year old and have been immunized with vaccinia. Numerous vesicular lesions with a red base appear, but the disease is fairly benign. **Eczema vaccinatum** occurs in individuals with atopic dermatitis. When immunized, they develop **Kaposi's varicelliform eruption.** Treatment is with **vaccinia immune globulin** (VIG).

Today, the vaccinia virus is being studied as a candidate for a pluripotent recombinant vaccine. Investigators hope that recombinant DNA techniques can be used to cause the virus to express a large number of nonvaccinia antigens and that the recombinant virus can be used to immunize against diseases as varied as measles, mumps, diphtheria, tetanus, and pertussis.

Other Orthopoxviruses and Associated Diseases. The lesions of **cowpox** and **buffalopox** are usually localized on the hand, but **monkeypox** is a generalized eruption similar to smallpox.

Characteristics of Parapoxviruses

Milker's nodule virus and **orf virus** are examples of parapoxviruses that can cause human disease. Milker's nodule virus is also called paravaccinia or pseudocowpox virus. Unlike infection with vaccinia or cowpox virus, however, infection with milker's nodule virus does not protect against smallpox.

Diseases Due to Parapoxviruses

Milker's nodule begins 5–7 days after contact with lesions on the teats or udders of infected cattle. A red papule develops and gradually becomes a firm purple nodule that itches. In most cases, the nodule resolves spontaneously in 1–2 months.

Humans usually are infected with the orf virus when they come in contact with infected sheep or goats, but the virus can also be spread on fomites. The infection is called **orf, contagious pustular dermatitis,** or **ecthyma contagiosum.** It begins with the appearance of a macule at the site of viral entry 3–6 days after contact. The lesion becomes papular and erythematous and characteristically has a red center surrounded by a white ring within an area of inflammation. Other manifestations may include fever, lymphadenopathy, and localized pain. The disease lasts from 3 to 24 weeks. The virus can be grown in cell culture, and electron microscopy can be used to identify virions in the lesion. There is no specific treatment.

Characteristics of Molluscipoxviruses

Only one molluscipoxvirus has been identified: the **molluscum contagiosum virus.** This virus is unique among the poxviruses in that it cannot be cultivated in chicken egg chorioallantoic membranes and it cannot be replicated in cell cultures. Humans are the only known host of the virus. The virus is transmitted by direct contact with infected patients and possibly on towels and washcloths. In adults, molluscum contagiosum is often transmitted during sexual contact.

Diseases Due to Molluscipoxviruses

Patients with **molluscum contagiosum** may have from 1 to 20 epidermal lesions that appear 14–50 days after contact with the virus. Although the lesions can appear almost anywhere except the soles of the foot or the palms of the hand, they are seen most often in the genital region in adults and on the trunk, face, or extremities in children. Lesions are 2–5 mm in diameter and are painless, dome-shaped, waxy papules that may be white, pink, or yellow. In the center of each lesion is a pore through which a white core can be seen. Microscopic examination of the lesion reveals a mass of hypertrophied and hyperplastic epidermis and the presence of virions within acidophilic cytoplasmic inclusions that are known as molluscum bodies.

The lesions of molluscum contagiosum can be removed by surgery, cautery, or cryotherapy. This treatment is primarily for cosmetic reasons and to prevent spread to other individuals.

Characteristics of Yatapoxviruses

Two yatapoxviruses have been shown to cause human disease. One is called **yabapox virus** or **Yaba**

monkey tumor virus and was first reported in Yaba, Nigeria. The other is called **tanapox virus** and was first seen in patients living along the Tana River in Kenya.

Diseases Due to Yatapoxviruses

People who handle monkeys are at risk of developing **yabapox.** Infection is characterized by the formation of a histiocytoma about 4 months after inoculation with the virus. The benign tumor grows to about 40 mm in diameter and eventually sloughs off spontaneously.

Among the poxviruses that cause human disease, tanapox virus is the only one that is disseminated by an arthropod vector. In most cases of **tanapox,** a single umbilicated papule appears after 3–4 days of fever, headache, and backache. The papule soon becomes a nodule that is 10–15 mm in diameter and is surrounded by red and edematous skin. The lesion heals in about 6 weeks and leaves a scar.

Papovaviruses
Classification, Structure, and Viral Replication

The family *Papovaviridae* is divided into two genera, known as *Papillomavirus* and *Polyomavirus.* The papillomaviruses cause a wide variety of human warts and are also associated with the occurrence of cervical carcinoma. Although infections with polyomaviruses are usually subclinical, a polyomavirus called JC virus causes a fatal demyelinating disease (progressive multifocal leukoencephalopathy) in immunosuppressed patients.

The papovaviruses have attracted much interest as models of oncogenesis in laboratory animals. Only recently, however, has it been possible to transform cultured cells with these viruses, and it still is not possible to establish productive infections in cultured cells.

The papovaviruses are small, nonenveloped, icosahedral viruses that contain a covalently closed, circular dsDNA genome. Their general scheme of replication is shown in Fig. 20–4. The nucleocapsid of papillomaviruses is about 55 nm in diameter and encloses a genome of about 8 kbp. In contrast, the nucleocapsid of polyomaviruses is about 45 nm in diameter and encloses a genome of about 5 kbp. Each nucleocapsid is an icosahedron constructed from 72 capsomers.

Papillomaviruses are replicated within the cell nucleus. The papillomavirus genome contains 5–7 early (E) and 2 late (L) open reading frames. E1 is involved in replication of the viral genome, while E2 modulates viral transcription. The E6 and E7 proteins of oncogenic papillomaviruses promote cell transformation by binding to tumor suppressor proteins. E6 binds to tumor suppressor protein p53, while E7 binds to the retinoblastoma (Rb) protein and p107. Binding of E6 to p53 promotes oncogenesis by increasing the rate at which this suppressor of oncogenesis is degraded. L1 encodes the major capsid protein of the papillomaviruses, and L2 codes for the minor capsid protein.

In replicating cells within the basal layer of the epidermis, only early papillomavirus genes are expressed. The products of these genes cause epithelial hyperplasia, but the nonintegrated viral genome is replicated very slowly. The viruses are replicated rapidly, however, in cells that form the outer layer of the epithelium.

The human polyomaviruses JC and BK are related to simian virus 40 (SV40), which has been well studied because of its propensity for integrating its genome into that of the host cell. Although SV40 and other animal polyomaviruses cause tumors in their hosts, there is no evidence that human polyomaviruses are oncogenic in humans.

Characteristics of Papillomaviruses

General Features. About 70 types of human papillomavirus (HPV) have been identified by DNA hybridization techniques. Although a common antigen derived from the major capsid protein of HPV has been used to produce antisera for diagnostic purposes, the inability to culture HPV in standard cell cultures has prevented the development of a serotyping system. Nevertheless, the genotyping system now available has shown that HPV organisms are extremely tissue-specific and are associated with the development of particular types of warts. As shown in Table 20–4, for example, plantar warts are caused by genotypes 1, 2, 4, and 63, but flat warts are caused by genotypes 3, 10, 27, 38, 41, and 49.

Mechanisms of Pathogenicity. HPV organisms infect the stratum germinativum, where they locate within the basal cells. Only early viral genes are expressed in these cells, but as the basal cells begin to mature and move to the epithelial surface, viral gene products cause the cells to hypertrophy. When the cells become terminally differentiated, late viral proteins are synthesized and complete virions are produced. In cells that are producing virions, the nucleus degenerates and a large vacuole develops. The virions are shed when dead keratinocytes are sloughed from the surface of the skin.

Hypertrophy of the epithelium leads to acanthosis and the appearance of a papilloma 3 months to 2 years after the infection begins. When a papilloma is cross-sectioned and examined, findings include hyperkeratosis of the stratum corneum and stratum lucidum, parakeratosis of the stratum granulosum, acanthosis of the stratum spinosum, and the presence of koilocytes (vacuolated, virion-producing cells) within the stratum spinosum.

Most warts resolve spontaneously. This is believed to be due to the development of cell-mediated immunity against HPV, but most evidence supporting this hypothesis is circumstantial and anecdotal. During the time of resolution, the tissue surrounding the warts contains a lymphomonocytic infiltrate.

The putative relationship between HPV and human cancers is discussed in Chapter 22. Briefly, it

TABLE 20–4.   The Papillomaviruses and Their Associated Diseases

Site of Infection	Disease	Human Papillomavirus Types
Anogenital region	Anogenital warts.	Most common are types 6 and 11; others include 30, 42, 43, 44, 51, 54, 55, and 70.
	Cervical carcinoma.	Most common are types 16 and 18; others include 31, 33, and 35.
	Cervical intraepithelial neoplasia.	Most common are types 16, 18, and 31; there are many others.
Mouth	Focal epithelial hyperplasia.	Types 13 and 32.
	Oral warts.	Most common is type 11; others include 6, 7, 16, and 32.
Respiratory tract	Respiratory warts.	Types 6 and 11.
Skin	Butchers' warts.	Most common are types 2 and 7; others include 1, 3, 4, 10, and 28.
	Common warts.	Most common are types 1, 2, and 4; others include 26, 27, 29, 41, 57, and 65.
	Epidermodysplasia verruciformis.	Most common are types 2, 3, 5, 8, 9, 10, 12, 14, 15, and 17; there are many others.
	Flat warts.	Most common are types 3 and 10; others include 27, 28, 38, 41, and 49.
	Plantar warts.	Most common are types 1 and 2; others include 4 and 63.

appears that the HPV types responsible for benign papillomas are replicated as plasmids. When the genome or a portion of the genome of an oncogenic HPV is integrated into that of a host cell, the cell is transformed and becomes cancerous.

Diseases Due to Papillomaviruses

Epidemiology.   Investigators believe that HPV is passed from person to person by direct contact. Pregnant women who have anogenital warts can transmit HPV to their offspring during childbirth, with the result that infants develop warts or recurrent respiratory papillomatosis. Adults can acquire anogenital warts via sexual contact. It is not known if HPV can be transmitted via fomites. The virions are resistant to heat, and steam sterilization is needed to inactivate the organisms on medical instruments.

Diagnosis.   Of the various types of warts shown in Table 20–4, common warts and plantar warts are the most frequently seen types in the general population. **Common warts** occur most often on the hands or feet and are rarely found on mucous membranes. The warts are rough, exophytic hyperkeratotic pap-

ules that are well demarcated. Most are quite small, but some may become as large as 1 cm in diameter. Meat handlers sometimes develop **butchers' warts,** which are a special type of common wart. **Plantar warts** occur most often on the plantar surface (sole) of the foot, although they occasionally occur on the palm of the hand. Plantar warts are much deeper than common warts, and shaving them reveals punctate, bleeding blood vessels.

Anogenital warts, or **condylomata acuminata,** are flesh-colored or gray and are often attached to the skin by a short, broad peduncle. They occur most often on the shaft of the penis of circumcised men, in the preputial cavity of uncircumcised men, and in the perianal area of homosexual men. In women, anogenital warts occur most often at the posterior introitus, although the labia majora and minora and the clitoris are other sites frequently affected. Some patients experience burning or itching, but anogenital warts are usually asymptomatic. Individuals infected with HPV type 16, 18, or 31 may develop **cervical intraepithelial neoplasia,** which may later progress to **cervical carcinoma.**

About 4% of warts are called **flat warts** or **juvenile warts** because they have a smooth surface, are only slightly elevated, and occur primarily in children, usually on the face, neck, or hands.

Epidermodysplasia verruciformis may be a genetically linked disease and is characterized by cutaneous warts disseminated over much of the body. Warts in areas exposed to the sun become cancerous in about one-third of affected patients.

Most warts can be diagnosed on clinical grounds, but anogenital warts may be confused with the lesions of molluscum contagiosum, and epidermodysplasia verruciformis may mimic flat warts or tinea versicolor. When histologic confirmation of HPV papillomas is needed, the presence of koilocytes is diagnostic. Polymerase chain reaction (PCR) assay, dot blot hybridization, and Southern blot hybridization have all been used to confirm the presence of HPV within tissues; PCR is by far the most sensitive and specific of these tests.

Treatment.   Many warts remit spontaneously after a few years, but for cosmetic or medical reasons it may be advantageous to remove papillomas. Cutaneous warts can be surgically excised or removed by cryotherapy, by the application of salicylic and lactic acid paint, by use of 10% glutaraldehyde with 5-fluorouracil, or by use of podophyllum resin. Similar methods have been used to treat anogenital warts.

Characteristics of Polyomaviruses

Two polyomaviruses are known to cause human disease: **BK virus** and **JC virus.** BK and JC were the initials of the first patients in whom the viruses were described. The viruses cause latent infections of the kidneys, usually beginning in early childhood. In the USA, 60–80% of adults have antibody to one or both of the viruses. Primary infections are usually asymptomatic, but reactivation of latent virions in immuno-compromised patients may be life-threatening.

Diseases Due to Polyomaviruses

Immunocompromised patients who are infected with BK virus may develop **progressive multifocal leukoencephalopathy.** Because this disease often heralds the development of AIDS and occurs in up to 4% of patients who already have AIDS, it is classified as an AIDS-defining disease. BK virions multiply within oligodendrocytes, especially within the cerebral white matter. This results in decreased myelin production and in demyelination. Patients exhibit rapidly progressing focal neurologic defects, including aphasia, ataxia, cognitive impairment, cranial nerve deficits, hemiparesis, and visual field deficits. Most patients deteriorate rapidly to dementia and coma, and death occurs within 6 months. However, a few patients develop a condition that waxes and wanes over 2–3 years.

BK and JC viruses infect the kidneys of 10–45% of renal transplant recipients. Most of these recipients shed virions in their urine and are asymptomatic, but a few develop ureteral ulceration and stenosis.

Laboratory diagnosis of disease caused by BK and JC viruses can include culturing the organisms, but this may take months. Urine can be examined microscopically for the presence of characteristic cells with an enlarged nucleus and a large, basophilic intranuclear inclusion. BK and JC viruses can also be detected in the urine using polymerase chain reaction technology. The diagnosis of progressive multifocal leukoencephalopathy must be established by brain biopsy, which reveals the presence of many asymmetric foci of demyelination in the cerebral white matter. Viral cytopathic effects can also be seen in infected oligodendrocytes.

There is no established treatment for progressive multifocal leukoencephalopathy. Among the drugs that have been used with at least some success are cytosine arabinoside, interferon alfa, idoxuridine (5-iodo-2′-deoxyuridine, or IUDR), and zidovudine.

Parvoviruses
Classification, Structure, and Viral Replication

Human parvoviruses are found in two genera of the family *Parvoviridae.* The genus *Dependovirus* contains viruses that infect humans but are replicated in cells coinfected with adenoviruses or herpesviruses. Thus, human dependoviruses are often known as adeno-associated viruses. Dependoviruses cause no human diseases. The only parvovirus known to be pathogenic in humans is parvovirus B19, which is classified within the genus *Erythrovirus.*

Although hepadnaviruses have a smaller genome than parvoviruses, the parvoviruses have the smallest nucleocapsids of all human viruses. Their icosahedral nucleocapsids are 18–26 nm in diameter and enclose a linear segment of ssDNA that is about 5 kb in length. Because the amount of information they carry is limited by their genome size, the parvoviruses seem to require some help in replicating themselves. Thus, human parvoviruses are replicated only in dividing cells (in the S phase) or in the presence of specific helper viruses. The replication scheme of parvoviruses is shown in Fig. 20–5.

Characteristics of Parvovirus B19

General Features. Parvovirus B19 is an almost ubiquitous virus that causes erythema infectiosum in children, aplastic crisis in patients with chronic anemia, and hydrops fetalis in fetuses.

Mechanisms of Pathogenicity. About 1 week after a patient is infected with parvovirus B19, viremia reaches a peak and the patient begins shedding virions in respiratory secretions. The virions multiply within the bone marrow and destroy erythroid precursor cells. By day 10 of infection, no erythroblasts are seen in the bone marrow, and no reticulocytes are seen in the blood. This is not a problem in otherwise healthy individuals, because the average life span of circulating erythrocytes is about 120 days, and these individuals will show no overt signs of anemia. However, because the erythrocytes circulate for only 15–20 days in patients who suffer from a form of chronic hemolytic anemia such as sickle cell anemia, thalassemia, or hereditary spherocytosis, these patients will experience an aplastic crisis. By days 17–24, parvovirus has disappeared from the blood, IgM antibody to parvovirus has peaked, and IgG antibody levels are rising. At this time, many patients develop a characteristic rash and arthralgia that are probably due to immune complexes. The rash disappears in about 10 days, and most patients recover without incident.

Diseases Due to Parvovirus B19

Epidemiology. Parvovirus B19 infections are usually acquired during childhood, and up to half of the individuals infected with the virus are asymptomatic. Erythema infectiosum, the most common of the diseases caused by this virus, is mild but highly contagious. It usually occurs between the ages of 4 and 10 years, and 80% of cases occur before the age of 15. The virus is normally spread via respiratory secretions to close contacts, but some patients are infected when they receive transfusions of blood or blood products. When epidemics occur, the secondary attack rate in homes and schools is 25–50%. Hydrops fetalis occurs when a woman is infected during pregnancy and passes the virus to her fetus transplacentally; however, most transplacental parvovirus B19 infections are harmless.

Diagnosis
(1) History and Physical Examination
(a) Erythema Infectiosum. Erythema infectiosum, also called **fifth disease,** is a biphasic disease. About 8–11 days after being infected, the typical patient experiences chills, fever, itching, malaise, and myalgia, which last for about 3 days. This is the invasive phase of the disease. Although hemoglobin levels

may drop about 1 g/dL at this time, patients without chronic anemia will have no symptoms of anemia. The disease remits and is followed during days 17–24 by the appearance of a characteristic rash, which is initially red and maculopapular and looks similar to rubella. During the first 1–4 days, the rash is seen only on the face, particularly on the forehead and chin and behind the ears. The skin around the mouth remains pale, while the cheeks become red, giving rise to the term "slapped cheek syndrome." The rash now spreads to the extensor surfaces of the arms and thighs and then to the trunk, buttocks, and the flexor and distal portions of the extremities. As the rash spreads, the center of coalesced regions of the exanthem fade to give the rash a lace-like or serpiginous pattern. Although the rash fades in about 10 days, it may reappear sporadically during the next few weeks or months upon bathing or prolonged exposure to sunlight.

(b) Transient Aplastic Crisis. When infected with parvovirus B19, some patients with chronic hemolytic anemia have a 2- to 4-day prodrome of fever and malaise, which may be accompanied by headache, nausea, vomiting, and abdominal pain. Patients may not develop a rash. Instead, they show signs of aplastic crisis during the invasive phase of infection, including lethargy, pallor, weakness, a precipitous drop in hemoglobin level, absence of reticulocytes in the blood, and few or no erythroblasts in the bone marrow. Physical examination may also show signs of congestive heart failure. Most patients recover in 7–10 days.

(c) Other Parvovirus Infections. Although transplacental parvovirus infections are often asymptomatic, some infants infected in utero develop hydrops fetalis. Women infected with the virus may develop a prominent arthropathy, particularly in the hands, wrists, and knees. Immunosuppressed patients may develop chronic anemia due to parvovirus B19.

(2) Laboratory Analysis. Erythema infectiosum is generally diagnosed on clinical grounds alone. When a precise virologic diagnosis is needed, enzyme immunoassay or radioimmunoassay can be used to detect IgM antibody to parvovirus B19 and a rise in IgG antibody titers. Viral DNA can be detected by polymerase chain reaction assay or dot blot hybridization. In patients with aplastic crisis, viral antigen can be detected by enzyme immunoassay.

Treatment. There is no specific treatment for erythema infectiosum. Patients with aplastic crisis may need to receive blood transfusions.

Hepadnaviruses

The first four letters of hepadnavirus ("hepa") were taken from the word hepatitis and the next three letters ("dna") denote that hepadnaviruses are DNA viruses. The hepatitis B virus (HBV) is a member of the family *Hepadnaviridae* and the genus *Orthohepadnavirus.* Historically, HBV has been the primary cause of serum hepatitis—that is, hepatitis that occurs after human serum is injected through the skin.

The earliest reports of serum hepatitis were among individuals in Bremen who, in 1833, received smallpox vaccine that contained human lymphatic fluid. During the 19th and 20th centuries, serum hepatitis became more frequent as human blood and its by-products were used for transfusions, for immunotherapy, or for immunization with vaccines such as yellow fever vaccine. Drug addicts sharing needles also spread the disease, as did the early practices of reusing syringes and needles, often without any attempt to clean them. The causative agent of serum hepatitis remained elusive until 1956, when B. S. Blumberg and associates reported the presence of an unusual antigen in the blood of an Australian aborigine. This so-called Australia antigen was at first thought to be a host antigen, but subsequent studies showed that it was associated with the occurrence of serum hepatitis. The antigen was renamed several times and is now called hepatitis B surface antigen.

Today, HBV is known to be just one of several hepatitis viruses capable of being disseminated by percutaneous injection of infected human blood or serum. Worldwide, an estimated 200 million people are chronic carriers of the virus, and about 1 million die each year from HBV infection. In much of the world, HBV is passed from mother to infant, resulting in lifelong chronic infection. Many of those chronically infected with the virus develop hepatocellular carcinoma. Thus, HBV infection is a major worldwide health problem.

Characteristics of Hepatitis B Virus

General Features. HBV is an icosahedral virus that contains a circular, partially double-stranded DNA genome, is surrounded by an envelope derived from the host cell, and has the smallest genome of all known DNA animal viruses. The replication of HBV is described in an earlier section of this chapter (see Specific Replication Schemes and Fig. 20–6). The nucleocapsid of HBV contains a polymerase that serves as both a DNA polymerase and a reverse transcriptase. The completed virion has a diameter of 42 nm, but many smaller particles (22 nm) known as **Dane particles** are released during viral replication, along with tiny filaments ranging in size from 20 to 200 μm. Although Dane particles and filaments contain HBsAg, they are not infectious, because they do not contain the HBV genome.

As shown in Tables 20–5 and 20–6, several antigens and antibodies are associated with HBV, and their presence in the blood can help identify whether a patient has primary hepatitis, subclinical hepatitis, or chronic active hepatitis. The HBV envelope contains **hepatitis B surface antigen** (HBsAg), while the HBV core contains **hepatitis B core antigen** (HBcAg) and a truncated form of the major core peptide known as **hepatitis B e antigen** (HBeAg). Tests are available to identify the presence of these three antigens, as

TABLE 20–5. Significance of Detecting Antigens and Antibodies Associated With Hepatitis B Virus (HBV) Infection

Laboratory Finding	Clinical Significance
Hepatitis B surface antigen (HBsAg)	First marker of HBV infection. Indicates the presence of active infection. Duration of positivity roughly correlates with severity of hepatitis.
Hepatitis B core antigen (HBcAg)	Not routinely assayed. Its primary significance is as an antigenic target for anti-HBc antibody.
Hepatitis B e antigen (HBeAg)	Appears just after and disappears just before HBsAg in self-limiting infections. Indicates that infection is active, that complete virions are in the blood, and that the patient is highly infectious.
DNA polymerase	Not routinely assayed. Appears late during the incubation period and disappears when hepatic disease begins.
HBV DNA	Indicates that high viremia is present and that the patient is highly infectious.
Anti-HBs antibody	Indicates immunity to HBV owing to previous infection or immunization. Appears in patients who spontaneously recover from HBV infection. Appearance of anti-HBs antibody during viremia results in development of an immune complex disease with manifestations including rash and arthritis. Immune complexes may also cause polyarteritis nodosa and membranous glomerulonephritis.
Anti-HBc antibody	Indicates present or past HBV infection. Tests for IgM antibody to HBc can be used to identify patients with acute HBV infection.
Anti-HBe antibody	Appears weeks to months after HBeAg and detectable circulating virus disappear from the blood. Its presence indicates low infectivity.

markers, some of which act as alleles (mutually exclusive alternatives). Almost all forms of HBsAg contain a group-specific determinant known as *a*. This determinant is combined with one of each of the pairs of markers known as pair *d* and *y* and pair *r* and *w*. Thus, an HBsAg may be *adw* or *ayr* but never *ady* or *arw*. The *w* marker is fairly heterogeneous and has been classified into a series of subdeterminants, and additional determinants (such as *g, q,* and *x*) have occasionally been identified. The genetic markers are significant for two reasons. First, they have been used as an epidemiologic tool to identify the path of transmission of HBV among patients. Second, rare individuals carry HBV organisms that lack the *a* determinant of HBsAg. Because antibody that protects against HBV is directed against the *a* determinant, these organisms can be transmitted to individuals who are considered HBV-immune.

HBsAg is the first HBV antigen that can be detected in patients with primary hepatitis. The appearance of HBeAg and DNA polymerase in the blood soon after indicates that complete virions are now in the blood. Just before active disease begins, anti-HBc antibody appears, and this persists throughout the acute phase and convalescence. The serum concentrations of HBsAg and complete virions drop sharply during acute hepatitis; HBeAg levels are elevated until the acute phase ends, but detectable DNA polymerase and HBV DNA typically disappear midway through the acute phase of hepatitis. HBsAg levels finally become undetectable during early convalescence, and anti-HBs antibody can be detected shortly thereafter. Weeks to months later, anti-HBe antibody appears in the blood. Table 20–6 contrasts these test results with the test results in two other groups: patients with subclinical hepatitis and patients with chronic active hepatitis.

While some patients are infected with HBV alone, other patients are found to have combined hepatitis B and hepatitis D infections. The **hepatitis D virus (HDV),** which is the smallest RNA animal virus known, acts as a satellite virus for HBV, which is the smallest DNA animal virus known. HDV is a single-stranded, negative-sense RNA virus that was originally called

well as **DNA polymerase** and **HBV DNA,** in blood samples from patients.

Early in the incubation period of primary hepatitis, patients produce enveloped virions and a variety of incomplete viral particles heavily impregnated with HBsAg. The HBsAg contains several genetic

TABLE 20–6. Comparison of Antigens and Antibodies Detected in Three Forms of Hepatitis B Virus (HBV) Infection

Laboratory Finding*	Primary Hepatitis			Subclinical Hepatitis	Chronic Active Hepatitis
	Prodrome	Clinical Disease	Convalescence		
HBsAg present	Yes	Yes	No	No	Yes
HBeAg present	Yes	Yes	No	No	Variable‡
DNA polymerase present	Yes	Variable†	No	No	Variable‡
HBV DNA present	Yes	Variable†	No	No	Variable‡
Anti-HBs present	No	No	Yes	Yes	No
Anti-HBc present	Variable	Yes	Yes	Yes	Yes
Anti-HBe present	No	No	Yes (late)	No	Variable‡

* See Table 20–5 for a description of the antigens and antibodies in this column.
† These antigens typically disappear midway through the acute phase of primary hepatitis.
‡ Although most patients with chronic active hepatitis show positive results in tests for HBeAg, DNA polymerase, and HBV DNA, some patients show negative results in these tests but positive results in the anti-HBe antibody test.

the **delta agent** and is now classified in the genus *Deltavirus.* It carries a 1700-base genome that encodes only a single protein: the **hepatitis D antigen** (HDAg). HDV has been compared to subviral agents that are called viroids and virusoids and infect plants. These subviral agents are nucleic acid fragments that act like viruses but do not encode a capsid or coat. The RNA of HDV can be replicated in a variety of human cells in the absence of HBV, but it is only when HBV is present that the virions of HDV are produced. This is because the HDV core must be packaged within a coat of HBsAg. Thus, individuals who have anti-HBs antibody and are immune to HBV are also immune to HDV.

Mechanisms of Pathogenicity. Exposure to HBV can result in primary hepatitis or subclinical hepatitis. Many patients recover completely, but others develop chronic persistent hepatitis (CPH) or chronic active hepatitis (CAH), and CAH may lead to cirrhosis or primary hepatocellular carcinoma. Thus, a discussion of the pathogenicity of HBV disease must consider factors that lead to (1) immunity from infection, (2) recovery from primary disease, (3) hepatocellular damage during acute and chronic disease, (4) viral persistence, and (5) extrahepatic disease.

The immune response plays a major role in all of these processes. Individuals with anti-HBs antibody are protected from infection, but the cellular response appears to be the critical factor both in recovery from infection and in the production of cellular damage. Patients recover from primary infection when they develop a vigorous CD8$^+$ T cell–mediated response to HBcAg and HBeAg. These same cytotoxic T cells are also responsible for most of the cellular damage that occurs during primary hepatitis B infection. It appears that the initial infecting dose of HBV plays a major role in determining whether the cellular response results in recovery from disease or in hepatic damage in patients with normal immune responses. Those who are heavily infected tend to develop more severe disease, while those who are infected with few virions tend to recover from primary infection, often with few symptoms. Regardless of the infecting dose of HBV, if the patient fails to mount an effective T cell response (as occurs with infants and immunosuppressed patients), there is little liver damage, but primary disease is followed by CAH.

CAH involves a long-term regenerative type of liver damage in which necrotic foci develop in the liver, the damaged region is repaired, more necrotic foci develop, and so forth. Ultimately, this cyclic process results in cirrhosis and may be at the heart of the relationship between HBV infection and the development of hepatocellular carcinoma. The origin of hepatocellular damage during CAH is less well understood than that during acute hepatitis, but it appears to be due primarily to antibody-dependent cellular cytotoxicity (ADCC) directed against hepatocytes that express HBcAg. There is also some evidence that accumulation of large amounts of HBcAg in the cytoplasm of chronically infected cells has some direct cytotoxic effect. The critical role of the immune response in the pathology of CAH is consistent with findings in patients who have been treated with corticosteroids to stem the progress of immune-mediated liver damage. Investigators believe that corticosteroids directly stimulate the replication of HBV. Thus, when patients receive corticosteroids, HBV organisms are rapidly replicated within hepatocytes, resulting in a great increase in HBV antigen expression. When the corticosteroids are withdrawn, some patients develop fulminant reactivation disease because there is an intense immune response to the high density of viral antigens in infected cells.

Anti-HBs antibodies may combine with HBsAg during the incubation period of hepatitis B infection, resulting in a serum sickness–like disease that is accompanied by rash, urticaria (hives), fever, arthralgia, and arthritis. Similar immune complexes formed later in disease may cause polyarteritis nodosa and membranous glomerulonephritis.

Diseases Due to Hepatitis B Virus

Epidemiology. HBV infection is a disease of young adults in the USA. The Centers for Disease Control and Prevention estimates that about 300,000 people acquire primary HBV infection each year. About 10,000 of them are hospitalized with acute disease, 300 die, and 18,000–30,000 become chronic carriers of the virus. Another 4,000–5,000 people die annually from the effects of chronic HBV infection (cirrhosis and hepatocellular carcinoma). Thus, the number of deaths from chronic HBV infection is 13–17 times higher than that from acute HBV infection.

Experimental HBV infections have been established in some primates, but humans are the only known natural reservoir of HBV. Although HBV has been found in a wide variety of body fluids, studies of the patterns of transmission have identified infectious HBV organisms only in blood, serum, saliva, and semen. Thus, HBV is not transmitted via the fecal-oral route, as are hepatitis A and hepatitis E viruses.

In the USA, the usual means of transmission of HBV are via percutaneous injection of human blood, sexual contact with an HBV-infected individual, and possibly mucous membrane contact with infected blood. Those at highest risk of infection are intravenous drug users, health care workers, sexual contacts of HBV-infected persons, patients who have received multiple blood transfusions or undergone hemodialysis, individuals who are institutionalized, and infants born to HBV-positive mothers. Blood transfusion was once the most frequent source of infection, but because blood products are now tested for HBV, intravenous drug users are currently the population at highest risk. Individual cases have been suspected of being acquired via contact with virus-contaminated toothbrushes, razors, baby bottles, toys, eating utensils, endoscopes, and instruments used in tattooing or ear piercing.

In countries where HBV is widespread, the most common means of transmission is from infected mothers to their newborn infants. Maternal transfer of HBV can occur during the third trimester of pregnancy, but it occurs most often during parturition, when the infant comes in contact with the mother's blood, and by unknown means during the first 2 months postpartum. In some countries in Southeast Asia, most adults are seropositive for HBV and 8–15% are chronic carriers.

Diagnosis

(1) History and Physical Examination. Fig. 20–11 depicts the various outcomes of HBV infection in two groups, the first consisting of adults with normal immune function and the second consisting of infants and immunosuppressed patients.

(a) Primary Hepatitis. Symptoms and signs of primary hepatitis begin 60–110 days after the patient is infected with HBV. In 10–20% of cases, there is an immune complex–derived prodrome of fever, urticaria, arthralgia, rash, and arthritis. The prodrome usually lasts 2–10 days but may persist for several weeks. The onset of jaundice is frequently preceded by malaise, loss of appetite, nausea, fever, vomiting,

and headache. These are signs that the liver is becoming involved. At this time, the urine begins to darken and the stools become light or clay-colored.

The acute phase of hepatitis B ranges widely in severity from almost asymptomatic to fulminant and rapidly fatal. Although the skin and sclerae may be jaundiced, most patients are anicteric. Many experience intense itching, as well as abdominal discomfort and pain in the upper right quadrant. The liver is enlarged, often as much as 15 cm in vertical breadth, and levels of serum transaminase, bilirubin, and total gamma globulin are elevated. Granulocytopenia with a relative increase in lymphocytes may also be noted.

Although acute hepatitis may persist for as long as a year, most patients with anicteric and icteric hepatitis B infection recover completely within weeks (adults in 4–6 weeks and children in about 2 weeks). Rarely, a patient develops fulminant hepatitis, in which case death may occur within 10 days and is due to hepatic failure and encephalopathy. Fulminant hepatitis is often associated with coinfection by HBV and HDV.

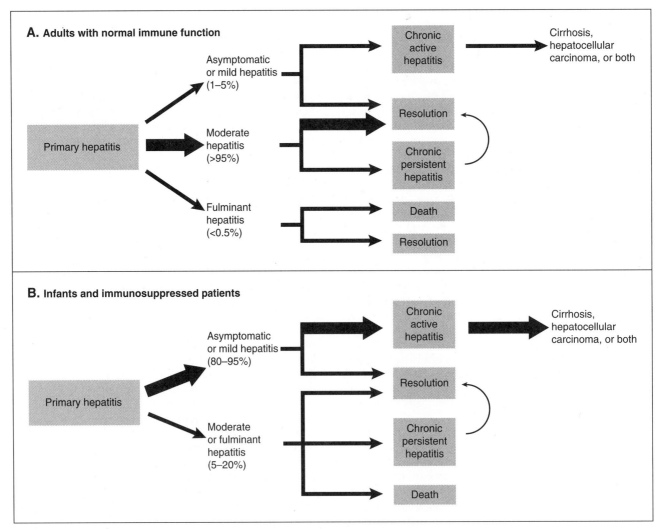

FIGURE 20–11. The outcomes of hepatitis B infection. Thick arrows indicate common outcomes and thin arrows indicate less common outcomes in adults with normal immune function **(A)** and in infants and immunosuppressed patients **(B)**.

(b) Chronic Hepatitis. Although most patients recover completely from primary infection, 1–10% of adults and 80–95% of infants become chronically infected, either with **chronic persistent hepatitis** (CPH) or **chronic active hepatitis** (CAH). In one large study, 70% of adults with chronic hepatitis developed CPH and 30% suffered from CAH.

Patients with CPH usually have no clinical signs of HBV infection, and most develop no significant hepatic damage. CPH is evidenced primarily by the persistence of HBsAg in the blood and may be accompanied by elevated levels of serum transaminase and bilirubin.

Patients with CAH show signs of continuous hepatic damage and regeneration that eventually result in cirrhosis, hepatocellular carcinoma, or both. CAH is characterized by the presence of HBsAg in the blood; elevated levels of serum transaminase, bilirubin, and gamma globulin; low levels of serum albumin; and prolonged prothrombin time. Liver biopsy reveals portal inflammation, fibrotic septa, and areas of hepatic necrosis. Some patients experience persistent or intermittent jaundice and rapidly progressing hepatic damage, with cirrhosis and death occurring within a year. Others experience a more gradual process, with slowly generating hepatic damage and no jaundice, but many of the patients in this group subsequently develop hepatocellular carcinoma.

(c) Combined Hepatitis B and Hepatitis D Infection. Two patterns of combined hepatitis B and D infection occur: coinfection and superinfection. In the USA, intravenous drug users are at greatest risk.

Depending on the size of the inoculum and the ratio of HBV to HDV in the inoculum, a patient who is **coinfected** (simultaneously infected) with both viruses may develop a single episode of combined HBV-HDV primary hepatitis or may develop HBV infection followed by HDV infection. Coinfection is more severe than infection with HBV alone.

Patients already infected with HBV may become **superinfected** with HDV. Because the hepatocytes of HBV-infected patients already contain HBsAg, the incubation period for HDV is shortened to about 3 weeks, and most patients develop severe primary hepatitis. This is a dangerous disease with a high mortality rate (up to 20%).

(2) Laboratory Analysis. A diagnosis of hepatitis can be made on clinical grounds and by showing that the patient has elevated levels of serum transaminase and bilirubin. A specific viral diagnosis, however, depends on detection of the antigens and antibodies associated with specific hepatitis viruses. Most of these are detected by radioimmunoassay, enzyme immunoassay, or reverse passive hemagglutination assay. HBV DNA can also be detected by dot blot hybridization, liquid hybridization, polymerase chain reaction, or a branched-chain DNA assay. Table 20–6 compares the serum antigen and antibody patterns seen in primary hepatitis, subclinical hepatitis, and chronic active hepatitis due to HBV. Coinfection or superinfection with HDV can be demonstrated by detecting HDAg or HDV RNA.

Differential Diagnosis. Infection caused by hepatitis B is often difficult to distinguish from infection caused by herpesviruses, yellow fever virus, and other types of hepatitis virus. The characteristics of type A, B, C, D, and E hepatitis viruses are compared in Table 20–7.

Treatment. Although bed rest is recommended for some patients with primary hepatitis, most can be

TABLE 20–7. A Comparison of the Characteristics of Hepatitis Virus Types A, B, C, D, and E

Characteristic	Hepatitis A	Hepatitis B	Hepatitis C	Hepatitis D	Hepatitis E
Classification	Picornavirus.	Hepadnavirus.	Flavivirus.	Deltavirus.	Calicivirus.
Mode of transmission	Fecal-oral route.	Via body fluids (blood, serum, saliva, and semen), sexual contact, and transplacental route.	Via body fluids and sexual contact.	Via body fluids and sexual contact.	Fecal-oral route.
Usual incubation period	3–5 weeks.	8–16 weeks.	5–10 weeks.	8–16 weeks for coinfection with hepatitis B; about 3 weeks for super-infection.	1–8 weeks.
Mortality rate for primary disease	0–0.2%.	0.3–1.5%.	Unknown.	2–20%.	1–2% overall; 10–20% in pregnant women.
Chronic disease develops	No.	Yes (in 1–10% of adults and 80–95% of infants).	Yes (in 10–60% of patients).	Yes (common in concert with chronic hepatitis B infection).	No.
Associated with hepatocellular carcinoma	No.	Yes.	Yes.	No.	No.
Vaccine available	Yes.*	Yes.†	No.	Yes.†	No.

* Hepatitis A vaccine is used only in high-risk individuals.
† Hepatitis B conjugate vaccine protects against infection with both hepatitis B and hepatitis D.

as active as they deem comfortable. Primary hepatitis does not respond to drug therapy. Corticosteroids should not be used to treat HBV disease, because when the drugs are withdrawn, the patient experiences a "flare" of hepatitis that can be life-threatening.

The only drug currently licensed in the USA for use in treating CAH is interferon alfa. Under 40% of patients show a short-term response, and far fewer experience long-term benefits from this treatment. Patients with extensive hepatic damage may undergo liver transplantation. Transplant results have been disappointing, however, with a 1-year survival rate of about 50% among these patients (compared with greater than 90% among liver transplant patients with alcoholic or cholestatic liver disease). Some transplant centers have reported increased survival rates and less frequent recurrence of HBV infection when transplant recipients were given immune globulin (anti-HBs antibody) in high doses both preoperatively and postoperatively. Antibiotics that inhibit reverse transcriptase or DNA polymerase have not proved effective in treating HBV infection.

Prevention. A plasma-derived hepatitis B vaccine was introduced in the USA in 1981 and was later replaced by **hepatitis B conjugate vaccine,** which consists of recombinant HBs particles produced in yeasts. This new vaccine is routinely used to immunize high-risk individuals against HBV infection, and the Centers for Disease Control and Prevention now recommends that it be given to infants and children in combination·with other childhood vaccines. Hepatitis B conjugate vaccine elicits high titers of anti-HBs antibody in more than 90% of those who receive three doses. It is 85–99% effective in recipients under the age of 50 years (including neonates), but only about 50% of recipients over the age of 60 seroconvert after immunization. The vaccine has also been shown to be effective in halting perinatal transmission of HBV from mothers to their infants.

HBV is transmitted via body fluids, so health care personnel should follow universal precautions when handling potentially infectious materials. If a nonimmune individual is exposed to HBV via a needle stick, **hepatitis B immune globulin** (HBIG) or pooled **immune serum globulin** (ISG) should be administered as soon as possible. Immune globulin administered as late as 48 hours after exposure to HBV probably does not protect against infection.

Because HDV is transmitted in a manner identical to HBV and HDV is enclosed within a coat of HBsAg, measures that prevent transmission of HBV will also prevent infection with HDV. Individuals immune to HBV are also immune to HDV.

Selected Readings

Berns, K. I. Parvovirus replication. Microbiol Rev 54:316–329, 1990.
Buller, R. M., and G. J. Palumbo. Poxvirus pathogenesis. Microbiol Rev 55:80–122, 1991.
Chisari, F. V. Analysis of hepadnavirus gene expression, biology, and pathogenesis in transgenic mice. Curr Top Microbiol Immunol 168:85–101, 1991.
Dubochet, J., et al. Structure of intracellular mature vaccinia virus observed by cryoelectron microscopy. J Virol 68:1935–1941, 1994.
Garcia-Blanco, M. A., and B. R. Cullen. Molecular basis of latency in pathogenic human viruses. Science 254:815–820, 1991.
Gershon, A. A., et al. Intracellular transport of newly synthesized varicella-zoster virus: final envelopment in the *trans*-Golgi network. J Virol 68:6372–6390, 1994.
Ginsberg, H. S., and G. A. Prince. The molecular basis of adenovirus pathogenesis. Infect Agents Dis 3:1–8, 1994.
Khanna, R., S. R. Burrows, and D. J. Moss. Immune regulation in Epstein-Barr virus–associated diseases. Microbiol Rev 59:387–405, 1995.
Lau, J. Y., and T. L. Wright. Molecular virology and pathogenesis of hepatitis B. Lancet 342:1335–1340, 1993.
Luppi, M., and G. Torelli. The new lymphotropic herpesviruses (HHV-6, HHV-7, and HHV-8) and hepatitis C virus (HCV) in human lymphoproliferative diseases: an overview. Haematologica 81:265–281, 1996.
Matthews, J. T., B. J. Terry, and A. K. Field. The structure and function of the HSV DNA replication proteins: defining novel antiviral targets. Antiviral Res 20:89–114, 1993.
Miller, G. The switch between latency and replication of the Epstein-Barr virus. J Infect Dis 161:833–844, 1990.
Moss, B. Regulation of vaccinia virus transcription. Annu Rev Biochem 59:661–688, 1990.
Munholland, J. M., et al. Cell specificity of transcription regulation by papovavirus T antigens and DNA replication. EMBO J 11:177–184, 1992.
Samulski, R. J. Adeno-associated virus: integration at a specific chromosomal locus. Curr Opin Genet Dev 3:74–80, 1993.
Siegel, G. Molecular biology and pathogenicity of human and animal parvoviruses. Behring Inst Mitt 85:6–13, 1990.
Sock, E., et al. Large T antigen and sequences within the regulatory region of JC virus both contribute to the features of JC virus DNA replication. Virology 197:537–548, 1993.
Terrault, N. A., and T. L. Wright. Therapy for chronic hepatitis B infection. Adv Exp Med Biol 394:189–205, 1996.
Young, N. S. Parvovirus infection and its treatment. Clin Exp Immunol 104(supplement 1):26–30, 1996.

CHAPTER TWENTY-ONE

RNA VIRUSES

Arenaviruses, Astroviruses, Bunyaviruses, Caliciviruses, Coronaviruses, Filoviruses, Flaviviruses, Orthomyxoviruses, Paramyxoviruses, Picornaviruses, Reoviruses, Retroviruses, Rhabdoviruses, and Togaviruses

CLASSIFICATION AND REPLICATION OF RNA VIRUSES

RNA viruses have been divided into five major classes according to the structure and polarity of their genomes (see Chapter 19 and Table 19–3). Class I RNA viruses are positive-sense (messenger polarity) single-stranded RNA (ssRNA) viruses. Direct transcription of the viral genome yields a single polyprotein that is cleaved to yield the individual viral proteins. Class II RNA viruses are negative-sense ssRNA viruses. The genome of these viruses must be copied to a series of positive-sense strands, which are then used as messages for viral protein synthesis. Class III RNA viruses contain multiple segments of negative-sense ssRNA. Each segment contains one gene that must be copied as a positive-sense strand to synthesize proteins. Class IV RNA viruses contain multiple nonoverlapping double-stranded RNA (dsRNA) segments, each of which carries the information for a single message. Finally, class V RNA viruses are ssRNA retroviruses that are diploid. The RNA of these retroviruses must be copied to DNA by reverse transcriptase to produce progeny virions.

General Concepts of Replication

Several generalizations can be made concerning the replication of RNA viruses. First, replication is not under strict temporal control. Instead, whenever positive-sense RNA is available, proteins are synthesized. In some cases, all classes of proteins are synthesized from the onset of the replicative cycle. Second, positive-sense RNA genomes can be used directly as messenger RNA (mRNA), but negative-sense genomes must be transcribed into positive-sense strands for protein synthesis. This requires that the virion contain an RNA-dependent RNA polymerase, since host cells do not have a replicase that will transcribe negative-sense RNA. Third, because

their genomes can be directly used as mRNA, positive-sense RNA viruses are transfective. That is, naked RNA from these viruses can be used to infect host cells. Fourth, all RNA viruses except retroviruses and paramyxoviruses are replicated entirely within the cytoplasm. Retrovirus replication involves converting RNA to DNA and then back to RNA. The retrovirus DNA is inserted into the cellular genome as part of the replicative process. Paramyxoviruses, in contrast, must go through a nuclear phase because they borrow a portion of the host mRNA strands in the construction of their own mRNAs. Finally, all RNA viruses except retroviruses are haploid.

Specific Replication Schemes
Class I RNA Viruses

Class I RNA viruses consist of **astroviruses, caliciviruses, coronaviruses, flaviviruses, picornaviruses,** and **togaviruses.** The last two types of viruses are the most completely studied members of the class.

Fig. 21–1 shows the general replicative scheme of poliovirus, an example of a picornavirus. The poliovirus genome is a single positive-sense RNA strand that is about 7400 base pairs (bp) long and has a viral protein (VP) called VPG attached covalently to the 5′ end. Once the poliovirus RNA enters the host cell cytoplasm, it is used as a single mRNA to produce a 2200-amino-acid polyprotein (see Fig. 21–1A). The polyprotein is subsequently cleaved by a viral protease to yield the individual viral proteins.

Replication of the viral RNA begins about 1 hour after uncoating. Poliovirus RNA polymerase 3D copies the entire positive-sense strand to yield a negative-sense strand, and the strands are separated. The negative-sense strand now forms a partially double-stranded replicative intermediate (see Fig. 21–1B) that consists of a single negative-sense strand

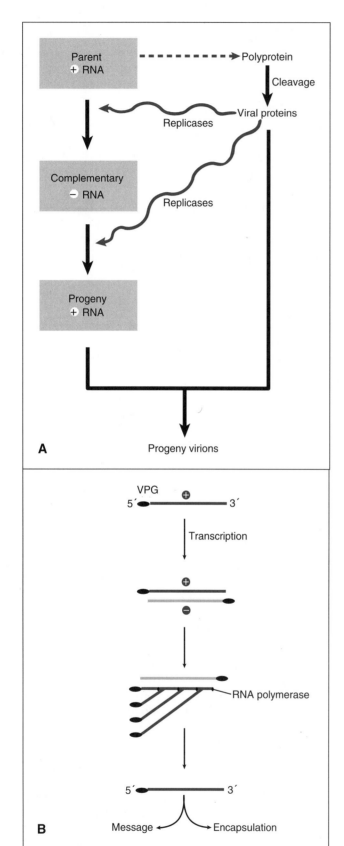

and multiple positive-sense strands of varying lengths. Thus, about 500,000 positive-sense strands can be constructed from about 10,000 negative-sense RNA strands within each infected cell. These positive-sense strands can be used as transcripts or can be encapsulated to form new virions.

The virions are constructed initially from three viral proteins: VP1, VP3, and VP0. During the maturation process, VP0 is cleaved to yield VP2 and VP4. The accumulation of capsid proteins causes translation to be prematurely terminated. As a result, during the latter parts of the replicative cycle, the polyprotein constructed is much smaller and consists primarily of precursors of the capsid proteins.

Togaviruses follow a similar replicative scheme but exhibit an interesting variation (Fig. 21–2). During the early phase of replication, only a portion of the genome is translated to produce a polyprotein. One of the cleavage products is a polymerase that transcribes the entire positive-sense strand genome to produce a negative-sense copy. The copy is then used to produce two types of positive-sense RNA. Many large strands, which are copies of the entire genome, are constructed to be used as genomes for new virions. Smaller RNA pieces are also made, and these serve as mRNA to produce a polyprotein that will be cleaved to yield viral structural proteins.

Class II RNA Viruses

Class II RNA viruses include **filoviruses, paramyxoviruses,** and **rhabdoviruses.** Each virion encloses a single piece of negative-sense ssRNA. Because the host cell cannot transcribe negative-sense RNA, the genome of these viruses is not transfective, and the viral capsid must carry an RNA-dependent RNA polymerase.

The prototypic class II RNA virus is vesicular stomatitis virus (VSV), an example of a rhabdovirus. In addition to the viral genome, each VSV virion contains multiple copies of three proteins: N (about 1250 copies), NS (about 460 copies), and L (about 50 copies). In the cell cytoplasm, VSV replicates as outlined in Fig. 21–3. A complex of N protein, NS protein, L protein, and the viral genome produces individual RNA messages, and these are subsequently capped by a viral enzyme. The proteins synthesized replicate the viral genome and form the structure of the nucleocapsid. As excess N protein accumulates in the cell

---

FIGURE 21–1. Replication of poliovirus (a class I RNA virus). As shown in diagram **A,** the viral genome is read in its entirety to produce a polyprotein. This protein is then cleaved to produce individual viral proteins. The viral proteins produce negative-sense RNA copies, which are subsequently copied to produce progeny positive-sense RNA. Diagram **B** illustrates the means by which the viral genome is replicated. First, positive-sense RNA strands to which a viral protein called VPG is attached are transcribed to produce negative-sense RNA strands. Next, each negative-sense strand is transcribed to produce multiple positive-sense strands, each of which has VPG at its 5′ end and an RNA polymerase at its 3′ end.

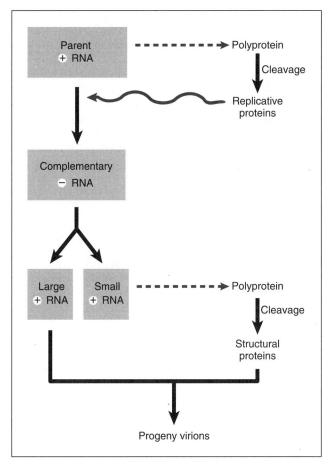

FIGURE 21–2. Replication of togavirus (a class I RNA virus). During the early phase of replication, only a portion of the genome is translated to produce a polyprotein. In a later phase, the negative-sense RNA is read to produce two types of positive-sense RNA. Large RNA is encapsulated to produce progeny virions, and small RNA is translated to produce a second polyprotein.

cytoplasm, it binds to termination signals in the genomic RNA. This allows a viral enzyme to make full-length copies of the viral genome. A positive-sense RNA copy is made first, and this copy is then transcribed by a viral enzyme to produce many negative-sense genomic copies. Finally, negative-sense RNA is encapsulated along with copies of N, NS, and L proteins.

Class III RNA Viruses

Class III RNA viruses consist of **arenaviruses, bunyaviruses,** and **orthomyxoviruses.** These viruses have segmented negative-sense RNA genomes. Each genomic segment encodes a single viral protein. Because these viruses contain negative-sense RNA, their genomes cannot transfect host cells, and their nucleocapsid contains an RNA-dependent RNA polymerase. Class III viruses are one of two groups of RNA viruses that have a nuclear phase as part of their replicative cycle.

The segmented genome of class III viruses allows an unusual genetic process to occur when closely related viruses coinfect a host cell. The RNA frag-

ments can become commingled, resulting in hybrid virions that have a gene from another virus. If the virus is functional, a new virus is created. This is the basis for the "genetic shift" that generates new influenza A strains responsible for periodic influenza pandemics (see the discussion of influenza virus, below).

The replicative cycle of influenza virus, a well-studied example of a class III RNA virus, is shown in Fig. 21–4. The ribonucleoprotein core of the virus migrates to the nucleus, where eight negative-sense RNA segments must be transcribed to construct complete positive-sense copies and mRNA. The viral RNA polymerase uses the 5′ ends of cellular mRNA as primers to initiate viral mRNA synthesis. The transcription of each viral mRNA strand halts about 20 bp short of the end, at the polyadenylated tail. Thus, the viral mRNAs contain a 5′ terminus that is pirated from cellular mRNA, but the copies of the positive-sense strand are 20 bp shorter at their 3′ ends than are their corresponding negative-sense originals. This process is the reason that class III RNA viruses replicate within the cell nucleus. They must

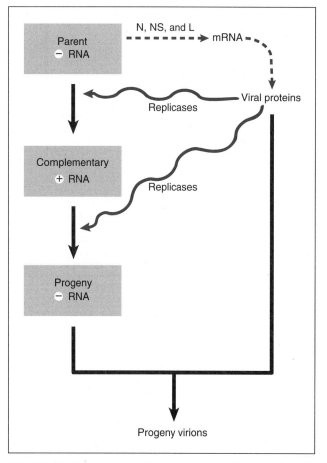

FIGURE 21–3. Replication of vesicular stomatitis virus (a class II RNA virus). The viral genome is transcribed by three proteins (N, NS, and L) to produce mRNA. The resulting proteins copy the RNA to a positive-sense strand and then to a negative-sense strand. After this, negative-sense strands are encapsulated to produce progeny virions.

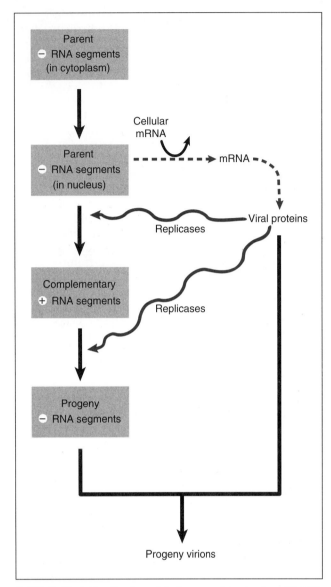

FIGURE 21–4. Replication of influenza virus (a class III RNA virus). The class III RNA viruses have a segmented negative-sense RNA genome. The viral RNA migrates to the nucleus, where it will be used to produce an mRNA from each segment. Cellular mRNA is used as a primer to produce viral mRNA segments, with the 5′ terminus of each viral mRNA being pirated from host mRNA. Viral proteins are then used to make positive-sense RNA copies of the genome. These copies are subsequently transcribed into negative-sense RNA fragments for encapsulation.

have mRNAs to serve as primers, and cellular mRNA is synthesized within the nucleus. In contrast, replication of complete negative-sense RNA strands does not require that a primer be available. Each negative-sense strand is copied entirely as positive-sense RNA, and this transcript is used to produce negative-sense RNA strands. Finally, the progeny negative-sense strands are encapsulated, and the nucleocapsid buds through sites in the host cell membrane that are rich in matrix protein, hemagglutinin, and neuraminidase.

Class IV RNA Viruses

Reoviruses constitute the class IV RNA viruses. The best-known reovirus is the rotavirus, which is responsible for epidemics of diarrhea among children worldwide. Reoviruses have a double capsid that encloses an RNA polymerase, a protein to cap mRNA, and 10 segments of dsRNA.

Reoviruses enter host cells via viropexis and are only partially uncoated. The viral replication cycle (Fig. 21–5) begins when the outer capsid is partially removed within cellular phagosomes and the resulting subviral particles are released into the cytoplasm. This process allows the viral RNA polymerase to come into contact with the encapsulated RNA segments, and positive-sense RNA copies are synthesized. The resulting mRNA fragments are capped but are not spliced or polyadenylated. Twelve proteins are synthesized from the 10 segments. (This is possible because one RNA segment encodes a second protein in a different reading frame, and another segment contains an internal initiation codon.) Some of the positive-sense strands are now transcribed to yield negative-sense RNA strands with which they will permanently associate to form progeny dsRNA. Finally, some of the newly synthesized negative-sense RNA strands are used to make additional mRNA segments. The dsRNA segments will spontaneously associate initially with core proteins and later with capsid proteins to form progeny virions. During this process, the parental dsRNA segments never leave the nucleocapsid.

Class V RNA Viruses

Retroviruses constitute the class V RNA viruses. These viruses are unique in that their replication involves the formation of DNA copies from viral RNA. When the term "retrovirus" is used, it is generally in reference to members of the subfamily *Oncovirinae* of the family *Retroviridae.*

The replicative cycle of retroviruses is presented in Fig. 21–6. Retroviruses contain two identical strands of positive-sense ssRNA. These strands are capped and polyadenylated at the 3′ terminus, and they are thought to be held together via base pairing between palindromic sequences near their 5′ ends (see Fig. 21–6A). Because of the unique replicative needs of retroviruses, the RNA of these viruses is not transfective. Retroviruses carry two enzymes within their nucleocapsid: an integrase and a reverse transcriptase (an enzyme that transcribes RNA to DNA). The retrovirus reverse transcriptase is both a DNA polymerase and a ribonuclease (RNase H).

The retrovirus genome contains four genes: *gag,* which encodes nucleocapsid proteins; *pol,* which encodes reverse transcriptase and integrase; *pro,* which encodes protease; and *env,* which encodes glycoprotein spike components. The *gag* and *pol* genes are translated into precursor proteins that are cleaved to yield two final products each.

As Fig. 21–6B shows, the linear viral RNA is transcribed in the cytoplasm to make a copy of negative-sense DNA shortly after uncoating. The RNase H activity of the reverse transcriptase then degrades the parent RNA strand, and a positive-sense DNA copy of the genome is constructed. The resulting linear

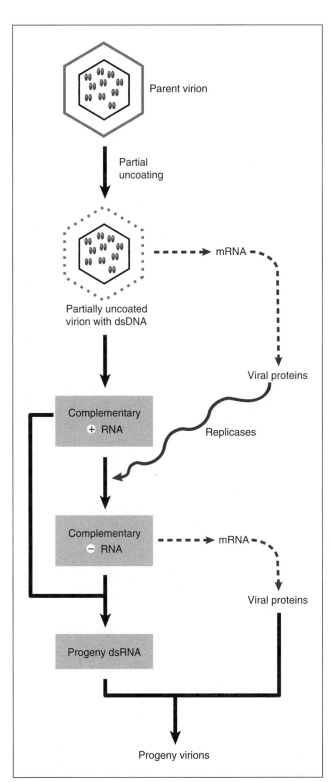

FIGURE 21–5. Replication of reoviruses (class IV RNA viruses). Reoviruses have a double capsid that encloses 10 segments of double-stranded DNA (dsDNA). Replication begins with partial degradation of the outer coat and production of positive-sense RNA copies of the dsDNA segments found within the capsid. After individual proteins are produced, these proteins transcribe the RNA, first to positive-sense RNA strands and then to double-stranded RNA (dsRNA). The negative-sense RNA strands formed during this process are used to synthesize capsid proteins.

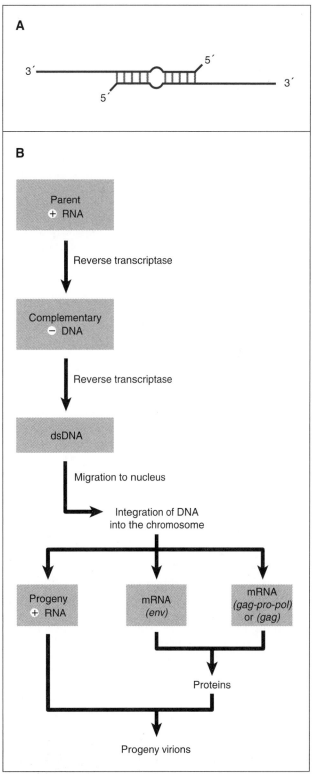

FIGURE 21–6. Replication of retroviruses (class V RNA viruses). As shown in diagram **A,** the genome consists of two identical positive-sense RNA strands that are held together by base pairing of palindromic sequences near their 5′ ends. As shown in diagram **B,** the viral reverse transcriptase first makes a negative-sense DNA copy of the viral RNA and then converts this to double-stranded DNA (dsDNA). The DNA migrates to the nucleus, where it becomes a provirus by being integrated into the chromosome. The integrated provirus is read to produce at least three positive-sense RNA species. The incomplete species are used as mRNA, and full-length copies are encapsulated to produce progeny virions. The progeny virions contain all four genes (*env, gag, pro,* and *pol*).

dsDNA segment now moves to the cell nucleus, where it is integrated into one of several discrete sites within the host chromosome to become a provirus. The provirus will be flanked by terminal repeats that are between 250 and 1200 bp in length.

Once the viral genome is integrated into the host chromosome, it can be transcribed by cellular enzymes. At least three groups of RNA products are seen. In the first group are transcripts that are full-length and can be encapsulated to produce progeny virions. In the second group are transcripts that contain only the *env* gene because the other genes have been spliced out. Finally, in the third group are transcripts that contain the *gag* gene or the *gag-pro-pol* gene complex and are capable of producing polyproteins that will later be cleaved. Some retroviruses also produce oncogenic gene products. These are discussed in Chapter 22.

CLASS I RNA VIRUSES

Tables 19–3 and 19–4 outline the characteristics and associated diseases of the RNA viruses in class I and other classes.

Astroviruses
Characteristics of Astroviruses

The family ***Astroviridae*** consists of icosahedral nonenveloped viruses. The name was derived from the fact that astroviruses look like five- or six-pointed stars when viewed from certain angles. The astrovirus capsid is 28–30 nm in diameter and encloses a 7.2-kb linear segment of positive-sense single-stranded RNA. The organisms can be isolated in human embryonic kidney cell or human colon carcinoma cell cultures.

Diseases Due to Astroviruses

Astroviruses are disseminated by the fecal-oral route. The organisms can be passed directly from person to person or can be consumed in contaminated food or water. The peak incidence of infection is during the winter months.

Infection in adults and older children is usually asymptomatic. In young children and in immunosuppressed and elderly patients, however, astrovirus infection causes **mild gastroenteritis** after an incubation period of 1–4 days. Symptoms and signs include watery diarrhea, abdominal discomfort, malaise, and vomiting. These manifestations commonly resolve in 1–4 days. Because astrovirus gastroenteritis is mild and self-limited, most patients are merely diagnosed as having an unidentified viral gastroenteritis. When a precise diagnosis is needed (for example, in cases involving immunosuppressed patients), viral antigens in the feces can be detected by enzyme immunoassay, or the viruses can be cultivated in human colon carcinoma cells.

Gastroenteritis caused by astroviruses is treated symptomatically, with administration of fluids and electrolytes as needed.

Caliciviruses
Classification and Structure

The family ***Caliciviridae*** consists of small (27–40 nm), nonenveloped icosahedral viruses. Each virion encloses a single strand of positive-sense RNA that is 7.5–7.7 kb long. The term *calix* means "cup," and the name "calicivirus" is derived from the numerous cup-shaped depressions seen on the surface of each virion in negatively stained electron micrographs. Two caliciviruses that cause human disease—namely, Norwalk virus and hepatitis E virus—are discussed below. Hepatitis F virus, a newly discovered hepatitis virus, is similar in its clinical presentation and epidemiology to both hepatitis E and hepatitis A viruses and is just beginning to be studied.

Characteristics of Norwalk Virus

General Features. Norwalk virus is more rounded than other caliciviruses and is relatively resistant to inactivation by heat, stomach acid, and water chlorination. Its name stems from the fact that it was the cause of a large outbreak of gastroenteritis among teachers and children in a school in Norwalk, Ohio. Several serotypes of the virus have been identified.

Mechanisms of Pathogenicity. During gastrointestinal infection, the tips of the villi in the jejunum slough off, giving them a blunt appearance. The lamina propria is infiltrated by mononuclear cells and polymorphonuclear leukocytes. Patients experience delayed gastric emptying and transient malabsorption.

Studies have shown that some individuals who ingest Norwalk virus do not develop infection and have no demonstrable antibody to the virus. When challenged with the virus again, these same individuals continue to resist infection. Those who develop disease on the first challenge with virus recover and develop antibody. These individuals become resistant to infection for only a few months, after which time they again become susceptible to infection. Thus, it appears that unidentified factors unrelated to antibody are most effective in preventing Norwalk virus infections, and antibody confers only short-term protection at best.

Diseases Due to Norwalk Virus

Epidemiology. Norwalk virus infections are acquired by the fecal-oral route and can cause gastroenteritis in individuals of any age. Outbreaks can sometimes be traced to a single common source, such as a sewage-polluted water supply, shellfish taken from a contaminated body of water, or salad or food served in a particular cafeteria or restaurant. Affected patients shed virions for about 2 days after symptoms begin, and secondary spread within a household is common. In the USA, up to 40% of all cases of gastroenteritis are attributed to Norwalk virus.

Diagnosis. Manifestations of **gastroenteritis**

("stomach flu" or "winter vomiting disease") begin about 24–48 hours after exposure, last for 12–60 hours, and may include nausea, vomiting, abdominal cramps, and diarrhea. Children tend to suffer from extensive vomiting, while adults are more likely to experience diarrhea. Some patients develop a low-grade fever accompanied by myalgia.

In most cases, the diagnosis is based on clinical findings. When a more precise viral diagnosis is needed, various techniques can be used. Immune electron microscopy, used extensively in the past, is now being replaced by enzyme immunoassays that detect the presence of Norwalk virus antigens in stool samples. Enzyme immunoassay or radioimmunoassay can also be used to detect rising titers of antibody to the virus, and polymerase chain reaction (PCR) assays are being developed. Norwalk virus has not been replicated in cell cultures.

Treatment and Prevention.   Gastroenteritis is treated symptomatically. Transmission of the virus can be reduced by adequate chlorination of water supplies and by proper personal hygiene (including thorough hand washing).

Characteristics of Hepatitis E Virus

General Features.   Hepatitis E virus is morphologically similar to Norwalk virus but is less stable under adverse environmental conditions. Like Norwalk virus, hepatitis E virus has not been cultivated in cell cultures. Purified viruses are prepared from the bile of experimentally infected monkeys and chimpanzees.

Mechanisms of Pathogenicity.   Hepatitis E virus causes a form of hepatitis similar to that caused by hepatitis A virus. The most prominent pathologic characteristic is cholestasis. The mechanisms responsible for liver damage and cholestasis are not well understood.

Diseases Due to Hepatitis E Virus

Epidemiology.   Hepatitis E virus is transmitted via the fecal-oral route. Most infections are acquired by drinking feces-contaminated water. Unlike hepatitis A, hepatitis E is not passed to household contacts at high frequency (10–20% for hepatitis A versus about 2% for hepatitis E). Hepatitis E virus is the most important cause of epidemic hepatitis in Asia. Clusters of cases often occur during the rainy season, when flooding causes water supplies to become contaminated.

The mortality rate associated with hepatitis E is 1–2% overall but is as high as 10–20% in infected pregnant women. The disease is extremely dangerous when acquired during the third trimester of pregnancy.

Diagnosis.   In its clinical presentation, **hepatitis E** is similar to hepatitis A. Children are usually asymptomatic. Most cases of icteric disease occur in young adults (age 15–40 years) and have their onset 1–8 weeks after exposure to the virus. There is no chronic form of hepatitis E, and infection does not predispose

patients to develop cirrhosis or hepatocellular carcinoma.

Laboratory diagnosis of hepatitis E involves excluding hepatitis A, B, and C. Immune electron microscopy can be performed to identify viral particles in feces. IgG and IgM antibodies to hepatitis E antigens can be detected by enzyme-linked immunosorbent assay (ELISA) by the time that symptoms of hepatitis are evident. A PCR assay has been developed to detect the presence of viral RNA in serum and fecal material. However, the ELISA and PCR tests for hepatitis E are not yet commercially available in the USA.

Treatment and Prevention.   Treatment of hepatitis E is supportive and palliative. Prevention depends on maintaining a potable water supply.

Coronaviruses
Characteristics of Coronaviruses

Coronaviruses are common pathogens of mammals and birds but cause only mild infections in humans. Their name comes from their appearance under electron microscopy. Each virion is surrounded by a layer of club-shaped peplomers that give the organism the appearance of a sun surrounded by a solar corona.

Coronaviruses are the largest of the spherical RNA viruses. The nucleocapsid is helical and encloses a single strand of RNA that is 27–33 kb long. The nucleocapsid lies within a pleomorphic envelope that is 60–220 nm in diameter. The nucleocapsid is constructed from N protein (nucleoprotein) and is loosely attached to the envelope by a transmembrane protein known as M. The M protein is not matrix protein. The peplomers consist of viral S (spike) protein and serve as adhesins. As such, coronavirus peplomers cause cell fusion and agglutinate erythrocytes.

The family ***Coronaviridae*** consists of two genera: ***Coronavirus*** and ***Torovirus.*** The HCV-0229E and HCV-OC43 strains of *Coronavirus* are known to cause common colds in humans. Other strains of *Coronavirus* and strains of *Torovirus* are thought to be the occasional causes of gastroenteritis. Little is known about how coronaviruses cause disease. The viruses replicate within the cytoplasm of nasal epithelial cells and do not spread to the blood.

Diseases Due to Coronaviruses

Human coronaviruses cause about 15% of **common colds** in the USA. Immunity is strain-specific and short-lived, so the viruses seem to cycle locally, with new outbreaks occurring every 2–4 years, usually during the winter. All ages are affected.

Patients develop nasal discharge and malaise 2–5 days after being exposed to an infective dose of virus. Most patients do not suffer from cough or sore throat. The disease runs its course in about 1 week, and patients shed virions for about the same length of time. Because the disease is so mild, definitive viral diagnosis is rarely needed. When such an identification is needed, enzyme immunoassay can be used to demonstrate the presence of organisms in nasal aspirates or on nasal swabs.

There is no specific treatment for coronavirus infections.

Flaviviruses

Classification and Structure

The flaviviruses are icosahedral, enveloped, and about 40–50 nm in diameter. The envelope contains glycoprotein peplomers, while the nucleocapsid encloses a single strand of positive-sense RNA. The flavivirus genome ranges in size from 9.5 to 11 kb and is infectious even when not enclosed within the nucleocapsid. Flaviviruses are replicated within perinuclear foci, are assembled within the cisternae of the endoplasmic reticulum, and escape the host cell via cell lysis.

At one time, viruses were classified by their means of transmission. Viruses that were arthropod-borne ("arbo") were called **arboviruses.** The arboviruses were then further grouped by other characteristics. The group A arboviruses eventually were reclassified within the family *Togaviridae* and genus *Alphavirus* (discussed in a later section), while most group B arboviruses were classified within the family ***Flaviviridae*** and the genus ***Flavivirus.*** The family *Flaviviridae* contains two additional genera: the genus ***Pestivirus,*** which consists of several nonarboviruses that cause diseases in animals but not in humans; and the genus ***Hepatitis C virus,*** which consists solely of the agent of acute and chronic hepatitis C. A new virus, designated as hepatitis G virus, is the cause of acute and chronic disease similar to but milder than that caused by hepatitis C virus. The hepatitis G virus is reported to be a flavivirus, but it is not known where it fits into the flavivirus taxonomic scheme. A virus previously designated as hepatitis GB-C is probably identical to hepatitis G.

Members of the family *Flaviviridae* are some of the most important viral pathogens in tropical and subtropical countries and include yellow fever virus, dengue virus, and various encephalitis viruses (see Table 19–4). Only the flaviviruses that cause human disease are discussed here.

Characteristics of Flaviviruses

General Features. The flavivirus capsid is constructed from a single protein, and its membrane contains glycoprotein spikes that serve as adhesins. Flaviviruses may enter host cells when their peplomers interact with host cell receptors, or their entry may be augmented by antibody. The attachment of nonneutralizing antibody to the flavivirus envelope can accelerate entry of flaviviruses into host cells via adherence to Fc receptors on target cells.

Mechanisms of Pathogenicity. Yellow fever virus is replicated within Kupffer cells in the liver, where its presence is evidenced by massive necrosis

of hepatocytes. This causes patients to become icteric, and a marked decrease in the rate of formation of prothrombin causes clotting disorders. Severely ill patients may suffer from extreme jaundice, gastrointestinal hemorrhaging, and hypotensive shock. Patients who develop petechiae and ecchymoses become thrombocytopenic and leukopenic.

Infections with dengue virus usually lead to a syndrome of fever, arthritis, and rash. However, a particularly dangerous form of disease, called hemorrhagic fever, develops in some patients—particularly children who have previously been infected with type 1, 3, or 4 dengue virus or who have received maternal antibody against these types of virus. When these patients become infected with type 2 dengue virus, the organisms are opsonized but not neutralized by cross-reacting antibody. As a result, the organisms rapidly and heavily infect monocytes and other immunocompetent cells and cause a fulminating hemorrhagic disease.

Encephalitis viruses can cause severe infection that is sometimes accompanied by cerebral edema, congestion, and hemorrhage in the brain. Neuronal necrosis can be extensive in cases involving Japanese encephalitis virus. Patients infected with tick-borne hemorrhagic viruses develop a form of encephalomyelitis that is characterized by extensive involvement of the anterior horn cells and looks like poliomyelitis.

The pathogenesis of hepatitis C is poorly understood but is believed to be analogous to that of hepatitis B (see Chapter 20).

Diseases Due to Flaviviruses

Epidemiology. Flavivirus infections occur mainly within the tropical and subtropical regions of the world, although there are exceptions. For example, St. Louis encephalitis occurs in temperate regions of North America. Yellow fever virus, perhaps the most notorious of the flaviviruses, is found only in tropical regions of Africa and South America. Dengue virus is found throughout the tropics worldwide, where it infects millions of individuals annually.

Viruses of the genus *Flavivirus* are transmitted to humans via arthropod bites. Table 21–1 groups these viruses by their associated disease states. Yellow fever, Japanese encephalitis, St. Louis encephalitis, and dengue are disseminated via the bites of mosquitoes and are seen more frequently than flavivirus infections that are spread by ticks. This pattern is not unexpected, since the feeding habits, relative mobility, and prevalence of mosquitoes makes them more likely than ticks to be vectors of epidemic diseases. Birds are usually the key nonhuman reservoirs for flaviviruses, but there are exceptions. Dengue virus and yellow fever virus are largely maintained in the wild within monkey populations, and Japanese encephalitis is frequently spread to humans from virus-infected pigs.

In South America, yellow fever is maintained in a jungle transmission cycle. The virus is transmitted among nonhuman primates via several mosquito vec-

TABLE 21-1. Arthropod-Borne Flaviviruses and Their Associated Diseases, Vectors, and Reservoirs

Disease	Virus	Vector	Nonhuman Reservoir
Encephalitis	Japanese encephalitis virus.	*Culex tritaeniorhyncus* and other *Culex* mosquitoes.	Birds and pigs.
	Kunjin virus.	*Culex* mosquitoes.	Birds.
	Louping ill virus.	*Ixodes* ticks.	Sheep and birds.
	Murray Valley encephalitis virus.	*Culex* mosquitoes.	Birds.
	Powassan virus.	*Ixodes* ticks.	Small mammals.
	Rocio virus.	*Aedes* and *Psorophora* mosquitoes.	Birds.
	St. Louis encephalitis virus.	*Culex* mosquitoes.	Birds.
Fever with arthritis, myalgia, and rash	Dengue virus.*	*Aedes* mosquitoes.	Monkeys.
	West Nile fever virus.	*Culex* mosquitoes.	Birds.
Hemorrhagic fever	Dengue virus.*	*Aedes* mosquitoes.	Monkeys.
	Kyasanur Forest disease virus.	*Haemaphysalis* ticks.	Rodents.
	Omsk hemorrhagic fever virus.	*Dermacentor* ticks.	Rodents.
	Yellow fever virus.	*Aedes* and *Haemagogus* mosquitoes; perhaps *Amblyomma* ticks.	Monkeys.

* Some patients infected with dengue virus have fever with arthritis, myalgia, and rash, while others have hemorrhagic fever.

tors, and humans are rarely infected. In Africa, where there are at least 200,000 cases of yellow fever each year, the virus is acquired predominantly via an urban cycle and is spread among people in villages and towns via *Aedes aegypti*. During the past 10 years, the incidence of yellow fever has been at its highest level since the World Health Organization began monitoring yellow fever in 1948. In Nigeria alone, epidemiologists estimate that more than 1 million residents suffered from yellow fever between 1984 and 1993.

Hepatitis C virus is the most prevalent "non-A, non-B" hepatitis virus and is a more common cause of chronic disease than is hepatitis B virus. In the USA, an estimated 21% of all cases of community-acquired hepatitis are due to hepatitis C virus, and about 1.4% of the population is infected with this virus. The epidemiologic patterns of hepatitis B and C viruses are similar. The US population most commonly infected with hepatitis C consists of intravenous drug users, who acquire the virus by sharing needles. Hepatitis C is probably also spread via sexual intercourse and from mother to fetus during pregnancy. It is likely that other means of transmission occur, since 40–50% of patients with hepatitis C have no identifiable risk factors for infection.

Diagnosis

(1) History and Physical Examination. Arthropod-borne infections fall into one of the three categories shown in Table 21–1. Hepatitis C infection may be acute or chronic.

(a) Encephalitis. Arthropod-borne infections are often subclinical. Acutely ill patients develop a fever that appears suddenly and is accompanied by headache and vomiting. Signs of meningeal involvement, including stiff neck, develop quickly and are followed by evidence of neuronal damage, such as ataxia, convulsions, drowsiness, paralysis, psychoses, or coma.

Among the encephalitides caused by flaviviruses, the most important are **Japanese encephalitis,** which is extremely common throughout Asia and has a mortality rate of 20–30%, and **St. Louis encephalitis,**

which occurs in the Americas and is not common but has a mortality rate of about 8%, making it an extremely dangerous disease. Many of the patients who recover from encephalitis are left with neurologic sequelae.

(b) Fever With Arthritis, Myalgia, and Rash. Patients with **dengue** or **West Nile fever** usually suffer from fever, arthritis, myalgia, and rash. The disease typically begins with a low-grade fever that lasts for 1–3 days. The patient then develops anorexia; headache; conjunctival injection, characterized by redness of the eyes; and eye, bone, and muscle pain. At this time, the patient appears quite flushed. The temperature quickly rises to 39–40 °C (102–104 °F) and remains elevated for 3–6 days. Because bone and muscle pain may become extremely severe in cases of dengue, the disease is commonly called **breakbone fever.** Many patients develop a flat or slightly raised rash on days 2–5 of disease, and 20–70% of patients develop a petechial rash on the last day of fever. Patients with the early rash typically complain of itching of the palms and soles and a loss of taste, and they are found to be granulocytopenic and thrombocytopenic. Most patients who do not develop hemorrhagic fever survive.

(c) Hemorrhagic Fever. Flavivirus diseases that may be manifested as a hemorrhagic fever include **dengue, yellow fever,** and, more rarely, **Kyasanur Forest disease** and **Omsk hemorrhagic fever.**

Children who have antibodies to type 1, 3, or 4 dengue virus and are later infected with type 2 dengue virus may develop hemorrhagic fever. These children typically become acutely ill 2–6 days after onset of a nonspecific fever. Manifestations of dengue hemorrhagic fever include cyanosis, dyspnea, ecchymoses, epistaxis, hematemesis (vomiting of blood), hepatomegaly, melena (black stools), and petechiae. Patients are markedly hypotensive and exhibit hemoconcentration. The mortality rate is about 8%.

The severity of yellow fever ranges from subclinical infection to disease that is fatal within 5 days. Acutely ill patients (about 15% of those infected) generally experience an abrupt onset of fever, muscle pain, anorexia, and vomiting, and these manifestations last 1–7 days. The disease is so named because jaundice is noted in some patients, beginning about the third day of illness. Findings in severely ill patients include bleeding from the gastrointestinal tract, gums, and nose. Mortality rates have varied widely in individual epidemics of yellow fever. The overall mortality rate is estimated to be 5%, but the rate in severely ill patients ranges from about 50% to 85%.

(d) Hepatitis C. Hepatitis C begins 6–8 weeks after exposure to body fluids contaminated with the hepatitis C virus. About 75% of those infected do not develop clinically apparent disease. In symptomatic patients, the manifestations of acute hepatitis C are similar to but less severe than those of acute hepatitis B. Most patients have little or no jaundice, and the mortality rate is only about 1% in those with fulminant disease. From 10% to 80% of patients infected with hepatitis C virus develop chronic infection, and this sometimes leads to cirrhosis (20–35% of patients), hepatocellular carcinoma, or both.

(2) Laboratory Analysis. Arthropod-borne flavivirus diseases can be best confirmed by isolating the viruses from the blood as early as possible during disease. The individual virus species and strains can then be characterized by serologic methods. The best methods utilize plaque reduction in cell cultures as a sign of viral neutralization. Flavivirus diseases can also be diagnosed by showing that the patient has a rising titer of antibody to a particular virus. Enzyme immunoassays are available for several of the flaviviruses.

Hepatitis C infection can be confirmed by serologic tests. Those currently available are enzyme immunoassays that detect the presence of antibody to hepatitis C virus about 3 months after the onset of infection. PCR-based tests can be used to confirm the diagnosis or to monitor the efficacy of treatment regimens.

Treatment and Prevention. No specific treatment is available for arthropod-borne flavivirus infections. Chronic hepatitis C has been treated with interferon alfa, but most patients who improve during treatment relapse when the drug is withdrawn.

Japanese encephalitis has been successfully controlled in Japan by the combination of draining rice paddies where *Culex* mosquitoes breed; raising pigs in areas that are farther removed from human living quarters; and immunizing children, horses, and pigs with a formalin-killed vaccine. Yellow fever is controlled in some areas by mosquito eradication and by use of **yellow fever vaccine.** No vaccines are available for the other arthropod-borne flaviviruses.

Methods to control the spread of hepatitis C include the testing of donated blood for the presence of antibody to hepatitis C virus and the counseling of individuals to avoid activities that increase the risk of infection (intravenous drug use, sharing of needles, and so forth).

Picornaviruses
Classification and Structure

The picornaviruses are so named because they are small ("pico") RNA ("rna") viruses. The picornaviruses are nonenveloped icosahedral viruses that contain a single strand of positive-sense RNA. The picornavirus genome is polyadenylated at the 3' end and has a viral protein known as VPG attached to its 5' end. The picornavirus genome can serve directly as a messenger and is infectious when introduced alone into appropriate host cells. The entire viral genome is read to produce a single polyprotein, which is subsequently cleaved to yield the four protomers (VP1, VP2, VP3, and VP4) needed to construct capsids.

The family ***Picornaviridae*** is divided into five genera. Three of these are pathogenic for humans: the genus ***Enterovirus,*** which includes 68 viruses known to infect humans; the genus ***Rhinovirus,*** which includes over 100 serotypes of viruses responsible for common colds; and the genus ***Hepatovirus,*** which includes the agent of hepatitis A.

Characteristics of Enteroviruses

General Features. The enteroviruses include a large number of viruses that are spread via the fecal-oral route, although some are spread by other types of close contact. These viruses are replicated initially in the oropharynx. They then pass through the stomach to the intestine, where they undergo a new round of replication. Included among the enteroviruses are **poliovirus** types 1–3; **coxsackievirus** types A1–A22, A24, and B1–B6; **echovirus** types 1–9, 11–27, and 29–34; and **enterovirus** types 68–71. The coxsackieviruses were named after Coxsackie, New York, where they were first identified. The echoviruses were isolated originally from asymptomatic patients and were deemed "orphan" viruses because they had no "parent" disease. "Echo" is an acronym for enteric cytopathogenic human orphan virus.

Mechanisms of Pathogenicity. Most enteroviruses enter the body via the fecal-oral route and are replicated initially within the oropharynx. In the case of polioviruses, this initial replicative round takes place in lymphoid cells. Virions from the oropharynx enter the saliva, pass safely through the stomach, and enter a second replicative round within the intestine. This round of replication may produce gastrointestinal symptoms, but some organisms released by intestinal cells spill into the blood, producing an asymptomatic form of primary viremia.

The primary viremia scatters organisms throughout the body, allowing enteroviruses to infect target cells specific for the species involved. The specific targets are governed largely by the availability of receptors that recognize enterovirus adhesins. Polioviruses infect neurons, particularly the anterior horn cells of the spinal cord, eventually leading to the generation of lesions throughout the brain and spinal cord. Targets of other enteroviruses include cardiac tissue, conjunctivas, meninges, muscles, skin, and liver. Viral replication within the target cells produces secondary viremia and gives rise to the symptoms associated with specific enteroviruses.

Diseases Due to Enteroviruses

Epidemiology. Enteroviruses are some of the most common viruses in the world. In countries with poor public hygiene and sanitation, they can be isolated from as many as 80% of young children at any time. In contrast, when proper sewage disposal methods are followed and water is consistently potable, infection rates tend to be low. Enteroviruses are extremely stable, and patients tend to shed them for weeks to months once infection reaches the intestine. Thus, patients can easily infect family members. The soiled diapers of infants sometimes serve as a source of infection, and the organisms can even be transmitted on the feet of flies. Coxsackieviruses responsible for respiratory infections and acute hemorrhagic conjunctivitis may be spread via respiratory droplets.

Polioviruses are an interesting epidemiologic problem. In countries where water sanitation is poor, young children are often infected early in life, usually resulting in diarrhea or asymptomatic infection. When such countries have experienced major improvements in sanitation procedures, the average age of initial infection with the viruses has increased and the prevalence of poliovirus infections has decreased. However, the incidence of paralytic poliomyelitis in those infected with the viruses has actually increased. This is because the risk of developing paralytic poliomyelitis following poliovirus infection increases with age. For this reason, paralytic poliomyelitis was a disease more commonly seen in countries with better water sanitation. The universal immunization of children with polio vaccines has helped to alter this epidemiologic pattern.

Diagnosis
(1) History and Physical Examination. Table 21–2 lists the major diseases caused by enteroviruses.

TABLE 21–2. Enteroviruses and Their Associated Diseases

Infection Site	Disease	Most Common Enteroviral Agents
Central nervous system	Meningitis.	Many enteroviruses.
	Poliomyelitis.	Poliovirus 1, 2, and 3.
	Other paralyses.	Enterovirus 70 and 71.
Eyes	Acute hemorrhagic conjunctivitis.	Enterovirus 70; coxsackievirus A24.
Heart	Myocarditis.	Coxsackievirus B.
Muscles	Pleurodynia.	Coxsackievirus B.
Respiratory tract	Common colds.	Coxsackievirus A21, A24, and B; echovirus 11.
Skin and mucosae	Hand-foot-and-mouth disease.	Coxsackievirus A6 and A16; enterovirus 71.
	Herpangina.	Coxsackievirus A.
	Maculopapular exanthemas.	Echovirus 9 and 16.

(a) Central Nervous System Disease. Although many enteroviruses cause aseptic **meningitis** and several enteroviruses can cause paralysis, **poliomyelitis** is the most important paralytic disease caused by enteroviruses. Poliomyelitis is a biphasic disease. Patients initially develop minor illness 6–20 days after ingesting polioviruses. Patients with minor illness suffer from constipation, coryza, headache, moderate fever, sore throat, and vomiting. These symptoms last for 2–6 days, after which the disease may disappear completely, abate for 3–4 days, or progress directly into the second phase. In this phase, patients have signs of aseptic meningitis that may progress to spinal or bulbar paralytic poliomyelitis. Early manifestations of paralytic disease include muscle pain and stiffness, weakness, muscle spasms, and hyperesthesia. Spinal poliomyelitis most severely affects the muscles innervated from the spinal cord, while bulbar poliomyelitis most severely affects the cranial nerves. Bulbar disease can cause respiratory paralysis, requiring that the patient receive mechanical ventilatory support.

(b) Eye Infections. Enterovirus 70 and coxsackievirus A24 are the two viruses most commonly associated with **acute hemorrhagic conjunctivitis.** This disease was first recognized in 1969 and infected 50 million people during its first 2 years of recognition. Patients, who are usually adults, develop acute conjunctivitis about 24 hours after being infected. Subconjunctival hemorrhaging is common, and some patients develop **keratitis.** A number of patients in an outbreak of hemorrhagic conjunctivitis in southern India developed myeloradiculitis.

(c) Myocarditis. Coxsackievirus B causes myocarditis in patients of all ages, including newborn infants and young adults. Manifestations include chest pain, fatigue, fever, and cardiac arrhythmia. Most cases of myocarditis are self-limited, but some patients develop life-threatening cardiomyopathy. Other coxsackieviruses and some echoviruses have also been implicated as occasional causes of myocarditis.

(d) Pleurodynia. Pleurodynia, a disease of the muscles, is also called **Bornholm disease, epidemic myalgia,** or **devil's grip.** It is primarily caused by coxsackievirus B but is occasionally attributable to coxsackievirus A or echoviruses. Pleurodynia begins abruptly in most cases, although about one-fourth of patients experience a flu-like prodrome. The disease is characterized by severe paroxysmal chest pain that is usually felt over the lower ribs or sternum. Despite the name of the disease, the pleurae are not involved. Chest pain is accentuated by coughing and is described as a stabbing or catching pain that is absent between paroxysms. In many patients, the pain radiates to the neck, scapula, or shoulder. Other manifestations may include cough, fever, frontal headache, diarrhea, abdominal pain, anorexia, nausea, and vomiting. Most patients recover in 3–4 days, but the disease may last up to 2 weeks.

(e) Respiratory Tract Infections. A wide variety of enteroviruses cause colds and sore throats, usually occurring as summer epidemics of mild respiratory disease.

(f) Skin and Mucosal Infections. Coxsackievirus A9 and A16 and the very similar enterovirus 71 cause **hand-foot-and-mouth disease.** This mild disease, which occurs most often in children, presents initially as a sore throat or sore mouth. Vesicular eruptions can be seen on the buccal mucosa, hard palate, gingivae, pharynx, and lips. The vesicles break down to yield shallow whitish lesions with a red areola. Many children also have a few vesicular lesions on the hands (usually in the periungual areas) and on the heel margins. Lesions are occasionally seen on the palms and soles. The disease typically resolves without incident in 4–8 days, although it is accompanied in rare cases by aseptic meningitis or myocarditis.

Herpangina occurs primarily during the summer and usually affects children under 7 years of age. Affected patients develop 10–20 grayish-white vesicles on the anterior tonsillar pillars, the uvula, and the edge of the soft palate. Each lesion is about 1–2 mm in diameter and is surrounded by red areolae. As older vesicles rupture, new vesicles appear, the ruptured vesicles enlarge, and the pharynx becomes extremely red. Other manifestations typically include anorexia, fever, dysphagia, excessive salivation, malaise, and sore throat, sometimes accompanied by abdominal pain and vomiting. Patients recover spontaneously in about 1 week.

Enteroviruses cause a variety of **maculopapular exanthems,** some of which can be mistaken for rubella, roseola, or rubeola.

(g) Other Diseases. Enteroviruses are responsible for a wide variety of other diseases, the most important of which are systemic neonatal infections. Coxsackievirus B and echovirus 11 cause neonatal encephalomyocarditis, and echovirus 11 can cause hepatitis in newborn infants. Enteroviruses have also been linked to juvenile-onset insulin-dependent diabetes and to hemolytic-uremic syndrome.

(2) Laboratory Analysis. Infection with an enterovirus can be confirmed by cultivating the virus in monkey or human cell lines. Antibody-mediated virus neutralization techniques are used to determine the virus type. Enzyme immunoassays are available for identification of antibodies to some enteroviruses in serum samples from infected patients. Polymerase chain reaction tests are available for diagnosis of poliovirus infections.

Treatment and Prevention. Supportive measures should be instituted. There are no specific treatments for enterovirus infections.

Poliomyelitis is prevented by administration of **oral polio vaccine** at 2, 4, and 6 months of age and again upon entry to elementary school. The vaccine induces immunity within the gastrointestinal tract, so it prevents infection. However, because some children who have received the oral vaccine have developed disease from the vaccine itself, children in some countries receive a single dose of **inactivated polio vaccine** before receiving the oral vaccine. The inactivated vaccine is injected intramuscularly. It does not prevent infection, but it blocks development of paralytic disease. Only Sweden, Iceland, and Holland use the inactivated polio vaccine exclusively.

Characteristics of Rhinoviruses

General Features. There are more than 100 serotypes of human rhinoviruses. These viruses are responsible for about 50% of all common colds. Rhinoviruses are about 25–30 nm in diameter and differ from other picornaviruses in that they are destroyed at a pH of less than 3. Rhinoviruses are replicated optimally at a temperature of 33–35 °C and are rapidly inactivated at 37 °C. This temperature sensitivity restricts most rhinovirus replication to the upper airways, where temperatures are low.

Mechanisms of Pathogenicity. Rhinoviruses attach to intercellular adhesion molecule 1 (ICAM-1) and are taken into respiratory epithelial cells. Rhinoviruses are replicated in the cell cytoplasm and are released via cytolysis. Their presence in the respiratory mucosa elicits the production of kinins that are thought to be responsible for much of the inflammation and mucus production seen during a cold. Inflammatory processes up-regulate the expression of ICAM-1, and this increases the rate of invasion of epithelial cells by rhinoviruses. Eventually, the infection is controlled by antibodies, of which IgA is probably the most important.

Neutralizing antibodies adsorb to type-specific viral antigens located on the surface of the rhinoviruses. These antigens are hypervariable, with little cross-reactivity between strains. Although cross-reacting antibodies could adsorb to rhinovirus adhesins for ICAM-1, the fact that these adhesins are located within narrow crypts makes them inaccessible to the antibodies. This problem has made production of a vaccine against colds extremely difficult. Another problem is that immunity against rhinoviruses tends to be short-lived, as is usual for mucosal immunity.

Human rhinoviruses do not infect lower animals naturally, although experimental infections have been produced in chimpanzees and gibbons.

Diseases Due to Rhinoviruses

Epidemiology. Rhinovirus infections are found most commonly in children and occur most frequently in the early fall and late spring. About half of those infected develop symptoms of a cold. Only a small number of rhinovirus serotypes tend to affect a community at any time.

The most common routes of rhinovirus infection are probably via hand contact and self-inoculation. Infected patients shed rhinoviruses during illness and continually contaminate their hands with mucinous secretions. When they touch other people or handle objects, they transmit the organisms to the hands of others, who then inoculate themselves when they touch their own face. Spread probably also occurs via respiratory droplets, but this mechanism is believed to be responsible for only a small proportion of colds in a population.

Diagnosis. About 2–3 days after exposure, patients develop symptoms of the **common cold,** such as watery nasal discharge, cough, sneezing, headache, and mildly sore throat. There is little or no fever unless a secondary infection, such as bacterial sinusitis or otitis media, is also present. The amount of virus shed is proportional to the severity of rhinorrhea. Colds caused by rhinovirus generally run their course in a week or less. In rare cases, individuals develop tracheobronchitis or atypical pneumonia.

Other than during epidemiologic studies, laboratory diagnosis of rhinovirus infection is rarely pursued. A specific diagnosis can be made by using nasal specimens to inoculate human fibroblast cell lines or human embryonic kidney cells. Cytopathic effects can be seen within a week, and antibody viral neutralization tests can confirm the rhinovirus type.

Treatment and Prevention. Treatment for rhinovirus infections is entirely symptomatic. Some studies have shown that use of antipyretic agents may actually increase viral shedding.

Hand washing is probably the most effective preventive measure. There is no vaccine for rhinovirus infections. Given that there are more than 100 serotypes of the virus, that antibody is not cross-protective, and that immunity is short-lived, a vaccine is not likely to be seen in the near future.

Characteristics of Hepatoviruses

General Features. Hepatitis A virus was originally classified as an enterovirus (enterovirus 72) but was later placed within a separate genus named *Hepatovirus.* Hepatitis A virus is 27 nm in diameter and is similar to the other picornaviruses in its morphology.

Mechanisms of Pathogenicity. Hepatitis A virus first infects the intestine and then infects the parenchymal cells of the liver, where it is believed to establish a persistent, noncytolytic infection. Before the onset of clinical illness, the viral organisms are in highest concentration in the feces, probably because they are being replicated within and shed from the intestinal epithelium.

The liver damage seen during hepatitis A is similar to that seen during active hepatitis B. Because the hepatitis A replicative cycle is noncytolytic and little damage is seen until the immune response becomes active, most of the damage to the liver is thought to be immune-mediated. Many investigators believe that cytotoxic T lymphocytes are the critical agents of hepatic damage during hepatitis A, but the pathogenic process is not well described. Hepatitis A infection does not lead to chronic disease, and patients have no increased risk of cirrhosis or hepatocellular carcinoma.

Diseases Due to Hepatoviruses

Epidemiology. Although serum transmission of hepatitis A can occur, the virus is most often spread via the fecal-oral route. Thus, hepatitis A is common and endemic wherever sanitation is poor and water supplies are readily contaminated with human waste. In the USA, where hepatitis A occurs sporadically, the virus is commonly spread among individuals in institutions and among infants in daycare centers. Sources of infection include poorly prepared food, contaminated swimming pools and wells, and shellfish grown in sewage-contaminated water. Intravenous drug users are at risk of infection from contaminated needles.

Hepatitis A tends to occur in epidemics. In undeveloped countries, most patients are children and adolescents. In industrialized countries with excellent sanitation, the highest attack rate is in the age group of 15–30 years. During epidemics in the USA, attack rates as high as 200 per 10,000 school children have been reported.

Diagnosis. Patients develop **hepatitis A** from 2 to 6 weeks after ingesting contaminated food or water. Clinically, hepatitis A is virtually indistinguishable from hepatitis B.

During the first and second week of infection, patients with hepatitis A complain of upper right quadrant abdominal pain, anorexia, lassitude, myalgia, nausea, and vomiting. Symptoms suggesting an upper respiratory tract infection are occasionally present. During the third week, icterus develops in some patients and is generally preceded by the appearance of dark urine. Icterus is more common in older patients, affecting about two-thirds of adults. In addition to causing the skin and sclerae to become yellow, icterus generally causes the feces to become pale. Many patients have mild pruritus. The liver is moderately enlarged, and about 20% of patients exhibit splenomegaly.

Patients with viral hepatitis have elevated serum levels of alanine and aspartate transaminase. The diagnosis of hepatitis A can be confirmed by demonstrating the presence of IgM antibodies to hepatitis A virus in serum samples tested by enzyme immunoassay or radioimmunoassay. Antibody appears coincident with symptoms and disappears 3–6 months later.

Acute hepatitis A usually lasts about 4 weeks, and most patients recover completely in 4 months. Although alcohol ingestion or heavy exercise shortly after recovery can cause a relapse of acute hepatitis, there is no chronic form of the disease. The mortality rate associated with hepatitis A is 0.1% overall, with death occurring in about 0.5% of patients who have acute primary hepatitis. Complete recovery confers lifelong immunity.

Treatment and Prevention. Treatment of hepatitis A is symptomatic.

Prevention of hepatitis A involves a two-pronged approach. First, the spread of infection is diminished by paying scrupulous attention to personal hygiene. Hand washing is extremely important, as are proper sewage disposal and water decontamination. Second, individuals at high risk of infection and travelers to endemic areas should be immunized with **hepatitis A vaccine.** The killed vaccine is usually administered in two doses, given 1 month apart, and immunity lasts several years.

Togaviruses

Classification and Structure

The family *Togaviridae* consists of two genera: *Alphavirus,* which includes viruses previously categorized as group A arboviruses; and *Rubivirus,* which consists solely of the rubella virus. The togaviruses are icosahedral enveloped viruses that contain a single strand of positive-sense RNA that is 10–12 kb long.

Characteristics of Alphaviruses

General Features. The alphaviruses can be divided into two major groups, based on the types of diseases that they cause. Three alphaviruses (Table 21–3) cause encephalitis in horses and humans, while the rest cause a disease whose hallmarks are fever, arthritis, myalgia, and rash.

Mechanisms of Pathogenicity. The alphaviruses are introduced into the skin by the bites of mosquitoes. The organisms multiply within capillary endothelial cells, blood monocytes, and tissue macrophages. After an initial round of replication, they disseminate hematogenously to specific target organs. During the viremic phase of infection, the patient suffers from prodromal symptoms. Depending on the viral species, the organisms may be found in the muscles, skin, joints, or brain, where they may produce myositis, rash, arthritis, or encephalitis, respectively. The viruses that cause encephalitis invade and damage neurons directly. Findings on microscopic examination of infected neural tissue include neuronal necrosis, neuronophagia, and an intense inflammatory response to the presence of the organisms.

Diseases Due to Alphaviruses

Epidemiology. *Culex* mosquitoes are usually responsible for the spread of eastern, western, and Venezuelan equine encephalitis viruses (EEE, WEE, and VEE viruses), although *Aedes* mosquitoes have also been implicated in the spread of EEE virus. Small birds are the usual reservoirs for WEE and EEE viruses, and rodents commonly harbor VEE virus. Hu-

TABLE 21–3. Alphaviruses and Their Clinical Presentations

Clinical Presentation	Alphaviruses
Encephalitis	Eastern equine encephalitis virus, western equine encephalitis virus, and Venezuelan equine encephalitis virus.
Fever with arthralgia, myalgia, and rash	Chikungunya virus, Mayaro virus, o'nyong-nyong virus, Ross River virus, and Sindbis virus.

mans and horses become involved when mosquito populations that generally feed on birds or rodents expand and begin to feed on larger animals. EEE and WEE are found throughout the Americas, but VEE is confined to tropical and subtropical areas (including Florida).

The nonencephalitic alphaviruses are found primarily throughout tropical regions of the Old World, where they are disseminated by a wide variety of mosquitoes. O'nyong-nyong virus is unique in that it is the only alphavirus disseminated by anopheline mosquitoes and is found only in eastern Africa. Chikungunya virus is widespread and has caused large epidemics in India, Africa, and Southeast Asia. Primates serve as reservoirs for this virus, and a wide variety of *Aedes* mosquitoes transmit chikungunya. Ross River virus is found in rural Australia, and infections due to Sindbis virus occur throughout Europe, Africa, and Asia. Only Mayaro virus is found in the New World, where it has been the cause of disease in the Amazon basin.

Diagnosis. Most infections with alphaviruses are asymptomatic. In symptomatic patients, either encephalitis or a syndrome characterized by fever, arthritis, myalgia, and rash is seen.

(1) History and Physical Examination

(a) Encephalitis. After several days of fever, patients develop nuchal rigidity and drowsiness. Subsequent manifestations may include confusion, convulsions, paralysis, and coma. The overall mortality rate in patients with encephalitis is 10–20%, with EEE virus causing the most severe disease. Many of those who survive are left with permanent neurologic damage, such as mental retardation, seizures, deafness, blindness, or paralysis.

(b) Fever With Arthritis, Myalgia, and Rash. About 2–3 days after the patient is bitten by an infected mosquito, there is an abrupt onset of chills, fever, myalgia, and severe polyarthritis of the small joints. The fever tends to be high, and the fingers are most severely affected by the arthritis. Most patients also develop a maculopapular rash. Individual patients variously develop backache, headache, photophobia, or retro-orbital pain. Many of those who recover continue to suffer from arthritis for months or years.

(2) Laboratory Analysis. During the viremic phase of disease, alphaviruses can be grown in cell cultures and identified. Among the cell culture systems used are Vero cells, BHK-21 cells, and C6/36 mosquito cells. Alphavirus species can be identified by immunofluorescence, enzyme immunoassay, or hemagglutination inhibition techniques.

Treatment and Prevention. There are no specific treatments for alphavirus diseases. Equine encephalitides can be partially controlled by immunizing horses against the diseases. Mosquitoes and mosquito breeding sites should be eradicated, and efforts should be made to avoid unnecessary exposure to mosquitoes.

Characteristics of Rubivirus

General Features. Rubella virus is the only rubivirus. It is morphologically similar to the alphaviruses but has a slightly smaller genome. Rubella virus causes rubella, a childhood disease also known in the USA as German measles. Although rubella is generally a mild disease in children, infection during pregnancy can spread to the fetus and cause congenital rubella syndrome, a life-threatening disease.

Mechanisms of Pathogenicity. Rubella virus enters via the respiratory route and multiplies within the draining lymph nodes. Viremia results and disseminates the virus further. Organisms can subsequently be found within lymphocytes and within the synovial fluid of patients who develop arthritis.

When a pregnant woman is infected and develops viremia, the organisms spread to the fetus. Transplacental infection is most dangerous when it occurs during the first trimester of pregnancy. Rather than causing rapid cytolysis, rubella virus causes cell division to slow, and a small number of cells in the infected tissue die. When this occurs during the first trimester, it can affect critical stages of organ development and cause fetal defects.

Diseases Due to Rubivirus

Epidemiology. Patients are most infectious beginning about 5 days before the rash of rubella appears and continuing for about 10 days, although some patients shed organisms in their respiratory secretions for a much longer period. Rubella is less contagious than the other childhood exanthematous diseases, so a single exposure to a patient carries a low risk of infection. Because of its relatively low contagiousness, many children are never infected with rubella virus. In the USA, an estimated 15–20% of women of childbearing age are not immune to the virus and are therefore at risk of becoming infected and transmitting the infection transplacentally during pregnancy.

Diagnosis

(1) History and Physical Examination. From 12 to 23 days after exposure to rubella virus, **rubella** may begin with anorexia, conjunctivitis, headache, a low-grade fever, malaise, and mild respiratory symptoms. This prodrome is more commonly seen in adults and adolescents than in young children. Patients may develop prominent lymphadenopathy, usually of the auricular, posterior cervical, and suboccipital nodes. When the lymphadenopathy is at its height, patients usually develop a pink maculopapular rash that starts on the face and then spreads generally downward over the trunk and extremities. Because the older portions of the rash fade as the leading edge spreads downward, the rash is said to "run out the feet." Often, the rash lasts for only 2 or 3 days, giving rubella the common name 3-day measles. Patients generally begin to feel better at the time that the rash appears. About half of the young children with rubella do not develop a rash.

Most patients with rubella recover without incident, but about 1 in 6000 develops acute rubella encephalitis as a complication, and about one-third of adult women with rubella develop a self-limiting form of arthritis.

The most dangerous aspect of rubella is its propensity to cause **congenital rubella syndrome.** About 20% of infants infected in utero during the first trimester are born with severe congenital abnormalities, including neurosensory deafness, blindness (often involving cataract formation), congenital heart disease, and mental retardation (often due to microcephaly).

(2) Laboratory Analysis. The key to diagnosis of rubella is identification of antibodies to the rubella virus in serum samples from patients. Antibody can be detected using enzyme immunoassays, latex agglutination tests, or hemagglutination inhibition tests.

Three groups of patients are likely to seek antibody testing: women who are considering immunization against rubella; pregnant women who have been exposed to rubella or have developed a rash during the first trimester; and infants who are born with clinical signs that suggest congenital rubella syndrome. Adults should have serial serum samples tested for a rise in the titer of IgG antibodies to rubella. Infants should have a single sample tested for the presence of IgM antibodies to rubella. If congenital rubella syndrome is suspected, a sample of cord blood from the newborn infant should be tested for antibody. Because some manifestations of congenital rubella syndrome do not develop until years after birth, a definitive diagnosis of this syndrome is helpful for preparing management strategies.

Treatment and Prevention. There is no specific treatment for rubella. The key to prevention is administration of a live, attenuated **rubella virus vaccine** (strain RA27/3), usually in combination with vaccines against measles (rubeola) and mumps. Although the vaccine is not known to be teratogenic, it is generally recommended that it not be administered during pregnancy. Rubella vaccine is about 95% effective in preventing disease.

CLASS II RNA VIRUSES

The class II RNA viruses include filoviruses, paramyxoviruses, and rhabdoviruses. An outline of these viruses and their associated diseases is presented in Table 19–4.

Filoviruses

Characteristics of Filoviruses

General Features. Filoviruses were first isolated from patients and monkeys involved in an epidemic in Marburg, Germany, in 1967. Thirty-one patients were infected with the causative agent, which originated from a shipment of monkeys from Uganda, and seven patients died. Although investigators suspected the agent to be a rhabdovirus because of its general morphology, further studies showed that it was distinct from rhabdoviruses. Because of its long and filamentous shape, it was called a filovirus (from *filo,* meaning "threadlike").

In addition to Marburg virus, the family ***Filovi-***

ridae includes Ebola and Reston viruses. Although most organisms in this family are 80 nm wide and 800–1400 nm long, individual virions as long as 14,000 nm have been seen. Each nucleocapsid encloses a single strand of negative-sense RNA that is 19 kb long. The nucleocapsids are composed of seven proteins and are enveloped.

Filoviruses enter host cells via phagocytosis and are replicated within the cell cytoplasm. Elongated inclusion bodies form, and the organisms escape the cell via budding through the plasma membrane.

Mechanisms of Pathogenicity. Filoviruses tend to concentrate heavily within the adrenal glands, kidneys, liver, and spleen and are reported to cause alterations in endothelial arachidonate metabolism. Early in disease, patients are leukopenic, but they later develop neutrophilia. During the hemorrhagic stage of disease, the platelets of patients become completely dysfunctional, but the source of this dysfunction is not known. Progress in establishing the means by which filoviruses cause disease has been slow. This is because filoviruses are biosafety level 4 agents. Working with them is extremely dangerous, and few facilities are available to conduct research.

Diseases Due to Filoviruses

Epidemiology. In the 1967 epidemic of Marburg disease, the Marburg virus was transmitted from monkeys to humans and from human to human, but the precise mechanism of transfer was never established. Since that time, cases of Ebola disease have occurred in Zaire, Sudan, the Ivory Coast, Uganda, and Kenya. There seems to be no doubt that reusing contaminated needles was involved in the spread of Ebola virus in Zaire and Sudan. Other risk factors were the care of patients with Ebola disease, contact with the body secretions of patients, preparation of bodies of Ebola victims for burial, and sexual contact with exposed individuals. There is some evidence that the Reston virus, which is prevalent among cynomolgus monkeys in the Philippines and Indonesia, is transmitted among monkeys via respiratory secretions; however, it is not known if Ebola virus can be transmitted among humans in this fashion. The Reston virus does not cause disease in humans. Although Marburg virus was clearly spread from monkeys to humans, investigators have not determined where the Ebola virus came from or how humans were first infected with this virus.

The strains of Ebola virus seen in Zaire and Sudan have been found to differ antigenically. The Zaire strain (Ebola-Z) appears to be more virulent than the Sudan strain (Ebola-S). Ebola-Z in 1976 killed 290 of 318 patients (a 91% mortality rate), while Ebola-S in 1976 killed 140 of 250 patients (56%) and in 1979 killed 22 of 34 (65%).

Diagnosis. After an incubation period of 7–10 days, the patient with **Ebola disease** is suddenly struck with arthralgia, fever, headache, lethargy, myalgia, and weakness. During the second and third days of illness, the patient develops a sore throat, which makes swallowing difficult, and also begins to vomit and experience extreme abdominal pain. By the fifth day of illness, there is profuse bleeding from the mucosae, including the gastrointestinal tract, and blood is found in the vomitus and stool. The patient becomes rapidly hypovolemic, and death is generally due to hypovolemic shock.

The manifestations of **Marburg disease,** another form of hemorrhagic fever, are similar.

Laboratory diagnosis of Ebola and Marburg disease can be performed only under conditions of strict isolation and containment. The filoviruses can be recovered from body fluids and will replicate in Vero cells. They can be identified by direct immunofluorescence and by their characteristic morphology under electron microscopic examination.

Treatment and Prevention. There is no treatment for filovirus infections other than administering supportive care to maintain life.

Because filoviruses are believed to be monkey viruses and because wild cynomolgus monkeys so often are infected with filoviruses, the importation of monkeys has become greatly regulated. To prevent the spread of filoviruses to humans, protocols have been established for handling monkeys that are caught in the wild. When humans become infected, they must be strictly isolated, and clinical specimens must be handled in the manner prescribed for biosafety level 4 agents.

Paramyxoviruses
Classification and Structure

In the past, the members of a group of viruses consisting mostly of respiratory viruses with hemagglutinins were called **myxoviruses.** When it became apparent that there were fundamental structural and replicative differences among the myxoviruses, the influenza viruses were taxonomically separated from the others to form the new family *Orthomyxoviridae* (discussed later in this chapter), and the remaining viruses formed the family ***Paramyxoviridae.***

Paramyxoviruses are enveloped viruses that contain a single helical nucleocapsid. The enveloped virion is 150–300 nm in diameter, and the helical nucleocapsid is about 1 μm long when extended to its full length. The nucleocapsid, which is constructed of nucleoprotein (known as N or NP), contains transcriptases (designated L and P) and a single strand of negative-sense RNA that is 15–16 kb long. Outside this is a matrix protein (M) and an envelope. In all paramyxoviruses except the measles virus, the envelope contains several small membrane proteins in addition to containing two key glycoproteins: F, which is the fusion protein; and HN, which is a combined hemagglutinin and neuraminidase. HN serves as the attachment protein for host cells and is known as G in the pneumoviruses, in which it has no hemagglutinating or neuraminidase activity.

Paramyxoviruses replicate within the cell cytoplasm and escape the cell by budding through the cytoplasmic membrane. Because F is inserted within the cell membrane, cells infected with paramyxoviruses tend to merge with adjacent cells and form syncytia (giant cells). Cells infected with paramyxoviruses other than pneumoviruses can adsorb erythrocytes to their surfaces because HN is expressed on the surface of infected cells.

The paramyxoviruses have been divided into two subfamilies. The subfamily *Paramyxovirinae* consists of three genera: *Morbillivirus* (measles virus); *Paramyxovirus* (human parainfluenza virus types 1 and 3); and *Rubulavirus* (human parainfluenza virus types 2, 4a, and 4b and the mumps virus). The subfamily *Pneumovirinae* has a single genus, *Pneumovirus,* which consists of the human respiratory syncytial viruses.

Characteristics of Morbillivirus

General Features.   Morbillivirus is the cause of measles. Measles was first shown to be transmissible in 1758, when a Scottish physician transmitted the disease to volunteers by injecting them with blood samples taken from measles patients. The human measles virus has several nonhuman relatives, among which are the viruses that cause distemper in dogs and rinderpest in cattle.

The genome of measles virus is smaller than that of the other paramyxoviruses and encodes only six genes. The envelope of the virus contains a hemagglutinin protein (H) and a fusion protein (F), but there is no neuraminidase activity.

Mechanisms of Pathogenicity.   The measles virus infects its host via the respiratory route and is initially replicated in the mucosal epithelium. The organisms spread to the draining lymph nodes, where they are again replicated, and then enter the blood, causing primary viremia. This begins the dissemination of organisms to secondary lymphoid organs and is followed in several days by secondary viremia, which disseminates the virus further. The F and H proteins act as viral adhesins for host cells by binding to CD46.

During viremia, the virus can be found free in the blood and within macrophages. Circulating and alveolar macrophages that are infected with the virus are weakened by the infection. Within lymphoid tissue, the presence of the virus is evidenced by the formation of multinucleated giant cells. The secondary viremia spreads the virus to epithelia throughout the body, including the epithelia of the alimentary canal, bladder, conjunctivas, oropharynx, respiratory tract, and skin. The viremia persists until the rash of measles begins, but viruria continues for several days thereafter.

About days 9 and 10 of infection, the respiratory and conjunctival epithelia necrose, producing the prodromal signs of cough, coryza, conjunctivitis, and Koplik's spots. About day 14, the cell-mediated immune response (CMIR) begins, and an attack of viral foci in capillaries and small blood vessels produces the characteristic rash of measles. Eventually, the virus is eliminated by the activity of cytotoxic T lymphocytes and other components of the CMIR, and the patient usually recovers without sequelae.

Complications are most likely to occur in patients who develop secondary infections, are malnourished, or are immunosuppressed. Infection with the measles virus increases susceptibility to secondary infection in several ways. Damage of the respiratory and conjunctival epithelia leaves these surfaces at risk of infection by other agents. The entry of virions into macrophages depresses the function of these cells and causes patients to experience demonstrable T cell anergy. Anergy may also result from binding of measles virus to CD46, a process that markedly down-regulates the production of interleukin-12 by monocytes. In children who are malnourished, an infection with measles virus diminishes the rate of intestinal absorption. As a result, hepatic vitamin A stores are depleted, and the children may develop corneal xerophthalmia, corneal ulceration, and blindness.

Measles can also cause three types of central nervous system disease. The first is acute postinfectious measles encephalitis, an autoimmune demyelinating disease. The second is subacute measles encephalitis, a disease that occurs in children with no cytotoxic T lymphocyte response and is the result of unchecked replication of measles virus in the brain. The third is subacute sclerosing panencephalitis, a disease that occurs years after measles and is due to limited replication of measles virus in the brain. Patients with panencephalitis have high titers of neutralizing antimeasles antibody in their cerebrospinal fluid. This antibody apparently causes antigenic modulation of the replication of virions. The expression of M, F, and H proteins is halted, and almost no L protein is made. Measles RNA is replicated, and many defective measles virus nucleocapsids can be found in neurons. These nucleocapsids are slowly transferred from cell to cell in the brain. How this causes subacute sclerosing panencephalitis is not clear, but the process is invariably fatal.

Diseases Due to Morbillivirus

Epidemiology.   Measles occurs as winter and spring epidemics in temperate climates, usually in 2- or 3-year cycles. Infection occurs most often in children, but maternal antibody appears to protect infants younger than 6 months of age from infection. There is no asymptomatic carrier state, and there are no nonhuman reservoirs of the virus. Measles is highly contagious, especially during the prodromal phase, when the patient is coughing extensively. The respiratory secretions are filled with virus, and the organisms can persist on the skin or environmental surfaces for some time within droplets.

Worldwide, measles causes 1–2 million deaths each year. This represents a case fatality rate of 3–6% in undeveloped countries. In industrialized nations, widespread mandatory immunization has reduced measles to a clinical curiosity.

Diagnosis

(1) History and Physical Examination. Nine or more days after exposure, **measles** begins with a prodrome consisting of cough, coryza, conjunctivitis (with photophobia), fever, and Koplik's spots. The latter are pinpoint grayish-white spots that are surrounded by a red areola and occur on the buccal mucosa. The characteristic rash of measles appears about day 14, and it is often at this time that the fever begins to fall. The measles rash is macular and blotchy. It starts behind the ears and on the forehead and neck, and it then spreads during a 3-day period to the chest, trunk, and limbs. As the lower lesions appear, the upper lesions fade, leaving a brownish discoloration that will eventually disappear. Many patients recover without incident in about 1 week. Some, however, are not so fortunate.

About 5–10% of patients develop bronchiolitis, laryngitis, or tracheobronchitis. Some of these patients then develop giant cell pneumonia, which can lead to secondary bacterial pneumonia. The risk of pneumonia is higher in older patients. Others with respiratory symptoms develop secondary bacterial mastoiditis, otitis media, or sinusitis.

About 0.1% of patients develop encephalomyelitis 3–4 days after recovering from measles. Manifestations may include confusion, seizures, and coma. Death occurs in 15–25% of the patients with encephalomyelitis, and half of the survivors have permanent neurologic sequelae.

About 1 in 300,000 patients develops subacute sclerosing panencephalitis, usually 5–7 years after recovering from measles. The disease is heralded by myoclonus, personality changes, and signs of focal neurologic deficits, such as memory loss, poor judgment, inappropriate behavior, gait difficulties, and paralysis. Patients suffer a gradual loss of consciousness and eventually become comatose and die.

(2) Laboratory Analysis. At one time, measles was one of the most easily recognized infectious diseases. Today, because measles has become uncommon in the USA, diagnosis may require laboratory confirmation. Urinary sediment and nasal smears can be examined for the presence of syncytia that contain inclusions. Once the rash begins, antibody can be detected by enzyme-linked immunosorbent assay or immunofluorescence techniques.

Findings in subacute sclerosing panencephalitis include electroencephalographic changes and the presence of antibody to measles virus in cerebrospinal fluid and serum. If a brain biopsy is performed, the tissue will exhibit gliosis, neuronal degeneration, perivascular round cell infiltration, and the presence of Cowdry intranuclear inclusion bodies that can be seen by hematoxylin-eosin staining.

Treatment and Prevention. There is no specific treatment for measles. Symptoms and secondary bacterial infections should be managed appropriately.

Attenuated **measles vaccine** should be administered to all children between the ages of 12 and 15 months. The vaccine produces a 95–98% seroconversion rate in this age group but only a 50% rate in 6-month-old children. Boosters are given between the ages of 4 and 6 years.

Characteristics of Paramyxoviruses

General Features. The genus *Paramyxovirus* includes parainfluenza virus (PIV) types 1 and 3. Although PIV types 2, 4a, and 4b are classified with mumps virus in the genus *Rubulavirus,* the various types of PIV cause respiratory illnesses that share many clinical characteristics and will therefore be discussed together here.

Virions in the genus *Paramyxovirus* are composed of a single strand of negative-sense RNA that encodes six genes. The PIV genome and replicative proteins L and P are enclosed within a helical nucleocapsid that is constructed from NP. The entire structure lies within a lipid envelope that contains HN and F glycoproteins.

Mechanisms of Pathogenicity. PIV virions infect the respiratory epithelium and spread from cell to cell in the nose and pharynx. This early round of replication causes nasal congestion and pharyngitis, and some patients become viremic. The organisms may now spread to the laryngeal and tracheal epithelia, causing patients to develop croup. In these patients, the lamina propria, adventitia, and submucosa become edematous and infiltrated with cells. The presence of F protein on the surfaces of infected cells causes nearby cells to fuse, and in this manner multinucleated giant cells are formed. Possibly because of the secondary effects of infection, the beating of cilia on the epithelium may be diminished. If the virus subsequently spreads to the lungs, lymphocytes will infiltrate into the tissues around the bronchioles, the bronchiolar epithelium will necrose, and mucus and cellular debris will collect within the bronchioles. There is no persistent immunity to PIV, so reinfection is common.

Diseases Due to Paramyxoviruses

Epidemiology. The various types of PIV are worldwide in their distribution. They are shed for about 7–10 days during active disease and are spread rapidly among children via respiratory droplets. PIV 1 and 2 cause croup, usually in children between the ages of 2 and 5 years. PIV croup often occurs as autumn epidemics in alternating years. PIV 3 causes bronchiolitis and pneumonia, primarily in infants under 1 year of age. PIV 3 is continuously endemic. PIV 4 is a rare cause of colds in children of all ages.

Diagnosis. Most PIV disease is caused by PIV 1 and 2. Patients are young children who develop a low-grade fever, coryza, bronchitis, and pharyngitis. About 24–48 hours later, these children develop signs and symptoms of **croup.** The cough of croup is brassy, and the child's voice becomes hoarse. Many experience only mild disease that resolves in 3–7 days, but some develop stridor and respiratory distress secondary to upper airway obstruction.

Bronchiolitis is seen in about 2–3% of children with PIV infections. It is sometimes accompanied by pneumonia and is clinically similar to disease caused by respiratory syncytial virus.

PIV antigens in nasal aspirates can be rapidly identified using immunofluorescence or an enzyme immunoassay. Alternatively, PIV organisms can be cultured in a variety of continuous cell lines. The cytopathic effect is minimal, but the cells infected with PIV will adsorb guinea pig erythrocytes. The strain involved can be further identified by hemagglutination inhibition or by immunofluorescence.

Treatment and Prevention.   In children with PIV infections, the airway must be adequately maintained. Cool mist therapy may help, but some children will require intubation. There is no specific antiviral therapy, and there is no PIV vaccine.

Characteristics of Rubulaviruses

General Features.   The rubulaviruses include parainfluenza virus types 2, 4a, and 4b (discussed above) and mumps virus. The rubulaviruses contain a genome that encodes seven genes. Like the paramyxoviruses, the rubulaviruses have HN and F proteins within their envelope and have a nucleocapsid that contains the NP, L, and P proteins.

Mechanisms of Pathogenicity.   The mumps virus enters via the respiratory tract and multiplies within the mucosal epithelium and within local lymphocytes. This primary round of replication results in viremia and the subsequent dissemination of virions to target organs. The salivary glands and central nervous system are the primary targets of mumps virus, but the testicles, mammary glands, myocardium, and pancreas may also be infected.

The hallmark of mumps is swelling due to parotitis. Microscopic examination of the infected salivary gland reveals that interstitial edema is present and that monocytes have infiltrated the interstitial stroma. The lumen of the duct is filled with necrotic debris and polymorphonuclear leukocytes.

In testicular lesions, there is a diffuse interstitial edema. Macrophages and polymorphonuclear leukocytes infiltrate the tissues, and the epithelium of the testicular tubules may necrose.

Mumps virus may also cause meningitis or meningoencephalitis. In most patients, organisms are found only in the meninges, but the neurons of some patients are infected, producing encephalitis.

Diseases Due to Rubulaviruses

Epidemiology.   Mumps is a uniquely human disease. It is found worldwide, causes springtime epidemics in temperate climates, and is spread via contact with droplets of saliva. Patients begin shedding virions 1–2 days before the onset of symptoms and continue to shed them for 7–10 days. Mumps is the least communicable of the childhood respiratory diseases, so many individuals reach adulthood with no immunity to the virus. Mumps virus is not teratogenic, but there have been reports of stillbirths to mothers infected during their first trimester of pregnancy.

Diagnosis

(1) History and Physical Examination.   In about 30% of individuals with **mumps,** the disease is asymptomatic. In the remainder, symptoms begin 14–25 days after exposure and include anorexia, headache, low-grade fever, malaise, and myalgia. About 1–2 days later, the patient notices an "earache" that is due to pressure from a swollen parotid gland. In about 75% of patients, both parotid glands are affected, but swelling in the second gland does not begin until about 1–5 days later. The patient's temperature at this time is 38–40 °C (100.4–104 °F) but begins to fall when the swelling reaches its zenith. The swollen glands are tender and cause severe discomfort. The orifices of Wharton's or Stensen's ducts may swell and hemorrhage, and this makes drinking sour liquids and chewing painful. In most cases, the parotitis of mumps lasts a total of 9–13 days, during which time the swelling increases for 1–3 days, remains maximal for 1–3 days, and then subsides.

About 20% of postpubertal males with mumps develop epididymo-orchitis, a condition in which one or both testicles swell to 3–4 times their original size. Accompanying manifestations include nausea, vomiting, and pain that subsides after 3–5 days. The swelling is bilateral in about one-fourth of affected patients and may remain for weeks. Although most patients experience some testicular atrophy, sterility is rare.

Up to 10% of patients with mumps develop a transient form of meningitis evidenced by fever, headache, lethargy, nausea, and mild nuchal rigidity. Patients with mumps meningitis recover in 3–10 days.

Other complications of mumps include encephalitis or meningoencephalitis (affecting 1 in 6000 patients), pancreatitis (50 in 1000 patients), neurosensory deafness (1 in 15,000 patients), mastitis, arthritis, myocarditis, nephritis, and oophoritis.

(2) Laboratory Analysis.   Classic mumps parotitis is usually diagnosed on clinical grounds alone. If laboratory confirmation is needed, antibody testing or culture can be performed. During the first week of infection, IgM antibodies to the NP protein can be detected. Patients usually show a fourfold rise in the titer of antibody to mumps virus during convalescence. The virus can be cultured from samples of blood, cerebrospinal fluid, saliva, or urine. The organisms will grow in a medium containing H292 cells (a continuous cell line that was derived from mucoepidermoid carcinoma of the human lung).

Treatment and Prevention.   There is no specific therapy for mumps. Patients should be given supportive care as needed.

Children should be immunized with live, attenuated **mumps vaccine** between the ages of 12 and 15 months. The vaccine is usually administered in combination with measles and rubella vaccine. Although it is not teratogenic, the vaccine is contraindicated in pregnant women.

Characteristics of Pneumoviruses

General Features.   Pneumoviruses differ from the other paramyxoviruses in that they have no hemagglutinin or neuraminidase proteins inserted in their envelope. Instead, pneumoviruses have an attachment protein known as G. Thus, the presence of pneumoviruses in cultured cells cannot be detected by hemadsorption techniques. Other than the lack of HN, the proteins of pneumoviruses are similar to those of other paramyxoviruses: an F protein is inserted in the envelope, along with several small membrane proteins; an M protein provides the envelope with shape; the nucleocapsid is constructed from N protein; and the nucleocapsid contains L and P proteins as well as a single segment of negative-sense RNA. The genome of the pneumoviruses is larger than that of the other paramyxoviruses and encodes 10 genes.

The genus ***Pneumovirus*** consists of one virus pathogenic for humans, the respiratory syncytial virus (RSV). RSV is the most important respiratory pathogen of early childhood, causing about 50% of cases of bronchiolitis and 25% of cases of pneumonia during the first few months of life. RSV is a human pathogen with no natural nonhuman reservoirs, although chimpanzees have been experimentally infected with the virus. Cattle have their own strains of RSV, but these have not been shown to infect humans.

Mechanisms of Pathogenicity.   RSV is replicated within the epithelial cells and macrophages in the mucosae of the eyes and nose. The virions may circulate in the blood within peripheral blood leukocytes, but there is no disseminated form of RSV disease. RSV organisms may subsequently infect the lower lung fields and bronchioles, where their presence is marked by the development of scattered atelectasis and bronchiolar obstruction.

The mechanisms responsible for RSV bronchiolitis and pneumonia are somewhat controversial, but many investigators believe that they involve immune-mediated damage. This hypothesis arose from clinical trials performed years ago using a formalin-inactivated RSV vaccine. Instead of being protected against disease, immunized children developed much more severe disease than did unimmunized cohorts. Investigators found that antibody was made in response to the vaccine but that the antibody was nonneutralizing. This led some to propose that infants develop more severe disease when infected with RSV because maternal nonneutralizing antibody binds to the virions and produces an Arthus-type reaction. This hypothesis made sense and seemed consistent with the outcome of the vaccine trials, but laboratory studies failed to confirm the hypothesis. Currently, processes mediated by IgE and cytotoxic T lymphocytes are under scrutiny for their role in RSV disease. Infection with RSV does not confer long-term immunity, and reinfection is common.

Diseases Due to Pneumoviruses

Epidemiology.   RSV is a worldwide cause of bronchiolitis and pneumonia in children, especially those under the age of 6 months. In temperate climates, outbreaks of RSV disease tend to occur from mid winter to late spring. The attack rate of RSV is about 50% during the first year of life, and most infants have been infected by the age of 2 years. When a child in the house develops RSV disease, all of the family members will become infected, but only infants will become severely ill.

Infants with RSV disease often have to be hospitalized, and nosocomial spread of RSV is common. Typically, adults who care for an infant with RSV disease are infected and develop coldlike symptoms. The adults in turn infect other infants to whom they give medical care. Infants with RSV disease shed virions for about 3 weeks. RSV is a fairly hardy virus and can survive within droplets on the skin or on environmental surfaces for at least 30 minutes. The key to halting nosocomial spread of RSV disease is for medical personnel to wash their hands well between consultations with patients and to wear goggles and a mask.

Diagnosis

(1) History and Physical Examination.   In older children and adults, **respiratory syncytial virus infection** causes coldlike symptoms, such as fever and rhinitis, sometimes accompanied by pharyngitis and mild tracheobronchitis.

About 40% of infants who are between the ages of 6 weeks and 6 months and are experiencing their first RSV infection develop bronchiolitis and pneumonia. Bronchiolitis begins with a low-grade fever, coryza, and cough and rapidly progresses to cyanosis, dyspnea, and expiratory wheezing. Infants may exhibit rales, and death from anoxia sometimes occurs. Infants who develop pneumonia are listless and have a cough and rapid heart rate. Their breathing is accompanied by retraction of the intercostal muscles, and fine moist rales can be heard. Radiographs reveal the presence of patchy consolidation. Most infants recover in 1–3 weeks, but death occurs in severe cases.

(2) Laboratory Analysis.   An enzyme immunoassay can be used to detect the presence of RSV antigens in detergent-solubilized nasal aspirates. Alternatively, immunofluorescence can be used to demonstrate the presence of RSV antigens on cells washed from the nose or throat. When viral isolation is needed, nasal aspirates can be used to inoculate HeLa or HEp-2 cells. Within 3–10 days, syncytia appear and are found to contain acidophilic cytoplasmic inclusions. The presence of RSV in cell cultures can be further confirmed by immunofluorescence.

Treatment and Prevention.   Hospitalized infants suffering from RSV disease should be placed in respiratory isolation to prevent spread of RSV to other infants. Patients should be given supportive care as needed to prevent anoxia. The severity and duration of RSV illness can be reduced by treatment with ribavirin. The drug is administered by nebulizer in an oxygen tent, hood, ventilator, or mask. It is given 12–18 hours per day for 3–6 days.

There is no vaccine for the prevention of RSV disease.

Rhabdoviruses

Characteristics of Rhabdoviruses

General Features. Over 150 members of the family *Rhabdoviridae* have been described, but most infect arthropods. Rhabdoviruses that infect humans have been divided into two genera: *Vesiculovirus,* which includes the vesicular stomatitis virus; and *Lyssavirus,* which includes rabies virus, Duvenhage virus, Lagos bat virus, and Mokola virus.

Rhabdoviruses that infect humans are bullet-shaped viruses that typically measure 70 nm by 170–200 nm. Each virion contains a single strand of negative-sense RNA that is 11–12 kb long. A bullet-shaped lipid envelope surrounds a helical nucleocapsid, and a matrix protein maintains the shape of the virion.

Rhabdoviruses replicate in the cell cytoplasm, where their presence is evidenced by inclusion bodies called Negri bodies. The viruses gain their envelope when they bud through the plasma membrane of the host cell.

Mechanisms of Pathogenicity. Rabies virus is the key human rhabdovirus. The virus is typically acquired via an animal bite and is replicated locally within muscle fibers and possibly within other cells. The glycoprotein spike found on the viral envelope (encoded by the G gene) is the viral adhesin, and it binds to acetylcholine receptors on host cells. The viral organisms migrate to the neuromuscular junction and are replicated within neuronal cells. Then the organisms travel via retrograde intra-axonal transport and infect nerves throughout the central nervous system. Eventually, the organisms infect motor, sensory, and autonomic nerves and return to the peripheral organs. Throughout this process, there is little inflammation or similar evidence of an immune response to the virus. However, the immune response is known to play a role in at least some patients. Those who develop a cellular response (a type IV immune response) to rabies virus have signs of encephalitis and die more rapidly.

The means by which rabies virus affects nerve function are not known. The nerves are heavily infected, yet there appears to be little damage. Studies using animal models suggest that there may be changes in expression of nerve receptors for neurotransmitters. The limbic system is heavily infected fairly early, leading to increased cortisol production and aggressive behavior. This promotes transmission of the virus, because the saliva is also heavily infected, and aggressive animals tend to bite. Later in the disease, the cortical system is affected more severely, leading to coma and respiratory arrest.

Diseases Due to Rhabdoviruses

Epidemiology. Rabies and vesicular stomatitis are the two rhabdovirus infections with the highest incidence in humans.

The World Health Organization has estimated that about 50,000 deaths each year are due to rabies.

The disease occurs throughout the world and is transmitted most often by the bite or scratch of a rabid animal, although aerosol transmission by bats has been reported. About 90% of human cases are acquired through the bite of a rabid dog, but cats are also a common source of rabies. Most cases of rabies occur in rural areas where domestic animals can come into contact with rabid wild animals. The wildlife reservoirs of rabies vary geographically. In much of the USA, skunks are the key wild reservoir of the virus, although foxes and raccoons are common sources of the virus on the East Coast. In Europe, foxes and bats carry rabies most often. In South and Central America, vampire bats commonly spread the virus to cattle.

Vesicular stomatitis is usually a disease of cattle, but it is occasionally spread to humans, probably via the bites of blackflies, mites, mosquitoes, and sandflies.

Diagnosis

(1) History and Physical Examination

(a) Rabies. Rabies usually begins 14–90 days after being bitten by a rabid animal, although some patients have experienced much longer incubation periods. The prodrome consists of anorexia, chills, fever, emotional lability, malaise, and paresthesia around the bite site. Then the patient shows signs of furious rabies, paralytic rabies, or both.

Furious rabies is marked by muscle hypertonicity, anxiety, and episodes of aggressive behavior that require restraint. Patients experience aerophagia, hydrophobia, seizures, and hallucinations that alternate with periods of lucidity. Those with hydrophobia suffer from painful spasms of the inspiratory and laryngeal muscles at the sound, sight, smell, touch, or thought of water. During each seizure, the heart rate increases dramatically and may result in cardiac arrest. Saliva production increases dramatically, with some patients producing up to 1.5 L of saliva per day. Death due to furious rabies usually occurs after 5–7 days.

Paralytic rabies, or **dumb rabies,** affects fewer than 20% of patients and may occur alone or after furious rabies. Paresthesia progresses to flaccid paralysis of the limbs and then to a fatal paralysis of the respiratory muscles. Patients experience delirium and may become comatose. Death generally occurs after about 2 weeks.

(b) Vesicular Stomatitis. Affected patients develop vesicular lesions in the mouth, accompanied by diarrhea, headache, fever, malaise, and myalgia. The disease resolves spontaneously in 7–10 days.

(c) Other Diseases. Duvenhage virus, Lagos bat virus, and Mokola virus can cause disease that is indistinguishable from rabies.

(2) Laboratory Analysis. Animals suspected of having rabies should be killed and their brain tissue examined for rabies virus antigen by immunofluorescence techniques. Touch impressions of the cerebellum, hippocampus, and medulla should also be examined. Infected cells will show the presence of Negri bodies. In patients, the diagnosis of rabies is generally made solely on clinical grounds. Postmortem examinations should include polymerase chain reaction assays and immunofluorescence of corneal impressions, saliva, and tissue from skin biopsy.

Vesicular stomatitis virus infections can be confirmed by serologic tests.

Treatment and Prevention. Only one patient (in 1977) has ever been known to survive rabies. Thus, it is imperative to prevent its occurrence. An individual bitten by a rabid animal must have the wound cleansed with soap and water and irrigated with **human rabies immune globulin** (HRIG). Then the patient should be given an injection of HRIG and be immunized with **rabies vaccine.** The treatment should begin within 8 days of being bitten. The current vaccine consists of an inactivated rabies virus obtained from human diploid cells. The vaccine is administered on days 0, 3, 7, 14, and 28. This procedure is highly effective in preventing rabies. The other key to prevention is to make certain that all dogs and cats are properly immunized against rabies.

There is no specific treatment for vesicular stomatitis.

CLASS III RNA VIRUSES

The class III RNA viruses include arenaviruses, bunyaviruses, and orthomyxoviruses. An outline of these viruses and their associated diseases is presented in Table 19–4.

Arenaviruses
Characteristics of Arenaviruses

General Features. Arenaviruses are so named because their capsids often enclose cellular ribosomes that look like grains of sand (*arena* means "sand") within the virions. Arenaviruses are circular enveloped viruses that contain two helical nucleocapsids. The viral particles are usually between 110 and 130 nm in diameter, but larger virions are sometimes seen. The arenavirus genome consists of two linear single-stranded RNA segments, designated L (large) and S (small). The L segment is 7.2 kb long, while the S segment is 3.4 kb long. Most of each segment is negative-sense, but a portion of each is positive-sense, giving rise to the term "ambisense" to describe the genome. Each RNA segment is circularized by hydrogen bonding at the ends of the strands.

Arenaviruses are replicated within the cytoplasm of host cells and escape via budding through the cytoplasmic membrane. Many defective virions, known as defective interfering particles (DIPs), are produced during arenavirus replication. Each DIP is an incomplete virion that can bind to cellular receptors and interfere with entry and replication of complete virions. Influenza viruses (which are orthomyxoviruses) also produce many DIPs during replication.

The family ***Arenaviridae*** contains only a single genus, ***Arenavirus.*** Within this genus are two complexes or serogroups of viruses. The **LCM-LAS complex** consists of the lymphocytic choriomeningitis (LCM) virus and the Lassa virus. The **Tacaribe complex** consists of a set of New World viruses with three lineages. Lineage A includes Flexal, Parana, Pichinde, and Tamiami viruses; lineage B includes Amapari, Guanarito, Junin, Machupo, Sabia, and Tacaribe viruses; and lineage C includes Latino and Oliveros viruses. The Tacaribe virus infects only rodents, but the other viruses are believed to infect humans.

Mechanisms of Pathogenicity. The means by which arenaviruses cause disease has been studied extensively in mice infected with LCM virus. Newborn mice infected with this virus demonstrate no immune response and develop a persistent asymptomatic infection. In contrast, older mice infected with LCM virus develop meningoencephalitis as a result of the activity of cytotoxic T lymphocytes against the virus. Thus, LCM is an immune-mediated disease in mice.

The role of the immune response in human disease is not so clear-cut. Antibody has been shown to protect against Junin and Machupo viruses, while a cell-mediated immune response has been shown to be involved in recovery from Lassa fever. The destructive effect of cytotoxic T lymphocytes seen in mice infected with LCM virus has not been shown to occur in humans.

Little is known of how arenaviruses cause human disease. Patients with Lassa fever develop necrotic foci in the liver, and some patients bleed extensively from the mucosae. This bleeding disorder has been shown to be due to a platelet dysfunction that blocks the release of dense granules and adenosine triphosphate during the secondary wave of in vitro platelet aggregation. The arachidonate-dependent primary wave of aggregation is not altered.

Diseases Due to Arenaviruses

Epidemiology. Arenaviruses are rodent viruses that are occasionally spread to humans who come into contact with the urine of infected rodents. Lassa fever is unusual in that about 20% of patients are infected from human sources. Lassa fever occurs in western Africa, particularly in Nigeria, and the natural reservoir of the virus is a feral mouse (*Mastomys natalensis*). LCM is found primarily in the USA, Argentina, Brazil, western Europe, and central Siberia, and the virus is spread in the urine of the common house mouse (*Mus musculus*). Members of the Tacaribe group of New World viruses are found in South America, where they cause hemorrhagic fever. Guanarito virus, the agent of Venezuelan hemorrhagic fever, is acquired through contact with the urine of the cotton rat (*Sigmodon hispidus*), while the other members of the Tacaribe group are found among voles of the *Calomys* species.

Diagnosis
(1) History and Physical Examination
(a) Lassa Fever. Lassa fever begins gradually with fever and malaise 7–18 days after being infected with Lassa virus. By the fourth day of illness, the patient has a cough accompanied by joint and lumbar

pain. During the next 24 hours, the patient develops a frontal headache, sore throat, and retrosternal chest pain and may also experience vomiting and diarrhea. About 4–8 days after symptoms begin, severely ill patients develop a tender abdomen and rales suggestive of pneumonitis, and about 10% develop pleural effusions. Subsequent manifestations in those with life-threatening disease may include facial and neck edema (due to capillary leakage); bleeding from the mucosae; fine tremors, confusion, and seizures (due to encephalopathy); and damage to the eighth cranial nerve, which causes temporary hearing loss or permanent sensorineural deafness.

Pregnant women who are infected with Lassa virus can transmit the infection to their offspring in utero or via breast-feeding. Maternal death, stillbirth, and infant death are common.

(b) Lymphocytic Choriomeningitis. Most individuals who are infected with LCM virus are asymptomatic or have a mild to moderate febrile illness with no central nervous system disease. Only about 15% of infected patients develop choriomeningitis. In these patients, anorexia, fever, malaise, myalgia, nausea, and weakness begin about 1–3 weeks after infection. Patients typically complain of severe retro-orbital headache accompanied by photophobia, and about half of them also suffer from arthralgia, chest pain, pneumonitis, sore throat, and vomiting. Severely ill patients exhibit nuchal rigidity and are found to have encephalopathy in one-third of cases and aseptic meningitis in two-thirds. Recovery from LCM may be slow, but most patients recover completely.

(c) Hemorrhagic Fever. Viruses of the Tacaribe group are responsible for various forms of hemorrhagic fever, the best known of which are Argentinean hemorrhagic fever (caused by Junin virus), Bolivian hemorrhagic fever (Machupo virus), and Venezuelan hemorrhagic fever (Guanarito virus). These diseases begin insidiously with anorexia, fever, malaise, and myalgia. Subsequent manifestations include constipation; nausea and vomiting; erythema of the face, neck, and trunk; petechiae under the arms; conjunctivitis; photophobia; and severe retro-orbital headache. Patients may also develop acute neurologic disease or pulmonary edema. About 50% of patients bleed from the skin or mucosae and experience epistaxis and hematemesis. About 70% of patients become hypotensive, and this is the usual cause of death. In those who survive, recovery takes 3–6 weeks, during which time many patients suffer from alopecia, autonomic instability, weakness, and weight loss.

(2) Laboratory Analysis. Arenaviruses are biosafety level 4 agents. Clinical samples must be handled and transported with extreme care to central facilities with proper containment. In such facilities, the viruses can be cultured in Vero E6 or BHK-21 continuous cell lines, and their presence can be confirmed in 2–3 days by immunofluorescence or enzyme immunoassay. A single serum sample can be tested for the presence of IgM antibody, or paired serum

samples can be tested for a rising titer of IgG antibody to viruses. Antibody is detected by immunofluorescence using "spotslides" of acetone-fixed, gamma-irradiated Vero E6 cells that have been infected with arenaviruses. Acetone fixing inactivates the organisms.

Treatment and Prevention. Patients with arenavirus diseases must be isolated. Symptoms such as hypotension and shock must be managed appropriately. Lassa fever can be treated with ribavirin. When this drug is administered during the first 6 days of illness, it results in a 5-fold to 10-fold reduction in the case fatality rate. Argentinean hemorrhagic fever has been treated successfully during the first week of illness with high-titer convalescent-phase plasma.

There are no vaccines against arenaviruses.

Bunyaviruses
Characteristics of Bunyaviruses

General Features. The bunyaviruses were so named because of their similarity to the Bunyamwera virus. The family ***Bunyaviridae*** includes four genera: ***Bunyavirus,*** with more than 160 viruses; ***Hantavirus,*** with 6 viruses; ***Nairovirus,*** with more than 30 viruses; and ***Phlebovirus,*** with more than 50 viruses. In addition, because the bunyaviruses have a segmented genome, hybrid viruses containing genetically reassorted genes are sometimes seen.

Bunyaviruses are the largest group of **arboviruses.** Members of only one genus (the hantaviruses) are not vector-borne. The bunyaviruses are circular viruses that are 90–100 nm in diameter. Their lipid envelope contains glycoprotein peplomers designated G1 and G2 and encloses three helical nucleocapsids. Each nucleocapsid contains a segment of negative-sense single-stranded RNA. The three RNA strands are designated L (large), M (medium), and S (small) and are 7, 4, and 1–2 kb long, respectively. In some genera, the S RNA segment is ambisense. The nucleocapsid contains two proteins: the nucleocapsid protein (N) and a transcriptase (L).

Mechanisms of Pathogenicity. Bunyaviruses are responsible for a variety of clinical conditions including dengue-like syndromes, encephalitis, and hemorrhagic fever. The mechanisms of pathogenicity are poorly understood but are believed to be analogous to those of similar diseases caused by alphaviruses and flaviviruses.

Diseases Due to Bunyaviruses

Epidemiology. Bunyaviruses tend to be geographically localized diseases. In general, members of *Bunyavirus* are transmitted to humans by mosquitoes; members of *Phlebovirus* are spread by gnats, sandflies, and ticks; members of *Nairovirus* are spread by ticks; and members of *Hantavirus* are spread by contact with the urine of rodents.

Several of the bunyaviruses are significant pathogens in nonindustrialized countries. Rift Valley fever, for example, is mosquito-borne and is widespread in Africa, where it has infected hundreds of thousands and has caused hundreds of deaths. Sandfly fever is common in the Middle East, India, and Central and South America, where it is spread via the bites of sandflies. Crimean-Congo hemorrhagic fever is a zoonotic disease that is disseminated by ticks and is widespread in Africa, Asia, and the Middle East. Oropouche fever, which is acquired via the bite of a midge, is common and widespread in Brazil. Hantaan virus, a hantavirus, is a common cause of hemorrhagic fever with renal failure in northeastern Asia and is acquired from contact with the waste of bats, rats, mice, and some birds.

In the USA, *Aedes triseriatus,* a large black mosquito, transmits La Crosse virus to about 300,000 people each year and causes encephalitis in about 100 of those infected. Sinnombre virus, a hantavirus, is acquired through contact with the urine of infected deer mice and is seen most frequently in the Southwest.

Diagnosis. The diseases briefly reviewed here are representative of the many types of infections caused by bunyaviruses.

(1) History and Physical Examination

(a) California Encephalitis. Several closely related viruses cause California encephalitis. Of these, La Crosse virus is the most important. Most infected individuals are asymptomatic, but a small proportion (less than 1%) develop encephalitis and suffer from fever, headache, drowsiness, nuchal rigidity, and vomiting. Most patients recover completely, with no neurologic sequelae or deficits.

(b) Crimean-Congo Hemorrhagic Fever. The onset of disease is abrupt, with fever, headache, and severe pain in the back and abdomen. Patients soon begin to bleed through the skin and mucosae, and this leads to pulmonary edema and shock. Other common manifestations include hematemesis, hematuria, hemorrhagic skin rash, melena, leukopenia, and thrombocytopenia. The mortality rate ranges from 5% to 50%, depending on the quality of supportive care that is provided.

(c) Hantavirus Infections. Hantaan virus, a hantavirus found in northeastern Asia, causes hemorrhagic fever with renal disease. Patients present with fever, lumbar abdominal pain, and proteinuria. This is followed by the appearance of petechiae and either gastrointestinal bleeding or hemorrhagic pneumonia. In the recovery stage, patients develop renal tubular disease with oliguria. The mortality rate is 1–10%. Belgrade virus causes a similar but milder disease; Puumala virus causes a milder disease with many of the same manifestations but without hemorrhage; and Seoul virus causes a milder disease with liver involvement instead of renal involvement.

In the USA, sinnombre virus (meaning "no name" virus) is the cause of a life-threatening respiratory disease. This disease appeared first in the Four Corners region of the Southwest and is called Four Corners fever or Muerto Canyon fever. Patients present with fever, myalgia, and influenza-like symptoms.

They soon develop dyspnea and rapidly progressive pulmonary edema. Clinical findings include hypoxia, thrombocytopenia, hemoconcentration, hypoproteinemia, leukocytosis, and diffuse bilateral interstitial pulmonary infiltrates. During the initial epidemic of the disease, 56% of the patients died.

(d) Oropouche Fever. Oropouche fever, a disease found primarily in Brazil and northern South America, is characterized by arthralgia, fever, headache, myalgia, and prostration. The disease is mild, and all patients recover spontaneously.

(e) Rift Valley Fever. From 2 to 6 days after being bitten by an infected sandfly, patients develop fever, severe headache, myalgia, photophobia, and retro-orbital pain. The disease then progresses in one of three manners. Some patients develop a mild form of encephalitis with no long-term effects; others develop retinitis, which may lead to permanent loss of central vision; and still others develop hemorrhagic fever. The mortality rate in patients with hemorrhagic fever is 5–10%.

(f) Sandfly Fever. Sandfly fever is seen most commonly in tourists and other individuals who are traveling through areas where sandfly fever is endemic. Patients develop a self-limited dengue-like syndrome of conjunctivitis, fever, headache, leukopenia, myalgia, and retro-orbital pain.

(2) Laboratory Analysis. Bunyaviruses can be cultivated in Vero E6 or BHK-21 cell lines. Viral replication within these cells can be detected by immunofluorescence, enzyme immunoassays, or hemagglutination tests. The viruses can then be serotyped by hemagglutination inhibition or virus neutralization techniques.

Treatment and Prevention. Hemorrhagic fever should be treated with blood transfusions and other supportive measures to prevent shock. There are no specific antiviral therapies effective against bunyaviruses, nor are there vaccines to prevent infection.

Orthomyxoviruses
Characteristics of Orthomyxoviruses

General Features. Orthomyxoviruses are helical enveloped viruses that contain six, seven, or eight negative-sense single-stranded RNA fragments. Each RNA segment is associated with an RNA polymerase complex. The shape of the envelope is maintained with matrix (M1) protein, and the envelope is spanned by ion channels constructed from tetramers of M2 protein. The envelope contains numerous copies of hemagglutinin (H) and neuraminidase (N) glycoproteins, which are sometimes referred to as HA and NA proteins.

In the family *Orthomyxoviridae,* there are three genera: *Influenzavirus A,B,* consisting of influenza type A and B viruses; *Influenzavirus C,* consisting of influenza type C virus; and a third genus that is yet unnamed but includes Thogoto virus and Dhori virus, which are tick-borne viruses. Influenza A virus is one of the most common causes of infectious disease–related deaths. Because it is the cause of epidemic and pandemic disease and because the other viruses are so similar, the discussion below will center on influenza A virus.

Mechanisms of Pathogenicity. Influenza viruses attach via the H protein to sialic acid receptors and are phagocytosed. Within endosomes, the pH reaches 5.5, and this changes the conformation of the H protein and allows the viral envelope to fuse with the endosomal membrane. Protons also pass through the M2 channels in the envelope and cause the nucleocapsid to be released into the cytosol by dissociating the M1 protein from the nucleoprotein. The viral genome goes to the nucleus, where transcription and viral RNA replication will occur.

Influenza viruses initially infect the ciliary columnar epithelium of the airway, causing tracheobronchitis to develop. Viral multiplication within cells in the epithelium results in impaired mucociliary clearance and bronchospasms. The viruses can be eliminated by being enmeshed within the mucous blanket, where they attach to sialoglycoproteins. The beating of respiratory cilia moves the organisms to the pharynx, where they can be swallowed or expectorated. The organisms counteract this by using neuraminidase to cleave sialic acids in the mucous blanket and by inhibiting ciliary activity. The organisms then can travel to the lungs within the thinned secretions. Once in the lungs, they are protected by mannose-binding lectins and by alveolar macrophages. Antibody to H protein neutralizes influenza viruses and promotes their phagocytosis, but antibody to N protein is nonneutralizing.

The key to the occurrence of influenza pandemics has been the ability of influenza viruses to infect various animal hosts and undergo antigenic change. Between pandemics, the viruses undergo point mutations in or near the receptor-binding pocket of the H protein. These mutations cause just enough antigenic variation to allow the viruses to find nonimmune subjects. This process is known as **antigenic drift.** A pandemic occurs soon after a pig is coinfected with human and avian influenza viruses. Some mixing of the RNA segments occurs, producing mostly defective viruses. However, in rare situations, a new H protein is obtained by the human virus, and the new influenza virus strain is able to cause disease in humans. This process is known as **antigenic shift.** Because the H protein is new to the human population, the entire population lacks immunity to the virus, and a pandemic begins.

Diseases Due to Orthomyxoviruses

Epidemiology. Influenza A occurs in annual epidemics throughout the world and has been responsible for several major pandemics. The 1917–1918 pandemic, for example, killed about 20 million people—more people than were killed during World War I. Epidemiologists believe that this pandemic was so deadly because many patients with primary viral pneumonia developed secondary bacterial pneumo-

nia and antibiotics against the bacteria had not yet been developed.

Influenza pandemics usually begin in Southeast Asia or China, where individuals live in close proximity to domesticated animals. The recombinant virus usually acquires its H protein from a duck influenza virus but sometimes acquires it from a swine virus. The new strain may spread across the globe within days or weeks. Spread is rapid because influenza has a short incubation period (1–4 days) and patients shed huge amounts of virus in their respiratory droplets.

The best indicator of an influenza epidemic is the number of unexpected deaths ("excess deaths") that are attributable to the disease. When the fatalities due to influenza are monitored, epidemic years yield 10,000–50,000 excess influenza deaths annually in the USA. The elderly are the group at greatest risk of death, but children are the ones most likely to develop influenza. Influenza-related death occurs in about 10–15% of patients who are over 65 years but only 1–2% of those under 45 years of age.

Diagnosis

(1) History and Physical Examination. From 1 to 4 days after exposure to influenza virus, patients develop fever (temperature of 39–40 °C or about 102–104 °F), chills, severe headache with retro-orbital pain, conjunctival injection, a slightly productive cough, myalgia, and prostration. Most people recover in about 1 week.

The course of influenza tends to be more severe in patients who are elderly, have an underlying cardiopulmonary or other chronic disease, or are in their third trimester of pregnancy. Findings in these patients may include a persistent cough and fever, marked prostration, pneumonia with rales, leukopenia, and impaired gas exchange. Some patients develop secondary bacterial pneumonia due to *Staphylococcus aureus, Haemophilus influenzae, Streptococcus pneumoniae,* or *Streptococcus pyogenes.*

Rare complications of influenza include Guillain-Barré syndrome and Reye's syndrome.

(2) Laboratory Analysis. In most cases, influenza is diagnosed simply on the basis of clinical signs. When laboratory confirmation is needed, respiratory secretions can be used to inoculate MDCK cells if the samples are taken during the first 5 days of disease. The replication of influenza viruses within these cells can be detected by hemagglutination, hemadsorption, or immunofluorescence. The virus can subsequently be typed by hemagglutination inhibition. When more rapid diagnosis is needed, viral antigens in respiratory epithelial cells can be detected by immunofluorescence.

Treatment and Prevention. Symptomatic treatment includes rest, fluids, and antipyretic agents as needed. Reye's syndrome has been associated with aspirin use in children, so acetaminophen should be administered instead to young patients.

Amantadine or rimantadine can reduce the severity of disease if administered during the first 48 hours of infection. These drugs are teratogens, so they should not be used during pregnancy.

Influenza can be prevented by administering **influenza vaccine,** preferably during the late autumn, before influenza season begins. The current vaccine contains viruses inactivated with formalin or β-propiolactone and is trivalent (A/H1N1, A/H3N2, and B). The vaccine is recommended for patients with chronic underlying diseases of the endocrine system, heart, kidneys, or lungs; residents of long-term care facilities and nursing homes; and individuals over the age of 65 years. Guillain-Barré syndrome is a rare complication of immunization, affecting 1 per 100,000 people immunized with vaccine containing A/H1N1.

Amantadine or rimantadine has been given prophylactically to individuals exposed to influenza. In some cases, these drugs have been administered to patients who are in high-risk categories and have been vaccinated but require protection against influenza during the 2-week period before immunity develops.

CLASS IV AND CLASS V RNA VIRUSES

The class IV RNA viruses consist of reoviruses, while the class V viruses consist of retroviruses. An outline of these viruses and their associated diseases is presented in Table 19–4.

Reoviruses
Classification and Structure

Members of the family **Reoviridae** are nonenveloped icosahedral viruses with nucleocapsids that are 70–80 nm in diameter. Reoviruses are unusual in that the virion consists of two concentric nucleocapsids that surround an inner core. The core contains 10–12 segments of double-stranded RNA and several enzymes needed to replicate the reovirus genome. Reoviruses are relatively resistant to heat, low pH, and proteolysis.

The first reoviruses isolated were not associated with human disease, so they were called respiratory enteric orphan ("reo") viruses. Since that time, reoviruses from three genera have been shown to be human pathogens: the genus **Coltivirus,** which includes Colorado tick fever virus and Eyach virus; the genus **Orbivirus,** which includes Kemerovo virus, an agent of meningoencephalitis in Siberia; and the genus **Rotavirus,** which includes human rotavirus, a cause of diarrhea epidemics in children. The genomes of *Coltivirus, Orbivirus,* and *Rotavirus* contain 12, 10, and 11 RNA fragments, respectively. Because of the clinical importance of Colorado tick fever virus and rotavirus, the discussion below focuses on these agents.

Characteristics of Coltiviruses

Coltiviruses have a genome of about 27 kb contained in 12 double-stranded RNA segments. Two coltiviruses—Colorado tick fever virus and Eyach virus—cause human disease by mechanisms that are not well understood. Colorado tick fever virus is unusual in that it infects human erythrocytes. The virus replicates in the bone marrow, heart, lungs, lymph nodes, and spleen, and some virions can be found in the meninges and brain. Viral replication in bone marrow may be responsible for the leukopenia that is seen during the disease, and persistence within erythrocytes may protect the viral organisms from antibody.

Diseases Due to Coltiviruses

Epidemiology. In Europe, coltiviruses are a rare cause of meningoencephalitis. In the USA, there are several hundred cases of Colorado tick fever each year, and 75% of affected patients are male adults. Colorado tick fever is found in mountainous states in the western USA, particularly California, Colorado, Idaho, Montana, Nevada, Utah, Washington, and Wyoming. The range of the virus is controlled largely by the range of its nonhuman reservoir (the golden-mantled ground squirrel) and its major vector (the tick *Dermacentor andersoni*). Most cases occur in April and May at low altitude and in June and July at higher elevations.

Diagnosis
(1) History and Physical Examination. The early manifestations of **Colorado tick fever** are generally similar to those of dengue fever. About 4 or 5 days after being bitten by an infected tick, the patient develops chills, fever, severe backache, a retrobulbar headache, nausea, and loss of appetite. The throat and conjunctivas are red, and some patients develop a petechial or macular rash. Children may develop bleeding disorders with hemorrhage or may suffer from meningitis. By the third day of disease, leukopenia and thrombocytopenia are sometimes present. The acute phase of disease usually remits after 2–3 days. In about half of the cases, however, the disease flares again after 2–3 days of remission. The recrudescent disease lasts 3–4 days, and then patients gradually recover over several weeks. Recovery confers lasting immunity, and deaths due to Colorado tick fever are extremely rare.

(2) Laboratory Analysis. Colorado tick fever virus can be detected in erythrocytes by direct immunofluorescence. Antibody to the virus can be detected in serum samples from the patient after the first week of illness, and the organisms can be isolated after inoculating blood into mice.

Treatment and Prevention. Supportive care is given as needed. There is no specific treatment for Colorado tick fever, nor is there a vaccine to prevent infection.

Characteristics of Rotaviruses

General Features. Rotaviruses were first discovered as a cause of diarrhea in 1973. Since that time, investigators have found many rotaviruses that cause diseases in animals and in humans. There are six virus serogroups, designated A through F. Most human rotaviruses are in serogroup A, but a few have been found within groups B and C.

Mechanisms of Pathogenicity. Rotaviruses are passed from person to person via the fecal-oral route. The organisms bind to receptors on mature villous epithelial cells in the intestine and are replicated within these cells. The entry of rotaviruses into the cells is facilitated by proteolytic cleavage of the capsid protein VP4. This protein produces VP5 and VP8, which are believed to serve as adhesins. Most of what is known about subsequent events has come from studies of animal models of rotavirus infection. The infection begins in the proximal small intestine and spreads caudally. The intestinal wall is thinned, and there is significant loss of chyle. The villi become stunted and shortened, and the tips of villi are denuded. Although reticulumlike cells infiltrate the lamina propria, there is no evident inflammation. It appears that the destruction of mature villous tip cells leads to carbohydrate malabsorption. Thus, the diarrhea associated with rotavirus infection is believed to be osmotic diarrhea.

Diseases Due to Rotaviruses

Epidemiology. Rotaviruses are a worldwide cause of diarrhea, usually in children between the ages of 6 and 24 months. In the USA, from 65,000 to 70,000 children are hospitalized each year with diarrhea due to rotavirus, and about 200 die. Worldwide, from 850,000 to 1,000,000 deaths each year are attributed to rotavirus infection.

In one study of children hospitalized with diarrhea, rotavirus was responsible for the diarrhea in 21% of those under 6 months old, 68% of those 6–24 months old, and 8% of those over 24 months old. In another study, 92% of neonatal rotavirus infections were found to be asymptomatic. During illness, infants shed rotaviruses for 3–7 days at a rate of about 10^{11} virions per gram of feces. Although adults in the home of an infant with rotavirus diarrhea will often become infected and shed the organisms, most infected adults are asymptomatic. Why do the majority of adults and neonates remain asymptomatic when infected with rotavirus? It appears that adults have relatively few receptors for rotaviruses on their intestinal villi, whereas neonates lack intestinal proteases. In the absence of proteases to cleave VP4, entry of the viral organisms into intestinal epithelial cells is inefficient. Circulating antibody does not protect against disease, and breast-feeding does not appear to be protective.

Diagnosis. About 1–3 days after ingesting rotaviruses, patients develop **diarrhea** and vomiting that last for 4–5 days. Disease tends to be more severe in malnourished children and those with concomitant rotavirus and *Escherichia coli* infections.

Electron microscopy of fecal samples was generally used in the past to diagnose rotavirus infections. Newer enzyme immunoassays and latex agglutination techniques are now used to identify rotaviruses in the feces. The organisms can also be isolated in MA104 (monkey kidney) or CaCo-2 (human colon carcinoma) continuous cell lines. Viral replication within these cells can be confirmed by immunofluorescence.

Treatment and Prevention. Management of children with diarrhea consists of rehydration, restoration of acid-base balances, and other supportive measures. There is no specific antiviral treatment. Several rotavirus vaccines have entered clinical trials, but none has shown great promise in preventing rotavirus disease.

Retroviruses

Because the class V viruses, retroviruses, are associated with leukemia and acquired immunodeficiency syndrome (AIDS), these viruses are discussed with the oncogenic and immunosuppressive viruses in Chapter 22.

Selected Readings

Charlton, K. M. The pathogenesis of rabies and other lyssaviral infections: recent studies. Curr Top Microbiol Immunol 187:95–119, 1994.

Coffin, J. M. Retroviral DNA integration. Dev Biol Stand 76:141–151, 1992.

Cullen, B. R. Mechanism of action of regulatory proteins encoded by complex retroviruses. Microbiol Rev 56:375–394, 1992.

Dinulos, M. B., and D. O. Matson. Recent developments with human caliciviruses. Pediatr Infect Dis J 13:998–1003, 1994.

Esolen, L. M., et al. Apoptosis as a cause of death in measles virus–infected cells. J Virol 69:3955–3958, 1995.

Garcin, D., and D. Kolakofsky. Tacaribe arenavirus RNA synthesis in vitro is primer-dependent and suggests an unusual model for the initiation of genome replication. J Virol 66:1370–1376, 1992.

Gosztonyi, G. Reproduction of lyssaviruses: ultrastructural composition of lyssaviruses and functional aspects of pathogenesis. Curr Top Microbiol Immunol 187:43–68, 1994.

Greenberg, H. B., H. F. Clark, and P. A. Offit. Rotavirus pathology and pathophysiology. Curr Top Microbiol Immunol 185:256–283, 1994.

Haseltine, W. A. Molecular biology of the human immunodeficiency virus type 1. FASEB J 5:2349–2360, 1991.

Jenison, S., et al. Characterization of human antibody responses to Four Corners hantavirus infections among patients with hantavirus pulmonary syndrome. J Virol 68:3000–3006, 1994.

Liebert, U. G., et al. Antigenic determinants of measles virus hemagglutinin associated with neurovirulence. J Virol 68:1486–1493, 1994.

Mast, E. E., and K. Krawcynski. Hepatitis E: an overview. Annu Rev Med 47:257–266, 1996.

O'Neill, R. E., and P. Palese. *Cis*-acting signals and *trans*-acting factors involved in influenza virus RNA synthesis. Infect Agents Dis 3:77–84, 1994.

Pogue, G. P., C. C. Huntley, and T. C. Hall. Common replication strategies emerging from the study of diverse groups of positive-strand RNA viruses. Arch Virol Suppl 9:181–194, 1994.

Richards, O. C., and E. Ehrenfeld. Poliovirus RNA replication. Curr Top Microbiol Immunol 161:89–119, 1990.

Robertson, S. E., et al. Yellow fever: a decade of reemergence. JAMA 276:1157–1162, 1996.

Rocaniello, V. R., and R. Ren. Poliovirus biology and pathogenesis. Curr Top Microbiol Immunol 206:305–325, 1996.

Sharara, A. I., et al. Hepatitis C. Ann Intern Med 125:658–668, 1996.

Shaw, M. W., N. H. Arden, and H. F. Maasab. New aspects of influenza viruses. Clin Microbiol Rev 5:74–92, 1992.

Shepley, M. P., and V. R. Rocaniello. A monoclonal antibody that blocks poliovirus attachment recognizes the lymphocyte homing receptor CD44. J Virol 68:1301–1308, 1994.

Tillman, M., et al. Neuroglial-specific factors and the regulation of retrovirus transcription. Adv Neuroimmunol 4:305–318, 1994.

Wimmer, E., and A. Nomoto. Molecular biology and cell-free synthesis of poliovirus. Biologicals 21:349–356, 1993.

CHAPTER TWENTY-TWO

ONCOGENIC AND

IMMUNOSUPPRESSIVE VIRUSES

Human Immunodeficiency Virus, Human T Cell Lymphotropic Virus, and Other Viruses

GENERAL PRINCIPLES OF VIRAL ONCOGENESIS

As early as 1908, investigators studying avian leukemia demonstrated that viruses could cause cancer. Many hoped that a viral etiology would be confirmed for most or all types of cancer. It has become apparent, however, that malignant lesions occur when the expression of genes which regulate cell growth or cell differentiation are altered and that viruses are merely one of many agents capable of precipitating changes in gene expression.

The cellular origins of human carcinoma, leukemia, lymphoma, and sarcoma are outlined in Table 22–1. About 15% of cases of human cancer are thought to be due to viral agents listed in Table 22–2.

Oncogenic viruses are capable of producing tumors in animals and of transforming cells in culture. The ability to transform cells is considered to be the in vitro correlate of oncogenesis. Infection of cells with oncogenic viruses does not, however, always result in transformation of the host cell. Oncogenic viruses that enter host cells may establish a latent infection with no observable effects on the host cell, may transform the cell, or may establish an infection that produces viral progeny which are released when the cell is lysed.

RNA tumor viruses transform and produce viral progeny within the same cells. In contrast, **DNA tumor viruses** produce lytic infections only in permissive cells, and they transform nonpermissive cells. These differences are reflected in real differences in how DNA and RNA viruses transform cells. The genomes of RNA tumor viruses are integrated into the host cell chromosome, where they become **proviruses.** The genomes of some DNA tumor viruses (adenoviruses, hepadnaviruses, and polyomaviruses) are integrated into the chromosome, but the genomes of others (herpesviruses and papillomaviruses) persist as episomal elements.

Eukaryotic cells contain two important sets of genes that are involved in inducing or blocking cell transformation. The first set consists of **proto-oncogenes,** and the second consists of **tumor suppressor genes.** Proto-oncogenes, which are also called **c-onc genes,** encode growth factors, growth factor receptors, intracellular signal transducers, and nuclear transcription factors, all of which allow cells to grow normally. Some retroviruses contain viral genes that are called **v-onc genes** and correspond to the c-onc genes of host cells.

Viruses can transform host cells through proto-oncogenes in several ways. First, the virus may introduce a v-onc gene that causes the cell to produce excess amounts of the oncogene product. If, for example, the v-onc gene encodes platelet-derived growth factor (PDGF), excess production of this growth factor may cause the cells to multiply without restraint. Second, the virus may integrate into the chromosome just upstream from a c-onc gene, causing the gene to no longer be subject to normal down-regulation processes. Third, the virus may cause a c-onc gene to be transposed to a new site, such as just downstream from a strong promoter. Fourth, the viral genome may contain a gene that produces a protein which trans-activates a c-onc gene. Fifth, the c-onc gene may mutate when the viral genome recombines with the host chromosome, resulting in a permanently up-regulated c-onc gene. In each of these scenarios, the net result is overproduction of the oncogene product and unrestrained cellular multiplication.

Tumor suppressor genes normally down-regulate growth and act as a balance to the positive growth signals produced by the c-onc gene products. Some viruses produce proteins that bind to and inactivate tumor suppressor genes. The net result is cell transformation and the loss of growth control.

In the final analysis, cell transformation and tumor production are multifactorial processes. Viruses

TABLE 22–1. Characteristics and Cellular Origins of Various Types of Cancer

Type	Cellular Origin
Carcinoma	A solid tumor of epithelial cell origin.
Leukemia	A cancer of circulating leukocytes.
Lymphoma	A solid tumor of leukocyte origin.
Sarcoma	A solid tumor of mesenchymal origin.

often carry multiple proto-oncogenes and may exert several types of effects on c-*onc* and tumor suppressor genes. Alterations in expression of these genes are not the only steps in tumorigenesis. For optimal growth, a tumor must be able to evade host cell defenses, be able to establish metastatic foci, become independent of host factors that regulate tissue growth, establish a blood supply adequate for survival, and avoid programmed cell death (apoptosis).

ONCOGENIC AND IMMUNOSUPPRESSIVE RETROVIRUSES

Although hepatitis C virus (see Chapter 21) has been linked epidemiologically with the development of hepatocellular carcinoma in some populations, the only RNA viruses that are known to directly cause cancers in humans are members of the family *Retroviridae.* Retroviruses have played a significant role in the development of virology. In 1966, Francis Peyton Rous was awarded a Nobel prize for his discovery in 1910 that avian sarcoma was caused by an infectious filtrable agent—an agent now called Rous sarcoma virus and known to be a retrovirus. Subsequent Nobel prizes have been awarded for the discovery of reverse transcriptase in retroviruses; the discovery that the ability of some retroviruses to cause cancers involves oncogenes; and the development of poly-

TABLE 22–2. Oncogenic and Immunosuppressive Viruses and Their Associated Diseases

Virus	Disease
RNA viruses	
Hepatitis C virus	Primary hepatocellular carcinoma.
Human immunodeficiency virus	Acquired immunodeficiency syndrome (AIDS).
Human T cell lymphotropic virus	Adult T cell leukemia or lymphoma; and tropical spastic paraparesis.
DNA viruses	
Epstein-Barr virus	Burkitt's lymphoma; nasopharyngeal carcinoma; and some non-Burkitt's B cell lymphomas.
Hepatitis B virus	Primary hepatocellular carcinoma.
Human herpesvirus 8	Kaposi's sarcoma and non-Hodgkin's lymphoma in patients with AIDS.
Human papillomaviruses	Cervical and anogenital carcinoma; and squamous cell carcinoma.

merase chain reaction (PCR) assays and other new molecular biologic techniques that followed from the discovery of reverse transcriptase.

Retroviruses are spherical enveloped viruses with a genome consisting of two copies of linear positive-sense RNA. Each virion contains the enzyme **reverse transcriptase,** which allows it to make DNA copies from the viral RNA. Thus, the flow of information is backward ("retro") because it goes from RNA to DNA and back to RNA.

The family *Retroviridae* consists of seven genera, three of which are known to be involved in human infection: *Lentivirus, Oncovirus,* and *Spumavirus.* The only lentiviruses known to be pathogenic in humans are human immunodeficiency virus types 1 and 2 (HIV-1 and HIV-2), which cause acquired immunodeficiency syndrome (AIDS). Many oncoviruses cause cancer in animals, but only human T cell lymphotropic virus type I (HTLV-I) is known to cause cancer in humans. Spumaviruses are referred to as "foamy" viruses and are seen primarily as contaminants of primary tissue cultures.

Human Immunodeficiency Virus (HIV)

Since the first report of AIDS in 1981 and the discovery of HIV in 1983, AIDS has become pandemic. In many areas of the world, it is now the number one killer of young adults.

F. Barre-Sinoussi and his colleagues who worked in the laboratory of Luc Montagnier at the Pasteur Institute were the first to report that they were able to isolate a virus that contained reverse transcriptase from a patient with persistent lymphadenopathy syndrome (LAS). At the time, it was not known that LAS was associated with AIDS. During the same year, Robert Gallo and his coworkers reported that they had isolated human T cell lymphotropic virus (HTLV) from patients with AIDS. It soon became apparent, however, that the virus isolated by Barre-Sinoussi and colleagues was not HTLV, because it killed lymphocytes. The virus isolated by workers at the Pasteur Institute was first known as lymphadenopathy-associated virus (LAV), but soon other workers isolated similar viruses from AIDS patients and called them HTLV-III and AIDS-associated retrovirus (ARV). In 1986, the International Committee on Taxonomy of Viruses determined that the viruses called LAV, HTLV-III, and ARV were the same virus, and this organism was given its present name, the human immunodeficiency virus (HIV).

Although the first clinical report of AIDS was in 1981, retrospective serologic studies have shown that sera collected in central Africa from as early as 1959 exhibited antibodies to HIV, and HIV itself has been isolated from sera collected in 1976. Some epidemiologists believe that the first cases of AIDS in Europe appeared around 1960 in individuals who had spent some time in central Africa. In some central African countries, between 20% and 30% of young adults are now infected with HIV. These observations and others have led to the widespread belief that HIV ap-

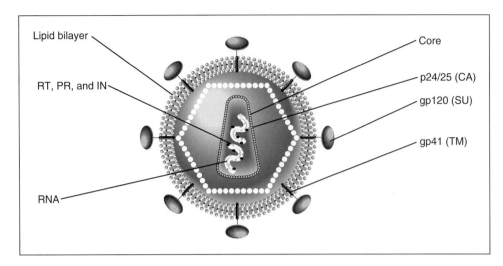

FIGURE 22–1. Structure of human immunodeficiency virus type 1 (HIV-1). The major structural proteins and the key intracellular enzymes are identified by location. RT = reverse transcriptase; PR = protease; IN = integrase; TM = transmembrane protein; SU = surface protein; and CA = core antigen.

peared first in central Africa, that it may be descended from another lentivirus known as simian immunodeficiency virus (SIV), that HIV infection spread slowly in the central African population for many years, and that changes in social structure (such as urbanization) and sexual practices have allowed the virus to spread rapidly from its remote origins.

During recent years, a second type of HIV was discovered in central Africa. The original HIV, which is responsible for most infections worldwide, was renamed HIV-1, and the newer type was called HIV-2. Additionally, at least five subtypes of HIV have been identified. These subtypes differ from one another by as much as 30–35% in the sequences of their *gag* and *env* genes.

Characteristics of HIV

General Features. The general structure and genome of HIV are depicted in Figs. 22–1 and 22–2, and the key viral proteins are listed in Table 22–3.

HIV is an enveloped virus that is 80–100 nm in diameter. Inside the viral core is an RNA-nucleoprotein complex that contains a diploid copy of positive-sense single-stranded RNA. Each RNA strand is 9.2 kb

long and encodes nine proteins. A molecule of cellular transfer RNA (tRNA) is base-paired to a site near the 5′ end of each RNA strand, and each strand contains a 3′ polyadenylated tail and a 5′ cap. Three structural genes are found in the HIV genome: the ***gag* gene,** which encodes the core proteins of the virus; the ***pol* gene,** which encodes reverse transcriptase; and the ***env* gene,** which encodes the envelope peplomer proteins. Because the products of these genes are modified by proteolytic cleavage, the three genes are used to produce at least eight separate structural proteins and enzymes.

The core contains three key enzymes: **reverse transcriptase, protease,** and **integrase.** These are all enclosed within a cone-shaped capsid that is constructed from the p24/25 capsid protein, which is a *gag* gene cleavage product. A second *gag* cleavage product known as p16/17 serves as the matrix protein.

The viral envelope surrounds the matrix protein and core of the HIV virion. The envelope contains several key glycoproteins that promote entry of the virus into host target cells. The most important of these are gp120, which serves as the primary adhesin for cellular receptors, and gp41, which makes it possible for the viral envelope to fuse with host cell

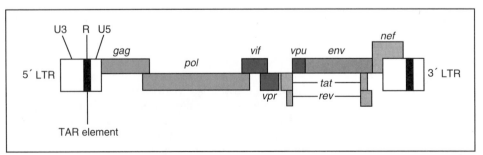

FIGURE 22–2. Organization of the genome of human immunodeficiency virus type 1 (HIV-1). LTR = long terminal repeat; and TAR = *trans*-activating response. The characteristics and functions of genes and gene products are described in Table 22–3. (Source: Greene, W. C. The molecular biology of human immunodeficiency virus type 1 infection. N Engl J Med 324:308–317, Copyright 1991, Massachusetts Medical Society. Redrawn and reprinted by permission of The New England Journal of Medicine.)

TABLE 22–3.   Genes and Gene Products of the Human Immunodeficiency Virus (HIV)*

Gene	Protein	Gene Product Designation[†]	Function
Structural genes			
gag	CA (core antigen)	p24/25	Capsid structural protein.
	MA (matrix)	p16/17	Myristilated matrix protein.
	NC (nucleocapsid)	p9	RNA binding protein.
		p6	RNA binding protein; assists in viral budding.
pol	RT (reverse transcriptase)	p66/51	RNA-dependent DNA polymerase and RNase H.
	PR (protease)	p15	Processes viral proteins by cleaving them after translation.
	IN (integrase)	p32	Integrates viral cDNA into host genome.
env	SU (surface protein)	gp120	Adheres to cellular receptors.
	TM (transmembrane)	gp41	Fuses with target cell membrane.
Regulatory genes			
tat	Tat	p14	Causes gene *trans*-activation.
rev	Rev	p19	Regulates viral rRNA expression.
nef	Nef	p27	Down-regulates CD4 and interleukin-2 expression.
vpr	Vpr	p18	Causes gene *trans*-activation (weak *trans*-activator).
Accessory genes			
vif	Vif	p23	Assists in viral infectivity.
vpu	Vpu	p15	Helps with viral release from host cells.

* Not listed in this table are gp160, p63/55, and p40, which are precursor proteins or intermediate cleavage products.
† The number indicates the approximate molecular weight in kilodaltons.

membranes. The envelope also contains several host proteins, including class I and class II major histocompatibility proteins.

Replication of HIV. The replication scheme of retroviruses is described in Chapter 21 and shown in Fig. 21–6. Briefly, the viral RNA genome is copied by the reverse transcriptase to produce complementary provirus DNA, which then migrates to the nucleus, where it is integrated into the chromosome. Unless the cell is activated, the provirus remains latent. This is because RNA polymerase II, which is needed to produce viral mRNA, is active only within replicating cells.

A variety of cytokines, monokines, and viral *trans*-activating proteins can cause HIV replication to begin. Examples of agents that activate HIV replication are interferon-gamma (IFN-γ), granulocyte-macrophage colony-stimulating factor (GM-CSF), two tumor necrosis factors (TNF-α and TNF-β), and three interleukins (IL-3, IL-4, and IL-6). Inducing agents cause transcription factors, such as NF-κB, to be released from their cellular inhibitors. When NF-κB is released from IκB, it migrates to the nucleus, where it initiates HIV replication by binding to κB enhancer elements within the HIV long terminal repeat (LTR) section. The integrated genome is read to produce three major classes of mRNA (9.2 kb, 4.5 kb, and 2 kb), and variations in RNA splicing produce additional RNA species.

The replication of HIV is controlled in part by expression of three key HIV regulatory proteins, known as Tat, Rev, and Nef. **Tat** is a *trans*-activating protein that binds to the *trans*-activating response (TAR) region found within the LTR segment and near the 5′ ends of all HIV RNA transcripts. Tat prevents premature termination of transcription and causes a thousandfold increase in the efficiency of transcription of the HIV promoter. **Rev** is a phosphoprotein that binds to the *env* gene in the 9.2-kb and 4.5-kb RNA transcripts and allows them to migrate into the cell cytoplasm, where they will be translated. **Nef** is a myristilated protein that appears to be essential for replication of HIV within macrophages and monocytes. Its most important effects may be related to its ability to down-regulate the expression of CD4 and IL-2 by these cells.

Mechanisms of Pathogenesis. Cells that express the CD4 antigen are the primary targets of HIV. Thus, helper T cells and cells of the monocyte-macrophage lineage are most often infected by HIV. Some HIV strains preferentially infect T cells, and others primarily infect macrophages and monocytes. The infection cycle begins when the virus attaches to the CD4 molecule via the envelope glycoprotein gp120. HIV strains that are tropic for T cells require the chemokine receptor known as CXCR5 (formerly known as fusin) as a coreceptor, while HIV strains that infect macrophages and monocytes use the chemokine receptor CCR5 (also known as CC-CCR5) as a coreceptor. CXCR5 is the natural receptor for chemoattractant stromal cell–derived factor, while CCR5 recognizes two macrophage inflammatory proteins (MIP-1α and MIP-1β) and RANTES (the term is an acronym for "regulated on activation normal T cells expressed and secreted"). Other members of the CC family of chemokine receptors have also been shown on occasion to serve as coreceptors for HIV. In addition, it appears that CXCR4 can serve as the primary receptor for HIV-2.

CD26 has been shown to cleave the V3 loop of gp120 to expose the fusogenic domain of gp41. Once gp41 is available to a yet-unidentified cell surface structure, the viral membrane fuses with the host cell membrane, and the core is liberated into the cytoplasm. There are, however, other means by which HIV enters host cells. Studies have indicated that HIV enters several CD4$^-$ cells in vivo, including bowel and renal epithelial cells, brain astrocytes, and brain oligodendrocytes. Moreover, studies using in vitro models have demonstrated that galactosylceramide, Fc receptors, and complement receptors act as HIV receptors in some CD4$^-$ cells. Nonneutralizing antibody promotes the entry of HIV into CD4$^-$ cells by acting as a bridge between HIV and Fc receptors in a process known as antibody-dependent enhancement.

The major feature of AIDS is the loss of immune responsiveness, and the hallmark of the disease is the depletion of circulating CD4$^+$ T lymphocytes. When circulating CD4$^+$ T cell counts dip to below 400 cells per microliter, patients become immunodepressed and are susceptible to a wide variety of opportunistic infections, many of which are rare in individuals with normally functioning immune systems. Patients also often suffer from neurologic disease that is subcortical initially but eventually leads to severe mental deterioration. Many patients develop diarrhea that cannot be attributed to normal gastrointestinal pathogens. This condition may lead to severe malabsorption and wasting that can be fatal. Thus, the pathogenesis of HIV disease is complex, and an explanation of how HIV causes disease must account for a wide variety of clinical conditions that occur during AIDS.

(1) The HIV Infection Cycle. HIV is transmitted via body fluids that contain infected cells, usually semen or blood. When sexually transmitted, the virus probably multiplies first within tissue macrophages and submucosal lymphocytes in the genital tract or rectum. The organisms soon travel to the draining lymph nodes, where they are again replicated. From 2 to 4 weeks after infection, the patient may suffer from symptoms that are similar to those of mononucleosis. At this time, HIV infection may be detected by the presence of virus in the blood and decreased CD4$^+$ T cell counts. The viremia and symptoms both decline in about 1 month as a result of antibody and cellular immune processes. A period of clinical latency begins and may last 5–10 years. During this period, the virus is produced by only a tiny fraction of circulating T cells, although many HIV-infected CD4$^+$ T cells can be found within lymph nodes. Eventually, viral replication is activated, CD4$^+$ T cells are depleted, and the patient becomes immunosuppressed.

(2) HIV Infection and the Origin of Immunosuppression. Two of the most pressing questions about the pathogenesis of HIV infection concern how CD4$^+$ cells are depleted and what factors are responsible for immunosuppression.

The depletion of CD4$^+$ cells has been attributed to a variety of direct and indirect mechanisms. HIV replication has been shown to be directly cytolytic in T cells and macrophages, and new cells can be infected directly by the formation of syncytia between infected and uninfected cells. Infected cells can also be destroyed by immune processes that are directed against HIV and include cytotoxic T lymphocyte–mediated cytolysis, antibody-dependent cellular cytotoxicity (ADCC), antibody-mediated lysis, and complement-mediated lysis. Moreover, in vitro studies have shown that HIV gp120 can induce apoptosis by cross-linking CD4 molecules.

There is some evidence that HIV may infect stem cells. This would make it difficult for the body to replace T cells that have been destroyed by the virus. Stem cell destruction may also be responsible for the presence of pancytopenia in many patients with AIDS. At least two other factors may be involved in the immunosuppressive effects of HIV. First, at least during the early phases of HIV infection, it appears that memory T cells are preferentially destroyed by HIV. Second, during the late phases of infection, the differentiation of Th0 cells to Th1 and Th2 cells becomes dysregulated. Th1 cells are responsible for delayed-type hypersensitivity responses, while Th2 cells secrete cytokines that assist in the production of antibody. During the late phases of HIV infection, there is a profound loss of Th1 cells. Shortly thereafter, the CD4$^+$ T cell count drops precipitously, and the patient develops clinically apparent AIDS.

(3) HIV Infection and Neurologic Disease. The origin of neurologic disease in patients with AIDS is another topic of considerable concern. In studies using simian immunodeficiency virus, investigators have shown that lentiviruses cross the blood-brain barrier by passing through the fenestrae of endothelial cells. It appears that certain HIV strains are neurotropic and are more likely to cause neurologic disease than are the so-called nonneurotropic strains. Once the neurotropic organisms invade the central nervous system, they infect glial cells (astrocytes and oligodendrocytes) and neurons. The invasion of these cells is probably facilitated by interactions between gp120 and CD4, since glial cells and neurons can express CD4. However, it appears that CD4$^-$ cells are also infected and that galactosylceramide is probably the receptor for HIV in these cells.

Investigators have suggested three mechanisms to explain neurologic disease in HIV patients: HIV infection alters cytokine production by infected cells; HIV or its products damage neurons; and HIV infection elicits autoantibodies.

First, the ability of HIV-infected cells to produce certain cytokines appears to be altered significantly. For example, increased levels of quinolinic acid, an excitotoxin that is probably produced by macrophages and microglial cells, have been found in the cerebrospinal fluid of HIV-infected patients with neurologic disease. HIV-infected monocytes have also been reported to produce increased amounts of transforming growth factor beta (TGF-β). TGF-β induces the production of TNF-α, and increased levels of this factor have been linked to disorders of the central nervous system. TNF-α has also been shown to destroy rodent neuronal cells and human brain cells in vitro.

Second, some HIV proteins have been shown to be toxic to neurons. For example, gp120 causes damage to cultured brain cells, possibly by altering membrane permeability to calcium and by activating tyrosine kinase. An HIV membrane epitope known as peptide T competes for receptors with several neurotropic factors that are needed by the nerve cells to grow, maintain function, and communicate with one another. Tat and gp41 are also neurotoxic and may act by altering membrane conduction.

Third, antibody directed against myelin basic protein has been detected in HIV-infected patients with dementia, and the levels of this antibody have tended to correlate with the severity of dementia seen.

(4) HIV Infection and Gastrointestinal Disease. The origin of gastrointestinal disease and wasting in patients with AIDS is not well understood. In the lamina propria, HIV can multiply within macrophages. In the bowel mucosa, the organisms can also multiply within enterochromaffin cells, the cells responsible for normal bowel motility and function.

Diseases Due to HIV

Epidemiology. Worldwide, at least 14 million individuals are currently infected with HIV, and an estimated 5000 new infections occur each day. About 70% of all HIV-infected individuals live in sub-Saharan Africa, and about 15% live in southern and southeastern Asia.

HIV is spread by three principal routes: via homosexual and heterosexual intercourse, via contact with blood and blood products, and via perinatal transmission from mother to infant. In each case, the viral organisms are transmitted within body fluids that contain HIV-infected cells.

Sexual intercourse is the most common route of spread, accounting for about 80% of all HIV infections. Semen contains about 10^6 leukocytes per ejaculate, and between 0.01% and 5% of these leukocytes contain organisms in HIV-infected men. Semen is an excellent vehicle for transmission of HIV because it contains factors that seem to increase cell-to-cell contact. If an HIV-infected man also has a sexually transmitted disease (STD) such as gonorrhea, syphilis, or chancroid, the number of leukocytes in the semen will be elevated and the risk of transmitting HIV will be concomitantly increased. If the nonpenetrating partner has lesions of STD on the genitourinary mucosa, the risk of acquiring HIV infection is also greatly increased. Although the squamous and columnar epithelia of the vaginal tract are naturally resistant to infection by HIV, the presence of open lesions on the mucosa removes this barrier to infection.

In sub-Saharan Africa, where heterosexual intercourse is the primary mode of HIV transmission, the prevalence of STD is thought to contribute significantly to heterosexual spread of HIV. In the USA, homosexual intercourse is the most common mode

of sexual transmission of HIV. Overall, the risk of acquiring HIV from a penetrating sexual partner is about 0.1% per episode of vaginal intercourse and 1% per episode of anal intercourse. The presence of an STD increases the risk of each by 10-fold. The risk of transmitting HIV from female to male during intercourse is about one-half the risk of passing the virus from male to female.

The second most common route of HIV transmission is via blood or blood products. This may occur during blood transfusions, during administration of blood products to hemophiliacs, or when syringes and needles are used by more than one person. From 3% to 5% of patients with AIDS have acquired their infections from tainted blood in a blood transfusion. Methods now used to screen blood have reduced the risk in the USA to 1 in 225,000 units of blood transfused. In hemophiliacs receiving factors VIII and IX, the practice of heating these blood products has virtually eliminated the risk of HIV infection. Thus, the major risk from blood is now via practices that involve the use of nonsterile needles and syringes.

In the USA, 5–10% of HIV infections are attributed to the sharing of needles and other paraphernalia by intravenous drug users. The transmission of HIV is increased by the practice of flushing blood back into the syringe (a practice known as "booting") to use all of the drug. In some countries where medical supplies are limited, HIV probably has been transmitted when medical personnel reuse needles and syringes in the care of multiple patients. HIV is also occasionally transmitted when medical personnel accidentally stick themselves with a needle that has been used to draw blood from an HIV-infected patient. The risk of HIV transmission via needle stick is about 1 per 300 episodes.

Blood transmits HIV because blood contains HIV-infected CD4$^+$ cells. Blood samples from asymptomatic HIV-infected individuals have been shown to contain about 5000 infected cells per milliliter, while blood samples from patients with AIDS may contain up to 500,000 infected cells per milliliter. Blood also contains free virions, but most of these are noninfectious.

The third major route of HIV transmission is perinatal transmission. Various studies have shown that between 11% and 60% of infants born to HIV-positive women are themselves HIV-infected. Most are probably infected during or just after birth via contact with amniotic fluid, blood, or genital secretions. In some cases, HIV has been transmitted to the fetus transplacentally or to the infant via breast-feeding. Factors that increase the risk for perinatal transmission include advanced or severe disease in the mother, low titers of HIV-neutralizing maternal antibody, and premature delivery.

Diagnosis
(1) History and Physical Examination. About 7% of individuals infected with HIV admit to no history of high-risk activity, and a few patients have been infected under unusual circumstances. Most of those

whose infections are not adequately accounted for have merely been interviewed inadequately.

(a) HIV Seroconversion Illness. Two to four weeks after being infected with HIV, about 50% of patients develop a fever and experience a mononucleosislike illness that lasts 1–4 weeks. Manifestations may include night sweats, arthralgia, depression, diarrhea, generalized lymphadenopathy, malaise, mucocutaneous ulceration, myalgia, sore throat, lethargy, and a rash on the trunk. Some patients with seroconversion illness experience signs of encephalitis or mild meningitis and may present with complaints of headache, photophobia, and retro-orbital pain. The symptoms and signs resolve when the patients develop antibodies to HIV.

(b) HIV Latency. About 50% of individuals who are infected with HIV do not experience seroconversion illness. These individuals and the patients who have recovered from seroconversion illness enter a prolonged period of latency that may last 5–10 years. During this time, HIV organisms can be found within circulating lymphocytes and lymphoid tissue, and the patient can pass the organisms to others through blood and semen. Lymphadenopathy in the axillas and groin may wax and wane, and mild splenomegaly may be noted. Patients nearing the end of latency may develop **progressive generalized lymphadenopathy** (PGL), which is also called **lymphadenopathy syndrome** (LAS) and is often accompanied by signs of autoimmune disorders such as Guillain-Barré syndrome, idiopathic thrombocytopenia, Reiter's syndrome, and Sjögren's syndrome.

(c) Symptomatic HIV Infection and AIDS. The extensive activation of viral replication within CD4+ cells initiates a drop in circulating CD4+ T cell counts and begins the downward spiral toward AIDS and death. When peripheral CD4+ T cell counts drop below 400 cells per microliter, the patient experiences a gradual onset of symptoms that are sometimes referred to as the **AIDS-related complex** (ARC). ARC does not have a precise clinical definition but is generally described as the clinical complex of diarrhea, fever, night sweats, oral candidiasis, and weight loss. Patients with ARC usually acquire relatively mild opportunistic infections at this time, but both the severity and the frequency of infections increase as CD4+ T cell counts decrease. The relationship between cell counts and the progression of HIV infection is depicted in Fig. 22–3.

AIDS is considered to begin when the patient becomes severely immunosuppressed, usually coinciding with CD4+ counts of 200 or below. At this time, the tempo of the disease increases dramatically, and peripheral CD4+ counts drop rapidly. The most commonly seen AIDS-associated infection is interstitial cell pneumonia caused by the parasite *Pneumocystis carinii*. Other AIDS-associated infections include bacillary angiomatosis and peliosis hepatis due to *Bartonella (Rochalimaea) henselae* and *Bartonella (Rochalimaea) quintana;* enteritis due to *Cryptosporidium;* encephalitis, enteritis, and retinitis due to cytomegalovirus; interstitial pneumonitis due to Epstein-Barr virus; systemic infections due to *Mycobacterium avium-intracellulare;* and encephalitis due to *Cryptococcus neoformans,* JC virus, and *Toxoplasma gondii.*

Patients with AIDS may also suffer from peripheral neuropathy and various forms of cancer, including Kaposi's sarcoma, non-Hodgkin's lymphoma, and papillomavirus-associated genital cancer. Kaposi's sarcoma was once an indolent skin cancer seen almost exclusively in elderly individuals of Mediterranean descent. In the early 1980s, the AIDS epidemic was heralded by the sudden appearance of an aggressive form of Kaposi's sarcoma in homosexual men with lymphadenopathy syndrome. Recent studies using polymerase chain reaction technology have shown that Kaposi's sarcoma and non-Hodgkin's lymphoma in AIDS patients are likely due to a newly identified herpesvirus known as human herpesvirus 8 (HHV-8) or Kaposi's sarcoma–associated herpesvirus (KSHV). This type of herpesvirus appears to be spread principally via anal intercourse.

About half of AIDS patients develop severe dementia during the final months of life. AIDS-associated neurologic disease begins as encephalopathy, motor dysfunction, and myelopathy. Affected patients find it difficult to concentrate or remember, and they suffer from tremor and a loss of balance that resembles Parkinson's disease. Radiographs show atrophy of the cerebrum and widening of the sulci. AIDS-associated dementia may be exacerbated by neurologic disorders such as progressive multifocal leukoencephalopathy.

Perhaps the most devastating condition associated with AIDS is inexorable wasting accompanied by diarrhea. This condition occurs when no gastrointestinal pathogens can be detected but is thought to be due to the presence of HIV in the gastrointestinal tract. As the condition progresses, there is a gradual drop in albumin and transferrin levels and an increase in nausea and anorexia. Death generally occurs when the patient's weight reaches 60–70% of ideal body weight.

(2) Laboratory Analysis
(a) HIV Seroconversion Illness. In patients with acute seroconversion illness, a temporary reduction in circulating CD4+ and CD8+ T cell counts is followed by CD8+ lymphocytosis. HIV can be found in body fluids, including blood and cerebrospinal fluid. Because patients have no antibodies to HIV at this time, confirmation of HIV infection is based on methods that do not identify antibodies. Polymerase chain reaction (PCR) assays identify viral nucleic acid in peripheral blood leukocytes and are the simplest, fastest, and most sensitive tests to demonstrate HIV directly. Some PCR assays can estimate total viral load and can distinguish between HIV-1 and HIV-2. When PCR is not available, an enzyme immunoassay (EIA) can be used to detect the presence of circulating HIV p24/25 (core antigen), or the virus can be cultivated in mitogen-activated peripheral blood leukocytes from a donor who is HIV-negative. HIV seroconversion illness generally ends when antibodies to

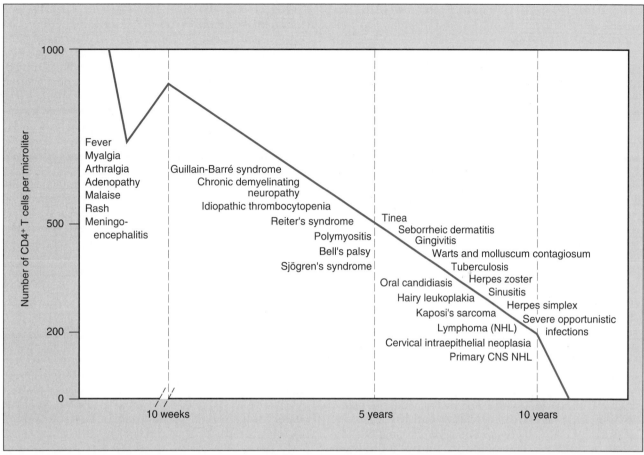

FIGURE 22–3. Relationship between CD4+ T cell counts and the progression of human immunodeficiency virus (HIV) infection. NHL = non-Hodgkin's lymphoma; and CNS = central nervous system. Severe opportunistic infections include infections with *Bartonella* (*Rochalimaea*), *Cryptococcus, Cryptosporidium, Listeria, Mycobacterium avium-intracellulare, Nocardia, Pneumocystis, Toxoplasma,* cytomegalovirus, Epstein-Barr virus, and JC virus. (Source: Stewart, G. J. The challenge: clinical diagnosis of HIV. MJA 1993;158:31–34. © Copyright 1993, The Medical Journal of Australia. Redrawn and reproduced with permission.)

HIV appear in the blood and circulating viral counts diminish radically.

(b) HIV Latency. Antibodies to HIV usually appear within about 1 month of infection but may appear as late as 3 months. The standard method to screen patients at this time is an EIA that uses recombinant HIV antigens to capture antibodies. When a serum sample yields positive results in the EIA, the same sample is retested once or twice by the same method. About 0.1% of positive results in the EIA for HIV infection are false-positive results. For this reason, samples from all patients with positive results in the EIA must be tested for HIV using a second, more sensitive test called the Western blot test. The rate of false-positive results in this test is about 1 per 100,000 samples tested. Based on the World Health Organization guidelines, the results of a Western blot test can be considered positive only if the sample is found to contain antibodies against the following: at least two envelope proteins (gp41, gp120, or gp160); one envelope protein and at least one Gag protein (p16/17, p24/25, p40, or p63/55); or one envelope protein and one Pol protein (p32, p51, or p66). If results are equivocal, the test must be repeated.

(c) Symptomatic HIV Infection and AIDS. Patients with symptomatic HIV infection exhibit CD4+ T cell counts of 400 cells per microliter and below. Patients with AIDS exhibit CD4+ T cell counts under 200. The virus can be detected in body fluids by PCR, and antibodies can be detected by EIA and Western blot tests. The reappearance of p24/25 antigen in the blood is associated with a poor prognosis because it indicates that HIV organisms are overcoming the immune response.

Treatment and Prognosis. A small percentage of patients develop AIDS during the first 2 years of infection, and about 5% of those who are HIV-positive develop AIDS in each succeeding year. Once an AIDS-defining condition begins, the median survival time is about 20 months. In many cases, death is not due directly to the effects of HIV but occurs as a consequence of overwhelming opportunistic infections. Thus, there are two goals of treatment: to decrease the virus burden by use of antiviral drugs and to prevent or promptly treat opportunistic infections.

The first line of attack against HIV continues to be the dideoxynucleoside analogues that inhibit reverse transcriptase, but the armamentarium has been expanded with the introduction of nonnucleoside reverse transcriptase inhibitors and protease inhibitors (see Chapter 19).

The oldest and most widely used dideoxynucleoside analogue is zidovudine (azidothymidine, or AZT). When used alone, AZT reduces the incidence and severity of opportunistic infections, but it does not appear to halt the progress of AIDS. The effectiveness of AZT monotherapy is also limited by the infidelity of reverse transcription, which rapidly produces mutants resistant to the action of AZT. Clinical studies have shown that half of patients who have severe HIV infection and are treated with AZT for 6 months harbor virus strains that are 10 times more resistant to AZT than were the original strains. In contrast, patients who are asymptomatic and are treated with AZT require about 2 years of therapy to develop the same level of resistance. The response to data derived from these and other studies has been to recommend that most patients initially receive combination therapy with AZT plus didanosine or with AZT plus zalcitabine. Trials are under way to evaluate regimens that include lamivudine and stavudine.

For patients who cannot tolerate AZT, didanosine monotherapy has proved to be an acceptable alternative. A protease inhibitor can be added to the regimen for patients who are at high risk of rapid disease progression. This includes patients with rapidly falling CD4$^+$ cell counts and rapidly rising plasma levels of HIV RNA. Indinavir appears to be the best-tolerated protease inhibitor and has shown good potency. Other protease inhibitors now available include saquinavir and ritonavir.

Combination therapy should be initiated in HIV-positive patients with CD4$^+$ T cell counts under 500 cells per microliter or CD4$^+$ percentages under 25. Some experts suggest delaying therapy in patients with CD4$^+$ T cell counts between 350 and 500 cells per microliter until plasma levels of HIV RNA reach at least 5000–10,000 HIV RNA copies per milliliter. Antiviral therapy should be halted when CD4$^+$ T cell counts drop below 50 cells per microliter.

A complete discussion of drugs to prevent and treat opportunistic infections is beyond the scope of this chapter. However, one of the most important advances in the management of HIV-infected patients has been the success in preventing and treating interstitial cell pneumonia caused by *P. carinii.* Trimethoprim-sulfamethoxazole (TMP/SMX) is generally indicated to prevent pneumonia in patients who have ARC and a CD4$^+$ T cell count under 300, as well as in patients with a CD4$^+$ T cell count under 200. TMP/SMX also prevents opportunistic infections with *Listeria, Nocardia,* and *Toxoplasma.* If TMP/SMX cannot be used, aerosolized pentamidine can be substituted and offers good protection against pneumonia caused by *Pneumocystis.*

Plasma levels of HIV RNA are measured to track the efficacy of antiretroviral treatments. Levels should be determined 3–4 weeks after initiating therapy and then every 3–6 months. A drop of at least 0.5 log$_{10}$ in the HIV RNA titer must be seen for any treatment regimen to be considered effective. The CD4$^+$ T cell count is determined at the same time as the plasma HIV RNA level and can be used as a prognostic indicator. The median survival time is about 3 years for patients with a CD4$^+$ count of around 200. Those whose counts drop to 50 generally die within a year.

Prevention. Unfortunately, there is no vaccine to prevent HIV infection, and there are numerous problems in developing one. First, the mutation rate of HIV is high, and any vaccine must be effective against all of the major HIV antigenic variants. Because of the poor fidelity of reverse transcription, new variants are continually appearing. Second, vaccines are effective against viruses that enter the body as free organisms. HIV enters its victims within host cells. Some infected host cells contain replicating HIV and exhibit HIV antigens on their surface, but many more contain latent HIV organisms that express no surface antigen. The latter cells would be missed by immune responses against the virus. HIV can also spread from cell to cell via formation of syncytia, a process that protects the viruses from antibody. Thus, any HIV vaccine developed is more likely to be a tool in reducing virus burden, rather than an effective measure for preventing infection.

In the absence of an effective HIV vaccine, the current approach to prevention of HIV infection is twofold: to ensure that medical facilities screen all body fluids and tissues intended for transfusion or transplantation and to encourage individuals to change high-risk behavior.

Several measures are recommended to reduce sexual transmission of disease. Individuals should limit the number of sexual partners. Persons who have multiple sexual partners should use condoms. This is especially important among those practicing anal sex. All forms of STD (syphilis, gonorrhea, and so forth) should be treated immediately. This reduces the rate of transmission of HIV infection from the infected partner and also reduces the degree of susceptibility to HIV infection.

The spread of HIV infection among intravenous drug users can be reduced if the practice of sharing needles and syringes is avoided. Educational programs have not been very effective. In some countries, intravenous drug users are registered and are provided free disposable syringes and needles.

Health care professionals and laboratory workers must dispose of needles properly and practice other universal precautions to prevent the spread of HIV and other infections. Medical personnel who test positive for HIV should not continue to perform invasive procedures on patients.

Persons who are at high risk of HIV infection should voluntarily be tested for HIV, especially if they have had unusual opportunistic infections. Individuals who test positive for HIV should receive counseling to help them determine what precautions they should take to reduce the risk of passing HIV to intimate contacts.

Human T Cell Lymphotropic Virus (HTLV)

Human T cell lymphotropic (or leukemia) virus types I and II are so-called C type viruses that infect CD4$^+$ cells of humans. HTLV-I infection is associated with the occurrence of two rare human diseases: adult T cell leukemia or lymphoma (ATLL) and tropical spastic paraparesis. HTLV-II does not routinely cause disease but may be associated with hairy cell leukemia.

Characteristics of HTLV

Although many retroviruses contain oncogenes, HTLV-I does not. Instead, HTLV produces two regulatory genes that influence the generation of leukemia.

The first regulatory gene, called *tax,* encodes a protein (Tax) that is a *trans*-activator both of viral genes and of host cell genes. Tax interacts with enhancer sequences on the host chromosomes and causes the synthesis of IL-2 and the IL-2 receptor to be increased. The promotion of this autocrine loop causes infected T cells to proliferate. Tax also upregulates the expression of two cellular oncogenes, *fos* and PDGF. Together, these processes are believed to start the infected cell along a path that ends with the development of leukemia.

The second regulatory gene, called *rex,* encodes a protein (Rex) that regulates the splicing of mRNA and promotes the production of viral progeny. Rex inhibits the production of itself and Tax because it promotes the export (to the cytoplasm) of unspliced RNA, and spliced RNA fragments are needed to produce Rex and Tax. Thus, Rex may cause the virus to undergo latency and productive cycles.

Diseases Due to HTLV

Epidemiology. HTLV-I is most prevalent in tropical countries, but it is found worldwide. The areas of greatest endemicity are in equatorial Africa, the Caribbean, southern Japan, Papua New Guinea, Siberia, and parts of South America.

HTLV-I is spread by three principal routes: via transmission from mother to infant, via sexual intercourse, and via contact with blood. In most countries of high endemicity, transmission of infection from mother to infant appears to be the most prevalent mode of spread and may occur perinatally or via breast-feeding. If the virus is transmitted to sexual partners, it is usually passed from male to female rather than the other direction. In Western industrialized countries, HTLV is primarily an infection of intravenous drug users. In the USA, about 5% of drug users are infected with HTLV. In most cases, the agent is HTLV-II, whose association with human disease is not well established.

Diagnosis

(1) History and Physical Examination

(a) Adult T Cell Leukemia or Lymphoma. ATLL begins 20–40 years after infection with HTLV-I and occurs in only a tiny proportion (1–4%) of those infected. Most patients are between 30 and 50 years of age. Bone lesions, hepatosplenomegaly, hypercalcemia, and lymphadenopathy are common manifestations, and leukemic cell infiltrates in the skin are sometimes seen. Patients are immunosuppressed and tend to develop opportunistic infections. Most die within a year of the onset of disease, but some patients experience a chronic course of disease that resembles non-Hodgkin's lymphoma.

(b) Tropical Spastic Paraparesis. Tropical spastic paraparesis is a progressive demyelinating disease that occurs most often in women between 20 and 50 years of age. The long motor neuron tracts in the spinal cord are affected. Patients initially suffer from lumbar pain that radiates down the legs. This progresses to weakness of the lower limbs and urinary incontinence. Patients may also suffer from dysesthesia and visual changes. Although tropical spastic paraparesis resembles multiple sclerosis in many ways, it does not remit.

(2) Laboratory Analysis. Patients with suspected HTLV infection can be tested with an enzyme immunoassay using genetically cloned HTLV antigens. Positive results must be confirmed by Western blot tests for HTLV-I and HTLV-II antigens. Viral nucleic acid in lymphocytes can be detected with a combination of polymerase chain reaction and Southern blot tests. Viral culture is difficult and is not routinely practiced.

On histologic examination of specimens from patients with ATLL, circulating CD4$^+$ leukemic cells are found to have a characteristic pleomorphic lobular appearance and have large, convoluted nuclei.

Treatment and Prognosis. ATLL is a fatal disease. Although current treatment consists of managing opportunistic infections, various antiviral agents are being tested for efficacy. In some patients, combined treatment with interferon alfa and zidovudine has been effective. At least one group has reported success in treating ATLL with monoclonal antibody directed against IL-2 receptors.

Prevention. Measures taken to prevent HIV infection (see above) will also prevent HTLV infection.

ONCOGENIC HEPADNAVIRUSES

Hepatitis B virus (HBV), a DNA virus discussed in detail in Chapter 20, is associated with a high risk of **primary hepatocellular carcinoma.** About 250,000 new cases of hepatocellular carcinoma are identified worldwide each year, and the locales of highest incidence correspond with the areas of highest incidence of hepatitis B and hepatitis C. Of the two viral agents, HBV is considered to be the most common cause of hepatocellular carcinoma. In one study of 22,000 men, carriers of hepatitis B surface antigen (HBsAg) were found to be more than 200 times as likely as noncarriers to develop hepatocellular carcinoma, and more than half of the carriers died of carcinoma or cirrhosis. In over 80% of patients with hepatocellular carcinoma, a portion of the HBV genome can be found integrated into the host cell genome.

The means by which HBV produces hepatocellular carcinoma are poorly understood. Truncated segments of the HBV genome are integrated into the host genome 20–50 years before carcinoma becomes clinically apparent. At least some of these segments contain a *trans*-activating protein encoded by the X gene. Based on results in studies of nonhuman hepadnaviruses, investigators have hypothesized that this gene *trans*-activator deregulates expression of nearby cellular oncogenes by activating protein kinase C.

When possible, hepatocellular carcinoma is treated by surgically resecting the diseased portion of the liver. Many patients have received liver transplants, but recurrence of carcinoma in these patients is not uncommon. A variety of other treatments, such as transcatheter arterial embolization, ultrasound-guided percutaneous ethanol injection, and chemotherapy, have been used when surgery is not possible. The survival rate depends on the stage of the cancer when discovered, the condition of the uninfected portion of the liver, the site of the tumor, and whether metastasis has occurred. The prognosis is poor if disease is advanced or inoperable.

ONCOGENIC HERPESVIRUSES

Epstein-Barr virus (EBV) has been associated with the development of three human cancers: Burkitt's lymphoma, nasopharyngeal carcinoma, and some non-Burkitt's B cell lymphomas. Because the links between EBV and the first two types of cancer are the best demonstrated, this section focuses on these cancers.

Human herpesvirus 8 (HHV-8) is a newly discovered herpesvirus that is found within the cells of Kaposi's sarcoma and non-Hodgkin's lymphoma in patients with AIDS.

Epstein-Barr Virus and Burkitt's Lymphoma

As described in Chapter 20, EBV is a herpesvirus that infects human B lymphocytes. In most parts of the world, infected individuals develop infectious mononucleosis. Burkitt's lymphoma is a B cell lymphoma that occurs mainly in western Africa and Papua New Guinea. EBV has been associated with the African form of the disease, but a strong correlation has not been found with the Papua New Guinea form. In western Africa, Burkitt's lymphoma occurs in tropical areas below 1500 m of elevation, where falciparum malaria is endemic.

Although a direct causal relationship between EBV and Burkitt's lymphoma has not been established, it has been shown that each lymphoma cell in affected patients contains multiple episomal copies of the EBV genome, appearing as closed circles. These cells produce Epstein-Barr nuclear antigen 1 (EBNA-1), and many express other antigens (EA, VCA, and MA antigens). However, they do not express EBNA-2 and latent membrane protein (LMP), the two antigens that are usually recognized by anti-EBV cytotoxic T lymphocytes (CTLs). This pattern of viral antigen expression may protect EBV-infected B cells from destruction by CTLs.

The unrestrained multiplication of EBV-infected B cells and their lack of differentiation are believed to be due to a genetic translocation that is typically seen in these cells. The c-*myc* oncogene, which is normally located on chromosome 8, is translocated to one of three chromosomes that contain immunoglobulin genes (usually chromosome 14, but sometimes chromosome 2 or 22). In experimental studies, mice that contain these translocations were reported to develop Burkitt's lymphoma. Mutations in tumor suppressor gene p53 have also been reported in patients with Burkitt's lymphoma.

The precise mechanisms by which EBV causes Burkitt's lymphoma are not fully understood. Some have proposed that at least three steps are involved. First, EBV stimulates B cells to divide while arresting their differentiation. Second, infection with *Plasmodium falciparum,* an agent of malaria, acts as an environmental cofactor. Various investigators have suggested that repeated *P. falciparum* infections may impair CTL function or may accelerate B cell division by acting as a persistent mitogenic stimulus. Third, once the relatively undifferentiated and EBV-infected B cells are multiplying and are avoiding CTL activity, chromosomal translocation of the c-*myc* gene may complete cell transformation by causing c-*myc* to be constitutively activated.

Burkitt's lymphoma usually presents as a large tumor of the jaw. It primarily affects children between the ages of 4 and 7 years, and over 80% of cases occur in those between 3 and 12 years. Children at highest risk exhibit high titers of antibodies to the EBV viral capsid antigen (VCA). The tumors often are associated with the premolar and molar teeth and cause these teeth to become loose. In some cases, the tumor extends from the maxilla into the orbit. When the disease is advanced, it may extend into the brain or spinal cord. Most patients also develop abdominal tumors, and breast and testicular tumors are reported. Burkitt's lymphoma is confirmed histologically by showing that the tumor is an undifferentiated lymphoblastic lymphoma.

Patients with Burkitt's lymphoma respond well to treatment with alkylating chemotherapeutic agents, particularly cyclophosphamide. Treatment with cyclophosphamide results in total remission in about 40% of patients and partial remission in another 40%.

Epstein-Barr Virus and Nasopharyngeal Carcinoma

Nasopharyngeal carcinoma is the most common form of cancer found in Cantonese populations living in southern China and other locations throughout the world. The incidence of nasopharyngeal carcinoma is also high in Eskimo populations and northern African populations. In other groups, nasopharyngeal carcinoma is rare.

Each malignant cell from nasopharyngeal carcinoma contains multiple copies of EBV DNA in episomal form. The means by which EBV may transform nasal epithelial cells are unclear. In fact, EBV does not infect epithelial cells in vitro. Virions that are coated with antiviral secretory IgA may infect the nasal epithelium via the IgA transport pathway. Once inside epithelial cells, the virions produce no progeny, but infected cells exhibit EBNA-1 on their surface. The strong association of nasopharyngeal carcinoma with people of Cantonese and Eskimo descent suggests that a host genetic factor may be involved in development of this type of cancer.

Nasopharyngeal carcinoma is treated with radiation therapy. About 40% of treated patients survive 5 years, and 33% survive 10 years.

Human Herpesvirus 8 and Malignant Neoplasms

Using polymerase chain reaction technology, investigators have recently identified the genome of human herpesvirus 8 (HHV-8) within the cells of **Kaposi's sarcoma** and **non-Hodgkin's lymphoma** in patients with AIDS. Because of its association with Kaposi's sarcoma, HHV-8 is also called Kaposi's sarcoma–associated herpesvirus (KSHV). Antibody tests have demonstrated that AIDS patients with Kaposi's sarcoma have antibodies directed against HHV-8 antigens but that most AIDS patients without Kaposi's sarcoma lack these antibodies. Moreover, the virus can be found in the peripheral blood leukocytes and semen of AIDS patients with Kaposi's sarcoma but not in other AIDS patients. Investigators believe that HHV-8 is transmitted during anal intercourse and is the cause of Kaposi's sarcoma. At this time, it is not known how HHV-8 might be directly involved in the generation of Kaposi's sarcoma or non-Hodgkin's lymphoma.

A variety of treatment regimens, including chemotherapy and fractionated radiotherapy, have been used to treat Kaposi's sarcoma. Most patients experience only a palliative benefit from treatment.

ONCOGENIC PAPILLOMAVIRUSES

Human papillomaviruses (HPV) are members of the family *Papovaviridae* and are capable of producing a variety of warts (see Chapter 20 and Table 20–4). These growths regress spontaneously in most cases, but they occasionally develop into carcinoma.

Only a small number of HPV serotypes cause cancer. **Cervical carcinoma,** the most common form of cancer in women living in developing countries, is primarily associated with HPV types 16 and 18 but has also been linked with other types. The virus is sexually transmitted, and the risk of cervical carcinoma increases as the number of sexual partners increases. HPV type 6 has been associated with the development of **anogenital carcinoma** subsequent to condyloma acuminatum, and types 5, 8, and 14 have been associated with **squamous cell carcinomas** that develop from epidermodysplasia verruciformis.

Although the oncogenic properties of some animal papovaviruses are well understood, little is known about how HPV serotypes cause cancer. Two processes appear to be involved: the integration of the HPV genome into the host genome and the participation of an environmental cofactor.

Individuals with warts caused by HPV type 16 or 18 may develop a precancerous condition known as cervical intraepithelial neoplasia, but only a small proportion of cases of neoplasia progress to cervical carcinoma. A key difference between benign and cancerous virus-infected cells is that the HPV genome is episomal in benign cells, but at least a portion of the HPV genome is integrated into the genome of cancerous cells. HPV has seven early open reading frames (ORFs) designated as E1 through E7 and two late ORFs designated as L1 and L2. E2 modulates viral transcription and suppresses the expression on E6 and E7. E6 binds to and accelerates the degradation of the host p53 suppressor gene product. E7 binds to and inhibits the retinoblastoma protein and p107, both of which are tumor suppressor proteins. When the HPV genome is integrated into the host genome, E2 is disrupted. As a result, E6 and E7 are fully expressed. Other possibly oncogenic events have been reported, but much remains to be learned of how HPV initiates malignant transformation.

The hypothesis that an environmental cofactor is needed for efficient cell transformation is based on epidemiologic studies in patients with HPV lesions. Some studies have shown that the incidence of cervical carcinoma is much higher in HPV-infected patients who smoke than in those who do not smoke. Others have shown that malignant transformation of laryngeal papillomas in patients with HPV type 6 infection occurs only after the papillomas have been irradiated.

Cervical carcinoma, the most frequently encountered form of HPV-associated cancer, is usually treated with surgery (hysterectomy) and pelvic irradiation.

Selected Readings

Bates, P. Chemokine receptors and HIV-1: an attractive pair? Cell 86:1–3, 1996.

Carpenter, C. J., et al. Antiretroviral therapy for HIV infection in 1996: recommendations of the international panel. JAMA 276:146–154, 1996.

Dictor, M., et al. Human herpesvirus 8 (Kaposi's sarcoma–associated herpesvirus) DNA in Kaposi's sarcoma lesions, AIDS Kaposi's sarcoma cell lines, endothelial Kaposi's sarcoma simulators, and the skin of immunosuppressed patients. Am J Pathol 148:2009–2016, 1996.

Gill, P. S., et al. Treatment of adult T cell leukemia-lymphoma with a combination of interferon alfa and zidovudine. N Engl J Med 332:1744–1748, 1995.

Hines, J. F., A. B Jensen, and W. A. Barnes. Human papillomaviruses: their clinical significance in the management of cervical carcinoma. Oncology (Huntingt) 9:279–285, 1995.

Lazo, P. A., et al. Genetic alterations by human papillomaviruses in oncogenesis. FEBS Lett 300:109–113, 1992.

Levy, J. A. Pathogenesis of human immunodeficiency virus infection. Microbiol Rev 57:183–289, 1993.

Liang, X. H., et al. Bcl-2 proto-oncogene expression in cervical carcinoma cell lines containing inactive p53. J Cell Biochem 57:509–521, 1995.

Luppi, M., and G. Torelli. The new lymphotropic herpesviruses (HHV-6, HHV-7, and HHV-8) and hepatitis C virus (HCV) in human lymphoproliferative disease: an overview. Haematologica 81:265–281, 1996.

Moore, P. S., et al. Primary characterization of a herpesvirus agent associated with Kaposi's sarcoma. J Virol 70:549–558, 1996.

Peto, M., et al. Epidermal growth factor induction of human papillomavirus type 16 E6/E7 mRNA in tumor cells involves two AP-1 binding sites in the viral enhancer. J Gen Virol 76:1945–1958, 1995.

Ressing, M. E., et al. Human CTL epitopes encoded by human papillomavirus type 16 E6 and E7 identified through in vivo and in vitro immunogenicity studies of HLA-A*0201-binding peptides. J Immunol 154:5934–5943, 1995.

Sherman, M. Hepatocellular carcinoma. Gastroenterologist 3:55–66, 1995.

Tahara, H., et al. Telomerase activity in human liver tissues: comparison between chronic liver disease and hepatocellular carcinoma. Cancer Res 55:2734–2736, 1995.

Takada, S., et al. Disruption of the function of tumor suppressor gene p53 by the hepatitis B virus X protein and hepatocarcinogenesis. J Cancer Res Clin Oncol 121:593–601, 1995.

Vousden, K. Interactions of human papillomavirus transforming proteins with the products of tumor suppressor genes. FASEB J 7:872–879, 1993.

Waldman, T. A. Lymphokine receptors: a target for immunotherapy of lymphomas. Ann Oncol 5(supplement 1):13–17, 1994.

Whitby, D., et al. Detection of Kaposi's sarcoma–associated herpesvirus in peripheral blood of HIV-infected individuals and progression to Kaposi's sarcoma. Lancet 346:799–802, 1995.

zur Hausen, H. Human papillomaviruses in the pathogenesis of anogenital cancer. Virology 184:9–13, 1991.

PARASITES AND

PARASITIC DISEASES

CHAPTER TWENTY-THREE

OVERVIEW OF PARASITOLOGY

AND ANTIPARASITIC AGENTS

CLASSIFICATION AND STRUCTURE OF PARASITES

Earlier sections of this book focused on organisms that are microscopic and prokaryotic. Even the largest bacteria are too small to be seen with the naked eye, and all bacteria differ greatly from the cells that make up the human body. The differences between bacteria and human cells provide excellent targets for antibiotic action and allow antibacterial agents to be selectively toxic. The parasites, in contrast, are **eukaryotes** and contain structures and organelles that are similar to those found within human cells. Parasites are even more like human cells than are fungal cells because, like humans, parasites are animals. Thus, they do not have the plantlike cell walls found in fungi. Developing effective and safe antibiotics against parasites has proved to be difficult, and most antiparasitic drugs have some adverse effects against humans.

The parasites that cause human infections can be divided into two major groups: **protozoan parasites,** which each consist of a single cell and are the focus of Chapter 24; and **helminths (worms),** which each consist of multiple cells and are the focus of Chapter 25.

As shown in Table 23–1, protozoan parasites that infect humans include members of the phyla **Apicomplexa** (the sporozoans), **Ciliophora** (the ciliates), and **Sarcomastigophora** (the flagellates and amebas). The **sporozoans** are found in the blood, tissues, or intestine and all reproduce both sexually and asexually. The most important are *Plasmodium, Pneumocystis,* and *Toxoplasma,* which are the agents of malaria, pneumonia, and toxoplasmosis, respectively. Although there are many **ciliates,** the only one that causes human disease is *Balantidium coli,* an agent of dysentery. The phylum Sarcomastigophora includes **flagellates** that are found in blood (*Trypanosoma*), lymphatic tissue (*Leishmania*), or the gastrointestinal tract (*Dientamoeba* and *Giardia*); two free-living **amebas,** *Acanthamoeba* and *Naegleria;* and the obligate amebic parasite *Entamoeba histolytica.* The importance of the protozoan parasites is underscored by the following facts: (1) approximately 10% of the world's population is infected with *E. histolytica,* the

agent of amebiasis; (2) malaria is the number one cause of infectious disease–related deaths worldwide; and (3) pneumonia caused by *Pneumocystis carinii* is the leading cause of death in patients with acquired immunodeficiency syndrome (AIDS).

Helminths are members of the phyla **Acanthocephala** (the thorny-headed worms), **Aschelminthes** (the roundworms), and **Platyhelminthes** (the flatworms, including tapeworms and flukes). Humans are primarily infected with the various **nematodes, cestodes,** and **trematodes** listed in Table 23–1. In fact, hundreds of millions of individuals are infected with hookworms (*Ancylostoma* and *Necator*), the common roundworm (*Ascaris*), schistosomes (*Schistosoma*), whipworms (*Trichuris*), and lymphatic filariae (*Brugia* and *Wuchereria*). Although many infections with helminths are mild, some are life-threatening. As a result, the human suffering and economic costs of these infections are staggering.

TECHNIQUES USED TO IDENTIFY PARASITES

Humans become infected when the parasites or their eggs are ingested, when free-living larvae of parasites pass through the mucosae or skin, or when organisms are introduced through the bite of a vector. After they enter a human host, the parasites develop and establish infections within a target organ or tissue. Most parasites that enter the host via ingestion of feces-contaminated food or water (the fecal-oral route) go through their life cycle in the gastrointestinal tract. In contrast, parasites that enter directly through the skin or are introduced by a vector may infect the blood or blood vessels or may establish infections in subcutaneous tissues or major organs, including the bone marrow and lymphatic tissues.

Because of the size and complexity of parasites, laboratory diagnosis of parasitic infections primarily involves finding the parasites in infected tissues, body fluids (including sputum), or stool samples and then visually identifying them. Diagnosis of parasitic infections is a labor-intensive process. Even in this day of highly specific and sensitive tests involving polymerase chain reaction assays and DNA hybridization technology, most parasites are identified using a microscope. If the infecting agent is a protozoan

TABLE 23–1.   Taxonomic Classification of the Endoparasites of Humans

Classification	Common Name	Examples
Protozoan parasites		
Phylum Apicomplexa	Sporozoans	*Babesia, Cryptosporidium, Isospora, Plasmodium, Pneumocystis,* and *Toxoplasma.*
Phylum Ciliophora	Ciliates	*Balantidium.*
Phylum Sarcomastigophora		
Subphylum Mastigophora	Flagellates	*Dientamoeba, Giardia, Leishmania, Trichomonas,* and *Trypanosoma.*
Subphylum Sarcodina	Amebas	*Acanthamoeba, Entamoeba,* and *Naegleria.*
Helminths		
Phylum Aschelminthes		
Class Nematoda	Roundworms	*Ancylostoma, Ascaris, Brugia, Capillaria, Dracunculus, Enterobius, Loa, Necator, Onchocerca, Strongyloides, Toxocara, Trichinella, Trichuris,* and *Wuchereria.*
Phylum Platyhelminthes		
Class Cestoda	Tapeworms	*Diphyllobothrium, Dipylidium, Echinococcus, Hymenolepis, Multiceps,* and *Taenia.*
Class Trematoda	Flukes	*Clonorchis, Echinostoma, Fasciola, Fasciolopsis, Heterophyes, Metagonimus, Opisthorchis, Paragonimus,* and *Schistosoma.*

parasite, the clinical sample must be stained and examined microscopically for the presence of trophozoites (feeding forms) or cysts (dormant forms) of the organism. If the infecting agent is a helminth, diagnosis may involve finding worm ova or larvae in the stool, finding microfilariae in the blood, or locating adult worms in the subcutaneous tissues or gastrointestinal tract.

Examination of Enteric Specimens

Diagnosis of parasitic infections may be difficult when it involves finding protozoa or worm ova within stool samples. This is because some parasites are shed into stools intermittently, the number of organisms in the stool may be small, and parasites and ova in stool samples can become distorted and unrecognizable if the patient is taking antidiarrheal agents. For these reasons, the way that a specimen is collected and handled may determine whether a correct diagnosis can be made.

A stool sample will yield the best results if it is examined 30 minutes or less after it is collected. Unfortunately, this is not generally possible, so most specimens must be properly preserved to ensure that ova and parasites will not degenerate. If the sample is to be shipped to an outlying laboratory to be examined later, it should be preserved in polyvinyl alcohol (PVA). This will keep the sample stable for about 1 month. Laboratories that examine stool samples on site often preserve specimens with merthiolate-iodine-formalin (MIF) fixative, which both preserves and stains the samples.

Standard stool specimens are not always reliable indicators of intestinal parasitic infections. Occasionally, intestinal parasites must be located by purging stools with a saline solution or by taking a biopsy of the intestinal wall. In some cases, parasites that infect the small intestine can be located by obtaining a sample from the duodenum via intubation. In other cases, the patient is asked to swallow an enteric capsule that is suspended from one end of a string. The other end of the string is fastened to the patient's cheek. After 4 hours, the capsule is drawn out by the string,

and the bile-stained mucus at the distal end of the capsule is examined microscopically for organisms.

Although diagnosis of intestinal parasites generally involves microscopic identification of the organisms in clinical samples, some parasites can be cultivated in vitro. For example, *Entamoeba histolytica* can be cultivated in TYI-S-33 medium or Locke egg-serum medium, and diagnosis of *Schistosoma* infections may be aided by hatching ova that are found in stool samples.

Concentration Techniques

When ova or parasites in the specimen are expected to be scarce, it is sometimes necessary to concentrate stool samples to optimize the technician's ability to locate and identify a parasitic agent. Flotation or sedimentation techniques can be used and are designed to separate parasitic ova and cysts from most of the fecal matter on the basis of differences in specific gravity. **Flotation techniques** cause the ova and parasites to float to the top of the liquid, where they can be collected on a slide. A common flotation technique uses a zinc sulfate solution with an adjusted specific gravity of 1.180. **Sedimentation techniques** do not yield as clean a preparation as do flotation techniques, but they are gentler in their effects on some parasites. The most widely used sedimentation technique concentrates the ova and parasites within a layer of formalin located below a layer of ether or ethyl acetate.

Staining Procedures

Samples from fresh and preserved stool and samples from concentrated stool preparations can be placed on slides and stained to find microscopic enteric parasites. If fresh stool specimens are available, a small sample can be mixed with saline on a slide and examined as a wet mount under a coverslip. The sample can also be mixed with D'Antoni's iodine solution, which will increase the technician's ability to identify parasites. If permanent slides are to be made from stool specimens, a small amount of the specimen should be placed on a slide and a smear can be made using an applicator stick. Once the sample is dried, the sample can be stained with Gomori's trichrome stain or with iron hematoxylin stain. When fresh stools are used, the smear should be fixed before the slide dries and before staining the sample. Once stained, the slide can be examined first under high-dry magnification to locate parasites and then under oil immersion to determine the species. Some ova are large enough to be readily identifiable when examined through the high-dry objective.

Examination of Blood, Tissue, and Other Samples

Infections with *Babesia, Plasmodium, Trypanosoma,* and microfilariae (*Brugia, Loa, Onchocerca,* and *Wuchereria*) are identified by examining blood films. Infections with *Leishmania, Toxoplasma,* and *Trichinella* are identified by examining tissue samples for the presence of microscopic parasites. *Naegleria* and *Trypanosoma* can be found within the cerebrospinal fluid of patients with meningoencephalitis, and *E. histolytica, Paragonimus westermani,* and *Pneumocystis carinii* can be found in the sputum of patients with pulmonary infections caused by these agents.

Making and Examining Blood Films

Blood samples are best taken from a fingertip or earlobe to ensure that the sample is peripheral blood. The skin is cleansed thoroughly with alcohol to remove fats and oils, and then an incision is made in a manner that will allow the blood to flow freely.

Blood films should be made on microscope slides that have been scrupulously cleaned with alcohol to remove any residual dust and oil. Two types should be made: a **thick film,** which allows for rapid confirmation of the presence of parasites in the blood, and a **thin film,** which is used to identify the species of parasite. A thin film should contain only one layer of blood cells. A drop of blood is placed on the slide and a second slide is held at a 30-degree angle and drawn up so that it touches the drop of blood. The upper slide is then drawn quickly across the other slide to allow the blood to be pulled down the slide in a manner that gives the spread blood a feathered edge. The slide is air-dried, fixed with absolute methyl alcohol, air-dried again, and then stained with Giemsa stain. A thick film is made by placing three drops of blood near the end of a slide. The tip of a second slide is used to stir the blood for about 30 seconds to make an area about 2 cm in diameter. The dried blood on the slide is then laked with buffer to remove hemoglobin, and the slide is stained with Giemsa stain without prior fixation.

Examining Tissue Samples

Tissue impression procedures are sometimes used to detect *Leishmania* or *Toxoplasma* in bone marrow, lymphatic tissue, or liver biopsies. A piece of tissue believed to be infected is pressed against a clean microscope slide, fixed, and stained with Giemsa stain. Lung biopsy samples can be similarly impressed to locate *P. carinii,* but such samples should be stained with Grocott-Gomori methenamine–silver nitrate stain.

In cases of suspected *Leishmania* infection, needle biopsy can be used to obtain spleen, liver, or bone marrow specimens. The specimens can then be stained, cultured, or inoculated into animals to demonstrate the presence of *Leishmania.*

Examining Cerebrospinal Fluid Samples

Cerebrospinal fluid is collected by spinal puncture and should be examined immediately. Because parasites may be scarce in cerebrospinal fluid, it may be necessary to centrifuge the specimen. The centrifuged specimen can then be examined for the presence of parasites by wet mount.

IMMUNITY TO PARASITIC INFECTIONS

The characteristics of parasites and parasitic diseases differ greatly. Some parasites cause acute infections, as is the case with *Plasmodium* species, which cause malaria. However, most parasitic infections last for many years. The liver fluke *Clonorchis sinensis,* for example, lives within its human host for 20–25 years. Parasites can be microscopic or enormous in size. The average length of the adult fish tapeworm *Diphyllobothrium latum* is 10 m, and that of the adult pork tapeworm *Taenia solium* is 5 m. Some parasites live entirely within the intestinal lumen, while others live within small blood vessels, in subcutaneous tissues, in the central nervous system, or within macrophages and monocytes. Often, when nematodes migrate through the body, the patient suffers from signs and symptoms of allergy, including hives (urticaria) and asthma. Taken together, these observations suggest that the immune responses in parasitic infections are complex and differ greatly from the immune processes that ameliorate and prevent the average bacterial or viral infection. While a detailed discussion of the various immune responses is beyond the scope of this book, it is appropriate to present a brief review of some basic immunologic principles and see how they relate to parasitic infections.

Parasites that live within the intestine may lie entirely within the lumen or may invade the intestinal wall. Unless tissues are invaded, there is little antibody response to the presence of parasites. Immunity to intestinal protozoa seems to be related to the ability of activated macrophages to kill them by a contact-dependent but antibody-independent mechanism. Some studies have shown that the critical macrophage product that kills protozoa is nitric oxide. Some intestinal protozoa are sensitive to complement-mediated damage, but studies have shown that virulent strains of *Entamoeba histolytica* are impervious to complement-mediated killing. These virulent strains kill neutrophils and macrophages that have not been activated.

A multistep immune process is believed to cause

TABLE 23-2.   Actions, Indications, and Adverse Effects of the Major Antiparasitic Agents

Agent	Mechanism of Action	Indications	Adverse Effects
Antiprotozoal drugs			
Amphotericin B	Binds to membrane steroids.	Leishmaniasis; meningoencephalitis due to *Naegleria* or *Acanthamoeba*.	Anorexia, dyspepsia, epigastric pain, fever, headache, hypotension, malaise, nausea, renal toxicity, tachypnea, and vomiting occur in most patients receiving intravenous amphotericin B. The severity of adverse effects is dose-related.
Atovaquone	Ubiquinone analogue; inhibits electron transport.	Alternative treatment for *Pneumocystis carinii* pneumonia.	Diarrhea, fever, headache, insomnia, nausea, rash, and vomiting occur in about 10% of patients.
Chloroquine	Inhibits nucleic acid synthesis.	Malaria chemoprophylaxis and treatment; amebiasis (kills trophozoites).	Central nervous system stimulation, gastrointestinal upset, headache, pruritus, and rash are uncommon and mild effects.
Clindamycin	Inhibits protein synthesis.	Combined with quinine to treat babesiosis.	Colitis and hypersensitivity reactions are common.
Diloxanide furoate*	Unknown.	Amebiasis (kills cysts).	Excessive flatulence is an uncommon effect.
Eflornithine hydrochloride	Inhibits ornithine decarboxylase; blocks synthesis of polyamines.	African trypanosomiasis; alternative treatment for cryptosporidiosis, leishmaniasis, or malaria.	Anemia, hearing loss, leukemia, loose stools, nausea, and thrombocytopenia are uncommon effects.
Emetine hydrochloride	Blocks protein synthesis by halting peptide chain elongation.	Amebiasis (kills trophozoites in lumen and tissues).	Various cardiovascular effects, including electro-cardiographic changes and myocardial damage, are common.
Furazolidone	Metabolic inhibitor.	Giardiasis.	Nausea, pruritus, and vomiting are uncommon effects. Acute hemolysis sometimes occurs in patients with glucose-6-phosphate dehydrogenase deficiency.
Iodoquinol	Unknown.	Amebiasis (kills cysts); infections with *Balantidium coli* or *Dientamoeba fragilis*.	Abdominal cramps, acne, nausea, pruritus ani, rash, and thyroid enlargement are uncommon effects.
Mefloquine	Inhibits nucleic acid synthesis.	Malaria chemoprophylaxis.	Anorexia, diarrhea, dizziness, headache, myalgia, nausea, rash, tinnitus, and vomiting are uncommon effects. Asthenia, bradycardia, emotional disturbances, pruritus, and vertigo occur in fewer than 1% of patients.
Meglumine antimoniate*	Unknown.	Leishmaniasis.	Cardiotoxicity, nausea, and vomiting are common.
Melarsoprol*	Inhibits metabolism by altering sulfhydryl groups on enzymes.	African trypanosomiasis.	Abdominal pain, albuminemia, angioedema, arthralgia, hypotension, peripheral neuropathy, rash, and vomiting are common. Potentially fatal reactive encephalitis occurs in 3–5% of patients.
Metronidazole	Inhibits the production of hydrogen by the pyruvate phosphoroclastic reaction.	Amebiasis; giardiasis; infections with *Trichomonas vaginalis* or *B. coli*.	Minor gastrointestinal upset is common. The drug may be teratogenic.
Nifurtimox*	Generates oxygen-derived free radicals.	American trypanosomiasis (Chagas' disease).	Abdominal pain, anorexia, headache, insomnia, myalgia, nausea, rash, vertigo, and vomiting occur in 40–70% of patients.
Paromomycin	Inhibits protein synthesis.	Amebiasis (kills cysts); giardiasis.	Abdominal pain, diarrhea, and nausea are common.

Continued

TABLE 23–2. **Actions, Indications, and Adverse Effects of the Major Antiparasitic Agents** (*Continued*)

Agent	Mechanism of Action	Indications	Adverse Effects
Antiprotozoal drugs (*continued*)			
Pentamidine isethionate	Unknown; may inhibit oxidative phosphorylation, glucose metabolism, nucleic acid synthesis, protein synthesis, or dihydrofolate reductase activity.	*P. carinii* pneumonia; early Gambian sleeping sickness; alternative treatment for some infections with *Leishmania.*	Pain at the injection site, followed by tissue necrosis and abscess formation, is common. Arrhythmia, hypotension, nausea, vomiting, and tachycardia are also common.
Povidone-iodine	Detergent and iodination reactions.	Infections with *T. vaginalis.*	Allergy is rare.
Primaquine phosphate	Unknown.	Malaria treatment (kills tissue forms of *Plasmodium ovale* and *Plasmodium vivax*); combined with clindamycin to treat *P. carinii* pneumonia.	Abdominal discomfort, headache, methemoglobinemia, nausea, and pruritus are common. Acute hemolysis sometimes occurs in patients with glucose-6-phosphate dehydrogenase deficiency. The drug may be teratogenic.
Pyrimethamine	Inhibits dihydrofolate reductase activity.	Combined with sulfadiazine to treat toxoplasmosis or infections with *Isopora belli.*	Eosinophilic pneumonitis occurs rarely in individuals taking the drug for chemoprophylaxis. Hematologic disorders are common in patients being treated. The drug may be teratogenic.
Quinacrine hydrochloride	Inhibits nucleic acid synthesis.	Alternative treatment for giardiasis.	Cinchonism (with altered hearing, blurred vision, headache, nausea, tinnitus, and vomiting) is common. Toxic psychoses are reported in 1.5–2% of patients.
Quinidine gluconate	Inhibits nucleic acid synthesis.	Malaria treatment in chloroquine-resistant infections with *Plasmodium falciparum.*	Cardiotoxicity and hepatotoxicity are common.
Sodium stibogluconate*	Unknown.	Leishmaniasis.	Cardiotoxicity, nausea, and vomiting are common.
Spiramycin*	Inhibits protein synthesis.	Toxoplasmosis.	Gastrointestinal upset is reported.
Suramin*	Metabolic inhibitor.	Early Rhodesian sleeping sickness; alternative treatment for early Gambian sleeping sickness.	Central nervous system effects, including hyperesthesia of palms and soles, paresthesias, peripheral neuropathy, and photophobia, are common. Loss of consciousness and seizures are reported in 0.3% of patients.
Tetracycline	Inhibits protein synthesis.	Infections with *B. coli* or *D. fragilis;* alternative treatment for chloroquine-resistant infections with *P. falciparum.*	Signs of gastrointestinal upset, including anorexia, diarrhea, flatulence, and nausea, are common. Photosensitivity is an uncommon effect. Use by pregnant women and young children causes deposits in bones and teeth of fetuses and children.
Trimethoprim-sulfamethoxazole	Blocks folic acid synthesis.	*P. carinii* pneumonia; infections with *I. belli.*	Anorexia, nausea, and vomiting occur in 3.5% of patients. Hypersensitivity reactions occur in fewer than 0.5% of patients.
Trimetrexate glucuronate*	Inhibits dihydrofolate reductase activity.	Alternative treatment for *P. carinii* pneumonia.	Bone marrow suppression, elevated aspartate and alanine transferase levels, leukopenia, and thrombocytopenia are common.
Trisulfapyrimidine*	Blocks folic acid synthesis.	Toxoplasmosis.	Adverse hematologic effects, gastrointestinal upset, hypersensitivity reactions, jaundice, and renal damage are uncommon effects.

Continued

TABLE 23–2. Actions, Indications, and Adverse Effects of the Major Antiparasitic Agents (*Continued*)

Agent	Mechanism of Action	Indications	Adverse Effects
Anthelmintic drugs			
Albendazole	Inhibits glucose uptake by inhibiting assembly of tubulin; causes depletion of glycogen and adenosine triphosphate (ATP) stores.	Cysticercosis; echinococcosis; adult worm infections with *Ancylostoma, Ascaris, Capillaria, Enterobius, Necator, Strongyloides,* or *Trichuris.*	Abdominal pain, constipation, diarrhea, dizziness, and nausea are uncommon effects.
Diethylcarbamazine citrate	Accelerates immune-mediated destruction of parasites by increasing adherence of granulocytes to microfilariae.	Infections with microfilariae of *Brugia malayi, Brugia timori, Loa loa,* or *Onchocerca volvulus.*	Dizziness, headaches, nausea, vomiting, and weakness are common.
Ivermectin*	Causes flaccid paralysis of worm by blocking the function of neuromuscular junctions that are dependent on gamma-aminobutyric acid (GABA).	Infections with *L. loa* or *O. volvulus;* alternative treatment for infections with *Strongyloides* or *Wuchereria.*	Fever, headache, muscle aches, pruritus, and swollen glands are uncommon effects.
Mebendazole	Inhibits glucose uptake by interfering with tubulin assembly; causes depletion of glycogen and ATP stores.	Infections with *Ancylostoma, Capillaria, Necator, Strongyloides, Trichinella,* or *Trichuris.*	Abdominal pain (transient), diarrhea, fever, and pruritus are uncommon effects.
Metrifonate*	Paralyzes worm by blocking the function of cholinergic nerves.	Alternative treatment for infections with *Schistosoma haematobium.*	Abdominal discomfort, diarrhea, headache, vertigo, vomiting, and weakness are uncommon and transient effects.
Niclosamide	Inhibits mitochondrial oxidative phosphorylation.	Adult tapeworm infections with *Diphyllobothrium latum, Dipylidium caninum, Hymenolepis diminuta, Hymenolepis nana, Taenia saginata,* or *Taenia solium.*	Abdominal pain, malaise, and nausea occur in about 10% of patients. The drug is not recommended for pregnant women.
Oxamniquine	Unknown, but paralyzes musculature of worm.	Alternative treatment for infections with *Schistosoma mansoni.*	Dizziness, orange discoloration of urine, and somnolence are common. Eosinophilia, fever, transient pulmonary infiltrate, and vomiting are uncommon effects. The drug is not recommended for patients with epilepsy, congestive heart failure, or renal failure.
Paromomycin	Inhibits protein synthesis.	Alternative treatment for some infections with tapeworms.	Abdominal pain, diarrhea, and nausea are common.
Piperazine citrate	Causes reversible muscle paralysis of worm by hyperpolarizing nerve endings.	Alternative treatment for infections with *Ascaris* or *Enterobius.*	Allergic reactions, diarrhea, nausea, and vomiting are uncommon effects.
Praziquantel	Causes tetanic paralysis of worm by causing efflux of intracellular calcium.	Infections with *Clonorchis, Echinococcus, Echinostoma, Fasciola, Fasciolopsis, Heterophyes, Opisthorchis, Paragonimus,* or *Schistosoma;* alternative treatment for infections with *Taenia* species (including cysticercosis), *D. caninum, D. latum, H. diminuta,* and *H. nana.*	Abdominal pain, diarrhea, dizziness, fever, headache, lassitude, malaise, moderate increases in alanine and aspartate transaminase levels, nausea, and pruritus are common but mild and transient.
Pyrantel pamoate	Paralyzes worm by depolarizing neuromuscular junctions.	Infections with *Ascaris.*	Abdominal pain, anorexia, diarrhea, dizziness, drowsiness, headache, nausea, rash, and vomiting are common.
Suramin*	Unknown in worms.	Combined with diethylcarbamazine as alternative to treat infections with adult *O. volvulus.*	Central nervous system effects, including hyperesthesia of palms and soles, paresthesias, peripheral neuropathy, and photophobia, are common. Loss of consciousness and seizures are reported in 0.3% of patients.
Thiabendazole	Inhibits assembly of microtubules.	Cutaneous larva migrans; infections with *Ancylostoma braziliense, Dracunculus medinensis,* or *Trichinella spiralis.*	Anorexia, dizziness, drowsiness, nausea, and vomiting are common.

* Investigational drug, available in the USA through the Centers for Disease Control and Prevention.

the expulsion of worms that live primarily within the lumen of the gut. After antibody and mast cell products damage the worms, the effector molecules secreted by T cells cause goblet cells to proliferate and increase their secretion of mucus. When the damaged worms are enveloped within globules of mucus, they are unable to attach to the intestinal wall, and they are expelled by peristalsis.

The invasion of tissue by parasites elicits the production of antibodies that include IgM, IgG, and IgE. In many cases, IgE is the critical antibody that will eliminate the parasite in conjunction with eosinophil degranulation. IgE molecules directed against worm antigens are fixed to mast cells that degranulate when they come into contact with the worms in tissues. Effectors released during mast cell degranulation produce the signs and symptoms of allergy that are often seen during worm migration or in the presence of large worm burdens. One of these effectors is a chemotactic factor for eosinophils, which acts in conjunction with chemotactic parasite antigens to attract eosinophils into sites of worm infection. The movement of inflammatory cells into these sites is augmented by an increased vascular permeability that is caused by mast cell degranulation. Simultaneously, T cells activated by worm antigens release eosinophil stimulation promoter, which causes eosinophils to proliferate and results in eosinophilia. Eosinophils collect around the worm, and the IgG-coated worm is killed by antibody-dependent cellular cytotoxicity (ADCC), probably through the release of a substance called eosinophil major basic protein. The adult forms of Schistosoma counteract this process by covering themselves with a layer of host antigens, which camouflages them from antischistosomal antibodies.

Schistosoma and Paragonimus are unusual in that the eggs produced by these flukes cause immune response–dependent pathologic changes in the tissue of patients. The eggs deposit in tissues, where they elicit a cell-mediated immune response. This forms granulomas around the flukes, similar to the granulomas seen in tuberculosis. Although adult forms of Paragonimus cause signs and symptoms of disease, the ova of Schistosoma are totally responsible for the disease known as schistosomiasis. The penetration of cercariae (larvae) of Schistosoma through the skin also elicits a cell-mediated response and results in a skin rash similar to that caused by poison ivy.

Protozoa that invade the blood and tissues present special challenges to the immune system because they typically go through immunologically distinguishable developmental phases. For example, Plasmodium parasites exist at different times within the human host in the form of sporozoites, trophozoites, schizonts, merozoites, macrogametocytes, and microgametocytes. Each of these forms has its own set of antigens. Additionally, some of these forms occur inside erythrocytes or may be found within hepatic parenchymal cells. It is not surprising, then, that infected patients do not develop a lasting protective immunity against malaria.

Trypanosoma parasites also go through a developmental cycle and are found as amastigotes within macrophages or as trypomastigotes in the blood. Other tissue parasites that go through developmental cycles include Babesia, Leishmania, Pneumocystis, and Toxoplasma. In general, the protozoa that live within macrophages are killed when the macrophages are activated, while the protozoa that live in the blood are susceptible to antibody-mediated processes, particularly complement-mediated lysis, opsonization, and interference with entry into the host cells in which they would go through developmental stages. Trypanosoma brucei has an unusual way of dealing with the threat of the immune response. Throughout the course of infection, the trypanosome undergoes antigenic variation. Patients typically exhibit extremely high levels of IgM antibodies to the various antigens. But because the antigens are changed often, this IgM response is futile.

ANTIPARASITIC AGENTS

The antiparasitic agents can be divided into two major groups: **antiprotozoal drugs** and **anthelmintic drugs.** Two agents—paromomycin and suramin—have been used against both protozoa and helminths.

For the antiprotozoal drugs, the most common mechanism of action is inhibition of nucleic acid synthesis. For the anthelmintic drugs, there are two common mechanisms. Some drugs affect the nervous system of worms and cause them to undergo spastic or flaccid paralysis, while other drugs inhibit glucose transport by interfering with microtubule polymerization.

Many of the antiparasitic drugs have significant adverse effects on patients. Table 23–2 lists the available drugs, along with their mechanisms of action, indications, and side effects.

Selected Readings

Camacho, M., et al. The amount of acetylcholinesterase on the parasite surface reflects the differential sensitivity of schistosome species to metrifonate. Parasitology 108:153–160, 1994.

Carter, N. S., and A. H. Fairlamb. Arsenical-resistant trypanosomes lack an unusual adenosine transporter. Nature 361:374, 1993.

Gherardi, R. K., et al. Organic arsenic–induced Guillain-Barré–like syndrome due to melarsoprol: a clinical, electrophysiological and pathological study. Muscle Nerve 13:637–645, 1990.

Krauth-Siegel, R. L., and R. Schonek. Flavoprotein structure and mechanism. 5. Trypanothione reductase and lipoamide dehydrogenase as targets for a structure-based drug design. FASEB J 9:1138–1146, 1995.

Molina, J. M., et al. Disseminated microsporidiosis due to Septa intestinalis in patients with AIDS: clinical features and response to albendazole therapy. J Infect Dis 171:245–249, 1995.

Pepin, J., et al. Risk factors for encephalopathy and mortality during melarsoprol treatment of Trypanosoma brucei gambiense sleeping sickness. Trans R Soc Trop Med Hyg 89:92–97, 1995.

Stadnyk, A. W., and J. Gauldie. The acute phase protein response during parasitic infection. Immunol Today 12:A7–A12, 1991.

Titus, R. G., B. Sherry, and A. Cerami. The involvement of TNF, IL-1, and IL-6 in the immune response to protozoan parasites. Immunol Today 12:A13–A16, 1991.

Van-Voorhis, W. C. Therapy and prophylaxis of systemic protozoan infections. Drugs 40:176–202, 1990.

CHAPTER TWENTY-FOUR

PROTOZOAN PARASITES

Acanthamoeba, Babesia, Balantidium,
Cryptosporidium, Dientamoeba, Entamoeba,
Giardia, Isospora, Leishmania, Naegleria,
Plasmodium, Pneumocystis, Toxoplasma,
Trichomonas, and *Trypanosoma*

The protozoan parasites can be divided into two major groups, the first consisting of lumen-dwelling protozoa and the second consisting of blood- and tissue-dwelling protozoa. Table 24–1 lists the clinically significant members of these groups and the drugs used to treat the infections they cause.

LUMEN-DWELLING PROTOZOA

Most of the lumen-dwelling parasites that are pathogenic for humans infect the gastrointestinal tract and cause diarrheal disease. Members of five protozoan groups are known to be significant causes of diarrheal disease: amebas (*Entamoeba histolytica*), ciliates (*Balantidium coli*), flagellates (*Dientamoeba fragilis* and *Giardia lamblia*), sporozoans (*Cryptosporidium parvum* and *Isospora belli*), and microsporidia (*Enterocytozoon bieneusi*). At one extreme is *E. histolytica,* which infects perhaps 10% of the world's population, while at the other extreme are the microsporidia, which are known to cause disease only in patients with acquired immunodeficiency syndrome (AIDS).

The amebas also include two species that are free-living and cause meningoencephalitis. *Naegleria fowleri* causes primary amebic meningoencephalitis in immunocompetent individuals, and *Acanthamoeba* species cause encephalitis in immunosuppressed patients. *Acanthamoeba* species also cause keratitis, usually in individuals who wear contact lenses.

One flagellate, *Trichomonas vaginalis,* is a common worldwide cause of vaginitis. The organism is transmitted sexually and is similar to a commensal found in the gastrointestinal tract of humans, *Pentatrichomonas hominis.*

Amebas
Classification, Structure, and Life Cycle

The amebas are members of the phylum Sarcomastigophora and the subphylum Sarcodina. The **ob-** **ligately parasitic amebas,** found only within the body of a human or animal host, include members of the genera *Entamoeba, Endolimax,* and *Iodamoeba.* The **free-living amebas,** which include *Naegleria* and *Acanthamoeba,* are found in the environment and only occasionally cause human infections. *Naegleria* is an unusual ameba in that it has a flagellate stage.

Amebas typically are seen in one of two stages. Actively feeding amebas are called **trophozoites** (from *trophē,* which means "nourishment," and *zōon,* which means "animal"), while resting amebas are called **cysts.** The relative resistance of cysts to environmental conditions is demonstrated by the fact that they can survive for about 60 days in water at near-freezing temperatures, while trophozoites under the same conditions survive only about 96 hours. Amebic trophozoites move by extending their pseudopodia. This form of **ameboid movement** results from polymerization and depolymerization of microfilaments within each pseudopodium. Amebas use their pseudopodia not only for motility but also to engulf and phagocytose the particles upon which they feed.

Parasitic amebas are transmitted between hosts primarily via the fecal-oral route. When a person ingests food or water that contains amebas, trophozoites are killed as they pass through the stomach, but the amebic cysts are unharmed by stomach acids. When cysts reach the lower portions of the small intestine, they begin the process of excystation. The cyst wall is broken down, and a transitional multinucleated form called a **metacystic ameba** is released. Each nucleus forms the core for a single trophozoite, and the newly formed trophozoites travel to the large intestine, where they begin to multiply by mitosis and cellular fission.

Fig. 24–1 depicts the typical structures of amebic trophozoites and cysts. The single parasitic ameba known to be consistently pathogenic in humans is

427

TABLE 24–1. Recommended Antiparasitic Drugs for the Treatment of Human Endoparasitic Infections

Parasite	Effective Treatments
Lumen-dwelling protozoa	
Acanthamoeba species	Amphotericin B.
Balantidium coli	Tetracycline,* iodoquinol, or metronidazole.
Cryptosporidium parvum	No effective treatment.
Dientamoeba fragilis	Iodoquinol or tetracycline.
Entamoeba histolytica	
Asymptomatic infections	Iodoquinol,* paromomycin, or diloxanide furoate.†
Symptomatic infections	Metronidazole followed by iodoquinol.
Enterocytozoon bieneusi	No effective treatment.
Giardia lamblia	Metronidazole,* quinacrine, furazolidone, or paromomycin.
Isospora belli	Trimethoprim-sulfamethoxazole; or pyrimethamine plus sulfadiazine.
Naegleria fowleri	Amphotericin B.
Trichomonas vaginalis	Metronidazole.
Blood- and tissue-dwelling protozoa	
Babesia species	Clindamycin plus quinine.
Leishmania species	Sodium stibogluconate,† meglumine antimoniate,† amphotericin B, or pentamidine.
Plasmodium species	
Plasmodium malariae, Plasmodium ovale, Plasmodium vivax, and chloroquine-sensitive *Plasmodium falciparum*	Chloroquine phosphate, chloroquine sulfate, quinine sulfate, or quinidine gluconate.
Chloroquine-resistant *P. falciparum*	Quinine sulfate; quinidine gluconate; quinine plus tetracycline; quinidine plus tetracycline; quinine plus a parenteral antifolate antibiotic; or quinidine plus a parenteral antifolate antibiotic.
Pneumocystis carinii	Trimethoprim-sulfamethoxazole* or pentamidine.
Toxoplasma gondii	Pyrimethamine plus sulfadiazine or trisulfapyrimidine;* spiramycin;† or clindamycin.
Trypanosoma species	
Trypanosoma brucei gambiense	
Hemolymphatic disease	Pentamidine.
Neurologic disease	Eflornithine* or melarsoprol.†
Trypanosoma brucei rhodesiense	
Hemolymphatic disease	Suramin.†
Neurologic disease	Eflornithine* or melarsoprol.†
Trypanosoma cruzi	Nifurtimox.†

* Antiparasitic drug of choice.
† Investigational drug, available in the USA through the Centers for Disease Control and Prevention.

Entamoeba histolytica. There are, however, other amebas found within the gastrointestinal tract. Diagnosis of amebic disease rests primarily on observing amebas in fecal samples and differentiating *E. histolytica* from the nonpathogenic amebas. Trophozoites are examined for the appearance of their **nucleus,** including the distribution of **chromatin** around the nuclear membrane, and for the size and position of the **karyosome,** or **nucleolus.** The cytoplasm is examined for the presence of bacteria and host cells, and wet mounts of fresh trophozoites are used to determine the extent of movement of motile trophozoites. Cysts are examined for the number and morphologies of nuclei, the presence of **chromatoid bars,** and the presence of **vacuoles.** Finally, the size of the ameba can be an important diagnostic clue. Of the intestinal amebas, only *Entamoeba coli* (a nonpathogen) and *E. histolytica* (a pathogen) are large amebas (see Fig. 24–1).

Characteristics of *Entamoeba histolytica*

General Features. The general morphologies of the trophozoites and cysts of *Entamoeba histolytica* are depicted in Fig. 24–1. Any population of amebas will contain some variants, so amebas in a sample are determined to be *E. histolytica* if most conform to the standard *E. histolytica* size and morphology.

The trophozoites of *E. histolytica* are 12–60 μm in diameter, with most being about 20 μm. Trophozoites are found in diarrheal stools. When fresh trophozoites are observed by wet mount microscopy on a warm slide, they move quickly and progressively, but nonpathogenic amebas are sluggish and seem to wander aimlessly. When stained appropriately, such as with trichrome, hematoxylin, or Lawless's stain, the cytoplasm of *E. histolytica* trophozoites looks "clean," with no cytoplasmic bacteria. In contrast, the cytoplasm of *Entamoeba coli* trophozoites looks "dirty" and contains many vacuoles and bacteria. *E. histolytica* is referred to as a **hematophagous ameba** because it sometimes phagocytoses erythrocytes. The pseudodopodia of *E. histolytica* are clear and translucent ("hyaline"), and their cytoplasm is referred to as ectoplasm. The most critical identifying feature of *E. histolytica* is its nucleus. The single nucleus contains a small, centrally located karyosome (see Fig. 24–1) and a clearly defined nuclear membrane that is lined on its inner aspect by a uniform layer of packed chromatin granules.

E. histolytica cysts are generally found in formed stools. The cysts are smaller than trophozoites and are usually 10–20 μm in diameter. Most cysts are spherical and have a hyaline cyst wall, but ovoid and irregular cysts are sometimes seen. Once again, the key to identification lies in examining the nuclei. *E. histolytica* cysts contain from one to four nuclei, so cysts that look like those of *E. histolytica* but contain more than four nuclei are considered to be *E. coli* cysts. The cyst nuclei generally look like the trophozoite nuclei, but many more atypical nuclei (with eccentric karyosomes or uneven chromatin) are seen among the cysts than among the trophozoites. *E. histolytica* cysts, particularly those with only one or two nuclei (immature cysts), may also contain one or more chromatoid bars with rounded or square ends. Chromatoid bars are crystalline RNA. *E. histolytica* cysts often contain a glycogen granule that can be stained with iodine.

Mechanisms of Pathogenicity. Humans are in-

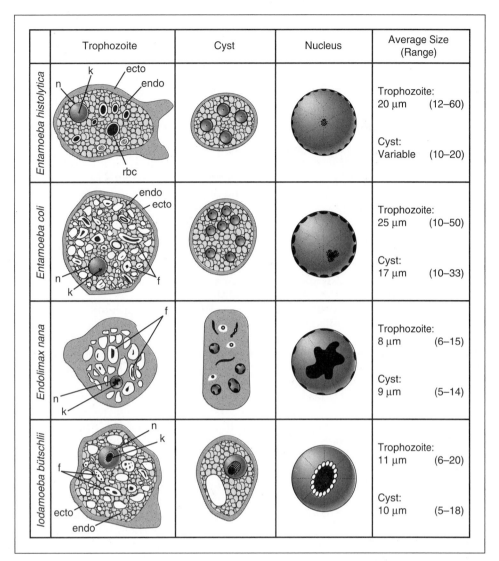

	Trophozoite	Cyst	Nucleus	Average Size (Range)
Entamoeba histolytica	k, ecto, n, endo, rbc			Trophozoite: 20 μm (12–60) Cyst: Variable (10–20)
Entamoeba coli	endo, ecto, n, k, f			Trophozoite: 25 μm (10–50) Cyst: 17 μm (10–33)
Endolimax nana	f, n, k			Trophozoite: 8 μm (6–15) Cyst: 9 μm (5–14)
Iodamoeba bütschlii	n, k, f, ecto, endo			Trophozoite: 11 μm (6–20) Cyst: 10 μm (5–18)

FIGURE 24–1. A comparison of the trophozoites, cysts, nuclei, and sizes of four species of ameba. *Entamoeba histolytica* is pathogenic, while the other three amebas (*Entamoeba coli, Endolimax nana,* and *Iodamoeba bütschlii*) are nonpathogenic. n = nucleus; k = karyosome; endo = endoplasm; ecto = ectoplasm; rbc = red blood cell; and f = food vacuole.

fected with *E. histolytica* when they ingest cysts in food or water. The cysts travel through the stomach to the lower small intestine, where they excyst. The trophozoites then travel to the large intestine, where they may be excreted or may establish a persistent infection.

Amebic trophozoites adhere to mucosal surfaces via a **lectin** that recognizes *N*- and *O*-linked oligosaccharides, particularly galactose (Gal) and *N*-acetyl-D-galactosamine (GalNAc). About 10% of *E. histolytica* strains are virulent, and virulence seems to correlate with the presence of the Gal-GalNAc lectin on the surface of the amebas. The lectin allows the amebas not only to adhere to the mucosa but also to adhere to and destroy polymorphonuclear leukocytes (PMNs). When the lectin is blocked with antibody, the amebas are rapidly destroyed by PMNs. Amebas kill the host cells to which they adhere via a calcium-dependent process that involves an extracellular product of the ameba—possibly phospholipase A, cysteine prote-

ase, a pore-forming protein called amebapore, or a combination of these. The Gal-GalNAc lectin is also involved in transmitting signals to the ameba, and it protects the ameba from complement-mediated lysis by blocking assembly of the C5b-9 membrane attack complex.

Amebas destroy cells from the outside and also engulf particles. These processes allow the amebas to invade the mucosa and enter the submucosa, where they are able to spread and erode the tissue. The amebas enter through a small opening on the mucosa but then generate a large submucosal ulceration. The combination of a narrow invasion pore and a large ulceration typically looks like a flask or urn in cross-section. Sigmoidoscopic examination may reveal that the mucosa looks fairly normal but has occasional small (10–12 mm) openings that mark the presence of the ulcerations. If the ulcerations are large and become interconnected, the overlying mucosa may slough off.

Invasive amebic infections may become chronic, leading to the formation of granulomatous material around a nidus of amebas in the bowel wall. The resulting amebomas are palpable masses that can be mistaken for annular carcinoma. More commonly, the amebas penetrate the abdominal wall and establish ectopic infections. The most common ectopic infection site is the liver, where a single amebic abscess usually forms. The amebas travel to the liver hematogenously, and most of the trophozoites probably do not survive within the liver. Other sites of ectopic amebic abscesses include the lungs, pericardium, peritoneum, brain, and kidney. Most abscesses in these sites arise from hematogenous spread of the amebas, but peritoneal infections may result from direct extension of an intestinal abscess, and some lung infections result from direct extension of a liver abscess.

No protective anamnestic immune response is generated against E. histolytica. There may be some PMN response in the intestine, but virulent amebas destroy PMNs. In general, there is little inflammatory response to the presence of amebas in the mucosa, and most of the cellular response seen is regenerative. The presence of PMNs in the stools of patients with amebic dysentery is usually a sign that there is a bacterial superinfection. Chronic infections involve a macrophage-type response that constructs a granuloma (ameboma) around the amebas. Virulent amebas are not killed or neutralized by antibody and complement, but invasive amebiasis elicits a vigorous (but ineffective) antibody response that can be monitored as a sign of disease progression. It appears that recovery from amebiasis occurs when activated macrophages kill amebas via a process that requires cell-to-cell contact but not antibody.

Diseases Due to *Entamoeba histolytica*

Epidemiology. *E. histolytica* is spread from person to person primarily via the fecal-oral route. The amebas may be ingested in food or water contaminated with human feces, but the amount of contamination needed to reliably transmit the organisms is small. The amebas can be transmitted on contaminated fingers of humans and on the feet of flies and cockroaches. Some transmission also occurs during anal intercourse, and surveys have indicated that up to 30% of male homosexuals have been infected with *E. histolytica.*

About 10% of the world's population is estimated to be infected at any one time with *E. histolytica.* Of those infected, fewer than 10% suffer from clinically apparent disease. This is in part because at least 90% of *E. histolytica* strains are not virulent. Virulent and avirulent strains are not morphologically distinguishable, but they can be differentiated by zymodeme (isozyme) electrophoretic patterns and by the presence or absence of the Gal-GalNAc lectin. Some host factors are probably involved in predilection to disease. For example, patients treated with corticosteroids may develop a more severe form of amebic colitis than they previously experienced. This suggests that there is an immune component to susceptibility to severe disease. Yet it appears that patients with AIDS are not susceptible to disease when infected with avirulent strains of *E. histolytica.*

Amebiasis is most common in tropical and subtropical countries where sanitation is poor, "night soil" (human waste) is used as fertilizer, and the population suffers from dietary deficiencies. The prevalence in some countries exceeds 50%. In the USA, the prevalence is between 1% and 5%.

The *E. histolytica* infective stage is the cyst. Patients with acute colitis or dysentery are not an epidemiologic problem, because they shed only trophozoites. Patients with chronic infections intermittently pass trophozoites or cysts, but infected individuals who are asymptomatic pass only cysts. Thus, the most important link in the epidemiologic chain is not the patient with diarrhea but the asymptomatic or chronically infected individual who passes formed stools.

Diagnosis. Patients with intestinal *E. histolytica* infections fall into four major groups: those without symptoms, those with acute amebic colitis, those with fulminant amebic colitis, and those with ameboma.

(1) History and Physical Examination. Patients with **acute amebic colitis** may suffer from **nondysenteric colitis** or from **amebic dysentery.** The name "dysentery" literally means "sick gut," a condition that was described by Hippocrates some 2400 years ago. Dysentery is characterized by blood and mucus in the stools. Patients without these manifestations have nondysenteric colitis.

Acute amebic colitis begins from 1 to 14 weeks after an individual has ingested cysts of *E. histolytica.* Symptoms and signs include cramping, abdominal pain, and diarrhea alternating with constipation. Stools are mushy, watery, and foul-smelling, and they may contain blood and mucus. The abdomen is tender, and the liver may be slightly enlarged. Bacterial superinfection is common and is heralded by moderate leukocytosis. The disease lasts up to 4 weeks in about 85% of patients. Some patients develop intestinal perforations secondary to erosion of the mucosa by an ulcer. The onset of this condition may be dramatic, with the rapid occurrence of peritonitis and abdominal rigidity, or it may be gradual, leading to abdominal distention, ileus, and the collection of gas in the peritoneum. The most common complication, however, is the hematogenous dissemination of amebas and the establishment of hepatic abscesses.

Fulminant amebic colitis is an uncommon disease that occurs mainly in children. Profuse bloody diarrhea is accompanied by fever and abdominal pain. Patients may experience intestinal perforations and often have a concurrent hepatic abscess.

An **ameboma** is a granuloma surrounding an amebic nidus, usually in the cecum or rectosigmoid region. The mass is palpable, can be seen on x-rays, and may be confused with carcinoma. The ameboma may be painless or tender, and some patients suffer from concurrent chronic amebic colitis.

The most common severe complication of amebiasis is the development of **amebic hepatic abscesses.** The amebic trophozoites enter the liver through the portal vein. As a result, about 90% of abscesses are in the right lobe of the liver. Only about half of the affected patients recall having suffered from amebic colitis prior to their attack of hepatic disease. The hepatic abscesses may be associated with an acute or subacute course. While symptoms of acute disease usually last for 10 days or less, those of subacute disease may last up to 6 months. Manifestations typically include cough, fever that peaks in the afternoon, night sweats, weight loss, anemia, leukocytosis, a tender and enlarged liver, and pain that originates in the right upper quadrant and is often referred to the right shoulder. Between 10% and 15% of patients have no abdominal pain and present only with a low-grade fever. About one-third of patients suffer from diarrhea.

There are numerous complications of amebic hepatic abscesses. In about 20–35% of cases, an abscess extends into the contiguous lung lobe and causes pleural effusions with pleuritic pain and cough. If the abscess ruptures into the pleural cavity, it causes empyema, with the sudden onset of severe pleuritic pain and respiratory distress. The most dangerous complication of amebic hepatic abscess is spread of the amebas into the pericardium, usually from a left lobe liver abscess. Shock may ensue, leading to death in about 40% of patients.

(2) Laboratory Analysis. The diagnosis of intestinal amebiasis depends on identifying *E. histolytica* trophozoites, cysts, or both in stool specimens. The use of antidiarrheal agents and enemas makes diagnosis difficult because it destroys trophozoites and damages cysts. When amebas are hard to find, their recovery can be increased by obtaining a scraping or biopsy from the edge of an amebic ulceration during colonoscopy. Fresh, unstained specimens can be examined by wet mount for the presence of progressively motile amebas. Fresh samples can be stained with trichrome stain or iodine to visualize the nuclei in trophozoites and the nuclei and chromatoid bars in cysts. Stool sample concentrates can be stained with iron hematoxylin stain. Biopsy samples should be stained with periodic acid–Schiff (PAS) stain.

Although cultures of clinical samples are not performed routinely, *E. histolytica* can be cultivated in TYI-S-33 medium. Serologic tests can also be used to diagnose invasive amebiasis (dysentery). In 85–95% of patients with dysentery, antibody develops and can be detected by enzyme-linked immunosorbent assay (ELISA), agar gel diffusion, or counterimmunoelectrophoresis (CIE). Results in these tests become negative 6–12 months after resolution of amebiasis. Indirect hemagglutination (IHA) tests are not as useful, because patients remain IHA-positive for as long as 10 years. In cases of suspected amebic colitis, invasive radiologic studies should not be performed, because they place the patient at risk of colonic perforation.

Ectopic amebiasis can be diagnosed with noninvasive radiographic techniques such as magnetic resonance imaging, computed tomography, and ultrasonography. Serologic tests for amebas will also be positive, and patients typically exhibit leukocytosis and anemia. Although eosinophilia accompanies many invasive parasitic diseases, it is not found in cases of ectopic amebiasis. If the patient has a pulmonary infection, the amebas may be seen in the sputum. Amebas are not usually found within fluid drawn from amebic hepatic abscesses but are seen in the parenchyma itself. Amebas can be found in stool samples from about one-third of patients with amebic hepatic abscesses.

Treatment. There are two types of antiamebic drugs: luminal amebicides and tissue amebicides. Luminal amebicides can be used to treat patients with asymptomatic infections. Tissue amebicides should be used to treat dysentery and hepatic abscesses and can be given either alone or in combination with a luminal amebicide. The key luminal amebicides are iodoquinol, paromomycin, and diloxanide furoate (see Table 24–1). Metronidazole is the mainstay of treatment for invasive amebiasis, since it kills both luminal and tissue amebas and it concentrates in the liver. Ornidazole and tinidazole (two better-tolerated nitroimidazoles) are not available in the USA but are the preferred drugs in some countries. Other tissue amebicides include dehydroemetine, emetine hydrochloride, tetracycline, erythromycin, and chloroquine. Chloroquine is effective only against amebas in the liver, while tetracycline and erythromycin will not eliminate luminal and hepatic amebas. Corticosteroids should not be used, because they may cause the patient to develop a life-threatening form of colitis.

Prevention. Amebiasis is generally acquired from feces-contaminated water or food. The key to prevention is to break the transmission cycle. Travelers to areas with poor sanitation should boil or iodinate water before drinking it or using it to make ice, to brush teeth, or to wash dishes, vegetables, salads, and fruits. Vegetables fertilized with "night soil" must be thoroughly cooked. Asymptomatic patients who shed cysts should be excluded from food preparation until they have been treated and shown to be free of infection.

In some countries, a drug called Entero-Vioform (iodochlorhydroxyquin) is sold as a prophylaxis against amebiasis. This drug is ineffective and causes severe eye disease, so it should not be used.

Characteristics of *Naegleria fowleri*

General Features. *Naegleria fowleri* is a free-living ameba. It is found in warm brackish water and in soil and occasionally causes primary amebic meningoencephalitis (PAM), a fatal disease. *N. fowleri* differs from the strictly parasitic amebas in that it has a flagellate stage and is therefore considered to be an **ameboflagellate.** In the flagellate stage, *Naegleria* is somewhat sluglike in shape and has two prominent flagella. Forms of the organism seen in water include cysts and ameboid and flagellated trophozoites. Only the ameboid forms are seen in the tissues and cerebrospinal fluid of infected humans.

Mechanisms of Pathogenicity. Most infections have occurred after an individual has been swimming in brackish water, but some have occurred after swimming in warm pools that contained chlorinated water. The amebas are believed to enter through the nose during swimming, pass through the olfactory epithelium and cribriform plate, and travel along the olfactory nerve to the olfactory bulb. The amebas invade the gray matter of the olfactory lobes and cerebral cortex, where they cause hemorrhage and necrosis. Some focal demyelination of the brain and spinal cord also occurs.

Diseases Due to *Naegleria fowleri*

Epidemiology. Close to 150 cases of PAM have been described since the first case was reported in 1965. Because the amebas flourish when water is warm, cases usually occur during the summer. Most victims are healthy young people who become ill after swimming. The majority of the cases have occurred in Australia, Czechoslovakia (now the Czech Republic and Slovakia), and the USA, but individual cases have been reported in a number of countries. In the USA, most cases of PAM have occurred in Florida, Texas, and Virginia.

During one 3-year period in Czechoslovakia, sixteen young people died of PAM after swimming in the same heated and chlorinated indoor swimming pool. Other sources of infection have been ponds, lakes, streams, and water used in religious purification rites. *Naegleria* is a common organism. In one survey, a single water sample was taken from each of 26 lakes in Florida. Half of these samples contained *Naegleria*, with some containing one ameba per 25 mL of water.

Diagnosis

(1) History and Physical Examination. Up to 8 days after the patient is exposed to amebas, **primary amebic meningoencephalitis** (PAM) begins with headache and fever. This prodrome is followed in a few days by nausea, vomiting, stiff neck, and other signs of meningoencephalitis. The olfactory lobe is usually affected most severely at first, causing disturbances in the senses of taste and smell. The cerebellar, frontal, and temporal areas also become severely affected. Manifestations include a positive Kernig's sign, seizures, and personality changes. Patients usually become irrational shortly before lapsing into a coma, and death follows closely thereafter. The entire clinical course lasts 3–7 days.

(2) Laboratory Analysis. The cerebrospinal fluid (CSF) of patients is cloudy and contains many neutrophils and some erythrocytes. Neutrophils in the CSF, low glucose levels, increased spinal pressure, and the absence of bacteria are suggestive of *Naegleria* infection in a patient with fulminant meningitis. Amebas may be seen in fresh (unrefrigerated) CSF samples. These can be put into distilled water to convert them to their ameboflagellate stage. Ameboflagellate forms begin to appear in about 1 hour, with maximum exflagellation occurring after 4–5 hours. Cysts are never found in clinical samples.

Unfortunately, definitive diagnosis of PAM often

occurs postmortem with the demonstration of amebas in the brain and CSF. Rounded amebas that are 10–11 μm in diameter are found in the gray matter of the brain, just ahead of the advancing margin of hemorrhage and necrosis. The nucleus of each ameba contains a large karyosome, and unusual phagocytic structures known as amebostomes can be seen.

Treatment and Prognosis. In only 3 of the 150 reported cases of PAM have the patients survived. Two survivors were treated with amphotericin B administered both intravenously and intrathecally. The combination of amphotericin B and rifampin has proved effective against experimental *Naegleria* infections in mice.

Prevention. *Naegleria* populations can be controlled in swimming pools by keeping the chlorine level at or above 0.5 mg/L at all times.

Characteristics of *Acanthamoeba*

Acanthamoeba is a free-living ameba whose name is derived from the thorny or spiked shape of its pseudopodia (*akantha* in Greek means "thorn"). *Acanthamoeba* is seen in soil, water, and air. Ameboid trophozoites and cysts are found throughout the environment, but *Acanthamoeba* is not an ameboflagellate.

At least six species of *Acanthamoeba* have been associated with human disease. *Acanthamoeba castellani* and *Acanthamoeba rhysodes* cause meningitis in immunosuppressed patients and keratitis in individuals who wear contact lenses. *Acanthamoeba astronyxis* and *Acanthamoeba palestinensis* cause only meningitis, and *Acanthamoeba hatchetti* and *Acanthamoeba polyphaga* cause only keratitis. Meningitis caused by *Acanthamoeba* is a chronic, granulomatous form of disease and is referred to as granulomatous amebic encephalitis (GAE) to distinguish it from the acute meningitis caused by *Naegleria*.

Diseases Due to *Acanthamoeba*

Epidemiology. Unlike primary acute meningoencephalitis (PAM) due to *Naegleria*, GAE due to *Acanthamoeba* does not occur as a consequence of swimming. Instead, the key risk factor is the immune status of the patient. Patients with GAE are immunosuppressed or have a debilitating condition such as lymphoma or poorly controlled diabetes. Investigators believe that the amebas enter through the lungs or abrasions and travel to the brain through the blood.

The majority of cases of amebic keratitis occur in individuals who wear contact lenses and have either suffered eye trauma or have used nonsterile wash solutions to clean their lenses. In about 90% of reported cases, the patients have been wearing soft lenses. About two-thirds of these were infected when they used home-made saline solutions, and most of the rest were infected when they rinsed their lenses with tap water.

Diagnosis

(1) History and Physical Examination. Although the course of **granulomatous amebic encephalitis** (GAE) is usually prolonged, some AIDS patients with *Acanthamoeba* infections have experienced fulminating disease that was indistinguishable from PAM. Disseminated *Acanthamoeba* infections have also been seen in patients with AIDS.

Non-AIDS patients with GAE have neurologic signs and symptoms similar to those seen in patients with PAM. The major difference is that GAE usually lasts weeks to months. In a few patients, it has lasted for several years. The disease may begin with granulomatous infections of the gastric wall, lung, skull, middle ear, scalp, or orbit. The amebas probably enter the brain through the blood and initiate infection deep within the brain. As the amebas move toward the surface of the brain, a granulomatous response is elicited. The clinical signs of encephalitis match the area of the brain that is infected at that time.

Patients with **amebic keratitis** usually wear contact lenses and have no underlying medical condition other than mild trauma to the eye. Manifestations of keratitis include inflammation, severe pain, a neutrophilic exudate, and gradual ulceration of the cornea. Early signs include the development of a superficial punctate keratitis and edema. If the disease persists, the eye may become perforated. The extreme pain of amebic keratitis is believed to be due to infection of nerves by the amebas.

(2) Laboratory Analysis.   A diagnosis of GAE is confirmed by identifying the trophozoites of *Acanthamoeba* species in CSF or the trophozoites and cysts in brain tissue. The trophozoites are slow-moving, are 11–47 μm in diameter, and have acanthopodia (spiked pseudopodia). The trophozoites and cysts can be stained with immunofluorescence methods to confirm their identity.

Amebic keratitis is diagnosed by finding *Acanthamoeba* trophozoites or cysts in corneal scrapings. The samples are examined directly by microscopy and are cultured in vitro. Then immunofluorescence techniques are used to determine the ameba species.

Treatment and Prognosis.   There is no satisfactory treatment for GAE. The current recommendation is to treat patients with amphotericin B. The fatality rate of GAE approaches 100%.

Amebic keratitis has been treated successfully with a diamidine drug (such as propamidine or dibromopropamidine isethionate) used in combination with neomycin. It has also been treated successfully with a combination of oral itraconazole, topical miconazole, and surgical debridement of lesions. When treatment is not successful, the possibility of secondary bacterial infection of the eye should be investigated.

Ciliates

Characteristics of *Balantidium coli*

Balantidium coli (Fig. 24–2) is the only ciliate that causes human disease. *B. coli* trophozoites vary in size. Small trophozoites are 42–60 μm in length, while large trophozoites are usually 90–120 μm but are

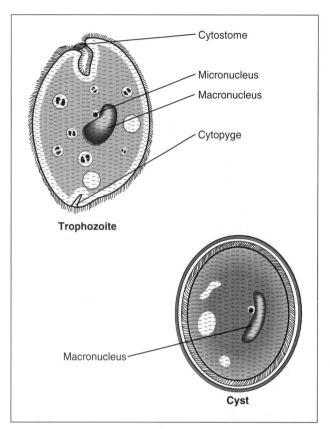

FIGURE 24–2. The trophozoite and cyst of *Balantidium coli*.

occasionally as large as 200 μm. Each trophozoite is covered with a layer of cilia, has a cytostome (mouth-like opening) and a cytopyge (excretory pore) at opposite ends, and has a macronucleus and a micronucleus. The larger, kidney-shaped macronucleus is easily seen in stained preparations, but the micronucleus is difficult to see. Two contractile vacuoles can be seen within the cytoplasm.

B. coli trophozoites can be found in the mucosa and submucosa of the cecum and terminal portion of the ileum. Their cilia give them a rotary motion that is similar to the movement of a thrown football. This motion, along with the extreme plasticity of the organisms, allows them to bore into the mucosa. Mucosal invasion is also facilitated by the production of an extracellular hyaluronidase by *Balantidium*.

B. coli cysts are 50–72 μm in diameter, have a double cyst wall, have no cytostome or cytopyge, and exhibit only a single nucleus (the macronucleus). Newly formed cysts have cilia, but the older cysts do not. The cysts are resistant to environmental conditions and can survive outside the body for several weeks.

Diseases Due to *Balantidium coli*

Epidemiology.   *B. coli* cysts are the infective form of the organism. Humans become infected when they ingest cysts in food or water contaminated with human or hog feces. In countries with temperate climates and good sanitation, humans usually acquire the infection from other humans. In the tropics, hogs are an important source of *B. coli*. Balantidiasis is rare in the USA but is occasionally seen among closed populations, such as among residents in mental hospitals. Balantidiasis is most common in tropical and subtropical countries, especially those in which humans and hogs live in close proximity.

Diagnosis. *Balantidium* infections range in severity from asymptomatic carriage to severe **dysentery** that mimics amebic dysentery. *Balantidium* penetrates the mucosa and forms small nests that are seen as mucosal abscesses. The abscesses progress to become ulcerations with red, undermined edges. The ulcerations may be limited in scope or may lead to massive areas of necrosis. Secondary bacterial infection can lead to an intense inflammatory response.

Patients with **acute balantidiasis** suffer from colitis with 6–15 liquid stools per day. The stools typically contain blood, mucus, and pus. *Balantidium* infections remain in the intestine and do not spread to the liver or other ectopic sites.

A diagnosis of balantidiasis is best confirmed by observing *Balantidium* trophozoites and cysts in wet mounts made from stool samples. The use of standard stains, such as trichrome, is sometimes less effective because the parasites often stain very darkly.

Treatment. The drug of choice for balantidiasis is oxytetracycline. Balantidiasis also responds well to treatment with iodoquinol or metronidazole.

Lumen-Dwelling Flagellates
Characteristics of *Dientamoeba fragilis*

Dientamoeba fragilis is found in the intestine as an ameboid trophozoite. The organism has no cyst stage. Until recently, *D. fragilis* was thought to be an ameba, but ultrastructural studies have shown that it contains structures usually found only within flagellates.

The trophozoite of *D. fragilis* (Fig. 24–3) usually contains two nuclei and is said to be in arrested telophase. Each nucleus contains three to five chromatin granules, and there is no peripheral chromatin along the nuclear membrane. The cell cytoplasm is usually vacuolated and contains debris. The trophozoites

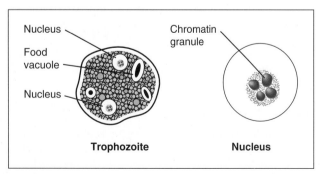

FIGURE 24–3. The trophozoite and nucleus of *Dientamoeba fragilis*.

range from 3 to 18 μm in diameter, but most are between 9 and 12 μm.

Diseases Due to *Dientamoeba fragilis*

D. fragilis lives in the human intestinal lumen and is carried by about 20% of the world's population. In some countries, more than 50% of the populace is infected with *D. fragilis*. Most infected individuals are asymptomatic. The route of infection is unknown, but since the organism has been seen within *Enterobius* (pinworm) eggs, it may be passed within the eggs of nematodes.

Between 15% and 27% of individuals infected with *D. fragilis* are symptomatic, and the most common clinical condition is intermittent, long-standing **diarrhea** and fatigue. In about 20% of patients, the stools contain blood, mucus, or both. Eosinophilia may be present and appears to coincide with the presence of nematodes. Symptoms are often more severe in children than in adults and may include abdominal pain, anorexia, flatulence, intermittent diarrhea, malaise, fatigue, and lack of proper weight gain. The diagnosis is confirmed by identifying the trophozoites in stool samples.

D. fragilis infections are treated with iodoquinol or tetracycline.

Characteristics of *Giardia lamblia*

Giardia lamblia is the most frequently isolated human intestinal protozoan and is a common cause of diarrhea in humans, dogs, and cats. The organism was first described in 1681 by Antonie van Leeuwenhoek, who discovered the parasite in his own feces. Although *Giardia* was long suspected to be a human pathogen, it was not until the 1970s that epidemiologic evidence convinced most scientists that the organism was a significant cause of diarrhea in humans.

General Features. *Giardia* has a simple life cycle, existing only in the form of flagellated trophozoites and semidormant cysts. The cysts are resistant to environmental conditions and have about 20% of the metabolic activity that trophozoites have. They are the infective form of the organism and are the form most often found in stool samples from infected patients.

The trophozoites and cysts of *G. lamblia* (Fig. 24–4) are possibly the most easily recognized among the protozoa. The trophozoite is 10–12 μm long and 5–7 μm wide, is bisected by two central axostyles, and has two nuclei, four pairs of flagella, and a pair of centralized parabasal bodies. The nuclei are equal in size and content, and both are transcriptionally active. Most of the ventral surface is occupied by a large sucking disk that is believed to be the critical organ of attachment to the host intestinal mucosa. The flagella propel the trophozoite in a jerky motion similar to that of a falling leaf. The *Giardia* cyst is oval and 9–12 μm long, and it may contain two or four nuclei. The internal structures seen in the trophozoite are arranged in a "jumble" within the cyst.

Mechanisms of Pathogenicity. The means by

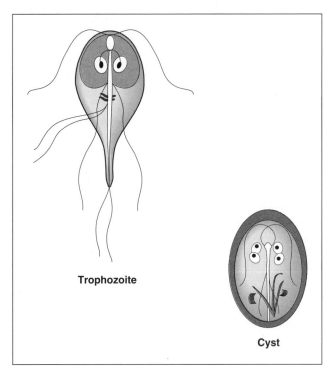

FIGURE 24–4. The trophozoite and cyst of *Giardia lamblia*.

Trophozoite

Cyst

augment recovery from infection, and activated macrophages can kill *Giardia* in mice. Recovery from giardiasis does not confer lasting immunity, and reinfection is common.

Diseases Due to *Giardia lamblia*

Epidemiology. Giardiasis is a cosmopolitan disease, but it occurs more frequently where sanitation is poor. Humans are infected when they ingest the cysts of *Giardia*. The organism is generally spread from person to person via contaminated surface water, but it can also be spread via anal intercourse, ingestion of contaminated food, or hand-to-mouth contact. Epidemics of giardiasis often begin in children in day-care centers. The children may have an asymptomatic infection and spread it to their parents. In some cases, disease is spread from animals to humans. Beavers are most closely linked to human cases.

Worldwide, the regions of greatest risk are Mexico, western South America, the former Soviet Union, tropical Africa, and southeastern and southern Asia. In the USA, giardiasis is most common in the western states and often occurs among campers who drink water from streams and ponds. Water-borne infections are more common in cooler climates, probably because the cysts survive for only about 4 days at 37 °C but can survive and remain infective for more than 2 months at 4 °C.

Diagnosis

(1) History and Physical Examination. Infection with *Giardia* can be asymptomatic, can cause acute disease, or can develop into chronic recurrent diarrhea with malabsorption.

Acute giardiasis begins 9–15 days after the patient ingests *Giardia* cysts. Although infection can begin after the ingestion of a single cyst, about one-third of volunteers who ingested 10–25 cysts developed giardiasis, and all patients who ingested 100 or more cysts did so. The length of the incubation period is related to the number of cysts that the patient ingests. Patients initially feel nauseated and experience some gastrointestinal uneasiness. This is followed by the development of an explosive, foul-smelling, frothy diarrhea that is accompanied by abdominal distention and belching. Patients may develop lactose intolerance, and stool samples are found to contain fat. The acute phase of giardiasis generally lasts 3–4 days.

Most patients recover from acute giardiasis, but some develop **chronic recurrent diarrhea,** which may last 2 years or longer and is often accompanied by headache, lassitude, myalgia, and weight loss. The stools may contain excess fat, and patients may suffer from malabsorption of fat, vitamins A and B_{12}, lactose, and xylose.

(2) Laboratory Analysis. The diagnosis is confirmed by demonstrating the presence of *Giardia* in stool samples. Symptoms of giardiasis begin 1–7 days before cysts can be found in the stool. Because the organisms are shed intermittently, a series of three

which *Giardia* produces diarrhea are not known. Cysts pass through the stomach to the duodenum, where they excyst, possibly under the influence of pancreatic secretions. Within 30 minutes, the excysted organism divides into two binuclear trophozoites. The trophozoites live in the lumen of the intestine and attach to the intestinal mucosa. The primary attachment organ is the ventral sucking disk, but a lectin may play a secondary role in attachment. In infected humans, the mucosa is only rarely invaded, and extraintestinal giardiasis is unknown.

In infected mice, superficial invasion of the mucosa has been associated with steatorrhea (an excessive amount of fat in the feces), but mucosal invasion is also a rare event. *Giardia* trophozoites adhere tenaciously to the mucosa, leaving a mark on the mucosal wall. Some investigators have postulated that this tenacious adhesion irritates the bowel and induces diarrhea. Others have noted that giardiasis often results in disaccharidase deficiencies and that deficiencies in lactase, xylase, and sucrase may initiate osmotic diarrhea. Infection causes shortening or flattening of the intestinal villi, and this may also contribute to the diarrheal state. The trophozoites tend to aggregate in groups on the intestinal wall, and some investigators have suggested that this mechanically obstructs the absorption of fats and fat-soluble vitamins. Finally, a few investigators, noting that there seems to be variation in virulence among isolates, have suggested that some *Giardia* strains produce an enterotoxin.

Recovery from giardiasis is believed to be primarily related to development of secretory IgA against the parasite. T cell–mediated immunity may

stool samples should be taken on alternating days or spaced within a 10-day period. The organisms are fragile, so the best results are obtained by fixing fresh samples and then staining them with trichrome or iron hematoxylin stain. Fresh (unfixed) stool samples can be examined in wet saline preparations for the presence of motile trophozoites. However, unless the patient has acute diarrhea, stool samples are likely to contain only cysts.

If *Giardia* cannot be found in stool samples, fluid from the duodenojejunal junction can be obtained via endoscopy and examined. The duodenal string test can also be used as needed to collect duodenal samples. If these methods are unsuccessful, a biopsy of tissue from the duodenojejunal junction should be taken. The biopsy specimen is used to make an imprint smear, which is subsequently stained with Giemsa stain and examined for the presence of *Giardia* trophozoites.

Treatment and Prognosis. In the USA, metronidazole is the antiparasitic drug used most often to treat giardiasis. When administered for 5 days, it is about 90% effective. In countries where it is available, tinidazole is widely used because it is as effective as metronidazole, is better tolerated, and can be administered in a single dose. Quinacrine is effective when given for 5–10 days, but it is not tolerated as well as metronidazole, making patient compliance more difficult. Furazolidone and paromomycin are less effective than the nitroimidazoles or quinacrine but are sometimes used to treat children or pregnant women.

Patients who relapse after completion of one of the above regimens usually respond to a second course of treatment with the same drug or an alternative drug.

Prevention. Water that may contain *Giardia* cysts must be treated to make it potable. Sand filtration is an effective means of removing *Giardia* cysts. Cysts can also be killed by boiling water for 1 minute or by adding 2–4 drops of household bleach or 0.5 mL of 2% tincture of iodine to each liter of water to be used for drinking. The water should be allowed to sit for at least 1 hour if the water is warm or overnight if the water is cold.

Characteristics of *Trichomonas vaginalis*

Trichomonas vaginalis is a member of the family Trichomonadidae. The organisms in this family received their name because they were each thought to possess three flagella. The family is now divided into three genera: *Tritrichomonas* has three flagella; *Trichomonas* has four flagella; and *Pentatrichomonas* has five flagella. Three species are found in humans: *Pentatrichomonas hominis* is an intestinal commensal; *Trichomonas tenax* is a nonpathogenic inhabitant of the mouth; and *T. vaginalis* is a sexually transmitted pathogen of the genitourinary tract.

General Features. *T. vaginalis* is the largest of the human trichomonads and is the only one known to cause human disease. The organism has no cyst form. Trophozoites (Fig. 24–5) range from 5 to 29 μm in length, but most are about 13 μm long. Each trophozoite has a single nucleus and four anterior flagella that extend upward from a V-shaped structure known as the pelta. A parabasal body lies next to the nucleus, and an undulating membrane lies between the costa and a recurrent flagellum. The anterior flagella propel the organism, and the undulating membrane causes the trophozoite to rotate as it moves. A sharp rod called the axostyle transects the parasite and extends outward from the posterior end. The axostyle, costa, and single nucleus are key characteristics used to identify *T. vaginalis*.

Mechanisms of Pathogenicity. *T. vaginalis* infections are generally asymptomatic in men but cause vaginitis in women. The mechanism of mucosal damage is not well understood, but investigators have identified at least four proteins that mediate adherence of *T. vaginalis* to host cells. Once the trichomonads attach to the mucosa, they kill epithelial cells in a contact-dependent process that does not involve phagocytosis. The trichomonads also produce a factor that causes cells to detach from the mucosa. The killing and detachment of cells may cause the vaginal mucosa to erode significantly, resulting in discomfort and the production of a vaginal discharge.

Diseases Due to *Trichomonas vaginalis*

Epidemiology. Each year, an estimated 200 million individuals are infected with *T. vaginalis,* a sexually transmitted parasite. The fact that men are usually asymptomatic is an important factor in the dissemination of disease. In the USA, 10–30% of

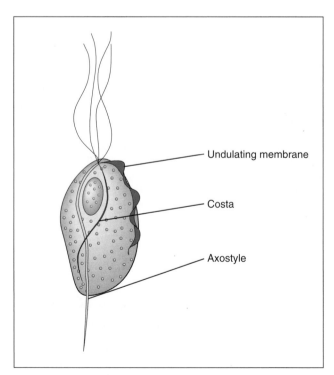

FIGURE 24–5. The trophozoite of *Trichomonas vaginalis*.

women and 5–15% of men are infected. In some tropical countries, infection rates approach 40%. Conditions that raise vaginal pH (such as pregnancy, menstruation, trauma, and bacterial infections) are believed to increase susceptibility to infection with *T. vaginalis.*

Diagnosis.   Often, the only signs of infection in men are the generation of a thin discharge and the presence of dysuria and nocturia. There may be pain if the prostate and epididymis become infected.

Most women infected with *T. vaginalis* develop persistent **vaginitis,** characterized by itching, chafing, and burning of the vaginal mucosa. In some cases, the vaginal discharge is purulent. The vaginal mucosa may look normal or may be hyperemic with bright red punctate lesions. Infected women occasionally develop **cystitis** and often develop **urethritis,** with accompanying dysuria and increased urinary frequency.

The diagnosis is usually confirmed by demonstrating the presence of organisms in a wet film or in a Papanicolaou smear. The organisms can be collected through a speculum on a cotton-tipped applicator, placed in saline, and observed via phase-contrast microscopy. There is no need to differentiate them from other trichomonads, because *T. vaginalis* is the only trichomonad that will infect the human genital tract. Standard protozoan stains (such as trichrome and iron hematoxylin) are not used, because the organisms stain poorly.

Trichomonas can also be cultured in modified Diamond's medium, where the organisms can be easily found after 2–4 days of incubation.

Treatment and Prognosis.   Trichomoniasis responds to treatment with metronidazole. Patients and their sexual contacts must be treated. Otherwise, reinfection is likely.

Intestinal Sporozoans

Characteristics of *Cryptosporidium parvum*

Cryptosporidium is a member of the phylum Apicomplexa (see Chapter 23 and Table 23–1) and has two reproductive cycles: **gametogony** (a sexual cycle) and **schizogony** (an asexual cycle). The genus *Cryptosporidium* is found within the family Cryptosporiidae, and its members are related to the parasites that cause isosporiasis and toxoplasmosis. Although the genus includes four species, *Cryptosporidium parvum* is the only species that causes human disease.

C. parvum undergoes gametogony and schizogony within the intestinal epithelium of humans and other mammalian hosts. Gametogony produces the infective form of the organism, the **oocyst.** Each oocyst is oval, is 4–6 μm in length, and contains from one to six **sporozoites.** Schizogony takes place within a vacuole inside host cells at the microvillous surface of the mucosa. In human hosts, the mechanism by which *Cryptosporidium* causes diarrhea is not well understood but probably is related to parasitic damage to the mucosa. The importance of the immune

system is evidenced by the unusual susceptibility of AIDS patients to severe cryptosporidiosis.

Diseases Due to *Cryptosporidium parvum*

Epidemiology.   *C. parvum* infects a wide variety of mammals. In the past, epidemiologists believed that most infections in humans were acquired from kittens, puppies, rodents, and calves. However, evidence derived from improved methods to detect the organism and from recent outbreaks of cryptosporidiosis indicates that spread from human to human is an important means of transmission.

In day-care centers, person-to-person spread may occur via the fecal-oral route. In many large-scale outbreaks, spread is via contaminated water. In a water-borne outbreak in Milwaukee, Wisconsin, an estimated 281,000 people were infected, and 7 died. The infective stage of *C. parvum* is the oocyst, and public health officials found that organisms in this stage are unusually resistant to standard chlorination and sand-filtering techniques used by community water treatment facilities.

Cryptosporidiosis is extremely common in tropical countries with poor sanitation and may be a common cause of traveler's diarrhea. It is the most frequent cause of diarrhea in AIDS patients.

Diagnosis.   In immunocompetent individuals, *C. parvum* causes watery **diarrhea** that is commonly associated with cramping, nausea, and vomiting. In some cases, mucus is seen in the stool. The diarrhea usually persists for several days to 2 weeks, but malnourished children may suffer from protracted diarrhea.

In individuals with AIDS, *C. parvum* can cause a life-threatening form of watery diarrhea. Patients may lose as much as 17 L of fluid in a day. The severity of the diarrhea seems to be generally related to the degree of immunosuppression. In some cases, the organism invades the biliary duct and causes fever, jaundice, right upper quadrant pain, and vomiting. In rare cases, AIDS patients have developed pulmonary cryptosporidiosis.

Cryptosporidiosis can be diagnosed by demonstrating the presence of *C. parvum* oocysts in diarrheal stool samples or the presence of *C. parvum* schizonts and gametocytes in tissue biopsies taken from the intestine. The preferred method is to concentrate the organisms in stool samples by using a flotation technique and then to identify the organisms by phase-contrast microscopy or staining methods. Standard stains used to identify intestinal protozoa do not stain *Cryptosporidium* adequately, so the samples should be stained with acid-fast stains, with auramine-rhodamine stains, or by use of fluorescein-conjugated monoclonal antibodies.

Treatment.   Patients should be rehydrated as needed. There is no adequate specific treatment for cryptosporidiosis. Spiramycin was used in the past, but recent studies have shown that it is ineffective in halting the disease.

Characteristics of *Isospora belli*

Isospora belli differs from *Cryptosporidium parvum* in that it infects only humans. Like *Cryptosporidium*, *Isospora* goes through sexual and asexual reproductive cycles in the intestinal mucosa. Gametogony results in the formation of *Isospora* **oocysts,** the infective organisms. Each oocyst is 20–33 μm long by 10–19 μm wide and contains one or two **sporocysts.** When sporocysts pass from the host, each one develops in 4–5 days and generates four **sporozoites.** When oocysts pass from the host, they can remain viable and infective for months as long as they are in water.

Multiplication of *Isospora* within the intestinal epithelium results in destruction of much of the intestinal mucosa. Villous atrophy is accompanied by fat malabsorption.

Diseases Due to *Isospora belli*

Isospora is transmitted via the fecal-oral route. In most cases, the infection is thought to be acquired from feces-contaminated water. Infected individuals may be asymptomatic, may have a self-limiting form of **diarrhea,** or may suffer from diarrhea and fat malabsorption that lasts months to years.

Infected patients usually pass from 6 to 10 watery or soft and mushy stools per day. In some cases, stools are foul-smelling and frothy and are accompanied by weight loss and malabsorption of fats and fat-soluble vitamins. Patients with AIDS suffer from profuse diarrhea that is accompanied by weight loss, anorexia, and weakness. The diagnosis is confirmed by identifying the oocysts of *Isospora* in wet mounts.

Diarrhea caused by *Isospora* is treated by rehydrating patients as needed and by administering a combination of trimethoprim plus sulfamethoxazole or a combination of sulfadiazine plus pyrimethamine.

Microsporidia

The microsporidia are obligately intracellular parasites that are considered to be primitive because they lack many of the intracellular organelles usually seen in eukaryotic cells. Although several members of the order Microsporida have been identified as isolated causes of human disease, the most common one is *Enterocytozoon bieneusi.*

In AIDS patients, microsporidia cause intractable diarrhea, accompanied by anorexia and nausea. Patients typically pass from four to eight watery stools per day and are often dehydrated and have signs of malabsorption. The diagnosis can be confirmed by demonstrating that microsporidia are present in Giemsa-stained touch impressions or sections of biopsy material. Alternatively, the diagnosis can be made by examining cytocentrifuged material from stools that have been stained with modified trichrome stain (a stain modified to contain 10 times the usual amount of the chromotrope 2R component).

There is no satisfactory treatment for microsporidiosis.

BLOOD- AND TISSUE-DWELLING PROTOZOA

Table 24–1 lists the clinically significant parasites that are blood- and tissue-dwelling protozoa. These protozoa infect erythrocytes, reticuloendothelial cells, or the central nervous system. *Leishmania* and *Trypanosoma* are flagellates, and *Babesia, Plasmodium,* and *Toxoplasma* are sporozoans. Although *Pneumocystis* is traditionally considered to be a sporozoan, some investigators classify it as a yeast rather than a parasite.

The blood- and tissue-dwelling protozoa are some of the most prevalent causes of severe disease in the world. Each year, for example, species of *Leishmania* cause cutaneous, mucocutaneous, or visceral infection in approximately 400,000 people; species of *Trypanosoma* cause Chagas' disease in about 24 million and sleeping sickness in another 100,000 people; and species of *Plasmodium* cause malaria in an estimated 400 million to 500 million people and are responsible for about 2.5 million deaths. Indeed, malaria is the number one cause of infectious disease–related deaths. For purposes of comparison, human immunodeficiency virus (HIV) is projected to cause infections in 40 million and deaths in 1 million people per year during the early 21st century.

Blood- and Tissue-Dwelling Sporozoans
Characteristics of *Plasmodium*

General Features. Numerous *Plasmodium* species cause infections in animals, but only four species infect humans: *Plasmodium falciparum, Plasmodium malariae, Plasmodium ovale,* and *Plasmodium vivax.* As indicated above, *Plasmodium* causes malaria, the number one killer among infectious diseases. The name of malaria (from the Italian *mala aria,* meaning "bad air") was based on the commonly held belief that the disease was caused by miasmas drifting out of swamps.

The hallmark of malaria is the cyclic nature of the disease. The febrile paroxysms of malaria wax and wane with a predictable periodicity. The duration of the cycles and the relative severity of the disease caused by each species are reflected in names that have been given to each type of malaria. A severe form of malaria that follows a 48-hour fever cycle (with paroxysms occurring on days 1 and 3 of each cycle) is caused by *P. falciparum* and is known as **malignant tertian malaria** or **falciparum malaria.** A milder form that follows a similar cycle and is caused by *P. vivax* is called **benign tertian malaria** or **vivax malaria.** Disease that has a 72-hour fever cycle and is caused by *P. malariae* is called **quartan malaria** or **malariae malaria.** *P. ovale* was discovered in 1922 and does not have a cycle-based disease name but is called **ovale malaria.**

Mechanisms of Pathogenicity. The key to understanding the pathogenesis of malaria lies in the relationship between the progression of disease and the life cycle of the malarial parasite.

(1) The Life Cycle of *Plasmodium.* The life cycle is presented in Figs. 24–6 and 24–7. When an infected *Anopheles* mosquito feeds on a human, *Plasmodium* **sporozoites** enter the blood and travel to the liver. Within minutes, the sporozoites invade hepatic cells (hepatocytes) and begin an asexual developmental cycle called **hepatic schizogony.** A large, polynucleated developmental form called a **schizont** develops within each infected hepatocyte. Eventually, the schizont cytoplasm divides to encase each nucleus and produce the **merozoites** that will leave the liver and invade erythrocytes. Both the amount of

time needed to produce merozoites and the number of merozoites produced within each hepatocyte vary with the *Plasmodium* species. For example, each *P. falciparum* sporozoite generates 40,000 merozoites in 5.5–7 days, while each *P. vivax* sporozoite generates about 10,000 merozoites in 6–8 days (Table 24–2). The release of merozoites from hepatocytes ends the **exoerythrocytic cycle** and begins the series of **erythrocytic cycles** that are responsible for the febrile paroxysms of malaria.

P. vivax and *P. ovale* generate an additional devel-

FIGURE 24–6. The generalized life cycle of *Plasmodium* within the human host. (Source: Brown, H. W. Basic Clinical Parasitology, 3rd ed. New York, Meredith Corporation, 1969. Redrawn and reproduced, with permission, from Appleton and Lange.)

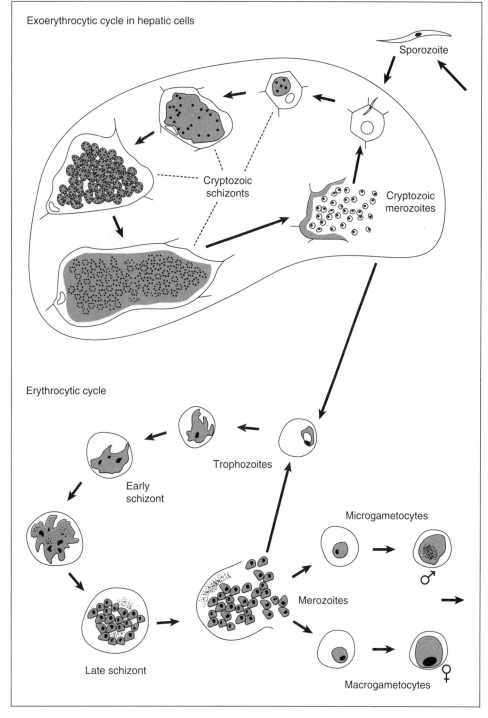

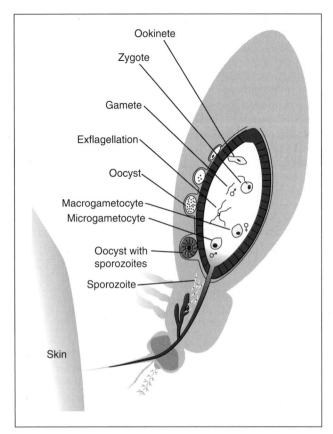

Ookinete
Zygote
Gamete
Exflagellation
Oocyst
Macrogametocyte
Microgametocyte
Oocyst with sporozoites
Sporozoite
Skin

FIGURE 24–7. The generalized life cycle of *Plasmodium* within the *Anopheles* mosquito. (Source: Brown, H. W. Basic Clinical Parasitology, 3rd ed. New York, Meredith Corporation, 1969. Redrawn and reproduced, with permission, from Appleton and Lange.)

opmental form within hepatocytes. This form, known as a **hypnozoite** (meaning "sleeping animal"), is believed to be responsible for relapses of malaria. *P. falciparum* and *P. malariae* do not form hypnozoites and do not relapse. The concepts of relapse and recrudescence are discussed further below.

Once merozoites enter the circulation, they adhere to and invade erythrocytes. Only some of the erythrocyte receptors for plasmodia have been found. For example, studies have shown that the Duffy antigen is a receptor for *P. vivax* merozoites, and Duffy-negative erythrocytes are impervious to infection with *P. vivax*. Both glycophorin A and human erythrocyte band 3 have been implicated as receptors for *P. falciparum* invasion of erythrocytes. Each malarial species invades a discrete subset of erythrocytes. While *P. falciparum* invades all erythrocyte forms, *P. vivax* and *P. ovale* infect only reticulocytes, and *P. malariae* is restricted to senescent red blood cells. This affects the extent of parasitemia because reticulocytes and senescent red blood cells each represent no more than 2% of the total erythrocyte pool.

Inside the erythrocytes, the malarial parasites undergo **erythrocytic schizogony** (see Fig. 24–6). Initially, each parasite has a chromatin spot and a large vacuole, giving it the appearance of a signet ring. The so-called **ring forms** enlarge to become ameboid **trophozoites** and then **schizonts**. The schizonts subsequently undergo cytokinesis to produce **merozoites.** The number of merozoites produced within each infected erythrocyte depends on the *Plasmodium* species (see Table 24–2) and ranges from 6 to 36. The simultaneous release of merozoites from large numbers of erythrocytes initiates the malarial febrile paroxysm.

TABLE 24–2.   A Comparison of the Characteristics of Four Types of Malaria

Characteristic	Falciparum Malaria	Vivax Malaria	Ovale Malaria	Malariae Malaria
Incubation period	8–25 days	8–27 days	9–17 days	15–30 days
Primary hepatic schizogony				
Merozoites produced per sporozoite	40,000	10,000	15,000	2,000
Duration	5.5–7 days	6–8 days	9 days	13–16 days
Hypnozoite production	No	Yes	Yes	No
Erythrocytic schizogony				
Erythrocytes invaded	All erythrocyte forms	Reticulocytes	Reticulocytes	Senescent red blood cells
Merozoites produced per red blood cell	8–36	12–24	6–16	6–12
Periodicity of paroxysms	48 hours	43.5–46 hours	48 hours	72 hours
Parasitemia	Up to 70%	Usually <1%	<1%	<1%
Disease				
Duration of fever	16–36 hours	2–10 hours	2–10 hours	11 hours
Duration of primary disease	2–3 weeks	3–8 weeks	2–3 weeks	3–24 weeks
Duration of untreated infection	6–18 months	1.5–5 years	1.5–5 years	1–53 years
Recrudescence	Yes	Yes	Yes	Yes
Relapse	No	Yes	Yes	No
Extent of anemia	++++	++	+	++
Central nervous system involvement	++++	±	±	±
Nephrotic syndrome	+	±	−	+++

A small proportion of the trophozoites produce male and female gametes, which are called **microgametocytes** and **macrogametocytes,** respectively. The gametocytes will not develop further unless they pass into a mosquito, where they mature and combine to produce a **zygote** (see Fig. 24–7). The mosquito is the definitive host of the malarial parasites because it is inside this host that *Plasmodium* goes through a sexual developmental cycle known as **sporogony.** Within the mosquito gut, the microgametocyte exflagellates to produce male gametes. These merge with macrogametocytes to produce zygotes. The zygotes implant in the gut epithelium and develop into **oocysts,** which in turn fill up with **sporozoites.** The sporozoites migrate to the salivary gland and are injected into the skin of humans when the mosquito feeds. Only female mosquitoes take blood meals, and the *Plasmodium* sexual cycle takes place only within *Anopheles* mosquitoes.

Because *P. falciparum* can infect all forms of erythrocytes and because each round of *P. falciparum* replication produces so many merozoites, this *Plasmodium* species produces much higher levels of parasitemia and causes more severe malaria than the other *Plasmodium* species. More than one ring form can often be seen within individual erythrocytes infected with *P. falciparum,* but only one of the intracellular parasites will mature in each cell. Falciparum malaria is unique in that only ring forms and gametocytes are seen in the peripheral circulation in all but moribund patients. This is because erythrocytes infected with the ameboid trophozoites and schizonts of *P. falciparum* adsorb to the endothelium of the deep microvasculature. Erythrocytes infected with these *P. falciparum* forms develop knobs that contain a protein called *P. falciparum* erythrocyte membrane protein 1 (PfEMP-1). Investigators believe that PfEMP-1 mediates adherence to the microvascular wall by recognizing endothelial receptors. Among the candidates for the pertinent endothelial receptor are CD36, intercellular adhesion molecule 1 (ICAM-1), endothelial leukocyte adhesion molecule 1 (ELAM-1), and vascular cell adhesion molecule 1 (VCAM-1).

(2) Pathogenic Processes in Malaria. The coordinated release of merozoites from erythrocytes is the proximal cause of the malarial febrile paroxysm (Fig. 24–8). In addition to releasing merozoites, the lysis of infected erythrocytes releases hemoglobin, malarial metabolites, and an insoluble product of hemoglobin metabolism known as **hemozoin** or **malarial pigment.** These substances are antigenic and pyrogenic. The severity and duration of each paroxysm is directly related to the extent of parasitemia and the number of erythrocytes that are lysed.

Anemia is an important component of malaria. The single greatest cause of malarial anemia is the coordinated lysis of infected erythrocytes, but infected and uninfected erythrocytes may also be destroyed by phagocytosis and complement activation. Hemozoin released from infected erythrocytes collects in the spleen and liver, where its accumulation causes iron store depletion and further development

of anemia. When anemia becomes profound, the patient may suffer from disease that involves multiple systems.

Infection with *P. falciparum* is unique in that it is associated with a wide range of complications, including cerebral malaria, dysenteric malaria, renal tubular necrosis, an intense form of hemoglobinuria known as blackwater fever, hyperreactive malarial splenomegaly, and algid malaria, with the latter characterized by collapse of the vascular system and shock. These disease states are largely related to the hyperparasitemia that develops during falciparum malaria. In addition, at least some of the disease states are produced when erythrocytes containing *P. falciparum* trophozoites and schizonts accumulate in the visceral microvasculature. When the microcirculation becomes occluded with infected erythrocytes, the tissues become anoxic, and this gives rise to symptoms that are consistent with damage to the affected organ. Cerebral malaria is believed to involve both parasite-induced ischemia and the production of tumor necrosis factor alpha (TNF-α). TNF-α, whose level of production is directly related to the severity of cerebral malaria, up-regulates the expression of ICAM-1, a receptor for *P. falciparum* cytoadherence. Patients with hyperreactive malarial splenomegaly develop enormous spleens, a phenomenon that is thought to result from an overproduction of IgM antibody coupled with a net reduction in T lymphocytes.

Malarial parasites protect themselves from the immune response in part by being antigenically polymorphic. Immunity against the *Plasmodium* species is strain-specific, and several of the dominant *Plasmodium* antigens have been shown to be hypervariable. Not only do these antigens vary from isolate to isolate, but individual parasites change their antigens during the course of an infection. The changes in expression of antigens appear on the surfaces of schizont-infected erythrocytes. These changes are genetically predetermined, but the appearance of antimalarial antibody is a selective pressure that may hasten the change. Antigenic polymorphism seems to be more prevalent in vivax malaria than in falciparum malaria.

Diseases Due to *Plasmodium*

Epidemiology. Malaria is spread by the bites of anopheline mosquitoes and is common throughout the tropics. In Africa alone, about 200 million people are infected and over 1 million die of malaria every year. In areas where high proportions of the population are Duffy-negative (primarily in western Africa), *P. ovale* is found instead of *P. vivax.* Elsewhere, *P. falciparum* and *P. vivax* are the predominant malarial species. In some regions of southern Africa, more than 80% of human malarial infections are caused by *P. falciparum.* In African children, falciparum malaria is believed to act as a cofactor in the development of Burkitt's lymphoma.

At one time, malaria was common throughout temperate, subtropical, and tropical areas of the

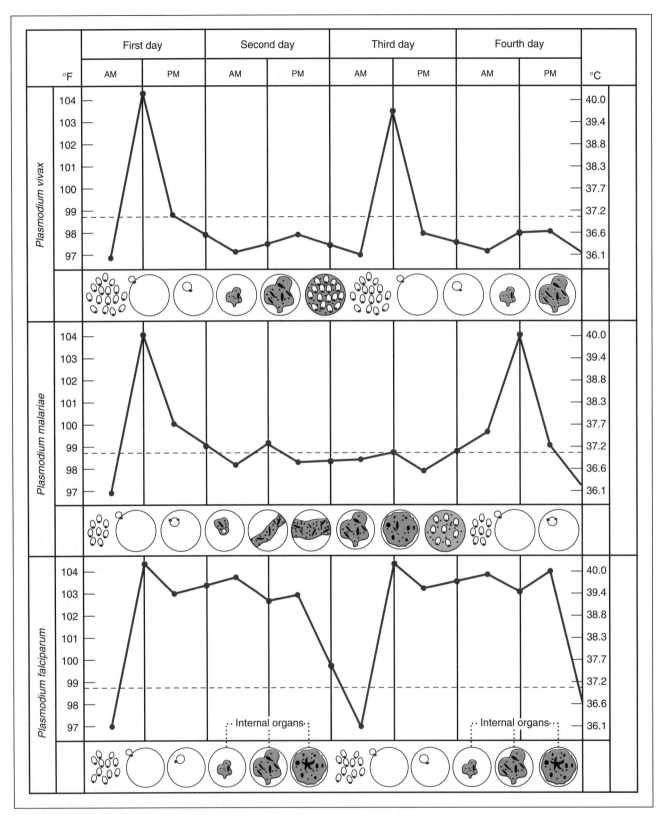

FIGURE 24–8. A comparison of the paroxysmal febrile cycles of malaria caused by three species of *Plasmodium*. The release of merozoites from infected erythrocytes signals the onset of a spike in fever. (Source: Brown, H. W. Basic Clinical Parasitology, 3rd ed. New York, Meredith Corporation, 1969. Redrawn and reproduced, with permission, from Appleton and Lange.)

world, but disease eradication schemes have largely eliminated malaria from industrialized temperate countries. In the USA, there are occasional localized outbreaks of malaria of very limited scope, but almost all patients who develop malaria have a history of travel outside the country.

Some population groups have been found to be resistant to infection with certain *Plasmodium* species or to develop less severe disease. As mentioned above, Duffy-negative individuals are resistant to vivax malaria. People who have Southeast Asian ovalocytosis (characterized by an abnormal erythrocyte band 3 protein) are relatively resistant to developing malaria, as are people with hemoglobin S and people who are deficient in glucose-6-phosphate dehydrogenase. Patients with sickle cell trait develop significantly less severe falciparum malaria, possibly because the increased sickling of parasitized erythrocytes that have adhered to the microvasculature kills the parasites.

Malaria is occasionally transmitted via blood transfusions. Affected patients may develop primary acute disease, but no relapses will follow, because hypnozoites are not passed in blood.

Diagnosis

(1) History and Physical Examination. The clinical manifestations of malaria usually begin 8–30 days after malarial parasites are introduced through the bite of a mosquito. Nevertheless, the first acute attack of malaria may not occur until 6–12 months after exposure to *P. vivax* or even longer after exposure to *P. malariae* or *P. ovale.*

The malarial prodrome lasts a week or more, during which time the patient suffers from a variety of nonspecific flu-like symptoms, such as anorexia, malaise, irregular fever, and vague pains of the bones and joints.

The acute phase begins dramatically with an attack of severe shaking chills that lasts an hour or longer. The skin becomes pale, the temperature rises to 40 °C (104 °F) or more, and the patient becomes agitated, flushed, and disoriented. Other manifestations may include vomiting, convulsions, severe headache, and muscle and joint pain. The duration and intensity of febrile paroxysms vary with the *Plasmodium* species (see Fig. 24–8), as does the periodicity of paroxysms. The fever generally remains high for 2–10 hours in patients with vivax and ovale malaria, but it may remain high much longer in patients with falciparum or malariae malaria. Although vivax malaria and falciparum malaria are both considered to be forms of tertian malaria, vivax paroxysms may be spaced only 43.5–46 hours apart, and patients with early falciparum malaria may suffer from nonperiodic fevers. It is for this reason that falciparum malaria is sometimes known as **subtertian malaria.**

The paroxysm ends when the patient begins to sweat profusely and the temperature drops rapidly. At this time, the patient is weak and falls asleep. When the patient awakens, he or she feels much better until the next paroxysm begins. Patients with acute falciparum malaria may have little time to rest between the end of one paroxysm and the onset of the next one. If the disease is untreated, the cycle of paroxysms will continue for weeks, and the duration of primary illness will vary with the type of malaria (see Table 24–2). Most deaths are due to falciparum malaria, but some are due to vivax malaria.

Most malarial complications occur in patients with falciparum malaria. The most dangerous complication is **cerebral malaria.** Affected patients have a severe headache that rapidly progresses to drowsiness and confusion and then to coma. Although cerebral malaria is often fatal, those who recover usually have no neurologic sequelae. **Algid malaria** is characterized by the rapid development of hypotension, hypothermia, generalized vascular collapse, and intractable shock. In **blackwater fever,** patients develop black urine in association with massive intravascular hemolysis. Although blackwater fever is usually seen in patients with falciparum malaria, it has been reported in patients with vivax or malariae malaria. Affected patients usually have experienced several previous bouts of malaria, and the blackwater fever is thought to be an autoimmune phenomenon. **Renal tubular necrosis** and **nephrotic syndrome** can occur during either falciparum or malariae malaria. Renal disease in falciparum malaria is believed to be secondary to tissue anoxia, while that seen during malariae malaria is believed to be due to deposition of antigen-antibody complexes in the glomerular basement membrane. Other complications seen in patients with falciparum malaria include **dysenteric malaria, pulmonary edema,** and rapidly progressive disease that is due to **hyperparasitemia.** In some cases of hyperparasitemia, up to 70% of the patient's erythrocytes are infected with *P. falciparum.*

(2) Laboratory Analysis. Diagnosis of malaria still rests on observing the parasites in Giemsa-stained blood films. Thick films are used to demonstrate the presence of *Plasmodium* organisms, and thin films are used to speciate the organisms. It is more difficult to make the diagnosis in samples taken immediately after a paroxysm has begun, because cell-free merozoites are present and are not easy to identify. Expert laboratory technicians usually have no difficulty in recognizing the other developmental forms of particular *Plasmodium* species. For example, *P. falciparum* is identified by the presence of multiply infected erythrocytes, the presence of more than one chromatin dot on some ring forms, the absence of mature trophozoites and schizonts in the peripheral circulation, the appearance of Maurer's dots on erythrocytes that contain trophozoites, and the presence of the unique crescent-shaped gametocytes.

Other tests for malaria are available, but none of them have proved to be as useful or cost-effective as microscopic examination of blood films. One of the most promising tests is a manual dipstick assay that detects the presence of a *P. falciparum* antigen known as histidine-rich protein 2 (HRP-2). This assay is extremely sensitive, specific, and easy to use. Unfortunately, it detects only *P. falciparum* and is not quantitative. Polymerase chain reaction assays and fluorescence tests are expensive and require high-tech equipment that is usually not available in laboratories located in tropical underdeveloped countries. The fluorescence tests also cannot distinguish among malarial species.

Treatment. For many years, chloroquine was the mainstay of malarial treatment and was particularly effective against strains of *P. falciparum* infection. Unfortunately, most regions with falciparum malaria now have a high prevalence of chloroquine-resistant *P. falciparum* strains, making it necessary to use alternative drugs.

Antimalarial drugs can be divided into two groups: drugs that are effective against blood forms of the parasites (blood schizonticides) and drugs that kill hepatic forms (tissue schizonticides). Of the drugs available in the USA, only primaquine is a tissue schizonticide.

Patients with acute malaria caused by *P. malariae, P. ovale, P. vivax,* or chloroquine-sensitive strains of *P. falciparum* are usually treated with a 3-day course of oral chloroquine phosphate or intravenous chloroquine sulfate. Alternatively, oral quinine sulfate or intravenous quinidine gluconate can be used. Supportive measures may include replacement of fluids and electrolytes. Most patients who have vivax or ovale malaria are also given primaquine to kill hypnozoites and prevent relapse. However, primaquine is contraindicated in patients who are deficient in glucose-6-phosphate dehydrogenase, because it may cause hemolysis in these patients.

Patients who contract falciparum malaria in an area where chloroquine resistance is known to occur are assumed to be infected with a chloroquine-resistant strain of *P. falciparum.* These patients are treated with one of the following: (1) quinine sulfate; (2) quinidine gluconate; (3) quinine or quinidine plus tetracycline; or (4) quinine or quinidine plus an antifolate drug regimen, usually pyrimethamine combined with sulfadiazine or sulfadoxine. Primaquine has also been used experimentally with some success in treating these patients. In rare cases, patients with extremely high parasitemia have received erythrocyte replacement therapy using a red blood cell separator.

Prognosis. It is a common misconception that malaria is "incurable" and persists for the life of the patient. Untreated *P. falciparum* infections may last from 6 to 18 months and be characterized by long periods of low-level parasitemia. *P. malariae* infections can last even longer, with extremely low levels of parasitemia that have resulted in recurring disease as long as 53 years after the initial bout of disease. In each of these two situations, the patient who has recurring disease is said to suffer from malarial **recrudescence.** Disease that recurs after a period of no parasitemia is called a malarial **relapse.** Relapse occurs only in patients infected with *P. vivax* or *P. ovale,* because only these malarial parasites produce the hypnozoites that are believed to be the source of the malarial relapse. As Table 24–2 shows, untreated *P.*

vivax and *P. ovale* infections may last up to about 5 years.

Recovery from malaria does not confer lasting protective immunity, and **reinfection** is common. Indeed, some patients develop **quotidian malaria** (daily fever cycles) because they are simultaneously infected with two or more *Plasmodium* strains or species, each following a different paroxysmal cycle. In areas of malaria endemicity, many individuals develop a condition called **premunition.** These individuals have persistent low-level parasitemia but appear to be resistant to attacks of acute malaria.

Prevention. No vaccine is currently available, but efforts to develop a malaria vaccine continue. Malaria prevention currently focuses on mosquito eradication, use of repellents, and chemoprophylaxis. People traveling to countries where there is little or no chloroquine resistance may take a tablet of chloroquine each week, beginning 1 or 2 weeks before entering the area and continuing for 4 weeks after leaving the area. People traveling to countries where chloroquine resistance is prevalent may take mefloquine at the same schedule used for chloroquine. A variety of other antimalarial drugs have been used in specific vicinities. Primaquine or doxycycline has been used successfully as chemoprophylaxis in some areas where chloroquine resistance occurs.

Characteristics of *Babesia*

Most cases of babesiosis in humans are caused by *Babesia microti,* a parasite that usually infects rodents and is transmitted to humans via tick bites. In Europe, some humans have been infected with *Babesia bovis,* a parasite that is responsible for the deaths of millions of cattle worldwide. At least 15 other species of *Babesia* are known to cause diseases in animals, including sheep, dogs, cats, and camels.

Babesia species develop asexually (via schizogony) within mammalian erythrocytes, and then they pass through two developmental cycles (gamogony and sporogony) within their definitive hosts, ticks. The presence of *Babesia* in erythrocytes is identified by the propensity of the parasites to form rings and tetrads ("Maltese crosses") without generating malarial pigment.

Diseases Due to *Babesia*

Epidemiology. Most cases of babesiosis have occurred in Europe and the USA. US cases have been reported primarily in Nantucket, Martha's Vineyard, Long Island, Shelter Island, and Connecticut. A few cases have also been reported in California. Most cases have been acquired via tick bites, but at least one transfusion-related case has been described. The vectors of babesiosis are *Ixodes scapularis* (a vector of Lyme disease and human granulocytic ehrlichiosis), *Rhipicephalus sanguineus* (the brown dog tick), *Rhipicephalus bursa,* and various *Boophilus* ticks. In several cases, patients have been reported to suffer from both babesiosis and Lyme disease, and *I. scapularis* ticks have been found to carry both *Babesia* and *Bor-*

relia. Because *I. scapularis* can also carry *Ehrlichia,* it is possible that a patient could suffer from a combination of babesiosis, Lyme disease, and ehrlichiosis.

Diagnosis. From 10 to 20 days after a tick bite, **babesiosis** typically begins with shaking chills, fever, malaise, arthralgia, myalgia, and weakness. Most patients develop palpable hepatosplenomegaly and mild to moderate hemolytic anemia. Unlike patients with malaria, patients with babesiosis do not develop periodic febrile paroxysms. The disease usually resolves spontaneously in several weeks. However, in patients who have been splenectomized, babesiosis follows a fulminating course, with anemia, fever, jaundice, and renal failure sometimes leading to death.

The diagnosis of babesiosis may be complicated if the patient has concomitant Lyme disease or ehrlichiosis. Laboratory confirmation of babesiosis requires that the characteristic ring forms and Maltese crosses be identified in Giemsa-stained blood films. The number of parasites in the blood can be very low in patients with intact spleens, making laboratory diagnosis difficult. Multiple peripheral blood smears may have to be examined to locate the parasites.

Treatment. Human babesiosis has been treated successfully with a combination of clindamycin and quinine. This combination ameliorates symptoms and causes the parasites to disappear from blood films. Chloroquine provides symptomatic relief but does not affect the degree of parasitemia.

Characteristics of *Toxoplasma gondii*

General Features. *Toxoplasma gondii* is the cause of toxoplasmosis, one of the most common protozoan infections in the world. Most human infections are benign, but toxoplasmosis can be fatal in immunocompromised patients and in neonates. Congenital toxoplasmosis is a frequent cause of chorioretinitis (also called retinochoroiditis), blindness, hydrocephaly, and mental retardation. The definitive host of *T. gondii* is the cat, but a wide variety of animals (including humans) can support the asexual cycle of the parasite.

Mechanisms of Pathogenicity. *T. gondii* infects the intestine of the cat, where it develops into **schizonts** and **gametocytes**. The gametocytes subsequently yield **oocysts** that each contain two **sporocysts.** Humans and other animals (including cats) that ingest mature oocysts develop an initial intestinal infection that yields rapidly multiplying trophozoites known as **tachyzoites.** The crescent-shaped tachyzoites enter the mesenteric lymph nodes and then spread throughout the body. Wherever they lodge, tachyzoites proliferate and cause tissue destruction. Intracellular multiplication of the tachyzoites kills the host cell and elicits a cellular response. Together, these processes lead to the development of areas of focal necrosis. In addition, some *T. gondii* parasites form **tissue cysts** that contain hundreds of slowly multiplying trophozoites known as **bradyzoites.** The tissue cysts may persist for years in muscles and in the central nervous system. Eventually, the cysts die and calcify.

The greatest effects of *T. gondii* are on the eye and brain. Chorioretinitis is probably due to the combined effects of direct damage from tachyzoite multiplication and a hypersensitivity response to the presence of tissue cysts in the eye. Central nervous system disease is related to the formation of necrotic foci in the brain.

Diseases Due to *Toxoplasma gondii*

Epidemiology. Human toxoplasmosis is acquired by transplacental transmission, by ingesting oocysts shed by cats, or by eating meat that contains tissue cysts.

A woman who was infected with *Toxoplasma* prior to her pregnancy is not at risk of passing the infection to her fetus. However, primary infection during pregnancy places the infant at risk. Infants born to mothers who are infected during the first or second trimester of pregnancy often are stillborn or are born with encephalomyelitis, hydrocephaly, microcephaly, or chorioretinitis. Although only about 20% of infants born to mothers who are infected during the third trimester have clinically apparent toxoplasmosis at birth, most of the infants later develop chorioretinitis.

Oocysts are fairly resistant to environmental conditions and have been shown to survive through two Midwestern winters in the soil. The oocysts are not infective when they are initially shed by cats, but they become infective within 1–5 days. For this reason, pregnant women who have cats in their homes should ask that another member of the family change the cat litter every day.

Tissue cysts are frequently found in meat. In the USA, a survey of meat sold in grocery stores revealed that *Toxoplasma* tissue cysts were present in 25% of pork samples and 10% of beef and mutton samples. The tissue cysts can be killed if the meat is well cooked. *Toxoplasma* infection is extremely common wherever people eat raw or undercooked meat. In Paris, for example, one survey showed that 87% of adults in their childbearing years had antibodies to *T. gondii,* indicating that they had been infected with the organism. The risk of fetal complications due to toxoplasmosis in Paris was reported to be about 40 per 10,000 live births.

Isolated cases of toxoplasmosis have also been traced to raw milk and to blood transfusions, but these are rare events.

Diagnosis

(1) History and Physical Examination. In immunocompetent children and adults, most **acquired *Toxoplasma* infections** are asymptomatic. A small percentage of immunocompetent individuals develop symptoms that mimic mononucleosis and include fatigue, chills, fever, headache, myalgia, and lymphadenitis, sometimes accompanied by a rash. In rare cases, the infection progresses and causes clinically apparent encephalomyelitis, hepatitis, myocarditis, or chorioretinitis.

In immunocompromised children and adults, including patients with AIDS, most cases of toxoplasmosis represent a reactivation of earlier disease due to the conversion of cystic bradyzoites to tachyzoites. Tachyzoites can be found in the cerebrospinal fluid, and necrotic foci appear in the brain. Typical manifestations include ataxia, confusion, headaches, hemiparesis, and chorioretinitis. The most common diagnoses in immunocompromised patients are diffuse encephalopathy, meningoencephalitis, and cerebral mass lesions.

The findings in infants with **congenital toxoplasmosis** vary, depending on when the mother was infected (see above). Newborn infants with congenital disease may be febrile, may have convulsions, and typically suffer from hepatosplenomegaly and an interstitial plasma cell pneumonia similar to the pneumonia caused by *Pneumocystis carinii.* In most cases, congenital toxoplasmosis leads to mental retardation and either blindness or severe visual impairment.

(2) Laboratory Analysis. The diagnosis of *Toxoplasma* infection is usually confirmed serologically using an indirect fluorescent antibody (IFA) test, an enzyme-linked immunosorbent assay (ELISA), an immunosorbent agglutination (ISA) test, or the Sabin-Feldman dye test. The gold standard is the Sabin-Feldman dye test, but it is difficult to perform, requires live *Toxoplasma* organisms, and is available in only a few reference laboratories. In serum from infants, the presence of maternal IgG antibody may interfere with the diagnosis. Therefore, it is best to use an IFA test, ELISA, or ISA test that permits separation of IgM from IgG antibody.

In patients with classic symptoms of *Toxoplasma* infection, the diagnosis is confirmed if the IFA antibody titer is high (1 : 1000 or greater) and the IFA test detects the presence of IgM antibody. In the absence of symptoms, the diagnosis is confirmed if both the IFA titer and the IgM IFA titer are high.

Laboratory confirmation of toxoplasmosis is rarely made on the basis of cultivating the organisms from clinical samples. If necessary, however, clinical samples can be injected into mice or used to inoculate Vero cells or MRC5 fibroblasts.

Prenatal diagnosis can be made by testing fetal blood for IgM antibody to *Toxoplasma,* by culturing fetal blood or amniotic fluid, or by use of ultrasonography to detect fetal cerebral abnormalities.

Treatment. Toxoplasmosis is usually treated with the combination of pyrimethamine and trisulfapyrimidines for 1 month. Corticosteroids can be administered to reduce inflammation. Clindamycin or spiramycin has also been used to treat toxoplasmosis.

Prevention. *Toxoplasma* infection can be prevented by washing hands thoroughly after handling meat or changing cat litter, by changing cat litter daily, and by cooking meat thoroughly.

Characteristics of *Pneumocystis carinii*

Pneumocystis carinii has traditionally been classified as a member of the phylum Apicomplexa. Recent studies examining a wide variety of characteristics, including rRNA sequencing, mitochondrial gene sequencing, DNA homology with certain fungi, and ability to grow *Pneumocystis* on fungal media, have cast doubts on the classification of this organism as a parasite. One of the developmental forms of *P. carinii* is ameboid, and the organism forms cysts that are analogous in appearance to those made by some other Apicomplexa. Those who consider the organism to be a parasite refer to the cysts as **sporocysts,** the intracystic bodies as **sporozoites,** and the extracellular forms as **trophozoites.**

P. carinii causes interstitial plasma cell pneumonia, a disease that has historically occurred mainly in premature and malnourished infants. With the advent of the AIDS epidemic, *Pneumocystis* has become an important pulmonary pathogen in immunocompromised patients. The pathogenic mechanisms are not well described, but patients develop a diffuse pulmonary exudate and some develop diffuse interstitial fibrosis. The alveolar exudate contains *Pneumocystis* cysts and macrophages. Although *P. carinii* most often causes pulmonary infections, disseminated infections have been reported.

Diseases Due to *Pneumocystis carinii*

Epidemiology. In the USA, more than 75% of children are believed to be asymptomatic carriers of *P. carinii.* The organism rarely causes disease in immunocompetent children and adults but poses a threat to premature infants, malnourished infants between the ages of 6 weeks and 6 months, and immunocompromised patients. About 85% of patients with AIDS and about 20% of children with acute lymphoblastic leukemia develop *P. carinii* pneumonia. Epidemics of *Pneumocystis* disease often occur among patients in chronic disease wards and occasionally in hospital nurseries and in orphanages. Transmission is via the respiratory route.

Diagnosis
(1) History and Physical Examination. Infants develop **interstitial plasma cell pneumonia** up to 2 months after exposure to a person carrying *P. carinii.* Infection begins with weakness and a nonproductive cough and soon progresses to severe disease with cyanosis, pallor, tachypnea, and progressive dyspnea with periods of apnea. Fever is often absent. Radiographs usually show a patchy infiltrate that spreads out from the hilar areas. Disease is most severe in infants under 3 months of age, and the fatality rate is 30–40%.

Immunocompromised patients develop *P. carinii* pneumonia from 40 days to 1 year after exposure to a person shedding the organisms. Manifestations may include diarrhea, a nonproductive cough, weight loss, malaise, a low-grade fever, and progressive dyspnea. Patients generally do not have rales, and blood gas measurements demonstrate hypoxia without acidosis or hypercapnia. *P. carinii* rarely disseminates to other organs, but disseminated or ectopic infections have been reported. Some patients with *P. carinii* infection have cotton wool spots in the fundus of the eye.

(2) Laboratory Analysis. The diagnosis is confirmed by demonstrating the presence of *P. carinii* in the lungs of patients. In patients without AIDS, the organisms are best located by lung biopsy. In patients with AIDS, who typically have more cysts present in the lungs than do other patients, *P. carinii* can be located by transbronchial biopsy or touch prints. When transbronchial biopsy and bronchoalveolar lavage are combined, the sensitivity of detection of *P. carinii* approaches 100%. Samples can also be taken by percutaneous transthoracic needle aspiration. A variety of stains can be used, but Grocott-Gomori methenamine–silver nitrate stain is considered the best for visualizing *P. carinii*. There are no serologic tests to detect *P. carinii* infections.

Treatment. Trimethoprim-sulfamethoxazole (TMP/SMX) is the treatment of choice for *P. carinii* pneumonia, but many AIDS patients cannot tolerate this treatment. Pentamidine can be substituted for TMP/SMX, but the two regimens should not be used together. In cases of mild pneumonia, an aerosolized form of pentamidine can be used. This delivers the drug directly to the infection site, allows less drug to be used, and results in fewer drug-induced complications. In cases of severe pneumonia, aerosolized pentamidine is not effective. Other drugs that have been used to treat pneumonia in AIDS patients include trimetrexate gluconate (investigational), eflornithine, and a combination of trimethoprim plus dapsone. Corticosteroids can be used as adjunctive therapy in selected patients.

Prevention. Aerosolized pentamidine can be used to prevent *P. carinii* pneumonia. The recommendations for chemoprophylaxis in children vary with the age of the child. Adults who have a CD4+ T lymphocyte count below 200 cells per microliter or a CD4+ T lymphocyte measurement under 20% should receive chemoprophylaxis.

Hemoflagellates

Two groups of hemoflagellates are known to cause human disease: the leishmania and the try-panosomes. Each organism passes through a developmental cycle within an insect vector and enters the circulation as a flagellated organism.

The hemoflagellates can pass through up to four developmental forms (Fig. 24–9) known as **amastigote, promastigote, epimastigote,** and **trypomastigote.** Originally, these forms were known, in order, as **leishmania, leptomonas, crithidia,** and **trypanosoma.** The *Leishmania* and *Trypanosoma* species were named after the original designation for the developmental form most often found in the tissue of infected patients. *Leishmania* species exist in two forms: as amastigotes in animal tissue and as promastigotes within the insect vector. *Trypanosoma brucei* exists in three forms: as amastigotes and trypomastigotes in animals and as epimastigotes in the vector. *Trypanosoma cruzi* exists in all four forms.

The *Leishmania* species cause cutaneous, mucocutaneous, or visceral leishmaniasis. *T. brucei* causes African sleeping sickness, and *T. cruzi* causes Chagas' disease.

Characteristics of *Leishmania*

General Features. The classification of the *Leishmania* species is in constant flux as new methods are used to identify patterns of interrelatedness among the leishmania. Currently, the leishmania are divided into two subgenera, called *Leishmania* and *Viannia,* based on where the organisms develop within the insect vector. The individual species are grouped within complexes of closely related organisms. Table 24–3 lists the complexes and the diseases they cause. The leishmania can also be divided into three groups on the basis of geographic distribution and clinical manifestations: the Old World cutaneous and mucocutaneous leishmania; the New World cutaneous and mucocutaneous leishmania; and the agent of visceral leishmaniasis, *Leishmania donovani.*

Mechanisms of Pathogenicity. Cutaneous and mucocutaneous forms of leishmaniasis are primarily localized leishmanial infections, although there is mounting evidence that more dissemination of the organisms occurs than was formerly believed. The

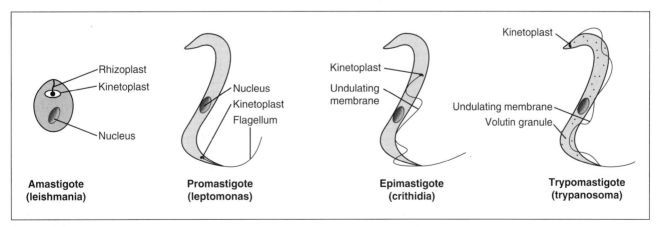

FIGURE 24–9. The developmental forms of parasites in the family Trypanosomatidae. *Trypanosoma* and *Leishmania* are human pathogens in this family. (Source: Brown, H. W. Basic Clinical Parasitology, 3rd ed. New York, Meredith Corporation, 1969. Redrawn and reproduced, with permission, from Appleton and Lange.)

TABLE 24-3. Diseases Caused by the Major *Leishmania* Complexes

Complex	Disease	Geographic Distribution	Reservoir
Leishmania aethiopica	Cutaneous and diffuse cutaneous leishmaniasis.	Ethiopia, Kenya, former Soviet Union, Uganda, and southern Yemen.	Rock hyrax.
Leishmania braziliensis	Cutaneous and mucocutaneous leishmaniasis.	Argentina, Belize, Bolivia, Brazil, Colombia, Costa Rica, French Guiana, Guatemala, Honduras, Mexico, Panama, Paraguay, Peru, and Venezuela.	Dogs and rodents.
Leishmania donovani	Cutaneous leishmaniasis, dermal leishmanoid, and visceral leishmaniasis.	Africa and Asia (*L. donovani*); Africa, Europe, Mediterranean basin, and southwestern Asia (*Leishmania infantum*); and Central and South America and southwestern USA (*Leishmania chagasi*).	Humans (in India); and dogs and rodents (outside India).
Leishmania guyanensis	Cutaneous leishmaniasis.	Brazil, French Guiana, Guyana, and Surinam.	Rodents and other small mammals.
Leishmania major	Cutaneous leishmaniasis.	Afghanistan, Africa, Middle East, and former Soviet Union.	Dogs and small rodents, including gerbils.
Leishmania mexicana	Cutaneous and diffuse cutaneous leishmaniasis.	Belize, Guatemala, Mexico (Yucatán peninsula), and southwestern USA (central Texas).	Anteaters, dogs, opossums, rodents, and sloths.
Leishmania tropica	Cutaneous leishmaniasis.	Afghanistan, India, Middle East, Turkey, and former Soviet Union.	Humans, dogs, and rats.

leishmania multiply within tissue macrophages and endothelial cells at the skin site where they are introduced via the bite of an infected sandfly. The promastigotes introduced by the sandfly rapidly convert to the amastigote form. The intracellular multiplication of amastigotes destroys the cells that host the parasites. This elicits a granulomatous response, which causes a nodule to form. Continued parasite-induced damage causes the nodule to ulcerate, and secondary bacterial infection may prolong the ulcerative stage. Eventually, a cell-mediated immune response activates macrophages that lyse amastigotes and control the infection. Species that cause mucocutaneous disease may disseminate to the mucosae, particularly the nasal and oral mucosae, where amastigote multiplication and the granulomatous response can cause destructive lesions to form.

Visceral leishmaniasis occurs when parasites in the *L. donovani* complex disseminate from the original infection site to the spleen and liver. Reticuloendothelial cells throughout the body are infected, but the presence of leishmania in the spleen and liver causes massive hypertrophy. Amastigotes may also be found in the bone marrow, where their presence can cause anemia and leukopenia. Patients may develop glomerulonephritis as a result of the deposition of immune complexes in the basement membrane of the kidney.

Recovery from leishmanial diseases is related to the development of a cellular response that generates interferon-gamma and interleukin-2. *L. donovani* is also subject to lysis by activated complement components generated via the alternative pathway.

Diseases Due to *Leishmania*

Epidemiology. The leishmania are found in tropical and subtropical regions where sandflies exist (see Table 24-3 and Fig. 24-10). *Lutzomyia* sandflies are the predominant vectors of New World leishmania, whereas *Phlebotomus* sandflies are the vectors of Old World leishmania. Stable or dog flies (*Stomoxys* species) can also transmit leishmania mechanically, and the parasites can be transmitted via direct contact with cutaneous or mucocutaneous lesions. About 12 million people throughout the world have leishmaniasis, and an estimated 400,000 new cases occur each year.

Diagnosis
(1) History and Physical Examination
(a) Cutaneous Leishmaniasis. Cutaneous leishmaniasis is caused by Old World and New World leishmania. In the Old World, cutaneous leishmaniasis has a variety of names—including **Oriental sore, Baghdad boil,** and **Aleppo boil**—and the prevalent agents of infection are members of the *Leishmania aethiopica, Leishmania major,* and *Leishmania tropica* complexes. In the Americas, various forms of cutaneous leishmaniasis are known as **chiclero ulcer** and **pian bois,** and the prevalent agents are members of the *Leishmania braziliensis* and *Leishmania mexicana* complexes.

Cutaneous leishmaniasis begins as a papule at the site of a sandfly bite. The incubation period may be as short as a few weeks (as occurs with *L. major*) or as long as 3 years (as occurs with *L. aethiopica* and *L. tropica*). The papule turns red, itches intensely,

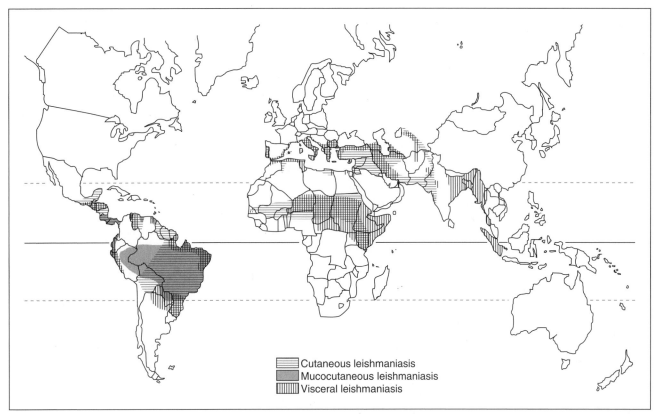

FIGURE 24–10. The geographic distribution of cutaneous, mucocutaneous, and visceral leishmaniasis. (Redrawn and reproduced, with permission, from Markell, E. K., M. Voge, and D. T. John. Medical Parasitology, 7th ed. Philadelphia, W. B. Saunders Company, 1992.)

becomes a pustule, and then ulcerates. *L. major* lesions tend to be covered with a serous exudate, making them moist, while *L. aethiopica* and *L. tropica* lesions are dry. The cutaneous lesions tend to heal spontaneously in a few months, but they may leave a prominent scar. *L. mexicana,* the agent of chiclero ulcer, often causes distinctive destructive lesions on the pinna of the ear.

Variations from the typical pattern of infection are seen in anergic patients and in hypersensitive patients. Patients who are selectively unresponsive to leishmanial antigens and are infected with *L. aethiopica* or with *Leishmania pifanoi* (a member of the *L. mexicana* complex) may develop a disseminated form of disease called **diffuse cutaneous leishmaniasis.** These anergic patients have normal immune responses to all but leishmanial antigens, and they develop nodular or plaque-like thickenings of the skin that resemble the lesions of lepromatous leprosy. Patients who are hypersensitive to leishmanial antigens and are infected with any of the species that cause cutaneous leishmaniasis may develop **leishmaniasis recidivans,** a condition in which satellite lesions form around a central healing leishmanial lesion. This condition is thought to occur because the leishmania are not completely cleared by the immune response.

(b) Mucocutaneous Leishmaniasis. Mucocutaneous leishmaniasis is sometimes called **espundia** or **uta** and is usually caused by members of the *L.* *braziliensis* complex. Rare cases of mucocutaneous leishmaniasis have been reported in Ethiopia and the Sudan and have been attributed to *L. aethiopica, L. donovani,* or *L. tropica.*

Patients develop one or more primary cutaneous lesions that are generally much larger than the single primary lesion caused by the agents of cutaneous leishmaniasis. Up to 20% of patients subsequently develop metastatic lesions on the oral and nasal mucosae. In some patients, the mucocutaneous lesions occur when the cutaneous lesions are still present. In others, the mucocutaneous lesions occur years after the primary lesions disappear. The lesions slowly spread to include the entire nasal mucosa and the mucosa of the hard and soft palates. Eventually, they disfigure and destroy the nasal septum and all of the soft parts of the mouth and nose. Some forms of mucocutaneous leishmaniasis are nonulcerative and produce hypertrophy of the upper lip and nose ("tapir nose"). If death occurs, it is generally as a result of secondary bacterial infections.

(c) Visceral Leishmaniasis. Visceral leishmaniasis is also known as **kala-azar** (Hindi for "black poison") or **Dumdum fever** (for a city just outside Calcutta). The name kala-azar is apt because the disease can cause blackening of the skin on the forehead, over the temples, and around the mouth. Kala-azar is caused by members of the *L. donovani* complex, which includes *Leishmania archibaldi, Leishmania chagasi, L. donovani,* and *Leishmania infantum.* Most patients infected with these organisms are asymptomatic or suffer from only mild disease. Among those with severe disease, however, the untreated fatality rate is high.

Kala-azar begins from 2 weeks to 18 months (but usually 2–4 months) after the patient is bitten by an infected *Phlebotomus* sandfly. The onset may be insidious or acute, depending on the *Leishmania* strain involved. Patients with a subacute onset generally present with abdominal swelling that has occurred without any obvious disease other than a period of vague malaise. When the onset is acute, patients suffer from malaria-like or typhoid-like symptoms, including anorexia, diarrhea, fever, malaise, and weight loss. The fever may be erratic or periodic, resembling the periodicity of malaria. Eventually, the fever assumes a two-a-day (dromedary) or three-a-day periodicity. Anemia, hepatosplenomegaly, and generalized lymphadenopathy develop. As the liver and spleen continue to enlarge, the patients begin to waste (cachexia) and ascites fluid may collect in the peritoneum. Death may occur within weeks in acutely ill patients or may occur as late as 3 years after the onset of disease.

There is no primary cutaneous lesion in kala-azar. Some patients, however, develop **dermal leishmanoid.** Patients with this skin condition are often those who have been treated for kala-azar or who have had no severe symptoms of kala-azar. The lesions of dermal leishmanoid may mimic the butterfly rash of systemic lupus erythematosus or may resemble the nodular lesions of leprosy.

(2) Laboratory Analysis.   Cutaneous and mucocutaneous forms of leishmaniasis are diagnosed by examining Giemsa-stained aspirates or biopsies taken from the margin or base of a lesion. Samples should be taken from the most recent lesion, because healing lesions may contain no detectable parasites. Touch impressions of biopsies should show amastigotes (Leishman-Donovan bodies) located within skin macrophages. Amastigotes are easily recognized because of the characteristic "frying pan" arrangement of the kinetoplast and nucleus. Specimens from patients can also be used to inoculate Novy-MacNeal-Nicolle (NNN) medium, which should result in the growth of promastigotes.

Kala-azar should be suspected in patients who live in areas where the disease is endemic, have typical symptoms, and have hypergammaglobulinemia, rheumatoid factor, and immune complexes. Definitive diagnosis involves identifying *Leishmania* amastigotes in reticuloendothelial tissues or venous buffy coat films. Tissue samples are usually obtained via sternal marrow aspiration, but they can be obtained via splenic puncture (which is considered risky) or via liver puncture (which is less productive). Samples should be used to inoculate hamsters intraperitoneally, and the liver and spleen of the hamsters should be examined for leishmania after 2–3 months. Samples taken via splenic aspiration are also sometimes used to inoculate Schneider's *Drosophila* medium,

Roswell Park Memorial Institute (RPMI) medium 1640, or NNN medium.

Treatment.   Leishmanial infections are treated with sodium stibogluconate or meglumine antimoniate, both of which are investigational drugs in the USA and must be obtained from the Centers for Disease Control and Prevention. Amphotericin B has been used as an alternative treatment for mucocutaneous leishmaniasis, and pentamidine has been used to treat kala-azar that fails to respond to conventional therapy.

Prevention.   Direct contact with cutaneous and mucocutaneous lesions should be avoided because it spreads the lesions to other sites on the body or to other persons. There is no commercial vaccine for the prevention of leishmaniasis. In some endemic areas, individuals are protected from disfiguring cutaneous lesions by inoculation of an innocuous site with serous exudate from the lesion of a person with active cutaneous leishmaniasis. About 2% of those who undergo this procedure develop progressive lesions that require treatment, but the procedure confers immunity for life against the inoculated strain. Other preventive approaches focus on control of sandflies.

Characteristics of *Trypanosoma brucei*

In the 1850s, David Livingstone described a disease that was spread from grazing and large game animals to humans and was called *nagana*. He believed that the disease, now commonly known as sleeping sickness, was caused by an infectious agent spread via the bites of tsetse flies. Sir David Bruce later showed that the agent was a trypanosome, and the species was named *Trypanosoma brucei* after Bruce.

General Features.   Three virtually indistinguishable subspecies of *T. brucei* have been described. *Trypanosoma brucei* subspecies *gambiense* causes Gambian (west African) sleeping sickness, *Trypanosoma brucei* subspecies *rhodesiense* causes Rhodesian (east African) sleeping sickness, and *Trypanosoma brucei* subspecies *brucei* causes mild infections in game animals and is not known to cause human disease. Pathogenic trypanosomes infect the blood, lymphatic tissue, and central nervous system. Gambian disease tends to follow a chronic course, with many remissions and exacerbations, and is fatal after months to years of disease. Rhodesian disease, in contrast, is an acute disease in which the central nervous system is invaded early and death generally occurs within 9 months.

Mechanisms of Pathogenicity.   The tsetse fly is infected with the **trypomastigote** form of *T. brucei* when it takes a blood meal from an infected animal. Once infected, the tsetse fly is infected for life. The trypomastigote develops in about 3 weeks into an **epimastigote** and then into the infective metacyclic form of the trypanosome.

Human infections begin when the **metacyclic trypomastigote** is introduced into the victim through the bite of a tsetse fly. The metacyclic trypomastigote quickly converts to a **mature trypomastigote** within the vicinity of the bite, and mature trypomastigotes are the form seen in body fluid throughout disease. The key to understanding the different disease courses is to remember that Gambian disease is chronic, while Rhodesian disease is acute. Table 24–4 compares the two.

Trypomastigotes divide longitudinally via binary fission. After a period of localized multiplication, the trypanosomes begin to spread. The trypomastigotes of *T. b. gambiense* tend to accumulate in the lymphatic system, with few being seen in the blood at this time, while those of *T. b. rhodesiense* are found primarily within the blood. Hyperplasia of the cervical lymph nodes, especially during Gambian disease, causes prominent cervical lymphadenopathy. Headaches soon begin and are probably due to blockage of blood and cerebrospinal fluid flow by amastigotes in the central nervous system. Eventually, trypomastigotes accumulate in the central nervous system and cause the form of meningoencephalitis commonly known as sleeping sickness. The mechanisms responsible for central nervous system disease are unclear.

Molecular studies have shown that surface glycoprotein antigens called **variant-specific glycoproteins** (VSGs) are expressed by the trypomastigotes and form a continuous coat over each of them. Each trypanosome has about 1000 VSG genes in its genome, and most of these are located near the ends (telomeres) of the chromosomes. Only one of these genes is expressed at any time, and the expression of a particular VSG is identified as the **variable antigenic type** (VAT) of the organism. Infection is initiated by organisms of a single VAT. As the immune response develops against the VSG expressed on that VAT, there is a genetic rearrangement that results in the expression of a new VSG. This is why the symptoms of trypanosomiasis wax and wane. The immune response greatly reduces the level of parasitemia, but then a new VAT population of trypanosomes appears and causes a relapse of disease. The sequential appearance of waves of VAT populations causes the patient to develop extremely high levels of circulating IgM.

Diseases Due to *Trypanosoma brucei*

Epidemiology. The geographic distributions of Gambian and Rhodesian trypanosomiasis are depicted in Fig. 24–11.

T. b. rhodesiense is transmitted to humans via the bites of tsetse flies (*Glossina* species) that feed primarily on large grazing animals, particularly the bushbuck, hartebeest, and domestic ox. The tsetse flies are found chiefly in rather open "bush" areas where grazing occurs. Rhodesian sleeping sickness occurs sporadically, with occasional epidemics. Because it follows an acute course, human carriers are believed to play little or no role in the transmission of this disease.

T. b. gambiense is transmitted to humans through the bites of *Glossina palpalis* and *Glossina tachinoides,* species of tsetse flies that are found primarily along streams near human habitations. Gambian sleeping sickness often assumes a subacute course, and asymptomatic human carriers are the reservoirs for infection. Game animals are not believed to serve as significant reservoirs for Gambian disease.

Diagnosis

(1) History and Physical Examination. Patients infected with *T. brucei* often develop a **trypanosoma chancre** at the site of a tsetse fly bite. This ulcerated lesion, which contains trypomastigotes, is seen most commonly in non-Africans. Other signs of **African trypanosomiasis,** or **sleeping sickness,** may appear days to weeks after infection; the incubation period

TABLE 24–4. A Comparison of the Characteristics of Gambian Trypanosomiasis and Rhodesian Trypanosomiasis

Characteristic	Gambian Trypanosomiasis	Rhodesian Trypanosomiasis
Vectors	*Glossina palpalis* and *Glossina tachinoides* (tsetse flies).	Various *Glossina* species (tsetse flies).
Risk areas	Streams near human habitations.	Open "bush" areas.
Reservoirs	Asymptomatic humans.	Large grazing animals, including the bushbuck, ox, and hartebeest.
Pattern of occurrence	Endemic.	Sporadic.
Infective stage	Metacyclic trypomastigote.	Metacyclic trypomastigote.
Incubation period	Weeks to months.	From 1 to 2 weeks.
Hemolymphatic disease		
Extent of lymphadenopathy	Prominent.	May be unremarkable.
Trypomastigotes in blood	Few.	Many.
Trypomastigotes in lymph nodes	Many.	Few.
Febrile attacks	Moderate.	Intense.
Neurologic disease		
Duration	From 1 to 3 years, with exacerbations and remissions.	Usually under 1 year.
Severity	Subacute course, with some patients developing chronic lesions of the central nervous system.	Acute course, with early death.

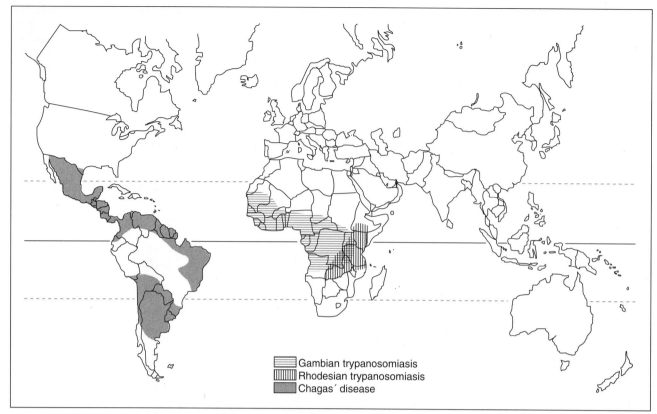

FIGURE 24–11. The geographic distribution of Gambian trypanosomiasis, Rhodesian trypanosomiasis, and Chagas' disease. These diseases are caused by *Trypanosoma brucei* subspecies *gambiense, Trypanosoma brucei* subspecies *rhodesiense,* and *Trypanosoma cruzi,* respectively. (Redrawn and reproduced, with permission, from Markell, E. K., M. Voge, and D. T. John. Medical Parasitology, 7th ed. Philadelphia, W. B. Saunders Company 1992.)

is typically shorter and the onset more acute in non-Africans.

Patients with hemolymphatic disease suffer from anorexia, confusion, lethargy, and malaise. **Winterbottom's sign** (prominent cervical lymphadenopathy) is usually present in patients with **Gambian trypanosomiasis** but is often absent in those with **Rhodesian trypanosomiasis.** The fever at this time is irregular and is accompanied by chills. Some febrile patients develop a rash that is similar in appearance to erythema multiforme. The fever lasts up to a week, and then it remits for several weeks. When the fever recurs, it is accompanied by parasitemia. The patient may pass through a series of such attacks and eventually remit, or central nervous system disease may follow.

In patients with Gambian disease, the recognizable onset of meningoencephalitis may be 6 months to a year after the onset of infection. In patients with Rhodesian disease, central nervous system manifestations develop shortly after the onset of infection. Patients with meningoencephalitis exhibit a wide variety of motor and sensory changes. They become progressively apathetic, confused, and somnolent, and they stop eating and soon become emaciated. **Karandel's sign** is positive: when pressure is initially applied to the hands or over the ulnar nerve and is then removed, the patient experiences severe pain.

Eventually, moribund patients slip into a coma. The progression from infection to coma takes months (usually less than a year) in patients with Rhodesian sleeping sickness, but it may follow a remittent course and take years in those with Gambian sleeping sickness.

(2) Laboratory Analysis. The diagnosis can be confirmed by demonstrating the presence of trypomastigotes in blood, cerebrospinal fluid, or lymph node aspirates. During the invasive and lymphadenopathy stages of disease, *T. b. rhodesiense* is most likely to be found in the blood, while *T. b. gambiense* is best found in lymph node aspirates. Identification of trypanosomes in cerebrospinal fluid indicates that the patient is suffering from central nervous system disease.

Patients with African trypanosomiasis have extremely high levels of IgM, owing to the antigenic variation expressed by trypanosomes. Immunologic tests available to detect antitrypanosomal antibodies include complement fixation and immunofluorescent antibody tests. Cerebrospinal fluid from patients with trypanosomal meningoencephalitis yields positive results in the immunofluorescent antibody test.

Treatment and Prognosis. Early (hemolymphatic) Gambian trypanosomiasis is treated with pentamidine, while hemolymphatic Rhodesian trypanosomiasis is treated with suramin. Once meningoencephalitis is present, Gambian and Rhodesian diseases are both treated with eflornithine (drug of choice) or melarsoprol. Suramin and melarsoprol are investigational drugs, available in the USA through the Centers for Disease Control and Prevention. Patients treated with melarsoprol may have a Jarisch-Herxheimer reaction, and some patients develop reactive encephalopathy or hemorrhagic encephalopathy.

Prevention.   There is no vaccine or chemoprophylactic regimen to prevent African trypanosomiasis. Preventive efforts have focused primarily on the elimination of tsetse flies and the avoidance of their bites.

Characteristics of *Trypanosoma cruzi*

General Features.   *Trypanosoma cruzi* is the cause of American trypanosomiasis, or Chagas' disease. *T. cruzi* differs from its African counterparts in several ways. First, *T. cruzi* exhibits all four of the developmental forms of trypanosomes. Second, *T. cruzi* is transmitted to humans through the feces of triatomid bugs (Fig. 24–12). Third, the parasites preferentially infect cardiac, smooth, and skeletal muscle; reticuloendothelial cells; and neuroglial cells. Fourth, the parasites do not pass through waves of antigenic variation, so Chagas' disease is not a remittent disease, and there is no accompanying elevation of serum IgM levels.

Mechanisms of Pathogenicity.   Metacyclic trypomastigotes enter the skin after a triatomid bite. An intense inflammatory response develops, and trypomastigotes enter histiocytes, adipose cells, muscle cells, and polymorphonuclear leukocytes. Within these cells, the trypomastigotes become **amastigotes** and multiply locally. Trypomastigotes that are formed escape the host cells and travel to the draining lymph nodes, where they multiply again as amastigotes. The organisms then spread hematogenously to the liver, spleen, various muscles, and the central nervous system. Amastigotes multiply within Kupffer cells in the liver and within macrophages in the spleen. In the heart and other muscles, **pseudocysts**

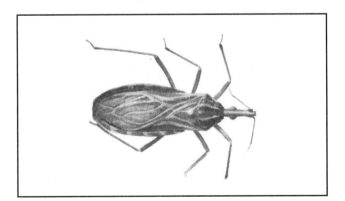

FIGURE 24–12. A triatomid bug. Triatomids transmit Chagas' disease through their feces. (Reproduced, with permission, from Markell, E. K., M. Voge, and D. T. John. Medical Parasitology, 7th ed. Philadelphia, W. B. Saunders Company, 1992. Photograph by Zane Price from material furnished by Dr. Ralph A. Barr.)

are formed around pockets of multiplying amastigotes. In the central nervous system, amastigotes and trypomastigotes attract a lymphocytic response, causing small granulomas to form around the parasites in the brain substance.

Cardiomyopathy results from multiplication of amastigotes in the heart and from the inflammatory response to these amastigotes. Some of the damage to the heart muscle may be related to the formation of autoantibodies directed against the endocardium, blood vessels, and striated muscle. *T. cruzi*–infected macrophages are thought to secrete cytokines that promote the generation of this autoimmune response. *T. cruzi* damages the autonomic nervous system of the heart or the gastrointestinal system in some patients. This damage can cause the heart to dilate tremendously or can cause the patient to develop megacolon or megaesophagus.

Diseases Due to *Trypanosoma cruzi*

Epidemiology.   The most important reservoirs of *T. cruzi* infection are dogs and cats, but other animals (including opossums and armadillos) are known to be naturally infected. *T. cruzi* infection is usually spread to humans when infected triatomid bugs feed on humans and defecate when they feed. The bite of the infected bug irritates the patient's skin, and when the patient scratches the bite, the trypanosomes are introduced into the skin. In areas where Chagas' disease is prevalent, *T. cruzi* is occasionally spread directly from person to person via blood transfusions.

Chagas' disease is found only in the Americas, with cases reported as far north as Texas and California and as far south as Argentina and Chile (see Fig. 24–11). The disease is rare in the USA. It is most common in Brazil, where about 20–30% of bloodsucking triatomids are infected with *T. cruzi*. Disease prevalence is highest in homes that have dogs or cats infected with *T. cruzi*.

Diagnosis

(1) History and Physical Examination.   At the site of entry of *T. cruzi* into the skin, a **chagoma** develops and causes the area to become red and painful. The lesion can reach several centimeters in diameter and may persist for 2–3 months. Within 3 days of infection, the lymph nodes that drain the area of the bite become firm and palpable.

During the early weeks of **acute Chagas' disease,** patches of hard, nonpitting edema appear suddenly and then persist for days to months. In many patients, an area of nonpitting edema appears on one side of the face and is accompanied by conjunctivitis and swelling of the upper and lower eyelids **(Romaña's sign).** The unilateral facial edema may spread to involve the cheek and neck **(oculoglandular syndrome).**

Between 4 days and 2 weeks after infection begins, patients develop chills, fever, aches, pains, malaise, and exhaustion. Some patients develop generalized lymphadenopathy, and others develop a rash that fades after 7–10 days. The clinical course is more severe in children than in adults, and the level of parasitemia is highest in infants under 1 year of age. Severe infections are characterized by anasarca (generalized edema), high fever, and splenomegaly. Some infants develop meningoencephalitis, and about 40% of patients develop cardiac abnormalities. Within a few weeks, patients will die, remit, or enter a period of chronic Chagas' disease.

Chronic Chagas' disease is seen most commonly in adults and is often heralded by cardiomyopathy. The most common cardiac changes are partial or complete atrioventricular block, complete right bundle branch block, and premature ventricular contractions. Patients develop progressive congestive heart failure that is usually right-sided. Many suffer from fainting spells, and many die suddenly. A few patients develop autonomic nerve damage that can lead to megaesophagus or megacolon.

(2) Laboratory Analysis. The diagnosis of Chagas' disease can be confirmed by identifying the trypanosomes in stained blood films. Amastigotes can be seen within the chagoma and in biopsies of swollen lymph nodes or other infected tissues. The trypomastigotes may be difficult to find in older patients and may require the use of xenodiagnosis or antibody tests. In xenodiagnosis, laboratory-raised triatomids are allowed to feed on the patient and are subsequently examined for the presence of trypanosomes. Laboratory tests for antitrypanosomal antibodies include a radioimmunoassay and a complement fixation test called the Machado-Guerreiro test.

Treatment. Chagas' disease is treated with nifurtimox, a drug available in the USA through the Centers for Disease Control and Prevention. Alternative treatments include benznidazole (not available in the USA), allopurinol, and ketoconazole.

Prevention. Most efforts to prevent Chagas' disease have focused on the use of insecticides to control triatomids. This approach has been quite successful in some vicinities. There is no vaccine.

Selected Readings

Adam, R. D. The biology of *Giardia* species. Microbiol Rev 55:706–732, 1991.

Aldape, K., et al. *Naegleria fowleri*: characterization of a secreted histolytic cysteine protease. Exp Parasitol 78:230–241, 1994.

Aucott, J. N., and J. I. Ravdin. Amebiasis and "nonpathogenic" intestinal protozoa. Infect Dis Clin North Am 7:467–485, 1993.

Beadle, C., et al. Diagnosis of malaria by detection of *Plasmodium falciparum* HRP-2 antigen with a rapid dipstick antigen-capture assay. Lancet 343:564–568, 1994.

Bryan, R. T. Microsporidiosis as an AIDS-related opportunistic infection. Clin Infect Dis 21(supplement 1):S62–S65, 1995.

Carbajal, M. E., et al. Fibronectin-induced intracellular calcium rise in *Entamoeba histolytica* trophozoites: effect on adhesion and the actin cytoskeleton. Exp Parasitol 82:11–20, 1996.

Chatterjee, S., et al. A conserved peptide sequence of the *Plasmodium falciparum* circumsporite protein and antipeptide antibodies inhibit *Plasmodium berghei* sporozoite invasion of Hep-G2 cells and protect mice against *P. berghei* sporozoite challenge. Infect Immun 63:4375–4381, 1995.

Coggswell, F. B. The hypnozoites and relapse in primate malaria. Clin Microbiol Rev 5:26–35, 1992.

Dubois, P., and L. Pereira da Silva. Towards a vaccine against asexual blood stage infection by *Plasmodium falciparum.* Res Immunol 146:263–275, 1995.

Ficker, L. *Acanthamoeba* keratitis: the quest for a better prognosis. Eye 2(supplement):S37–S45, 1988.

Goodgame, R. W. Understanding intestinal spore-forming protozoa: cryptosporidia, microsporidia, isospora, and cyclospora. Ann Intern Med 124:429–441, 1996.

Green, S., et al. Activated macrophages destroy intracellular *Leishmania major* amastigotes by an L-arginine–dependent killing mechanism. J Immunol 144:278–283, 1990.

Grendon, J. H., et al. Descriptive features of *Dientamoeba fragilis* infections. J Trop Med Hyg 98:309–315, 1995.

Joiner, K. A., and J. F. Dubremetz. *Toxoplasma gondii:* a protozoan for the nineties. Infect Immun 61:1169–1172, 1993.

Lin, J. Y., et al. Tumor necrosis factor alpha augments nitric oxide–dependent macrophage cytotoxicity against *Entamoeba histolytica* by enhanced expression of the nitric oxide synthase gene. Infect Immun 62:1534–1541, 1994.

McCoy, J. J., B. J. Mann, and W. A. Petri, Jr. Adherence and cytotoxicity of *Entamoeba histolytica* or how lectins let parasites stick around. Infect Immun 62:3045–3050, 1994.

Mendis, K. N., P. H. Davis, and R. Carter. Antigenic polymorphism in malaria: is it an important mechanism for immune evasion? Immunol Today 12:A34–A37, 1991.

Pays, E., L. Vanhamme, and M. Berberof. Genetic controls for the expression of surface antigens in African trypanosomes. Ann Rev Microbiol 48:25–52, 1994.

Rabeneck, L., et al. Observations on the pathological spectrum and clinical course of microsporidiosis in men infected with the human immunodeficiency virus: follow-up study. Clin Infect Dis 20:1229–1235, 1995.

Reed, S. L. Amebiasis: an update. Clin Infect Dis 14:385–393, 1992.

Rotterdam, H., and P. Tsang. Gastrointestinal disease in the immunocompromised patient. Hum Pathol 25:1123–1140, 1994.

St. Georgiev, V. Management of toxoplasmosis. Drugs 48:179–188, 1994.

Sargeantson, S. W., and G. G. Crane. Analysis of the patterns of inheritance of splenomegaly and serum IgM levels in the Watut of Papua New Guinea. Hum Biol 63:115–128, 1991.

Tapia, F. J., G. Caceres-Dittmar, and M. A. Sanchez. Inadequate epidermal homing leads to tissue damage in human cutaneous leishmaniasis. Immunol Today 15:160–165, 1994.

Toney, D. M., and F. Marciano-Cabral. Membrane vesiculation of *Naegleria fowleri* amoebae as a mechanism for resisting complement damage. J Immunol 152:2952–2959, 1994.

Wolfe, M. S. Giardiasis. Clin Microbiol Rev 5:93–100, 1992.

al-Yaman, F., et al. Assessment of the role of the humoral response to *Plasmodium falciparum* MSP2 compared to RESA and SPf66 in protecting Papua New Guinean children from clinical malaria. Parasite Immunol 17:493–501, 1995.

Zilberstein, D., and M. Shapira. The role of pH and temperature in the development of *Leishmania* parasites. Annu Rev Microbiol 48:449–470, 1994.

CHAPTER TWENTY-FIVE

HELMINTHS

Cestodes, Nematodes, and Trematodes

The helminths are a large group of parasitic worms that include cestodes (tapeworms), nematodes (roundworms), and trematodes (flukes). Manifestations of helminthic disease vary, depending on both the type and the developmental form of the parasite. Although the mature (adult) form of most helminths does not produce severe disease, the eggs and larvae of some helminths can cause life-threatening disease. For example, most adult tapeworms are innocuous or cause only vague gastrointestinal symptoms, yet larval tapeworms can produce seizures and personality changes and may result in the death of the patient.

Helminths are among the most prevalent causes of disease in the world and are especially common in those tropical countries in which living conditions are squalid and water and food are often contaminated with human feces. Most helminths do not multiply directly within the human host, so patients who are removed from the source of infection will rid themselves of worms over time. Thus, it is often not necessary to treat patients with anthelmintic drugs unless they are severely ill. Chapter 23 provides information about the actions and effects of anthelmintic drugs, and Table 25–1 outlines specific treatments for cestode, trematode, and nematode diseases.

CESTODES
Classification and Structure of Cestodes

Cestodes are members of the phylum Platyhelminthes and the class Cestoda. Commonly called **tapeworms,** the cestodes must pass through one or more hosts during their life cycle. **Intermediate hosts** are hosts in which the parasite develops into a larval form. The **definitive host** is the host in which larvae develop into adult parasites. Table 25–2 provides information about the classification and hosts of the medically important tapeworms.

Cestodes have no alimentary or vascular tracts. They absorb nutrients through the **tegument,** a cuticle that encloses the worm. Cestodes are shaped like ribbons and consist of a **scolex** (a headlike organ) and a long chain of segments. Each segment is called a **proglottid,** and the chain of proglottids is called the **strobila.** The strobila is attached to the base of

the scolex at a region known as the **neck.** Because proglottids arise from the neck, any treatment meant to eradicate a tapeworm must also eliminate the scolex.

The scolex of the tapeworm has organs of attachment that are distinctive for each genus or species of worm. *Taenia* species, for example, have cuplike sucking disks by which they attach to the intestinal mucosa. At the anterior end of its scolex, *Taenia solium* also has a protrusion that is called a **rostellum** and is armed with **chitinous hooks** (Fig. 25–1). In contrast, the scoleces of *Diphyllobothrium* and related tapeworms have elongated suctorial grooves called **bothria.**

The proglottids of most tapeworms are hermaphroditic. Proglottids closest to the neck are relatively undifferentiated, but as the proglottids distance themselves from the scolex, they develop mature male and female reproductive organs. The segments farthest from the scolex are **gravid proglottids** and contain only a uterus distended with eggs. The shape and contents of the mature and gravid proglottids are used to differentiate among the various tapeworm species. For example, the gravid proglottids of *Taenia saginata* contain 15–30 pairs of lateral uterine branches, while those of *T. solium* (see Fig. 25–1) contain only 7–12 pairs. The gravid proglottids may break off and be found in stool samples from patients, or they may disintegrate while still attached to the strobila.

Life Cycle of Cestodes

Each tapeworm has a definitive host and one or more intermediate hosts. Tapeworms can persist within humans either as adults or as larvae, but few can persist as both. In other words, humans may serve as the definitive host or as an intermediate host, but they rarely serve as both.

Fig. 25–2 depicts the general life cycle of tapeworms. The adult worm lives within the gastrointestinal tract of its definitive host, where it attaches to the intestinal wall via its scolex. Adult taeniids and *Diphyllobothrium* may live as long as 20–25 years, while some of the smaller tapeworms live as adults for only a few months. Within the definitive host, the

TABLE 25–1. Recommended Antiparasitic Drugs for the Treatment of Human Helminthic Infections

Helminth	Effective Treatments
Cestodes	
Diphyllobothrium latum	Niclosamide or praziquantel.
Dipylidium caninum	Niclosamide or praziquantel.
Echinococcus species	Surgery plus albendazole;* surgery plus mebendazole; or surgery plus praziquantel.
Hymenolepis diminuta	Niclosamide or praziquantel.
Hymenolepis nana	Praziquantel or niclosamide.
Multiceps multiceps	Surgery.
Taenia saginata	Niclosamide or praziquantel.
Taenia solium	
Adult tapeworms	Niclosamide or praziquantel.
Cysticercosis	Albendazole plus dexamethasone; or praziquantel plus dexamethasone.
Trematodes	
Clonorchis sinensis	Praziquantel.
Echinostoma species	Praziquantel.
Fasciola hepatica	Praziquantel* or bithionol.
Fasciolopsis buski	Praziquantel* or niclosamide.
Heterophyes heterophyes	Praziquantel* or tetrachloroethylene.
Metagonimus species	Praziquantel.
Opisthorchis species	Praziquantel.
Paragonimus westermani	Praziquantel* or bithionol.
Schistosoma species	Praziquantel;* or metrifonate† for Schistosoma haematobium infection; or oxamniquine for Schistosoma mansoni infection.
Nematodes	
Ancylostoma braziliense	Thiabendazole.
Ancylostoma duodenale	Albendazole* or mebendazole.
Ascaris lumbricoides	Albendazole,* piperazine citrate, or pyrantel pamoate.
Brugia species	Diethylcarbamazine citrate* or ivermectin.†
Capillaria philippinensis	Mebendazole* or albendazole.
Dracunculus medinensis	Niridazole,† thiabendazole, or metronidazole.
Enterobius vermicularis	Albendazole* or piperazine citrate.
Loa loa	Diethylcarbamazine citrate* or ivermectin.†
Necator americanus	Albendazole* or mebendazole.
Onchocerca volvulus	Nodulectomy plus ivermectin;*† or nodulectomy plus diethylcarbamazine citrate.
Strongyloides stercoralis	Albendazole,* mebendazole, or ivermectin.†
Toxocara species	Corticosteroids plus antihistamines.
Trichinella spiralis	Thiabendazole plus corticosteroids; or mebendazole plus corticosteroids.
Trichuris trichiura	Mebendazole* or albendazole.
Wuchereria bancrofti	Diethylcarbamazine citrate* or ivermectin.†

* Antiparasitic drug of choice.
† Investigational drug, available in the USA from the Centers for Disease Control and Prevention.

gravid proglottids break off or disintegrate, and eggs and proglottids pass into the feces. Then one of two developmental pathways is followed, depending on the type of tapeworm.

The first developmental pathway is followed by tapeworms that have a uterine pore. The worm passes undifferentiated eggs that develop within water, and a ciliated **coracidium** is released from the egg into the environment. The coracidium is eaten by the first intermediate host, which usually is a copepod. Within the copepod, the larva develops into a **procercoid larva,** and the procercoid larva enters the second intermediate host (a fish) when the copepod is eaten. The procercoid larva becomes a **plerocercoid larva,** or **sparganum,** in the muscles of the fish, and it is this form that is infective for the definitive host.

The second developmental pathway is followed by the taeniid worms. The eggs of these tapeworms, which are passed fully differentiated in the feces, contain an embryo known as an **oncosphere.** Although only T. solium will develop an adult scolex that contains hooks, the oncospheres of both T. solium and T. saginata contain easily observable hooklets. Taeniid eggs are eaten by the intermediate host, and a vesicular larva develops within the tissues of the intermediate host. The definitive host is infected when it eats the vesicular larva along with the flesh of the intermediate host.

Fig. 25–3 shows several larval forms of tapeworms that infect humans. Procercoid and plerocercoid larvae, which are part of the Diphyllobothrium developmental series, are examples of **solid larvae.** Cysticercoid, cysticercus, coenurus, and echinococcus larvae have fluid-filled chambers and are therefore considered to be **vesicular larvae.**

Pathogenesis of Cestode Disease

Most humans who harbor **adult tapeworms** in their intestinal tract are unaware of their presence. Attachment of the adult worm to the mucosa elicits a mild inflammatory reaction, which may be responsible for mild to moderate abdominal discomfort and persistent diarrhea in some patients. In rare cases, the adult worm may obstruct the intestine, common bile duct, or pancreatic duct. Diphyllobothrium latum absorbs vitamin B_{12} from the host, and some patients infected with this worm develop a vitamin B_{12} deficiency that mimics pernicious anemia.

Larval tapeworms can cause serious disease, especially when the larvae encyst within the heart, liver, bone marrow, or brain and cause space-occupying lesions. There are four types of larval tapeworm disease: cysticercosis, coenurus disease, echinococcosis (hydatid disease), and sparganosis.

Cysticercosis is caused by the larvae (cysticerci) of T. solium, which are 0.6–1.8 cm in diameter. Patients are generally asymptomatic unless the cysticerci locate within the heart or central nervous system. In the heart, cysticerci may cause cardiac arrhythmia as a result of changes in electrical conduction. In the central nervous system, cysticerci are

TABLE 25–2.   The Medically Important Tapeworms

Family, Genus, and Species	Definitive Hosts	Intermediate Hosts	Larval Disease in Humans
Dilepididae			
Dipylidium caninum	Dogs, cats, and humans.	Dog, cat, and human fleas.	None.
Diphyllobothriidae			
Diphyllobothrium latum	Humans.	Copepods (first); fish (second).	None.
Other *Diphyllobothrium* species	Various mammals other than humans.	Humans, snakes, and amphibians.	Sparganosis.
Spirometra mansonoides	Dogs and cats.	Copepods (first); humans, other mammals, frogs, and snakes (second).	Sparganosis.
Hymenolepididae			
Hymenolepis diminuta	Humans and rats.	Grain beetles and flour moths.	None.
Hymenolepis nana	Humans, mice, and rats.	Fleas and grain beetles.*	None.
Taeniidae			
Echinococcus granulosis	Dogs and wolves.	Humans, pigs, camels, horses, cattle, sheep, elk, deer, and moose.	Cystic echinococcosis (hydatid disease).
Echinococcus multilocularis	Foxes, dogs, and cats.	Humans and rodents.	Alveolar echinococcosis.
Echinococcus oligarthrus	Dogs.	Humans and rodents.	Ocular echinococcosis.
Echinococcus vogeli	Bush dogs.	Humans, pacas, agoutis, and spiny rats.	Polycystic echinococcosis.
Multiceps multiceps	Dogs and wild canids.	Humans and many herbivorous animals.	Coenurus disease.
Taenia saginata	Humans.	Cattle and camels.	None.
Taenia solium	Humans.	Hogs, humans, cats, dogs, sheep, and deer.	Cysticercosis.

* For *H. nana,* an intermediate host is not required.

found most often in the subarachnoid space, where their presence elicits an inflammatory response. The inflammation may in turn be responsible for the development of arachnoiditis and obstructive hydrocephalus. Less common are intraventricular cysts and spinal cysts. Intraventricular cysts can cause ependymitis and hydrocephalus, while spinal cysts may be accompanied by radiculitis or spinal cord compression. In rare cases, patients develop racemose cysts, which are large lobulated cysts that lack a scolex and are usually found in the ventricular system or subarachnoid space. Because of their size, racemose cysts cause more severe disease. Although neurocysticercosis can be severe, it is often transient.

Coenurus disease is caused by the larvae of *Multiceps* tapeworms. These larvae are about 2 cm in diameter and preferentially locate within the central nervous system, where they cause lesions that are difficult to differentiate from racemose cysts but are generally associated with more severe manifestations. In some patients, coenurus larvae are also found in muscles and subcutaneous tissues. The larvae produce a factor that inhibits the ability of macrophages to act as accessory cells during the immune response.

Echinococcosis, or **hydatid disease,** is caused by the larvae of *Echinococcus* species. These larvae form vesicular cysts that are called hydatid cysts and vary in size, depending on their location. Most cysts develop in the liver and lungs, where they are usually about 1 cm in diameter after approximately 5 months. The cysts may accumulate large amounts of fluid and increase by 4–5 cm per year, eventually reaching the size of a small pumpkin. Hydatid cysts act as space-occupying lesions that can significantly disrupt organ function, cause pressure necrosis, and obstruct blood, lymph, or biliary flow. The cysts often leak a protein-filled fluid that elicits an IgE-mediated allergic response, and rupture of a large cyst can cause systemic anaphylaxis to occur. In addition to containing fluid, hydatid cysts contain millions of **protoscoleces,** which are also called **hydatid sand.** When the sand leaks from the cyst, each protoscolex can develop into a daughter hydatid cyst. Daughter cysts most often locate in the bone, brain, eye, heart, or kidney.

Sparganosis is caused by the larvae (spargana) of various *Diphyllobothrium* species that do not develop into adult forms in humans. The larvae are solid and are usually several centimeters long. Sparganosis is seen most often in people who use poultices containing snake or frog meat. The parasites enter via the poultice and affect the tissues where the poultice was applied to the skin or eye. The presence of spargana elicits a painful granulomatous response, characterized by the development of necrosis and accumulation of eosinophils. Individuals who eat raw frogs or snakes can develop neurosparganosis, a disease in which granulomas form around the sparganum in the frontoparietal lobes or the occipital lobes.

Dipylidium caninum
Characteristics of D. caninum

Dipylidium caninum is a tapeworm that is found worldwide, is usually harbored by dogs and cats, and

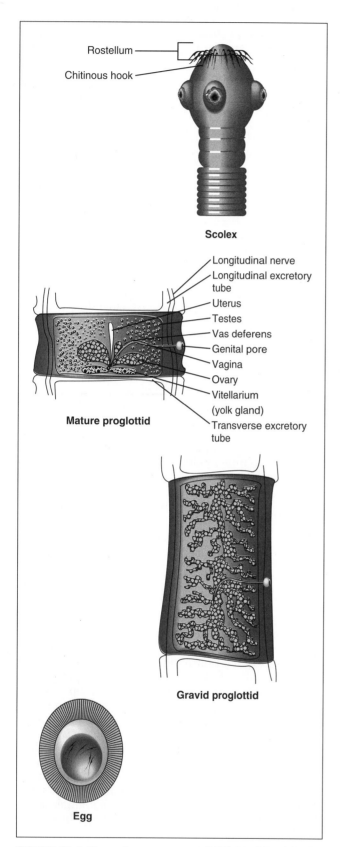

FIGURE 25–1. The scolex, mature proglottid, gravid proglottid, and egg of *Taenia solium*. (Source: Brown, H. W. Basic Clinical Parasitology, 3rd ed. New York, Meredith Corporation, 1969. Redrawn and reproduced, with permission, from Appleton and Lange.)

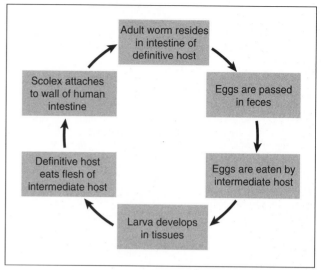

FIGURE 25–2. The general life cycle of tapeworms that infect humans.

occasionally infects humans. The adult worms are 10–70 cm long and are constructed from a series of barrel-shaped proglottids. The gravid proglottids eventually break into units that are called egg packets and contain from 5 to 30 eggs each. The egg packets are passed in the stool, where they are eaten by cat, dog, or human fleas that are in the larval stage of development. Within the fleas, cysticercoid larvae develop, and these are the infective forms for the definitive host.

Diseases Due to *D. caninum*

Humans are infected with *D. caninum* when they swallow dog or cat fleas, usually while cuddling a pet. Most human infections occur in children. Light infections are asymptomatic, but children with heavy worm loads may have abdominal pain, diarrhea, and pruritus ani. Laboratory confirmation involves identifying proglottids or egg packets in stool samples.

D. caninum infections are treated with niclosamide or praziquantel.

Diphyllobothrium Species
Characteristics of *Diphyllobothrium*

Diphyllobothrium latum, also called the **broad tapeworm** or **fish tapeworm**, is the principal *Diphyllobothrium* species that causes disease in humans. *D. latum* is a large tapeworm, reaching 3–10 m in length and having over 4000 proglottids. The tiny scolex is 2.5 mm long by about 1 mm wide and has suctorial grooves called bothria. The eggs of *D. latum* are 60–70 μm long by 40–50 μm wide, are passed from the uterine pore in the unembryonated state, and will develop an embryo after 11–15 days in cool fresh water. *D. latum* eggs are unusual among the tapeworm eggs in that they are operculated. A ciliated coracidium escapes from the egg into the water and is eaten by a copepod. Inside the copepod, the egg develops into a procercoid larva. If the copepod is eaten by a

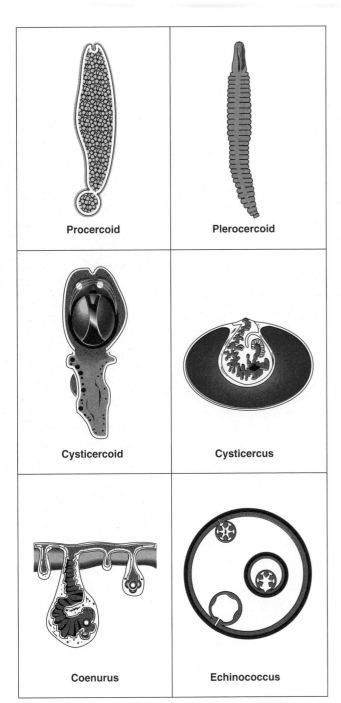

Procercoid

Plerocercoid

Cysticercoid

Cysticercus

Coenurus

Echinococcus

FIGURE 25–3. Larval forms of tapeworms that infect humans. Procercoid and plerocercoid larvae, which are characteristic of *Diphyllobothrium* and *Spirometra,* are solid larvae. The other larvae pictured are vesicular larvae. (Source: Brown, H. W. Basic Clinical Parasitology, 3rd ed. New York, Meredith Corporation, 1969. Redrawn and reproduced, with permission, from Appleton and Lange.)

fish, the larva will develop into a plerocercoid larva (sparganum) within the muscles of the fish.

Humans are the definitive host of *D. latum* and are infected when they eat raw or undercooked freshwater fish. The plerocercoid larva attaches to the wall of the human intestine and grows to maturity in about 3–5 weeks. When the adult tapeworm attaches to the jejunum, the patient may develop a deficiency

in vitamin B_{12} that resembles pernicious anemia. This vitamin deficiency is seen most often in Finland, leading some investigators to believe that it may have a genetic component.

Other *Diphyllobothrium* species and *Spirometra mansonoides,* a closely related tapeworm, cause a larval infection called sparganosis. As noted earlier, humans are usually infected via contact with frogs or snakes that contain spargana.

Diseases Due to *Diphyllobothrium*

Epidemiology. *D. latum* infection is found in cold climates where raw or undercooked freshwater fish are eaten. It is reported most commonly in the Baltic states, Finland, the former Soviet Union, central and southeastern Europe, northeastern China, Japan, Canada, the northern USA (Alaska and Minnesota), Chile, and Argentina. In North America, the fish most often associated with *D. latum* infection are burbot, pike, salmon, trout, and whitefish.

Sparganosis occurs most often in Indonesia, Vietnam, Japan, Korea, southern China, Thailand, the southern USA, and Australia, but it occurs sporadically in other areas as well.

Diagnosis. About 50% of patients infected with *D. latum* have no clinical signs of infection. Others suffer from vague digestive disturbances, including anorexia, heartburn, a sense of fullness, nausea, and vomiting. In some cases, low-level eosinophilia is noted. Definitive diagnosis is based on finding the operculated eggs or evacuated proglottids of *D. latum* in the feces.

Three forms of **sparganosis** are seen: ocular, subcutaneous, and neurologic. Ocular sparganosis occurs in individuals who have used eye poultices made from frog or snake meat. Massive swelling and edema of the soft tissues around the eye are accompanied by intense pain. If the worm locates under the conjunctiva, a nodule will form and the cornea may ulcerate. Subcutaneous sparganosis usually occurs under a site where a poultice has been applied to the skin. The worm elicits an intense inflammatory response, and the affected area becomes swollen and painful. If the lymphatic vessels are blocked, elephantiasis can develop. Neurosparganosis is rare but can be accompanied by severe neurologic symptoms. Diagnosis of sparganosis is usually made by excising the lesion and examining the sparganum.

Treatment. Infections with *D. latum* can be treated effectively with niclosamide. Praziquantel is an acceptable alternative.

Sparganosis does not respond to drug therapy. Cure is achieved when the sparganum is surgically excised. Some spargana are branching and are extremely difficult to remove, and spargana located in the central nervous system may be impossible to remove.

Echinococcus Species
Characteristics of *Echinococcus*

Echinococcosis is a larval tapeworm infection that can be caused by *Echinococcus granulosus, Echi-*

nococcus multilocularis, Echinococcus oligarthrus, or Echinococcus vogeli. Because most human disease is caused by E. granulosus, the discussion focuses on this organism.

The definitive hosts of E. granulosus are dogs and wolves, and intermediate hosts are pigs and large grazing animals, including camels, horses, cattle, deer, elk, sheep, and moose. Humans are only occasionally infected, but with disastrous results.

Dogs and wolves become infected when they eat the flesh of an intermediate host that contains hydatid cysts. The adult worms develop in the canid intestines and reach a length of only 3–6 mm. Dogs often become very heavily infected, and individual dogs may have up to 50,000 worms and shed a million Echinococcus eggs per day in their feces. The intermediate hosts, including humans, are infected when they ingest Echinococcus eggs in water or food contaminated with dog feces. The eggs hatch in the intestine, and embryos that are released penetrate the intestinal wall. The embryos most often locate in the liver or lung, and it is here that they develop into large cysts called hydatid cysts (see Pathogenesis of Cestode Disease, above).

Diseases Due to *Echinococcus*

Epidemiology. E. granulosus can be found throughout the world in regions where grazing animals are kept, but most cases of hydatid disease are reported in Australia, New Zealand, Argentina, southern Brazil, Uruguay, Chile, the Middle East, Canada, and grazing areas in the USA. E. multilocularis is more closely associated with foxes and field mice and is seen in central Europe, Russia, western China, western Alaska, the upper midwestern part of the USA, and the wheat-growing provinces of Canada. E. vogeli usually infects bush dogs and rodents in tropical forests in central and northern South America. The epidemiologic distribution of E. oligarthrus is unknown.

Diagnosis. The most prevalent form of echinococcosis is called **hydatid disease** or **cystic echinococcosis** and is caused by E. granulosus. About two-thirds of primary hydatid cysts are found in the liver, and many patients develop cysts in the lung. The cysts may go undetected for years until they become large enough to cause pressure necrosis and damage to surrounding tissue or to block the flow of blood, lymph, or bile. Hepatic hydatid disease causes the liver to become enlarged, and there may be clinical signs of hepatic dysfunction. Affected patients may initially be suspected of suffering from hepatocellular carcinoma. Patients with large pulmonary cysts may complain of shortness of breath, coughing, and chest pain. Leakage of cysts can cause allergic manifestations such as hives and asthma. Between 5% and 20% of patients with hydatid disease present initially only with allergic manifestations.

Cysts that develop secondary to leakage of hydatid sand (protoscoleces) may be found in a wide variety of sites, including long bones, eyes, central nervous system, heart, kidneys, and spleen. Fortunately,

fewer than 5% of patients develop cysts outside the lungs or liver. Because ocular and central nervous system cysts can cause severe clinical signs when quite small, these cysts are often identified in children. In contrast, lung and liver cysts tend to escape detection for years, with the result that most cases of pulmonary and hepatic hydatid disease are diagnosed in adults.

E. multilocularis causes **alveolar echinococcosis,** a disease in which the host tissue is extensively invaded by the primary cyst and metastases are common. The liver is the most prevalent site for primary cysts, but lung and brain metastases are frequently found. The mortality rate associated with alveolar echinococcosis is between 50% and 75%, and most patients are adults.

E. vogeli causes **polycystic echinococcosis,** a disease that is intermediate between cystic and alveolar echinococcosis in its clinical presentation.

Hydatid disease is usually detected initially by imaging studies. Computed tomography (CT), magnetic resonance imaging (MRI), and ultrasound techniques allow the physician to see the cyst in deep tissues, and CT and MRI provide details about the site and condition of the cyst. The cyst contents can be determined by means of a percutaneous fine-needle biopsy guided by CT or ultrasound. The aspirate will contain fluid and acellular hydatid membranes and may contain hydatid sand. Serologic tests are available, but their usefulness in diagnosis is controversial.

Treatment. A combination of surgery and drug therapy is the most effective method of treating hydatid disease. Albendazole or mebendazole has been used not only to treat surgical patients before and after surgery to prevent the development of metastatic cysts but also to treat inoperable patients. Albendazole is reported to be more effective than mebendazole. Praziquantel has also been used with some success. In some countries, treatment consists of draining the cysts via ultrasound-guided percutaneous puncture and replacing the fluid in the cyst with an agent (such as ethanol or cetrimide) that kills protoscoleces.

Hymenolepis Species
Characteristics of *Hymenolepis*

Hymenolepis nana is called the **dwarf tapeworm.** The adult forms reach a length of about 2 cm and are found in mice, rats, and humans. Children are the usual hosts for the worm, and the eggs are passed among children on their hands. Because the life cycle can be completed in a single host, autoinfection is common. Humans can also be infected by coming into contact with rodent droppings in food or water. The eggs are fragile, so passage of the eggs must occur soon after they have been shed. Although no intermediate hosts are required, fleas and grain beetles can serve as intermediate hosts, and humans can be infected when they swallow insects that contain H. nana cysticercoid larvae. The oncospheres are released in the intestinal lumen and burrow into the villous mucosa of the small intestine, where they develop into cysticercoid larvae. The larvae eventually rupture the villi and mature into adults in the intestinal lumen.

Children are occasionally infected with *Hymenolepis diminuta,* but this tapeworm is much less common than *H. nana.* The adult form of *H. diminuta* is usually found in rats, where it grows to a length of 10–60 cm. *H. diminuta* must pass through an arthropod intermediate host. More than 20 different insect species have been found to be natural intermediate hosts, but flour moths and grain beetles seem to be the most common sources for human infections.

Diseases Due to *Hymenolepis*

H. nana is found throughout the world and is common in central Europe and in South America. Children with light infections suffer from no ill effects. However, autoinfection can lead to heavy worm burdens, and children harboring several thousand dwarf tapeworms may suffer from weakness, loss of appetite, abdominal pain, diarrhea, vomiting, dizziness, headache, and allergic manifestations. Some patients develop anemia and low-level eosinophilia. Those with extremely heavy infection may have bloody diarrhea. The diagnosis of *H. nana* infection is confirmed by demonstrating the presence of eggs or proglottids in stool samples or on skin in the perianal region.

Most humans infected with *H. diminuta* are asymptomatic, but some develop vague gastrointestinal symptoms, including anorexia, abdominal pain, diarrhea, and nausea. Infection caused by *H. diminuta* is much less severe than that caused by *H. nana* because *H. diminuta* has no autoinfection cycle and also because it lives only 5–7 weeks. Thus, heavy worm burdens with *H. diminuta* are extremely rare. Diagnosis is based on identifying eggs and proglottids in stool samples.

H. nana and *H. diminuta* infections are treated with praziquantel or niclosamide.

Multiceps multiceps

Characteristics of *M. multiceps*

Multiceps multiceps is a tapeworm whose adult forms reach 40–60 cm in length and are found in the intestines of dogs and wild canids. *M. multiceps* eggs are passed in dog feces and are ingested by herbivorous animals or humans, who serve as intermediate hosts. In humans, disease is caused by the coenurus larva of *M. multiceps.* This larva is a bladder worm that reaches about 2 cm in diameter, has multiple scoleces budding from the germinal layer (Fig. 25–4), and preferentially locates within the central nervous system. In sheep and goats, infection with the coenurus larva causes a neurologic disease called gid.

Diseases Due to *M. multiceps*

Coenurus disease has been reported from a variety of countries, including the USA. In most cases, the

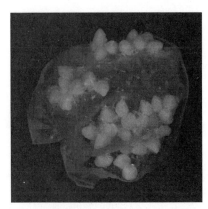

FIGURE 25–4. A cyst taken from a patient with *Multiceps multiceps* infection. (Courtesy of Armed Forces Institute of Pathology. AFIP photo 70-4295.)

larvae are implanted in the central nervous system, where they act as space-occupying lesions. The symptoms of disease depend on the site of implantation but may include loss of sensation, convulsions, diplopia, and syncope. In some cases, laboratory confirmation of coenurus disease can be made by surgically removing and identifying the coenurus larva. In other cases, surgical treatment is not possible.

Taenia Species

Characteristics of *Taenia*

Taenia saginata is the **beef tapeworm.** The adult worms may reach a length of 25 m, but most are between 4 and 10 m. Humans are the definitive host, and cattle serve as an intermediate host of *T. saginata.* Adults worms in the human intestine shed embryonated eggs that are 30–40 μm long by 20–30 μm wide. Cattle ingest the eggs, and a bladder larva called a cysticercus develops within the muscles of the cow. Humans become infected when they ingest undercooked or raw beef that contains larvae. The scolex of the cysticercus attaches to the intestinal mucosa, and the adult worm develops in the upper jejunum.

Taenia solium is called the **pork tapeworm.** While humans are the usual definitive host and hogs are the most important intermediate host of *T. solium,* other intermediate hosts include humans, cats, dogs, sheep, and deer. The adult form of *T. solium* is somewhat shorter than that of *T. saginata,* usually reaching a length of 4–8 m. Although the eggs of *T. solium* are indistinguishable from those of *T. saginata,* the two species of *Taenia* can be differentiated by the appearance of their scoleces and gravid proglottids. Unlike the scolex of *T. saginata,* the scolex of *T. solium* has a rostellum armed with chitinous hooks (see Fig. 25–1). The gravid uterus of *T. solium* has fewer pairs of lateral branches than does that of *T. saginata.* Each gravid proglottid of *T. saginata* contains 30,000–50,000 eggs, and a fully developed worm consists of 800–1000 proglottids.

The life cycle of *T. solium* is depicted in Fig. 25–5. Humans who are infected with adult worms pass *T. solium* eggs in their feces, and the eggs are eaten

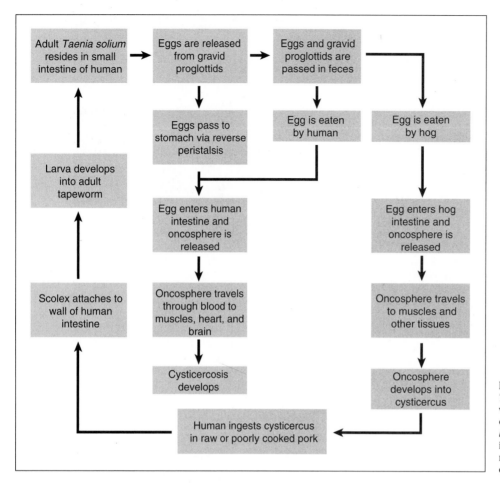

FIGURE 25–5. **The life cycle of** *Taenia solium,* **the pork tapeworm.** Humans who ingest cysticerci in meat develop adult *T. solium* infections, while those who ingest eggs or activate eggs via reverse peristalsis develop cysticercosis.

by hogs. Inside the hog intestine, the oncosphere is released from the egg. After the oncosphere penetrates the intestinal mucosa, it is carried by the blood to muscles and other tissues, where it then develops into a bladder larva known as a cysticercus. (At one time, cysticerci in muscle were considered to be a unique parasite and were known as *Cysticercus cellulosae.* Although cysticerci are now known to be larval forms of *T. solium,* the name *C. cellulosae* is sometimes still used.) Humans are usually infected when they eat raw or poorly cooked pork that contains cysticerci ("measly" pork). The scolex of the cysticercus attaches to the mucosa in the upper jejunum, where the worm then develops to maturity. The adult *T. solium* lives about 25 years. A person who harbors an adult tapeworm can develop cysticercosis when *T. solium* eggs pass from the jejunum into the stomach via reverse peristalsis. Cysticercosis can also result if a person ingests *T. solium* eggs in food or water containing human feces or if food or hands are contaminated with feces from the hands of a *T. solium* carrier.

Diseases Due to *Taenia*

Epidemiology. In 1973, epidemiologists estimated that about 45 million people throughout the

world were infected with *T. saginata.* In contrast, about 3 million were infected with *T. solium.*

The cycle of spreading *T. saginata* from human to cow to human is maintained wherever humans eat raw or undercooked beef and human sewage contaminates the pasture land or water used by cattle. Cysticerci are the infective form for humans, and eggs are the infective form for cattle. Other large grazing animals, such as camels, can also be infected with *T. saginata.*

In the USA, *T. saginata* infection is more common than *T. solium* infection. The latter infection is seen most frequently in Africa, India, China, Latin America, Southeast Asia, Spain, Portugal, and the Slavic countries. Adult *T. solium* infections occur among those who ingest cysticerci in pork, while cysticercosis develops in those who ingest *T. solium* eggs. Most people who are infected with *T. solium* have adult tapeworms, but a small but significant percentage of patients develop cysticercosis. Worldwide, cysticercosis is the most common parasitic disease of the central nervous system.

Diagnosis

(1) History and Physical Examination. Patients infected with adult *T. saginata* or *T. solium* tapeworms are usually asymptomatic or develop only mild gastrointestinal symptoms, such as increased or decreased appetite, chronic indigestion, vague abdominal discomfort, diarrhea, nausea, or vomiting. In most cases, the infection is first noticed by patients when they pass proglottids in their stool. In some cases, patients suffer from vertigo or epigastric pain. Appendicitis, intestinal obstruction, and pancreatic necrosis have been reported but are rare.

Patients infected with the larvae of *T. solium* develop **cysticercosis.** Although cysticerci are sometimes found in the muscles, viscera, eyes, or skin, they are found in the central nervous system in 60% of cases. Neurocysticercosis is the most common cause of acquired epilepsy in countries where *T. solium* is prevalent. Many patients with neurocysticercosis are asymptomatic or develop only transient symptoms, but some develop life-threatening disease. The incubation period for neurocysticercosis is about 3.5 years. In most cases, the disease is parenchymal and is evidenced by the development of focal epileptic seizures. Rare patients develop encephalitis, which is accompanied by mental disturbances and generalized seizures. Nonparenchymal neurocysticercosis can be intraventricular (about 15% of patients), subarachnoid, or spinal. As described earlier (see Pathogenesis of Cestode Disease), individuals who harbor racemose cysts in their central nervous system tend to develop more severe disease.

(2) Laboratory Analysis. Infections with adult *T. saginata* or *T. solium* tapeworms are confirmed by demonstrating the presence of proglottids and eggs in stool samples or on the skin in the perianal region. Cysticercosis is diagnosed by use of imaging techniques such as MRI and CT. Several enzyme-linked immunosorbent assay (ELISA) and Western blot techniques are now available, and these may assist in the diagnosis.

Treatment. For infections with adult *T. saginata* or *T. solium* tapeworms, niclosamide or praziquantel is used. For treatment of cysticercosis, some investigators have reported that albendazole is effective and that praziquantel may offer some benefit. When either drug is used, dexamethasone is given concurrently to ameliorate side effects and, possibly, to augment the effectiveness of the helminthicide. Other investigators have reported that patients treated with prednisolone alone fared better than those treated with the combination of albendazole or praziquantel plus a corticosteroid. Thus, the treatment of cysticercosis remains controversial.

TREMATODES

The trematodes can be divided into two large groups of worms. The **schistosomes,** or **blood flukes,** are diecious (have sexually distinct males and females) and are tube-shaped. Schistosomes infect the small blood vessels of the intestinal mesentery or bladder, and the deposition of their eggs throughout the human body causes granulomatous disease. The **lung, liver, and intestinal flukes,** in contrast, are monoecious (hermaphroditic) worms that are generally leaf-shaped and are flattened dorsoventrally.

Some of them live in the lungs, while others reside in the bile ducts or the tissues of the gastrointestinal tract, including the liver. Disease reflects the damage produced by the migration of flukes, obstruction of bile ducts, and cellular immune response to fluke antigens.

Trematodes cannot multiply within humans and must pass through one or more intermediate hosts. This has two key implications. First, the worm burden of each patient correlates directly with the number of worm larvae that enter the patient. A patient who moves away from an area of endemicity cannot become reinfected, and the worms in the body will eventually die. Second, the geographic distribution of each trematode is restricted by the availability of intermediate hosts. If a key intermediate host is not present in a geographic locale, the organism cannot be perpetuated.

Schistosomes

Worldwide, about 200 million individuals are infected with schistosomes. Of these, an estimated 20 million suffer from severe disease, another 90–100 million are symptomatic, and 200,000 die each year. Although there is a temptation to dismiss schistosomiasis as a tropical disease with no relevance to medicine in the USA, epidemiologists estimate that as many as 400,000 Americans are infected with schistosomes. All of these infections were acquired outside the USA. There is no indigenous schistosomiasis in North America, because the proper intermediate hosts are not available to allow the schistosomes to multiply.

Three species of *Schistosoma* are most commonly responsible for human disease: *Schistosoma japonicum* and *Schistosoma mansoni* infect the venules of the intestinal mesentery, and *Schistosoma haematobium* infects the venules of the bladder. Rarer causes of human infection include *Schistosoma malayensis* and *Schistosoma mekongi,* both of which infect the intestine, and *Schistosoma intercalatum,* which infects the rectum. Schistosomes live an average of 3–10 years, but infections persisting over 30 years have been reported.

Characteristics of Schistosomes

General Features. Schistosomes (Fig. 25–6) are diecious organisms. The males range from 0.6 to 2.2 cm in length, while the females range from 1.2 to 2.6 cm. The two sexes live in a perpetual symbiotic relationship, with the female lying within the elongated gynecophoral canal of the male. The male absorbs nutrients, stores them, and supplies them to the female as needed. The pairs live in the venules of the intestinal mesentery and bladder for years. Each day, the female leaves the male, ventures into a small blood vessel, dilates the vessel, lays from 200 to 11,000 eggs, and then withdraws to return to the male. The eggs are lodged temporarily in the venule, but they soon escape either to be swept into the

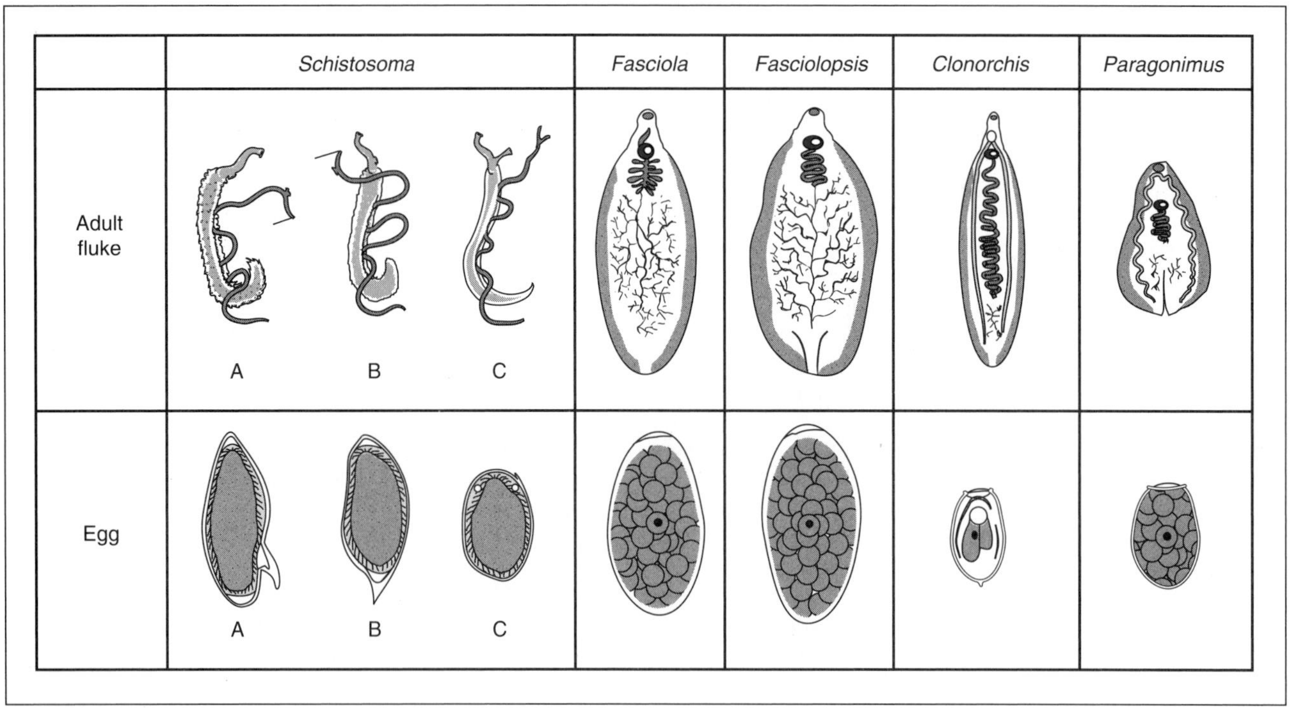

	Schistosoma			Fasciola	Fasciolopis	Clonorchis	Paragonimus
Adult fluke	A	B	C				
Egg	A	B	C				

FIGURE 25–6. The adult flukes and their eggs. The schistosomes pictured are *Schistosoma mansoni* **(A)**, *Schistosoma haematobium* **(B)**, and *Schistosoma japonicum* **(C)**.

circulation or to pass into the intestine or bladder and be excreted in the feces or urine.

The eggs of each species, which contain a larval form known as a **miracidium,** have a characteristic appearance that aids both in identification and in escape from the blood vessels. Fig. 25–6 shows the eggs of the three major *Schistosoma* species. *S. japonicum* eggs are only 55–85 μm in length and have a tiny lateral spine that is not easily seen; *S. mansoni* eggs are 114–180 μm and have a large lateral spine; and *S. haematobium* eggs are 112–170 μm and have a terminal spine. The spines of the two larger eggs puncture the venule, and the miracidium secretes an enzyme that degrades the vessel wall. Together these actions cause necrosis of vessel walls.

Life Cycle of Schistosomes.   Schistosomes do not multiply within humans. They go through a multiplication cycle in various species of freshwater snails. As shown in Fig. 25–7, the eggs of schistosomes pass out of the human body in the feces or urine. When an egg enters water, a ciliated miracidium is released. The miracidium penetrates into a snail to begin the schistosomal developmental cycle. Inside the snail, the miracidium begins a 90-day journey during which it initially becomes a **mother sporocyst** and is then transformed into **daughter sporocysts.** Each daughter sporocyst produces a multitude of **cercariae.** The cercariae break out of the snail and swim until they contact an appropriate definitive host.

The definitive host is often a human, but *S. japonicum* and *S. mansoni* can also infect rodents and small domestic animals. The definitive host is infected when wading or swimming in fresh water. The cercar-

iae burrow into the skin and produce a transient allergic reaction that is commonly called swimmers' itch.

Each cercaria remains in the skin for about 2 days, during which time it develops into a larval form known as a **schistosomulum.** The schistosomulum now goes through a migratory cycle that will take about 2 weeks. After it migrates into the small blood vessels, it is carried by the blood through the heart, lungs, and portal circulation. The schistosomulum is then transported into the sinusoids of the liver, where it develops into an adult worm and migrates to its final resting place in the venules of the intestinal mesentery or bladder.

Mechanisms of Pathogenicity.   Two key factors are involved in the pathogenesis of schistosomiasis: first, the ability of the worm to survive the patient's immune response and, second, the production of the symptoms and tissue damage associated with acute and chronic schistosomiasis.

(1) Evasion of the Immune Response.   In vitro studies, experimental studies using animal models of schistosomiasis, and clinical studies have shown that schistosomula and adult schistosomes are eliminated by an unusual type of antibody-dependent cellular cytotoxicity (ADCC) that involves IgE, IgA, macrophages, and eosinophils. The Fc region of IgE and IgA antibodies to *Schistosoma* adheres to receptors on the surface of eosinophils and macrophages. When these antibodies bind to schistosomal antigens, the bound effector cells release substances that are toxic to schistosomes, with the result that the worms are damaged or killed. Among the substances believed to be toxic are oxygen-derived free radicals (superox-

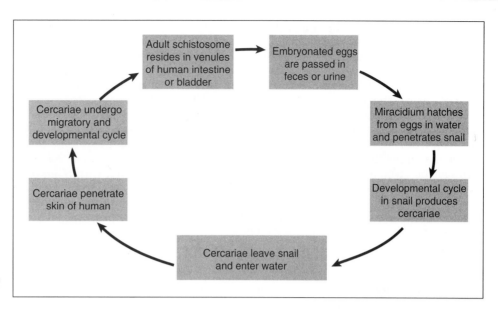

FIGURE 25–7. The life cycle of schistosomes that infect humans.

ide, hydroxyl radical, hydrogen peroxide, and singlet-excited oxygen) and two key products of eosinophils (peroxidase and major basic protein). The presence of schistosomes is heralded by the development of eosinophilia and the occurrence of hives and other IgE-mediated allergic manifestations. IgG2, IgG4, and IgM antibodies to *Schistosoma* block the effective expression of ADCC.

The schistosome evades immune processes in at least three ways: by antigen variation, by antigen mimicry, and by antigen cloaking.

(a) Antigen Variation. Each stage of schistosomal development involves the expression of a new set of schistosomal antigens. This is a common theme among parasites and is effective because it keeps the immune system "off guard." About the time that an effective immune response is generated against the antigens of one developmental stage of the parasite, that stage disappears and is replaced with a new stage that expresses its own antigens.

(b) Antigen Mimicry. Several schistosomal antigens have been shown to mimic host antigens. This mimicry protects adult schistosomes by ensuring that little or no antibody is made against their antigens. Two schistosomal surface proteins cross-react with the human immunodeficiency virus (HIV) regulatory proteins Nef and Vif, and some patients with schistosomiasis who are not infected with HIV express antibodies against these HIV proteins. There has been much speculation concerning what effect, if any, schistosomiasis might have on the occurrence of acquired immunodeficiency syndrome (AIDS) in areas such as Africa, where both diseases have a high prevalence.

(c) Antigen Cloaking. Fans of the long-running television series "Star Trek" and its successors will recognize the concept of cloaking. In this series, the Romulans held a strategic advantage in battle because they could cloak their starships with invisibility. Schistosomes are like Romulans. They lie for years within the venules of intestinal mesentery or bladder, unrecognized and unattended by the immune system because they make themselves invisible by cloaking their bodies with host proteins. This layer of "self" hides the schistosomes from the immune system. Interestingly, praziquantel, the antibiotic used most often to treat schistosomiasis, is believed to work in part by forcing the schistosomes to abrogate their cloak of invisibility and expose antigens that are easily recognized by the immune system. Two key antigens that are expressed are a 200-kD glycoprotein and a 27-kD protein with esterase activity.

(2) Pathogenic Processes. The initial manifestation of schistosomiasis is a pruritic rash that develops at the site where cercariae enter into the skin. This transient condition is an allergic reaction, probably involving both cell-mediated and IgE-mediated processes. More important are the events that occur during acute and chronic schistosomiasis. The associated symptoms, some of which may be life-threatening, are caused by the eggs of the schistosome.

When schistosome eggs are deposited in the venules of the intestinal mesentery or bladder, they necrose the vessel wall. Some pass out of the body, but others are swept back into the circulation. The eggs that remain in the body may deposit nearby, or they may be carried by the blood to the small blood vessels that supply the body organs. Wherever the eggs deposit, they elicit a granulomatous response. While the initial response involves neutrophils, the subsequent response involves macrophages and lymphocytes. The granulomas that are formed are sometimes called pseudotubercles because of their resemblance to the granulomas of tuberculosis.

The formation of granulomas around the eggs may be accompanied by localized necrosis, or the granulomas may act as space-occupying lesions in tissues. In some cases, they obstruct the blood supply to the area. Granulomas are most often found in the liver and spleen of patients with *S. japonicum* and *S. mansoni* infections and in the bladder of patients with *S. haematobium* infection. Other sites in which granulomas occur are the intestine (*S. mansoni* and *S. haematobium*), the lung (*S. haematobium*), and the central nervous system (*S. japonicum*). Ectopic granulomas tend to occur most frequently with *S. japonicum,* because the eggs of this species have smaller spines that allow them to travel with less obstruction through the circulatory system.

Tumor necrosis factor (TNF) contributes to the pathogenesis of schistosomiasis by acting as a key signal in granuloma formation and by stimulating the female schistosome to produce more eggs.

Diseases Due to Schistosomes

Epidemiology. The range of each species of *Schistosoma* is restricted by the presence of appropriate snails that act as intermediate hosts. In highly endemic areas, about 5–10% of the people are infected with schistosomes. Most cases of human schistosomiasis are caused by *S. japonicum, S. mansoni,* and *S. haematobium* and are found in Asia and Africa. Infections with *S. mansoni* occur in Africa, in three South American countries (Brazil, Surinam, and Venezuela), and in seven Caribbean islands, one of which is Puerto Rico. Schistosomiasis is not indigenous in the USA, but cases are sometimes found in New York City, which has a large Puerto Rican population.

Note that although swimmers' itch is commonly seen as the initial manifestation of schistosomiasis, it is not always caused by *Schistosoma* species. It can also be caused by any of a large number of related organisms whose adult forms live in ducks, shore birds, and semiaquatic mammals (such as muskrats). The cercariae of *Trichobilharzia* and *Schistosomatium,* for example, penetrate into the skin of swimmers and produce a pruritic rash, but these cercariae cannot develop into adults within humans, so the parasites die in the skin. Swimmers' itch caused by these "nonhuman" schistosomes is common in the USA.

Diagnosis

(1) History and Physical Examination. There are three clinically apparent phases of schistosomiasis: cercarial dermatitis, acute schistosomiasis, and chronic schistosomiasis.

(a) Cercarial Dermatitis. The penetration of cercariae through the skin results in a pruritic, edematous rash that peaks after 24–36 hours and generally lasts less than 4 days. This rash is sometimes called **swimmers' itch, clam diggers' itch,** or **sea bathers' eruption.** The rash is usually not accompanied by constitutional symptoms, but some patients with large-scale invasion suffer from fever, malaise, hives, and general gastrointestinal discomfort. The migration of schistosomula to the liver is usually clinically quiescent, but a few patients develop a cough when the larvae pass through the lungs. Some coughing patients spit up blood (hemoptysis).

(b) Acute Schistosomiasis. The acute phase of schistosomiasis begins about 1–3 months after infection, when the schistosomes reach the mesenteric or vesicular venules and begin laying eggs. Manifestations include generalized malaise, fever, hives, abdominal pain, and liver tenderness. Eggs that travel to ectopic sites may produce acute lesions, including lesions within the central nervous system. Acute schistosomiasis is most severe in patients with **Katayama fever,** a life-threatening condition named after a Japanese city and found in patients who are heavily infected with *S. japonicum.* Acute schistosomiasis is more likely to occur in travelers to an endemic region than in residents of the region.

(c) Chronic Schistosomiasis. The most significant cause of morbidity and mortality in patients with schistosomal infections is the chronic phase of the disease, which generally begins 5 or more years after infection is initiated. The severity of manifestations in this phase depends on the worm burden (number of worms present) and the sites of egg deposition. The most significant sites are the liver, spleen, intestinal tract, bladder, central nervous system, and lungs.

Hepatosplenomegalic schistosomiasis is the most frequent manifestation of schistosomiasis caused by *S. mansoni* and *S. haematobium* and is characterized by granulomas that form around eggs deposited in the liver and spleen. The most common sign is palpable enlargement of the left lobe of the liver. Hepatic granulomas amputate intrahepatic veins, and periportal granulomas cause a peculiar perilobar fibrosis known as pipestem fibrosis. The fibrosis leads to portal hypertension and the shunting of blood to the collateral circulation in the esophagus. The resulting esophageal varices (distended, tortuous veins) may bleed extensively and are often associated with profound anemia and ascites. In many cases, eggs are swept from the liver to the lung, where they cause pulmonary disease (see below). Hepatosplenomegalic schistosomiasis caused by *S. japonicum* predisposes patients to the development of hepatocellular carcinoma.

Gastrointestinal schistosomiasis is most often due to *S. mansoni* or *S. japonicum.* Granulomas develop in the intestine, causing cramping, abdominal tenderness, and the intermittent production of bloody, mucoid stools. Patients typically suffer from anemia and weight loss associated with loss of protein.

Urinary schistosomiasis occurs 3–6 months after infection begins and is usually caused by *S. haematobium* eggs that have deposited in the bladder wall, where they elicit the formation of ulcers and granulomas. Manifestations include painful urination (dysuria), urinary frequency, and blood in the urine (hematuria). Urinary schistosomiasis is so common in Egypt that a finding of mild hematuria is considered to be "normal" in boys. Urinary schistosomiasis predisposes patients to the development of squamous cell carcinoma of the bladder.

Neurologic schistosomiasis occurs when the eggs of *S. japonicum* migrate to the brain and spinal cord, forming granulomas that cause transverse myelitis, chronic meningitis, and focal seizures.

Pulmonary schistosomiasis is most often due to *S. haematobium* and is often secondary to hepatosplenomegalic schistosomiasis. The pulmonary bed fibroses, causing the patient to become dyspneic and suffer from a chronic cough that is accompanied by hemoptysis. Pulmonary dysfunction may cause the right ventricle to hypertrophy, a condition called cor pulmonale.

(2) Imaging Studies. Abdominal ultrasonography has become the standard for evaluation of the status of patients with abdominal schistosomal disease, particularly hepatosplenomegalic or urogenital disease. Ultrasound can be used to assess the presence and extent of pipestem fibrosis in patients with liver disease. Other helpful tools for evaluating schistosomiasis include CT scan, cystoscopy, and intravenous pyelography.

(3) Laboratory Analysis. Eggs can be identified microscopically in the feces or urine of patients. If necessary, biopsies can be performed to identify eggs in the tissues. The number of eggs is estimated to determine the worm burden and extent of infection.

Immunologic tests are available to identify the presence of schistosomal antigens in serum or urine samples. The most popular test is an ELISA that detects the presence of a schistosomal proteoglycan antigen (anodic antigen) that is released from the gut of adult schistosomes. Current immunologic tests can detect 1 ng of antigen, which corresponds to about seven eggs per gram of feces. Although tests are available to detect circulating antibody to *Schistosoma*, these tests cannot distinguish between new and old infections, so they are not useful for diagnosing disease in adult patients who live in endemic areas.

Treatment. Praziquantel is used to treat infections with all species of *Schistosoma*. The drug disrupts the integrity of schistosomal surface membranes, exposing antigens that elicit the attention of the immune system. In addition, the drug increases the entry of calcium into the schistosome and causes the worm to have tetanic contractions. Praziquantel cures 75–100% of patients and is 90% effective in reducing the number and viability of eggs shed by schistosomes. As an alternative to praziquantel, oxamniquine can be used to treat *S. mansoni* infections, and metrifonate can be used to treat *S. haematobium* infections. Metrifonate is an investigational drug in the USA and can be obtained from the Centers for Disease Control and Prevention.

Prevention. Improvements in sanitation have greatly reduced the incidence of schistosomiasis in some regions. In fact, *S. japonicum* infections are now rare in Japan. Penetration of cercariae can be inhibited by applying niclosamide lotion to the skin before entering water that may contain schistosomes. Investigators continue in their efforts to develop a vaccine to prevent schistosomiasis. Many of their efforts have concentrated on a vaccine that uses Sm28 protein, which is a glutathione-S-transferase. Vaccines utilizing this protein have proved effective in preventing disease in rodents.

Monoecious Flukes

There are three groups of monoecious trematodes: lung flukes, liver flukes, and intestinal flukes. The **lung flukes** are members of the genus *Paragonimus* and include many species that infect humans. Of these, *Paragonimus westermani* is the most important human pathogen. The **liver flukes** include members of the genera *Clonorchis, Dicrocoelium,* and *Opisthorchis,* which live in the distal portions of the biliary tree; they also include the much larger *Fasciola* flukes, which live in the common bile duct and the gallbladder. The two most important liver flukes are *Clonorchis sinensis* and *Fasciola hepatica.* The **intestinal flukes** are members of the genera *Echinostoma, Fasciolopsis, Gastrodiscoides, Heterophyes,* and *Metagonimus,* and the most common intestinal flukes are *Fasciolopsis buski* and *Heterophyes heterophyes.*

The monoecious flukes are leaf-shaped and flattened dorsoventrally. Each fluke is structurally complex and has a cecum, bladder, male and female sexual organs, and a nervous system. The flukes ingest nutrients through a mouth, and they are able to attach to host surfaces via a central ventral sucker and an oral sucker at the anterior end.

The monoecious flukes share a common life cycle. As shown in Fig. 25–8, the adult fluke resides in the human intestine, liver, or lung. Eggs are shed when the host defecates or spits. A ciliated **miracidium** hatches from the egg and penetrates the **first intermediate host,** which is a snail. Within the snail, the miracidium goes through a multiplication and developmental cycle that starts with a **sporocyst** and yields many **cercariae.** The cercariae burrow out of the snail and enter a species-specific **second intermediate host,** which may be a crustacean, fish, or water plant. Within this host, each cercaria encysts to become a dormant **metacercaria.** Humans enter the life cycle when they eat the second intermediate host either raw or undercooked. Table 25–3 summarizes some key aspects of the fluke life cycle.

Characteristics of *Paragonimus*

General Features. The lung flukes include about 10 species of *Paragonimus,* the most important of which is *Paragonimus westermani.* The adult *Paragonimus* is an oval-shaped trematode that is 0.8–1.6 cm long. Like other flukes, the worm has an oral and ventral sucker. The eggs have a discernible operculum (see Fig. 25–6) and are 80–120 μm long.

The adult forms of *P. westermani* live in the lungs, where they may reside for 10–20 years. The eggs are discharged into the bronchi and are subsequently expelled into the environment by coughing or spitting. The eggs may also be excreted in feces when the patient coughs and swallows. When an egg enters water, it releases a free-swimming miracidium. The miracidium enters a freshwater snail and develops into many cercariae, which eventually burrow out of

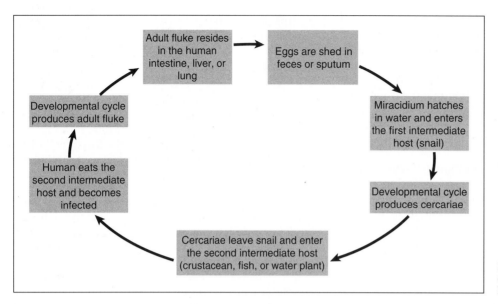

FIGURE 25–8. The life cycle common to intestinal, liver, and lung flukes that infect humans.

the snail and enter their second intermediate host, a crab or crayfish. The cercaria encysts, becomes a metacercaria, and enters a human who eats raw or pickled crustaceans. The larvae develop in the small intestine, penetrate into the abdominal cavity, and migrate to the abdominal wall or liver to develop further. In about 1 week, the fluke reenters the abdominal cavity. It may now penetrate the diaphragm and enter the lungs, or it may wander throughout the viscera. Inside the lungs, the fluke becomes an egg-laying adult in about 6 weeks.

Mechanisms of Pathogenicity. Symptoms associated with the invasive stage of *Paragonimus* infection are due to IgE-mediated allergic reactions to the presence of wandering immature flukes in the viscera. Subsequent manifestations of the acute and chronic stages of disease are caused by adult flukes and eggs in the tissues. Granulomatous cysts are constructed around the adult fluke and may also form around eggs deposited in the lungs. Lung flukes tend to wander, and many migrate and establish ectopic foci in the central nervous system, gastrointestinal tract, and subcutaneous tissues. Each cyst in the lung typically

encloses from two to four worms, and the cyst wall contains fibroblasts, macrophages, eosinophils, lymphocytes, and plasma cells. Bronchial arteries in the vicinity of a cyst may hypertrophy or rupture, and lung cysts may calcify.

Diseases Due to *Paragonimus*

Epidemiology. *P. westermani* infections are frequently seen in Japan, Korea, China, Taiwan, Southeast Asia, Papua New Guinea, northeastern India, Sri Lanka, and central Africa. In the Americas, *Paragonimus mexicanus* is found in Mexico, Central America, and the northern tier of South America. Worldwide, from 3 million to 4 million people suffer from paragonimiasis.

Paragonimiasis is prevalent in areas where abundant numbers of the first and second intermediate hosts are found and where raw or pickled crustaceans are ingested. For example, live crabs in sauce is a popular dish throughout Southeast Asia, and raw crayfish juice is sometimes used to treat measles, diarrhea, and hives in Korea and Japan. *Paragonimus*

TABLE 25–3.   Characteristics of the Most Common Lung, Liver, and Intestinal Flukes

Organism	Egg Size (μm)	Usual Route of Human Infection	Infection Site of Adult Flukes
Lung flukes			
Paragonimus westermani	80–120	Ingestion of metacercariae in crustaceans.	Lungs; some ectopic foci.
Liver flukes			
Clonorchis sinensis	29	Ingestion of metacercariae in fish.	Bile ducts.
Fasciola hepatica	130–150	Ingestion of metacercariae on water plants (such as watercress).	Common bile duct and gallbladder; various ectopic foci.
Intestinal flukes			
Fasciolopsis buski	130–140	Ingestion of metacercariae on water plants (such as bamboo shoots and water chestnuts).	Duodenum and jejunum; occasionally infects stomach and large intestine.
Heterophyes heterophyes	26–30	Ingestion of metacercariae in fish.	Walls of small intestine; various ectopic foci.

infection can also be acquired by eating the flesh of other hosts that contain *Paragonimus* larvae. In this fashion, wild boar and field rats serve as **paratenic hosts** (transfer hosts) in some cultures. Paragonimiasis is sometimes spread via eating or cooking utensils contaminated with larvae. The habit of spitting promotes spread because *Paragonimus* eggs are expelled in the sputum of infected people.

Diagnosis

(1) History and Physical Examination. During the migration of flukes, there may be transient IgE-mediated allergic symptoms such as hives and asthma. Depending on the worm burden, paragonimiasis may be asymptomatic or may result in acute and chronic disease.

Acute paragonimiasis occurs during the first 20 days of infection. Manifestations include diarrhea, abdominal pain, and hives, which are followed by fever, chest pain, cough, dyspnea, malaise, and night sweats that last for weeks. Because the eggs cannot be found in the sputum at this time, most acute paragonimiasis passes without being definitively diagnosed.

Chronic paragonimiasis begins about 6 months after the initiation of infection and generally takes the form of chronic bronchitis. The patient develops a dry cough that gradually becomes productive. The sputum is rust-colored or golden brown and contains *Paragonimus* eggs. Other manifestations may include chest pain, wheezing, shortness of breath, and hemoptysis. If numerous flukes have migrated to the lungs, the bronchi may be dilated (bronchiectasis), and the patient may suffer from bronchopneumonia accompanied by pleural effusion, empyema, and lung abscesses.

Wandering lung flukes may establish ectopic infections in the central nervous system, abdomen, or subcutaneous tissues. **Cerebral paragonimiasis** occurs in fewer than 1% of patients, primarily affects children, and may cause headache, vomiting, seizures, facial palsy, and paralysis. Cerebral paragonimiasis is sometimes fatal, but many patients recover spontaneously in 1–2 months. Those who recover may suffer from periodic neurologic sequelae. **Abdominal paragonimiasis** is a chronic colitislike disease that is associated with abdominal pain and bloody diarrhea. Patients with **subcutaneous paragonimiasis** develop subcutaneous nodules on the lower abdomen and inguinal region. The nodules are granulomas surrounding immature flukes.

(2) Laboratory Analysis. Confirmation of paragonimiasis rests on identification of eggs in sputum, feces, cerebrospinal fluid, or tissue biopsies; demonstration of eosinophilia; detection of antibody to *Paragonimus* in immunologic tests; and demonstration of granulomas on x-ray or CT scan.

Sputum from patients with lung disease contains many brown eggs. It also contains Charcot-Leyden crystals, which are elongated, double-pyramid crystals that appear in the sputum when eosinophils are present. The cerebrospinal fluid of patients with cerebral disease is turbid or bloody and contains many eosinophils. An ELISA is most often used for immunologic diagnosis because it is easier to perform than complement fixation tests. Nevertheless, the latter tests have proved useful for monitoring the progress of treatment, since they yield negative results 6–12 months after the flukes are eradicated. Chest films typically show pleural effusion accompanied by nodular cystic shadows or signs of calcified cysts.

Treatment and Prevention. Paragonimiasis is treated with praziquantel or, alternatively, with bithionol. Patients with cerebral disease should receive corticosteroids with praziquantel to prevent the occurrence of convulsions and coma. Paragonimiasis is not usually fatal, but death occurs in about 5% of patients with untreated cerebral disease.

Paragonimiasis can be prevented by avoiding the ingestion of raw or pickled crustaceans that are harvested in areas where the disease is endemic.

Characteristics of *Clonorchis* and *Opisthorchis*

General Features. *Clonorchis* and *Opisthorchis* are narrow flukes that live in the distal portions of the biliary tree. The species considered the most significant human pathogen is *Clonorchis sinensis,* also called the **Chinese liver fluke.** The adult form of *C. sinensis* is 1.0–2.5 cm long, lives for up to 30 years, and lays about 2400 eggs each day. The eggs are operculated and are about 29 μm long. The egg and adult fluke are illustrated in Fig. 25–6.

Clonorchis and *Opisthorchis* flukes follow the same life cycle. The embryonated eggs in bile pass into the intestine and are shed in feces. The egg is eaten by one of several specific water snails, and the miracidium hatches from the egg. The miracidium then passes through a replicative and developmental cycle that produces many cercariae from each miracidium. The cercariae break out of the snail and burrow under the scales of a fish (a carp) within 48 hours of leaving the snail. Under the scales, each cercaria encysts to become a metacercaria, and humans acquire the infection when they eat raw, smoked, pickled, or undercooked fish. The metacercaria excysts in the intestine and migrates up the biliary tree by passing through the ampulla of Vater and ascending the common bile duct.

Mechanisms of Pathogenicity. The symptoms of clonorchiasis and opisthorchiasis are due to the presence of flukes in the bile ducts. The flukes mechanically irritate the tissue and release excretions that damage the ducts. People who continually reinfect themselves by eating infected fish may carry thousands of flukes, resulting in blockage of the biliary tree and in fibrosis and destruction of the liver. Heavy infection causes marked hyperplasia of the small mucinous glands of the duct mucosa, as well as thickening and localized dilatation of the bile ducts. Hepatic damage elicits a host of effects, including tachycardia, anemia, jaundice, and liver hypertrophy. Portal hypertension may lead to ascites. The gallbladder and pancreatic duct may also become heavily infected.

Diseases Due to *Clonorchis* and *Opisthorchis*

Epidemiology. *C. sinensis* is found in China and nearby countries, including Taiwan, Japan, Korea, and Vietnam. An estimated 19 million people are infected with this organism and its close relatives, the *Opisthorchis* flukes. Many people are heavily infected and suffer from chronic symptoms of biliary obstruction and impairment of liver function. Moreover, long-standing *Clonorchis* infections have been statistically associated with the occurrence of primary hepatocellular carcinoma and cholangiocarcinoma.

People acquire clonorchiasis and opisthorchiasis when they eat fish that contain the metacercariae of liver flukes. In some parts of Asia, the practice of raising fish in ponds fertilized by night soil (human excreta) is common, as is the practice of eating raw or lightly cooked fish. Where these practices are prevalent, infection has been documented to occur at rates ranging from 3000 to 36,000 individuals per 100,000 population. Occasionally, human infections have been traced to ingestion of cysts in drinking water.

Diagnosis

(1) History and Physical Examination. People who are lightly infected with *Clonorchis* or *Opisthorchis* tend to be asymptomatic.

Patients who become heavily infected in a short time (over the course of less than 1 month) may suffer from acute illness characterized by facial edema, hives, sore muscles and joints, high fever, diarrhea, epigastric pain, and anorexia. About the time that the acute symptoms subside, eggs begin to appear in the feces and the patient becomes eosinophilic.

Patients who become heavily infected over a long period of time have an enlarged liver, mild hepatitis, and recurrent attacks of dull pain in the right hypochondrium. As the attacks recur over several years, the skin over the liver may have a hot sensation. The bile ducts become obstructed, leading to functional impairment of the liver. If the gallbladder is invaded, the patient may suffer from cholecystitis and cholelithiasis (gallstones). Gallbladder invasion is characterized by epigastric pain that is more severe immediately after eating. Patients may also suffer from acute pancreatitis.

(2) Laboratory Analysis. Clonorchiasis and opisthorchiasis are diagnosed by demonstrating the presence of eggs in stool samples, in duodenal aspirates, or in duodenal samples obtained by use of an enteric capsule. In the latter procedure, the patient is asked to swallow a gelatin capsule attached to a string and a 1-g weight. The part of the string that protrudes from the mouth is tied to the patient's neck. After 4 hours, the string and capsule are pulled up, and the mucus adhering to the capsule is examined for the presence of eggs. The status of liver disease can be monitored by use of abdominal ultrasonography.

Treatment and Prevention. Praziquantel cures almost 100% of patients. Clonorchiasis and opisthorchiasis can be prevented by cooking fish thoroughly before eating them. The use of night soil to fertilize fish ponds should be discouraged.

Characteristics of *Fasciola*

General Features. In humans, fascioliasis is most frequently caused by *Fasciola hepatica*. This fluke is also a parasite of sheep, cattle, deer, rabbits, and other herbivorous animals. Because of its close association with sheep, it is commonly called the **sheep liver fluke.** In infected humans, the fluke lives in the larger biliary passages and gallbladder. The adult fluke, shown in Fig. 25–6, is about 3 cm long and is easily recognized by its prominent cephalic cone. The egg, also shown in Fig. 25–6, is operculated and ranges from 130 to 150 μm in length.

Fasciola infection in humans is less frequently caused by *Fasciola gigantica*. This fluke, called the **giant liver fluke,** is a parasite of cattle, camels, and water buffaloes. It grows to a length of about 7.5 cm and has operculated eggs that range from 150 to 190 μm in length.

The embryonated eggs of *Fasciola* are shed in the feces, and the miracidium enters one of 21 species of lymneid freshwater snails. In the snail, the miracidium becomes a sporocyst, develops into multiple rediae and daughter rediae, and then produces many cercariae. The cercariae burrow out of the snail, encyst on water plants (particularly grasses or watercress) and become metacercariae. Humans are infected when they eat uncooked watercress. When a metacercaria excysts, the larval fluke burrows through the duodenal wall. It then migrates across the abdominal cavity and enters the biliary tree by burrowing through Glisson's capsule and the liver parenchyma. Some of the larvae fail to reach the liver. These larvae wander about the abdominal cavity and establish ectopic foci of infection.

Mechanisms of Pathogenicity. *F. hepatica* elicits eosinophilia and attracts an inflammatory response that damages the biliary tract. The production of IgE can result in hives and asthma.

F. hepatica is a large fluke, and a single fluke can cause significant symptoms by obstructing the biliary tree. Each adult fluke consumes about 0.2 mL of blood per day. Because the burrowing of the flukes through the liver damages the parenchyma, fascioliasis is sometimes called "liver rot." The tissues in the vicinity of the fluke are fibrotic, edematous, and inflamed. The combination of toxic fluke products and mechanical obstruction causes the parenchyma to atrophy, causes the biliary epithelium to become hyperplastic, and sometimes leads to periportal cirrhosis.

Organs other than the liver may be damaged when wandering flukes establish ectopic infections. In some patients, the ingestion of *Fasciola* leads to the deposition of larval flukes in the pharyngeal mucosa. This is thought to be responsible for halzoun, an unusual form of laryngopharyngitis associated with fascioliasis.

Diseases Due to *Fasciola*

Epidemiology. About 10 million people worldwide are infected with *F. hepatica*. This large fluke is cosmopolitan in its distribution, but there are locales where it is particularly common. Areas of high endemicity include southern France, Algeria, Cuba, and Latin America. Fascioliasis is usually acquired by eating uncooked watercress or other plants that contain the metacercariae of *F. hepatica*. However, halzoun is acquired by eating raw animal liver that contains *Fasciola*.

Diagnosis
(1) History and Physical Examination. Patients may have acute illness, chronic illness, or both. Acute fascioliasis is followed by a latent period that may last for years.

Manifestations of **acute fascioliasis** include fever, abdominal pain, and gastrointestinal disturbances, sometimes accompanied by nausea, loss of appetite, diarrhea, and flatulence. Hives and asthma may develop, and the liver gradually begins to enlarge. Patients with **halzoun** complain of difficulty in swallowing and of other symptoms associated with acute laryngopharyngitis.

Chronic fascioliasis is characterized by eosinophilia, an enlarged liver, fever, chills, and right upper quadrant pain that radiates to the scapula. Cholangitis, cholecystitis, or gallstones may also be present. Patients with **ectopic fascioliasis** have symptoms consistent with the presence of flukes in a specific organ. The brain, lungs, skin, intestinal wall, and testes have all been identified as sites of ectopic fascioliasis.

(2) Laboratory Analysis. Laboratory confirmation of fascioliasis involves identifying the eggs of the fluke in stool samples, duodenal aspirates, or bile. The use of an enteric capsule may facilitate the recovery of eggs. Leukocytosis and eosinophilia are found in patients with acute fascioliasis. Ultrasonography or cholangiography can be used to evaluate the status of liver disease or gallbladder disease, respectively.

Treatment. Praziquantel is the drug of choice for treatment of fascioliasis. Alternatively, bithionol can be used. Although triclabendazole has been used effectively in developing countries, it is not approved for use in the USA.

Characteristics of *Fasciolopsis*

General Features. The intestinal flukes include the huge *Fasciolopsis buski,* the medium-sized *Echinostoma* flukes, and the tiny *Heterophyes* and *Metagonimus* flukes. Of these, *F. buski* is the most important cause of human disease and is also the largest trematode that infects humans. The adult form (see Fig. 25-6) is about 7.5 cm long and up to 2 cm wide. It lives in the duodenum and jejunum but may also infect the stomach and large intestine. Its mouth is buried in the mucosa, and the fluke ingests intestinal contents and secretions.

The adult fluke produces between 21,000 and 28,000 eggs each day. The eggs range from 130 to 140 μm in length; are undeveloped; have a clear, thin shell; and have a terminal operculum. The eggs exit the human body via the feces and will hatch in water

in 3–7 weeks. The miracidium of *F. buski* penetrates into one of several specific freshwater snails. Inside the snail, the miracidium develops into many cercariae. The cercariae burrow out of the snail in 4–7 weeks and enter any of a wide number of water plants. Humans become infected when they eat plants that contain the metacercariae of *F. buski*. The inner wall of each metacercaria is digested in the human duodenum, and the larval fluke attaches to the intestinal mucosa, where it becomes an adult in 25–30 days. The adult lives about 6 months.

Mechanisms of Pathogenicity. Infections with *F. buski* may become quite heavy, with some patients harboring thousands of flukes. The adult flukes feed on intestinal contents and cause erosion, ulceration, and inflammation of the intestinal mucosa. Patients with heavy infections have signs of malabsorption, and hypoalbuminemia resulting from such heavy infections may cause edema, ascites, and wasting. Elicitation of eosinophils and IgE is accompanied by signs of allergy, including hives and asthma.

Diseases Due to *Fasciolopsis*

Epidemiology. An estimated 10 million individuals are infected with *F. buski*. This intestinal fluke is found most often in China, Taiwan, Vietnam, Thailand, Malaysia, Indonesia, India, and Bangladesh. Humans are infected when they eat bamboo shoots, water chestnuts, water caltrop, watercress, or other water plants that contain *F. buski* metacercariae. These plants are commonly grown in ponds fertilized with night soil, and the edible portions of the plants are typically peeled with the teeth, exposing the individual to metacercariae living on the outside of the plant. Hogs and dogs are also commonly infected with the adult form of *F. buski*.

Diagnosis. Infection with *F. buski* causes epigastric pain that is similar to the pain of an ulcer, is more severe in the morning, and is relieved by eating. Nausea and diarrhea are common. If the worm burden is heavy, there may be symptoms and signs of ascites, vitamin B_{12} deficiency, intestinal obstruction, wasting, and facial edema secondary to hives. The diagnosis is confirmed by identifying the eggs of *F. buski* in stool samples. These eggs look much like *Fasciola hepatica* eggs but can be differentiated by their distribution of yolk granules.

Treatment and Prevention. Praziquantel is the drug of choice for the treatment of *F. buski* infection. Niclosamide is an acceptable alternative.

To prevent infection, edible water plants should not be grown in ponds fertilized with night soil. Because hogs are often infected with *F. buski,* control of contamination of ponds is difficult in the Far East. Unslaked lime or copper sulfate can be used to reduce the amount of infestation in ponds. Whenever possible, water plants should be cooked or steeped in boiling water.

Characteristics of *Echinostoma*

The echinostomes are medium-sized flukes that sometimes cause intestinal disease. In their adult form, they are about 1 cm in length and are recognized by a distinctive horseshoe-shaped collar of spines around the oral sucker.

The first intermediate hosts of echinostomes are snails. The second intermediate hosts may be snails, fish, or water plants. Humans are most often infected when they eat raw snails that contain metacercariae.

Diseases Due to *Echinostoma*

Echinostoma infections occur primarily in Southeast Asia, although some cases have been reported in eastern Africa. The most important species, *Echinostoma ilocanum,* is found in the Philippines.

Most infections are asymptomatic, but heavily infected patients may suffer from epigastric pain, nausea, diarrhea, and eosinophilia. Infected children may become anemic. The diagnosis is based on the clinical history and the identification of eggs in stool samples.

Echinostoma infections are treated with praziquantel.

Characteristics of *Heterophyes* and *Metagonimus*

Heterophyiasis is caused most often by *Heterophyes heterophyes* or *Metagonimus yokogawai.* The adult forms of these flukes are 1.5 mm or smaller, and their eggs range from 26 to 30 μm in length. Snails serve as the first intermediate hosts, and the metacercariae are found in fish, particularly mullet. Humans become infected when they eat raw, pickled, or poorly cooked fish.

Diseases Due to *Heterophyes* and *Metagonimus*

Heterophyiasis is found most often in Asia, the Middle East, Spain, and Russia.

Patients are usually asymptomatic, but heavily infected individuals may suffer from epigastric pain, abdominal tenderness and discomfort, intermittent mucoid diarrhea, and eosinophilia. Although ectopic foci are seen most often in the heart and central nervous system, a few patients have developed granulomatous lesions around ectopic flukes that have penetrated the intestinal wall and entered the abdominal cavity. The diagnosis of heterophyiasis is based on clinical manifestations and the finding of eggs in stool samples.

Heterophyiasis is usually treated with praziquantel. Alternatively, tetrachloroethylene can be used.

NEMATODES

The nematodes are elongated, cylindrical worms that range in length from 2 mm (*Strongyloides stercoralis*) to about 1 m (*Dracunculus medinensis*). Nematodes have a mouth, digestive tract, and primitive nervous system, but they have no circulatory system. They have male or female reproductive organs (the sexes are usually separate), and the males are generally much smaller than the females. The life span of adult worms varies considerably. For example, while the female *Trichinella spiralis* is expelled from the

intestine after 4 or 5 weeks, the adult *Necator americanus* is believed to live as long as 18 years.

There are about 50,000 species of nematodes, but fewer than 20 routinely infect humans and cause disease. Most nematodes that infect humans have no intermediate hosts and are passed either directly from host to host or pass through a free-living cycle in the environment. Those which require an intermediate host generally pass through an insect, and humans are infected when bitten by an infected insect. In the case of *Trichinella* species, the same host acts as both the definitive and the intermediate host. Other ways that nematodes infect humans include ingestion of eggs, ingestion of larvae, ingestion of copepods containing larvae, and penetration of the skin by larvae in the environment.

Roundworms
Characteristics of *Ascaris*

General Features. *Ascaris lumbricoides,* commonly called the **human roundworm,** is a white worm that has a pinkish cast and superficially resembles the common earthworm (*Lumbricus*) in appearance. The males are 10–31 cm long, while the females are 22–35 cm.

Each female ascarid lays up to 200,000 eggs per day and will release up to 100 million eggs during its lifetime. The eggs (Fig. 25–9) are unembryonated when released and must spend 2–3 weeks in the soil before a mature embryo develops and the eggs become infective. Humans are infected when they ingest *Ascaris* eggs. The larvae hatch in the duodenum and begin a migratory cycle that will end with the worm returning to the intestine. This cycle (Fig. 25–10) is found among several of the intestinal nematodes. The larvae travel to the lungs hematogenously in 1–7 days after passing sequentially through the liver and heart. Once in the lungs, the larvae break out of the capillaries and into the alveoli. While in the lungs, they pass into the bronchioles and increase in size about fivefold to reach about 1.5 mm in length. The larvae crawl up the trachea to the pharynx, are swallowed, and then locate in the small intestine, where they mature. An adult ascarid begins laying eggs in about 2 months and lives for 12–18 months.

Mechanisms of Pathogenicity. *Ascaris* produces clinical signs when larvae are migrating and when large numbers of adult worms are established in the intestine. During the migratory phase, the larvae break out of the lung capillaries and cause some hemorrhaging in the lungs. The larvae also elicit an IgE-mediated immune response that is evidenced by eosinophilia and by the appearance of manifestations of immediate hypersensitivity, such as hives and asthma. The damage caused by adult ascarids is related to their number and size. Some people are infected with hundreds of ascarids, and this can lead to blockage of the intestine. Ascarids may also become excited in the presence of drugs used to treat other infections. When this occurs, the worms may bore into the peritoneum, migrate up the gastrointestinal

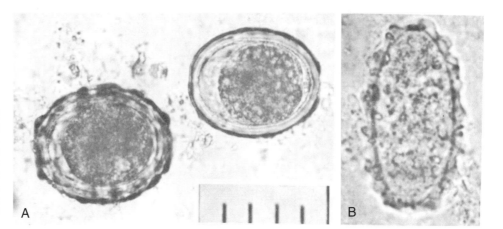

FIGURE 25–9. Embryonated (A) and unembryonated (B) eggs of *Ascaris lumbricoides.* Note that the egg in the middle is nearly decorticated. (Reproduced, with permission, from Markell, E. K., M. Voge, and D. T. John. Medical Parasitology, 7th ed. Philadelphia, W. B. Saunders Company, 1992.)

A   B

tract, and pass out through the nose or mouth, or the worms may bore through the skin of the abdomen or groin to escape.

Diseases Due to *Ascaris*

Epidemiology. *Ascaris* is common in tropical and temperate climates throughout the world. In 1947, investigators estimated that 18,000 tons of *Ascaris* eggs were shed each year in China alone. In 1989, the authors of an editorial in *Lancet* postulated that if all the ascarids infecting humans worldwide were placed end to end, they would encircle the earth 50 times. Currently, epidemiologists believe that about 1 billion individuals are infected with ascarids, making ascariasis one of the most frequently occurring infections in the world. Fortunately, the consequences of ascariasis are relatively mild in most cases. Fewer than 2000 people die each year from ascariasis, typically from intestinal obstruction.

Ascaris infections are most prevalent in children, especially those between the ages of 5 and 9 years. This is because young children frequently play in the dirt, where they come into contact with *Ascaris* eggs. The eggs can be found not only in soil but also in water and on vegetables grown in soil that contains human or swine feces. Humans are also susceptible to infection with the hog roundworm, *Ascaris suum.*

Diagnosis. In the presence of large numbers of migrating larvae, patients may suffer from transient allergic manifestations that include hives, edema of the lips, pneumonitis that mimics primary atypical pneumonia, and bronchopneumonia. These symptoms generally appear between 4 days and 2 weeks after *Ascaris* eggs are eaten. *Necator, Ancylostoma,* and *Strongyloides* (discussed below) produce similar but milder forms of pneumonitis during larval migration.

Most individuals who are infected with adult ascarids harbor between 10 and 20 worms and suffer no symptoms other than vague abdominal discomfort. Some patients, however, have been reported to harbor as many as 1000 adult worms. Children who are already living on a meager diet may become malnourished when carrying large numbers of ascarids, since 20 adult ascarids absorb 2.8 g of carbohydrate and 0.7 g of protein daily from the intestine. Findings in heavily infected patients, especially if they are young children, may include eosinophilia, hives, asthma, and potentially fatal abdominal obstruction.

The diagnosis of ascariasis is confirmed by identifying ascarids or their eggs in stool samples.

Treatment. Ascariasis is usually treated with albendazole or piperazine citrate. Pyrantel pamoate has also been used. Management of patients with intestinal blockage includes nasogastric suction followed by nasogastric administration of piperazine.

Characteristics of *Toxocara*

Toxocara canis and *Toxocara cati* are roundworms of dogs and cats, respectively, but they can cause larval roundworm infections in humans. *T. canis* is passed transovarially to puppies, and the adult worms become gravid in the dog intestine when the puppy is 5–6 weeks old. *Toxocara* eggs shed by infected puppies and kittens are extremely resistant to environmental conditions, and children frequently become infected when they ingest soil contaminated with animal feces. In some countries, adults have become infected by eating raw chicken livers that came from chickens raised with dogs.

When *Toxocara* eggs hatch in the human intestine, the larvae enter a migratory and developmental cycle. The larvae halt their development as second-stage larvae and then encyst in the tissues, never becoming adult worms. The migration of larvae causes hemorrhage, necrosis, and the development of eosinophilic granulomas around encysted larvae.

Diseases Due to *Toxocara*

Toxocariasis may occur as visceral larva migrans or as ocular larva migrans. Patients with **visceral larva migrans** have eosinophilia and usually suffer from hepatomegaly or nonspecific pulmonary dis-

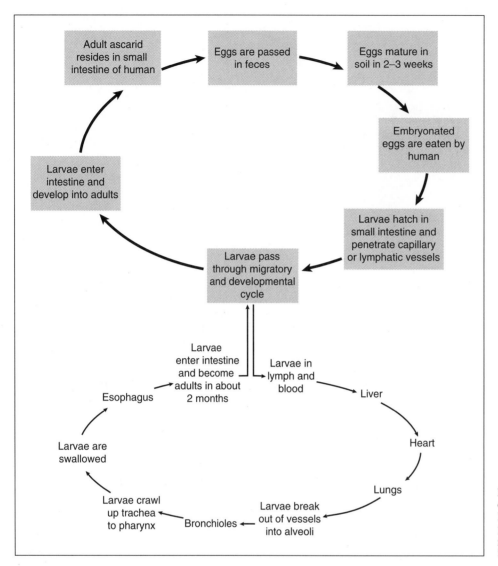

FIGURE 25–10. The life cycle of *Ascaris lumbricoides.* The lower portion of the life cycle presents details of the larval migratory and developmental cycle in humans.

ease. Some fatal cases have involved children with multiple granulomas in the brain, heart, and liver. **Ocular larva migrans** occurs when *Toxocara* larvae migrate to the eye, causing retinochoroiditis.

An enzyme-linked immunosorbent assay is available to detect antibodies to *T. canis,* but antibodies to some other roundworms can cause false-positive results. In patients with chronic eosinophilia, the diagnosis of visceral larva migrans is often reached by eliminating other possible causes and by noting the history of the patient. In some cases, for example, infected children have a history of pica (compulsive eating of nonnutritive substances) and exposure to a puppy.

Toxocariasis is treated by administering corticosteroids and antihistamines to reduce the immune-mediated damage that accompanies visceral or ocular larva migrans. Albendazole, mebendazole, or thiabendazole has been used as an adjunct to treat larva migrans, but clinical studies have not shown these drugs to be effective.

Hookworms
Characteristics of Human Hookworms

General Features. Two very similar worms cause human hookworm infections and are commonly considered together: *Ancylostoma duodenale* (the Old World hookworm) and *Necator americanus* (the New World hookworm). In addition, other *Ancylostoma* species that naturally infect dogs or cats can cause larval hookworm infections known as cutaneous larva migrans.

Hookworms have a whitish or pinkish hue, and the males are somewhat smaller than the females. The males of *A. duodenale* are about 1 cm long, and the females are about 1.3 cm. In comparison, the males of *Necator* species are about 0.5–0.9 cm long, and the females are about 1 cm. The mouth of *Ancylostoma* has well-developed teeth (Fig. 25–11), while that of *Necator* has cutting plates. The term "hookworm" is apt because the caudal end of the worm is curved into a characteristic hook shape.

an appropriate host. When stepped on by a bare human foot, the filariform larva penetrates the skin and enters a migratory phase that takes it through the heart and lungs and then into the gastrointestinal tract. The entire migratory phase takes about 1 week to complete. The adults live in the small intestine, where they attach to the mucosa via their buccal cavity and suck juices from host tissues. The adult *A. duodenale* lives 1–8 years, while the adult *Necator* species live 2–18 years. The females pass eggs daily. *Ancylostoma* females shed up to 20,000 eggs each day, while *Necator* females shed about half that amount.

Mechanisms of Pathogenicity. Hookworms produce clinical signs when they penetrate the skin, when they migrate, and when they reside as adults within the intestine.

Penetration of filariform larvae through the skin can elicit an allergic reaction at the entry site. This reaction, known as ground itch, is similar to swimmers' itch seen during penetration of the skin by schistosomes. Ground itch caused by *Necator* is more severe and occurs more commonly than that caused by *Ancylostoma*.

The larval migratory phase produces few symptoms unless a large number of larvae are involved. As with *Ascaris,* signs of pneumonitis are due to allergic reactions to the larvae and to the damage caused when larvae break out of capillaries and move into the lung.

In many cases, adult hookworm infections are unnoticed. However, heavy worm burdens can lead to hypochromic microcytic anemia. Each adult *Ancylostoma* ingests 0.15–0.26 mL of blood per day, while each adult *Necator* ingests about 0.03 mL. Patients with more than 500 worms develop severe anemia, and the problem is exacerbated in patients with iron-deficient diets.

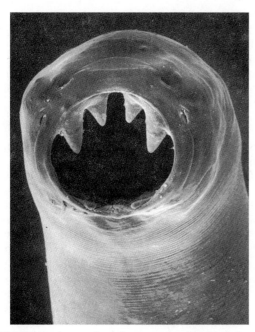

FIGURE 25–11. A scanning electron micrograph of the mouth of *Ancylostoma duodenale.* (Reproduced, with permission, from Markell, E. K., M. Voge, and D. T. John. Medical Parasitology, 7th ed. Philadelphia, W. B. Saunders Company, 1992.)

The life cycle of hookworms is presented in Fig. 25–12. Hookworm eggs pass into the soil in human feces, and a feeding larva called a **rhabditiform larva** hatches in 24–48 hours. The rhabditiform larva molts and becomes a nonfeeding larva that is covered with a loose sheath and is called a **filariform larva.** When there is moisture on the grass, the filariform larva crawls to the highest point that is covered with dew and extends itself, waiting to come into contact with

FIGURE 25–12. The life cycle of *Ancylostoma duodenale* and *Necator americanus,* two hookworms that infect humans.

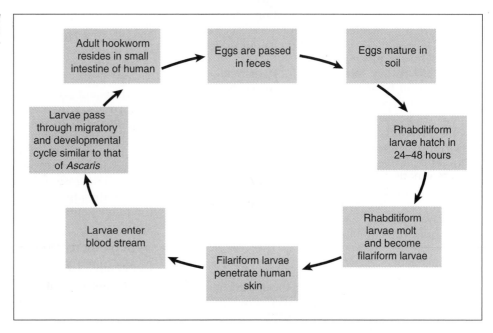

Diseases Due to Human Hookworms

Epidemiology. Throughout the world, hookworms are found in tropical and temperate climates where there is sufficient rainfall for the free-living larvae to thrive. The incidence of hookworm infection is highest in areas where there is sandy or loam soil, public sanitation is poor, people do not wear shoes, the climate is warm, and there is at least 75–125 cm (about 30–50 in) of rain per year. *Necator* infection is especially prevalent in the southern USA, Mexico, Central America, northern South America, Africa, and parts of India. *Ancylostoma* infection is most common in Europe, the Mediterranean, the western coast of South America, Southeast Asia, and parts of India and China.

An estimated 1 billion people are infected with hookworms. Humans are infected when their skin comes into contact with moist vegetation that contains the filariform larvae of hookworms. The usual site of entry is the bare foot or the hand. Individuals can also be infected when they drink water or eat food that contains the larvae.

Diagnosis

(1) History and Physical Examination. The penetration of hookworm larvae through the skin produces ground itch. The itching is accompanied by a maculopapular rash at the site of entry and subsides spontaneously within about 6 days. During the migration of larvae, some patients develop mild pneumonitis and allergic symptoms, but many patients are asymptomatic. About 30 days after the penetration of larvae, the presence of adult hookworms in the intestine may cause epigastric pain, nausea, vomiting, and diarrhea. Between days 30 and 45, individuals who have not previously been infected with hookworms and who are now infected with a large number of worms may experience fairly severe diarrhea and nausea accompanied by eosinophilia.

For most patients, hookworm disease is a chronic disease. Repeated infection over many years results in a heavy worm burden. Findings may include iron deficiency anemia, pica, poor appetite, nausea, vomiting, diarrhea or constipation, rapid pulse, and cardiac hypertrophy.

(2) Laboratory Analysis. Hookworm infections are diagnosed by identifying the eggs of *Necator* or *Ancylostoma* in stool samples. Concentration techniques may be needed to locate the eggs when small numbers are present. Rhabditiform larvae of hookworms are sometimes seen, and these must be differentiated from the larvae of *Strongyloides stercoralis*.

Treatment. Hookworm infections can be effectively treated with albendazole or, alternatively, with mebendazole. The anemia associated with chronic hookworm infection responds well to daily administration of ferrous sulfate.

Characteristics of Nonhuman Hookworms

Humans can be infected with the filariform larvae of hookworms that normally infect other animals. When this occurs, the larvae are unable to mature to adults, but they migrate for some time in the subcutaneous tissues and produce cutaneous larva migrans.

The most common causes of cutaneous larva migrans are *Ancylostoma braziliense* (a hookworm that infects dogs and cats) and *Ancylostoma caninum* (a hookworm whose adult forms are found only in dogs). Other causes include *Uncinaria stenocephala* (a hookworm that infects dogs and other animals) and *Necator americanus* (discussed above). *Strongyloides stercoralis* (discussed below) causes a similar condition known as larva currens.

The filariform larvae of nonhuman hookworms enter the skin but are unable to develop further. They wander aimlessly in the subcutaneous tissues, producing serpiginous tracks that are erythematous. Vesicles form along the skin as the tunnels advance, and the lesions then become dry and crusted. The larvae migrate up to 2.5 cm each day, but they rarely migrate more than about 5 cm from the site of entry. The duration of larval wandering may be as short as a few weeks or as long as a year. The migration elicits an eosinophilic response and results in intense itching. Scratching may cause the serpiginous tracks to become secondarily infected with bacteria. The larvae of *A. caninum* may migrate to the muscles and encyst.

Diseases Due to Nonhuman Hookworms

Epidemiology. Cutaneous larva migrans is found most often in the tropics and subtropics. In the USA, it occurs primarily in the southeastern region and Gulf states. Individuals who must crawl under houses, such as plumbers, are most likely to develop cutaneous larva migrans. Others who are often infected are people who sunbathe on beach sand and children who play in sandboxes that are accessible to cats.

Diagnosis. Typical manifestations of **cutaneous larva migrans,** also called **creeping eruption,** include itching and erythematous subcutaneous tracks formed by wandering hookworm larvae. The feet, legs, and hands of patients are the most common sites of infection, but plumbers often develop infections on the buttocks, elbows, knees, and shoulders. Allergy to the larvae may result in the development of a transient pulmonary infiltration. Secondary infection with bacteria may be noted in patients who scratch the skin lesions.

Treatment. Patients are commonly treated with thiabendazole. The advancing edge of the tunnel can be frozen with ethyl chloride to try to kill the larvae in the tissues. Lidocaine ointments can be used to ease itching, and antibiotics may be indicated for the management of secondary bacterial infections.

Strongyloides stercoralis
Characteristics of *S. stercoralis*

General Features. *Strongyloides stercoralis* is generally similar to hookworms in geographic distribution, clinical manifestations, and life cycle, but it is less prevalent, can exist as a free-living form in the environment, and has **rhabditiform larvae** that usually hatch from eggs in the intestinal mucosa. The adult females are typically about 2.2 mm in length, and the males are smaller. When *Strongyloides* lives in the environment, however, it reaches only about 1 mm in length.

As shown in Fig. 25–13, the life cycle of *Strongyloides* has three variations: a direct cycle, which is identical to the cycle of hookworms; an indirect cycle, which produces adults that live freely in the soil; and an autoinfection cycle.

The rhabditiform larvae of *Strongyloides* are

passed in stools. After they enter the soil, they develop into **filariform larvae.** These larvae may infect another human by penetrating the skin, or they may remain in the soil and develop into free-living adults. The adults mate and produce eggs, and the larvae that hatch may either infect a new host or enter another free-living cycle. The direct cycle is characteristic of temperate climates, while the indirect cycle is seen commonly in wet tropical countries. Patients can also be autoinfected when larvae that hatch in the intestinal mucosa develop into filariform larvae, penetrate the mucosa or the perianal skin, and establish a wandering developmental cycle. Via the autoin-

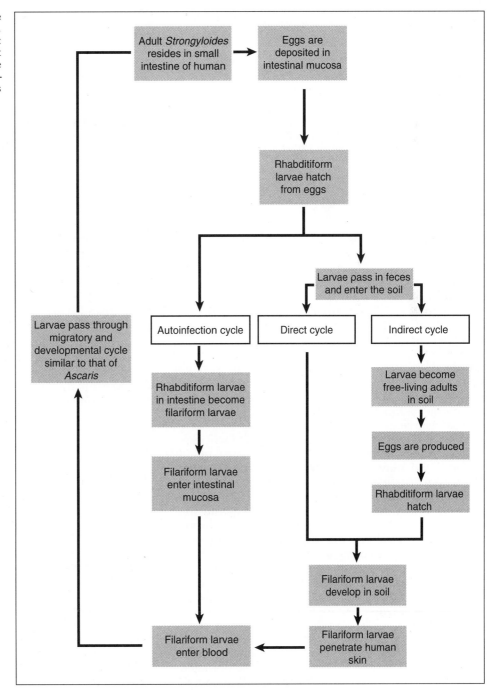

FIGURE 25–13. The life cycle of *Strongyloides stercoralis.* Three variations are presented: an autoinfection cycle; a direct cycle, which is identical to the cycle of hookworms; and an indirect cycle, which produces adults that live freely in the soil.

fection cycle, patients can repeatedly reinfect themselves and develop disease that persists for decades after moving away from a location where *Strongyloides* is endemic. In fact, persistence for 36 years has been documented.

Mechanisms of Pathogenicity. Penetration of larvae through the skin can produce ground itch, but this tends to be less severe than that seen with hookworm penetration. Larval migration after penetration can induce patchy pneumonitis, but many patients are asymptomatic. Occasionally, larvae migrate through the subcutaneous tissues, producing clinical manifestations similar to those of cutaneous larva migrans. The migration of *Strongyloides* larvae is much more rapid (5–10 cm per hour) than that of hookworm larvae, giving rise to the name larva currens for *Strongyloides* infection. The pathogenesis of larva currens is the same as that for cutaneous larva migrans.

When they reach the intestine, *Strongyloides* adults burrow into the mucosa. The worms are typically found in the duodenum and upper jejunum, but they may spread throughout the intestinal tract of patients who are heavily infected. Their presence elicits an eosinophilic response and may cause diarrhea with ulceration and sloughing of the mucosa.

Diseases Due to *S. stercoralis*

Epidemiology. *Strongyloides* is most common in tropical and subtropical regions where rainfall is heavy. Worldwide, an estimated 35 million individuals are infected. In the USA, *Strongyloides* infection occurs in the southeastern region and Gulf states. The usual mode of infection is via penetration of the skin by filariform larvae in the soil. Autoinfection is common, but larva currens is rare in the USA.

Diagnosis. The pneumonitis and ground itch associated with *Strongyloides* penetration and migration are generally unremarkable unless the patient is heavily infected. In some cases, wandering of larvae through subcutaneous tissues produces the serpiginous erythematous tracks of **larva currens.** Many patients with strongyloidiasis have no associated symptoms, but burrowing of adults into the intestinal mucosa can lead to ulceration and cause epigastric pain, nausea, vomiting, alternating diarrhea and constipation, and eosinophilia. The stool may contain occult blood, may become tarry as a result of heavy bleeding from the mucosa, or may be mucoid.

Autoinfection may lead to hyperinfection, a condition in which worms can be found throughout the body. Hyperinfection can be fatal when the worms disseminate to the viscera. Disseminated strongyloidiasis occurs most often in immunosuppressed patients.

The diagnosis of strongyloidiasis is confirmed by identifying the rhabditiform larvae of *Strongyloides* in stool samples. Eggs are rarely found.

Treatment. Albendazole is the drug of choice for treating strongyloidiasis, but mebendazole and ivermectin are suitable alternatives. Ivermectin is an investigational drug in the USA and can be obtained from the Centers for Disease Control and Prevention.

Enterobius vermicularis
Characteristics of *E. vermicularis*

General Features. *Enterobius vermicularis* is called the **pinworm** because the adult form has a sharp, pointed tail. The adult males are 2–5 mm long, while the adult females are 8–13 mm.

Humans are the only known host of pinworms. The adult worms live primarily in the cecum, although immature females and adult males can occasionally be found in the rectum. The worms sometimes wander to the stomach, esophagus, and nose. When females are fully gravid, they contain about 11,000 eggs. They migrate down the intestinal tract and exit from the anus to lay their eggs in the perianal region. Because they begin to dry out when they leave the intestine, the female pinworms often explode before they can finish laying their eggs. The eggs are fully embryonated and are infective within 4–6 hours. When humans ingest pinworm eggs, the first-stage larvae hatch in the duodenum, undergo several rounds of molting in the jejunum and upper ileum, and become mature adults in about 6 weeks.

Mechanisms of Pathogenicity. Pinworms are commensals in most individuals, but some children have symptomatic infections. In most cases, clinical manifestations represent an allergic reaction to pinworm secretions and excretions, which produce intense perianal itching. Eggs and worms encased within granulomas are sometimes found in the peritoneum of women and girls, but these granulomas have not been demonstrated to be responsible for clinically apparent disease.

Diseases Due to *E. vermicularis*

Epidemiology. Pinworms are found worldwide in temperate climates and are common even where sanitation is good. During the late 1960s, epidemiologists estimated that about 210 million individuals were infected with pinworms. Currently, the number is thought to be even higher. Humans can become infected with *Enterobius* (1) when they ingest the eggs after scratching their perianal region or handling contaminated fomites, (2) when they inhale pinworm eggs from the environment, or (3) when eggs in the perianal region hatch and the larvae crawl back into the anus. When one person in a house has pinworms, the eggs are distributed throughout the house, but the greatest concentration of eggs will be in the bedroom. Fortunately, the eggs are not hardy. After 2 days at 20–24.5 °C (68–76 °F), fewer than 10% of the eggs will be viable. On hotter days, most eggs will die within 3 hours.

Diagnosis. Children sometimes suffer from poor appetite, weight loss, abdominal pain, renewed bed-wetting, hyperactivity, and other vague constitutional symptoms, all of which are believed to result from sleep loss caused by perianal itching. Young girls may also suffer from vaginal itching due to migration of worms into the vagina from the perianal region.

Pinworm eggs are rarely found in the feces, and then only in small numbers. The usual method of finding the eggs is to loop some transparent tape over a microscope slide and then to lightly touch the perianal region with the gummed surface of the tape. The eggs will stick to the tape and can be seen easily without staining. Visualization of the eggs can be improved either by clearing the preparation with a drop of toluol or by placing a drop of iodine in xylol on the slide to clear and stain the background. Pinworm eggs are asymmetric, are 50–60 μm long by 20–32 μm wide, and contain a well-developed embryo.

Treatment. Pinworm infections can be treated with albendazole or piperazine sulfate. Itching can be alleviated by administering tap water enemas.

Trichuris trichiura

Characteristics of T. trichiura

General Features. *Trichuris trichiura* is called the **whipworm** because it is shaped like a bullwhip with a long lash (Fig. 25–14A). Adult whipworms range from 3 to 5 cm in length, and females are longer than males. Humans are the primary host of whipworms, but monkeys and hogs can also be infected.

Adult whipworms live in the cecum, where they attach to the mucosa via their anterior tip. Females shed from 3000 to 10,000 eggs each day. The distinctive barrel-shaped eggs have polar plugs (see Fig. 25–14B) and are unsegmented when they pass via the feces into the environment. They become infective after 3–4 weeks in warm, moist soil. When humans ingest the eggs, the larva escapes the egg in the upper small intestine, penetrates an intestinal villus, and develops into an adult in 30–90 days. Adult whipworms live 4–8 years.

Mechanisms of Pathogenicity. The attachment of a few whipworms to the mucosa produces no clinically apparent symptoms. When worm burdens become heavy, however, the mucosa may become inflamed and edematous. Each worm consumes about 0.005 mL of blood per day, and extremely heavy worm burdens can lead to anemia. In severe cases, bleeding at the sites of worm attachment also contributes to anemia. When the rectum becomes edematous, straining during defecation may result in rectal prolapse. Large numbers of worms may invade the appendix, causing appendicitis. Diarrhea may occur and

is sometimes due to secondary bacterial invasion of mucosa heavily infected with whipworms.

Diseases Due to T. trichiura

Epidemiology. The distribution of *Trichuris* is similar to that of *Ascaris,* with areas of highest prevalence being tropical and subtropical regions in which rainfall totals are high and the soil is contaminated with human feces. Worldwide, between 500 million and 800 million people are thought to be infected with *Trichuris.* In some Asian countries, up to 80% of the population may be infected. Humans become infected when they ingest whipworm eggs in the soil, and children are most often infected because they play in the dirt. The eggs can be introduced on dirty hands, on fomites (such as toys), and in food or water.

Diagnosis. Patients with light whipworm infections are usually asymptomatic. Some patients with heavy infections present with acute appendicitis. More frequently, those with heavy infections suffer from anemia, abdominal pain and tenderness, nausea, vomiting, weight loss, and frequent small stools streaked with blood. Young children commonly present with chronic dysentery, profound anemia, eosinophilia, and growth retardation. These children may become extremely anemic, and worm burdens of several thousand may be fatal. Occasional patients develop rectal prolapse, and the worms can easily be seen attached to the rectal mucosa.

The diagnosis of trichuriasis is confirmed by identifying the barrel-shaped eggs in stool samples. In some countries, the eggs of *T. trichiura* must be differentiated from similarly appearing eggs produced by *Capillaria philippinensis.*

Treatment. Whipworm infections respond to treatment with mebendazole or albendazole.

Capillaria philippinensis

Characteristics of C. philippinensis

Investigators believe that *Capillaria philippinensis* is acquired by eating fresh and brackish water fish infected with *Capillaria* larvae and that autoinfection also occurs. Some patients develop enormous worm burdens, with worms found primarily in the jejunum. Adult *Capillaria* worms are 4–5 mm in length.

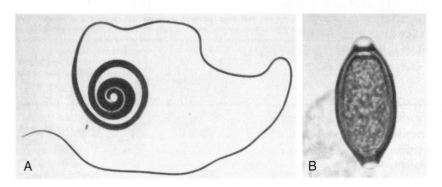

FIGURE 25–14. The adult *Trichuris trichiura* (A) and its egg (B). (Reproduced, with permission, from Markell, E. K., M. Voge, and D. T. John. Medical Parasitology, 7th ed. Philadelphia, W. B. Saunders Company, 1992.)

A

B

Diseases Due to *C. philippinensis*

Although *C. philippinensis* infection is found primarily in the Philippines, it is occasionally reported in Taiwan, Thailand, Egypt, Japan, and Iran. From 1967 to 1970, an epidemic in Luzon and Leyte in the Philippines infected 1400 people and caused 95 deaths.

Manifestations of infection include abdominal gurgling and pain, anorexia, protracted diarrhea, nausea, vomiting, and hypotension. Some patients develop wasting disease. The diagnosis is based on identifying *Capillaria* eggs in stool samples.

Capillaria infections are treated with mebendazole or albendazole. Because of the severity and protracted nature of the diarrhea, patients should be rehydrated with electrolyte solutions and be fed a high-protein diet.

Trichinella Species

Characteristics of *Trichinella*

General Features. *Trichinella spiralis* is the usual cause of trichinosis. *Trichinella nativa, Trichinella nelsoni,* and *Trichinella pseudospiralis* have also been found to cause human infection and are considered by some investigators to be subspecies of *T. spiralis.* The term "spiralis" refers to the coiled appearance of the encysted larval form of the worm (Fig. 25–15).

The adults of *T. spiralis* are small worms, with males averaging about 2 mm in length and females averaging 5 mm. The adults live for a few weeks in the intestine of the definitive host, where they mate and produce live young. The larvae travel via the lymphatic system and blood to various tissues, encyst in muscle fibers, and remain encysted until the flesh of the definitive host is eaten by another host, such as a human host. The larvae excyst in the intestine of the new host and penetrate into the intestinal

mucosa, where they mature to adults in 30–40 hours. Within weeks, the adult worms are rejected by the immune response.

Mechanisms of Pathogenicity. Adult *Trichinella* worms cause symptoms in only a minority of those infected. Some individuals develop diarrhea that may be due to damage caused by adult worms in the intestinal mucosa. The extent of intestinal damage and the severity and duration of diarrhea can be prolonged by the use of corticosteroids, which interfere with immune-mediated rejection of the worms.

Most of the clinical manifestations of trichinosis are attributable to the larval form of *Trichinella.* When larvae first enter the muscle, the muscle fibers become inflamed and degenerate. The migration of larvae before encystment causes vasculitis and is believed to be responsible for the splinter hemorrhages and periorbital edema that characterize trichinosis. Granulomas sometimes form around the encysted larvae, but most of the symptoms and signs of trichinosis (including pain, edema, and loss of muscle function) are due to immune-mediated damage of tissues in which the larvae encyst. Encysted larvae can live for years and even continue to survive after the cyst calcifies.

Diseases Due to *Trichinella*

Epidemiology. Trichinosis is found wherever humans eat undercooked or raw pork and pigs are fed raw pork scraps. In the USA, an estimated 2% of the overall population has been infected with *T. spiralis,* but the rate of infection is about 25 times as high in US immigrants from Southeast Asia. At one time, there were more people with trichinosis in the USA than in all of the other countries combined. Changes in farming practices have greatly reduced the incidence, and China is now the country with the most cases of trichinosis.

T. spiralis is found most commonly in temperate climates and can also infect rats and a variety of wild carnivores, including canids and bears. One recent well-known case in the western USA involved a hunter who developed acute trichinosis after eating cougar jerky. *T. nativa* is found predominantly in the arctic and northern temperate zones, where it infects humans, walruses, and bears. *T. nelsoni* is seen most commonly in the tropics, where it infects humans, jackals, hyenas, lions, and numerous other carnivores.

Diagnosis

(1) History and Physical Examination. The presence of adult *Trichinella* worms in the intestine is usually not accompanied by symptoms, but some patients develop diarrhea. The adult worms are rejected in 3–6 weeks.

The wandering of larvae before encystment in tissues does not always produce symptoms, but it can cause acute trichinosis, characterized by the clinical manifestations outlined in Table 25–4. The severity of illness is related to the number of invading larvae and the intensity of the immune response to the lar-

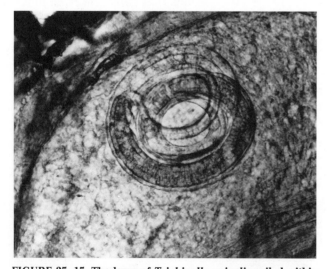

FIGURE 25–15. The larva of *Trichinella spiralis* coiled within the sheath of a muscle fiber. (Courtesy of Armed Forces Institute of Pathology. AFIP photo 76-9379.)

**TABLE 25–4. Clinical Manifestations of
Acute Trichinosis**

Common clinical signs

Conjunctivitis	Muscle spasms
Eosinophilia	Periorbital edema
Fever	Photophobia
Muscle pain	

Other clinical signs

Abdominal pain	Hypotension
Apathy	Nausea
Bronchitis	Peripheral edema
Cough with hemoptysis	Pleurisy
Deafness	Pneumonia
Delirium	Precordial pain
Diarrhea	Rash
Dicrotic pulse	Sore throat
Dysphagia	Thrombosis
Dyspnea	Tinnitus
Electrocardiographic changes	Vertigo
Headache	Vomiting

vae. The eosinophilia of trichinosis is greatest during the migratory phase and ranges from 10% to 90%.

Acute illness usually begins about 10 days after infection and persists for 10–14 days, although muscle pain may persist for up to 6 months. Rarely, patients suffer from prolonged muscle weakness or hemiplegia. The muscles most often infected are the diaphragm and the muscles of the chest, arms, and legs. Some of the more severe consequences of trichinosis include myocarditis, endocarditis, and meningitis. Between 10% and 20% of patients develop neurologic disease, and the untreated fatality rate among these patients is high. When death occurs, it is usually after 4–8 weeks and may be due to cerebral involvement, heart failure, pulmonary embolism, or pneumonia.

(2) Laboratory Analysis. Direct microscopic examination of biopsy specimens from the biceps, deltoid, and gastrocnemius muscles can confirm the presence of *Trichinella* larvae in muscle tissue beginning about 2–3 weeks after the onset of infection. The larvae can also be released from biopsy specimens by digestion techniques. A bentonite flocculation test and an enzyme-linked immunosorbent assay are available for detecting antibodies to *Trichinella* in serum samples.

Treatment. Trichinosis does not respond well to specific antiparasitic drugs. Some success has been reported when patients were treated with benzimidazole antibiotics, particularly thiabendazole and mebendazole. Corticosteroids may be lifesaving, particularly for patients with central nervous system disease, but their early use can prolong the intestinal phase of the disease.

Prevention. The incidence of trichinosis can be reduced by avoiding the practice of feeding raw pork scraps to domestic hogs and also by cooking pork thoroughly before human consumption. Unfortunately, rats that find raw scraps in garbage may continue the infection cycle, and cooking does not always eliminate *Trichinella.* For example, cooking pork in a microwave does not kill all *Trichinella* larvae, even when done according to the manufacturers' recommended guidelines.

Dracunculus medinensis
Characteristics of *D. medinensis*

General Features. *Dracunculus medinensis,* also called the **guinea worm,** is suspected by some biblical scholars to be the "fiery serpent of the Israelites." In addition to infecting humans, the worms infect dogs and other small mammals.

Female guinea worms reach 1 m in length and 0.9–1.7 mm in diameter, while the male worms are only about 2 cm long. Humans carry the adult worms in the body cavity or connective tissue. When the female worms become gravid, they migrate to the subcutaneous tissue, usually on the lower leg or foot. A papule forms over the worm's anterior end, which is just below the dermis. After the papule vesiculates and ulcerates, the uterus of the worm prolapses into the ulcerated lesion. When the patient's infected limb is placed into water, rhabditiform larvae are released from the worm. Release of larvae occurs intermittently over a period of about 3 weeks. The larvae are eaten by copepods and mature to an infective form in 2–3 weeks. Humans are infected when they drink water containing *Dracunculus*-infected copepods. The larvae penetrate the gastrointestinal tract and wander through the deep connective tissue for about 1 year until they become adults.

Mechanisms of Pathogenicity. The symptoms associated with *Dracunculus* infections are due primarily to allergic reactions to the presence of adult worms and to localized damage and inflammation during release of larvae. If the body of the elongated female worm is broken under the patient's skin, the patient may develop a secondary bacterial infection and suffer severe allergic reactions to the release of worm contents.

Diseases Due to *D. medinensis*

Epidemiology. *D. medinensis* infection is found in India, Pakistan, and parts of Africa. Of the estimated 5–10 million cases per year, about one-fourth to one-half occur in Nigeria. Humans become infected when they drink water that contains *Dracunculus*-infected copepods. The incidence of infection is highest in vicinities where water is drawn from wells that people step into.

Diagnosis. Patients with maturing worms may experience intermittent allergic symptoms, such as hives and asthma. The lesion of dracunculiasis is a tender red papule that becomes a painful ulcer and is usually located on the leg or foot (Fig. 25–16). When the lesion appears, the patient may suffer from accompanying clinical manifestations, including diarrhea, nausea, vomiting, and asthma. The lesion persists for 2–3 weeks, and then the worm withdraws and the lesion heals.

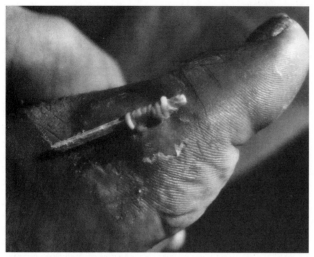

FIGURE 25–16. A female *Dracunculus medinensis* extending from an ulcer on the foot of a patient. (Courtesy of Armed Forces Institute of Pathology. AFIP photo 67-1563-6.)

The diagnosis is based on the typical appearance of the lesion and the finding of a characteristic adult worm in the lesion. If laboratory confirmation is needed, the lesion can be flooded with water and the effluent examined microscopically for the presence of *Dracunculus* larvae.

Treatment. Three drugs have been used to treat dracunculiasis, but none has been universally effective. Niridazole, thiabendazole, and metronidazole are the drugs of choice, and their effects may be related more to suppression of inflammation than to toxicity to the worm itself. Niridazole is an investigational drug in the USA and can be obtained from the Centers for Disease Control and Prevention.

Worms are often removed by winding them around a stick or by surgical procedures. Worm removal poses some risk, however, because if the worm breaks, the patient may develop a secondary bacterial infection or allergic symptoms.

Loa loa

Characteristics of *L. loa*

General Features. *Loa loa*, sometimes called the **African eye worm,** is an example of a microfilarial nematode. Like the species of *Onchocerca, Wuchereria,* and *Brugia* discussed below, *L. loa* produces nonfeeding larvae called **microfilariae** and must pass through a developmental cycle in an arthropod host.

L. loa is carried by *Chrysops,* a genus of mango fly. When an infected fly bites a human, the *L. loa* larvae migrate out of the fly's mouth and onto the human's skin. After entering the skin through the bite, the larvae go to the subcutaneous and deep connective tissues, where they mature to become adults. The adult worms live about 10 years. They migrate extensively and produce microfilariae that must be ingested by a mango fly to develop further. The adult female worms are 5–7 cm long, while the males are 2.0–3.5 cm.

Mechanisms of Pathogenicity. The wandering of adult *L. loa* worms produces few direct problems. When the worms migrate across the bridge of the nose or across the conjunctiva, however, they can become quite noticeable. Patients often have allergic reactions to the worms and their products and develop patches of subcutaneous edema known as Calabar swellings. When these swellings are excised, a worm is not usually found in the underlying tissues. Severe symptoms are rare but may occur when wandering adult worms enter sites not generally accessible to them.

Diseases Due to *L. loa*

Epidemiology. *L. loa* is found throughout the rain forest areas of central and western Africa and the Sudan. Infection is spread to humans by mango flies, which are closely related to deerflies found in the USA.

Diagnosis. Loiasis is often first recognized when the worm migrates across the eye (Fig. 25–17). Patients also periodically develop Calabar swellings, most often on the extremities. The swellings are generally preceded by pain and itching, arise rapidly, and last 1–3 days. Severe complications include cardiomyopathy, encephalopathy, renal disease, and pleural effusion.

Loiasis is generally diagnosed on the basis of clinical manifestations, since microfilariae may not appear until the patient has been infected for several years. When microfilariae are present, they can be identified in blood samples taken between 10 AM and 2 PM. Each *L. loa* microfilaria is sheathed and has nuclei that extend to the tip of the larva.

Treatment and Prevention. Diethylcarbamazine citrate is used to treat loiasis. Because this drug may cause massive extinction of microfilariae, anti-inflammatory drugs are given to control allergic reactions to the release of worm antigens. Ivermectin, an investigational drug in the USA, has also been used

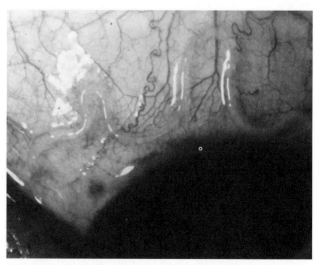

FIGURE 25–17. An adult *Loa loa* in the eye of a patient. (Courtesy of Armed Forces Institute of Pathology. AFIP photo 73-6654.)

with some success. When the worm crosses the conjunctiva, a few drops of 10% cocaine can be used to immobilize the parasite so it can be surgically removed.

Diethylcarbamazine has been used successfully as chemoprophylaxis against loiasis.

Onchocerca volvulus

Characteristics of O. volvulus

General Features. *Onchocerca volvulus* is best known as the cause of river blindness in humans. Blackflies (buffalo gnats) of the genus *Simulium* serve as the insect intermediate host. The blackflies ingest *Onchocerca* microfilariae when they bite an infected person, and the larvae subsequently develop into a form that causes disease in humans.

People become infected when an infected blackfly takes a blood meal. The larvae migrate through the subcutaneous tissues and then settle down in groups of two or more. Within a year, the adult worms are encapsulated and lie coiled within fibrous tissue capsules in subcutaneous and deep connective tissues, where they produce microfilariae. The female worms reach a length of 50 cm but are only about 0.5 mm in diameter. The males are considerably smaller, averaging about 5 cm in length. The microfilariae reach highest densities in the skin, but they also can be found occasionally in the blood, sputum, and urine.

Mechanisms of Pathogenicity. Infection is characterized by the formation of onchocercomas, which are subcutaneous nodules containing adult *Onchocerca*. Onchocercomas are not painful and are not a source of inflammation or significant tissue damage, but they serve as a haven where adult worms can produce microfilariae for years, and it is the microfilariae that are responsible for the severe manifestations of onchocerciasis.

Adult worms live 9–11 years, and microfilariae live about 2 years. The microfilariae wander through the subcutaneous tissues and the eyes and produce two clinically apparent manifestations, onchodermatitis and blindness. Onchodermatitis is an allergic response to the presence of microfilariae and may be due to deposition of immune complexes in tissues that contain large numbers of microfilariae. Repeated bouts of onchodermatitis cause the affected areas of skin to become atrophic and inelastic. The skin gradually begins to sag, causing characteristic features known as leonine facies and hanging groin. Treatment of onchocerciasis with diethylcarbamazine can cause huge numbers of microfilariae to die, and this intensifies the onchodermatitis. Chronic recurrent inguinal onchodermatitis can also cause patients to suffer from inguinal hernias.

River blindness occurs as a result of infection of the eye with *Onchocerca* microfilariae. The persistent presence of microfilariae in the cornea and anterior chamber elicits inflammatory processes that first cause punctate keratitis. After exudate collects, an abnormal skin fold (pterygium) grows out and extends over the cornea. The pupil becomes distorted and may become displaced by posterior adhesions (synechiae).

Diseases Due to *O. volvulus*

Epidemiology. Worldwide, an estimated 30 million people are infected with *O. volvulus*. Infection occurs primarily in Africa, Saudi Arabia, Yemen, Mexico, Central America, and South America, although sporadic cases have appeared in sites as unlikely as Great Britain. The limiting factor is the availability of *Simulium* species that can serve as intermediate hosts for the worms. The name "river blindness" arose from the association of simuliids with fast-moving streams where their larvae develop.

Diagnosis

(1) History and Physical Examination. Onchocerciasis is recognized by the development of onchocercomas and onchodermatitis. In Venezuela and Africa, **onchocercomas** are usually found on the trunk or limbs, and very few form on the scalp. In Guatemala and Mexico, however, the nodules generally develop on the scalp. The distribution of nodules may be related to biting habits of local simuliids. **Onchodermatitis** is heralded by the onset of red or purplish lesions that usually itch and are painful, hot, and edematous. The dermatitis subsides slowly and then recurs repeatedly for years. Each round of dermatitis leaves the skin more atrophic, causing the affected skin to sag. In Venezuela and Africa, many patients develop **hanging groin** (Fig. 25–18), a condition in which the inguinal skin may hang as low as the knees. In some areas of Africa, scrotal elephantiasis may also develop with this condition. In Guatemala and Mexico, patients more commonly develop **leonine facies,** characterized by long jowls.

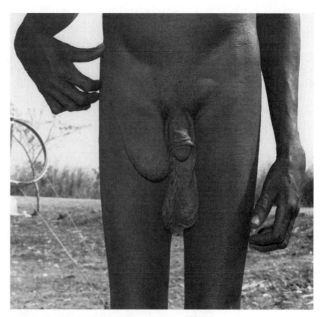

FIGURE 25–18. Hanging groin, a condition that results from repeated bouts of onchodermatitis. (Courtesy of Armed Forces Institute of Pathology. AFIP photo 70-3172.)

In some areas of endemicity, as many as 80–90% of children are infected with *Onchocerca.* As a result, 2–5% of the children suffer from **river blindness,** and the incidence of blindness among adults may exceed 14%. Eye lesions tend to be most severe in American forms of onchocerciasis.

(2) Laboratory Analysis. Nodulectomy can be used to demonstrate the presence of adult worms in onchocercomas. The microfilariae are best located by preparing skin snips. A tiny portion of skin is snipped off with a needle or scalpel, and the microfilariae are teased from the snip into a small amount of growth medium. The microfilariae can then be visualized via light microscopy. If skin snips yield negative results, the Mazzotti test can be used to presumptively confirm a diagnosis of onchocerciasis. In this test, the patient is given an oral dose of diethylcarbamazine. If microfilariae are present, intense pruritus will occur within hours.

Treatment. Ivermectin, the drug of choice, is investigational in the USA and can be obtained from the Centers for Disease Control and Prevention. The drug is effective in killing microfilariae and does so with much less toxicity than does diethylcarbamazine. Because ivermectin does not kill adult worms, patients should be retreated every 6 months.

Nodulectomy can be effective in eliminating adult worms from subcutaneous nodules and thereby lowering the patient's burden of microfilariae. However, some adult worms may persist outside the subcutaneous nodules and inside visceral nodules.

Wuchereria and *Brugia* Species
Characteristics of *Wuchereria* and *Brugia*

General Features. Elephantiasis is caused most commonly by *Wuchereria bancrofti* but can also be caused by *Brugia malayi* and *Brugia timori.* Other diseases caused by these worms include elephantoid fever and tropical pulmonary eosinophilia.

Adult forms of *Wuchereria* and *Brugia* live in the lymph nodes of humans and can survive for 4–5 years. The male worms are about 4 cm long, while the females reach a length of 8–10 cm. The females give birth to microfilariae, and these organisms circulate in the blood and are ingested by mosquitoes when they take a blood meal. During their developmental cycle in the mosquito, the microfilariae increase in length from under 300 μm to up to 2 mm.

A wide variety of *Aedes, Anopheles,* and *Culex* mosquitoes have been shown to act as intermediate hosts for *Wuchereria* and *Brugia.* When a mosquito feeds, the larvae crawl out the proboscis and onto the skin of the human host. They then enter the host through the hole made by the mosquito bite. The larvae migrate to the lymphatic vessels, develop into adults, and begin producing microfilariae in 8–12 months. In most areas of the world, microfilariae are found in greatest numbers in the blood during certain parts of the day (usually between 10 PM and 2–4 AM) and persist in the capillaries and small vessels of the lung during the rest of the day. The reasons for this are unknown, but some investigators believe that the periodicity is influenced by the levels of activity of the patient.

Mechanisms of Pathogenicity. The adult forms of *Wuchereria* and *Brugia* locate within the lymph nodes, where their presence elicits an inflammatory response involving eosinophils, macrophages, and plasma cells. Endothelial hyperplasia occurs as the inflammatory response seeks to eliminate the worms. The lymphatic vessels are damaged, causing increased vessel wall permeability and allowing lymphatic fluid to leak into the surrounding tissues. The adult worm eventually is killed and calcifies, but repeated blockage of lymphatic vessels coupled with cellular infiltration leads to the development of collateral lymphatic channels and edema in the surrounding tissues. The death of adult worms can lead to abscess formation. Elephantoid lesions contain a mixture of lymph and fibrotic tissue. Blockage of lymph flow can also result in the development of scrotal lymphocele.

Tropical pulmonary eosinophilia is probably due to the accumulation of microfilariae in lung tissues. This elicits an eosinophilic response that is meant to eradicate the organisms.

Diseases Due to *Wuchereria* and *Brugia*

Epidemiology. Worldwide, from 85 million to 100 million individuals are infected with *Wuchereria* and *Brugia.* These organisms are widely distributed throughout the tropics and subtropics in Asia, Africa, Micronesia, and the northern coast of South America. Most patients are infected through the bites of night-biting *Anopheles* and *Culex* mosquitoes and day-biting *Aedes polynesiensis.*

Diagnosis

(1) History and Physical Examination. The earliest clinical sign of *Wuchereria* or *Brugia* infection is **elephantoid fever.** Manifestations include high fever, chills, and urticaria, sometimes accompanied by lymphangitis and lymphadenitis. The epitrochlear and femoral nodes are most often affected. The nodes are swollen and tender, and the skin over them is hot and red. Recurrent attacks of lymphangitis and lymphadenitis lead to lymphedema. Some patients have early and repeated scrotal involvement and eventually develop scrotal lymphocele and chyluria.

Most patients infected with *Wuchereria* or *Brugia* develop no disease beyond elephantoid fever. A small percentage, however, develop clinically apparent **elephantiasis** after years of infection. The limbs, scrotum, breasts, and vulva are the areas most often affected. *Wuchereria* tends to affect the scrotum and legs, while *Brugia* usually affects the leg below the knee and is more likely to cause ulceration of the affected lymph nodes.

Patients with **tropical pulmonary eosinophilia** suffer from coughing and wheezing that produces little sputum, and they typically have persistent eosinophilia and high titers of IgE antibody. Other manifestations may include weight loss, adenopathy, and low-grade fever.

(2) Laboratory Analysis. The appearance of elephantiasis in a patient who has lived in a region where *Wuchereria* or *Brugia* is endemic usually confirms the presence of filarial elephantiasis. It is possible, however, for patients in some parts of Africa to develop a chemically induced form of elephantiasis from walking barefoot on soils rich in iron, aluminum, and kaolinite. By the time that elephantiasis develops, the adult worms usually are dead and microfilariae can no longer be found in the blood. In one survey of patients with elephantiasis, for example, only 4% of patients had microfilariae in their blood, but 30% had hydrocele. Thus, it is important to diagnose filarial infections before there is significant damage to lymphatic vessels.

The blood of patients with lymphocele or elephantoid fever should be examined for the presence of microfilariae. In most locales, the microfilariae are periodic in their appearance and are best located in blood samples taken between 10 PM and 2–4 AM. In the Pacific islands, microfilariae can be seen throughout the day but are found in greatest number between noon and 8 PM. The microfilariae of *Wuchereria* have a sheath and have nuclei that do not go to the tip of the tail.

Treatment and Prevention. Diethylcarbamazine or ivermectin can be used to treat disease caused by *Wuchereria* or *Brugia*. Although these drugs do not appear to significantly affect adult worms, they are effective in killing microfilariae. Ivermectin, an investigational drug in the USA, is available from the Centers for Disease Control and Prevention.

Elephantoid fever can be managed with antihistamines and salicylates used in combination. Reconstructive surgery may be necessary to correct the damage caused by elephantiasis.

In some locales, massive efforts have been launched to reduce the transmission of filariasis by use of ivermectin or diethylcarbamazine to kill microfilariae, and these efforts have been somewhat successful.

Selected Readings

Akhan, O., et al. Liver hydatid disease: long-term results of percutaneous treatment. Radiology 198:259–264, 1996.

Akuffo, H., et al. Ivermectin-induced immunoprecipitation in onchocerciasis: recognition of selected antigens following a single dose of ivermectin. Clin Exp Immunol 103:244–252, 1996.

Badawi, A. F., and M. H. Mostafa. Possible mechanisms of alteration in the capacities of carcinogen-metabolizing enzymes during schistosomiasis and their role in bladder cancer induction. J Int Med Res 21:281–305, 1993.

Capron, A., and J. P. Dessaint. Immunologic aspects of schistosomiasis. Annu Rev Med 43:209–218, 1992.

Capron, M. Dual function of eosinophils in pathogenesis and protective immunity against parasites. Mem Inst Oswaldo Cruz 87(supplement 5):83–89, 1992.

Carpio, A., et al. Is the course of neurocysticercosis modified by treatment with anthelmintic agents? Arch Intern Med 155:1982–1988, 1995.

Chang, K. H., et al. Cerebral sparganosis: analysis of 34 cases with emphasis on computed tomographic features. Neuroradiology 34:1–8, 1992.

DaSilva, L. C. Portal hypertension in schistosomiasis: pathophysiology and treatment. Mem Inst Oswaldo Cruz 87(supplement 4):183–216, 1992.

Donovan, S. M., et al. Imported echinococcosis in southern California. Am J Trop Med Hyg 53:668–671.

Erttmann, K. D., et al. Molecular cloning, expression, and localization of E1, an *Onchocerca volvulus* antigen with similarity to brain ankyrin. J Biol Chem 271:1645–1650, 1996.

Freedman, D. O., et al. Abnormal lymphatic function in presymptomatic bancroftian filariasis. J Infect Dis 171:997–1001, 1995.

Fukushima, T., et al. The metabolism of arachidonic acid to prostaglandin E_2 in plerocercoids of *Spirometra erinacei*. Parasitol Res 79:634–638, 1993.

Harinasuta, T., et al. Trematode infections: opisthorchiasis, clonorchiasis, fascioliasis, and paragonimiasis. Infect Dis Clin North Am 7:699–716, 1993.

King, C. L., et al. Interleukin-12 regulation of parasite antigen-driven IgE production in human helminth infections. J Immunol 155:454–461, 1995.

Kong, Y., et al. Characterization of three neutral proteases of *Spirometra mansoni* plerocercoid. Parasitology 108:359–368, 1994.

Lucey, D. R., and J. H. Maguire. Schistosomiasis. Infect Dis Clin North Am 7:635–653, 1993.

McManus, D. P., and M. Hope. Molecular variation in human schistosomes. Acta Trop 53:255–276, 1993.

Pearlman, E., et al. Interleukin-4 and T helper type 2 cells are required for development of experimental onchocercal keratitis (river blindness). J Exp Med 182:931–940, 1995.

Pitella, J. E. The relationship between involvement of the central nervous system in schistosomiasis mansoni and the clinical forms of the parasitosis: a review. J Trop Med Hyg 94:15–21, 1991.

Rakha, N. K., et al. Modification of accessory activity of sheep monocytes in vitro by a coenurus antigen from *Taenia multiceps*. Vet Immunol Immunopathol 30:293–304, 1992.

Rueda, M. C., et al. Changes in T cell subpopulations in mice during prolonged experimental secondary infection with *Echinococcus granulosus*. Biosci Rep 15:201–208, 1995.

Saenz-Santamaria, J., et al. Role of fine-needle biopsy in the diagnosis of hydatid cyst. Diagn Cytopathol 13:229–232, 1995.

Simonsen, P. E., et al. Selective diethylcarbamazine chemotherapy for control of bancroftian filariasis in two communities of Tanzania: compared efficacy of a standard dose treatment and two semiannual single-dose treatments. Am J Trop Med Hyg 53:267–272, 1995.

Sloan, L., et al. Evaluation of an enzyme-linked immunoassay for serodiagnosis of cysticercosis. J Clin Microbiol 33:3124–3128, 1995.

Sotelo, J., et al. Cysticercosis. Curr Clin Top Infect Dis 16:240–259, 1996.

Wyler, D. J. Schistosomes, fibroblasts, and growth factors: how a worm causes liver scarring. New Biol 3:734–740, 1991.

INDEX